Introduction to
CLINICAL
NUTRITION

Third Edition

Introduction to
CLINICAL NUTRITION

Third Edition

Vishwanath Sardesai

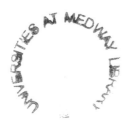

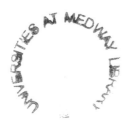

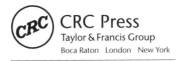

CRC Press
Taylor & Francis Group
Boca Raton   London   New York

CRC Press is an imprint of the
Taylor & Francis Group, an **informa** business

CRC Press
Taylor & Francis Group
6000 Broken Sound Parkway NW, Suite 300
Boca Raton, FL 33487-2742

© 2012 by Taylor & Francis Group, LLC
CRC Press is an imprint of Taylor & Francis Group, an Informa business

No claim to original U.S. Government works

Version Date: 20110714

International Standard Book Number: 978-1-4398-1818-3 (Hardback)

Visit the Taylor & Francis Web site at
http://www.taylorandfrancis.com

and the CRC Press Web site at
http://www.crcpress.com

Contents

PART II Special Nutritional Needs

PART III   Nutrition and Specific Disorders

PART IV Special Topics

Preface to the Third Edition

The explosive advances in clinical nutrition knowledge since the publication of the second edition of this book have made it necessary to make some changes in this new edition, including the addition of three new chapters. With the completion of the Human Genome Project in 2003 and the development of new technology, the number of genes of interest in clinical nutrition has expanded. The new research is expected to greatly advance our knowledge of nutrition and health.

It has been known for some time that diet and specific nutrients can affect gene function. The recognition that nutrients have the ability to interact and modulate molecular mechanisms underlying an organism's physiological functions has prompted a revolution in the field of nutrition. There is rapid development in the area of epigenetics—the study of inherited changes or gene expression caused by mechanisms other than changes in the underlying DNA sequences. Also, there are recent findings relative to the effects of nutrients and other environmental factors on telomere length and health—telomere is the region of repetitive DNA at the end of chromosomes. Hence, a new chapter has been added entitled Gene–Nutrient Interaction—Molecular Genetics, Epigenetics, and Telomeres.

The sequencing of the human genome, subsequent analysis of human genetic variations, and studies that associate gene variants with disease markers or other alterations have led to the promise of personalized medicine. It has also become apparent that people respond differently to diet depending on their genetic makeup, lifestyle, and other environmental factors. Scientists can now identify the various ways in which diet and some nutrients can affect individuals and how our genes are turned on or off by what we eat. With the growing awareness of the need for preventing disease, nutritional genomics and nutrigenetics—the study of gene and nutrient interaction—are anticipated to provide specific information for designing an optimum diet that allows each individual to maintain health and prevent disease. This is covered in the new chapter "Personalized Nutrition and Personalized Medicine."

The kidneys are the major excretory organs for the end products of the metabolic processes involved in the utilization of nutrients. A new chapter, "Nutritional Aspects of Kidney Disease," has been added. It covers those diseases that require careful dietary management. These are acute and chronic kidney diseases, nephrotic syndrome, and kidney stone diseases.

Consumers are increasingly interested in alternative medicine. There is a separate chapter on this topic. In addition, several supplements are described in some chapters. The supplements are those that have shown benefits in experimental and/or clinical studies. Because exercise or physical activity is a crucial component toward the prevention of disease, a section on its benefits has been included in the introductory chapter, and it is also discussed in other relevant succeeding chapters.

Among other changes, metabolic syndrome is added in the chapter on "Nutritional Aspects of Diabetes," and information on the popular Mediterranean diet is covered in the chapter entitled "Vegetarianism and Other Popular Nutritional Practices."

Each chapter is thoroughly revised and updated with the most recent information available. The book is divided into four major parts as before. The chapter on kidney disease is included in Part III, "Nutrition and Specific Disorders," and other new chapters are added in Part IV, "Special Topics."

The objectives of the third edition remain unchanged from those of the first two editions. The book is designed to serve as a textbook and reference source in clinical nutrition for medical students and students in osteopathic medicine and dentistry and practitioners in the fields of medicine, dentistry, nutrition, dietetics, nursing, pharmacy, and public health. The ultimate focus of this edition is to generate interest and enthusiasm in clinical nutrition among students and practitioners in an age that recognizes the growing need for prevention. Nutrition is a vitally important component not only of individual health but also to community well-being.

Preface to the Second Edition

Since the publication of the first edition of this book, the continued dramatic progress in nutrition knowledge required a critical review and evaluation of the entire text. The goal of this revised edition is to facilitate the study and understanding of this dynamic and challenging discipline. All chapters in this edition have been revised and updated to reflect our changing knowledge in this field. Excessive detail and redundancy have been minimized as far as possible without detracting from clarity and accuracy.

This book is divided into four parts as before. Three new chapters have been added, and some chapters have been expanded. Chapter 1, "Introduction: Fundamentals of Nutrition," now contains a new section on gene–nutrient interaction. This section along with the chapter's glossary will help clarify the terms used throughout the text.

Chapter 6, "Inorganic Elements (Minerals)," has a new section on diet and hypertension. Some minerals, such as sodium, potassium, and calcium, are known to affect blood pressure. Thus, in context, the role of nutrition as it relates to hypertension is considered.

A new chapter (Chapter 22, "Nutritional and Metabolic Effects of Alcohol") has been added because alcohol is interrelated with nutrition. Alcohol provides calories (an estimated 5%–6% of the calories that are consumed in the American diet) and affects the metabolism of nutrients. Therefore—although alcohol is not a nutrient—it has an important, if indirect, role in the field of nutrition.

Chapter 23, "Nutritional Epidemiology," is also new. Numerous initial findings in nutrition research continue to come from epidemiological studies as was true during the discoveries of several vitamins during the early part of the last century. Epidemiology is being used more extensively to determine the relationship between diet and disease. In several chapters, statements are made "based on epidemiological studies," cohort, or case-control "research designs." Therefore, the reader is provided with a chapter to help clarify the methods used and their applications in the field of clinical nutrition.

While the first edition was being written, the field of nutraceuticals was in its infancy; it has grown rapidly since 1998. Chapter 29, "Nutraceuticals," has been expanded to include several more functional foods, including biotechnology advances in the development of new foods, such as β-carotene-rich yellow rice.

"Alternative Medicine: Dietary Supplements" (Chapter 30) is new. In the first edition, some supplements were briefly discussed in "Vegetarianism and Other Popular Nutritional Practices." However, this content is now explored more fully in a new chapter. Interest in supplements has grown rapidly over the past few years. People want to have control of their health. They also use common and traditional herbs from many cultures and belief systems. Physicians should know about this field in general, the supplement law passed by Congress in 1994, the role of the U.S. Food and Drug Administration, and the benefits and consequences of some commonly used supplements including herbs. Are some supplements potions or poisons? The topic is discussed via an evidenced-based approach, as well as through a critical analysis of some products.

Selected clinical cases are presented in most chapters. All the patient cases (except one) are real, published in medical literature. Cases are essential because they allow the reader to apply the discussed principles. Analyzing cases helps students comprehend why nutrition principles are important in the health sciences and how nutrition principles are involved in day-to-day professional practices.

As was the first edition, this book is designed to be a textbook and reference source in clinical nutrition for medical students and practitioners in the fields of medicine, dentistry, dietetics, nursing, pharmacy, and public health. The ultimate focus of this edition is the clinical nutrition practices of these professionals and students—and, more importantly, the nutritional needs of their current and future patients.

Preface to the First Edition

It is impossible to overestimate the tremendously important role that nutrition plays in the maintenance of human health, longevity, and community well-being. Dietary factors have been implicated in the etiology of at least 4 of the 10 leading causes of death in the United States: heart disease, cancer, diabetes, and stroke. Nutrition is also crucial in many of the currently common problems such as obesity, hypertension, hypercholesterolemia, and osteoporosis. Since the advent of parenteral nutrition in clinical medicine, there has been renewed interest in nutrient requirements, especially the changes associated with bypassing the gastrointestinal tract.

Interest in nutritional information is not confined to the medical profession. Public interest in the subject is more evident today than ever before. Most individuals consider their physicians to be the primary source of such information, yet in a recent extensive study of office-based primary care physicians, 68% stated that they had received inadequate nutritional training in medical school, and 86% indicated that more nutritional information should be taught as part of the basic medical curriculum.

Because doctors are admittedly not being trained to give adequate advice in this critical field, their patients have turned to unqualified, unregulated, self-proclaimed experts in nutrition. This has caused a tremendous increase in food faddism and outright fraud. A report by the Surgeon General stated that nutrition fraud is the leading example of health fraud at the present time.

In 1985, the Committee of the Food and Nutrition Board of the National Academy of Sciences was commissioned to evaluate the status of nutrition training and education of the nation's physicians. Its report stated that "nutrition education programs in U.S. medical schools are largely inadequate to meet the present and future demand of the medical profession." The committee recommended that nutrition be a required course in every medical school in the United States and that a minimum of 25 classroom hours be devoted during preclinical years to the teaching of basic nutritional material. The National Nutrition Monitoring and Related Research Act of October 22, 1990, mandated that "students enrolled in U.S. medical schools, as well as physicians practicing in the United States, have access to adequate training in the field of nutrition and its relationship to human health."

Many medical schools have started to increase the number of hours for nutrition education, but a common concern among medical educators is how to teach all the materials currently known in the already overcrowded, information-dense curriculum. Another problem is the lack of a suitable nutrition textbook that covers, in sufficient detail, all of the important topics in medicine and focuses on the interaction of nutrition and disease. For example, to understand the significance of topics such as essential fatty acids, eicosanoids, and detoxication, both pertinent biochemistry and nutritional aspects have to be in one place.

This resource is written to serve as the collective textbook for medical students during the preclinical years by addressing the multidisciplinary requirements. It is based on a course that has proved extremely effective in teaching nutrition to medical students. Selected nutritional aspects as they relate to human health and disease and those which are generally covered during the first two years are included.

The science of nutrition deals with the processes by which components of food are made available to the body for meeting energy requirements, building and maintaining tissues, and, in more general terms, the maintenance of optimum functional health. Thus, nutrition is concerned with issues traditionally considered to be biochemical (e.g., digestion, absorption, transport, metabolism, biochemical nature, and the function performed by individual substances). The basic course material in this text is likely to be better received and understood after the students have been introduced to biochemistry, especially the metabolic aspects.

The book is divided into four major parts. The first chapter, "Introduction: Fundamentals of Nutrition," defines the terminology as used in the science of nutrition and briefly discusses the body's need for nutrients and its ability to adapt within limits to conditions of nutrient deficiency or excess. Since water is covered extensively in biochemistry and physiology courses, only its role as a nutrient is included in this chapter, instead of having a separate chapter for this topic.

Part I starts with an overview of digestion and absorption of macronutrients and is followed by a chapter that deals with the need for energy and energy-yielding substrates (carbohydrate, fat, and protein), the importance of protein in the diet (primarily to supply amino acids), and the effect of deficiency and excess of each of these macronutrients. Separate chapters cover the pertinent biochemistry and nutritional roles of essential fatty acids and the biochemistry of eicosanoids, their relation to various diseases, and strategies for dietary manipulation of eicosanoid formation. The chapter on eicosanoids (although actually not nutrients) follows essential fatty acids, which serve as precursors of these biologically active compounds. Individual inorganic elements and vitamins, including vitamin-like substances, are presented in detail in terms of chemistry, food sources, biochemical role, their physiology and metabolic interrelation, and the effects of deficiency and excess of each of the micronutrients.

Part II covers the special nutritional needs during pregnancy, lactation, and the life cycle in relation to physiological changes.

Part III deals with the assessment of nutritional status and focuses on the interaction of nutrition and some selected diseases (e.g., obesity, hyperlipidemia, osteoporosis, diabetes, genetic diseases).

Part IV covers topics of special interest. These include dietary fiber, antioxidants, vegetarianism, and other popular nutritional practices, toxicants occurring in food, additives, and how the body metabolizes many of the toxic substances present in the diet. The role of nutrients in biotransformation (detoxication mechanism) is also discussed. The chapter "Nutraceuticals" is included because of the recent increased interest in the health effects of some foods and their possible roles in the prevention of some chronic diseases. The health-promoting properties of many of these foods are attributed to their content of specific nonnutrient substances, most of which act favorably on the body's detoxication mechanisms. Therefore, this topic follows the chapter entitled "Nutritional Aspects of Biotransformation."

The science of nutrition, important as it is to human welfare, has had a very long history. Centuries ago, the relationship between nutrition and medicine began with the recognition by Hippocrates that food was the source of energy and body heat. Early physicians recognized the relation between certain foods and classical deficiency diseases such as scurvy and pellagra. Today, our knowledge of the fascinating role of nutrition is growing at a geometrical rate. To help all those involved in human health to keep pace with its growth is the purpose of this book.

This text should be useful not only for students in the field of traditional medical practice but also for those in osteopathic medicine, dentistry, and other health professions. It should be of particular interest to students who are directing their careers toward community medicine and family practice. Nutrition is a vitally important component not only of individual health but equally vital to community well-being.

Acknowledgments

Many people have contributed in a multitude of ways to the completion of this book. I am grateful to many colleagues and students for their comments and suggestions during the preparation of the manuscript. Letters were received from several readers of the second edition, and their comments are highly appreciated.

I wish to thank my son Amey and my nephew Mahesh Sardesai for their help with work that needed special computer expertise; and to thank Kevin Mallett of our Department of Surgery for his technical computer support; I also wish to thank Linda Draper, Reference Librarian of our Schiffman Medical Library, and Jana Thompkins, a graduate student in the School of Library and Information Science, for assisting in numerous literature searches.

I am deeply grateful to Amie Dozier, from the Medical Education Support Group, for preparing several excellent illustrations. I also greatly appreciate the assistance and advice by the editorial staff of CRC Press, Taylor & Francis, particularly Randy Brehm, Joselyn Banks-Kyle, and Kyle Meyer, during the completion of this project. I wish to express my sincere appreciation to Brenda Kennedy-Marable, administrative assistant of our department, for her generous help and encouragement over the many months required for the completion of the edition.

I wish to gratefully acknowledge the secretarial assistance of Kathryn Maysen. She did the work with care, accuracy, speed, and dedication.

Finally, I wish to thank my wife Sudha and children Amey and Gauri for their patience, understanding, and encouragement during this endeavor.

Part I

Biology and Biochemistry

1 Introduction
Fundamentals of Nutrition

To a man with an empty stomach, food is God.

M. Gandhi

The science of nutrition deals with the processes by which components of food are made available to an organism for meeting energy requirements, building and maintaining tissues, and in a more general sense, maintaining the organism in optimal functional health. Thus, nutrition is concerned with many issues traditionally considered to be biochemical (e.g., digestion, absorption, transport, metabolism, and biochemical functions performed by individual chemical substances).

1.1 TERMINOLOGY

Nutrients are the chemical substances needed for the growth and maintenance of normal cells, both in animals and plants. The present emphasis, however, is on human cells and tissues. *Clinical nutrition* is a medical specialty dealing with the relationship between disease and nutrition. Acute and chronic illnesses are caused by deficiencies or excesses of dietary components.

Malnutrition is a condition characterized by an inappropriate quality, quantity, digestion, absorption, or utilization of ingested nutrients. It includes *undernutrition*—low food intake (calorie deficiency) leading to growth suppression or other deficiency signs—and *overnutrition*—consumption of too much food and/or single nutrients leading to specific toxicities.

Some 45–50 chemical entities are now known to be required by humans, either preformed in food or added as an appropriate chemical substitute. These can be divided into six main categories: (1) carbohydrates, (2) fats, (3) proteins, (4) vitamins, (5) inorganic elements, and (6) water. Dietary fiber, although not classified as nutritionally essential, is important in maintaining good health. The term *essential* or *dietary essential nutrient* means that we must obtain the nutrient from our diet because either we lack the biochemical machinery to manufacture it or we cannot make enough of it.

Recommended Dietary Allowances (RDAs) are developed by the Food and Nutrition Board of the National Academy of Sciences.[17,23] RDAs are defined as the "levels of intake of essential nutrients considered, in the judgment of the Committee of Dietary Allowances of the Food and Nutrition Board, on the basis of available scientific knowledge to be adequate to meet the known nutritional needs of practically all healthy persons."[13] Nutrient allowances are categorized into 17 classifications based on age and sex. The recommended intakes of essential nutrients must, therefore, by definition, exceed the requirements of almost all individuals in the group. The Food and Nutrition Board normally meets every six years to consider currently available information and to update its recommendations. The RDAs are meant to apply only to a healthy population and should be met from the consumption of a wide variety of readily available foods. They should not be confused with nutrient requirements of individuals because these are too variable. Rather, an RDA represents an average level of daily intake of a nutrient, which over time approximates the RDA, and thus nutritional inadequacy will be rare in that population. RDAs do not provide the needs that have been altered as a result of disease states, chronic usage of certain drugs, or other factors that require specific individual attention.

The term *minimal daily requirement* (MDR) is the minimum amount of a nutrient from exogenous sources required to sustain normality (i.e., the absence of any biochemical hypofunction that is correctable by the addition of greater quantities of that nutrient).

Fortified is a term generally meaning that vitamins, minerals, or both have been added to a food product in excess of what was originally found in the product.[2]

Individuals consume food more for the satiation of energy needs than for individual nutrients. Therefore, to express the quality of any food in relation to its content of a specific nutrient, the term *nutrient density* is used. It is defined as the concentration of a nutrient per unit of energy (e.g., 1000 Cal) in a specific food. For any nutrient, the higher the nutrient density, the better the food source; for example, one whole green pepper contains 20 mg of vitamin C and provides 4 Cal, while one medium sweet potato also contains 20 mg of vitamin C but provides 100 Cal. Therefore, green pepper is a much better source of vitamin C than sweet potato.

Spices are plant products. They come from various woody shrubs, vines, trees, and aromatic lichens, as well as the roots, flowers, seeds, and fruits of herbaceous plants. Each spice has a unique aroma and flavor that derive from secondary compounds, chemicals that are secondary (not essential) to plants' basic metabolism. Most spices contain dozens of these secondary chemicals. These phytochemicals evolved in plants to protect them from their natural enemies (parasites, pathogens, and herbivores).

Spices enhance the flavor, color, and palatability of food and are used almost universally throughout the world. Most commonly used spices are potent inhibitors of bacterial growth and protect us from food-borne microorganisms. Spice plants have medicinal applications in some societies. These include use as topical or ingested antimicrobials, aids to digestion, treatment for high blood pressure, and sources of micronutrients.

1.1.1 METABOLISM

All cells have in common two major general functions: energy generation and energy utilization for growth and/or maintenance. These may be termed *metabolic reactions* or simply *metabolism*. *Anabolism* broadly refers to processes in which relatively large molecules such as proteins are biosynthesized from small nutrient materials such as amino acids. These reactions require energy, which is available in cells in the form of stored chemical energy in high-energy phosphate compounds. *Catabolism* is the degradation of relatively large molecules to smaller ones. Catabolic reactions serve to capture chemical energy (in the form of adenosine triphosphate [ATP]) from the degradation of energy-rich molecules. Catabolism also allows nutrients (in the diet or stored in cells) to be converted into the building blocks needed for the synthesis of complex molecules. *Intermediary metabolism* refers to all changes that occur in a food substance beginning with absorption and ending with excretion.

In adults, there is a delicate regulated balance between anabolic (synthetic) and catabolic (degradative) processes. In growing children, the input of nutrients and anabolism exceed catabolism so that the growth of tissues may occur. In the aging process or in wasting diseases, the catabolic processes exceed the anabolic ones.

1.1.2 HOMEOSTASIS

The body tends to maintain a state of equilibrium within its internal environment; this is often referred to as a dynamic equilibrium or *homeostasis* because it occurs despite changes in the external environment. The maintenance of equilibrium is governed by an adequate supply of nutrients, a balance between nutrients, a normal complement of enzyme systems, the secretion of hormones that regulate metabolic rates, and control by the nervous system. Homeostasis plays a vital role in the body because tissues and organs can function efficiently only within a narrow range of conditions.

1.2 NUTRITIONAL LABELING

Before 1990 nutritional labeling was required only for fortified foods and those for which nutrition claims were made. Uniformity in nutrition labeling accelerated in the United States with the passage of the Nutrition Labeling and Education Act in 1990 (NLEA Public Law 101–535).

This federal mandate preempted all existing state and federal laws and regulations and stimulated a planned schedule to achieve uniformity in the way that food content is named and quantified on all food products, including water.

Food labels contain standardized information on serving size, Cal content, and ingredients. Reference is also made to the amount of certain ingredients in comparison to recommended daily values. There are 14 mandatory per serving components of the nutrition label: total calories, total fat, saturated fat, *trans* fat, cholesterol, sodium, total carbohydrate, dietary fiber, sugars, protein, vitamin A, vitamin C, calcium, and iron. Percent of Recommended Daily Values for specific nutrients as recommended by the USDA/HHS is required in food labeling and is listed as a footnote at the bottom of the label.

The daily value indicated is based on an average caloric intake of both 2000 and 2500 Calories/day for an adult who performs at a light-to-moderate activity level. The actual daily value may be higher or lower depending on physical activity level.

1.3 THE NEED FOR A VARIETY OF FOODS

Recommended daily allowances should be met by a variety of foods for several reasons. Most foods contain more than one nutrient, but no single food item supplies all the essential nutrients in the amounts that are needed. Certain dietary components (e.g., carotenes, fiber, and possibly others) that are not considered "required" may nevertheless have a beneficial effect on body functioning. The greater the variety of foods, the less likely one can develop a deficiency or an excess of any single nutrient. Variety also reduces the likelihood of being exposed to excessive amounts of toxic substances that occur naturally in foods and to additives or contaminants that may be present in any single food item. A simple approach to adequate nutrition is to consume a variety of foods. Foods can be selected from each of the "Four Basic Food Groups" (Table 1.1). The foods from the milk group are major sources of calcium, protein, and riboflavin; items in the meat (and meat substitutes) group supply protein, fat, iron, and other minerals as well as several vitamins. Fruits and vegetables are rich in vitamin C and are precursors of vitamin A, while the bread and cereal group provides carbohydrates, several B vitamins, and iron.

In addition to the food from the basic food groups, other items (e.g., tea and certain spices) can provide nutrients and antioxidants that have been claimed to be good for health. Tea is a rich source of manganese and flavonoids, which have antioxidant properties. Black pepper is a good source of chromium.

TABLE 1.1
Four Basic Food Groups

Group	Food	Major Nutrients
Milk	Milk and other dairy products	Calcium, protein, riboflavin
Meat	Meat, poultry, fish, eggs	Proteins, fat, iron, other minerals
Fruits and vegetables	All varieties of fruits and vegetables, green and yellow vegetables	Vitamin C, vitamin A precursors
Bread and cereal	Bread, cooked cereal, dry cereal, rice, pasta	B vitamins, iron, carbohydrates

1.3.1 Fruits and Vegetables—More Matters

There is a growing body of evidence that fruits and vegetables offer even more health benefits than previously understood and may play roles in preventing several diseases. Also, in 2004, the Institute of Medicine, a federal advisory body, recommended that adult Americans increase their intake of potassium that helps lower blood pressure and is plentiful in many fruits and vegetables.

According to the Centers for Disease Control and Prevention (CDC), which is helping to develop the "More Matters" campaign along with the Produce for Better Health Foundation, about 90% of the U.S. population does not meet the government's recommendations for fruits and vegetables consumption.[5] One of the most popular vegetables (dish) in the country is french fries. Two-thirds of the adult population is overweight, and 90 million Americans suffer from chronic diseases. The hope is that by emphasizing "more" rather than a specific number, the new campaign will inspire people to, at least, add to their intake and expand the variety of foods they eat.

Recently reported benefits are given as follows:

- People who eat fruits and vegetables more than three times a day reduce their risk of having a stroke and dying from cardiovascular disease by nearly a quarter, compared with those who eat them less than once a day.
- Eating lots of fruits and vegetables may be one of the best ways to lose weight. For instance, a survey of 7356 adults found that those who ate at least 4.5 cups of fruits and vegetables a day were less likely to be obese than people who ate fewer, even if their diet was high in fat. Fruits and vegetables are key players in determining weight status.
- High consumption of produce may improve bone health, helping stave off osteoporosis. One recent study found an association between high intake of fruits and vegetables and bone mineral density in boys and girls ages 16–18, and a similar association involving fruit intake in women ages 60–83. Vitamin C and other antioxidants in fruits may play a role. Scientists are exploring the benefits of compounds found in fruits and vegetables.[30]

The guidelines for intake vary by age, sex, and level of activity for everyone over the age of 2 years. A 40-year-old woman, for instance, should eat 2–5 cups of vegetables and 1.5 cups of fruits daily if she exercises less than 30 minutes a day—more if she is more active. A 65-year-old man who exercises less than 30 minutes a day should eat 2.5 cups of vegetables and 2 cups of fruits.

According to the CDC, potatoes, corn, and peas make up 40% of vegetables that Americans consume. People are not eating enough dark green vegetables.

Caution: It is better to eat an actual fruit or vegetable rather than to take a pill containing an active compound of a fruit or a vegetable. In a study of 29,133 male smokers published in 1996, participants who took high doses of β-carotene actually had an 18% higher rate of lung cancer compared with the group that was not given supplements.

1.3.2 Red and Processed Meat—Less Is Better

A study was done recently on two groups of children: one group was in an African village that followed mostly fiber-rich meals of millet, legumes, and other vegetables; another group was in Italy that followed a typical Western diet rich in sugar, fat, and meat. Analysis of intestinal bacterial composition revealed that African children had lots of bacterial species that produced short-chain fatty acids, which are known to have beneficial effects, for example, causing less allergies and inflammation. In contrast, Italian children, though healthy, had bacterial profile that indicated greater risk for diarrhea, allergy, and inflammation. Though the researchers did not measure health outcomes directly, these findings arrive amid growing evidence that gut bacteria control important immune functions.

A second study of nearly 150,000 adults has found that eating too much red and processed meat increases a person's risk of colorectal cancer by up to 50%.[8,33] Researchers reported that the group that ate red meat the most over the long term (defined as an average of at least three ounces daily for men and two ounces for women) had a 30%–40% increased risk of cancer compared with those whose consumption was the lowest (less than 1.5 ounces daily for men and 1 ounce for women).

Another study of more than 90,000 women found that the more red meat the women consumed in their 20s, 30s, and 40s, the greater their risk for developing breast cancer in the next 12 years.[9] Those who consumed the most red meat had nearly twice the risk of those who ate red meat infrequently.

Eating red meat increases the chance of dying prematurely, according to a recent large study (on more than 500,000 middle-aged and elderly Americans) to examine whether regularly eating beef or pork increases mortality. The researchers reported that those who consumed about four ounces of red meat a day (the equivalent of about a small hamburger) were more than 30% likely to die during the 10 years they were followed, mostly due to heart disease and cancer. Sausage, cold cuts, and other processed meat also increased the risk.

The reason for the possible adverse effects of excess red meat (a source of good-quality proteins and some nutrients) consumption is unknown. Fat, nitrites in processed meat, growth hormones and antibiotics administered to animals, carcinogens produced during some types of cooking, or other factors may be involved. More research is needed to confirm the association. We do not know enough to recommend a maximum daily intake of red meat. But the findings provide motivation to choose smaller portions and leaner cuts and include more proteins from fish, poultry, beans, and nuts.[11]

1.4   THE NEED FOR ENERGY

The human body needs a continuous regulated supply of nutrients. Energy is required for all body processes, growth, and physical activity. Even at rest, the body requires energy for muscle contraction, active transport of molecules and ions, and synthesis of macromolecules and other biomolecules from simple precursors. For example, the heart pumps approximately 8000 L/day of blood in about 80,000 pulsations. The daily energy required for this heart function alone is estimated to be equivalent to lifting a weight of 1000 kg to a height of 10 m. In most processes, the energy is supplied by ATP. Energy is liberated when ATP is hydrolyzed to adenosine diphosphate (ADP) and inorganic phosphate. A resting human consumes about 40 kg of ATP in 24 hours. The amount of ATP in the body tissues is limited but is generated continuously from the fuel stores to supply the required energy. These fuel stores must be replenished via food intake.

1.5   THE NEED FOR DIGESTION, ABSORPTION, AND UTILIZATION OF NUTRIENTS

The body cannot use raw materials as they are found in ingested complex foods and beverages. Dietary elements need to be digested in the alimentary tract to substances that can cross the epithelial barrier. Absorption requires sufficient absorptive surface for contact, healthy mucosal cells for uptake, and an intact system for intracellular and extracellular transport. Most of these processes are energy dependent.

After absorption, the energy-yielding substrates and other nutrients are transported to the cells. The conversion of the substrates into energy involves a series of biochemical changes. Many of these changes require the assistance of enzymes; these are proteins produced by the cells of the body to be used by the same cells or other cells. Some enzymes do not act by themselves but require the assistance of coenzymes (e.g., active forms of some vitamins) or cofactors (e.g., minerals). Finally, the excess nutrients and their degradation products are eliminated via excretory pathways so that they do not accumulate and reach toxic levels. Therefore, the assimilation of dietary nutrients and their proper functions require the participation of several organs, enzymes, and biochemical processes. Defects in any of these steps can affect the availability of a nutrient and cause nutrient deficiency, toxicity of a metabolite, or some other health problem despite the consumption of an adequate diet.

Lactase-deficient individuals cannot hydrolyze lactose efficiently and are unable to consume milk without experiencing diarrhea.[27] The loss of small intestinal surface (as in surgical ablation or pathological atrophy) can compromise absorption. Some nutrients after absorption, if not metabolized properly, can be toxic. Given below are two examples of inborn errors of metabolism, one involving an essential nutrient, phenylalanine, and the other involving fructose.

Phenylketonuria (PKU) is an inherited autosomal recessive metabolic disorder that results from a deficiency of the enzyme phenylalanine hydroxylase, which catalyzes the transformation of phenylalanine to tyrosine.[16] Phenylalanine, therefore, is metabolized by an alternate pathway forming phenylpyruvic and phenyllactic acids and, as a result, there is a buildup of phenylalanine and phenylpyruvic and phenyllactic acids in the blood. These compounds act as toxins to the developing nervous system and cause mental retardation unless the disease is treated early. Phenylalanine is essential in the diet, so the disease can be treated nutritionally by restricting the amount of this amino acid to a level that is just sufficient to meet the requirement for growth and small molecule synthesis (Chapter 20). In addition, adequate amounts of tyrosine (which becomes an essential amino acid for a patient with PKU) must be supplied in the diet.

In hereditary fructose intolerance, the individual has a deficiency of the enzyme fructose-l-phosphate aldolase. When fructose-containing foods are ingested, there is accumulation of fructose-l-phosphate; this inhibits some important metabolic steps and causes hypoglycemia and other problems (Chapter 21). Fructose is not essential, so the disease can be treated by eliminating fructose-containing foods from the diet.

1.6 ENTERAL AND PARENTERAL NUTRITION

Many patients either cannot or should not use their gastrointestinal (GI) tract or cannot maintain an adequate oral intake because of anorexia and/or dysfunction of the GI tract. This is especially true of patients with severe infections or burns and those recovering from acute trauma and major surgical procedures who are also hypermetabolic and have increased energy and protein requirements. To meet their nutrient requirements, specialized nutritional feeding must be instituted as either enteral or parenteral feeding.[32,34]

1.6.1 ENTERAL FEEDING

Enteral nutrition is the provision of liquid formula diets by feeding tubes or mouth into the GI tract. It is essential for the maintenance of GI mucosal growth and function. Enteral feeding is indicated in patients with a normal GI tract who cannot or will not eat or in whom oral consumption is inadequate. Nutrients are delivered in a suitable (liquid) form through feeding tubes introduced at various points into the alimentary tract.

Several options exist for the route of tube feeding. The route is determined by the anticipated duration of tube feeding, the disrupted step(s) in the normal process of obtaining nutrients, and the risk of aspiration.[22] The name of the feeding route usually includes both the type of tube placement and the site of formula delivery. For example, nasogastric indicates nasal placement with gastric delivery of formula, whereas gastrostomy indicates ostomy placement with gastric delivery of formula. Metabolic complications of tube feeding include hyperglycemia, electrolyte abnormalities, and fluid imbalance. Regular biochemical determinations are needed to identify developing abnormalities and to allow correction before severe problems occur.

1.6.2 PARENTERAL FEEDING

Parenteral feeding is the administration of nutrients by the intravascular route. It is initiated when the GI tract should not be used or when, because of GI dysfunction, adequate enteral nutrition cannot be achieved. Total parenteral nutrition (TPN) is the administration of an individual's entire nutrient requirement. Nutrients have to be in a form that normally enters the circulation after digestion and absorption. When parenteral nutrition (PN) is necessary, the type of venous access must be selected. PN nutrient formulations may be administered via peripheral veins or central veins, depending on the anticipated duration of PN therapy, degrees of malnutrition, nutrient requirement, and availability of venous access.[24] Peripheral administration is considered when PN is expected to be necessary for fewer than 7–10 days and the patient has fairly low energy and protein needs because of minimal stress. An isotonic solution of glucose, amino acids, vitamins, and minerals can be administered via a peripheral vein for sufficient nitrogen balance; however, it cannot provide more than 600 Cal/day, which is not even adequate for the energy requirement at rest. Higher concentrations of caloric nutrients produce a hypertonic solution that can damage tissues at the site of entry and increase the risk of thrombosis. PN through a central vein is preferred for patients whose GI tracts are either nonfunctional or should not be used for more than 7–10 days and for patients who have limited peripheral venous access or have energy and protein needs that cannot be met with peripheral nutrition formulations. If TPN is to be prolonged, sufficient calories must be infused either as a lipid emulsion or as a hypertonic glucose solution, which requires a central venous catheter.

The bowel atrophies when nutrients are provided exclusively by vein. It has been shown that the addition of glutamine in TPN prevents the deterioration of gut permeability and preserves mucosal structure. There is also significant improvement in nitrogen balance with glutamine-containing TPN formulation in comparison to glutamine-free formulation during the first 3 days after abdominal surgery.[31] Glutamine is added in the TPN as a dipeptide such as glycyl-glutamine because glutamine itself is unstable under the high-temperature and high-pressure sterilization conditions.

The PN nutrition therapy may be associated with multiple metabolic complications. The most common abnormalities are hypokalemia, hypomagnesemia, hypophosphatemia, and hyperglycemia. Routine monitoring of these serum parameters to identify complications early is necessary to manage or prevent complications.[29]

1.7   ADAPTATION

The human body has a powerful ability to take care of itself under various conditions. It obtains what it needs from widely differing diets; within limits it protects itself from some toxic substances present in foods; and it tries to survive by adapting its metabolism when dietary nutrients are in short supply.

One of the main objectives of the living organism's existence with its environment is the maintenance of a favorable nitrogen economy. The metabolic activity of proteins or turnover (the process of breakdown and resynthesis) is a continuous process, constantly undergoing modulation to respond to the adaptive stresses placed upon the organism from the environment. Amino acids must be obtained to replace those lost by the inefficiencies of the turnover process (particularly for the essential amino acids). Energy substrates must be continuously available to fuel not only synthesis processes but also support the activity of these proteins whether it be hormonal, enzymatic, organ function, or locomotion. The body maintains all these vital functions at a relatively constant rate when dietary replacement is often intermittent or erratic.

The body has an amazing ability to adapt. Biological clocks are set to inform the individual that repletion of nutrients is required (e.g., hunger); however, if nutrients are not forthcoming, adaptation to endogenous fuel stores can be accomplished. Hormonal activity is precisely integrated to maintain continuous supplies of nutrients. Nutrition is indeed an endogenous event.

Under normal conditions, about 10% of dietary iron is absorbed, but when there is a deficiency of this nutrient, the absorption is more efficient. On the other hand, when there is an excess of iron in the body, the amount absorbed is curtailed substantially. Almost all the ascorbic acid (vitamin C) present in a normal diet is absorbed, but consumption of larger doses reduces its absorption efficiency. Long-term ingestion of larger doses of vitamin C causes induction of the enzyme involved in the catabolism of ascorbic acid. When the plasma level of ascorbic acid is at or below the normal range, there is very little ascorbic acid excreted in the urine because of its efficient reabsorption by renal tubules. The amount excreted increases when plasma levels of the vitamin are higher than normal. The body adapts to larger doses, and thus the daily requirements for the vitamin increases. Vitamin deficiency signs can appear when long-term ingestion of large doses of vitamin C is discontinued. It may take several weeks for the body to readjust itself for lower doses.

Whenever there is a shift in the quantity or the nature of the fuel supply, the enzymatic constitution changes so as to make the most efficient use of the material at hand. This is especially true of the liver, which plays a major role in balancing the flow of different metabolites. During starvation, the body has to adapt to substrate deprivation. It has to rely on its own fuel stores, and it stops synthesizing the enzymes required for the digestion of food and for handling the excesses of foodstuffs; instead, the amino acids are used for more pressing purposes.

At the beginning of starvation, glycogen is broken down to glucose, which is oxidized to provide energy.[7] The glycogen stores are limited and are totally dissipated within the first 3 days of fasting. Body fat then plays a major role as the source of energy. Some tissues (e.g., the brain, red blood cells) use only glucose as a source of energy. The brain cannot use fatty acids because these substrates do not readily cross the blood–brain barrier. Because fatty acids cannot be converted to glucose, those tissues that use only glucose for energy have to rely on body protein catabolism (amino acids) for the formation of glucose. Although body protein represents a substantial source of calories, there is no storage or depot protein, per se. Each protein molecule serves some important structural, contractile, or enzymatic function. Survival is not possible if 25%–33% of the body protein is lost.

After glycogen stores are depleted, skeletal muscle protein is used as a source of glucose for some tissues. During the first 3–5 days of starvation approximately 75 g of protein/day is used for energy. This is equivalent to about 300 g of muscle; at this rate, body protein can diminish quickly. Therefore, during fatty acid catabolism (and in the absence of carbohydrate catabolism) ketone bodies are synthesized and the brain adapts to use these metabolites as energy sources. Amino acids are still used to provide glucose to tissues that rely entirely on this substrate; however, the amount of protein required is only about one-third of that needed without this adaptation. Thus, to lengthen survival time, the body tries to conserve body protein and uses fat and fat-derived fuels as the major energy sources.

1.8   WATER AS A NUTRIENT

Water, sometimes called the "silent nutrient," is taken for granted in nutritional consideration.[15,18] A deficient intake, however, can produce death faster than that of any other nutrient. Total body water in humans varies from 55% to 65% of the body weight depending on body composition. Lean body tissues contain approximately 75% water, but adipose tissue has very little water. Therefore, the percentage of water is greater in lean individuals than in obese individuals.

Most of the body water is found within three major body compartments: intracellular fluid (within the cells) has about 70%, interstitial fluid (e.g., lymph) has about 20%, and blood plasma has about 7%. The latter two compartments together come under the extracellular fluid category. The remaining 3% of body water is in the intestinal lumen, cerebrospinal fluid, and other body compartments. The body controls the amount of water in each compartment mainly by controlling the ion concentrations in each compartment. Intracellular water volume depends primarily on intracellular potassium and phosphate concentration. Extracellular water volume depends primarily on extracellular sodium and chloride concentration.

The body has three sources of water: (1) ingested water and beverages, (2) the water content of solid foods, and (3) metabolic water, which is derived from the oxidation of carbohydrate, fat, and protein. The latter amounts to about 300–350 g/day in an average adult male. According to composite estimates, 100 g of starch yields 55 g of water, 100 g of fat yields 107 g of water, and 100 g of protein gives 41 g of water. Water is absorbed in the upper small intestine and is distributed by way of the lymph and blood into and from the various tissues and cells of the body. Eventually, water is excreted via the kidneys, sweat, expired air, feces, and so on.

Under ordinary conditions, the water balance between the cells and the fluids of the body is maintained at a constant level. The loss of water equals the intake and endogenous formation and is in the range of 2–4 L. Water intake is regulated mainly by "thirst," and the output is controlled by antidiuretic hormone and the kidneys. If excessive amounts of water are ingested, the kidneys excrete the excess. On the other hand, if the fluid intake is low, the kidneys excrete a more concentrated urine so that less water is lost from the body. Starvation or a carbohydrate-restricted regimen is associated with an acute loss of body water (e.g., 1–1.5 L), which represents the water normally held by glycogen storage in the tissues.

Water is vital to the body as a solvent and lubricant and as a medium for transporting nutrients and waste. It also has a role in regulating body temperature. A decrease in body water can result from either an inadequate intake or excessive excretion (e.g., sweating, vomiting, or diarrhea). Loss of electrolytes along with water may also occur under the latter condition.[14]

Normally, the total osmotic effects of the plasma, interstitial fluid, and the intracellular fluid are all the same. The osmotic effect is attributable mostly to inorganic ions but also to nonelectrolytes such as glucose, urea, and proteins. Consequently, gains or losses of electrolytes, especially sodium or potassium, or changes in their concentrations are usually followed by shifts of fluid to restore osmotic equilibrium.

Abnormalities of extracellular fluid volume are generally caused by net gains or losses of sodium and accompanying gain or loss of water. Volume depletion may result from unreplaced losses such as prolonged sweating, vomiting, diarrhea, or burn injury. A fluid volume excess tends to result from diseases such as kidney or heart failure, which prevent the excretion of sodium and water. Early signs of water loss include headache, fatigue, loss of appetite, flushed skin, heat intolerance, light-headedness, dry mouth and eyes, and a burning sensation in the stomach. Signs of more advanced dehydration include clumsiness, sunken eyes and dim vision, and delirium. The prevalence of kidney stones is higher in populations with low urine volume, which is related to fluid intake. Increased fluid intake to allow for urine volume of about 2 L/day can prevent or reduce the incidence of stone formation.

Although a multitude of factors determine water requirements under ordinary circumstances, a reasonable allowance is 1.5 mL/Cal for infants or 10%–15% of body weight/day. For adults, the corresponding values are 1 mL/Cal or 2%–4% of body weight/day.

Healthy people have no need to track their water intake. "Obey your thirst" is good advice. Patients with conditions such as nephrolithiasis and urinary tract infections may benefit from consciously increasing their fluid intake; patients who are at risk for hypertension should restrict their water consumption.

1.8.1 REQUIREMENT FOR ATHLETES

Of all nutritional concerns for athletes, the most critical is adequate water intake. An athlete's immediate need for water is to control body temperature and to cool working muscles. For several years the advice to athletes has been to drink as much liquid as possible to avoid dehydration. It is known that even as little as 1%–2% loss of body water affects performance. Heat illness such as heat cramps can progress to heat exhaustion and eventually heat stroke, which can be fatal. Reduced work capacity of muscle occurs around 5%–10% loss of body water.

New studies suggest that marathon runners should limit the amount of water they drink during the race or they may be faced with headache, collapse, confusion, memory loss, vomiting, seizures, and even death. These complications result from excess intake of water during exercise (exercise associated hyponatremia or water intoxication). The runners who develop problems tend to be slower and gain weight during the race. The kidneys cannot excrete excess water during intense exercise. As people keep drinking, the extra water moves into their cells including brain cells.[1,26] It can result in swelling of the brain, and the symptoms of hyponatremia are mainly neurological. Women are at higher risk for developing the condition. Patients are treated with 1.8% (hypertonic) saline, and recovery is generally quick.

The advice to race participants is to drink fluids safely and leave the event with some good memories of their achievements. They should be well hydrated before the race. Drinking according to the perception of thirst appears safe. Specific advice on hourly volume intake is not possible (because of individual variations) but would typically be between 400 and 800 mL/hr. The faster, larger athlete racing in hot weather will have higher requirements, whereas slower, smaller runners taking part in colder conditions will have lower requirements.

1.9 FOOD ALLERGY

An allergy may be defined as any unusual or exaggerated response to a particular substance, called an allergen, in a person sensitive to that substance. Allergies are the result of reactions of the body's immunological processes to "foreign" substances (chemical substances in items such as foods, drugs, and insect venom) or to physical conditions.[3,28] The reaction is caused by an allergen, either alone or coupled with a hapten,* which simulates the production of antibodies. Subsequent exposure to previously sensitized antibody-producing cells may precipitate an allergic reaction. The symptoms range from sneezing to vomiting, headaches to hives, edema to diarrhea, and many more, some minor and some quite serious. These effects are believed to be due to the release of histamine by an immunological reaction.

Allergies are classified into two broad classes: (1) immediate and (2) delayed. Immediate allergies, as implied by their name, are those that occur within minutes to an hour or so after the ingestion of the offending food. Delayed allergies occur hours (at least 4 hours) or days after exposure to the allergen. Immediate allergies are mediated by a specific class of antibodies known as immunoglobulin E or IgE. With the exception of celiac disease, which is an abnormal intestinal immune response to wheat, rye, and barley, the role of delayed hypersensitivity in adverse reaction to foods remains poorly understood.

Many individuals are particularly sensitive to certain foods, just as others are to pollen or other particles in the air they breathe. Some foods are more likely to produce allergic reactions than others, but practically all foods can produce an allergic reaction in some people. Proteins are often considered the causative agents, and undoubtedly they are in most cases, but there are some assertions in the literature that fats and even carbohydrates can be responsible. Many different foods have been associated with allergies. They all contain proteins, one or more of which enter the body across the intestinal epithelium and elicit an immune response; however, any major alteration in the protein such as heat denaturation usually results in the loss of its allergenic properties. For example, raw or pasteurized milk may cause an allergic reaction, but if the same milk is boiled—a process that denatures the proteins—the sensitive individual may be able to consume it without an allergic reaction.

About 90% of food allergies can be traced to proteins found in the so-called big eight: milk, eggs, fish, crustacea (crab, shrimp, lobster), peanuts, tree nuts, soybeans, and wheat. Also, some people are allergic to strawberries and other berries, citrus fruits, tomatoes, and chocolate. Foods that rarely cause allergic reactions include rice, lamb, gelatin, peaches, pears, carrots, lettuce, and apples.

Cross-reactions can develop in which sensitivity to proteins in one substance can trigger a reaction to another. This can occur not only within food groups but also with seemingly unrelated substances. For example, if an individual is allergic to soybean, that individual might react to other

---

* A hapten is a small molecule that cannot by itself stimulate antibody synthesis but can combine with a protein to stimulate antibody formation.

legumes. More surprisingly, if an individual is allergic to natural rubber latex proteins, that individual might react to bananas. You would not necessarily expect those two substances to have anything in common, but they must have something in common.

When a food substance is ingested, it encounters three lines of body defense. Enzymes in the mouth, stomach, and small intestine break down the substance into its component amino acids, sugars, etc., and decrease the probability that the body will react to the food substance immunologically. Acid in the stomach denatures the proteins of the food substance, thus changing other configurations and reducing immunologic reactivity. Immunoglobulin A or IgA antibodies in the GI tract specifically combine with the proteins, carbohydrates, etc., to severely curtail their absorption into and through the wall of the GI tract (villi, microvilli, etc.) before enzymatic hydrolysis takes place. In spite of the above defense mechanisms, small amounts of food proteins enter the blood in immunologically recognizable forms.

All of the major food allergens appear to be very stable to digestion in the GI tract. The reason for this is not completely understood though some of these indigestible proteins have a particularly stable three-dimensional structure. Proteins that are rich in cysteine residues are especially stable. Stability to digestion is now widely accepted as a useful, albeit not perfect, marker of food protein allergenicity.

The body's immune system provides protection against foreign proteins or antigens, including those in the diet. The blood contains substances that suppress immunologic reactions to the food components: white cells that have a suppressor function and antibodies that are specific for a particular food component. These substances help the body process food components that have entered the body fluids by inhibiting reactions that would be detrimental to the body.

Once these food substances are in the circulation, they can travel to any site in the body where there are specific antibodies to the substances bound to target-organ tissues. The specific food substance antigens then presumably attach to the specific antibodies and initiate antigen-antibody reactions on the surface of the target organ. The target organ responds by functioning abnormally, producing a symptom or a set of symptoms characteristic of a malfunction. Thus, a particular food can elicit symptoms in sensitive individuals that could be different for each person, depending on which target organ(s) are affected by that food.

Normally our bodies develop a tolerance to most of these foreign proteins. But people with food allergies mount an inappropriate immune response to these antigens, generating IgE antibodies. These antibodies latch onto the antigen and to the surface of the immune system's mast cells and basophils. These cells then release "mediators" such as histamine that lead to the allergic reaction, whether it be a stuffy nose, twitching bronchi causing asthma, a rash, or other symptoms.

Certain allergies tend to be hereditary in that they are passed on from parent to child. The word "atopy" is used to describe a group of allergic diseases that occur in humans and that are the result of genetic abnormality. And there may be other factors. For example, someone's bronchi may be a little more twitchy, and so different types of stimuli might cause a bronchospasm, which we would see as an asthmatic attack.

A small group of people suffers from exercise-induced allergies in which they develop allergic symptoms "only if they exercise either right before or right after eating the specific food in question." We do not know how it happens. Curiously, one of the foods that have been most commonly associated with it is celery, which is otherwise not a prominent allergenic food.

Approximately 100–200 people die from food allergies each year in the United States. Peanuts are responsible for about half of the annual deaths associated with allergies. Food allergies afflict 1%–2% of the overall population and as many as 5% of young children, though they sometimes outgrow the problem as they get older. In some cases, this may happen because of "gut closure," in which the gut becomes less permeable to the allergic molecules. But the reason for improvement in other children is not understood. Some adults who have tolerated certain foods for years suddenly become allergic to them. The mechanism for this is unknown. Some speculate that there may be as-yet-unknown "secondary events that either predispose someone to an allergic reaction effect or that might enhance the ability of an allergen to stimulate an immune response."

As many as 3 million Americans have an allergy to peanuts and usually also to tree nuts such as almonds and walnuts. According to the CDC, the percentage of U.S. children with a food allergy jumped 18% from 1997 to 2007, and there has been a fourfold increase in children's hospitalizations for food allergies in recent years. The cause of this rapid rise is not known, but some have suggested that dwindling exposure to dirt, soil, and animals has driven the increase. A study tested whether peanut-allergic children could be helped to tolerate this food by consuming a tiny amount (1/1000th of a peanut) and progressively increasing the amount. Children exhibited "long-term tolerance" of peanuts.[10] Others have used a similar technique to build tolerance of children severely allergic to milk with some success.

Severe food allergies are becoming more common, but the cause is not quite clear. Scientists are making progress, however, on identifying and determining the structure of the allergenic components of food. They are attempting to create hypoallergenic forms of food that will not elicit symptoms that can include mild itching, diarrhea, asthma, etc. Other than very small studies on oral immunotherapy, there are no therapeutic approaches at this point for food allergy. The best treatment after the offending food, or foods, is identified is to plan an adequate diet that does not contain the allergen.

Food intolerance is an adverse reaction to food that does not involve an immune response. Several basic mechanisms produce clinical manifestations of food intolerance. For example, the failure to digest lactose due to a deficiency of lactase leads not only to inefficient utilization of dietary lactose but also to a disordered GI physiology. Tyramine in cheese or red wine may provoke or exacerbate migraine. Monosodium glutamate provokes flushing, headache, and abdominal symptoms. Metabolic or biochemical abnormalities can alter the intermediary metabolism of a substance. Inborn errors such as PKU and galactosemia have this effect and are described in Chapter 21.

1.9.1 ALLERGIES—READ IT AND EAT

According to the nonprofit Food Allergy & Anaphylaxis Network, 300,000 people visit emergency rooms due to food-allergy-related reactions each year, and about 150 die. The most common culprits, accounting for 90% of all food allergies include milk, soy, eggs, fish, wheat, peanuts, tree nuts like almonds and walnuts, and shrimp and other crustacean shellfish. They are used in hundreds of products, but sometimes it is hard to tell which ones. Lunchmeat can contain milk, and wheat may be in candy. Under the new Food Allergen Labeling and Consumer Protection Act of 2004, any product labeled on or after January 1, 2006 must say if it includes any of the eight allergens, no matter how small the quantity. Shopping is made little easier. Anyone, including children, can read the labels and understand them. This should mean fewer visits to the emergency room.

1.9.2 CELL PHONE ALLERGY

Among the nonfood items, increased use of cell phones has led to prolonged exposure to nickel in phones. Menu buttons, decorative logos, and metallic frames around the liquid crystal display (LCD) are the most common sites where nickel is found on mobile phones. Symptoms of cell phone allergy include a red, bumpy, itchy rash in areas where the nickel-containing parts of a cell phone touch the face.[4] It can even affect the fingertips of those who text continuously on buttons containing nickel. In severe cases, blisters and itchy sores can develop. Nickel allergy affects an estimated 17% of women and 3% of men. Women typically develop cell phone rash more often because they are more likely to have been sensitized to nickel after ear piercing or had an allergic reaction to nickel-containing jewelry.

1.10   GUIDELINES FOR AMERICANS

On January 12, 2005, the sixth edition of the Dietary Guidelines for Americans (Dietary Guidelines), the federal government's science-based advice to promote health and reduce chronic disease through nutrition and physical activity, was released by the United States Department of Agriculture (USDA) and the Department of Health and Human Services (DHHS). The "Dietary Guidelines for Americans 2005," which has been published every five years since 1980, provide recommendations for Americans ages two years and over. They are based on the work of a committee of nutrition experts who regularly review existing published literature. The guidelines include the Food Guide Pyramid (Figure 1.1), which is widely used to educate consumers about ideal food consumption choice. The pyramid depicts, in terms understandable to the average person, daily recommended proportions from each major food group. The 2005 version places strong emphasis on consuming a nutrient-dense diet while staying within Cal needs and on physical activity. This focus stems from knowledge that the major causes of morbidity and mortality in the United States are related to a poor diet and a sedentary lifestyle.

Nutrients are reorganized into six categories (grains, vegetables, fruits, oils, milk, and meat and beans), plus a seventh "discretionary Cal allowance" category (e.g., solid fat, added sugars). Instead of the old pyramid, which had food groups arrayed like building blocks many found confusing, the new pyramid has rainbow-hued bands running vertically, each color representing a different food group. Orange represents grains, green is for vegetables, red stands for fruits, yellow means oils, blue represents dairy products, and purple stands for meat and beans. The width of the bands represents the relative proportions of each group that individuals should consume each day, with grains and vegetables predominating.

Exercise is a key to the new system and is represented by a person climbing steps toward the tip.

The USDA's website allows people to personalize the graphic to their individual caloric and physical activity requirements. The site features 12 different pyramids to meet individual needs.

An interactive version of the food pyramid that provides more information is available at www.mypyramid.gov/pyramid/index.html.

On January 31, 2011, the Secretaries of the USDA and DHHS announced the release of the seventh edition of the Dietary Guidelines for Americans. The "2010 Dietary Guidelines for Americans" places

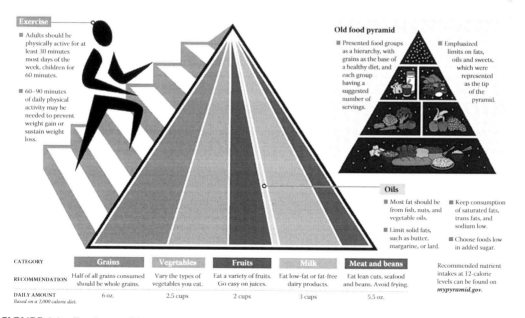

FIGURE 1.1   Food pyramid.

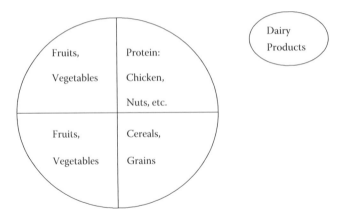

FIGURE 1.2   USDA's newest guidelines for Americans represented as a dinner plate.

strong emphasis on reducing Cal consumption and increasing physical activity. The guidelines include 23 key recommendations for the general population and 6 additional key recommendations for specific population groups such as women who are pregnant. Key recommendations are the most important messages within the guidelines in terms of their implications for improving public health. The recommendations are intended as an integrated set of advice to achieve overall healthy eating patterns.

More consumer friendly advice tools, including a next generation of food pyramid, will be released by the USDA and DHHS in the coming months. Given below is a preview of some of the tips that will be provided to help consumers translate the Dietary Guidelines into their everyday lives:

- Enjoy your food, but eat less.
- Avoid oversized portions.
- Make half of your plate fruits and vegetables.
- Use fat-free or low-fat (1%) milk.
- Compare sodium in foods like soup, bread, and frozen meals—and choose the foods with lower numbers.
- Drink water instead of sugary drinks.

The 2010 Dietary Guidelines are available at http://www.dietaryguidelines.gov.

On June 2, 2011 the USDA unveiled "My Plate," the new food icon, to help consumers make healthier food choices. My Plate—a simple circle designed to evoke a dinner plate—gives viewers a quick idea of what their meals would look like when they sit down at the table (Figure 1.2). The plate features four sections (quadrants). Half of the circle is filled with fruits and vegetables, another section features cereals and grains; and the rest contains protein source such as chicken and nuts. Off to the side, a small circle represents dairy—a glass of milk, a cup of yogurt, or other dairy product.

Many countries have their own ways to present information on healthful eating. In Guatemala, a traditional ceramic cooking pot called olla is filled with pictures of pineapple, fish, and bags of maize. Grenada illustrates food circled inside a cracked-open nutmeg. And in China, a five-tiered pagoda has distinct levels for starches, produce, protein, dairy, and oil!

1.11   EXERCISE FOR HEALTH

Many chronic diseases result from unhealthful eating and a sedentary lifestyle. Poor nutrition and inadequate exercise substantially increase the risk of maladies such as coronary heart disease (CHD), hypertension, stroke, diabetes mellitus, obesity, osteoporosis, and certain cancers and account for about 300,000 deaths in the United States each year. Regular physical activity over months and years produces long-term health benefits and reduces the risk of many diseases. Several recent studies reaffirm the dose-response relationship between the amount of physical activity performed and health risk. Thus, the most fit and active individuals generally have the best risk profile and reduced levels of early mortality and morbidity from a variety of diseases. For example, men and women who were healthy but less fit by treadmill testing had a higher risk of death from any cause over an eight-year follow-up compared with those who were moderately or highly fit. Data from the Nurses' Health Study found that physical activity of less than 3.5 hours/week and excess body weight accounted for 31% of all premature deaths; 59% of deaths were from cardiovascular disease; and 21% of deaths were from cancer.

Physical activity benefits children and adolescents, young and middle-aged adults, older adults, and those in every studied racial and ethnic group. In children and adolescents, regular physical activity improves cardiorespiratory and muscle fitness as well as bone health and contributes to favorable body composition. In adults, it reduces the risk of early death from chronic diseases. Exercise and physical activity deliver oxygen and nutrients to body tissues and help the cardiovascular system work more efficiently. Exercise can reduce the risk of hypertension (high blood pressure). It also causes the body to burn stored fat and prevent excess weight gain, and losing weight can improve insulin sensitivity and blood glucose levels. Also, fat-soluble toxins accumulate in body fat. Therefore, lowering excess body fat can reduce levels of toxicants in the body. These changes are all important for good health. It can improve ability to think and engage in activity needed for daily living. Generally, the longer and harder and more often the exercise, the greater are the health benefits, though the intensity may need to be varied or reduced to a more moderate level depending on individual constitution, quality of health, and seasonal temperatures. Unfortunately, the scientific knowledge about the benefits of exercise among the public and health professionals has not translated into a more active population. Only about 27% of adults in the United States engage in levels of activity sufficient to produce health benefits, and 40% do not participate in any regular physical activity.

The physical activity goal in the Healthy People 2020 report by the CDC is to increase the proportion of adults who engage in regular moderate exercise for at least 30 minutes, preferably daily. In 2008 the U.S. Department of Health and Human Services announced the Physical Activity Guidelines for Americans (PAGA). The guidelines are designed so people can easily fit physical activity into their daily plan and incorporate activities they enjoy. The contents of PAGA complement the Dietary Guidelines for Americans. Together, the two documents provide guidelines on the importance of being physically active and eating a healthy diet to promote good health and reduce the risk of chronic diseases. The guidelines describe the major research findings on the health benefits of physical activity. Guidelines are given for children and adolescents, adults, older adults, women during pregnancy and postpartum period, adults with disabilities, and people with chronic medical conditions. For more information visit www.health.gov/paguidelines.

Exercise causes lowering of catecholamines and triglycerides, reduction in insulin resistance, increase in high-density lipoprotein cholesterol, reduction in total and abdominal adipose tissue, and slowing of loss of bone mass. It also reduces blood levels of cortisol, a stress hormone that builds fat in the abdominal region making weight loss difficult. But the biological mechanisms underlying the effects are uncertain. A few of the recent findings on exercise and benefits are described below.

Genes have a role in physical activity. Exercise activates several genes in skeletal muscle and other tissues.[6] Skeletal muscle is known to adjust its composition to meet the acute and chronic demands placed on it—a process known as plasticity. When the demands for weight-bearing activity are lost, such as during bed rest or space flight, the muscle remodels into a weak muscle, and also a portion is lost because it recognizes that it is not needed. Conversely, if the work demand increases in a sedentary individual, the muscle changes its protein composition to allow energy to be used more efficiently when it contracts. Exercise also influences genes involved in stress and inflammation.

Studies have shown that people who are active (but not necessarily athletic) tend to have similar variations in several different genes. The genetic differences are subtle. One of the affected genes is thought to influence how people respond to fatigue, suggesting that for some people doing the same amount of exercise may be tiring—and less appealing—than for others, even though they may be equally fit. One gene expressed in muscle and brain is likely to have an impact on how physically easy and mentally rewarding exercise feels. Another gene is linked to how the body regulates energy, which can have an effect on the desire to exercise. Other clues on genes are found in the studies of identical twins. One study found that between identical twins 57% exercised while in nonidentical twins only 25% exercised despite varying environments. In another study, physical inactivity was found to be genetically related.

Just because some people have "fat genes" does not mean they will become overweight or obese. According to a new study, exercise can override fat genes.[20] Researchers in Great Britain studied 12 genetic variants known to increase the risk of obesity and tracked the physical activity levels of 20,430 people. They created a genetic summary score to quantify a person's risk of obesity and then examined whether an active life could reduce the genetic influence. According to their findings, genetic predisposition to increased body weight and obesity is attenuated by a physically active lifestyle.

The hippocampus, the brain region that is implicated in memory and spatial reasoning, shrinks a little bit each year in late adulthood, leading to impaired memory and increased risk for dementia. Hippocampus and medial temporal lobe volumes are longer in higher-fit adults, and physical activity increases hippocampal perfusion.

In a recent study 120 sedentary adults aged 55–80 years were recruited. Half of them were assigned to walk around a track for 40 minutes, 3 days a week for a year. Sixty other participants (control group) did toning workouts that included weight training, yoga sessions, and stretching for the same amount of time. After a year of toning, their hippocampi lost over 1% of their volume. In contrast, a year of aerobic exercise led to about a 2% increase in hippocampus volume, effectively reversing age-related loss of volume by 1–2 years.[12] They also did better on memory test than at the start of the study. In addition, the aerobic exercise group tended to have a higher level of brain-derived neurotrophic factor (BDNF), a compound that is associated with having a larger hippocampus and better memory.

Being in better shape to begin with is linked to better memory. The findings also support the concept that "starting an exercise regimen later in life is not futile for enhancing cognition or augmenting brain volume." And even though stretching might be good for physical flexibility and peace of mind for mental agility, aerobic exercise keeps the mind sharp and the brain healthy, not only by preventing natural age-related declines but also by enhancing and improving cognitive functions (e.g., learning, memory, multitasking).[13]

As human brains age they lose their ability to recall memories. Studies were done on women ages 65–75. Some were assigned resistance training, done once or twice weekly in which participants worked out with free weights and weight machines and did squats and lunges. Others were assigned toning and balance exercises, which the volunteers did twice a week. By the end of the year-long study, the women who weight-trained saw an improvement in their performance on cognitive tests of memory and learning as well as in executive functions such as decision making and conflict resolution.[21] Women who trained once a week improved their scores in executive reasoning by 12.6% while those who did toning and balance exercise showed no such improvement. The muscle strengthening exercise also helped the volunteers boost their walking speed, a commonly used indicator of overall health status in the elderly, as faster pace has been linked to lower mortality. In addition, studies have found that people who weight-train have an increase in blood levels of growth factor that is important for maintaining skeletal mass. This factor also promotes nerve growth, which could be another way that resistance training boosts mental function. In another brain function study on 3485 elderly people, scientists found that increased physical activity was associated with a lower incidence of dementia. Those who exercised at least three times a week were half as likely to have developed dementia compared with people who reported no physical activity.

Exercise improves insulin sensitivity. But when muscle cells metabolize glucose, oxygen free radicals, which cause cell damage, are produced (Chapter 25). Some people take antioxidant supplements that can counteract free radicals and protect cells from oxidative damage. To determine the effects of antioxidants on exercise, researchers compared insulin sensitivity and free radical levels in 40 young men; half of them were randomly assigned to receive antioxidant vitamins (vitamin C 1000 mg/day and vitamin E 400 IU/day). After four weeks of exercise, men who took the vitamins showed no change in free radical levels and no improvement in insulin sensitivity. Free radical levels increased and insulin sensitivity improved in those who did not take the vitamins. These studies suggest that free radicals, inevitable byproducts of exercise, are a natural trigger for exercise benefits.[25] Antioxidants, by efficiently destroying free radicals, short-circuit the body's natural response to exercise. It may be that free radicals are beneficial in small doses because they touch off the body's natural defense system, but harmful in high doses. The take-home message from these observations is that those who exercise should not take larger amounts of antioxidants. The advice does not seem to apply to fruits and vegetables even though they are rich in antioxidants; the many other substances they contain presumably outweigh any negative effect.

A study published recently presented a profile of exercise's impact on the human body's metabolites in plasma and revealed biological differences among more and less fit individuals. Scientists measured metabolites in 70 people before and after a 10-minute run on a treadmill.[19] They found an increase in some metabolites after exercise. Glycerol, which is released when fat is used for energy, increased during exercise with levels twice as high in fit people than those less fit. Niacinamide, a metabolite that increases insulin sensitivity, increased more than twice in leaner subjects as it did in larger individuals. And samples from 302 participants in the Framingham Heart Study (the large long-term study that began in 1948 by recruiting an Original Cohort of 5209 men and women from the city of Framingham, Massachusetts, to identify common contributors of cardiovascular disease) indicated that glycerol and glutamine also varied with resting heart rate, another measure of physical fitness.

The issue of how much exercise is required to maintain a normal weight is far from settled. Many people do not want to diet but do want to avoid gaining weight over time. Most Americans gain about 1–1.5 pounds a year after the age of 25. There is growing evidence that combining activities such as walking or cycling with nature boosts well-being. Just 5 minutes of exercise in a "green space" such as a park boosts mental health. National health guidelines suggest 30–60 minutes a day of exercise for better health. But numerous studies now show that one does not have to break a sweat to reap the most significant benefits of exercise.

Researchers reviewed 44 exercise studies and found that most of the benefits of exercise kick in with the first 1000 Calories of increased activity each week, which reduced the risk of dying during the various study periods by 20%–30%. Adults who exercised only once a week were 40% less likely to die during the 12-year study periods than those who did not exercise. Moderate exercise added nearly 2.5 years to life expectancy for patients compared with those who were sedentary. To burn 1000 calories a week, or about 145 Calories a day, most people need to increase their daily activity slightly. A 180-pound person could burn off about 100 Calories during 20 minutes of housework. Add in a 10-minute walk (50 Calories) or take the stairs four times a day (50 calories) to achieve the daily goal. The benefits of just a little exercise are presented in Table 1.2.

Exercise alone may not be enough to counteract the effects of too much sedentary life during the rest of the day. Researchers recently looked at the relationship between the time spent sitting—in

TABLE 1.2
Benefits of Very Little Exercise Demonstrated in Medical Studies

Activity	Benefit
55 flights of stairs a week	33% lower death rate
1 hour of gardening a week	66% lower risk of sudden cardiac death
Walking 1 hour a week	51% lower risk of coronary heart disease
Regular demanding household cleaning	Lowered heart attack risk by 54% in men and more than 84% in women
Exercising 30 minutes just 6 days a month	43% lower mortality

their cars, at their desks, in front of the TV—and dying from heart disease. They found that men who reported more than 23 hours a week of sedentary activity (other than sleeping about 8 hours daily) had a 64% greater risk of dying from heart disease than those who reported less than 11 hours a week of sedentary activity. Many of these men routinely exercised. They recommended hourly minibreaks, even 1 minute long throughout the day, to help movement of muscles and provide health benefits.

1.12 HEALTHY ADVICE

An appropriate diet is one that maintains an appropriate body weight, provides sufficient daily nutrient intake so that deficiency and excess are avoided, and minimizes the risk of subsequent disease.
   The following are some tips on eating wisely:

- Steam or bake foods instead of frying.
- Reduce intake of red meat.
- Include low-fat milk and yogurt.
- Eat more whole grain products.
- Reduce intake of refined sugar and eat more complex carbohydrates.
- Increase intake of fiber, such as apples, oatmeal, and legumes.
- Keep sodium intake to less than 2300 mg/day, about 1 teaspoon of salt.
- Include garlic, onion, and ginger.
- Consider eating meat analogs.
- Reduce number of yolks to five/week.
- Consider using tofu in place of eggs for baking.
- Include cabbage, cauliflower, soybeans, grapes, nuts, turmeric, parsley, and lettuce.
- Consider using fruits and vegetables regularly.
- Eliminate alcohol consumption, except for the occasional glass of red wine for those who are not pregnant.
- Whenever possible choose fresh, wholesome foods (or frozen) over prepackaged or canned ones.

Phenylketonuria—A Case

A four-and-a-half-year-old girl was admitted to a hospital because of retardation of development and a possible neurological problem. She began to sit up at 1 year of age and could use a few words. She learned to walk at the age of 2 years but did not develop further in language ability and gradually lost the few words she had acquired. She was stiff-legged and hypertonic. She had been hyperactive and noisy, frequently banging her head on the wall, slapping her face, voluntarily falling down, biting her tongue, and screaming. There had been no episodes of unconsciousness or convulsions.

   A physical examination revealed that she was an above-normal-weight child with extensive red scaling dermatitis of the forearm and legs and the characteristic odor of phenylacetic acid. She was extremely hyperactive, and her attention span was short. She grated her teeth together nearly continually and frequently uttered unrecognizable cries but no words. She responded to attention but did not play with toys or feed herself.

   A neurological examination showed that her muscular tone was somewhat increased generally and her reflexes were hyperactive. No objective evidence of sensory impairment was apparent. Electroencephalogram showed no seizure discharges. The blood and urine examinations were normal. Fasting serum phenylalanine was 42 mg/dL (normal 0.5–2 mg/dL). Acidified urine developed green color on addition of ferric chloride (positive for PKU).

She was placed on an artificial formula diet containing all of the amino acids in adequate amounts except phenylalanine. Her urinary phenylalanine fell promptly from 14 to about 3 mg/mg creatinine, and serum phenylalanine came down to 20 mg/dL. During the next 2 weeks, her urinary keto acids and serum phenylalanine continued to fall but her weight also declined. Phenylalanine in an oral dose of 90 mg/day was started on the 13th day, but the dose was increased to 500 mg/day in order for growth to resume. During the first few weeks of her dietary regimen, she showed some improvements in behavior. There was a moderate decrease in hyperactivity and increase in attention span. She also engaged in activities of her own choosing for periods as long as 15–20 minutes. The dermatitis disappeared after the first week of the diet, and her skin remained clear during her stay in the hospital. She was discharged after 13 weeks on this diet.

On a natural home diet, serum phenylalanine rose to 30 mg/dL, and phenylpyruvic aciduria and dermatitis recurred. She continued to grow normally during the following 22 months.

This case of PKU was one of the first to be investigated for the possible salutary effect of phenylalanine restriction in the diet.[36,37] PKU is characterized by reduced activity of phenylalanine hydroxylase (less than 2% of normal activity). The disease manifests between the third and sixth months of age and is characterized by mental retardation, abnormal electroencephalogram, dermatitis, hyperactivity, and reduced attention span. Although the exact pathogenesis of mental retardation in PKU is unknown, the accumulation of phenylalanine or its metabolites up to 5–10 times normal levels, or the deficiency of tyrosine or its products, or a combination of the two, cause irreversible damage to the central nervous system. High phenylalanine appears to interfere with decarboxylation of dihydroxyphenylalanine (DOPA) and 5-hydroxytryptophan, which could impair neurotransmitter synthesis. This effect causes hyperactivity, short attention span, and dermatitis, which can be reversed by reducing serum phenylalanine levels, as was seen with this case.

In PKU, phenylalanine levels are elevated and tyrosine levels tend to be depressed. The rational therapy, therefore, is to reduce phenylalanine to just enough for growth requirements and increase tyrosine intake to the level required for growth. Tyrosine becomes a dietary essential amino acid for patients with PKU. The estimated requirement for infants less than 6 months of age is 140 mg/kg of body weight/day. This drops with time to 70 mg at 2 years and about 20 mg/kg of body weight/day with maturity. The diet should be started as soon as possible, preferably by the time the child is 3 weeks old. The diet's effectiveness is remarkable. In almost every case, it can prevent the devastating array of symptoms described above.

REFERENCES

1. Almond, C. S. D., A. Y. Shin, E. B. Fortescue et al. 2005. Hyponatremia among runners in the Boston Marathon. *New Engl J Med* 352:1550.
2. Backstrand, J. R. 2002. The history and future of food fortification in the United States: A public health perspective. *Nutr Rev* 60:15.
3. Bayer, K., and S. Teuber. 2004. The mechanics of food allergy; what do we know today? *Curr Opin Allergy Clin Immunol* 4:197.
4. Berkovitch, L., and J. Luo. 2008. Cellphone contact dermatitis with nickel allergy. *J Can Med Assoc* 178:23.
5. Blanck, H. M., C. Gilespie, J. E. Kimmons et al. 2008. Trends in fruits and vegetable consumption among U.S. men and women 1994–2005. *Prev Chronic Dis* 5(2):A35.
6. Booth, F. W., and P. Darrell Neufer. 2005. Exercise controls gene expression. *Amer Scientist* 93:28.
7. Cahill Jr., G. F. 1976. Starvation in man. *Clin Endocrinol Metab* 5:397.
8. Chao, A., M. J. Thun, C. J. Connel et al. 2005. Meat consumption and risk of colorectal cancer. *J Amer Med Assoc* 293:172.
9. Cho, E. 2006. Red meat intake and risk of breast cancer among premenopausal women. *Arch Intern Med* 166:2253.

10. Clark, A. T., S. Islam, Y. King et al. 2009. Successful oral tolerance induction in severe peanut allergy. *Allergy* 64:1218.
11. Clark, N. 1991. How to pack a meatless diet full of nutrients. *Physician Sports Med* 19:31.
12. Erickson, K. I., M. W. Voss, R. S. Prakash et al. 2011. Exercise training increases size of hippocampus and improves memory. *Proc Nat Acad Sci* 108:3017.
13. Etgen, T., D. Sander, and U. Huntgeburth. 2010. Physical activity and incident cognitive impairment in elderly persons. *Arch Int Med* 170:186.
14. Goldberger, E. E. 1975. *Water: Electrolyte and Acid–Base Syndrome*. 4th ed. Philadelphia: Lea and Febiger.
15. Grandjean, A., and S. Campbell. 2009. *Hydration: Fluids for Life*. Washington, DC: International Life Sciences Institute.
16. Guttler, F. 1980. Hyperphenylalaninemia: Diagnosis and classification of the various types of phenylalanine hydroxylase deficiency in childhood. *Acta Paediatr Scand Suppl* 280:7.
17. Harper, A. E. 1989. Evolution of recommended dietary allowances—New direction? *Annu Rev Nutr* 7:509.
18. Kleiner, S. M. 1999. Water: An essential but overlooked nutrient. *J Amer Diet Assoc* 99:200.
19. Lewis, G. D., L. Farrell, M. J. Wood et al. 2010. Metabolic signatures of exercise and human plasma. *Sci Transl Med* 2(33):33–37.
20. Li, S., J. H. Zhao, J. Luan et al. 2010. Physical activity attenuates the genetic predisposition to obesity in 20,000 men and women from EPIC-Norfolk Prospective Population Study. *PLoS Medicine* 7(8):pii:e1000332.
21. Liu-Amrose, T., L. S. Nagmatsu, P. Graf et al. 2010. Resistance training and executive functions. A 12 month randomized controlled trial. *Arch Int Med* 170:170.
22. Monturo, C. A. 1990. Enteral access device selection. *Nutr Clin Pract* 5:207.
23. National Academy of Sciences. 1989. *Food and Nutrition Board of the National Academy of Sciences: Recommended Daily Allowances*. 10th ed. Washington, DC: National Academy of Sciences.
24. Perman, M., A. Crivelli, and M. Khouri. 2002. National prognosis in hospitalized patients. *Amer J Clin Nutr* 75:4265.
25. Ristow, M., K. Zarse, A. Oberbach et al. 2009. Antioxidants prevent health-promoting effects of physical exercise in humans. *Proc Nat Acad Sci* 106:8665.
26. Rosner, M. H., and J. Kirven. 2007. Exercise-associated hyponatremia. *Clin J Amer Soc Nephrol* 2:151.
27. Saavedra, J. M., and J. A. Perman. 1989. Current concepts in lactose malabsorption. *Annu Rev Nutr* 9:475.
28. Sampson, H. A., and A. W. Burks. 1996. Mechanisms of food allergy. *Annu Rev Nutr* 16:161.
29. Sheldon, G. F., R. P. Scott, and R. Sanders. 1978. Hepatic dysfunction during TPN. *Arch Surg* 113:504.
30. Sherman, P. W., and S. M. Flaxman. 2001. Protecting ourselves from food. *Amer Scientist* 89(2):142.
31. Shipley, S. G. 1996. Glutamine in total parenteral nutrition. *Nutr Today* 31(2):74.
32. Silberman, H. 1989. *Parenteral and Enteral Nutrition*. 2nd ed. Norwalk, CT: Appleton & Lange.
33. Sinha, R., A. J. Cross, B. I. Graubard et al. 2009. Meat intake and mortality: A prospective study of over half a million people. *Arch Intern Med* 169:562.
34. Souba, N. W. 1997. Nutritional support. *N Engl J Med* 136:41.
35. Stewart, K. J., A. C. Bacher, K. Turner et al. 2005. Exercise and risk factors associated with metabolic syndrome in older adults. *Amer J Prev Med* 28:9.

CASE BIBLIOGRAPHY

36. Armstrong, M. D., and F. H. Tyler. 1955. Studies in Phenylketonuria. I. Restricted phenylalanine intake in phenylketonuria. *J Clin Invest* 34:565.
37. Clinical Nutrition Cases. 1983. The dietary treatment of phenylketonuria. *Nutr Rev* 41:11.
38. de Freitas, O., C. Izumi, M. G. Lara, and L. J. Greene. 1999. New approaches to the treatment of phenylketonuria. *Nutr Rev* 57:65.

2 Digestion of Carbohydrates, Lipids, and Proteins

2.1 INTRODUCTION

Our normal food is a mixture of complex plant and animal materials that are composed largely of carbohydrates, fats, proteins, vitamins, and minerals. The bulk of these ingested nutrients consists of large polymers that must be reduced to simpler components before they can be absorbed and thus made available to all the cells in the body. The disintegration of naturally occurring foodstuffs into assimilable forms in the gastrointestinal tract constitutes the process of digestion and involves enzymes. The gastrointestinal tract is important in terms of both maintaining the nutritional status of the gut as well as providing nutrients to maintain the nutritional status and homeostasis of the whole organism. The majority of the enzymes involved in the digestive process are hydrolases (i.e., they split bonds of esters, glycosides, or peptides by the addition of water). The powerful hydrolytic enzymes of the digestive tract catalyze the degradation of large molecules present in food (e.g., starch or protein) into small molecules that can be readily absorbed such as glucose or amino acids. The digestive tract is under neurological and hormonal control. Fear, anger, irritation, and worry all may exert unfavorable influences in the digestive system, while the thought, smell, and presence of food cause secretion and motility necessary for digestion. Both types of changes are controlled via the nervous system of the body. Several areas of the digestive tract secrete hormones, which act as chemical messengers on other areas of the digestive tract to control the process of digestion.

We take food by mouth where it is homogenized, mixed, and lubricated by saliva secreted by salivary glands. One constituent of human saliva is amylase, which catalyses the hydrolysis of starch. Approximately 1.5 L of saliva is secreted daily. From the mouth, the food contents pass via the esophagus (a straight muscular tube about 25 cm long) to the stomach. The stomach consists of three anatomically and functionally distinct regions: (1) the fundus, an upper portion; (2) the body, the central portion; and (3) the antrum, a constricted portion just before entry into the small intestine. The body that makes up approximately 80%–90% of the stomach contains parietal cells and chief cells. In the stomach, the food contents come in contact with gastric juice with a pH ≤ 2. Gastric juice contains hydrochloric acid, mucins, and the enzymes pepsin and lipase. Hydrochloric acid is secreted by parietal cells and pepsin by the chief cells. Chyme, the acidic food content in the stomach, is intermittently introduced into the small intestine. The small intestine is divided into three sections: (1) the duodenum, which receives chyme from the stomach and the secretions from the gallbladder and the pancreas; (2) the jejunum; and (3) the ileum. Bile is formed and secreted continually by hepatocytes. Bile flows from the liver into the gallbladder, where it is concentrated, stored, and emptied into the duodenum when the partially digested contents of the stomach enter the duodenum. The alkaline content of pancreatic (about 1.5 L/day) and biliary secretions (0.5 L/day) neutralizes the acid of the chyme and changes the pH to the alkaline side necessary for the optimum activity of pancreatic and intestinal enzymes. Most of the breakdown of food is catalyzed by the soluble enzymes and occurs within the lumen of the small intestine; however, the pancreas is the major organ that synthesizes and secretes the large amounts of enzymes needed to digest the food. Secreted enzymes amount to about 30 g/day of protein in a healthy adult. The pancreatic duct joins with the common bile duct to form the ampulla of Vater; thus, pancreatic juice and bile empty into the duodenum at the same point.

When fat and products of protein digestion reach the small intestine, the duodenal and jejunal mucosa release cholecystokinin, a peptide hormone (Table 2.1). It stimulates the secretion of pancreatic juice rich in enzymes and also stimulates the contraction of the gallbladder and secretion of bile. The presence of acidic food in the small intestine causes the release of another peptide hormone, secretin, by the duodenal and jejunal mucosa; this stimulates secretion of pancreatic juice rich in bicarbonate and potentiates the action of cholecystokinin on the pancreas. The secretion of gastric juice is under the control of the hormone gastrin, a heptadecapeptide, and its release is stimulated by the presence of food in the stomach. Gastrin is secreted by the antral region of the gastric mucosa and by the duodenal mucosa. The main function of gastrin is to stimulate the secretion of hydrochloric acid into the stomach, but it also stimulates pepsin secretion and increases the motility of the gastric antrum. Gastric inhibitory peptide (GIP) consists of 43 amino acid residues. Its secretion by the K cells of the duodenum and jejunum is stimulated by the presence of glucose and lipids in the duodenum. GIP stimulates secretion of insulin and inhibits gastric secretion and motility. In addition to these hormones, there are several others (e.g., epidermal growth factor) of possible gastrointestinal significance. The discussion of their effects is beyond the scope of this chapter.

At the low pH of the gastric juice, proteins are denatured, and this allows the polypeptide chains to unfold and makes them more accessible to the action of proteolytic enzymes. Some digestion of protein occurs within the lumen of the stomach, and the acid environment also destroys most of the microorganisms swallowed or ingested with food. This protective action against many and varied microorganisms that accompany normal food intake constitutes the body's first and major defense against food-borne infection. It also aids in maintaining qualitative stability in the intestinal flora distal to the stomach. The absence of hydrochloric acid is termed *achlorhydria*. Achlorhydria may occur in pernicious anemia and in a number of other conditions. An average of 2–2.5 L/day of gastric juice is secreted, but the volume is reduced in atrophy of the gastric glands. The intestinal bacterial concentration increases in hypochlorhydria (i.e., abnormally small amounts of hydrochloric acid in the stomach) and may affect the absorption of some nutrients by bacterial binding or metabolizing nutrients. The bulk of digestion occurs distal to the second (descending) part of the duodenum. The final result of the action of digestive enzymes is to reduce the nutrients to forms that can be absorbed and assimilated.

There is little absorption of nutrients from the stomach although alcohol can be absorbed to a significant extent by this organ. Even water passes through the stomach to be absorbed subsequently in the intestine. The main organ for the absorption of nutrients is the small intestine, which has sites for the absorption of specific nutrients.

Intestinal absorption has been aptly termed the first common pathway since all food nutrients in the digestive tract are topologically still outside the body. They must traverse the barrier of intestinal absorptive cell membrane before it can be said that they are actually "inside" the body and available for metabolic purposes.[10] Absorption requires sufficient absorptive surface for contact, healthy mucosal cells for uptake, and an intact system of intracellular and postcellular transport for

TABLE 2.1
Gastrointestinal Hormones

Hormone	Site of Secretion	Biological Action
Gastrin (34 amino acids)	Gastric antrum; stimulated by the presence of food in the stomach	Increased secretion of hydrochloric acid, pepsin
Secretin (27 amino acids)	Duodenum, jejunum; stimulated by the presence of acid in duodenum	Increased secretion of pancreatic juice rich in bicarbonate
Cholecystokinin (33 amino acids)	Duodenum, jejunum; stimulated by the presence of digestion products of fat and protein in the duodenum	Increased secretion of pancreatic juice rich in enzymes; increased contraction of gallbladder

transferring nutrients into the body. Thus, loss of intestinal surface (e.g., from atresia, surgical ablation, or pathologic atrophy) will compromise absorption.

The basic functional unit of the small intestine consists of a crypt and villus. Intestinal epithelial cells originate by mitosis in the crypt base, where DNA and protein synthesis are highly active (Figure 2.1). However, they do not have fully formed microvilli or the biochemical machinery for hydrolysis and transport. The crypt epithelial cell is both morphologically and functionally immature until it migrates into the lower villus some 24 hours after its birth to assume the typical columnar shape with elongated finger-like microvilli. At this time, the oligosaccharidase activity first becomes detectable in the microvillar membrane. Further migration up the villus is associated with the maximal enzyme activity at the middle and upper villus levels and a slight decrease in the activity at the villus tip from which senescent cells are extruded. The life cycle of these cells is only a few days. The half-lives of oligosaccharidases are only a few hours. In general, younger more immature crypt cells secrete, while the "adult" cells in the upper third of the villus primarily absorb. Diarrhea, intestinal flu, infection, etc., can cause loss of some cells.

In a newborn baby, the length of the small intestine is about 200 cm. It elongates and grows in diameter with age, and by adulthood the length is 700–800 cm. The morphology of the intestine ideally meets the need for maximum surface area for digestion and absorption of nutrients. The luminal surface of the small intestine is so organized that the area available for contact with intestinal contents is greatly amplified by visible spiral or circular concentric folds with villi lined by absorptive columnar epithelial cells. The apical surface of each epithelial cell, in turn, is covered by microvilli that form the brush-border of each epithelial cell of the villus. The result of this folding is that the intestinal surface of an adult human covers an estimated area of 300 m^2, or about 600 times greater than its external surface area. The mucosal cells of the small intestine and stomach have a life of about 3–4 days. The cells are sloughed off from the tips of the villi and are replaced by new ones. This amounts to 20–30 g protein/day, which is reclaimed as amino acids after hydrolysis in the lumen.

About 90%–95% of the ingested foodstuffs along with water are absorbed in the small intestine. The unabsorbed residue then enters the large intestine, which is about 1.5 m long. The major functions of the large intestine are absorption of water, sodium, and other electrolytes present in the residue and temporary storage of unabsorbed contents and their elimination. The semiliquid intestinal contents gradually become more solid. During this period bacterial activity on the residual

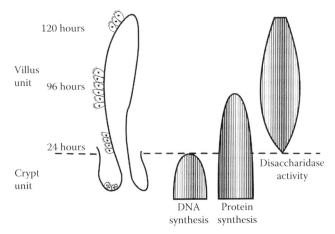

FIGURE 2.1 Correlation of functional activities with the location of the epithelial cells in the crypt-villus unit. The position of the shaded areas locates the site of the particular activity, and the width denotes the relative amount of each functional parameter. Note the tendency to sequential DNA synthesis, protein synthesis, and disaccharidase activity as epithelial cells migrate from crypt to villus and mature morphologically.

matter takes place with the production of gases including ammonia, carbon dioxide, methane, and hydrogen; lactic and acetic acids; and certain substances such as indoles and phenols that may have toxic properties.

Nutrients that are absorbed from the gastrointestinal tract are subsequently transported via either the portal circulation or the lymphatic system. Most of the water-soluble nutrients (amino acids, monosaccharides, glycerol, short-chain fatty acids, electrolytes, and water-soluble vitamins) are transported predominantly by the portal route. These nutrients enter the capillaries that feed into the portal vein, which carries blood draining from the splanchnic bed to the liver. The liver is unusual in that its major blood supply is the venous portal blood with the hepatic artery supplying only about one fourth of the liver's blood flow. The lymphatic system in the gastrointestinal tract plays a pivotal role in the transport of lipophilic substances. A substance transported by the system will enter the blood just before it goes to the heart and will enter the circulation throughout the body in the arterial blood, whereas the substances transported in the portal blood will first pass through the liver where they may be taken up and metabolized by the hepatocytes or returned to the venous circulation via the portal vein.

2.2 CARBOHYDRATES

2.2.1 DIGESTION AND ABSORPTION

From a quantitative point of view, carbohydrate is the major group of chemical substances metabolized by humans and most animals. Approximately 50% by weight of the American diet or 400–500 g/day for the average American male is carbohydrate. About 60% of the total digestible carbohydrate is in the form of starch largely derived from cereal grains and vegetables such as corn and potatoes. The other 40% is supplied in the form of sucrose, lactose, maltose, glucose, fructose, and other sugars. Some glycogen is ingested in meat.

Starch contains two polysaccharides, amylose and amylopectin, which are both polymers of glucose but differ in molecular architecture.[17] Amylose consists of 250–300 glucose units linked by α-1,4 glucosidic bonds (unbranched type). In amylopectin the majority of the units is similarly connected by α-1,4 glucosidic bonds, but has about one α-1,6 glucosidic bond for 30 α-1,4 linkages (branched type). Glycogen resembles amylopectin in structure but has a higher degree of branching.

The digestion of starch begins in the mouth when food is mixed with salivary α-amylase, but the hydrolysis stops in the stomach because of the change in pH and resumes in the duodenum where pancreatic α-amylase is secreted. Both salivary and pancreatic amylases are α-1,4 glucosidases and serve to hydrolyze only the internal 1,4 glucosidic bonds found in starch and glycogen. There is little activity at the 1,4 linkages adjacent to the branching points, and the α-1,6 bonds (or branch points) are not attacked by amylase. Consequently, the products of digestion by α-amylase on starch or glycogen are maltose, isomaltose, maltotriose (a trisaccharide), and α-limit dextrins (containing on the average eight glucose units with one or more α-1,6 bonds). The final digestive process occurs at the mucosal lining and involves the action of α-dextrinase (isomaltase), which hydrolyzes the 1,6 glucosidic bonds from limit dextrins and isomaltose, and glucoamylase, which acts on glucose oligomers containing four to nine glucose units. Maltase, another brush-border enzyme, breaks down maltose and maltotriose into glucose, which is the end product of starch and glycogen digestion. Sucrose and lactose are similarly hydrolyzed by sucrase and lactase, which are located on the brush-border, to their corresponding monosaccharides glucose and fructose and glucose and galactose, respectively.

Monosaccharides are absorbed from the intestinal lumen by passage through the mucosal epithelial cells into the bloodstream. The transport of glucose and galactose across the brush-border membrane of the mucosal cell occurs by an active, energy-requiring process that involves a specific transport protein SGLT1 and the presence of sodium ions. Fructose is absorbed by a facilitated diffusion process supported by GLUT5 that efficiently accommodates luminal fructose and functions independently of sodium ions. Glucose, galactose, and fructose exit from the enterocytes primarily via the GLUT2 transporter of the basolateral membrane. Other sugars (e.g., pentoses) are absorbed by simple diffusion through the lipid bilayer of the membrane. In a normal individual, the digestion and absorption of usable carbohydrates are 95% or more complete. Some sugars and sugar alcohols such as sorbitol are universally malabsorbed, and diarrhea ensues with the ingestion of ample medications, gums, and candies sweetened with these slowly absorbable sugars.

2.2.2 CARBOHYDRATE INTOLERANCE

Carbohydrate intolerance is characterized by malabsorption that leads to symptoms, particularly diarrhea, with excretion of acidic stools and carbohydrate in the feces following ingestion of sugars. It can be due to a defect in digestion and/or absorption of dietary carbohydrate. Di-, oligo-, and polysaccharides that are not hydrolyzed by amylase and/or small intestinal surface (brush-border) enzymes cannot be absorbed; they reach the lower tract of the intestine, which contains bacteria. Microorganisms can break down and anaerobically metabolize some carbohydrates, resulting in the formation of short-chain fatty acids, lactate, hydrogen gas, carbon dioxide, and methane. The presence of osmotically active carbohydrate and fermentative products within the lumen is associated with intestinal secretion of fluid and electrolytes until osmotic equilibrium is reached. These products also cause increased intestinal motility and cramps because of intraluminal pressure and distention of the gut, or because of the direct effect of degradation products on the intestinal mucosa. Some intestinal mucosal cells along with disaccharidases may be lost.

Disaccharidase deficiency is frequently encountered in humans.[22] The deficiency can be due to a single or several enzymes for a variety of reasons (e.g., genetic defects, injuries to mucosa, or physiological decline with age). Mucosal injury may arise from either tissue invasion and destruction of the epithelial cells by enteric microorganisms or cell injury caused by products of bacterial metabolism. Viral gastroenteritis damages the mucosa and destroys a significant proportion of disaccharidases of the brush-border cells. Mucosal damage does not usually affect sucrose hydrolysis probably because a high level of sucrase is normally present, but lactose hydrolysis is significantly reduced. Secondary deficiency may result due to a disease or disorder of the intestinal tract; these defects disappear when the disease is resolved. Such diseases include protein deficiency, celiac disease, tropical sprue, and intestinal infections. Brush-border enzymes are rapidly lost in normal individuals with severe diarrhea, causing temporary acquired enzyme deficiency. These patients suffering or recovering from a disorder cannot drink or eat significant amounts of dairy products (lactose) or sucrose without exacerbating the diarrhea. Lactase deficiency is most commonly observed (milk intolerance) in humans. There are three types of lactase deficiency: (1) inherited deficiency, which is relatively rare, in which symptoms of intolerance develop very soon after birth and disappear with feeding on a lactose-free diet; (2) secondary low-lactase activity, which can occur as a result of damage to the small intestine; and (3) primary low-lactase activity, which is a relatively common syndrome, particularly among African Americans, Asians, and South Americans. In these individuals, intolerance to lactose is not a feature of the early life of adults, but there is an age-related decline in lactase activity in susceptible individuals. In olden times nonhuman mothers' milk was *not* a readily available source of nutrients. But after cattle were domesticated 9000 years ago and people started to consume milk as well as its products, there was a need for continued lactase activity. Natural selection favored a mutation to keep the lactase gene switch on. Such a mutation is known to have arisen among an early cattle-raising people, the Funnel Beaker culture,* which flourished 5000 years ago in northern central Europe. People with a persistent active lactase gene have no problem

---

* The Funnel Beaker culture takes its name from the characteristic pottery made by those people. The distinctive pottery consists of a flared rim in the upper few inches of the vessel, so that the opening of the vessel is widest along the top rim. It is believed that this characteristic shape had a very practical purpose, which was to reduce the amount of milk lost during the milking process.

digesting milk and are said to be lactose tolerant.[2] Almost all Dutch people and 90% of Swedish people are lactose tolerant, but the mutation becomes progressively less common in Europeans who live at increasing distances from the ancient Funnel Beaker region. Recent studies have shown that some ethnic groups originally from this region who had settled in parts of Africa about 4500 years ago have lactose tolerance. Studies on lactose tolerance in different regions of the world suggest that adaptation to digest lactose throughout adult life is related to the development of dairying in these regions thousands of years ago.[19]

Approximately 75% of adults worldwide are lactase deficient (primary low-lactase activity). Lactose intolerance is highest in Native Americans and Asians and is slightly lower in Blacks, Jews, Hispanics, and Southern Europeans.[8] It is believed that 25% of Caucasians; 51% of Hispanics; 75% of African Americans, Jews, and Native Americans; and 90% of Asian Americans are lactose intolerant. Lactose content of some dairy products is listed in Table 2.2.

Sucrase–isomaltase deficiency is a rare inherited deficiency of sucrase and isomaltase. Individuals with this combined enzyme deficiency cannot hydrolyze sucrose and the disaccharide products of ingested starch. The deficiencies of these two enzymes coexist because sucrase and isomaltase occur together as a complex enzyme. This disorder is found in about 10% of Greenland Eskimos. Symptoms occur in early childhood and are the same as those described for carbohydrate intolerance. Osmotic diarrhea may be relieved by restricting both sucrose and starch.

Oligosaccharides such as raffinose (a trisaccharide containing glucose, fructose, and galactose) and stachyose (a tetrasaccharide containing two moles of galactose, one mole of glucose, and one mole of fructose) are ingested in small amounts in legumes (e.g., kidney beans, lentils, and navy beans) but cannot be hydrolyzed by intraluminal or intestinal enzymes. Although not nutritionally important, saccharides in legumes are acted upon by bacteria in the lower small intestine and colon to yield two or three carbon fragments, hydrogen, and carbon dioxide. Hence, depending on the bacterial population, ingestion of large quantities of legumes may increase flatus production.

The definitive diagnosis of a deficiency of a particular enzyme involved in carbohydrate digestion requires collection of a biopsy specimen from the small intestine and demonstration of a decreased activity of the enzyme. Because of the difficulty in obtaining a biopsy specimen, especially in children, indirect methods for the detection of enzyme deficiency are used. One involves the measurement of breath hydrogen.

Bacteria that produce hydrogen are normally located almost entirely in the colon. These bacteria produce little hydrogen during metabolism of substrates endogenous to the gut, but rather require a supply of ingested fermentable substrates, primarily carbohydrates. Therefore, hydrogen production occurs only when incompletely digested carbohydrates (and thus not absorbed in the small intestine) reach the colonic bacteria.[6] A certain proportion of hydrogen produced is absorbed and then

TABLE 2.2
Lactose in Common Dairy Foods

Food	Lactose (Percent)
Cow's milk	
Whole	4.7
Skim	5.0
Yogurt (low fat)	4.0–4.6
Cream	3.0
Cottage cheese	1.4
Hard cheeses	Trace
Ice cream (14% fat)	3.6
Milk chocolate	8.1
Butter	Trace

excreted in the breath air. Therefore, identification of specific enzyme deficiencies can be obtained by performing oral tolerance tests with the individual digestible carbohydrate. Measurement of hydrogen gas in the breath is a reliable test for determining the amount of ingested carbohydrate that is not absorbed, but rather is metabolized by the intestinal flora.

2.3 LIPIDS

2.3.1 DIGESTION AND ABSORPTION

Lipids include a wide variety of chemical substances such as neutral fat (e.g., triglycerides), fatty acids and their derivatives, phospholipids, glycolipids, sterols, carotenes, and fat-soluble vitamins. Fat constitutes about 90% of dietary lipids and provides energy in a highly concentrated form. It accounts for 40%–45% of the total daily energy intake (100 g/day in the average Western diet). The digestion of fat and other lipids poses a special problem because they are insoluble in water while the lipolytic enzymes, like other enzymes, are soluble in aqueous medium.[9,16] The problem is solved by emulsification, which is the intimate admixture of two phases, one dispersed in the other as fine droplets or micelles. In this context, the two phases are water and fat, the latter making up the micelles. Micelles tend to aggregate if they are not stabilized in some way; in the duodenum this role is performed by the bile salts. A bile salt molecule has two sides, one is hydrophobic and the other hydrophilic. So, one side tends to be associated with the aqueous phase and the other with the lipid phase. Such molecules are said to be amphipathic and are powerful emulsifying agents.

Little or no lipid digestion occurs in the mouth. There is some lipase in the stomach, but the acidic environment and the absence of bile salts prevent any significant digestion of fat in this organ. The forceful contraction of the stomach (antrum) breaks up lipids into fine droplets, and in the duodenum these droplets are exposed to the solubilizing effects of bile salts. A fat globule, which has an average diameter of about 100 Å, is reduced severalfold after emulsification, and the surface area is amplified about 10,000 times (Figure 2.2). Lipolytic enzymes cannot penetrate the lipid droplets but can function at the lipid–water interface. Emulsified triglycerides are readily attacked by lipase secreted in pancreatic juice. The bile salts and phospholipids present in bile normally adhere to the surface of triglyceride droplets, thereby displacing lipase from its substrate. This problem is overcome by colipase (a small protein with a molecular weight of 10,000), which binds to both the water–lipid interface and lipase, thereby anchoring and activating the enzyme. Colipase is secreted by the pancreas as procolipase (inactive) simultaneously with lipase in a 1:1 ratio and is activated by trypsin hydrolysis of an arginyl–glycyl bond in the N-terminal region and the removal of a small group (<12) of amino acids.

Pancreatic lipase attacks the ester linkages at the 1- and 3-carbons of the triglyceride, leaving a monoglyceride with the fatty acid esterified at the 2-carbon position of glycerol (Figure 2.3). This linkage can be cleaved by an esterase to release the third fatty acid molecule and glycerol, but is

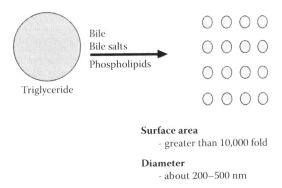

FIGURE 2.2   Emulsification of a fat droplet.

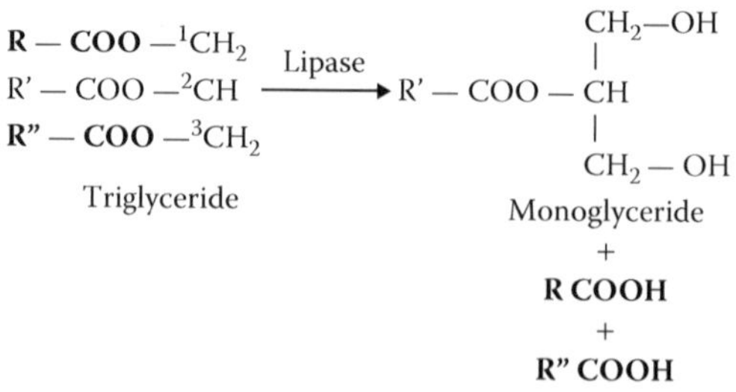

$$R - COO -{}^1CH_2$$
$$R' - COO -{}^2CH \xrightarrow{\text{Lipase}} R' - COO - CH$$
$$R'' - COO -{}^3CH_2$$

$$\begin{array}{c} CH_2-OH \\ | \\ R' - COO - CH \\ | \\ CH_2 - OH \end{array}$$

Triglyceride   Monoglyceride

+

R COOH

+

R″ COOH

FIGURE 2.3   The action of lipase on triglyceride. R = hydrocarbon chain.

not a necessary step for absorption. Monoglycerides, along with bile salts, play an important role in stabilizing and further increasing the emulsification of lipid in the small intestine. The emulsified lipid droplets (micelles) are further reduced in size, which enhances the digestion of fats and other lipids solubilized in the micellar particles.

Several other enzymes secreted in the pancreatic juice are involved in the digestion of certain lipids. For example, cholesterol esterase hydrolyzes cholesterol esters to cholesterol and fatty acids. Another less specific lipid esterase acts on short-chain triglycerides, monoglycerides, or other lipid esters (e.g., esters of vitamin A) with fatty acids. Phospholipids are hydrolyzed by phospholipase A_2, which is secreted as a proenzyme (inactive) and is activated by trypsin. Phospholipase A_2 releases the fatty acid at the 2-carbon of the phospholipid, leaving a lysophospholipid.

In normal individuals lipid absorption occurs in the upper part of the small intestine. Monoacylglycerol, fatty acids, and cholesterol leave the micelles at the brush-border of the epithelial cells of the intestinal mucosa and pass through the cell membrane by passive diffusion. The fate of the absorbed fatty acids depends on their size. Those with less than 10 carbon atoms pass directly from the mucosal cells into portal blood and are bound to albumin for transport as unesterified (free) fatty acids. The large fatty acids are reesterified with monoacylglycerol to the triglyceride level in the smooth endoplasmic reticulum. Some of the cholesterol that enters the mucosal cells from the micelles is also esterified. The newly synthesized triglycerides and cholesterol esters are complexed with a specific protein, cholesterol, and phospholipids to produce particles called chylomicrons, which are released from the mucosal cells by exocytosis and enter the lymph. Medium-chain triglycerides (MCTs) contain fatty acids with a chain length of 6 to 10 carbon atoms. These triglycerides (TGs) differ from long-chain triglycerides (LCTs) in the manner by which they are absorbed and transported from the gastrointestinal (GI) tract to organs. Both MCTs and LCTs are digested to their respective medium- and long-chain fatty acids (MCFAs and LCFAs, respectively) in the GI tract. Unlike LCFAs, which are repackaged as LCTs into chylomicrons for transport through the peripheral circulation, MCFAs, because they are water soluble, do not require chylomicron formation for their absorption and transport. MCTs are hydrolyzed more rapidly by lipase than are LCTs, do not require bile salts for absorption, and can also be absorbed as TGs. Once inside the intestinal epithelial cells, MCTs are rapidly hydrolyzed to MCFAs by specific lipase. After leaving the enterocyte, MCFAs enter the portal system where they are bound to albumin and transported to the liver where they are mostly oxidized for use as a source of energy (Figure 2.4). MCTs have been advocated in various situations including small intestinal disease or damage, short bowel syndrome (SBS), pancreatic and biliary insufficiency, and abetalipoproteinemia. Among disadvantages, MCTs do not stimulate chylomicron formation, and fat-soluble vitamins are, therefore, not transported out of the enterocyte. Coconut oil is a good source of MCFAs.

Although they play a critical role in delivering the fat digestion products to the mucosal cells in micellar form, the bile salts do not cross the mucosal barriers into the lymphatic system. Instead, they are reabsorbed in micellar form in the lower segment of the small intestine and are returned to the liver by the portal vein. This route is part of enterohepatic circulation and permits the bile salts to be salvaged for resecretion into the bile.

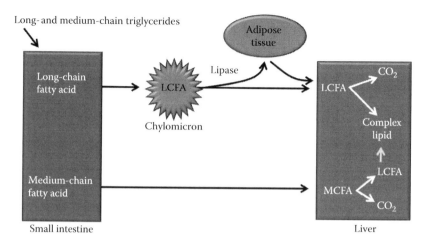

FIGURE 2.4   Absorption of long- and medium-chain triglycerides. Long- and medium-chain triglycerides are digested to their respective fatty acids in the gastrointestinal tract. Long-chain fatty acids (LCFAs) are packaged into chylomicrons for their transport to peripheral tissues, whereas medium-chain fatty acids (MCFAs) travel directly to the liver via portal circulation. As a result, LCFAs are mostly deposited into adipose tissue, whereas MCFAs are mostly oxidized to carbon dioxide in the liver, and small amounts are elongated to LCFAs and incorporated into complex lipid. (Modified from St-Onge, M. P. 2005. *Amer J Clin Nutr* 81:7.)

Short-chain fatty acids (SCFAs) are not dietary lipids but are formed by colonic bacterial enzymes from nonabsorbable carbohydrates. SCFAs in the stool are primarily acetate, propionate, and butyrate, whose carbon chain lengths are 2, 3, and 4, respectively. Butyrate is the primary nutrient for colonic epithelial cells. SCFAs are rapidly absorbed and stimulate sodium chloride and fluid absorption. Treatment with some antibiotics is associated with diarrhea due to depression of SCFAs, producing microflora resulting in decreased SCFAs level in the colon.

2.3.2   Lipid Malabsorption

In adults with a moderate fat intake, as much as 95% of the ingested triglycerides will be absorbed, but in infants 10%–15% of the dietary fat may escape absorption and be excreted. Steatorrhea, a condition in which there is excessive lipid appearing in the stool, accompanies many illnesses. Basically, lipid malabsorption may result from defective lipolysis in the intestinal lumen or defective mucosal cell metabolism. Defective lipolysis in the lumen of the small intestine may be due to bile salt deficiency caused by impaired hepatic formation, obstruction of the bile duct, or excessive bile salt loss. Bile salt deficiency results in poor micellar solubilization of lipid digestion products. Solubilization of lipid digestion products is an important step for their delivery to the intestinal epithelial cells. Bile salt deficiency does not affect the digestion of triglycerides. Therefore, the fats present in the stool are mainly lipid digestion products. Impaired lipolysis may result from lipase deficiency caused by pancreatic tissue damage or obstruction of the pancreatic duct. A reduction in intraduodenal pH can also result in altered lipolysis as pancreatic lipase is inactivated at pH <7. Approximately 15% of patients with gastrinoma have an increase in gastric acid secretion. This can result in steatorrhea secondary to acid inactivation of lipase. Similarly, patients with pancreatitis often have a reduction of bicarbonate secretion, and this can cause a decrease in intraduodenal pH. Defective mucosal cell metabolism may be caused by impaired resynthesis of triglycerides resulting from a mucosal cell disorder (e.g., tropical sprue).

The reesterified triglycerides require formation of chylomicrons to permit their exit from the small intestinal epithelial cell and their delivery to the liver via the lymphatics. Chylomicrons are composed of apolipoprotein B-48 (apo B-48), triglycerides, cholesterol, and phospholipids and enter the lymphatics, not the hepatic portal vein. Abetalipoproteinemia is a rare disorder of impaired synthesis of apo B-48 with abnormal erythrocytes (acanthocytosis), neurological problems, and steatorrhea. Lipolysis, micelle formation, and lipid uptake are all normal in patients with abetalipoproteinemia, but the reesterified triglycerides cannot exit from the epithelial cells because of the failure to produce chylomicrons. Small intestinal biopsies of these patients in the postabsorptive state reveal lipid-laden epithelial cells that become perfectly normal following a 3–4 day fast.

Patients with abetalipoproteinemia are treated with a low-fat diet containing MCTs. Coconut oil is rich in MCTs. In contrast to LCTs, MCTs do not require lipolysis or micelle formation. They are easily absorbed intact by the intestinal epithelial cells and released directly into portal circulation, thereby bypassing the defect of abetalipoproteinemia. Poor absorption of LCFAs can sometimes result in essential fatty acid deficiency. Steatorrhea is often associated with deficiencies of fat-soluble vitamins and, in particular, vitamin E deficiency. These vitamins require micelle formation and solubilization for absorption. Patients with steatorrhea require replacement with water-soluble forms of these vitamins.

2.4   PROTEINS

2.4.1   Digestion and Absorption

The total daily protein load to be digested includes about 70–100 g of dietary protein and 35–200 g of endogenous protein from digestive enzymes and sloughed cells. The overall process of proteolysis must occur without the body's own protein being digested.[14] A protected compartment for the hydrolytic process is provided by the lumen of the gastrointestinal tract. In addition, the secretory cells that synthesize proteases (except dipeptidases and aminopeptidases) are protected because these enzymes are formed and sequestered in storage granules in inactive forms, the zymogens, until needed. The subsequent transformation of the zymogens to the active enzymes occurs largely in the lumen of the gastrointestinal tract and involves, in part, changes in the molecular conformation. In almost all cases, a relatively small masking peptide is split off from the zymogen, which results in a catalytically active species of proteolytic enzyme. Protein digestion can be divided into gastric, pancreatic, and intestinal phases, depending on the tissue source of the enzymes.

2.4.1.1   Gastric

The digestion begins in the stomach where protein is denatured by low pH and is exposed to the action of proteolytic enzymes. The acidic environment also provides the optimum pH for pepsin activity. The zymogen pepsinogen, which is secreted by chief cells, is converted to pepsin in the acid medium (autoactivation) or by active pepsin (autocatalysis) by the removal of a peptide consisting of 44 amino acids from N-terminus. Although pepsin has a broad specificity, it attacks primarily peptide linkages in which the carboxyl group is donated by aromatic amino acid residues. Pepsin is an endopeptidase, and the products of its action consist of a mixture of oligopeptides.

2.4.1.2   Pancreatic

The proteolytic enzymes are synthesized in the acinar cells of the pancreas and secreted in pancreatic juice as zymogens. These include trypsinogen, chymotrypsinogen, proelastase, and the procarboxypeptidases. In the lumen of the small intestine, enteropeptidase (which used to be called enterokinase), a protease produced by duodenal epithelial cells, activates trypsinogen to trypsin (by scission of the hexapeptide). Trypsin, in turn, activates trypsinogen, chymotrypsinogen, proelastase, and the procarboxypeptidases to their respective active enzymes. Recently, enteropeptidase has been reported to be activated from an inactive precursor proenteropeptidase by duodenase, a newly discovered protease in the duodenum (Figure 2.5). Studies have also shown that the trypsin formed activates proenteropeptidase. Trypsin appears to be an inefficient activator of trypsinogen. Trypsin, chymotrypsin, and elastase are endopeptidases. Trypsin is specific for peptide linkages

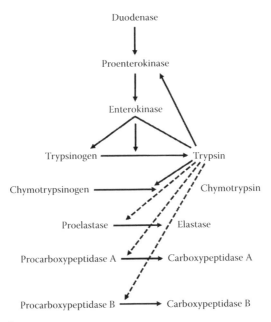

FIGURE 2.5 Activation of zymogens.

in which carboxyl is donated by arginine or lysine. The specificity of chymotrypsin is similar to pepsin. Elastase has a rather broad specificity in attacking bonds next to small amino acids such as glycine, alanine, and serine. Carboxypeptidases A and B attack the carboxyl terminal peptide bonds, thereby liberating single amino acids. The combined action of pancreatic peptidases results in the formation of free amino acids and small peptides of two to eight amino acid residues.

2.4.1.3 Intestinal

The luminal surface of small intestinal epithelial cells contains amino peptidases and dipeptidases. The end products of cell surface digestion are amino acids and di- and tripeptides. These are absorbed by the epithelial cells via specific amino acid or peptide transport systems. The di- and tripeptides are hydrolyzed within the cytoplasmic component before they leave the cell. The hydrolysis of most proteins is thus complete to their constituent amino acids. After active absorption by the intestinal mucosal cells, the amino acids are taken up primarily by the blood capillaries in the mucosa and are transported in the plasma to the liver and other tissues for metabolic use. A significant amount of the absorbed amino acids also appears in the lymph. The digestion and absorption of the majority of dietary proteins is about 95% complete in normal human subjects.

2.4.2 Defects in Protein Digestion and Absorption

Gastric proteolysis is not essential for protein digestion. Individuals with achlorhydria or total gastrectomy have normal protein digestion and absorption. Small intestinal function compensates for the lack of pepsin activity. Thus, the pancreatic and small intestinal diseases will be the major causes of protein malabsorption. However, the reserve capacity of the pancreas is substantial, and fecal loss of protein may not become significant in pancreatic insufficiency states until trypsin falls to about 10% of normal. There are two rare genetic disorders of protein digestion: enterokinase deficiency and trypsin deficiency. As can be expected from the important role each plays in the activation of zymogens, deficiency of either of them has far-reaching effects on the efficiency of protein digestion.

Hartnup disease is inherited as an autosomal recessive trait, and the gene has been mapped to chromosome 11qB. Homozygotes occur with a frequency of about 1 in 24,000 births. Heterozygotes show no clinical abnormalities. In patients with Hartnup disease, the intestinal and renal transport defect for neutral amino acids, including tryptophan, leads to niacin deficiency. Tryptophan is converted to niacin and normally supplies about one-half of the daily niacin requirements. Pellagra-like skin lesions, variable neurologic manifestations, and neutral or aromatic aminoaciduria characterize this disease. Hartnup disease ranks among the most common amino acid disorders in humans.

Cystinuria is one of the most common inborn errors with a frequency of between 1 in 10,000 and 1 in 15,000 in many ethnic groups. The disorder is transmitted as an autosomal recessive trait and results from impaired function of membrane carrier in the apical brush-border of renal tubular and small intestinal cells. Clinical manifestations include massive excretion of cystine and other dibasic acids in homozygotes with classic cystinuria. Cystine stones account for 1%–2% of all urinary tract calculi but are the most common causes of stones in children.

2.5 MALABSORPTION SYNDROMES

Disorders of malabsorption represent a broad spectrum of conditions with multiple etiologies and varied clinical manifestations. Mucosal damage, congenital or acquired reduction in absorptive surface, failure to produce enzymes, defects in ion transport, pancreatic insufficiency, impaired enterohepatic circulation, inflammation, infection, injury, or surgical removal of portions of the intestine may inhibit absorption of certain nutrients. Almost all of these clinical problems are associated with diminished intestinal absorption of one or more dietary nutrients, and they are often referred to as the malabsorption syndromes (MS). Malabsorption is also caused by a number of different diseases, drugs, or nutritional products that impair digestion, mucosal absorption, or nutrient delivery to the systemic circulation. Individuals suffering from MS display, in varying degrees, the following clinical manifestations: diarrhea, steatorrhea, progressive weight loss and muscle wasting, abdominal distension, and evidence of vitamin and mineral deficiencies such as macrocytic anemia due to inadequate folic acid and/or vitamin B_{12} absorption and iron-deficiency anemia. Diagnosis of MS is based on the results of absorption tests such as D-xylose absorption, fat content in stool on a defined diet, and the Schilling test for vitamin B_{12}. Biopsy of the small intestine and radiological examination are useful diagnostic tools. A urinary D-xylose test for carbohydrate absorption provides an assessment of proximal small intestinal mucosal function. D-xylose, a pentose, is absorbed almost exclusively in the proximal small intestine. The test is usually performed by giving 25 g D-xylose orally and collecting urine for 5 hours. An abnormal test (4.5 g excretion) primarily reflects the presence of duodenal/jejunal mucosal disease. Fluids and nutrient monitoring and replacement are essential for any individual with malabsorption syndrome. Hospitalization may be required to treat severe fluid and electrolyte imbalances.

2.5.1 Celiac Disease

Celiac disease,[15,20] also known as celiac sprue and gluten enteropathy, is an intolerance to ingested gluten, a protein present in wheat, rye, and barley, that results in immunologically mediated inflammatory damage to the small intestinal mucosa. A subfraction of gluten, gliadin, appears to be toxic to sensitive individuals.[25]

Until recently celiac disease was considered to be a rare disease occurring in 1 in 3345 people worldwide. However, recent studies have shown the worldwide prevalence to be 1 in 266. Population-based studies suggest that the prevalence in the United States is much greater, possibly affecting as many as 3 million Americans (approximately 1% of the U.S. population). First-degree relatives of individuals with celiac disease have a prevalence of between 4% and 12%.

Classic symptoms of celiac disease are diarrhea, weight loss, and malnutrition. However, only a small percentage of the total celiac disease population has these classic symptoms. Some patients may have symptoms related to low-grade malabsorption such as fatigue, anemia, bone changes, or skin rash. About 15%–25% of patients with the disease have dermatitis herpetiformis (DH), an intensely itchy blistering skin rash that occurs on the elbows, knees, and buttocks. Most patients with DH have no digestive symptoms of the disease. The clinical manifestations are highly variable, may present at any age, and involve multiple organ systems. Prolonged delays in diagnosis are common.[23]

More recently, it has been reported that symptoms of celiac disease may appear much later in life. A study was designed to identify risk factors for cancer and heart disease. Healthy participants provided health information and blood samples in 1974 and again in 1989. A small number of these participants developed new symptoms of celiac disease. Researchers retested blood samples of these individuals, collected several years back, this time for biomarkers related to celiac disease. They found these individuals had the condition, but none of them had been diagnosed with the disease. What causes late onset of the disease is not known. People may have a genetic predisposition to it, but scientists are not sure why gluten intolerance would develop after so many trouble-free years. The cause may be environmental factors such as antibiotics, vaccinations, bioengineered foods, chemicals, and pollutants, which had not been around 30 years back in the concentrations we now have.

The diagnosis of celiac disease in made by characteristic changes found in small intestinal biopsy and improves when a gluten-free diet is instituted. Mucosal flattening can be observed endoscopically as reduced duodenal folds or duodenal scalloping. Characteristic features found in intestinal biopsy include the absence of villi and crypt hyperplasia and increased intraepithelial lymphocytes. People with celiac disease have higher-than-normal levels of certain autoantibodies—proteins that react against the body's own cells or tissues—in their blood. The best available tests are the IgA antihuman tissue transglutaminase and IgA endomysial antibody that appear to have equivalent diagnostic accuracy. Biopsies of the proximal small intestine are indicated in individuals with a positive celiac disease antibody test. These tests are identifying many individuals with nonclassical gastrointestinal and extraintestinal symptoms.

Celiac disease may be linked to diabetes. Children with type 1 diabetes are more likely to have celiac disease than those without diabetes. About 1 in 20 people with type 1 diabetes has celiac disease. Both are autoimmune disorders. It is advisable that children be checked for celiac disease soon after being diagnosed with type 1 diabetes. A significant number of patients with autoimmune thyroid disease also have celiac disease, and autoimmune thyroid disease is more common in people with celiac disease than in the general population.[21] Organ-specific antibodies (i.e., thyroid antibodies) disappear after 3–6 months on a gluten-free diet. Patients with celiac disease have a higher incidence of malignancy and, therefore, should be monitored closely for any indication of lymphoma. The risk of lymphoma is increased between 50-fold and 100-fold in people with celiac disease as compared with normal individuals. Gastrointestinal carcinomas are also more common.

The treatment of patients with celiac disease consists of lifelong complete abstinence of gluten-containing foods. In the diet wheat, barley, and rye should be avoided. For most people with celiac disease, following a gluten-free diet will stop symptoms, heal existing intestinal damage, and prevent further damage. Improvements begin quickly, within a day of starting the diet. With supermarkets brimming with gluten-free breads, cereals, cakes, and cookies and restaurants serving gluten-free pastas and beer, it has become far less difficult to stay on a gluten-free diet.

Patients should be aware that 100% gluten avoidance may not be possible. Some processed foods may contain wheat, barley, or rye. Even naturally occurring gluten-free products may contain 20–200 mg gluten/kg. The Food Allergen Labeling and Consumer Protection Act (FALCPA), which took effect on January 1, 2006, requires food labels to clearly identify wheat and other common food allergens in the list of ingredients. FALCPA also requires the U.S. Food and Drug Administration to develop and finalize rules for the use of the term *gluten-free* on product labels. Evidence supports setting the threshold for gluten contaminants at 100 mg/kg, which is within the range found to allow for mucosal recovery in clinical and challenge studies.[1,11]

2.5.2 Cystic Fibrosis

Cystic fibrosis (CF) is inherited as an autosomal recessive trait.[12] In the United States, approximately 3.3% of the Caucasian population is a carrier of the defective allele, with an incidence of CF in this group of about 1 in 3500 live births. It is uncommon among Asians and African Americans. The defective gene is on chromosome 7, and the CF gene encodes a 1480 amino acid protein called cystic fibrosis transmembrane regulator (CFTR), which functions as a chloride channel throughout the body.[7] CFTR is found in a variety of tissues providing different functions depending on the site. For example, in the sweat glands it reabsorbs chloride, while in the lung it excretes chloride. Therefore, a dysfunctional misfolded or absent CFTR has different pathological consequences. CF is fundamentally a widespread disorder in epithelial transport affecting fluid secretion in exocrine glands and in the epithelial lining of the respiratory, gastrointestinal, and reproductive tracts. More than 700 mutations have been described in this gene. The most common mutation is the deletion of a single amino acid, phenylalanine, from the 508th position of CFTR protein. This deletion affects 70% of the patients. In many patients, this disorder leads to abnormal viscid mucus secretions that directly or indirectly cause the clinical manifestations. The most life-threatening clinical feature is related to pulmonary disease. The sticky, viscous mucus clogs the airway and encourages lung infections by bacteria.

Pancreatic insufficiency is a common consequence of CF, seen mostly in children and young adults. The defect in chloride secretion leads to desiccation of pancreatic secretion, accumulation of secretory material within the pancreatic duct, and ductal obstruction. The exocrine defect inhibits the secretion of digestive enzymes and bicarbonate into the duodenum. Without the enzymes, there is poor digestion of fats and to a lesser extent of carbohydrates and proteins. As a result, 85% of patients with CF exhibit steatorrhea, decreased absorption of fat-soluble vitamins, malnutrition, and failure to thrive. With blockage of the pancreatic duct, the enzymes that normally flow down in the intestine to participate in the digestion are trapped in the pancreas by ductal obstruction. Over time these enzymes accumulate and eventually begin to digest the pancreatic tissue. This leads to loss of functional tissue, and the pancreas eventually becomes scarred and fibrotic.

The most common symptoms of CF include persistent coughing, shortness of breath, excessive appetite but poor weight gain, and bulky stools. Respiratory infections increase with age. Diagnosis of CF is established by demonstration of increased chloride in sweat. Most patients with CF have chloride values between 60 and 110 milliequivalents/L.

The cornerstones of treatment for CF patients are antibiotics, drugs that open the airways in the lungs, and nutritional support. Nutritional abnormalities are mainly secondary to pancreatic insufficiency. Treatment with a high-protein, low-fat diet with adequate supplement of pancreatic enzymes and fat-soluble vitamins often helps. The treatment of CF disease has improved substantially during the last several years. The median age of survival in 2006 was 36.9 years compared to 25 years in 1985, 14 years in 1969, and 5 years in 1955. It is still the most lethal genetic disease in America affecting 30,000 people. In the next few years a stream of new small-molecule drugs armed squarely at repairing the thick mucus problem could reach patients. The drugs may offer the potential to not only improve the health of CF patients but also dramatically change the outlook for people newly diagnosed with the disease. Some of the drugs may be in pill rather than aerosol form, which could make life a lot easier for patients.

2.5.2.1 Alternative Medicine: Can Turmeric Alleviate Cystic Fibrosis?

CF is caused by mutations in the gene encoding CFTR and results in the production of a misfolded protein. CFTR is supposed to travel to a cell's surface to create openings or channels for chloride ions to exit the cell. But the misfolded protein, though functional, is prevented by the cell's quality control agent(s) from taking its right place on the cell surface and instead is trapped in the endoplasmic reticulum. Scientists reasoned that if the quality control agent is disabled it may be possible for CFTR to get to the cell surface to do its work. Many quality control agents require calcium for their functions. Several chemicals, including phenyl butyrate, have been studied as inhibitors of calcium

ATPase, but they also have adverse effects. Curcumin, a substance found in turmeric, which is a spice used to flavor curries and color mustard, is also an ATPase inhibitor.[13] Test-tube studies showed that CFTR got to the cell surface and functioned after addition of curcumin.

Researchers decided to administer the substance to mice with a CF-like disorder. Mice with this genetic mutation suffer much more severe gastrointestinal effects but fewer respiratory problems. They gave the animals 45 mg curcumin/kg body weight per day. The animals' gut problems largely disappeared. There were also changes in electrical potential across the nasal epithelium suggesting that the respiratory system was also improving. Only 10% of curcumin-treated mice died within 10 weeks compared with 60% of untreated mice, and survivors gained weight.

These are interesting findings, but it is not known whether curcumin will help patients with CF. There is a need to determine an optimal dose for humans and if there is any curcumin-drug interaction. Turmeric contains 2% curcumin. To get the dose of curcumin (45 mg/kg) one has to consume a lot of turmeric every day. Turmeric is a member of the Curcuma botanical group, which is part of the ginger family of herbs. It has long been used in folk medicines. It has anti-inflammatory, anti-oxidant, and anticarcinogenic properties. It may also be a neuroprotective agent.

2.5.3 TROPICAL SPRUE

Tropical sprue is a poorly understood syndrome that affects both visitors and natives in certain but not all tropical areas and is manifested by chronic diarrhea, steatorrhea, weight loss, and nutritional deficiencies, including those of folate and vitamin B_{12}. This disease affects approximately 5%–10% of the population in some tropical areas.[5] The etiology of tropical sprue is not known, but since it responds to antibiotics, the consensus is that tropical sprue may be caused by one or more infectious agents. The diagnosis is made by an abnormal small intestinal mucosal biopsy in an individual with chronic diarrhea and evidence of malabsorption and megaloblastic anemia, who is residing or has recently traveled in a tropical country. The biopsy may resemble and can often be indistinguishable from that seen in celiac disease. It may be due to the effect of bacterial toxin on the gut structure or to the secondary effect of vitamin B_{12} deficiency. Treatment is a prolonged course of broad-spectrum antibiotic, oral folate, and vitamin B_{12} injections until symptoms resolve.

2.5.4 INFLAMMATORY BOWEL DISEASES

Inflammatory bowel diseases (IBDs) are a group of chronic idiopathic, relapsing disorders of the gastrointestinal tract. They are common in developed countries. The prevalence in the United States is 20–200 per 100,000 people. Two of the most prevalent diseases are Crohn's disease (CD) and ulcerative colitis (UC). The cause of IBD is unclear; however, hypotheses for these disorders include a combination of genetic abnormalities, chronic infection, environmental factors, and abnormalities of immunoregulatory mechanisms.[3] CD is a chronic patchy, granulomatous inflammatory disease that can involve the entire gastrointestinal tract with discontinuous ulceration. The degree of colonic involvement is variable; however, the terminal ileum is most commonly affected. Patients usually present with abnormal pain, diarrhea, and weight loss. UC develops only in the large intestine. During active episodes, UC causes almost continuous diarrhea with malabsorption and losses of fluid and electrolytes.

IBD is diagnosed through a careful patient history, physical examination, and endoscopic and radiological studies. The area and extent of the intestine affected by IBD determine the type of and degree to which malabsorption occurs. Malnutrition is more likely to be a problem in people with CD of the small intestine than in people with CD of the colon or UC. Patients with active CD respond to bowel rest, total parenteral nutrition (TPN), or enteral nutrition. Enteral nutrition with elemental or peptide preparations appears to be efficacious. Fish oils, which contain ω-3 fatty acids, have had modest efficacy in the treatment of UC or CD.

Patients with CD experience a decrease in appetite, which can affect their ability to receive the daily nutrition needed for good health and healing. It is associated with diarrhea and poor absorption of necessary nutrients. No special diet has been proven effective for preventing or treating CD, but it is very important that people who have CD follow a nutritious diet and avoid any foods that seem to worsen symptoms.[18]

2.5.5 SHORT BOWEL SYNDROME

SBS is a descriptive term for a myriad of clinical problems that often occur following resection of varying lengths of the small intestine. The most common causes in the United States are CD, radiation enteritis, and mesenteric ischemia. SBS is characterized by maldigestion, malabsorption, dehydration, and both macronutrient and micronutrient abnormalities.[4] The severity of malnutrition depends on the site and extent of resection, the capacity for bowel adaptation, and the function of the residual bowel. To maintain adequate nutritional status TPN is required until the patient's remaining intestine begins to adapt to improve digestion and absorption of nutrients. This adaptive period may take several weeks to months to years. Adaptation is enhanced by stimulation of the enterocytes with nutrients, which can be achieved by frequent small, oral meals or feeding.

2.6 MICROORGANISMS

The human gastrointestinal tract contains more than 500 species of bacteria. Most are anaerobic. Relatively sterile sites include the stomach (where acid conditions are too hostile to support microorganisms) and the upper part of the small intestine. There are few bacteria in the lower part of the small intestine and very large population in the large intestine. They make up about 60% of the dry mass of the feces. Most bacteria are beneficial and perform a number of useful functions. These include fermentation of unused energy substrates, training the immune system, preventing the growth of harmful bacteria, and production of vitamins some of which (vitamin K, biotin) can be absorbed by the host. They potentially control the intestinal epithelial cell differentiation and proliferation through the production of SCFA. They play a major role in metabolizing dietary carcinogens. Some bacteria are harmful. They utilize nutrients and prevent their absorption. They produce toxic compounds that can damage the mucosa. Bacteria can also metabolize bile acids to carcinogenic compounds.

Most components of food consumed by humans are digested and absorbed in the upper gastrointestinal tract. There are only a few food ingredients that are not broken down and absorbed, which reach the large intestine. They are acted on by the bacterial enzymes, and some serve as nutritional substrates for bacteria. The metabolic products of these bacteria are, in turn, available to the intestinal cells. The microorganisms act on undigested carbohydrates (fiber) and produce SCFA and gases (hydrogen, methane, and carbon dioxide). The SCFA lower the pH in the large intestine. An acidic pH optimizes the growth conditions for favorable bacteria. In contrast, acid pH provides only suboptimal conditions for pathogenic bacteria. SCFA also have a vital role in nutrition of colonic epithelial cells. In the small intestine, SCFA have also been noted to increase the growth and differentiation of enterocytes. The SCFA are absorbed and inhibit cholesterol synthesis in the liver and may be responsible for the effect of dietary fiber on plasma cholesterol level.

The action of microorganisms on fat is probably simple hydrolysis and saturation of part of the unsaturated fatty acids. The nitrogenous materials that reach the large intestine may be undigested food residues, unabsorbed amino acids, or cellular detritus. Proteolysis by microorganisms results in amino acids. Since little or no absorption of amino acids takes place in the large intestine, these are attacked by bacteria to a varying degree in two general ways: 1) decarboxylation and 2) deamination. Several compounds are formed.

Primary bile acids are converted to secondary bile acids by bacteria in the colon. Some of these are potent colonic secretory agents, and their presence in the colon results in secretory diarrhea. The intestinal flora converts conjugated bilirubin to urobilinogen, some of which is absorbed and excreted in the urine. The flora also converts the remainder of the urobilinogen to stercobilinogen, which is excreted in the feces. The microorganisms also act on drugs, steroids, and many other compounds.

There is normally a balance between beneficial and harmful bacteria. Diarrhea may occur in up to 20% of patients receiving broad-spectrum antibiotics. Antibiotic-associated alteration of the normal intestinal flora can result in impaired fermentation of poorly absorbed carbohydrates, leading to osmotic diarrhea and reduced production of SCFA that normally enhance the colonic absorption of fluids. Decreased bacterial carbohydrate metabolism due to antibiotics may result in functional disturbances of the colonic mucosa. In the distal colon, one of the SCFA, butyrate, is an important source of energy for the mucosa through cellular oxidation. The beneficial microorganisms can be increased by a diet such as a vegetarian diet rich in dietary fiber as well as ingesting buttermilk, yogurt, and so on.

Under normal conditions, the intestinal mucosa prevents the bacteria colonizing the gut from invading systemic organs and tissues; however, under certain circumstances, it appears that the gut can serve as a reservoir for bacteria that cause systemic infections. Many bacterial infections in cancer patients and other immunocompromised patients may originate in their indigenous bowel flora.

Inborn Error of Enterokinase Deficiency—A Case

The patient was a girl born at term with birth weight of 3.4 kg. From birth she had diarrhea (6–10 watery stools/day) and failed to gain weight. She was admitted to a hospital at 3 weeks of age. Changes in feeding regimen failed to control the diarrhea, and at 3 months of age, her weight was 3.05 kg. At 4 months, she became severely ill and edematous. Her total serum protein was 3.2 g/dL (normal 6 g/dL), and her blood hemoglobin was 6.4 g/dL (normal 12 g/dL). Duodenal juice had low levels of amylase, lipase, and proteolytic activity. Fecal fat was 14 g in a single 24-hour specimen. Normal sweat sodium chloride excluded the possibility of CF.

Intravenous albumin and blood were given, and pancreatic extract was added to the feeds. Her general condition improved considerably. Barium meal and other follow-through were normal. Two further samples of duodenal juice were obtained at 7 and 12 months of age; amylase and lipase were normal, but very little proteolytic activity was detected in either sample. Withdrawal of oral pancreatic extract resulted in the recurrence of diarrhea and clinical manifestations, and substitution therapy was restarted.

The patient was reinvestigated at 13 months of age when her weight was 8.6 kg and height 72.4 cm (both just below third percentile). Oral pancreatic extract was stopped. Mean fecal fat was 3 g/day, total serum protein was 6 g/dL, albumin was normal, and blood hemoglobin was 11.2 g/dL. Jejunal biopsy was normal. Duodenal juice was analyzed for the activities of various digestive enzymes after the administration of intravenous cholecystokinin. Amylase and lipase activities were normal, but the activities of trypsin, chymotrypsin, and carboxypeptidase A were undetectable and enterokinase activity was extremely low. The addition of human enterokinase to the duodenal juice resulted in the appearance of normal levels of proteolytic enzymes within 35 minutes. The presence of normal amylase and lipase activity and the appearance of normal proteolytic activity after the addition of enterokinase in the duodenal juice suggest that this patient had normal pancreatic function but had a deficiency of enterokinase. This was the first reported case of enterokinase deficiency.

The clinical features of this patient were similar to those reported for patients with trypsinogen deficiency. It is possible that this patient as well as those with trypsinogen deficiency were deficient in the newly discovered enzyme duodenase. This case illustrates the key role of enterokinase (or duodenase) in the activation of pancreatic zymogens and how its deficiency can cause serious health problems.

REFERENCES

1. Akobeng, A. K., and A. G. Thomas. 2008. Systematic review: Tolerable amount of gluten for people with celiac disease. *Aliment Pharmacol Ther* 27:1044.
2. Albano, B., G. Lunkart, G. England et al. 2003. Gene-culture coevolution between cattle milk protein genes and human lactase genes. *Nat Genet* 35:311.
3. Baumgart, D. C., and W. J. Sandborn. 2007. Inflammatory bowel disease: Clinical aspects and established and evolving therapies. *Lancet* 369:1641.
4. Bernard, D. K. H., and M. J. Shaw. 1993. Principles of nutrition therapy for short-bowel syndrome. *Nutr Clin Pract* 8:153.
5. Binder, J. H. J. 2006. Causes of chronic diarrhea. *New Engl J Med* 355:236.
6. Bond, H., and M. D. Levitt. 1977. Use of breath hydrogen (H_2) in the study of carbohydrate absorption. *Am J Dig Dis* 22:379.
7. Breuer, W., N. Kartner, J. R. Riordan, and Z. Ioav Cabantchik. 1992. Induction of expression of the cystic fibrosis transmembrane conductance regulator. *J Biol Chem* 267:1045.
8. Buller, H. A., and R. J. Grand. 1990. Lactose intolerance. *Am J Med* 41:141.
9. Carey, M. C., D. M. Small, and C. M. Bliss. 1983. Lipid digestion and absorption. *Annu Rev Physiol* 45:651.
10. Caspray, W. F. 1992. Physiology and pathology of intestinal absorption. *Am J Clin Nutr* 55:299.
11. Collin, P., L. Thorell, K. Kaukinen, and M. Makim. 2004. The safe threshold for gluten contamination in gluten-free products. Can trace amount be accepted in the treatment of celiac disease? *Aliment Pharmacol Ther* 19:1277.
12. Davies, J., E. Alton, and A. Bush. 2007. Cystic fibrosis. *Brit Med J* 335:1255.
13. Egan, M. E., M. Pearson, S. A. Weiner et al. 2004. Curcumin, a major constituent of turmeric, corrects cystic fibrosis defects. *Science* 304:600.
14. Erickson, R. H., and Y. S. Kim. 1990. Digestion and absorption of dietary protein. *Annu Rev Med* 41:133.
15. Farrell, L. R. J., and C. P. Kelly. 2002. Celiac sprue. *N Engl J Med* 346:180.
16. Fridman, H. I., and B. Nylund. 1980. Intestinal fat digestion, absorption, and transport: A review. *Am J Clin Nutr* 33:1108.
17. Gray, G. M. 1975. Carbohydrate digestion and absorption: role of the small intestine. *N Engl J Med* 292:1225.
18. Hanauer, S. B., and S. Meyers. 1997. Management of Crohn's disease in adults. *Am J Gastroenterol* 92:559.
19. Lee, M., and S. D. Kransinski. 1998. Human adult onset lactase decline: an update. *Nutr Rev* 56:1.
20. Rodrigo, L. 2006. Celiac disease. *World J Gastroenterol* 12:6585.
21. Sategna-Guidetti, C., U. Voltau, C. Ciacci et al. 2001. Prevalence of thyroid disorders in untreated adult celiac disease patients and effect of gluten withdrawal: An Italian multicenter study. *Amer J Gastroent* 96:751.
22. Savaiano, D. A., and M. D. Levitt. 1987. Milk intolerance and microbe-containing dairy foods. *J Dairy Sci* 70:397.
23. Seraphin, P., and S. Mobarhan. 2002. Mortality in patients with celiac disease. *Nutr Rev* 60:116.
24. Swallow, D. M. 2003. Genetic influences on carbohydrate digestion. *Nutr Res Rev* 16:37.
25. Van Heel, D., and J. West. 2006. Recent advances in celiac disease. *Gut* 55:1037.

CASE BIBLIOGRAPHY

26. Hadorn, B., M. J. Tarlow, J. K. Lloyd, and O. H. Wolff. 1969. Intestinal enterokinase. *Lancet* 1:812.
27. Zamalodchikova, T. S., E. A. Sokolova, D. Lu, and J. E. Sadler. 2000. Activation of recombinant proenteropeptidase by duodenase. *FEBS Lett* 466:295.

3 Requirements for Energy: Carbohydrates, Fats, and Proteins

3.1 ENERGY

Energy is well recognized as a prime requirement for humans and other living organisms. The major dietary sources of energy-yielding substrates are carbohydrates, fats, and proteins.[1] After these food components are digested and the resulting nutrients are absorbed, they are converted, in part, to chemical energy in the form of adenosine triphosphate (ATP) and other high-energy compounds; ATP is the central chemical intermediate involved in many processes that require energy. Parts of the nutrients also are used, of course, for the growth and maintenance of body tissues. It is a common knowledge that if the food energy intake is inadequate to meet the body's energy requirements, loss of body weight occurs, body carbohydrate and fat stores are gradually decreased, and, because of the urgent drive for energy, the body protein itself is metabolized to supply energy. Severe emaciation and drastic metabolic alterations (e.g., acidosis, ketosis, loss of cations and nitrogen, dehydration) ensue and, if extended, may result in death.

3.1.1 CALORIES

The energy value of food is expressed in terms of a unit of heat, the kilocalorie (kcal). This represents the amount of heat required to raise the temperature of 1 kg (1000 g) of water by 1°C. This large calorie (Cal) used in nutrition should not be confused with the small calorie (cal), which is 0.001 Cal. The accepted international unit of energy is the joule (J). One kilocalorie is equal to 4.184 kJ. To convert energy from Calorie to kilojoule, the factor 4.2 may be used.

The energy value of food is obtained by combustion methods or by direct calorimetry using an oxygen bomb calorimeter. This instrument is a highly insulated boxlike container about 1 ft^3 in size. The bomb chamber itself consists of a thick-walled metal vessel equipped with a sample dish, electrodes for igniting the sample in an oxygen atmosphere, and a valve for introducing oxygen. This combustion chamber is surrounded with an outer chamber containing a measured amount of water, a stirrer, and a thermometer. The dried and weighed test sample of food is completely oxidized in an oxygen atmosphere, and the heat is transferred to the surrounding water and measured with an accurate thermometer. The heat production is calculated in terms of calories per gram (Table 3.1). The energy value of a food sample thus obtained is known as the heat of combustion.

Under physiological conditions, the nitrogen of protein is not oxidized, but is excreted mainly as urea; therefore, a deduction must be made in the case of proteins from the value obtained in the bomb calorimeter. The heat due to the excreted nitrogen amounts to 1.3 Cal/g protein oxidized in the tissue cell and must be subtracted from the heat of combustion of 5.65 Cal/g. In addition, a correction must be made for the efficiency of digestion, absorption, and metabolism for each class of nutrients. Carbohydrates are digested to the extent of about 98%, fat digestion is 95% efficient, and protein digestion is 92% efficient; hence, the coefficients of digestibility for these macronutrients are 0.98, 0.95, and 0.92, respectively. It should be noted that the caloric values of compounds within

TABLE 3.1
Physiologic Energy Value of Major Nutrients (Cal/g)[a]

	Carbohydrate	Fat	Protein	Alcohol[b]
Heat of combustion	4.1	9.45	5.65	7.1
Nitrogen unavailable			1.30	
Net heat of combustion	4.1	9.45	4.35	7.1
Digestion efficiency	0.98	0.95	0.92	
Physiological energy value	4.0	9.00	4.00	7.0

[a] The corresponding values in kilojoules per gram are 17 for proteins and carbohydrates, 38 for fat, and 30 for alcohol.

[b] No digestion required; small loss in urine and breath.

each class of nutrients vary to some extent. One gram of polysaccharide, for example, provides more calories per gram than the same amount of monosaccharide (4.1 and 3.8 Cal/g, respectively). There are similar variations among individual proteins and triglycerides. In addition, although these coefficients apply generally in the United States, other coefficients may be more appropriate in other countries, reflecting the digestibilities of the predominant foods.

The major dietary sources of energy-yielding substrates are broken down into intermediate energy sources, called "common denominators," because the primary source no longer can be distinguished. They are pyruvic acid, acetyl CoA, and α-ketoglutarate; these are further metabolized to yield carbon dioxide, water, and energy via the citric acid cycle. Alcohol is not a nutrient by definition, but its caloric value is given because the estimated contribution of alcohol to the average American diet is 5.5%–6% of the total calories based on national consumption figures. The share of dietary calories is much greater in the heavy drinkers—generally estimated to be more than half of their daily calorie intake.

3.1.2 BASAL METABOLISM

The basal metabolic rate (BMR) or resting metabolic rate is the metabolism of the body at rest. More exactly, it is defined as the heat production of the body when in a state of complete mental and physical rest and in the postabsorptive state. Because food, exercise, sleep, and external temperature all modify heat production, these factors must be excluded. Therefore, the individual is required to take the test after a 12-hour fast (i.e., in the postabsorptive state). The test is performed in a warm, comfortable, quiet room that has subdued lighting. The subject must be put in a resting condition and be informed about what is to be performed so that stress will not occur. Under such circumstances, the individual's metabolism is considered basal. The basal metabolism reflects the energy requirements for the maintenance and the conduct of those cellular and tissue processes, which are fundamental to the continuing activities of organisms (e.g., the metabolic activity of muscle, the brain, the liver, kidneys, and other cells, plus the heat released as a result of the mechanical work represented by the contraction of muscles involved in respiration, circulation, and peristalsis). Sodium ion transport may make a major contribution. BMR can be estimated at 20–25 Cal/kg body weight/day.

Basal metabolism varies from one individual to the next. It is also not constant throughout life. Both age and sex affect basal metabolism. From birth until two years of age, the rate is relatively high (more energy is required for rapid growth), and it continues to rise until adolescence. But from maturity on, most people undergo a slow reduction in their BMR throughout life. The decrease in the rate with aging is explained largely by decrease in lean body mass. Women have a lower rate than men because of their smaller body size, and it has also been shown to vary with the menstrual cycle. It increases by 7.7% in the postovulatory period and drops in the early stages of pregnancy and lactation. Body composition also affects the rate, with more energy being needed for the metabolic activities of muscle and glandular tissues than fatty tissues.

The BMR also depends on the thyroid hormone status and the sympathetic nervous system activity. In the early part of this century, the metabolic rate measurement was used to diagnose the underactivity and overactivity of the thyroid gland. In hypothyroidism, the rate may be as much as 40% lower than normal standards, and in hyperthyroidism the rate may be increased to 50%–75% above normal standards. Epinephrine causes an increase in metabolic rate. Fever increases heat production by approximately 13% of the BMR for each 1°C rise in body temperature. Muscular training, as in athletes, may be reflected in a slightly elevated BMR.

3.1.3 RESTING ENERGY EXPENDITURE

Resting energy expenditure (REE) is the energy expended in the postabsorptive state (2 hours after a meal) and is approximately 10% greater than BMR. It can be estimated by using the following formula:

$$\text{for men, REE} = 900 + 10W; \quad \text{for women, REE} = 700 + 7W$$

where W is the body weight in kilograms and REE is expressed in calories. The calculated REE is then adjusted for physical activity level by multiplying by 1.2 for sedentary individuals, 1.4 for moderately active individuals, or 1.8 for very active individuals. The final figure provides an estimate of total caloric need in a state of energy balance.

Energy expenditure can be determined more accurately by an indirect calorimetry that uses an analytical machine (often termed *metabolic cart*) to measure an individual's amount of oxygen consumed and carbon dioxide produced when standard conditions are maintained. It determines through a series of equations the energy expenditure, including stress, for that point in time, and then extrapolates it for 24 hours. Because the measurement is performed while the individual is at rest, activity is not included in the energy expenditure assessment. This computerized method for determining energy expenditure is especially valuable in the energy assessment of critically ill patients.

3.1.4 THERMIC EFFECT OF FOOD

The thermic effect of food (TEF) refers to the increase in energy expenditure above the BMR that occurs a few hours after the ingestion of a meal. It is also known as a specific dynamic action and is a consequence of the extra energy released incident to the digestion, absorption, and metabolism of the food. In the case of protein, the TEF amounts to approximately 30%, while for carbohydrate it is 6%, and for fat it is 4% of the energy value of the food ingested. Thus the ingestion of 25 g of protein that has 100 Cal (420 kJ) leads to 30 Cal (126 kJ) of extra heat; therefore only 70 Cal (294 kJ) of potentially useful energy can be derived from 25 g of protein. For a mixed diet, the TEF is estimated to be 6%–10% of the calories needed for basal metabolism and activity.

3.1.5 CALORIC DENSITY

Caloric density (CD) is the amount of energy contained per unit measure of food. Usually CD is expressed as the amount of Calories provided in 1 g of a given food. For example, 100 g of apple contain 52 Calories. This means that 1 g of apple contains 0.52 Calories. Therefore, the CD of an apple is 0.52.

For processed foods the CDs are higher. For example, CD for potato is 0.76, but for potato chips it is 5.31. The CDs (per ounce) for some common foods are presented in Table 3.2.

TABLE 3.2
Caloric Density of Selected Foods (per Ounce)

High-Caloric Density (Cal/oz)		Low-Caloric Density (Cal/oz)	
Peanut butter	185	Beans: kidney, lima	35
Bacon	162	Bananas	26
Salad dressing	160	Pea	25
Graham crackers	130	Grapes, apples	17
Salami, spare ribs	115	Oranges	13
Cheese	104	Carrots	12
Frankfurter	88	Squash	10
Ground beef	74	Green beans	10
Bread	72	Cantaloupes	10
Sirloin	62	Strawberries	8
Ham	52		

In general, foods from plant origin tend to have low CDs and foods from animal origin tend to have high CDs. Calorie dense foods provide more calories in a small amount of food, and foods with low CDs supply fewer total calories in a large amount of food.

CD as opposed to macronutrient content of foods is currently thought to be the key factor in the regulation of food intake. Under ad libitum conditions people tend to consume a constant weight of food rather than a constant quantity of energy. Diets based on low-CD foods are more healthy and effective for weight management.

3.1.6 CALORIC REQUIREMENT

The first law of thermodynamics states that energy cannot be created or destroyed, and there is no exception for living organisms. The total calories required for an individual vary considerably with surface area (which is related to height and weight), age, sex, and daily activity and is not the same for all periods of life of a given individual. The surface area is related to the rate of heat loss by the body—the greater the surface area, the greater the heat loss. The energy requirements and the efficiency with which food energy is utilized may also be influenced by genetic differences in the metabolic makeup of individuals.

A healthy 70-kg man stores approximately 70 g of liver glycogen, 200 g muscle glycogen, and 30 g glucose in body fluids, totaling 1200 Cal (5200 kJ), Available glucose stores can meet energy needs for only 12–18 hours. However, adipose tissue triglycerides (about 15,000 g) typically represent energy deposits of 135,000 Cal (56,484 kJ), more than 100 times the glucose energy reserves. Body proteins are unavailable for energy except under conditions of starvation or severe stress. For an adult to prevent the wasting of body tissues, the caloric intake of the food ingested must be equivalent to the total heat production during the same period. The amount of heat required is the sum total of energy needed for basal metabolism, specific dynamic action (or TEF), and physical activity. Sedentary adults require about 30 Cal/kg body weight/day (126 kJ) to maintain body weight, moderately active adults require 35 Cal/kg/day (147 kJ), and very active adults require 40 Cal/kg/day (168 kJ). On average, therefore, a 70-kg (154 pounds) young adult man requires between 2000 and 3000 Cal/day (8400 and 12,600 kJ/day). Young adult women require between 1800 and 2200 Cal (7560 and 9240 kJ). The higher value is needed by a person under more stress or with a higher degree of physical activity. The lower number would be required by a person whose physical activity is minimal, for example someone with a desk job. Over the years, the daily life in developed countries has been simplified by an increase in mechanization. Chopping wood was at one time a part of the daily routine of most Americans, but as industrialization progressed, this type of physical exertion was no longer necessary.

Energy requirement = basal metabolism + TEF + physical activity

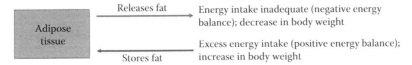

FIGURE 3.1   Energy balance.

Energy balance occurs when the number of calories absorbed equals the amount of energy expended for body processes and activities; hence, no weight gain or loss is occurring. When the amount of energy available to the adult body exceeds the capacity to expend it (i.e., a positive energy balance), weight gain results and excess energy is stored in the body as adipose tissue; each pound of adipose tissue contains 3500 Calories (14,700 kJ). In order to preserve health and prevent excessive weight gain, the continued storage of excess fat is discouraged.[28] Adipose tissue either stores or releases fat, depending on the energy balance. When the daily diet does not supply adequate calories to meet energy needs (i.e., a negative energy balance), the stored body fat is utilized (Figure 3.1). The lean body mass (muscle and organ tissues) may be utilized as a secondary source.

In the last century, the average American diet shifted from one based on fresh, minimally processed vegetable foods to one based on animal products and highly refined, processed foods. As a result, Americans now consume far more calories, refined sugar, and so on than is healthful.[10] Two out of every three adults in the United States are overweight compared to fewer than one in four in the early 1960s. The consequences include a substantial decrease in life expectancy and an increase in morbidity. Patients with excess body weight should be encouraged to shift from high-fat, calorie-dense foods to low-fat, low-CD foods. To lose 1 pound of body weight a week one has to consume 500 fewer Calories (2100 kJ) than one expends each day.

Rapidly growing children and adolescents require a high number of calories per unit body weight to allow for growth. The energy requirements for growth decline with increasing age. At the age of 3 months, an infant requires 28 Cal/kg (118 kJ/kg); at 9–12 months, an infant requires 6 Cal/kg (25 kJ/ g); at 2–5 years, one needs 2 Cal/kg (8 kJ/kg); and at 9–17 years, one needs 1 Cal/kg (4 kJ/ kg) for growth. Pregnancy and lactation impose additional energy requirements to compensate for the building of new tissues and the production of milk. With increasing age, the BMR and physical activities generally decrease; hence, a 10% reduction in energy allowance is proposed for adults over 50 years of age.

Illness often alters energy needs. Unstressed hospitalized patients at bed rest usually require 1.2 times their REE, whereas those who are stressed, febrile, and catabolic require 1.5–2 times their REE. Intestinal malabsorption decreases most utilizable energy to as little as 25% of ingested energy and may necessitate feeding by the parenteral route. In addition to febrile condition, other diseases such as burns increase one's energy requirement by varying amounts (40%–100%).

3.1.7 CALORIE INTAKE AND BODY WEIGHT

It is assumed that 1 pound of body weight equals 3500 calories. So, if a person eats an extra donut (125 Cal) daily in addition to his or her regular diet, the individual will gain 1 pound of weight in 4 weeks, 13 pounds in a year, 130 pounds in 10 years, and so on. But, this does not actually happen. The person gains 1 lb of weight in 4 weeks, and then the gain slowly declines and stabilizes. This is because as the body weight increases, extra energy is needed for metabolism and to carry it. For example, a person weighing 150 pounds expends about 50 calories to walk a mile. If the body weight is 152 pounds, the person may need little more than 50 calories to walk a mile. New research—based on studies of volunteers whose calorie consumption is observed in laboratory settings—suggests that the body's self-regulatory mechanisms tamp down the effects of changes in diet. The same thing applies, in reverse, to weight loss.[13]

The 3500 calorie rule makes sense in short time frames with small diet changes. But just as the body requires less fuel to power itself as weight declines, it requires more to create and sustain more weight. Scientists are working on formulas that attempt to more accurately predict long-term weight loss and gain due to changes in diet and exercise.

Many people who want to lose or gain weight follow food labels to calculate their caloric intake. Calorie counts listed on food labels are based on a system developed in the late nineteenth century by the American chemist W. O. Atwater.[36] Atwater calculated the energy content of food by burning small samples in controlled conditions and measuring the amount of energy released in the form of heat. He then subtracted a small amount of energy lost as indigested food in the feces and chemical energy lost as urea and other nitrogenous compounds in urine. Atwater estimated that carbohydrate and protein provide an average of 4 Cal/g and fat 9 Cal/g, respectively. These values have been used on food labels in the United States and other countries. Our bodies do not incinerate food. Food needs to be digested, absorbed, and metabolized. It can lower the number of calories extracted from food anywhere between 5% and 25%, depending on the type of food. Some argue that the caloric value for protein should be about 3.2 Cal/g instead of 4, a 20% reduction. This is because energy is required to convert protein to amino acids and ammonia to urea. Dietary fiber is given the value of 2 Cal/g on food labels. But fiber is resistant to digestion, and some energy derived from fiber is used by intestinal microorganisms. These factors reduce the available energy from fiber to about 1.5 Cal/g from 2 Cal/g, a 25% reduction.

Animal studies have suggested the beneficial effects of a hard (requires chewing) diet on obesity. Mice fed a hard diet from age 4 weeks had significantly lower body weight at age 36 weeks than did mice fed a normal diet. In addition, body weight gain from 4 to 9 weeks was significantly smaller in male (but not female) mice fed a hard diet than in those fed a soft diet. Researchers surveyed 45 Japanese female students (18–22 years old) about their eating habits and classified the food they ate according to how difficult it was to chew. They found that women who ate the hardest foods had significantly slimmer waist lines than those who ate the softest foods. Dietary hardness was a significant determinant of waist circumference in a group of free-living women.

Two individuals of the same weight may consume the same number of calories, and one may put on weight and the other may maintain the same weight. This may be because of genetic variations, hormones, or other factors. It is true that if one consumes more energy than required for maintenance the individual will put on weight, but the extent of weight gain depends on several factors, some of which are presented here.

3.2   RESPIRATORY QUOTIENT

During the course of oxidation of body fuels, oxygen is consumed and carbon dioxide is produced. The molar ratio of carbon dioxide produced to oxygen consumed is known as the respiratory quotient (RQ) and is characteristic of a given substrate. The measurement of RQ, therefore, provides a means of assessing the type of fuel component that is being metabolized.[28,30] For carbohydrate, the RQ is 1, and for fat it is approximately 0.7, as given by the following reactions:

$$C_6H_{12}O_6 (glucose) + 6O_2 \rightarrow 6CO_2 + 6H_2O$$

$$C_{16}H_{32}O_2 (palmitate) + 23O_2 \rightarrow 16CO_2 + 16H_2O$$

The RQ of protein is difficult to measure because protein is not oxidized completely in the body (the nitrogen of protein is eliminated in the urine); however, the RQ is usually taken to be 0.8. On the basis of analytical data for the average protein, it is generally estimated that 1 g of urinary nitrogen represents the metabolism of 6.25 g of protein, the utilization of 5.91 L of oxygen, and the production of 4.76 L of carbon dioxide. Therefore, by measuring the amount of urinary nitrogen produced, the quantity of protein oxidized can be estimated. The rest of the metabolic energy must be from a combination of fat and carbohydrate, and the percentage of each can be determined from the protein-corrected RQ. A normal adult who consumes a mixed diet has an overall RQ of 0.85. This value is increased by increasing the amount of carbohydrate in the diet, and it is reduced by increasing the amount of fat in the diet. When glucose is used to synthesize fat, the RQ increases to above 1.

The major endogenous source of fuel is the body fat that, on average, is about 15 kg in a 70-kg adult male. Stored glycogen in the liver and muscle amounts to about 200 g. On a short-term basis such as an overnight fast or acute exercise, glycogen is utilized first (RQ > 0.95). As the fast or exercise continues and glycogen is depleted, the oxidation of fatty acids becomes the major energy source, and the RQ decreases and approaches that of fat (RQ = 0.7). This mechanism allows the body to withstand long periods of low dietary energy. In untreated diabetes mellitus very little carbohydrate can be utilized by the body's cells because of insulin deficiency and the RQ is near 0.7.

Another way to determine the RQ is by measuring heat production (using a respiratory calorimeter or respirometer). This can be done at the same time as the measurement of oxygen consumption and carbon dioxide excretion.[6] This technique is useful to assess the energy expenditure and the type of fuel substrate oxidized under controlled conditions, such as when a subject walks on a treadmill or rides a stationary bicycle. It can also assess the RQ in stressed or hypermetabolic patients receiving intravenous glucose. Metabolic measuring carts (MMCs) have been developed and can be used at bedside. They measure the oxygen consumed and the carbon dioxide produced by the patient and then calculate RQ and energy expenditure. Measurements are made over periods of 10–20 minutes. The principal use of MMC is to monitor RQ for patients receiving total parenteral nutrition (TPN) and ascertain whether the patient can actually use the calories given. One of the problems of TPN is the development of fatty liver and subsequent liver dysfunction secondary to excess parenteral glucose. Glucose that is converted into fat and deposited in the liver is not available for energy by the rest of the body. Thus, for a patient with an RQ of 1.08, less than 70% of glucose is available for immediate use as energy. If the RQ is greater than 1, it indicates the patient is accumulating fat in the liver, and it is a signal to reduce glucose intake.

An additional benefit of the MMC for patients receiving TPN is that it can detect potential respiratory distress secondary to excess glucose.[21,22] TPN can aggravate respiratory dysfunction in some severely ill patients by increasing ventilation rate due to an increase in carbon dioxide production (e.g., RQ = 1 during glucose oxidation). This nutritionally induced increase comes at a time when the patient's pulmonary capacity is already compromised. Thus, judicial use of the RQ enables physicians to customize the nutrition regimen to meet the patient's energy need without exceeding the patient's capacity to utilize the energy in the form provided.

3.3 CARBOHYDRATES

The primary function of carbohydrates is to provide a source of energy, and about 50%–60% of the energy requirement comes from this source in the American diet. Carbohydrates such as glucose can be made in the body from both amino acids and glycerol (from fat). Therefore, there is no specific requirement for this nutrient in the sense used for essential amino acids. But a carbohydrate-free diet leads to ketosis and an excessive breakdown of tissue proteins, thus causing the loss of cations (especially sodium) and resulting in dehydration. Some carbohydrates therefore are necessary in the diet so that the oxidation of fatty acids can proceed normally. When carbohydrate is severely restricted in the diet, fat is metabolized faster than the body can take care of its intermediate products. The accumulation of these incompletely oxidized products leads to ketosis.

Individual tests with salts, proteins, fats, and carbohydrates showed that only carbohydrates in the diet produced sodium retention and the associated water retention. Diet mixtures containing 1500–2000 Cal (6300–8400 kJ) of proteins and fats, with or without salt, failed to prevent sodium and water excretion. The addition of as little as 50 g/day carbohydrate in the diet prevented ketosis and about 100 g/day stopped loss of water and electrolytes.

Most tissues can use a variety of sources for energy, but the brain and red blood cells are more restricted. Red blood cells depend entirely on glycolysis; the brain uses glucose but can be partially adapted to use ketone bodies. In an adult human, the brain and the red blood cells use about 180 g/day glucose.

The main source of carbohydrates in our diet is vegetable food. Of the animal products, only milk, oysters, and liver contain significant amounts of carbohydrates. In developing countries where vegetable foods are predominant, carbohydrates provide much of the energy, sometimes as high as 90%. It is estimated that in developed countries, carbohydrates provide, on the average, about 50% of calories. At least 55% of calories should be derived from carbohydrates.

The available carbohydrates in our diet that are digested and/or absorbed include starch (polymer of glucose), the disaccharides—sucrose (glucose–fructose), the milk sugar lactose (glucose–galactose), and maltose (glucose–glucose)—and the oligosaccharides related to maltose and isomaltose. A small contribution also comes from sugar alcohols and related substances that either occur naturally, or are added as sugar substitutes.[8] Sucrose substitutes include sorbitol, mannitol, and xylitol, which are derived from the monosaccharides glucose, mannose, and xylose, respectively. Although these compounds are absorbed more slowly, they are still metabolized by the body and provide 4 Cal/g. They are often inappropriately promoted as noncaloric sweeteners in dietetic candies and desserts.

Honey is a sweet viscous fluid produced by honeybees from the nectar of flowers. It is significantly sweeter than sugar and has attractive chemical properties for baking. Honey is a mixture of sugars and other compounds. With respect to carbohydrates, honey is mainly fructose (about 38.5%) and glucose (about 31%). The remaining carbohydrates include maltose, sucrose, and other complex carbohydrates. It also contains several vitamins including B1, B2, B6, niacin, and pantothenic acid. Essential minerals include calcium, copper, iron, magnesium, manganese, phosphorus, potassium, sodium, and zinc. Several different amino acids and antioxidants have been identified in honey. The specific composition of any batch of honey will depend largely on the mix of flowers consumed by the bees that produce the honey. Maple syrup is a sweetener made from the sugar maple tree sap. It contains about 67% solids of which about 80% is sucrose; the remainder is primarily fructose and glucose, with traces of other sugars. Molasses is a thick syrup by-product from the processing of the sugarcane or sugar beet into sugar. In some parts of the United States, molasses also refer to sorghum syrup.

High-fructose corn syrup (HFCS) was introduced in the 1970s. It is produced by processing cornstarch to yield glucose (bacterial *l*-amylase and glucoamylase) and its conversion to fructose by glucose isomerase. This fructose syrup mixture is then combined with regular corn syrup, which contains 100% glucose to get the right percentage of fructose and glucose. The final product is a clear liquid that is as sweet as sugar. The name high-fructose corn syrup is something of a misnomer. It is high in fructose only in relation to regular corn syrup (100% glucose), not to sucrose. The version of HFCS used in sodas and other sweetened drinks consists of 55% fructose and 45% glucose. The form of HFCS used in other products like breads, jams, and yogurt contains 42% fructose and 58% glucose and thus is actually lower in fructose than sucrose (a disaccharide), which has 50% fructose and 50% glucose joined by glycosidic linkage. Fructose and glucose in HFCS are free sugars.

HFCS is used in foods and beverages because of the many benefits it offers. In addition to providing sweetness at a level equivalent to table sugar (sucrose), the HFCS makes foods such as breads and breakfast cereals "brown" better when baked and gives cookies and snack bars their soft texture. It can help prevent freezer burn, so it is found in many frozen foods. It is easier to blend into beverages than refined sugar. It is also about 20% cheaper due to the relative abundance of corn, farm subsidies, and sugar tariffs in the United States. HFCS's usage leads to products with much longer shelf life. But HFCS may cause obesity and other health problems.

In 1966, sucrose held the number one slot, accounting for 86% of the sweeteners used. At present, HFCS is the leader, racking up more than $4.5 billion in annual sales and accounting for 55% of the sweetener market. That switch largely reflects the steady growth of HFCS, which climbed from zero consumption in 1966 to 62.6 pounds per person in 2001. Sugar is added to soft drinks, canned

TABLE 3.3
High-Fructose Corn Syrup Content per Serving in Commercial Products

Products	Teaspoons (Table Sugar Equivalent)
Sunkist soda	11 tsp.
Berkeley Farms low-fat yogurt with fruit	10 tsp.
Mott's applesauce	5 tsp.
Slim-Fast Chocolate Cookie Dough Meal Bar	5 tsp.
Ketchup	1 tsp.

fruits, dairy desserts and flavored yogurts, most baked goods, cereals, and jellies. Sugar is also added to products not thought of as "sweet" such as salad dressing, mayonnaise, ketchup, breads, crackers, and chips (Table 3.3). About two-thirds of all HFCS consumed in the United States are in beverages. Added sweeteners are important components of our diet, representing 318 calories for the average American or 16% of the daily caloric intake.

3.3.1 GLYCEMIC INDEX AND GLYCEMIC LOAD

Different carbohydrate-containing foods produce different blood glucose responses despite equivalent quantities of carbohydrate. The glycemic index (GI) is a ranking of carbohydrate-containing foods based on their immediate effects in an individual's blood glucose levels.[23] It is expressed as a percentage of the response to a standard food or carbohydrate. The glycemic response of different carbohydrate-containing foods was originally compared to glucose but was later studied with white bread. A high GI means that the dietary carbohydrate elevates blood glucose faster and to a higher level than a carbohydrate of lower GI. A GI of 70 or more is considered high, 56–69 is medium, and 55 or less is low. Carbohydrates in food have traditionally been classified as either "simple" (sugars) or "complex" (starches). Simple carbohydrates from commonly used foods tend to raise blood glucose more than do complex carbohydrates. Clearly, the glycemic response to 50 g of glucose is much greater than the response to a variety of foods providing 50 g starch. Although glucose, maltose, and sucrose produce large increases in blood glucose, fructose does not. Fructose produces only minimal increases in blood glucose concentrations in nondiabetic as well as diabetic subjects with reasonable glycemic control. Insulin is not necessary for fructose metabolism and evokes little increase in serum insulin concentration in a nondiabetic subject. Therefore, fructose may play a role as a sweetener for selected individuals with diabetes. However, one negative effect of high fructose intake is the potentially adverse influence on serum lipids.

Glycemic load (GL) is a new way to assess the impact of carbohydrate, which takes the GI into account but gives the relative indication of how much a particular serving of food is likely to increase the blood sugar levels.[17] It is calculated by multiplying a food's GI (as a percentage) by the number of available carbohydrate in grams in a given serving.

$$GL = \frac{GI}{100} \times \text{carbohydrates in grams}$$

A GL of 20 or more is considered "high," 11–19 is "medium," and 10 or less is "low." Because GL is related to the food's effect on blood sugar, low GL meals are often recommended for diabetic control and weight loss.

3.3.2 CARBOHYDRATES AND HEALTH

About 100 years back, carbohydrates contributed over 56% of the total calories in the American diet; starch supplied about 69% and sugars 31% of the total carbohydrates. In recent years, the calories contributed by carbohydrates have dropped to about 47%, and the use of starch decreased to 50% of total carbohydrates. The decreased intake of starch and increased sugar consumption have been incriminated in the cause of several chronic diseases such as coronary heart disease, hypertension, obesity, diabetes mellitus, and dental caries.

An elevated level of plasma triglycerides is a risk factor for heart disease. In humans, the fasting concentration of triglycerides increases when either starch or sugar is added to an experimental diet and also when carbohydrate replaces fat isocalorically. The carbohydrate induction of plasma triglycerides has been confirmed repeatedly; however, over a period of 3–4 months, adaptation occurs and the triglyceride level returns to near normal. People who subsist on diets high in starchy foods like rice and corn do not appear to have high plasma triglycerides unless they are obese. Sucrose at the present level of intake (i.e., 20%–25% of dietary energy) does not appear to have a specific triglyceride-inducing effect in normal people; however, among patients with triglyceridemia, a few are sensitive to carbohydrate intake. Individuals with this carbohydrate-induced hypertriglyceridemia respond well to a low-carbohydrate diet that restricts sugar more than starch.

Sucrose and other sweeteners are important components of our diet, representing 20%–25% of the daily caloric intake. About two-thirds of all HFCS consumed in the United States are in beverages. Some researchers have suggested that the use of HFCS in this country mirrors the rapid increase in obesity.[7,9,19] An extra can of soda a day, which is equivalent to 10–12 teaspoons of table sugar, can pile on 15 pounds in a year. The amount of soda we drink has more than doubled since 1970 to about 60 gallons per year, and so has the amount of HFCS we take in. This increased consumption may be one of the reasons that more people have gained weight.

Consumption of glucose increases secretion of insulin, which enables blood glucose to be transported into cells where it can be used for energy. It increases secretion of leptin that regulates appetite and fat storage, and suppresses secretion of ghrelin, an appetite stimulator. This results in hunger decline. Fructose does not stimulate secretion of insulin and does not increase leptin levels and decrease ghrelin production. This suggests that consuming a lot of fructose can contribute to weight gain. Whether fructose actually does contribute to weight gain has not been studied.

A study was done in overweight men and women (average age was 55 years) who were asked to consume either fructose-sweetened or glucose-sweetened drinks for 10 weeks. Drinks sweetened with fructose led to increases in the subjects' blood levels of low-density lipoprotein (LDL) and triglycerides, while the drinks sweetened with glucose did not. Another research group reported that drinking as little as one can of soda a day was associated with increased risk of several parameters linked to heart disease.

The World Health Organization (WHO) has recommended limiting intake of added sugar found in foods and beverages to no more than 10% of daily calories, a step the WHO said could help stop the worldwide rise in obesity that is fueling the growth of chronic diseases such as type 2 diabetes.[14] The U.S. Department of Agriculture suggests most of us limit our intake of added sugar to about 10–12 teaspoons a day. In 2001, the average consumption was 31 teaspoons a day. Reducing the intake of HFCS is a strategy worth considering. A healthful diet should provide 55%–65% of calories from carbohydrates, and a substantial contribution should be from complex carbohydrates.

The United States, with less than 5% of the world's population, is the largest soda consumer that accounted for one third of total soda consumption in 1999. According to the National Soft Drink Association, consumption of soft drinks is now over 600 12-oz. servings per person per year. Since the late 1970s, the soft drink consumption in the United States has doubled for women and tripled for men. The highest consumption is in men between the ages of 12 and 29 years: the average in that demographic is one-half gallon a day or 180 gallons a year. The amount spent per household in 2004 was nearly $850. On a nationwide basis, U.S. consumers spent more than $65 billion on soft drinks and consumed nearly 560 12-oz. servings per year. Soft drinks have replaced milk in the diet of many American children as well as adults.

The most common soft drink-associated health risks are obesity, nutritional deficiencies, tooth decay, diabetes, bone fractures, and heart disease. The relationship between soft drink consumption and body weight is so strong that researchers estimate that one extra drink a day gives a child a 60% greater risk of becoming obese.

Artificially sweetened "diet" drinks get touted as a healthy alternative to sugary drinks because they contain no calories or carbohydrates. But new research has shown that people who drank diet soda daily had a 48% increased risk of cardiovascular events compared to those who drank regular soda pop or no soda pop at all, even when accounting for smoking, physical activity, alcohol consumption, and calories consumed per day. The study included more than 2500 adults.

The participants filled out a questionnaire detailing their ethnic background and dietary and exercise habits. Researchers followed their health for a period of nearly 10 years. Diet soda does not contain sugar or calories of regular soda, but it has other health-draining chemicals like caffeine, artificial sweeteners, sodium, phosphoric acid, flavors, and other additives. Both regular and diet soda are high in phosphate and contain no calcium. This leads to lower calcium and higher phosphate levels in blood and may lead to osteoporosis and bone fractures. It is even more of a concern when parents give their growing—chemically vulnerable—children diet soda in an effort to avoid sugar. It is a good idea to cut back on soda consumption and substitute with (unsweetened) fruit juice and water.

Energy drinks are soft drinks and are classified as dietary supplements. They are promoted to increase energy levels, stamina, athletic performance, concentration as well as to lose weight. In addition to sugar or other sweeteners, they usually contain 70–80 mg caffeine for 8 oz. serving, more than double of cola drinks. They also contain guarana, a plant that contains caffeine, taurine (an amino acid), vitamins, and herbal supplements. Energy drinks are the fastest growing commodity in the U.S. beverage market and are consumed by 30%–50% of adolescents (12–18 year old). Together with children and young adults (19–25 years old), these age groups consume half of the energy drinks (on the) market.

Energy drinks[29] are unregulated and are available in grocery stores. According to a recent study, energy drinks have no therapeutic benefit and could adversely affect children's health, particularly those who consume large amounts or have health-related problems, especially those with cardiovascular, renal or liver disease, seizures, diabetes, mood and behavior disorders, and hyperthyroidism. They are at a higher risk for health complications from these drinks. The researchers encourage pediatricians and parents to talk to kids and teens about whether they should be drinking such beverages.

3.4   FAT

Fat provides a highly concentrated form of energy (9 Cal/g). In addition to being an important energy source, dietary fat serves as a carrier for fat-soluble vitamins and certain fatty acids that are essential nutrients. Fatty acids are needed to form cell structures and to act as precursors of prostaglandins. These needs can be met by a diet containing 20–25 g of fat, and there is no other specific requirement for fat as a nutrient.

Triglyceride is the principal form of fat that occurs both in foodstuffs and in the fat depot of most animals. There are over 40 fatty acids found in nature. They provide diversity and chemical specificity to natural fats, similar to that given to proteins by amino acids. Characteristically, fats are mixtures of triglycerides; no fat found in nature consists of a single triglyceride. Fatty acids of varying chain length occur naturally. They may be saturated (no double bonds), monounsaturated (one double bond), and polyunsaturated (two or more double bonds). The relative proportions and intake levels of these acids are of primary importance in determining their significance in nutrition and health.

With a few exceptions, natural food fats contain unbranched (i.e., the straight-chain type) and even-numbered carbon fatty acids of variable length. The fatty acid composition of various food fats is highly variable. Among the saturated fatty acids, palmitic acid (C 16) is widely distributed in nature and may contribute 10%–50% of the total fatty acids in any fat. Of the other saturated fatty acids, only myristic (C 14) and stearic acid (C 18)—up to 25% in beef fat—are comparable in distribution to palmitic acid, although they are not invariably present in every fat. Among the monounsaturated fatty acids, oleic acid (C 18:1) is the most widely distributed fatty acid in nature. In most fats, it forms 30% or more of the total fatty acids. The polyunsaturated fatty acids (PUFAs) are of special interest. Linoleic acid (C 18:2) and linolenic acid (C 18:3) cannot be synthesized in the body and are known as essential fatty acids (Chapter 4). Arachidonic acid (C 20:4) can be formed from linoleic acid.

Saturated fatty acids palmitic, myristic, and lauric (C 12) tend to increase blood cholesterol. Stearic, capric (C 10), and caprylic (C 8) acids tend to increase blood triglycerides. Monounsaturated fatty acids have no effect on blood cholesterol and triglycerides, and PUFAs decrease blood cholesterol and triglycerides.

Erucic acid (C 22:1) is a long-chain monounsaturated fatty acid and is the principal fatty acid (20%–25%) in rapeseed oil—one of the few vegetable oils that is easily grown in the temperate areas of the world such as Northern Europe and Canada. When large amounts of rapeseed oil (i.e., 50% of total energy) are fed to experimental animals, fatty changes occur in the heart muscle. This is because erucic acid enters the myocardial cell, but is oxidized more slowly than other fatty acids and so accumulates intracellularly in triglycerides. Some countries now limit the use of this oil to no more than 5% of the fat content. Rapeseed also contains high amounts of glucosinolates, which interfere with the formation of thyroxine and can cause thyroid disease. Through plant breeding, however, the content of erucic acid has been lowered to nearly zero and that of oleic acid increased. Also, glucosinolates are eliminated. Because the work on changing rapeseed species to meet consumer needs was first done in Canada, it is named canola. The advantages of canola oil include high oleic acid similar to that of olive oil and high linolenic acid as in soybean oil. It has the lowest amount of saturated fatty acids among all major oils.

Coconut oil has the highest percentage of saturated fatty acids of all common food oils (Table 3.4). They are primarily medium- and short-chain fatty acids. This is the reason coconut oil is very useful in the dietary treatment of certain digestive disorders. However, the high degree of saturation of coconut oil may raise blood cholesterol in some people.

Milk fat contains a relatively high proportion of short-chain fatty acids. These are water-soluble, are absorbed through the intestinal wall without being resynthesized to triglycerides, and are

TABLE 3.4
Content of Selected Fatty Acids in Vegetable Oils[a]

Oil	Oleic	Linoleic	Linolenic	Saturated
Canola	64.1	18.7	9.2	5.0
Coconut	7.0	2.0	0.0	86.0
Corn	28.0	54.0	1.0	17.0
Mustard[b]	13.0	19.9	10.8	4.9
Olive	75.0	9.0	0.0	15.0
Palm	38.0	9.0	0.0	53.0
Peanut	61.0	22.0	0.0	17.0
Rapeseed[b]	23.8	14.6	7.3	4.4
Sesame	40.0	44.0	2.0	14.0
Soybean	24.0	54.0	0.0	2.2
Safflower	16.4	77.0	0.0	6.6
Sunflower	21.0	66.0	0.0	13.0

[a] Values are percentages of total fatty acids.
[b] Contains high amounts of erucic acid.

transported in the portal vein directly to the liver where they are immediately converted to forms utilizable for energy. For this reason, they serve as a quick source of energy, which may be important especially early in life. Generally, fatty acids are approximately 51% saturated, 21% monounsaturated, and 3% polyunsaturated. Butter has about 60% saturated fatty acids, 31% oleic, and 0.3% PUFAs.

In some countries clarified butter or ghee is used. It is made from unsalted butter by slowly heating the butter over a low flame. The butter separates into three layers with oil on top, the water below, and the milk solids at the bottom. Butter is about 20% water. A little froth of casein proteins will collect atop the oil. This is skimmed, and the fat layer is collected, leaving the milk solids at the bottom. The lactose remains in the milky layer of water. Clarified butter is lactose free, can withstand high heat without breaking down, and is quite stable since proteins are removed.

Fatty acids that contain double carbon bond(s) can exist in either of two geometrically isomeric forms—*cis* and *trans* (Chapter 4). The natural unsaturated fatty acids exist in *cis* form. *Trans* fatty acids are produced in the hydrogenation process widely used in the food industry to harden unsaturated oils. They are also present in beef and milk fat. *Trans* isomers of PUFAs do not have essential fatty acid activity and lack the ability possessed by *cis* isomers of lowering the level of plasma cholesterol. *Trans* isomers formed during hydrogenation may play a role in atherosclerotic vascular disease.

An increase in dietary fat intake leads to obesity in animals and has been associated with higher incidence of overweight and obesity in many human studies. In recent years there has been a trend toward cutting calories and fat in the diet. For example, some eat only cereal with fat-free milk for breakfast and only salad without dressing for lunch. Studies in humans show that fat-soluble compounds with health-promoting properties such as carotenoids are better absorbed in the presence of fat.

3.4.1 NEED FOR FAT IN THE DIET

Some of the health-promoting components of food are fat soluble and require some fat to adequately absorb them. A recent study has shown that if we do not have fat in the diet the absorption of some of the wonderful substances in food is affected.[32] Researchers used 11 subjects and 2 diets: salsa and salad.

3.4.1.1 Salsa Test

Test subjects were given a meal of fat-free salsa and bread one day. The next day the similar meal was offered, but this time avocado was added to the salsa, boosting the fat content of the meal to about 37% of calories. Researchers found that (on the basis of blood levels) the individuals absorbed an average of 4.4 times as much lycopene and 2.6 times as much β carotene when avocado was added to the meal.

3.4.1.2 Salad Test

The salad for the first day included romaine lettuce, baby spinach, shredded carrots, and a no-fat dressing, resulting in a fat content of about 2%. For the second day, avocado was added and the fat content jumped to 42%. When the salad was consumed with avocado, the 11 test subjects absorbed seven times more the lutein and nearly 18 times more β-carotene than without avocado.

Lutein is a carotenoid found in green leafy vegetables and is linked with improved eye and heart health. Lycopene is found in tomato and some fruits and is being studied as a potential fighter of prostate and other cancers. β-carotene, which is found in colored fruits and vegetables, is used as a precursor of vitamin A and is also associated with lower cancer rates.

A study on rats by German researchers showed that the type of fat matters. They determined the absorption of vitamin E in the presence of pure vegetable oil or hydrogenated fat, which contains *trans* fatty acids. The *trans* fat slowed the absorption of vitamin E.

These are interesting observations. More systematic studies are needed using pure oil in place of avocado, which has several other components. The fat content of avocado ranges from 11% to 25%

and provides 128–233 Calories per 100 g (about 3.3 oz). No other fruit has an energy value as high as avocado. What should people who are watching their weight and the fat content of their diet do? The balance might be tricky. The best absorption from the salad in the aforementioned study occurred when individuals had dressing with about 28 g or about 2 tablespoons of fat. This translates to about 250 extra calories. It is best to consider the overall fat content of the meal. One does not have to add dressing if the meal contains a significant amount of fat such as in meat, fish, yogurt, or dessert.

3.4.2 Dietary Fat and Health

Foods contain combinations of saturated and unsaturated fats. Substantial quantities of saturated fats are found in dairy products, eggs, meats, and coconut and palm oils. Monounsaturated fats predominate in olive and canola oils, and PUFAs are found in nuts, seeds, seed oils, fish, and to a lesser extent in meats. Studies have shown that increasing the amount of PUFAs in the diet while reducing the saturated fatty acids promotes a modest drop in blood cholesterol. However, of greater importance than the increased PUFAs intake is the ratio of PUFAs to saturated fatty acids—the P/S ratio—in relation to coronary heart disease. Currently, the recommendation is for a P/S ratio ranging from 1:1 to 2:1. The basis for this recommendation is that some studies have demonstrated increased blood cholesterol levels when saturated fatty acids were high and that increasing linoleic acid counteracted this effect. However, PUFAs are particularly sensitive to lipid peroxidation, resulting in the generation of peroxides that can contribute to a spectrum of common chronic diseases. Vitamin E, an antioxidant, inhibits peroxide formation. Some vegetable oils are rich sources of this vitamin.

When highly unsaturated vegetable oils are heated at frying temperatures (365° F) for an extended period or even for half an hour a highly toxic compound, 4-hydroxy-2 *trans* nonenal (HNE) is formed. It is incorporated into fried foods in the same concentration as it forms in the heating oil. The compound is highly reactive with proteins, nucleic acids, and other biomolecules. HNE has been linked to a number of diseases including Parkinson's and Alzheimer's.

Dietary fat holds more than twice as many calories per gram as carbohydrate and protein, and it provides passive overconsumption of energy. This may explain why the prevalence of overweight worldwide is directly related to the percentage of fat in the diet and why low-fat diet has been consistently shown to provide moderate weight loss. Saturated fats tend to raise blood cholesterol and triglyceride concentrations, which are risk factors for cardiovascular disease. Reduction of saturated fat is important to control these lipids. A high intake of saturated fat from animal sources appears to increase the risk of some forms of cancer. Compared with individuals eating the least fat (25% of calories), those who are eating the highest amount (37% of calories) have been shown to have 10% greater risk for cataracts.

Fat constitutes, on average, 34% of calories in the U.S. diet. However, for optimal health, fat intake should not total more than 30% of calories.[11] Saturated and *trans* fatty acids should be limited to less than 10% of calories, and the PUFAs should be less than 10% of calories with monounsaturated fatty acids, the remainder of fat intake.

3.5 PROTEINS

The fundamental importance of proteins to the living cells and the human organism has long been appreciated; in fact, the very word *protein* was derived from the Greek word *proteos*, meaning "holding first place." Proteins are important in the structure of membranes, musculature, and connective tissues; for the transport of oxygen by hemoglobin and the transport of electrons by cytochromes; for the maintenance of fluid balance by serum albumin; in genetics as nucleoproteins; in defense mechanisms involving γ-globulins of blood, and in blood clotting by prothrombin and fibrinogen; and as enzymes in the catalysis of thousands of reactions.[3]

At any given time there are about 7000 different types of protein molecules in the average human body cell. About a third of these are embedded in the cells outer membrane. Some control the movement of the substances into and out of the cell. Some transmit signals from the exterior to the interior. Such proteins are frequently the targets of drugs. About half of the drugs currently on the market work by interacting with proteins in the cell membrane.

The importance of protein in the diet is primarily to act as a source of amino acids, some of which are essential (indispensable) dietary constituents because their carbon skeletons cannot be synthesized by mammals. Other amino acids are nonessential (dispensable) because they can be made within the mammalian tissues from carbon and nitrogen precursors.

There are 20 common amino acids found in tissue proteins. Eight amino acids are identified as absolutely essential for adult humans (Table 3.5).[12,16] In addition, infants require arginine and possibly histidine. The latter may also be required in small amounts in adults because prolonged histidine deficiency results in impaired hemoglobin formation. Two amino acids, cysteine and tyrosine, are made from the essential amino acids methionine and phenylalanine, respectively, and are considered semiessential. The requirements of methionine and phenylalanine are significantly reduced by the provision of cystine and tyrosine. The remaining amino acids can be synthesized from common intermediates in metabolism and thus are nonessential as dietary constituents. The terms *essential* and *nonessential* have no meaning in determining the relative importance that individual amino acids may have in metabolism. The nonessential amino acids may be of equal or greater significance for the organism in that they may participate in diverse cellular reactions and functions and provide precursors for the synthesis of many important cellular constituents. For example, glutamic acid (nonessential) has many important metabolic roles and if an organism suddenly were to lose its capacity to synthesize this amino acid, a serious disruption of key reactions of metabolism might result because the organism cannot wait until the next meal to replenish its supply.

Other amino acids occur in proteins in nature but these are made by modifying the side chain of an individual amino acid once the protein has been synthesized. Examples are hydroxyproline in collagen made by hydroxylation of certain proline residues in the collagen and 3-methyl histidine in the muscle made by methylation of certain histidine residues in these proteins. These derived amino acids are not used again for the de novo protein synthesis. When proteins containing them are broken down within the body, they are either metabolized (hydroxyproline) or excreted quantitatively (3-methyl histidine).

TABLE 3.5
Nutritional Classification of Common Amino Acids

Essential (Indispensable)	Semiessential	Nonessential (Dispensable)
Isoleucine	Tyrosine	Alanine
Leucine	Cystine	Aspartic acid
Lysine		Glutamic acid
Methionine		Glycine
Phenylalanine		Hydroxyproline
Threonine		Proline
Tryptophan		Serine
Valine		Cysteine
		Arginine[a]
		Histidine[b]

[a] Essential for infants.
[b] May be essential.

Proteins are essential structural components of all cells and are needed by the body to build and repair tissues, which are constantly undergoing breakdown and change. Proteins are important for maintaining the output of essential secretions such as digestive enzymes and peptide hormones. Body proteins are not static structures, but there is a continuous take-up and release of amino acids. In adults, the gains and losses are about equal, and the state is known as dynamic equilibrium. The liver is the key organ in the metabolism of proteins. It selectively removes amino acids from the portal circulation for the synthesis of its own proteins and for many of the specialized proteins such as lipoproteins, plasma albumins, globulins, and fibrinogen as well as nonprotein nitrogenous substances such as creatine. The liver is also the principal organ for the synthesis of urea. Amino acids are transported throughout the body by the systemic circulation and are rapidly removed from the circulation by various tissue cells. Similarly, amino acids and products of amino acid metabolism are constantly added to the circulation by the tissues. The amino acid pool available for any given tissue at any given time thus includes exogenous (dietary sources) and endogenous (tissue breakdown) sources. These sources are indistinguishable. The rate of protein replacement of the entire body is greater than the usual dietary intake and may be as high as 400 g/day, or about 3.5% of the protein in the body.

The rate of protein turnover varies widely in body tissues. The intestinal mucosa, for example, renews itself every 1–3 days—a fantastic rate of repletion; red blood cells have a life of about 120 days, and the skin is shed and replaced continuously. Muscle proteins have a much slower rate of turnover, but the size of the muscle mass in the body is so great that the net daily release of amino acids is considerable. The turnover rate of collagen is very slow and that of brain cells is negligible.

Human protein needs are known to be influenced by several factors (e.g., energy intake, nutritional and physiological state of the individual).[25,26] Assuming an adequate caloric intake in the average American diet, the recommended protein requirement for adults is 0.8 g/kg body weight/day. This amounts to about 56 g of protein for a 70-kg man and about 44 g/day for a 55-kg woman. Recommended allowances for children and adolescents decline from 2 g/kg body weight during the first year of life to 0.8 g/kg body weight at 18 years of age. In general, protein intake should constitute 12%–15% of the total caloric intake.

When energy intake is inadequate, protein intake must be increased because ingested amino acids are diverted into pathways of glucose synthesis and oxidation. In extreme energy deprivation, protein–energy malnutrition (PEM) may ensue. Protein needs increase during growth, pregnancy, lactation, and rehabilitation during treatment of malnutrition. Hospitalized patients with minimal stress who are well nourished need 1.0–1.2 g/kg body weight/day for the maintenance of lean body mass. The requirement for protein intake may be as high as 2 g/kg body weight/day for a patient in a hypermetabolic, hypercatabolic state secondary to trauma or burns. In addition, patients with renal or hepatic dysfunction may require a decrease in protein intake as a result of altered metabolism. Normal protein intake can precipitate or worsen uremia in patients with renal failure.

3.5.1 Amino Acid Catabolism

The amino acids that enter the free amino acid pool are incorporated into proteins; catabolized via transamination and oxidative reactions, leading to their elimination from the body as carbon dioxide, water, and nitrogen (principally as urea and ammonia); or converted to other physiologically important compounds such as nucleic acids, porphyrins, glutathione, and creatine. The continuous synthesis and the subsequent breakdown of protein within cells and organs enable the body to adapt to internal or external alterations. This overall process is usually referred to as protein turnover. The body has no special storage form of proteins to accommodate the excessive dietary intake of amino acids comparable to liver or muscle glycogen, or the deposition of fat as in carbohydrate or lipid metabolism, respectively. Hence amino acid catabolism is operating continually with substrates derived from excess dietary amino acids and from the turnover of tissue proteins.

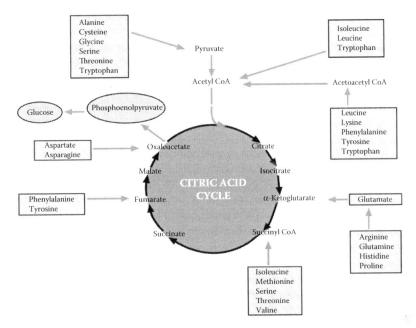

FIGURE 3.2 Catabolic disposition of carbon chains derived from amino acids.

The salient feature of amino acid catabolism involves the removal of α-amino groups by transamination and oxidative deamination, forming ammonia and the corresponding keto acids. A portion of free ammonia is excreted in the urine, but most parts are used in the synthesis of urea, which is quantitatively the most important route for disposing nitrogen from the body. The carbon skeletons of amino acids are funneled into seven molecules: pyruvate, acetyl CoA, acetoacetyl CoA, α-ketoglutarate, succinyl CoA, fumarate, and oxaloacetate (Figure 3.2). Amino acids that are degraded to acetyl CoA or acetoacetyl CoA are termed *ketogenic* because they can give rise to ketone bodies. In contrast, amino acids that are degraded to the other five molecules are termed *glucogenic*. The citric acid cycle intermediates and pyruvate can be converted to phosphoenolpyruvate and then to glucose.

3.5.2 Anabolism or Catabolism

Whether the ingested amino acid is utilized for the synthesis (anabolism) of new proteins or is deaminated and used for energy (catabolism) depends on several factors.

3.5.2.1 All-or-None Law

A very important point to keep in mind is the time factor with respect to the ingestion and utilization of proteins. Not only must all the essential amino acids be assimilated during the course of a day's dietary intake, but all must be ingested simultaneously if any is to be of benefit. This reflects two well-established facts concerning protein metabolism: (1) amino acids are not stored in appreciable quantities (as are carbohydrates and fats); and (2) the utilization of amino acids to form proteins occurs rapidly (within three hours) after the amino acids enter the bloodstream. For these reasons, a person receiving only tryptophan at one meal, for example, and all the other essential amino acids except tryptophan at the next meal will be in a negative nitrogen balance, as the essential tryptophan is not present at the crucial time. In this instance, tryptophan will be supplied by the endogenous catabolism of somatic proteins, causing a negative nitrogen balance. This results in a situation in which roughly one metabolic equivalent of tryptophan (endogenously derived) is available at some time during the day to be utilized with two metabolic equivalents of other essential amino acids. This excess quantity of amino acids would probably be deaminated, with the resulting α-keto acids then being utilized as an energy source, or stored as glycogen and depot lipid. The nonessential amino acids are also needed to maintain health. They differ from essential amino acids in that they may be synthesized endogenously if the essential amino acids are ingested in adequate quantities to provide nitrogen for transamination and certain carbon skeletal structures (e.g., the aromatic ring of tyrosine).

3.5.2.2 Caloric Intake

The body's first requirement is for energy-yielding substrates, and therefore, until energy requirements have been met by the intake of carbohydrates and fats, amino acids will be catabolized for energy and not used for protein synthesis. For most of the hungry people of the world, it is the total food that is lacking rather than protein specifically, so that the limitation of the nutritional value of that protein may be relatively unimportant. Even for growing children, it is generally the total food rather than protein that is inadequate. Thus, as the energy (calorie) content of the diet from carbohydrates and fats increases, the need for proteins decreases. This is referred to as protein sparing. Carbohydrates are somewhat more efficient than fats at protein sparing because carbohydrates can be used as an energy source by almost all tissues, whereas fat cannot be. Dietary protein in excess of requirements is utilized for energy.

3.5.2.3 Nutritional and Physiological State of the Individual

The rate of protein synthesis is high during growth and in tissue repletion following illness or injury. In a healthy adult, synthesis just balances tissue depletion when the caloric intake is adequate. The breakdown of proteins is increased immediately following injury, burns, and/or immobilization because of illness, fear, and anxiety.

3.5.2.4 Development of Specific Tissues

Some tissues are formed regardless of the overall nitrogen balance of the individual. The fetus and the maternal tissues are developed at the expense of the mother when the diet is inadequate. Also, rapidly growing tumors will use amino acids for synthesis at the expense of normal tissues.

3.5.2.5 Hormonal Control

The general control of protein metabolism depends a great deal upon the activity of several hormones. The growth hormone of the anterior pituitary gland causes a protein-anabolic effect during infancy and childhood if associated with the permissive activity of insulin. The androgens and estrogens have an anabolic effect during preadolescent and adolescent years; these hormones are, in part, responsible for the rapid growth phase of adolescence. Thyroxine demonstrates an apparently paradoxical activity in that it causes a net anabolism of proteins in physiological doses while large doses result in the catabolism of muscle tissues. The adrenocortical hormones increase the catabolism of body tissues by stimulating the breakdown of tissue proteins to yield glucose.

3.5.3 PROTEIN RESERVES

Although the body does not store proteins in the sense that it stores glycogen or fat, certain reserves are available from some tissues of the body for use in an emergency. Based upon animal studies, about 35% of the body proteins can be depleted. Thus, the vital functions of the organism may be protected for 30–50 days of total starvation. A well-fed human adult contains about 7 kg of protein, so a person can lose about 2.5 kg without a serious loss of function or threat to life; however, the use of these reserves eventually requires the restoration of these tissues to their normal protein composition.[33]

3.5.4 NITROGEN BALANCE

Nitrogen balance studies are based on the fact that proteins, on average, contain about 16% nitrogen; thus, 1 g of nitrogen is equivalent to 6.25 g of protein. Nitrogen balance is the term used to denote the qualitative and the quantitative adequacy of the protein portion of the diet. It is simply a difference between the amount of nitrogen ingested (mainly as proteins) and the amount of nitrogen excreted, with the difference being positive, negative, or zero (nitrogen equilibrium). The determination of nitrogen balance requires a careful estimation of intake (I) and all routes of nitrogen loss, namely in the urine (U), feces (F), and dermal losses (S). Fecal nitrogen includes that from undigested dietary proteins and protein fractions of desquamated cells of the intestinal mucosa, enzymes from digestive juices, and bacterial cells. The daily fecal nitrogen excretion is about 1 g but varies with the quality of dietary proteins. The difference between the nitrogen in the diet and fecal nitrogen is the amount of nitrogen absorbed and available for use.

The equation of nitrogen balance (B) is

$$B = I - (U + F + S)$$

A positive nitrogen balance is seen during infancy and childhood, during pregnancy, and in those recovering from illness or injury (if adequately nourished). A net deposition of protein occurs in body tissues with a reduction in urinary nitrogen (most of which is urea). A negative nitrogen balance can result following injury when there is a destruction of tissues and in major traumas or illnesses when the body's adaptive response causes an increased catabolism of body protein stores. It is also observed when the caloric and/or protein intake is inadequate. The normal adult is in nitrogen equilibrium with losses just balanced by intake.

3.5.5 NUTRITIONAL QUALITY OF PROTEINS

The effectiveness of food protein in supporting growth in the young organism and in tissue maintenance and repair in the adult depends primarily on the quantity and the quality (amino acid composition) of the protein. The digestibility of the protein and the efficient absorption of its constituent amino acids are other factors that can affect its utilization. The overall effectiveness of the food proteins or the fraction of absorbed nitrogen retained in the body is defined as the biological value of the protein. It is expressed in comparison with some other arbitrarily designated food proteins of high quality such as whole egg proteins. The term *biological value* is synonymous with the nutritional quality of proteins.

Several procedures for determining the biological value of proteins are used. One is the classical "rat growth" method and another is the nitrogen balance procedure. The biological value is expressed as the percentage of the absorbed nitrogen (N) retained (utilized by the individual). It is calculated as follows:

$$\text{Biological value} = \frac{\text{Food N} - (\text{Fecal N} + \text{Urinary N})}{\text{Food N} - \text{Fecal N}}$$

The biological value of eggs is considered to be 100, whereas that of white flour is approximately 50. In general, the value for animal proteins (80–100) is higher than that for cereal proteins (50–70); legumes give intermediate values.

Another common method of expressing the nutritional quality of protein is based on the amino acid composition or chemical score. This value is the amount of the most limiting amino acid in a test protein expressed as the percentage of the amount present in whole egg proteins:

$$\text{Chemical score} = \frac{\text{mg of limiting amino acid in 1 g of test protein}}{\text{mg of amino acid in 1 g of reference protein}} \times 100$$

TABLE 3.6
Composition of Essential Amino Acids

Protein Source	Amino Acid Content (%)				Score (Limiting AA)
	Lys	Saa	Thr	Try	
Ideal protein	5.5	3.5	4.0	1.0	100
Cereal	2.4	3.8	3.0	1.1	44 (Lys)
Legume	7.2	2.4	4.2	1.4	68 (Saa)
Milk powder	8.0	2.9	3.7	1.3	83 (Saa)
Mixture of cereal + legumes + milk powder	5.1	3.2	3.5	1.2	88 (Thr)

Lys = lysine; Saa = sulfur-containing amino acids; Thr = threonine; Try = tryptophan; Score = chemical score.

This value does not take into account the differences in digestibility; however, the chemical scores generally agree with biological values and have the advantage over the latter of requiring less time. The score, in theory, should be calculated for all the essential amino acids, and the lowest score should be taken. In practice, however, the scores are calculated only for lysine, the sulfur-containing amino acids, and tryptophan, as generally one of these is the limiting amino acid in the common foods.

Proteins with a low chemical score or biological value have to be consumed in a proportionately higher quantity to satisfy requirements. Apparently, protein requirements may be satisfied by x g of protein with a biological value of 100 or $2x$ g of a protein with a value of 50. Thus, in order to express the true protein value of food, both quality and quantity must be considered (Table 3.6). The product of the two factors is a convenient way of doing this. Most people in underdeveloped countries obtain their protein needs by eating adequate amounts of relatively poor-quality proteins; the amino acids that are not utilized for protein synthesis are metabolized for energy.

An ideal protein has 5.5% lysine while cereal protein has 2.4% lysine or about 44% lower than ideal protein (Table 3.6). Cereal protein therefore is considered 44% as efficient as the ideal protein; however, when cereals are mixed with legumes and milk powder, the efficiency of the mixture is much higher because of the complementary effect. The essential amino acids present in one protein balance the deficit or deficits of one or more proteins of lower biological value. For this reason, vegetarians should combine foods such as cereal grains with legumes (i.e., soybeans, peas, beans) or milk products to obtain a more complete protein source.

Complementary protein combinations are found in almost all cultures (Table 3.7). In the Middle East bread and cheese are eaten together. Mexicans eat beans and corn (tortillas). Indians eat rice and peas. Americans eat breakfast cereals with milk. This kind of supplementation works only when the deficient and complementary proteins are ingested together or within a few hours of each other.

3.5.6 Protein Needs in Disease

Individual diseases affect protein needs to different extents, and each disease process varies in intensity from individual to individual. In some of these conditions (fever, fracture, burns, and surgical trauma) body protein is lost extensively during the acute phase of the disease and needs to be regained during convalescence. For example, simple disuse atrophy during a short period of bed rest can cause a loss of 0.3 kg body protein. To this can be added losses related to the particular disease

TABLE 3.7
Complementary Protein Combinations

Food Group	Generally Limited in Amino Acids	Generally Good Source of Amino Acids
Nuts and seeds + legumes	Isoleucine, lysine Tryptophan, methionine	Tryptophan, methionine Isoleucine, lysine
Legumes + cereal grains	Tryptophan, methionine Isoleucine, lysine	Isoleucine, lysine Tryptophan, methionine
Cereal grains + leafy vegetables	Isoleucine, lysine Methionine	Tryptophan, methionine Tryptophan, lysine

process, such as 0.4 kg body protein after a gastrectomy, 0.7 kg after fracture of a femur, and 1.2 kg after 35% burn. These losses need to be regained during convalescence.

A large amount of protein has been considered necessary to improve performance, hence the popularity of highly promoted protein formulations. Muscle mass can be increased only by appropriate exercise. Scientific data suggests that muscular activity does not increase the body's need for protein beyond the amount consumed in a normal diet. A diet containing as much as 2.8 g protein/kg does not enhance physiological work performance during intense physical training.

Although excessive protein intake has not been proved to be harmful, there are several potential disadvantages to a very high protein intake. The protein in foods of animal origin is often accompanied by large amounts of fat. In the body excess protein (or amino acids) is not stored, but amino acids are deaminated and utilized for the supply of energy. There is a load on the liver to convert nitrogen to urea and on the kidney to excrete urea and other nitrogenous compounds in the urine. It is often accompanied by calcium excretion, increasing the risk of osteoporosis. Additional dangers of excess protein intake include greater risk of type 2 diabetes, possible ketosis, hyperuricemia with the threat of gout, and when protein contributes >35% of total energy intake, hyperaminoacidemia and hyperammonemia. Protein, while essential to build and repair tissues, is the least important nutrient as an energy source.

In some cases, administration of certain individual amino acids has been found to be of benefit.[31] Glutamine is an amino acid released by muscle and is used by enteral cells and immune cells for energy. In malnutrition and after trauma, muscle glutamine and protein synthesis are reduced and may result in enterocyte and immunocyte starvation. Glutamine enrichment of enteral or parenteral feedings normalizes muscle glutamine, restores protein synthesis, limits nitrogen loss, and improves outcome in critically ill patients who are postsurgery or in the intensive care unit. In addition, glutamine[5] significantly increases plasma concentrations of taurine, an amino acid with antihypertensive, antiarrhythmic, and positive inotropic effects.[4] This may be important for patients with chronic kidney disease, in whom low intracellular taurine concentrations are common and who are at high risk for cardiac events. Therefore, glutamine has been considered to be a nutrient that becomes conditionally essential in trauma and infection. The term *conditionally essential* applies when endogenous synthesis cannot meet metabolic needs. Arginine is another nonessential amino acid that is proposed as a nutrient for altering immune function and improving wound healing.

In some diseases protein must be restricted. An example is acute liver failure in which intake has to be restricted to avoid hepatic coma. In uremia, the capacity to excrete nitrogenous end products is limited and protein intake must also be restricted. In this illness sufficient protein must be provided to avoid depletion of tissue protein without exceeding the capacity of the patient to deal with the amino acid load. In the dietary management of uremia an intake of 0.5 g protein/kg body weight allows patients to resist intercurrent infections better than an earlier recommended intake of 0.25 g/kg.

3.5.7 PROTEIN–ENERGY MALNUTRITION

Protein synthesis, resistance to infection, and wound healing depend on the maintenance of adequate levels of protein and other nutrients. A deficiency involving both protein and energy sources is called protein–energy malnutrition.[27,33] The persons most often afflicted with PEM are young children under 5 years of age because of their demand for growth; however, adolescents and adults are also vulnerable groups for this type of malnutrition. A disease associated primarily with protein deficiency commonly occurs in children between the ages of 1 and 4 years. These children are usually in good health while they are breast-fed, but they become ill soon after they have been weaned. It is common in many developing countries and is a consequence of feeding the child a diet adequate in calories but deficient in proteins. The disease is known as kwashiorkor, which is derived from the Bantu word meaning "displaced child" (Figure 3.3). The disease becomes clinically manifest when amino acid requirements are increased by infection (e.g., malaria, gastroenteritis). The syndrome is characterized by poor growth, low plasma protein levels, edema, diarrhea, and increased susceptibility to infection. A fatty liver is common because of the reduced hepatic fat mobilization as a consequence of decreased lipoprotein synthesis.

A striking finding in kwashiorkor is the deceptive plump appearance of the young.[33] In the Caribbean, these patients are known as sugar babies because they are fed on a diet rich in starch and sugar. The name also evokes an image of round cheeks and bellies. The plumpness is not an expression of overeating but is due to edema. The normal plasma albumin level is about 4 g/dL, but patients with this disease may exhibit a level of about 1 g/dL, which causes a reduction in intravascular oncotic pressure. Plasma water decreases and accumulates in extravascular tissues. When these patients are put on restorative diet, their weight initially may decrease due to a loss of excess water.

An overall deficit in food intake, including both calories and proteins, can lead to the development of the syndrome known as marasmus,[33] which is derived from a Greek word and means "to

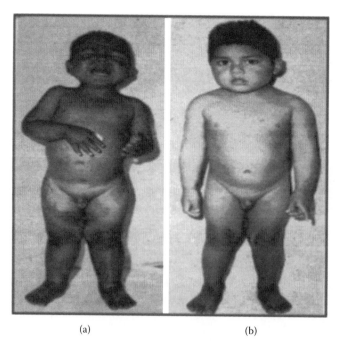

(a)   (b)

FIGURE 3.3 A 36-month-old child with severe edematous PEM and preservation of adiposity (kwashiorkor) (a) on admission to the hospital and (b) 4 months later when fully recovered. (Reproduced with permission from F. E. Viteri, University of California, Berkeley.)

waste." Although it is not restricted to any age group, it is most common in children under 1 year of age. The child is small for its age, looks emaciated, and in the extreme condition is reduced to skin and bones because of what is essentially a total absence of adipose tissues (Figure 3.4). This condition is also known as PEM, especially when seen in older children and adults.

Many children with PEM sometimes exhibit the features of marasmus with some degree of edema[33] (Figure 3.5); others may have many signs of kwashiorkor, but also appear to have much less adipose tissue. Patients who combine the features of kwashiorkor including edema and marasmus are diagnosed to have marasmic kwashiorkor.

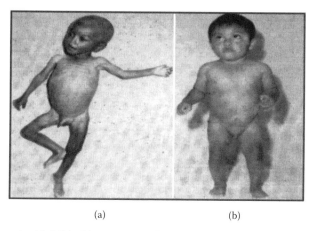

(a)   (b)

FIGURE 3.4   A 21-month-old child with severe nonedematous PEM (marasmus) on (a) admission to the hospital and (b) 4 months later when fully recovered. (Reproduced with permission from F. E. Viteri, University of California, Berkeley.)

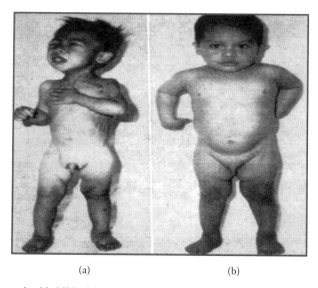

(a)   (b)

FIGURE 3.5   A 25-month-old child with severe edematous PEM superimposed on chronic caloric deficit. In addition to being edematous, he appears wasted (marasmus–kwashiorkor). Pictures were taken on (a) admission and (b) 4 months later when fully recovered. (Reproduced with permission from F. E. Viteri, University of California, Berkeley.)

Perhaps the most devastating result of both kwashiorkor and marasmus is the reduced ability of the affected individuals to fight infections. The diagnosis of PEM is different in adults than in children because adults are no longer growing in height. Therefore, undernutrition in adults causes wasting rather than stunting.

Protein–calorie malnutrition is the most common type of nutritional deficiency in hospitalized patients and is manifested by the depletion of both tissue energy stores and body proteins. Malnourished patients have prolonged hospitalization and are at a higher risk of developing complications during therapy. These nutrition-associated complications are the result of organ wasting and functional impairment and include weakness, decreased wound healing, altered hepatic metabolism of drugs, and infections.

3.6 USE OF BODY ENERGY SOURCES DURING HYPOMETABOLISM AND HYPERMETABOLISM

3.6.1 STARVATION—HYPOMETABOLISM

The metabolic fuels available in a normal 70-kg man at the beginning of a fast are 15 kg as fat, 6 kg as protein, and 0.4 kg as glycogen. During a 24-hour fast, energy needs are met by the consumption of liver glycogen stores and the conversion of up to 75 g of protein to glucose (gluconeogenesis). By 24-hour fasting, only 15% of glycogen stores remain. Gluconeogenesis increasingly provides the source of blood glucose. For this purpose, about 155 g of muscle protein must be degraded daily with a loss of nearly 25 g of nitrogen. The body has a total of about 1000 g of nitrogen, of which it cannot lose more than 25%–40% without the threat of death. The brain continues to use glucose as fuel exclusively.

To prevent the dissolution of excessive body proteins, glucose production and whole body glucose oxidation decrease. Endogenous fat stores become the body's major fuel, and the rates of adipose tissue lipolysis, hepatic ketone body production, and fat oxidation begin to increase. After 3 days of fasting, the rate of glucose production is reduced by half, and the rate of lipolysis more than doubles the value found at 12 hours of fasting. The increase in fatty acids delivery to the liver, in conjunction with the increase in the ratio of plasma glucagon to insulin, enhances hepatic ketone body production. By 7 days of fasting, plasma ketone body concentration increases 75-fold and ketone bodies provide 70% of the brain's energy needs. Ketone bodies are also used for energy needs by the muscle and the renal cortex. In contrast to fatty acids, ketone bodies can cross the blood–brain barrier and provide water-soluble fuels derived from water-insoluble adipose tissue triglycerides. The use of ketone bodies by the brain greatly diminishes glucose production from amino acids. Plasma ketone bodies and thyroid hormone inactivation inhibit protein breakdown and prevent a rapid protein loss. The body still cannot do entirely without glucose. The citric acid cycle must be maintained to produce ATP for synthetic reactions. Red blood cells, which derive their ATP only from glycolysis, are totally dependent on blood glucose. As fasting continues, the kidneys become an important site for glucose production. Glutamine released from the muscle is converted to glucose by the kidneys and accounts for almost half the total glucose production. The REE decreases by approximately 15% at 7 days of starvation.

Adaptation is maximal during prolonged starvation (> 14 days of fasting). At this time, adipose tissue provides more than 90% of the daily energy requirement. Total glucose production is decreased to about 75 g/day (from 150 g at 24 hours of fasting to 120 g at 3 days and 87 g at 7 days of fasting) and provides fuel for glycolytic tissues (40 g/day) and the brain (35 g/day). Muscle protein breakdown is decreased to less than 30 g/day, which causes a marked decrease in urea formation and nitrogen excretion. REE is decreased by approximately 25%. These metabolic changes, which occur during starvation, ensure that all tissues have an adequate supply of fuel molecules. Because of these adaptive mechanisms, adult humans are capable of going without food for incredible periods. For example, obese patients have fasted for as long as 236–249 days.

Thus, starvation involves metabolic alterations that enhance the chance of survival by increasing the use of body fat stores, by sparing the use of glucose, by minimizing nitrogen loss, and by decreasing energy expenditure.

3.6.2 STRESS—HYPERMETABOLISM

Stress includes injury, surgery, burns, and infections. It triggers a characteristic hypermetabolic state in which REE is increased along with body temperature.[4,24] The extent and the pattern of the metabolic changes vary with the type as well as the severity of injury or infection. However, stress exhibits certain common features. The demands of accelerated energy expenditure are met by skeletal muscle and visceral proteolysis to provide amino acid substrates for gluconeogenesis. Muscle proteolysis and gluconeogenesis are promoted by high levels of circulating catecholamines, glucagon, cortisol, and cytokines. The patient is resistant to insulin. The blood glucose and free fatty acids are elevated. However, ketogenesis is not accelerated as in fasting, and perhaps as a result of this, the body is less able to preserve protein stores in muscle.

A simple bone fracture causes a significant loss of nitrogen in the urine. For most people, the impact of injury on overall protein metabolism is minimal. However, in chronic illness or in patients otherwise weakened by age or other factors, the onset of a hypermetabolic state may produce a significant and dangerous loss of body proteins. In severe stress, when untreated, body protein catabolism may be sufficient to deplete 50% of body protein stores within 3 weeks. The process of PEM in such patients is associated with decreased cardiac and renal functions, fluid retention, intestinal mucosal atrophy, loss of intracellular minerals, diminished cell-mediated immune function, increased risk of infection, and eventual death. The greater the stress, the more body protein is broken down, the more nitrogen is excreted in the urine, and the greater is the need for protein.

Protein–Calorie Malnutrition and Anemia—A Case

A 2½-year-old female was admitted to a hospital as a desperately ill, conscious child with a blood pressure of 78/40 mmHg, a temperature of 37.2°C, a respiration of 28 min⁻¹, and pulse of 132 min⁻¹. She weighed 5.2 kg (50% normal weight for age) with moderate peripheral edema and extensive dermatosis. Her eyes showed scleral dryness and corneal clouding with incipient ulcerations. Her history revealed that she was reasonably well, but 2 months prior to admission, she had watery diarrhea, would not eat, and had lost weight. One month prior to admission, she developed swelling of her legs, increased weakness, and poor vision. These conditions worsened, and a week before admission, she developed skin sores and a nasal discharge.

A blood analysis showed that her hemoglobin was 6.5 g/dL, hematocrit was 24 vol%, platelets were 151,000 mm⁻³, and white cells were 29,800 mm⁻¹. Serum albumin level was 1.57 g/dL and vitamin A was 6 μg/dL. The child was diagnosed as having marasmus–kwashiorkor, xerophthalmia (vitamin A deficiency), and severe nutritional anemia. Cultures of blood, urine, and nasopharynx indicated that she had staphylococcal pneumonia, and sepsis with genitourinary infection.

She was treated with 100,000 IU of vitamin A intramuscularly and intravenous fluids with antibiotics. She continued to be septic for the first 3 days but began to improve on day 4. However, her hemoglobin level declined over the first week of treatment, during which her intake of protein was 1 g/kg body weight/day and her intake of energy was 100 Cal/kg body weight/day. The patient showed no evidence of hemorrhage. On day 7, she was given 100 mg of iron intramuscularly, and her dietary proteins and energy were increased to 2 g and 175 Cal/kg body weight/day, respectively. There was no improvement on hemoglobin level. On day 14, she was given 50 mL of packed red cells, which raised her hemoglobin to 7 g/dL. She did improve clinically, but her albumin level remained depressed at 1.7 g/dL. On day 28, her dietary protein was increased to 4 g/kg body weight/day. A few days later, her hemoglobin level rose to 12 g/dL.

This is a classical case of PEM that made the child susceptible to infection.[37] Also, the deficiency of vitamin A contributed to her eye condition. The patient was not only severely malnourished but—because of the infection—she was also in a hypermetabolic state, which caused the loss of her already limited body proteins. Antibiotics did control the infection and vitamin A did improve the condition of her eyes. Erythropoietin has a role in normal red cells production. The secretion of erythropoietin is dependent on adequate protein status. To start with, this patient was deficient in both protein and calories. The stress of infection worsened her protein status. Only after increasing the intake of protein and calories did the hemoglobin level start to rise.

This case illustrates a delayed but dramatic response to protein feeding in a child hospitalized for PEM. An adequate protein intake is required for an appropriate hemopoiesis.

REFERENCES

1. Anderson, C. E. 1977. Energy and metabolism. In *Nutritional Support of Medical Practice*, ed. H. A. Schneider, C. E. Anderson, and D. B. Cousin, 10–23. Hagerstown, MD: Harper and Row.
2. Bell, S. J., D. Bradley, R. Armour Forse, and B. R. Bistrian. 1997. The new dietary fats in health and disease. *J Am Diet Assoc* 97:280.
3. Bisborogh, S., and N. Mann. 2006. A review of issues of dietary protein intake in humans. *Int J Sport Nutr Exer Metab* 16:129.
4. Boelens, P. G., A. P. Houdijk, H. N. de Thomas et al. 2003. Plasma taurine concentrations increase after enteral glutamine supplementation in trauma patients and stressed rats. *Amer J Clin Nutr* 77:250.
5. Boelens, P. G., R. J. Nijveldt, A. P. Houdijk et al. 2001. Glutamine alimentation in catabolic state. *J Nutr* 131(suppl 9):2569S.
6. Brandi, L. S., R. Bertolini, and M. Calafa. 1997. Indirect calorimetry in critically ill patients: Clinical applications and practical advice. *Nutrition* 13:349.
7. Bray, G. A., S. A. Nielson, and B. M. Popkin. 2004. Consumption of high-fructose corn syrup in beverages may play a role in the epidemic of obesity. *Amer J Clin Nutr* 79:537.
8. Dills Jr., W. L. 1989. Sugar alcohols as bulk sweeteners. *Annu Rev Nutr* 9:161.
9. Forsche, R. A., M. L. Storey, D. B. Allison et al. 2007. A critical examination of the evidence relating high-fructose corn syrup and weight gain. *Crit Rev Food Science Nutr* 47:561.
10. Hill, J. O. 2006. Understanding and addressing the epidemic of obesity: An energy balance perspective. *Endocr Rev* 27:750.
11. Hu, F. B., and W. C. Willett. 2002. Optimal diets for prevention of coronary heart disease. *J Amer Med Assoc* 288:2569.
12. Jackson, A. A. 1983. Amino acids: Essential and nonessential. *Lancet* 1:1034.
13. Katan, M. B., and D. S. Ludwig. 2010. Extra calories cause weight gain—But how much? *J Amer Med Assoc* 303(1):65.
14. Krauss, R. M., R. H. Eckel, B. Howard et al. 2000. AHA dietary guidelines: Revision 2000: Statement for healthcare professionals from the nutritional committee of the American Heart Association. *Circulation* 102:2284.
15. Krebs, M. 2005. Amino acid-dependent modulation of glucose metabolism in humans. *Eur J Clin Invest* 35:351.
16. Laidlaw, S. A., and J. D. Kopple. 1987. New concepts of the indispensable amino acids. *Am J Clin Nutr* 46:593.
17. Liu, S., W. C. Willett, M. J. Stampfer et al. 2000. A prospective study of dietary glycemic load, carbohydrate intake, and risk of coronary heart disease in U.S. women. *Amer J Clin Nutr* 71:1455.
18. Malik, V. S., M. B. Schulze, and F. B. Hu. 2006. Intake of sugar-sweetened beverages and weight gain: A systematic review. *Amer J Clin Nutr* 84:304.
19. Manson, J. E., and S. S. Bassuk. 2003. Obesity in the United States. A first look at its high toll. *J Amer Med Assoc* 289:229.

20. Marakami, K., S. Sasaki, Y. Takahashi et al. 2007. Hardness (difficulty in chewing) of the habitual diet in relation to body mass index and waist circumference in free living Japanese women aged 18–22 years. *J Clin Nutr* 86:206.

21. McClave, S. A., C. C. Lowen, M. J. Kleber et al. 2003. Clinical use of respiratory quotient obtained from indirect calorimetry. *J Parenteral Enteral Nutr* 27:21.

22. McWhirter, J. P., and C. R. Pennington. 1994. Incidence and recognition of malnutrition in hospital. *Br Med J* 308:945.

23. Miller, J. B., S. Colagiuri, and K. Foster-Powell. 1997. The glycemic index is easy and works in practice. *Diabetes Care* 20:1678.

24. Naber, T. H. J., T. Schermer, A. de Bree et al. 1997. Prevalence of malnutrition in nonsurgical hospitalized patients and its association with disease complications. *Am J Clin Nutr* 66:1232.

25. Pellet, P. L. 1990. Protein requirements in humans. *Am J Clin Nutr* 51:723.

26. Pencharz, P. B., and R. D. Ball. 2003. Different approaches to define individual amino acid requirements. *Annu Rev Nutr* 23:101.

27. Rao, K. S. 1974. Evolution of kwashiorkor and marasmus. *Lancet* 1:709.

28. Ravussin, E., and C. Bogardus. 1992. A brief overview of human energy metabolism and its relationship to essential obesity. *Am J Clin Nutr* 55:242s.

29. Seifert, S. M., J. L. Schaechter, E. R. Hershorin, and S. E. Lipshultz. 2011. Health effects of energy drinks on children, adolescents, and young adults. *Pediatrics* 127:511.

30. Stein, T. P. 1985. Why measure the respiratory quotient of patients in total parenteral nutrition? *J Am Coll Nutr* 4:501.

31. Sullivan, D. H., S. Sun, and R. C. Walls. 1999. Protein–energy undernutrition among elderly hospitalized patients. A prospective study. *J Am Med Assoc* 281:2013.

32. Unlu, N. Z., T. Bohn, S. K. Clinton et al. 2005. Carotenoid absorption from salad and salsa by humans is enhanced by the addition of avocado or avocado oil. *J Nutr* 135:431.

33. Viteri, F. E., and B. Torun. 1980. Protein–calorie malnutrition. In *Modern Nutrition in Health and Disease.* 6th ed., ed. R. S. Goodhart and M. E. Shils, 697–720. Philadelphia: Lea and Febiger.

34. Waterlow, J. C. 1986. Metabolic adaptation to low intake of energy and protein. *Annu Rev Nutr* 6:495.

35. Woo, R., R. Daniels-Kush, and E. S. Horton. 1985. Regulation of energy balance. *Annu Rev Nutr* 5:411.

36. Zou, M. L., P. J. Moughan, A. Awati, and G. Livesey. 2007. Accuracy of the Atwater factors and related food energy conversion factors with low-fat, high-fiber diets when energy intake is reduced spontaneously. *Amer J Clin Nutr* 86:1649.

CASE BIBLIOGRAPHY

37. Clinical Nutrition Cases. 1979. The anemia of protein–calorie malnutrition and its response to dietary protein. *Nutr Rev* 37:81.

4 Role of Essential Fatty Acids

4.1 FATTY ACIDS

Fatty acids are chains of covalently linked carbon atoms, bearing hydrogen atoms, which terminate in a carboxylic group that is responsible for their properties as acids. The naturally occurring fatty acids are, for the most part, unbranched and acyclic, but complex structures with branched or cyclic chains do occasionally occur, particularly in lower biological forms. The total number of carbon atoms in a molecule is usually even although fatty acids containing odd-numbered carbon atoms also are found in nature. They have the basic formula $CH_3[CH_2]_nCOOH$, where n can be any number from 2 to 22 and is usually an even number. One method of classification of fatty acids is according to their chain length (i.e., the number of carbon atoms they contain). Fatty acids containing 2–4 carbon atoms are called short-chain fatty acids, while those with 6–10 and 12–24 carbon atoms are called medium-chain and long-chain fatty acids, respectively. Fatty acids can also be classified according to the number of double bonds between the carbon atoms (i.e., the degree of saturation): saturated, with no double bonds; unsaturated, with one double bond; and polyunsaturated fatty acids (PUFAs), with two or more double bonds. Fatty acids with two, three, four, five, and six double bonds are called dienoic, trienoic, tetraenoic, pentaenoic, and hexaenoic, respectively.

The carbon atoms of the fatty acids are numbered from the carboxyl group (Δ numbering system) or lettered (W or n numbering system):

Δ numbering system (carboxyl side)

16   4   3   2   1

$CH_3(CH_2)_{11}$ CH_2 CH_2 CH_2 COOH

1   13 14 15 16

W or n numbering system (W-side)

Fatty acids are abbreviated in the Δ nomenclature by listing the carbon number and position of double bonds ($C_a\Delta_b$). Thus, palmitic acid is abbreviated as C_{16}:0 or C_{16}:$0\Delta_0$, and palmitoleic acid as C_{16}:1 or C_{16}:1, Δ_9. The number after the Δ in this classification system signifies the position of the double bond relative to the carboxyl end. In palmitoleic acid the double bond is on the ninth carbon atom from the carboxyl group (i.e., it is between carbon atoms 9 and 10, counting the carboxyl carbon as carbon 1). In the W-numbering system, palmitoleic acid is abbreviated as C_{16}:1, W_7. This signifies that the fatty acid has 16 carbons and one double bond that is located seven carbon atoms away from the W carbon, counting the W carbon as carbon 1 (i.e., the double bond is between carbon atoms 7 and 8, counting from the W end).

$$CH_3-CH_2-CH_2-CH_2-CH_2-CH_2-CH=CH-(CH_2)_7COOH .$$
Palmitoleic acid

Most of the fatty acids in the blood and tissues of humans have 16, 18, and 20 carbon atoms, but there are a few with longer chains that exist in the lipids of the nervous system.

4.2 NEUTRAL FAT

The neutral fats are esters of one, two, or three fatty acid residues with glycerol and are called mono-glycerides, diglycerides, and triglycerides, respectively. Most triglyceride molecules contain two or more different fatty acid moieties (i.e., the fatty acids within one triglyceride are not often repeated) and have the general composition

$$
\begin{array}{l}
CH_2 - O - COR_1 \\
| \\
CH - O - COR_2 \\
| \\
CH_2 - O - COR_3
\end{array}
$$

where R_1COOH, R_2COOH, and R_3COOH are fatty acid chains that may or may not all be the same.

4.3 PROPERTIES OF FAT

The chemical and physical properties of fat are influenced by the fatty acids they contain. Saturated fatty acids (SFA) up to 10 carbon atoms in their structure are liquid and those containing more than 10 carbon atoms are solid at room temperature. Unsaturated and PUFAs are liquid at room temperature.

4.3.1 IODINE NUMBER

Fatty acids in fat will combine with iodine in proportion to the number of double bonds that they contain. This property of fatty acids is the basis of a test to determine the degree of unsaturation of a fat or iodine number. Iodine number is expressed as the grams of iodine absorbed by 100 g of fat; the higher the iodine number, the greater the unsaturation in fat. Thus, coconut oil, composed largely of SFA, has an iodine number of 8–10. Butterfat has an iodine number ranging from 36 to 38, while linseed oil has an exceedingly high iodine number of 177–209. Iodine numbers for common vegetable oils are as follows: corn oil, 115–124; olive oil, 79–90; peanut oil, 85–100; and soybean oil, 130–138.

4.3.2 RANCIDITY

Most fats on exposure to air develop an unpleasant odor and flavor as a result of a slight hydro-lysis of fat, leading to the liberation of volatile fatty acids having rather unpleasant odors. It is known as rancidity. The double bonds in fatty acids also make them vulnerable to deterioration as a result of oxidation. Light, heat, moisture, and bacterial action are all factors that lead to bring about rancidity. Besides their disagreeable properties, the rancid fats and oils may have distinctly unphysiological effects by oxidizing a number of essential dietary substances, for example, vitamin A, carotenes, and linoleic acid. The rate of production of rancidity varies with the type of fat as well as being influenced by air, moisture, etc. There are substances present in fat that inhibit the auto-oxidation. These are called antioxidants and occur in different concentrations in various natural fats. The occurrence of antioxidants explains why some fats keep better than others. Compounds possessing this property include certain phenols, naphthols, and quinones. The most common natural antioxidant is perhaps vitamin E. Addition of antioxidants (e.g., butyl-ated hydroxyanisole, butylated hydroxytoluene) is necessary if the fat is to be kept for long periods without deterioration.

4.3.3 HYDROGENATION

The unsaturated or PUFAs can be hydrogenated by gaseous hydrogen in the presence of a catalyst such as active nickel. Hydrogenation is used for converting liquid oils into solid fats in the manufacture of shortenings and margarines. The extent to which the melting point may be increased depends upon the completeness of hydrogenation.

4.3.4 *TRANS* FATTY ACIDS

Fatty acids that contain double bonds can exist in either of two geometric isomeric forms; this is known as *cis* and *trans* isomerism. Thus, oleic acid is a *cis* form and elaidic acid is its *trans* isomer. Unsaturated fatty acids in naturally occurring fats are in *cis* form (i.e., the hydrogen atoms are on the same side of the double bond). When these unsaturated and PUFAs are hydrogenated to make margarine and shortening anywhere from 8% to 70% of the double bonds occur in a *trans* form (i.e., the hydrogen atoms are on the opposite side of the double bond). These *trans* fatty acids account for 5%–8% of the fat in the American diet.

$$H-C-(CH_2)_7CH_3 \qquad CH_3-(CH_2)_7-C-H$$
$$\parallel \qquad\qquad\qquad \parallel$$
$$H-C-(CH_2)_7COOH \qquad H-C-(CH_2)_7COOH$$

$$cis \qquad\qquad\qquad trans$$

$$\text{oleic acid} \qquad\qquad \text{elaidic acid}$$

Although hydrogenation offers advantages to the product (e.g., controlled consistency and improved stability), questions have been raised about the nutritional and biological effects of the high amount of *trans* fatty acids in the diet, since, at least in rats, the *trans* fatty acids cannot fulfill the role of essential fatty acids (EFA). They have different biological functions than their *cis* isomers. There is evidence that they can interfere with the biosynthesis of arachidonic acid from linoleic acid (discussed below) through competition for Δ_6 desaturase and also affect the desaturation of stearic and palmitic acids to their respective monounsaturated acids. They also can be incorporated into the phospholipid fractions of cells. Dietary *trans* fatty acids raise low-density lipoprotein (LDL) cholesterol and lower high-density lipoprotein (HDL) cholesterol in healthy human subjects.

4.3.5 CONJUGATED LINOLEIC ACID

Conjugated linoleic acid (CLA) occurs naturally in food products derived from ruminant sources (e.g., beef, lamb, dairy) because of the process of bacterial isomerization of linoleic acid (present in foodstuffs for these animals) in the rumen. CLA is also found in a variety of other foods, including seafood and turkey. The double bonds in CLA are conjugated and not separated by a methylene group as in linoleic acid. Several recent reports suggest that CLA may have biochemical and physiological properties that may offer protection against certain chronic diseases[22] (e.g., cancer, heart disease). Estimate of CLA intake ranges from 0.3 to 1.5 g/day depending on the consumption of foods of animal origin. CLA has been a widely advertised nutritional supplement. However, extensive research is needed to determine the benefits and possible adverse effects of CLA and its isomers.

4.4 DIETARY SOURCES AND HEALTH EFFECTS OF *TRANS* FATTY ACIDS

Due to fermentation in ruminant animals such as cows, relatively low levels of *trans* fatty acids occur naturally in meat and dairy products. This was the major source of *trans* fatty acids in the diet of humans until the beginning of the last century.

After the introduction of hydrogenation, margarines and hydrogenated fat are being used in increasing amounts because of their high level of PUFAs and public fear that saturated fats (usually animal fat) are associated with coronary heart disease (CHD). Consumers buy these products, usually considered to be "cholesterol free," to lower blood cholesterol intake, theoretically reducing the risk of heart disease. Hydrogenated fat is used in numerous products, including crackers, cookies, and other baked products; margarine; and fried snacks such as potato chips. Many restaurants and fast-food chains use shortening for deep-fat frying rather than naturally occurring saturated fats.

The content of *trans* fatty acids generally increases with the extent to which a vegetable oil has been hydrogenated. For example, a hard stick of vegetable margarine may contain high amounts of *trans* fatty acids, whereas lightly hydrogenated oils usually contain 5% or less of these acids.

Trans fatty acids account for 5%–8% to the fat in the American diet or 8.5–13.5 g/day. However, the intake may be much higher for persons consuming large amounts of commercial baked products and fried foods. Conversely, individuals who are concerned with total fat in the diet for health reasons are likely to reduce such foods and significantly decrease the intake of these fatty acids. A medium-size helping of French fries contains 5–6 g, a doughnut contains 2 g, and an ounce of crackers contains 2 g of *trans* fatty acids.

Research conducted since the 1960s had produced conflicting data on the effect of *trans* fatty acids on plasma cholesterol. But in 1990 a study in normolipemic male and female subjects showed that a diet high in saturated fat (lauric, myristic, palmitic) increased plasma LDL level by 18 mg/dL, whereas a *trans* diet increased LDL levels by 14 mg/dL when compared to the control (oleic acid) diet.[11] The *trans* diet resulted in a 4 mg/dL decrease in HDL level compared to the saturated and oleic acid diets. The *trans* diet used in the study contained 33 g of *trans* fatty acids/day, which is about four times the amount present in the average U.S. diet. A follow-up study supplying half the *trans* intake of the first study also showed a rise in LDL and a decrease in HDL. Several other clinical trials also produced similar results; however, only the diets with high *trans* fatty acids showed a decrease in HDL concentration. Two studies also showed a rise in plasma lipoprotein (a) with relatively high consumption of *trans* fatty acids. Like LDL, the concentration of lipoprotein (a) in plasma is directly associated with increased risk for CHD.

On a per calorie basis, *trans* fats currently appear to increase the risk of CHD more than any other macronutrient at low levels of consumption (1%–3% of energy intake). The major evidence came from the Nurses' Health Study (NHS)—a cohort study that has been following 120,000 female nurses since its inception in 1976. Researchers analyzed data from 900 coronary events from the NHS population during 14 years of follow-up and determined that a nurse's CHD risk roughly doubled for each 2% increase in *trans* fat calories consumed (instead of carbohydrate calories).[18] By contrast, it took a more than 15% increase in saturated fat calories (instead of carbohydrate calories) to produce a similar increase in risk. Eating non-*trans* unsaturated fats instead of carbohydrates reduced the risk of CHD rather than increasing it. Replacing 2% of food energy from *trans* fat with non-*trans* unsaturated fat reduced the risk of CHD by more than half (53%). By comparison, replacing a larger 5% of food energy from saturated fat with non-*trans* unsaturated fats reduced the risk of CHD by 43%.

Trans fat behaves like saturated fat by increasing plasma LDL cholesterol but unlike saturated fat it has the additional effect of decreasing plasma HDL cholesterol levels. The net increase in LDL/HDL ratio with *trans* fat is about double that due to saturated fat.

There are reports suggesting that the intake of both saturated and *trans* fats may promote the development of Alzheimer's disease, prostate and breast cancer, type 2 diabetes, increase in weight gain and abdominal fat, liver dysfunction, and risk of ovulatory infertility. But there is less scientific consensus that *trans* fats specifically increase the risk of chronic health problems, other than CHD. Both metabolic and epidemiological studies have shown that the consumption of *trans* fatty acids increases the risk of CHD.[14] It is estimated that 30,000 premature deaths per year in the United States are due to the consumption of partially hydrogenated vegetable fat.

Several countries have begun passing laws regulating the amount of *trans* fat allowed in foods. In March 2003, Denmark became the first country to introduce laws strictly regulating the sale of foods containing *trans* fats, a move which effectively bans partially hydrogenated oils. The limit is 2% of fats and oils used for human consumption. This approach has made Denmark the only country where it is not possible to consume more than a gram of industrially produced *trans* fat per day even with a diet that may include prepared foods. It is estimated that the Danish government's efforts to decrease *trans* fat intake from 6 g to less than 1g/day over 20 years will decrease by 50% the deaths from ischemic heart disease.

As of January 1, 2006, the U.S. Food and Drug Administration (FDA) requires manufacturers to list the amount of *trans* fat on the nutrition facts panel of foods and some dietary supplements. The new law is mandatory, effective January 1, 2008, across the board even for companies that petitioned for exemption. However, unlike in many other countries *trans* fat levels of less than 0.5 g per serving can be listed as 0 g *trans* fat on the label. The FDA estimates that *trans* fat labeling would prevent from 600 to 1200 cases of CHD and 250 to 500 deaths each year. This benefit is expected to result from consumers choosing alternative foods lower in *trans* fats as well as from manufacturers reducing the amount of *trans* fats in their products. Critics of the plan have expressed concern that the 0.5 g per serving threshold is too high. Many consumers would assume that the products contain no *trans* fat. A person eating multiple products during the day may still consume a significant amount of *trans* fat. In May 2006, Tiburon, California became the first city in the United States where all restaurants voluntarily use *trans*-fat–free oils, and on December 5, 2006, New York became the first large city to strictly limit fats in restaurants. The restaurants were banned from using most frying and spreadable fat containing *trans* fat above 0.5 g per serving on July 1, 2007.

Since December 2005, Health Canada has required that food labels list the amount of *trans* fat in the nutrition facts section for most foods. Products with less than 0.2 g of *trans* fat per serving may be labeled as free of *trans* fats. On January 1, 2008, Calgary became the first city in Canada to ban *trans* fats from restaurants and fast-food chains. *Trans* fat present in cooking oils may not exceed 2% of the total fat content. In September 30, 2009, British Columbia became the first province in Canada to restrict the *trans* fat content of oils and spreadable margarines to 2% of total fat content of the food.

4.5 SATURATED FATTY ACIDS

There is no requirement for SFA in the diet since they can be synthesized endogenously. The most commonly consumed are myristic (C14), palmitic (C16), and stearic (C18) acids. The first two tend to increase plasma cholesterol, with palmitic acid having the most effect. The SFA occur mainly in foods of animal origin. Among vegetable fats, coconut oil consists of almost 86% SFA (mostly of the medium-chain length), and palm oil is about 56% SFA. The average American diet provides approximately 15% of the calories in the form of saturated fat.

4.6 MONOUNSATURATED FATTY ACIDS

As with SFA, there is no requirement for monounsaturated fatty acids (MUFA) in the human diet, but MUFA in the American diet provide approximately 20% of the calories. Oleic acid is the most commonly occurring MUFA and is the most concentrated in olive oil, but animal fats also contain substantial amounts of these fatty acids. MUFA have no effect on plasma cholesterol.

The liver is the main organ responsible for the endogenous synthesis of MUFA by the interconversion with saturated fatty acids. Monodesaturation at the Δ_9 position is the rule, and in humans the double bond cannot be introduced between carbon atoms 1 and 6 starting from the W carbon. There are only two SFAs available for desaturation: palmitic and stearic acids. An enzyme system, Δ_9 desaturase, in liver microsomes (endoplasmic reticulum) catalyzes the conversion of palmitate via palmitoyl CoA to palmitoleic acid. The conversion of stearic acid to oleic acid is also accomplished by the same enzyme system. Oxygen and either NADPH or NADH are necessary for this reaction. The enzyme system is specific for introducing the double bond in the Δ_9 position of SFA. Palmitoleic acid can be abbreviated as $C_{16}:1(W_7)$ or $C_{16}:1\Delta_9$ and oleic acid as $C_{18}:1(W_9)$ or $C_{18}:1\Delta_9$. MUFAs with double bonds occurring before the Δ_9 position are not synthesized to a significant extent by animals because the required desaturase is absent, and the trace amounts found in animal tissue lipids probably arise from the diet.

4.7 ESSENTIAL FATTY ACIDS

EFAs are those that cannot be biosynthesized in adequate amounts by animals and humans and that are required for growth, maintenance, and proper functioning of many physiological processes.[8,20,21] These fatty acids have one or more double bonds situated within the terminal seven carbon atoms (counting from the W end) and cannot be made de novo; therefore, these must be supplied in the diet. Linoleic ($C_{18}:2$, $W_{6,9}$), linolenic ($C_{18}:3$, $W_{3,6,9}$), and arachidonic acid ($C_{20}:4$, $W_{6,9,12,15}$) are generally considered to be essential, although linoleic acid can be converted by mammals to arachidonic acid (Figure 4.1).

Mammalian tissues contain four series of PUFAs. The four families can be recognized by the location of the first double bond from the terminal methyl group (Table 4.1). Two types can be synthesized by animals, namely, those fatty acids in which all double bonds lie between the seventh carbon from the terminal methyl group (W) and the carboxyl group. Such fatty acids may be made by alternate desaturation and chain elongation commencing with palmitoleic (W_7) acid and oleic (W_9) acid. The other two types of PUFAs are necessarily derived from dietary linoleic (W_6) and linolenic (W_3) acids. These four precursors are alternately desaturated (two hydrogen atoms are removed to create a new double bond) and elongated by the addition of two carbon atoms (by the enzyme system called elongase). The desaturations are catalyzed by Δ_6, Δ_5, and Δ_4 desaturases to form the principal PUFAs found in animal tissues (Figure 4.1).

Additional double bonds are always inserted between the preexisting double bonds and the carboxyl group, and since the chain elongation always proceeds by the addition of two carbon units to the carboxyl terminus of the fatty acyl chain, the position of the first double bond (counting from the methyl, W, end of the precursor fatty acid) remains unaltered through all transformations. Therefore, all transformation products of oleic acid possess the W_9 configuration of oleate itself and are recognized as members of the W_9 series family. Nervonic acid $C_{24}:1$ (W_9), a component of nerve

	C16:0 Palmitic	C18:0 Stearic		
Δ_9 Desaturase	↓	↓		
	C16:1,W_7 Palmitoleic	C18:1,W_9 Oleic	C18:2,W_6 Linoleic	C18:3,W_3 Linolenic
Δ_6 Desaturase	↓	↓	↓	↓
	C16:2,W_7	C18:2,W_9	C18:3,W_6 γ-Linolenic	C18:4,W_3
Elongase	↓	↓	↓	↓
	C18:2,W_7	C20:2,W_9	C20:3,W_6 DGLA	C20:4,W_3
Δ_5 Desaturase	↓	↓	↓	↓
	C18:3,W_7	C20:3,W_9 Mead	C20:4,W_6 Arachidonic	C20:5,W_3 EPA
Elongase	↓	↓	↓	↓
	C20:3,W_7	C22:3,W_9	C22:4,W_6	C22:5,W_3
Δ_4 Desaturase			↓	↓
			C22:5,W_6	C22:6,W_3 DHA

FIGURE 4.1 Biosynthesis of the polyunsaturated fatty acids. DGLA = dihomo-γ-linolenic acid; EPA = eicosapentaenoic acid; DHA = docosahexaenoic acid.

TABLE 4.1
Some Unsaturated Fatty Acids of Importance in Human Nutrition

Common Name	Systematic Name	Structural Formula
Palmitoleic	Hexadecenoic (W_7)	$CH_3(CH_2)_5CH = CH(CH_2)_7COOH$
Oleic	Octadecenoic (W_9)	$CH_3(CH_2)_7CH = CH(CH_2)_7COOH$
Linoleic	Octadecadienoic ($W_{6,9}$)	$CH_3(CH_2)_4CH = CHCH_2CH =$ $CH(CH_2)_7COOH$
Linolenic	Octadecatrienoic ($W_{3,6,9}$)	$CH_3CH_2CH = CHCH_2CH =$ $CHCH_2CH = CH(CH_2)_7COOH$
γ-Linolenic	Octadecatrienoic ($W_{6,9,12}$)	$CH_3(CH_2)_4CH = CHCH_2CH =$ $CHCH_2CH = CH(CH_2)_4COOH$
Dihomo-γ-linolenic	Eicosatrienoic ($W_{6,9,12}$)	$CH_3(CH_2)_4CH = CHCH_2CH =$ $CHCH_2CH = CH(CH_2)_6COOH$
Arachidonic	Eicosatetraenoic ($W_{6,9,12,15}$)	$CH_3(CH_2)_4CH = CHCH_2CH =$ $CHCH_2CH = CHCH_2CH =$ $CH(CH_2)_3COOH$
	Eicosapentaenoic ($W_{3,6,9,12,15}$)	$CH_3CH_2(CH =$ $CHCH_2)_5CH_2CH_2COOH$
	Docosahexaenoic ($W_{3,6,9,12,15,18}$)	$CH_3(CH_2CH = CH)_6CH_2CH_2COOH$
Vaccenic	Octadecenoic (W_7)	$CH_3(CH_2)_5CH = CH(CH_2)_9COOH$
Nervonic	Tetracosenoic (W_9)	$CH_3(CH_2)_7CH = CH(CH_2)_{13}COOH$

tissue lipid, is derived by chain elongation of oleate. Vaccenic acid C_{18}:1 (W_7), which occurs in small amounts in animal lipids, is formed by chain elongation of palmitoleic acid. Similarly, linoleate and linolenate give rise to the W_6 and W_3 families, respectively, of PUFAs.

The same enzyme systems catalyze the equivalent steps in W_7, W_9, W_6, and W_3 fatty acid pathways, and there is competition among substrates for these enzymes. The critical enzyme in these reactions is Δ_6 desaturase, which exhibits the greatest affinity for species with the greatest number of double bonds in the C_{18} substrate (provided that the substrate concentrations are equal). Thus, linolenic acid C_{18}:3 (W_3) is desaturated at the highest rate, followed by linoleic acid C_{18}:2 (W_6) and oleic acid C_{18}:1 (W_9). In the presence of either of these two dietary acids little desaturation of oleate occurs. Linolenate effectively inhibits the desaturation of linoleate (at equal concentration). In the absence of members of the W_3 or W_6 families, however, oleate is desaturated and the members of the W_9 family, particularly C_{20}:3 (W_9; Mead acid) appear in the tissues. This explains the well-documented finding that in essential fatty acid deficiency a trienoic acid [largely C_{20}:3 (W_9)] increases dramatically in the tissues, but it decreases with a diet containing the EFA. *Trans* fatty acids appear to compete with Δ_6 desaturase but cannot fulfill the role of EFA.

There is also competition for the desaturase enzyme, the chain elongation enzymes, and the acetyl transferases involved in the formation of phospholipids (which require PUFAs). Thus, the dietary fatty acids are important regulators of tissue fatty acid composition not only because they are precursors but also because of their ability to affect the alteration in fatty acid synthesis of other families. It also seems probable that a lower member of a family may be able to compete with some of its products for enzyme sites and therefore limit the extension of its own family. Furthermore, there is a limit to the indefinite extension of a family because of a phenomenon called retroconversion. In this reaction, long-chain, highly unsaturated fatty acids are shortened by two carbons and, in some cases, hydrogenated.

Because of competition, retroconversion, and so on, each family has characteristic end products that accumulate in tissue lipids while the intermediates are usually found in much smaller, often trace amounts. Thus, for oleate and palmitoleate, the major PUFAs are the trienes C_{20}:3 (W_7) and

C_{20}:3 (W_9), respectively. For linoleate, the major PUFAs are arachidonic acid with four double bonds (tetraene) and some dihomo-γ-linolenic acid (DGLA). For linolenate, eicosapentaenoic acid (EPA) and docosahexaenoic acid (DHA) are the main end products. The 22-carbon hexaenoic acid is the most unsaturated fatty acid commonly found in the lipids of higher animals.

4.7.1 FUNCTIONS

The biological functions of EFA include stimulation of growth, maintenance of skin and hair growth, regulation of cholesterol metabolism, and maintenance of cell membrane integrity. EFA and other PUFAs derived from them play a major and vital role in the properties of most biomembranes. In the phospholipids (Figure 4.2), the SFAs preferentially occupy a position on the 1-carbon and the PUFAs on the 2-carbon of glycerol moiety, although MUFA can also take the 1- or 2-carbon position.

Of utmost importance for the proper functioning of most membranes is the control of liquid crystal–gel transition temperature, which is significantly influenced by the structure of the phospholipid fatty acids. The PUFAs are necessary components of most biomembranes. Their major function in this role appears to be the regulation of the physical properties of membrane lipids, leading to proper transport abilities and osmotic characteristics. Membrane proteins (e.g., receptors, enzymes, ion channels) are highly sensitive to the lipid environment. The physical properties affect the ability of the phospholipid to perform structural functions such as the maintenance of the normal activity of membrane-bound enzymes (e.g., adenyl cyclase and Na^+/K^+ ATPase). Several cellular functions such as secretion, signal transmission, and susceptibility to microorganism invasion depend on membrane fluidity. One of the examples of the role of fatty acids in membrane function can be illustrated in the "pink egg white" disease of chickens. This is caused by ingestion of the seeds of the genus *Sterculia* and certain other plants that contain cyclopropane fatty acids such as sterculic acid. The eggs laid by these hens have a faulty yolk membrane, which allows the yolk pigment to leak into the white portion. The yolk also has a peculiar consistency that damages the acceptability of the egg. To function normally, the membrane apparently needs oleic acid, which is formed by desaturation of stearic acid. The desaturation process is inhibited by sterculic acid, which causes an accumulation of stearic acid and a deficiency of oleic acid in the membrane. The resulting change in the ratio of unsaturated to SFA leads to loss of transport selectivity of the yolk membrane.

The highly unsaturated fatty acids EPA and DHA are particularly concentrated where there is a requirement for rapid activity at the cellular level, such as may be required in transport mechanisms in the brain and its synaptic junctions and in the retina where only the long-chain PUFAs derived from EFA are found. A few specific functions of EFA are given below.

4.7.1.1 Skin

Linoleic acid in the skin maintains the integrity of the epidermal water barrier. The physical structure of this water barrier is ascribed to sheets of stacked bilayers that fill the epidermis. These lipid bilayers contain large amounts of sphingolipids, which contain linoleate-rich ceramides. In EFA deficiency, linoleic acid is replaced by oleic acid and results in severe water loss from the skin.

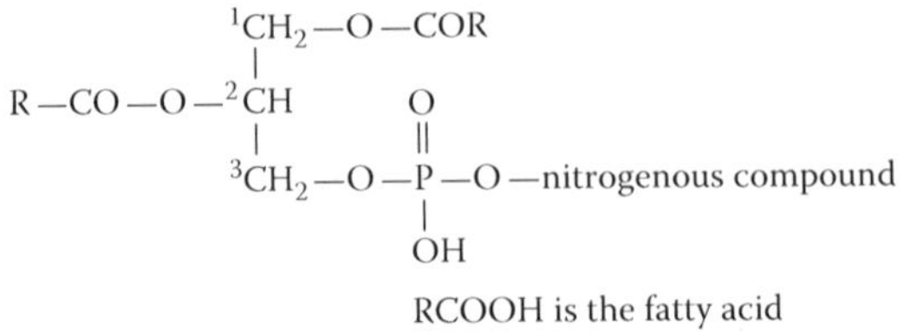

$$
\begin{array}{l}
^1CH_2-O-COR \\
\quad\quad\quad | \\
R-CO-O-{}^2CH \quad\quad O \\
\quad\quad\quad | \qu\quad\quad\quad || \\
\quad\quad{}^3CH_2-O-P-O-\text{nitrogenous compound} \\
\quad\quad\quad\quad\quad\quad | \\
\quad\quad\quad\quad\quad\quad OH
\end{array}
$$

RCOOH is the fatty acid

FIGURE 4.2 General structure of a phospholipid.

4.7.1.2 Infection and Immunity

An increased susceptibility to infection is a common clinical problem for patients undergoing fat-free hyperalimentation. Certain PUFAs are known to be effective in killing viruses that have a lipid component in the envelope, but the mechanism by which EFA deficiency causes infections is not clear. There is a reduction in immune response in EFA deficiency. The EFA may affect immune function via membrane structural changes and/or via altered availability of chemical mediators such as prostaglandins and related compounds derived from EFA in lymphoid cell membranes. Patients with acquired immune deficiency syndrome (AIDS) exhibit significant reductions of 20- and 22-carbon fatty acids derived from EFA. Normalization of these PUFAs levels in patients with AIDS may be a worthwhile therapeutic aim.

4.7.1.3 Eicosanoids

DGLA, arachidonic acid, and EPA are the precursors of biologically active compounds that include prostaglandins, thromboxanes, prostacyclins, and leukotrienes. These compounds participate in many physiological and pathological processes and are potent regulators of cell function.

4.7.1.4 Specific Role for ω_3 Fatty Acids

ω_3 fatty acids are important components of structural lipids in many tissues, particularly in the brain and retina. Biological structures involved in fast movement or signal transmission appear to have a requirement for the highly unsaturated fatty acid, DHA. The retinal rod outer-segment disk membrane in which rhodopsin rests, the major phospholipid, contains 40%–60% of the total fatty acid as DHA. In the cerebral cortex of humans, DHA accounts for approximately one-third of the fatty acid content of phospholipids.

4.7.2 DEFICIENCY OF ESSENTIAL FATTY ACIDS

Since adults have adequate stores of EFA it is difficult to produce deficiency signs. Young, especially low-birth-weight infants, have limited body stores of EFA and are more susceptible to deficiency. In human infants, the deficiency signs include dermatitis (Figure 4.3) involving dryness, desquamation,

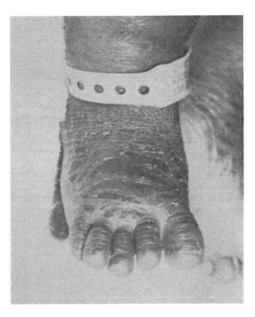

FIGURE 4.3 Dermatitis of essential fatty acids deficiency in a child maintained by total parenteral nutrition without fat. (Reproduced with permission from Holman, R. T., University of Minnesota.)

and thickening of the skin, often accompanied by unsatisfactory growth,[9] fatty liver, and impaired water balance. The skin symptoms and water loss are both examples of a general derangement of membrane structure and consequent function. There is an increase in capillary permeability and fragility. Erythrocytes become more fragile and susceptible to osmotic hemolysis. A deficiency of EFA results in a decreased rate of synthesis of phosphatidylcholine—a constituent of HDL—and hence affects the formation of HDL and leads to a breakdown of the cholesterol transport process. There are also accumulations of triglycerides and cholesterol in the liver. It has been suggested that the formation of bile acids from cholesterol requires EFA because cholesterol ester with EFA is a better substrate than cholesterol itself. Furthermore, EFAs apparently participate in the formation of a cholesterol–phosphatidylcholine–bile acid complex that is secreted in the bile. Presumably, the phosphatidylcholine involved in this process must contain its usual component of PUFAs derived from EFA in carbon 2 of the glycerol moiety. Linolenic acid-derived fatty acid $C_{22}{:}6(W_3)$ is the most abundant fatty acid in the cerebral gray matter and retina. When this fatty acid level is reduced in the brain of rats maintained on low–linolenic acid diets, these animals show decreased physical activity and learning ability.

The most common cause of EFA deficiency in humans in all age groups is the long-term intake of fat-free parenteral nutrition (PN).[6] It is commonly administered as a continuous infusion of a glucose-containing solution. This results in a constant elevation of serum insulin and depresses the release of fat from adipose stores. Normal adults have a little more than 1000 g of EFA, which could otherwise sustain dietary needs for more than 6 months. Because of the block in the release of EFA, continuous fat-free PN seems to provide optimal conditions for the development of deficiency. In these patients, plasma-free fatty acids are derived from glucose and these do not include EFA. Glucose-free PN containing only amino acids and fat does not produce EFA deficiency. Many people with severe fat malabsorption develop EFA deficiency.

Premature infants on fat-free PN develop very rapid clinical signs of EFA deficiency[8,9] (Figure 4.3) as well as biochemical changes in the plasma (triene to tetraene ratio above 0.4) as early as 2–3 days of life. In the neonate, signs of deficiency may become apparent in 5–10 days, whereas in adults the biochemical evidence of deficiency is generally seen 2 weeks after the initiation of PN. By the end of 7 weeks, all patients exhibit clinical signs of deficiency. The administration of linoleic acid reverses both clinical and biochemical abnormalities.

The first case involving linolenic acid deficiency in humans was described in 1982. A 6-year-old girl sustained an accidental gunshot wound to the abdomen, requiring multiple small intestinal resections. She was maintained on PN, which included a safflower oil emulsion rich in linoleic acid but poor in linolenic acid. After 5 months, she experienced episodes of numbness, paresthesia, weakness, inability to walk, leg pain, and blurred vision. Serum analysis revealed very low levels of linolenic acid and other PUFAs derived from it. The PN was then changed to include soybean oil emulsion, which contains both linoleic and linolenic acids. Within 3 months, all of the symptoms of deficiency disappeared. Recently, more cases of W_3 fatty acid deficiency have been reported. The observed clinical symptoms were scaly and hemorrhagic dermatitis, hemorrhagic folliculitis, and impaired wound healing.

Patients with Zellweger syndrome and other disorders of peroxisomal biogenesis have a profound deficiency of DHA.[12] In the brain, the DHA concentration is only 20%–30% of the normal value. In the retina, DHA may be nearly absent. In contrast, the levels of arachidonic acid are usually within normal limit in these tissues. Erythrocytes from patients with Zellweger syndrome have very low DHA concentrations, and arachidonic acid values are either normal or only slightly decreased. The crucial role of DHA in cell membranes, particularly in neuronal tissues and retinal photoreceptor cells make it likely that its deficiency may be the cause of severe dysfunction in these tissues. Clinical symptomatology in peroxisomal disease including psychomotor retardation, dysmyelination, and visual impairment could, at least in part, be due to DHA deficiency. DHA treatment provides some benefits in children with disorders of peroxisomal biogenesis.

EFA deficiency, especially of W_3 fatty acids may be responsible for the heightened depressive symptoms associated with low plasma cholesterol. Recent studies show a correlation between low levels of DHA and certain behavioral and neurological conditions associated with aging, such as dementia, depression, memory loss, and visual problems.

4.7.3 REQUIREMENTS

An adequate dietary intake of EFA decreases the formation of trienes (fatty acids with three double bonds, derived from oleic acid) and increases the formation of tetraenes (arachidonic acid with four double bonds, derived from linoleic acid). This is a consequence of competitive inhibition among families of PUFAs for desaturase. Normally, the ratio of trienes to tetraenes in plasma is below 0.4, but in EFA deficiency, the ratio is above 0.4. In humans, the optimal dietary linoleate that can maintain the ratio near normal level is 1%–2% of total calories. This may be adequate to prevent symptoms attributable to the membrane function of EFA. Physiological and metabolic functions that depend on eicosanoid formation may show an optimal response with a dietary linoleate intake level of about 10% of total calories. An absolute requirement cannot yet be given, but because no untoward effects have been reported up to this level (10% of calories), the tendency is to consider it as optimal in the light of present information. The average daily intake of linoleic acid in the American diet is about 10 g.

During pregnancy the approximate accumulation of EFA is estimated to be about 620 g, which includes the demand for uterine, placental, mammary gland, and fetal growth and increased maternal blood volume. To meet these needs, 4%–5% of the expected caloric intake in the form of EFA is recommended. Approximately 4%–5% of the total energy in human milk is present as linoleic acid and linolenic acid and 1% as long-chain PUFAs that are derived from these acids; this amounts to about 6% of total energy as EFA and their metabolites. To meet these needs, an additional 2%–4% of energy in the form of EFA is recommended during lactation. Normal growth of infants depends on an adequate supply of EFA. Formula that is fed to infants should contain at least 2% of the total fatty acids as linoleic acid (0.95% of calories) and a ratio of linoleic:linolenic acid similar to that of human milk.[4]

The quantitative requirement for linolenic acid in humans is not known, but on the basis of its derived products found in the body and some observations on elderly patients treated by gastric tube feeding, linolenic acid requirements should be about 0.2%–0.3% of total energy. Also, there is a role of W_3 fatty acids in the development of neural tissue and visual function. The fatty acid derived from linolenic acid, DHA, is found in high concentrations in the structural lipids of the brain and retina, where it is the major PUFAs. Selective incorporation mechanisms appear to supply the fetal brain with the relatively high levels of DHA that are needed for brain development. Human milk lipids contain significant amounts of DHA, with the level dependent on maternal diet. Therefore, it is recommended that foods containing linolenic acid be included in the diet of pregnant and lactating women. Infants may be susceptible to EFA deficiency because the high growth rates of both brain and body increase the demand for these nutrients. Most synthetic formulas provide no long-chain PUFAs, which may influence the development of the young denied the benefits of human milk.

It is important to maintain an appropriate balance of ω_6 and ω_3 fatty acids in the diet as these two groups work together to promote health. A healthy diet should contain a ratio of ω_6 to ω_3 fatty acids between 4 and 8:1. The typical American diet tends to contain 14–25 times more ω_6 than ω_3, and it is believed that this imbalance is a significant factor in the rising rates of diseases such as inflammatory disorders. Increasing intake of ω_3 fatty acids has been shown to prevent certain chronic diseases such as heart disease and arthritis.

EFA deficiency in developed countries is rare; in poorly nourished populations of some developing countries, however, the circumstances may be different. The growth of infants will be poor when the intake of both protein and other nutrients is not adequate, but the tissue level of EFA generally remains normal. When a high-protein diet is initiated such as one based on powdered skim milk, rapid growth resumes. Because brain development requires EFA, its deficiency can cause permanent brain damage. Thus, the diet to correct the deficiency of one nutrient must be carefully chosen with respect to other nutrients.

4.7.4 EFFECT OF EXCESS ESSENTIAL FATTY ACIDS

Not much is known about the adverse effect of high doses of EFA in the diet. The enzyme Δ_6 desaturase is susceptible to feedback from both linoleic and arachidonic acids, and the intake of linoleic acid in excess of 12% of calories tends to suppress arachidonic acid synthesis further. Dietary EFA depresses the activity of some enzymes such as fatty acid synthetase and glucose-6-phosphate dehydrogenase, but we do not know whether this action is beneficial or harmful.

A high intake of PUFAs may be an environmental factor in some types of cancer. As the intake of PUFAs increases, the antioxidant capacity of the body is challenged. The oxidation of excess PUFAs results in the formation of peroxidized free radicals that can damage and destroy cells, cellular components, and other body proteins. The end result is the formation of lipofuscin pigment granules that are polymers of peroxidized PUFAs. Lipofuscin seems to be associated with the aging process because the amount of this pigment increases with age. Vitamin E works as an effective antioxidant and inhibits the oxidation of PUFAs. Vegetable oils generally are rich in this vitamin, but PUFAs in the body have a longer half-life than vitamin E, and therefore, the requirement of the vitamin is increased with excess intake of PUFAs.

Several hazardous effects have been reported in newborn infants receiving intravenous lipids. A reduced clearance rate in small-for-age infants as well as in premature infants (i.e., born before 32 weeks of gestation) is observed. When lipids are metabolized in vivo, free fatty acids are generated that can competitively displace bilirubin from the albumin-binding site and increase the risk of kernicterus in jaundiced newborns.

4.7.5 FOOD SOURCES

The most prevalent W_6 fatty acid is linoleic acid. It is present in almost all vegetable oils such as corn oil, soybean oil, safflower oil, and sunflower oil. Common fatty acids found in most land plants are generally not chain elongated above the 18 carbon level. Borage seed oil is the richest source of γ-linolenic acid (GLA) among vegetable oils. GLA makes up around 24% of the oil. Black currant seed oil contains 17% GLA and evening primrose oil contains 8% GLA. The advantage of GLA is that it bypasses the Δ_6 desaturase enzyme. Arachidonic acid is found in foods of animal origin. Linolenic acid is present in only small amounts in soybean oil, rapeseed oil, and leafy vegetables such as spinach, kale, and romaine lettuce. Flaxseed oil is a rich source of linolenic acid. It contains 50%–60% of linolenic acid. Linolenate-derived fatty acids make up a large part of PUFAs in marine fish oils and fat. Varieties of fish rich in W_3 fatty acids include salmon, mackerel, sardines, scallops, oysters, and red caviar. Cold water vegetation such as phytoplankton and algae synthesize the first member of the W_3 family, linolenic acid, and the fish that feed on these marine plants convert this fatty acid to higher members including the two most abundant components of this class, EPA and DHA. The fatty acids present in marine cellular and subcellular membranes reflect their dietary sources. Cultured fish, unless their diet contains fish oil, do not provide the levels of W_3 acids found in wild commercial fish. For example, analysis of cultured salmon marketed in Seattle had about 50% of the W_3 fatty acids as compared to commercial salmon.

The intake of total ω_3 fatty acids in the United States is about 1.6 g/day (0.7% of energy intake) and of this linolenic acid accounts for 1.4 g/day and only 0.1–0.2 g/day comes from EPA and DHA. The major food sources of linolenic acid are vegetable oils, principally canola and soybean oils. Although some linolenic acid is converted to EPA and DHA, the extent of this conversion is modest. Some investigators reported a 15% conversion, whereas others found only 0.2% conversion. Fish are the major sources of EPA and DHA. Table 4.2 shows the linolenic acid content of selected vegetable oils, nuts, and seeds, and Table 4.3 gives the ω_3 content (EPA + DHA) in some fish.

TABLE 4.2
Linolenic Acid Content of Selected Vegetable Oils, Nuts, and Seeds

Source	Content (g/Tablespoon)
Olive oil	0.1
Walnuts	0.7
Soybean oil	0.9
Canola oil	1.3
Walnut oil	1.4
Flaxseeds	2.2
Flaxseed (linseed) oil	8.5

TABLE 4.3
ω_3 Fatty Acids (EPA and DHA) in Fish

Fish	Content per 3-Ounce Serving (before Cooking)
Salmon	1.7–1.8 g
Shrimp	0.27 g
Clam	0.24 g
Crab	0.34–0.4 g
Scallop	0.17 g
Lobster	0.07–0.41 g
Oyster	0.37–1.17 g

4.7.6 DIETARY ω_3 FATTY ACIDS AND HEALTH

The beneficial role of fish and fish oils rich in W_3 fatty acids has been studied in the prevention of many diseases (e.g., inflammatory diseases, CHD, cancer). Fatty acids in carbon 2 (of glycerol moiety) in membrane phospholipids are the precursors of eicosanoids (described in Chapter 5), which are important mediators of inflammation, cytokine synthesis, and cell communication. The Western diet contains an excess of W_6 and low levels of W_3 fatty acids. The W_6-derived eicosanoids exhibit proinflammatory activity whereas W_3-derived eicosanoids are less active in this respect. Thus, W_3 fatty acid supplementation can alter the balance of W_6 to W_3 eicosanoids to produce decreased proinflammatory activity. Evidence from biochemical and clinical studies suggests that W_3 PUFAs have a modest beneficial effect in arthritis.

W_3 fatty acids are known to decrease plasma triglycerides and very low-density lipoproteins but increase LDL. They have a variable effect on HDL cholesterol. The consumption of fish has been shown in numerous studies to be associated with decreased mortality from CHD.

Each year about 220,000 Americans experience sudden death, collapsing and dying within an hour, often before they get to a hospital. In most cases, an abnormal heart rhythm arising from heart disease is believed to be the cause. In about 50% of the cases, the victim is unaware of the heart disease. There is no chest pain or previous heart attack. Instead, sudden death is the first symptom of the problem. Prevention of heart disease is really the only way to reduce the mortality from sudden death. Two new studies show that people who eat substantial amounts of fish are greatly protected from sudden unexpected death caused by severely abnormal heart rhythm.[1]

In the first study, researchers looked at the experience of about 22,000 male doctors who enrolled in the Physicians' Health Study in 1982. They were all free of heart disease at the time. They volunteered to give blood samples. Over the next 17 years, 94 of the men who had not subsequently been diagnosed with heart disease died suddenly. The researchers chose 184 surviving members of the study and compared them with those victims. In particular, they compared the baseline blood W_3 fatty acids. The men who died suddenly had the lowest amounts of ω_3 fatty acids in blood than those who did not.

All men were divided into four groups based on the concentration of W_3 fatty acids in blood. The men in the highest quartile had an 81% lower risk of sudden death than those in the lowest quartile.

In the second study, investigators used dietary information gathered in five interviews between 1980 and 1994 to estimate the fish intake of 85,000 female nurses. Like the doctors, they volunteered to be questioned and followed over many years as part of the Nurses' Health Study, which began in 1976. The researchers found that higher fish intake was associated with lower CHD risk in women.[10] Of the 1513 cases of CHD (484 deaths and 1029 nonfatal myocardial infarctions) reported during the 16-year follow-up, CHD was likely to occur in the group with fish intake of <1 per month. Those who ate fish once a week had a 30% lower risk of heart attack or death than those who never ate fish, and those who ate fish five times a week had a 34% lower risk. The data also indicated that like mortality from CHD, all-cause mortality was lowest among groups of women who ate the most fish.

A European study published in 1999 showed that fish oil supplements reduced the risk of sudden death in people who had previously survived a heart attack. The W_3 fatty acids appear to have a specific antiarrhythmic effect by incorporation into phospholipids of heart cell membranes in the functionally critical carbon-2 position. In the event of severe physiological stress, such as that caused by the loss of blood supply to a portion of the heart early in an ischemic attack, the EPA or DHA is released from phospholipids and protects the heart cell locally from participating in the genesis of propagation of ventricular tachycardia, which can result in cardiac arrest and sudden death. W_3 fatty acids may have the unique ability to stabilize contractile heart cells electrically and thus protect against sudden death from arrhythmias. Also, the eicosanoids formed from EPA have a more favorable spectrum of biological activities.

Results of these studies indicate that even in people with no history of CHD, high blood ω_3 fatty acid levels can lower their risk of future CHD death. The link to arrhythmias is the most substantiated, but fish oils also have other heart-friendly effects, such as lowering the levels of triglycerides in the blood, reducing inflammation, slowing coronary artery thickening, and reducing the tendency of blood to clot.

In September 2004, the FDA allowed the following "qualified" health claim for certain foods containing fish oils: "Supportive but not conclusive research shows that consumption of EPA and DHA ω_3 fatty acids may reduce the risk of coronary heart disease." The FDA action marks the second time the agency has allowed a qualified health claim for a conventional food product: earlier the same year, the agency granted a claim linking walnuts and certain other nuts to a reduction in heart disease risk.

The American Heart Association recommends that healthy adults, especially those at higher risk for heart disease, eat a variety of fish—preferably oily fish such as salmon, mackerel, sardines, herring, and trout—at least twice weekly. The heart association also recommends increasing intake of α-linolenic acid (ALA)-rich foods such as walnuts, flaxseeds, and canola and soybean oils. People with preexisting heart disease should try to consume 1 g of W_3 oils each day, preferably from food. Individuals who have to lower blood triglycerides may need 2–4 g daily, which will presumably mean supplements; the content of W_3 fatty acids in fish vary from 0.25 to 0.8 g per 3-ounce serving.

Fish intake is associated with lower risk of prostate cancer. A recent study has shown that consumption of fish constituting at least a moderate part of the diet significantly lowers the risk of prostate cancer. It has been suggested that fish oil might also be of value in slowing the progression of established prostate cancer. The mechanism for the beneficial effects of fish in protecting against cancer is not clear. It may be that the people who eat more fish are likely to eat less of the other forms of animal fat. There is evidence of an association between nonfish animal fat and prostate cancer risk as there is between such fat and other forms of cancer.[17] It is more likely that there may be specific protective properties of fish oil, in relation to its W_3 fatty acids.

Population studies in Chicago have reported that people 65 and older who ate fish once weekly or more were 60% less likely to develop Alzheimer's disease than those who never or rarely ate fish.[13] The meals included tuna sandwiches, fish sticks, and shellfish. This could be because DHA is crucial for the proper working of brain cells and is destroyed during the course of Alzheimer's disease. Mice with an Alzheimer's-like condition performed better in memory tests when fed DHA than when fed safflower oil, which does not contain ω_3 fatty acids. Mood too has been linked to levels of fish oil consumption suggesting that a lack of ω_3 fatty acids contributes to some abnormalities therein.

Depression is associated with lower levels of ω_3 fatty acids in red blood cell membranes.[3] Some studies have found that countries with the highest rate of depression ate the least amount of fish, while those with the lowest rate of depression ate the most fish. Several small clinical trials have reported that fish oils helped improve psychiatric symptoms. One study found that bipolar patients given fish oils showed improvements in symptoms, and another study showed that supplements of EPA were more effective than placebos at improving the mood of depressed patients.[23]

ω_3 fatty acids may also protect the eyes. A study of 681 American men showed that those who ate fish twice a week had a 36% lower risk of macular degeneration,[7] the leading cause of blindness in old age. The men who ate not only more ω_3 fatty acids but also fewer ω_6 fatty acids got the most benefit. In the other study, which followed 2335 Australian men and women over 5 years, people who ate fish just once a week reduced their risk by 40%. Macular degeneration starts with blurring in the center of what the eye sees. It progresses to blindness slowly or quickly depending on the type of disease. About 6%–8% of people age 75 and older have an advanced form of the disease.

There are also data suggesting ω_3 fatty acids may be helpful for a raft of other ills such as aggression, attention deficit disorder, autoimmune disease, and breast cancer. Fish and fish oils thus qualify as functional foods.

Fish such as salmon and albacore tuna are considered the optimal dietary source of ω_3 fatty acids. The acceptable daily intake for these fatty acids is 1.6 g for men and 1.1 g for women although more may be recommended for certain conditions such as heart disease and arthritis. It is difficult to reach the acceptable intake even by eating fish every day. And, because fish can contain mercury and other unsafe pollutants there are limits to the amount of fish that should be consumed particularly for women who are pregnant or breastfeeding as well as for children.[15] Mercury, as one of these pollutants, is a known toxin to the human nervous system and is linked to learning and behavioral problems in children. In adults, mercury can cause memory loss and other health problems.

For those who do not eat fish, have limited access to a variety of fish, or cannot afford to purchase fish, a fish oil supplement may be considered. The best fish oil supplements contain 1 g/capsule, which provide 440 mg of ω_3 fatty acids. The most common fish oil capsules in the U.S. provide 180 mg EPA and 120 mg DHA. The recommended dosage is one to two capsules per day for adults. The possible side effects are relatively minor. These include dyspepsia as well as an unpleasant after taste. Worsening glycemic control has been reported in diabetic patients taking large doses exceeding 3 g. ω_3 fatty acids exert a dose-related effect on lowering bleeding time. However, there are no documented cases of abnormal bleeding as a result of supplements. But the supplements should be used cautiously by people who have a bleeding disorder, or who take blood-thinning medications.

With the increasing popularity of vegetarian diets and mounting focus on mercury in seafood, and other increasing chemical contaminants being found in oceans as a result of human sewage and farm runoff, the safer choice for many has become flaxseed oil, which contains ALA. We can make

EPA and DHA from ALA, but the process is slow. Researchers at Dow Agrosciences inserted the algae genes required to make DHA into canola seeds.[2] The enzymes that these genes produce allow the canola plant to synthesize DHA from arachidonic acid. Such plants produce canola oil that is enriched with DHA. Monsanto genetically engineered a soybean plant enriched in stearidonic acid (SDA). SDA is a short-chain ω_3 fatty acid, which humans can use as a precursor to make EPA and DHA. According to researchers at Monsanto, SDA is more stable than fish oil and has an excellent taste profile.

Linolenic Acid Deficiency—A Case

A 59-year-old woman, after a cerebrovascular stroke, received by nasogastric feeding a 200-g nutrient powder mixed in skim milk and water as her sole nutrition. After 4 years on this diet, she developed a very thin, atrophic skin with scaly dermatitis on her shoulders, face, and forearms, together with multiple small excoriations.[24]

Analysis of her blood count showed normal values for hemoglobin, blood count, electrolytes, glucose, etc. Her plasma and erythrocyte lipid analysis showed that W_6 fatty acids were normal, eicosatrienoic acid (W_9) was slightly elevated, which is strongly elevated in EFA deficiency, and all W_3 fatty acids were low. The patient was supplemented with 10 mL of cod-liver oil and 10 mL of soybean oil. After 4 weeks, the scaly dermatitis disappeared and the skin became less atrophic. There were no excoriations, and old ones had disappeared. W_3 fatty acids were normalized in both plasma and erythrocyte lipids. W_6 fatty acids were slightly lower than normal and eicosatrienoic acid (W_9) was very low. Reexamination after 22 weeks showed the same normal fatty acid pattern with no scaly dermatitis, no excoriations, and no skin atrophy.

From the initial diet linolenic acid intake in this patient was extremely low, providing 0.02% of total calories. Supplementation with cod-liver oil and soybean oil increased the intake of linolenic acid, which provided 0.8% of total calories. This gave a rapid mobilization of skin changes as well as the normalization of W_3 fatty acids in plasma and erythrocytes. It was not possible to assess changes in neurologic and visual functions because the patient had brain damage. This is the first case of linolenic acid deficiency reported in human adults. The same investigator has described several more cases with similar clinical manifestations.[25]

REFERENCES

1. Albert, C. M., H. Campos, M. J. Stampfer et al. 2002. Blood levels of long-chain n-3 fatty acids and the risk of sudden death. *N Engl J Med* 346:113.
2. Arnold, C. 2008. Fish out of water. Plunging salmon population means "heart healthy" fish oil compounds may soon be in your veggies. *Chem Eng News* 86(32):39.
3. Bruinsma, K. A., and D. L. Taren. 2000. Dieting, essential fatty acid intake and depression. *Nutr Rev* 58:98.
4. Hansen, A. E. et al. 1958. Essential fatty acids in infant nutrition: III. Clinical manifestations of linoleic acid deficiency. *J Nutr* 66:565.
5. Hibbeln, J. R., L. R. Nieminen, T. L. Blasbalg et al. 2006. Healthy intakes of n-3 and n-6 fatty acids: Estimations considering worldwide diversity. *Amer J Clin Nutr* 85:1483S.
6. Hirono, H., H. Suzuki, Y. Igarashi, and T. Konno. 1979. Essential fatty acid deficiency induced by total parenteral nutrition and medium chain triglycerides feeding. *Am J Clin Nutr* 30:1670.
7. Hodge, W. G., D. Barns, H. M. Schachter et al. 2007. Evidence for the effect of omega-3 fatty acids on progression of age-related macular degeneration: A systematic review. *Retina* 27:216.
8. Holman, R. T. 1988. George O. Burr and the discovery of essential fatty acids. *J Nutr* 118:535.

9. Holman, R. T., and S. Johnson. 1983. Essential fatty acid deficiencies in man. In *Dietary Fats and Health*, ed. E. G. Perkins and W. J. Visek, 247–266. Champaign, IL: American Oil Chemists' Society.

10. Hu, F. B., L. Bronner, W. C. Willet, M. J. Stampfer, K. M. Rexrode, C. M. Albert, D. Hunter and J. E. Manson. 2002. Fish and omega 3 fatty acid intake and risk of coronary heart disease in women. *J Am Med Assoc* 287:1815.

11. Katan, M. B. 2000. *Trans* fatty acids and plasma lipoprotein. *Nutr Rev* 58:188.

12. Martinez, M. 1996. Docosahexaenoic acid therapy in docosahexaenoic acid-deficient patients with disorders of peroxisomal biogenesis. *Lipids* 31:S145.

13. Morris, M. C., D. A. Evans, J. L. Bienias et al. 2003. Consumption of fish and n-3 fatty acids and risk of incident Alzheimer's disease. *Arch Neurol* 60:940.

14. Mozaffaria, D., M. B. Katan, A. Ascherio et al. 2006. *Trans* fatty acids and cardiovascular disease. *New Engl J Med* 354:1601.

15. Mozaffarian, D., and E. B. Rimm. 2006. Fish intake, contaminants and human health: Evaluating the risks and the benefits. *J Amer Med Assoc* 296:1885.

16. Mussner, M. J., K. G. Parhofer, K. von Bergmann et al. 2002. Effects of phytosterol ester-enriched margarine on plasma lipoproteins in mild to moderate hypercholesterolemia are related to basal cholesterol and fat intake. *Metabolism* 51:189.

17. Norrish, A. E., C. M. Skeaff, G. L. B. Arribas et al. 1999. Prostate cancer risk and consumption of fish oil. A dietary biomarker-based case–control study. *Br J Cancer* 81:1238.

18. Oomen, C. M., M. C. Ocke, E. J. M. Feskens et al. 2001. Association between *trans* fatty acids intake and a 10-year risk of coronary heart disease in the Zutphen elderly population-based study. *Lancet* 357:746.

19. Rosenberg, I. H. 2002. Fish-food to calm the heart. *N Engl J Med* 346:1102.

20. Sardesai, V. M. 1992. The essential fatty acids. *Nutr Clin Pract* 7:179.

21. Sardesai, V. M. 1992. Nutritional role of polyunsaturated fatty acids. *J Nutr Biochem* 3:154.

22. Watkins, B. A., and Y. Li. 2000. Conjugated linoleic acid. The present state of knowledge. In *Handbook of Nutraceuticals*, ed. R. E. Wildman, 445–476. Boca Raton, FL: CRC Press.

23. Young, G., and J. Conquer. 2005. Omega-3 fatty acids and neuropsychiatric disorders. *Reprod Nutr Dev* 45:1.

CASE BIBLIOGRAPHY

24. Bjerve, K. S. 1987. Alpha linolenic acid deficiency in adult woman. *Nutr Rev* 45:15.

25. Bjerve, K. S. 1989. *n*-3 fatty acid deficiency in man. *J Int Med* 225(Suppl.):171.

5 Eicosanoids

A variety of compounds with diverse physiological and pharmacological activities are formed in the body; as a group, these compounds are referred to as eicosanoids, reflecting their origin from 20-carbon (eicosa) polyunsaturated fatty acids (PUFAs).[27] These short-lived, highly potent mediators participate in the normal physiology of virtually every organ system and have been implicated as playing important roles in the pathophysiology of many life-threatening illnesses. Several of these compounds (or their synthetic derivatives) show considerable promise as therapeutic agents for treating or preventing problems encountered in critical care medicine. Agents that inhibit the formation of these biologically active mediators are also used for some beneficial effects. The PUFAs are present as constituents of cell membrane phospholipids. In most species, including humans, the tissue phospholipid content of arachidonic acid (ArA) is much higher than that of the other 20-carbon PUFAs and, therefore, the eicosanoids derived from ArA dominate over those formed from other PUFAs.[26]

In humans, ArA is derived from dietary linoleic acid, or is ingested as a dietary constituent and is then incorporated into membrane phospholipid. Normally, the concentration of free ArA (and other 20-carbon PUFAs) in the cell is very low, but it is released in response to widely divergent physical, chemical, and hormonal stimuli. The biosynthesis of eicosanoids depends primarily on the availability of free 20-carbon PUFAs.

The eicosanoids include the prostaglandins (PGs), thromboxanes (TXs), prostacyclins (PGIs), leukotrienes (LTs), lipoxins, and products generated by the action of cytochrome P450 on fatty acids. Eicosanoids work like hormones but with some very important differences. Unlike hormones, which are produced in one tissue and then transported to the target organ, they act locally in the cells in which they are formed and quickly disappear because of their rapid inactivation. In general, eicosanoids bind to receptors in target cell plasma membranes in various tissues and stimulate or inhibit the synthesis of other messengers.

5.1 PROSTAGLANDINS

5.1.1 CHEMISTRY AND NOMENCLATURE

PGs are 20-carbon carboxylic acids, and they have the same basic carbon skeleton of the hypothetical parent compound, prostanoic acid (Figure 5.1). There are several types of PGs and all have a five-membered ring (carbon atoms 8 and 12 as counted from the carboxyl group are bound to each other), two aliphatic chains, a terminal COOH group, a $C_{13}:C_{14}$ double bond, and a 15-hydroxyl group. The letter designations refer to specific chemical substitution on the cyclopentane ring. The letters E and F are derived from the early observations that PGs could be separated by ether extraction of tissue homogenates in phosphate (*fosfat* in Swedish) buffer. Those soluble in ether belong to the E series, whereas those soluble in the aqueous phase belong to the F series. The E series is characterized by the presence of 11-hydroxy and 9-keto groups. The F series has two hydroxyl groups, one at the 9 position and the other at the 11 position. The A series is derived from the E series by the loss of water from the cyclopentane ring, and the B series is derived from A by the isomerization of the ring double bond from the $C_{10}:C_{11}$ to the $C_8:C_{12}$ position. The D series has a hydroxyl group at C_9 and a keto group at C_{11} (i.e., the opposite substitution to the E series). Figure 5.2 illustrates the differences in ring structure for various PGs.

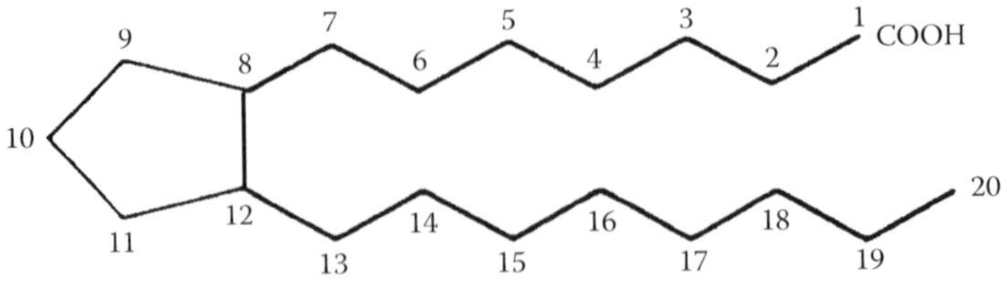

FIGURE 5.1   Prostanoic acid.

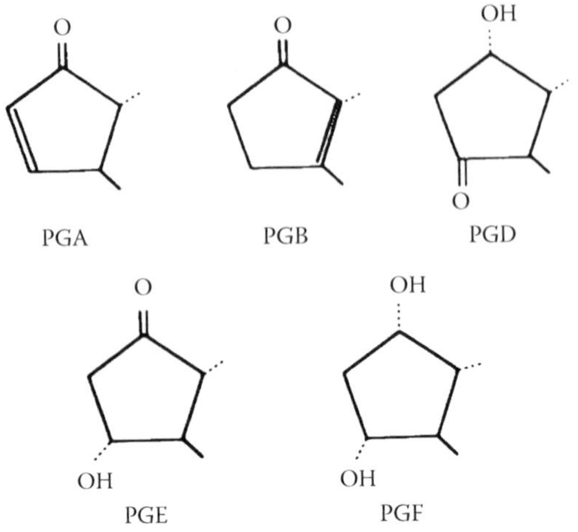

FIGURE 5.2   Structural differences between prostaglandins of the A, B, D, E, and F series.

The subscripts 1, 2, and 3 refer to the number of double bonds present in the side chains of each molecule. The α and β designations refer to the position of the 9-hydroxyl group with respect to the cyclopentane ring; α signifies that the substitution is oriented on the same side of the ring as the aliphatic chain bearing the COOH group, whereas the β-substituent is oriented on the side of the ring bearing the alkyl side chain. The PGs with α subscript occur naturally and compounds with β-configuration are produced synthetically.

5.1.2   BIOSYNTHESIS

The essential prerequisite for PG (and other eicosanoid) formation is the availability of precursor PUFAs. Normally, most of the precursor fatty acids are found esterified at the 2-carbon position of glycerol (of the membrane phospholipid). Perturbance of the cell membrane, including a slight chemical or mechanical stimulus, activates phospholipase A_2—a membrane-bound enzyme that is found in virtually every cell type and organ in the body and liberates the precursor from phospholipid. This appears to be the rate-limiting step because the free fatty acid is readily converted to PGs (and related compounds).

The synthesis is carried out by a membrane-bound PG synthetase complex, which has two components: the cyclooxygenase (Cox) component catalyzes the cyclization of carbon atoms 8 and 12 of the fatty acid to form PGG, and the peroxidase component quickly converts PGG to PGH, which is accompanied by the formation of superoxide. Once formed, PGH is acted upon by a series of enzymes that produce biologically active PGs, TXs, and PGIs. PG synthetase is found in every mammalian cell, but a specific PGH-metabolizing enzyme (or enzymes) is located in each tissue and produces a particular type of PG (or related component) that regulates the function of the tissue with its specific biological activity. In other words, most cells become highly selective in their

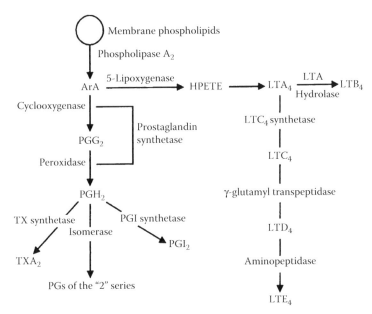

FIGURE 5.3 Formation of eicosanoids. ArA, arachidonic acid. When DHGL is the substrate (in place of ArA), the products formed are PGG_1, PGH_1, PGs of the "1" series, and TXA_1; when EPA is the substrate, the products are PGG_3, PGH_3, PGs of the "3" series, TXA_3, and PGI_3. In the lipoxygenase pathway, EPA produces LTB_5, LTC_5, LTD_5, and LTE_5; the products of Mead acid are LTA_3, LTC_3, LTD_3, and LTE_3.

metabolism of PGH to the biologically active product. This selectivity is usually linked to the function of the cell and its communication with cells that carry receptors for that specific PG, TX, or PGI. All the metabolites of the PGH are referred to as prostanoids, although TX and PGI do not have the true prostanoic acid skeleton.

PGH is converted to PGE, PGF, or PGD by their individual isomerases. The formation of PGF from PGE is catalyzed by PG 9-keto reductase. Figure 5.3 gives the pathway for the formation of PGs of the "2" series using ArA as a substrate; with dihomo-γ-linolenic acid (DHGL) as the substrate, PGs of the "1" series are formed, and with eicosapentaenoic acid (EPA) as the substrate, PGs of the "3" series are formed.

Receptors mediating the actions of PGs and other prostanoids were recently identified and cloned. They are G protein-coupled receptors with seven transmembrane domains. There are eight types and subtypes of prostanoid receptors that are encoded by different genes but as a whole constitute a subfamily in the superfamily of the rhodopsin-type receptors.

5.1.3 CATABOLISM

PGs are rapidly metabolized by a variety of tissues to compounds with little or no biological activity. The lungs, liver, and kidneys are the major sites for this degradation. Infused PGs disappear from the blood after one passage through the lungs. The metabolic steps include dehydrogenation of the C_{15} hydroxyl group, which is essential for biological activity; a reduction of C_{13} double bond; β-oxidation of the carboxyl side chain; and ω hydroxylation at C_{20} followed by ω-oxidation of the alkyl side chain.

5.1.4 PHYSIOLOGICAL ACTIONS

PGs play important roles in several aspects of human physiology.[4,15,19] A few of the relevant actions to the normal physiological and pathological conditions are given below.

5.1.4.1 Reproduction

The greatest number and the highest concentrations of individual PGs are found in seminal fluid. The PG content of human semen is sufficiently high to cause dilatation of the cervix and to facilitate sperm transport to the ovum. Decreased concentrations of PGE_2 have been found in semen of men who are infertile despite having a normal sperm count and motility. PGE_1 and PGE_2 increase the plasma luteinizing hormone concentration and this may have a role in ovulation and menstruation. $PGF_{2-\alpha}$ has oxytocic properties and promotes labor. Administration of this PG to women at any stage of pregnancy causes a powerful contraction of the uterus and the expulsion of the fetus. This PG has been used to cause abortion or to induce labor.

5.1.4.2 Gastrointestinal Tract

There are PGs that stimulate the contraction of intestinal smooth muscle. Relatively large amounts of PGs are present in the gastrointestinal mucosa; PGs of the E series inhibit gastric acid secretion in humans and prevent the formation of gastric and intestinal ulcers. Several synthetic metabolically stable analogs of PGs have been used as cytoprotective agents.

5.1.4.3 Vascular

PGs of the E series are powerful vasoconstrictors, as is $PGF_{2-\alpha}$. PGE_2 functions in the fetus to maintain the patency of the ductus arteriosus, which serves to bypass the nonfunctioning lung in the fetus. At birth, the ductus undergoes constriction and permanent closure via the elevation of the partial pressure of oxygen. This allows the normal circulation to occur. In some premature infants, the ductus arteriosus may not respond to oxygen, and this lack of response may be corrected by the administration of the inhibitor of PG production. In infants with pulmonary atresia and other disorders where ductal flow is necessary while these patients are being prepared for corrective surgery, PGE_1 infusion provides a means to keep the ductus arteriosus open.

5.1.4.4 Inflammation

PGs occur around inflamed tissues. The involvement of PGs of the E type in inflammation is demonstrated by their proinflammatory effects and their generation in a variety of inflammatory situations, which are curtailed by anti-inflammatory drugs.

5.1.4.5 Central Nervous System

Both PGE_1 and PGE_2 increase body temperature, especially when administered into the cerebral ventricles. Pyrogens release interleukin 1, which in turn promotes the synthesis and release of PGE_2. The synthesis is blocked by aspirin and other antipyretic compounds.

5.2 THROMBOXANES

The TXs are classified into the 1, 2, or 3 series, depending on the number of double bonds. The endoperoxide PGH is metabolized by TX synthetase to TXA (Figure 5.3). The enzyme is present in high concentrations in platelets; TXA has a very short half-life (~ 30 seconds) and breaks down nonenzymatically to the stable TXB, which is biologically inactive. The product formed from PGH_1 is TXA_1, but it is not of much significance because PGH_1 is a poor substrate for the enzyme. PGH_2 and PGH_3 are converted to TXA_2 and TXA_3, respectively. TXA_2 is a potent vasoconstrictor and stimulates platelet aggregation. TXA_3 is less potent as a vasoconstrictor than TXA_2 and has little platelet-aggregating ability.

A mutation in the first intracellular loop of the TX receptor has been linked to a bleeding disorder characterized by a selective defect in the signal transduction and aggregation of platelets induced by TX agonists.

5.3 PROSTACYCLINS

Like PGs and TXs, PGIs are classified into the 1, 2, and 3 series, depending on the number of double bonds. PGI is derived from PGH by the action of PGI synthetase (Figure 5.3). The enzyme is present mainly in the vascular endothelium, but the lungs and stomach are also capable of synthesizing PGI. PGI has a half-life of 2–3 minutes and breaks down nonenzymatically to the stable compound, 6-OXO-PGF$_{1-\alpha}$. PGH$_1$ does not have the Δ_5 double bond and therefore cannot be converted to PGI$_1$. PGI$_2$ and PGI$_3$ are the most potent inhibitors of platelet aggregation and are also powerful vasodilators. Thus, TXA$_2$ produced by platelets and PGI$_2$ (as well as PGI$_3$) produced by endothelial cells have diametrically opposite effects.[21]

PGI$_2$ synthesis is increased in several human diseases in which evidence of platelet activation is present, including severe peripheral arterial disease and unstable coronary artery disease, thus implying a homeostatic role for this eicosanoid.

5.4 LEUKOTRIENES

The name leukotriene reflects its discovery in leukocytes and the conjugated triene structure that produces their characteristic ultraviolet absorption spectrum. Several different LTs are found in the tissues, and they are identified by lettered suffixes A, B, C, D, and E, which refer to the order in which they are formed and also to the character of the substituents. The subscripts denote the number of double bonds present. They are formed by the action of 5-lipoxygenase on ArA, EPA, or Mead acid. DHGL acid lacks the Δ_5 double bond and thus cannot react with the enzyme. This enzyme cannot metabolize these fatty acids in the free form; instead, they must be linked to a membrane-bound protein called 5-lipoxygenase activating protein (FLAP). The 5-lipoxygenase catalyzes the conversion of ArA to 5-hydroperoxyeicosatetraenoic acid (HPETE), which, in turn, is rapidly converted to an unstable epoxide LTA$_4$. Two metabolic routes are available to LTA$_4$; one is the enzymatic conversion by LTA hydrolase to LTB$_4$, and the other is the addition of glutathione by LTC$_4$ synthetase (a specific glutathione-S-transferase) to form LTC$_4$. This can be further metabolized to LTD$_4$ by γ-glutamyl transpeptidase with the loss of glutamic acid. The subsequent removal of glycine by aminopeptidase produces LTE$_4$ (Figure 5.3). Mononuclear cells and neutrophils are the main sources of LTB$_4$, although certain other cell types such as tracheal mucosal cells are capable of synthesizing this eicosanoid. Eosinophils and monocytes are major sources of the cysteinyl LTs (LTC$_4$, LTD$_4$, and LTE$_4$), which make up the biological mixture previously known as the slow-reacting substance of anaphylaxis. With the substrate EPA, the LTs of the "5" series are formed: LTA$_5$, LTB$_5$, LTC$_5$, LTD$_5$, and LTE$_5$. With the substrate Mead acid, LTA$_3$ is formed by the action of 5-lipoxygenase. LTA$_3$ is a poor substrate for hydrolase, and thus no LTB$_3$ is formed; however, LTA$_3$ can be converted to LTC$_3$, LTD$_3$, and LTE$_3$.

5.4.1 METABOLISM OF LEUKOTRIENES

The metabolism and the inactivation of LTB$_4$ involve ω oxidation to give 20-OH and 20-COOH LTB$_4$ that can undergo β-oxidation to give the final products carbon dioxide and water. LTC$_4$, LTD$_4$, and LTE$_4$ are oxidatively metabolized with complete loss of activity.

5.4.2 PHYSIOLOGICAL ACTIONS

The two groups of LTs—LTB$_4$ and the cysteinyl LTs—differ in their biological activity.[10] LTB$_4$ is a potent chemotactic agent attracting neutrophils and macrophages and causing aggregation at sites of infection or injury. It also causes lysosomal enzyme release and the generation of superoxide in neutrophils and has an important role in inflammatory conditions and tissue damage. Synthetic LTB$_3$ has actions similar to LTB$_4$ and is equally potent in its biological activity. The LTB$_5$ is 10- to

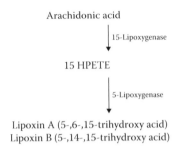

FIGURE 5.4   Formation of lipoxins.

100-fold less active than LTB$_4$. The cysteinyl LTs are potent vasoconstrictors and bronchoconstrictors. They increase permeability in postcapillary venules and stimulate mucus secretion. These LTs also induce pathophysiological responses similar to those with asthma. These products can cause tissue edema and migration of eosinophils and can stimulate airway secretion.

5.5   LIPOXINS

In addition to 5-lipoxygenase (which is involved in the generation of LTs), there are two other lipoxygenases in mammalian tissues: 12-lipoxygenase and 15-lipoxygenase. The 15-lipoxygenase is predominant in neutrophils while 12-lipoxygenase is concentrated in platelets. The 15-lipoxygenase converts ArA to 15-HPETE. The action of 5-lipoxygenase (present in the same or neighboring cells) on HPETE and on reduction yields two trihydroxy (5-, 6-, 15-; and 5-, 14-, and 15-) compounds with four conjugated double bonds. These are isomers that are designated lipoxin A and lipoxin B, respectively (Figure 5.4). The biological properties of these compounds include the contraction of lung parenchymal strips, the alteration of microvasculature, and the generation of superoxide anion in polymorphonuclear leukocytes. Levels of lipoxin A are elevated in bronchoalveolar lavage fluid in some patients with lung disease and may play a role in the modulation of the inflammatory process.

5.6   CYTOCHROME P450–DERIVED PRODUCTS

Cytochrome P450 catalyzes the oxidative transformation of a large number of lipophilic endogenous and xenobiotic substrates. It also metabolizes ArA[5] via three types of reactions (Figure 5.5). Olefin epoxidation leads to the formation of four (5,6-; 8,9-; 11,12-; and 14,15-) epoxyeicosatrienoic acids (EETs). The EETs can undergo hydrolysis by epoxide hydrolase to form the corresponding dihydroxyeicosatrienoic acids (DHTs). The allylic oxidation of ArA leads to the formation of six monohydroxy eicosatrienoic acids (HETEs). ω and ω_1 hydroxylation of ArA gives rise to 20-HETE and 19-HETE, respectively, and 20-COOH-ArA may arise from the metabolism of 20-HETE.

The EETs and their hydrolytic metabolites (DHTs) possess several biological activities. These include the stimulation of hormone release from endocrine cells, the inhibition of Cox activity, vasodilation, and the inhibition of TX-induced platelet aggregation. Among the EETs, 5,6-EET appears to be the most potent vasodilator. HETEs inhibit Na$^+$/K$^+$ ATPase and renin release, 20-HETE is a potent vasoconstrictor, and 20-HETE and 19-HETE have prohypertensive properties and are implicated in the development of hypertension in rats.

Much of the information on these cytochrome P450-derived metabolites has come from in vitro systems; however, recent work has identified some of these compounds in human platelets, kidney cortex, and urine. The urinary excretion of EETs increases during pregnancy and pregnancy-induced hypertension. In rats, about 92% of the total rat liver EETs are found in cellular phosphatidylinositol, esterified to the 2-carbon position of the glycerol moiety. This is in contrast to the Cox and

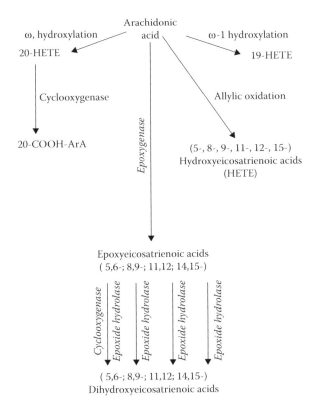

FIGURE 5.5   Arachidonic acid metabolism by cytochrome P450-dependent reactions.

lipoxygenase products that are formed after the release of free fatty acids from phospholipids, are quickly inactivated, and are not stored in tissues. The presence of EETs in phospholipid suggests that they may have a role in cell membrane functions. Thus far, the findings on cytochrome P450-derived products have come from ArA as a substrate. It is likely that other 20-carbon PUFAs may substitute for ArA as substrates for cytochrome P450. The relative importance of this pathway within the family of eicosanoids and the differences in biological actions among the metabolites derived from different PUFAs are not known. Research in this field should contribute to our understanding of the importance of cytochrome P450 products of ArA metabolism in human physiological and pathophysiological processes.

5.7   INHIBITORS OF EICOSANOID BIOSYNTHESIS

A number of compounds are known to interact at one or more of the many steps involved in the formation of eicosanoids.[31] The first step in the biosynthesis of these compounds is the release of PUFAs from membrane-bound phospholipid by phospholipase A_2. The steroidal anti-inflammatory agents (i.e., corticosteroids) inhibit phospholipase A_2 and block the release of PUFAs. This prevents the biosynthesis of all eicosanoids. The main naturally occurring corticosteroids are cortisol and corticosterone. Several synthetic corticosteroids have been developed and are used clinically (e.g., dexamethasone and prednisolone). Drugs blocking prostanoid synthesis from 20-carbon PUFAs are usually preferred over the more powerful steroids because of their undesirable systemic effects.

The nonsteroidal anti-inflammatory drugs (NSAIDs) such as aspirin, indomethacin, and ibuprofen are potent inhibitors of the enzyme Cox. These inhibitors block the synthesis of PGG and hence PGs, TXs, and PGIs. It is this specific action that accounts for the anti-inflammatory, antipyretic, and analgesic properties of these drugs. Aspirin acts by acetylating a serine residue at the active site of Cox and makes the inhibition irreversible. Therefore, the PGs and other prostanoids can only be formed again after the new enzyme is synthesized. The other NSAIDs act reversibly on Cox.

TXA_2 contributes to the intravascular aggregation of platelets and the formation of thrombus or hemostatic plug. PGI_2 inhibits the action of TXA_2. Too much TXA_2 generation or too little PGI_2 production may cause thromboembolic diseases. One way to reduce the level of TXA_2 is to use substances that specifically inhibit TX synthetase. Drugs such as imidazole and its analog, dazoxiben, are known to inhibit the enzyme in vitro, but convincing data to support their use clinically are not yet available. The commonly used drug for reducing TXA_2 is aspirin. Theoretically, aspirin inhibits the formation of PGG and hence of all prostanoids (e.g., PGs, TXs, and PGIs). Therefore, it should not be of benefit; however, there is an advantage in using aspirin to reduce the level of TXA_2. Platelets are nonnucleated and have no ability to synthesize new enzymes. Therefore, the aspirin effect should persist for the life of platelets in circulation (8–10 days). In other tissues, notably the vascular endothelium, the recovery of prostanoid biosynthesis is rapid because these cells have the ability to synthesize new enzymes. When aspirin is administered daily in low doses (less than 100 mg), the formation of TXA_2 is inhibited much more than that of PGI_2 and other prostanoids. Continued intake of low doses of aspirin should show a cumulative inhibition of TXA_2 formation without substantially affecting the production of PGI_2.

Patients with vascular disease and arthritis may receive low-dose aspirin and another NSAID. It has been recently reported that the concomitant administration of ibuprofen, an NSAID present in Motrin and Advil, interferes with the inhibitory effect of aspirin on platelet Cox. It is believed that ibuprofen may clog a channel inside the enzyme and prevent aspirin from reaching its active site. Thus, treatment with ibuprofen in patients with cardiovascular risk may limit the cardioprotective effect of aspirin. Other NSAIDs, acetaminophen, diclofenac, and rofecoxib, do not affect aspirin action.

Aspirin is one of the most important and cost-effective drugs for the secondary prevention of cardiovascular disease.[6] It reduces the rate of arterial thrombotic events in high-risk patients by at least 25%. Aspirin inhibits platelet activation and reduces thrombotic complications; however, some patients are resistant to the therapeutic effects of aspirin and may experience a thrombotic event due to pharmacologic resistance or some other clinical failure. This aspirin resistance represents the failure of aspirin to prevent arterial thrombotic events in patients who are compliant with therapy prescribed by their cardiologists or other healthcare professionals. Amid the uncertainty, doctors are increasingly testing patients for resistance and prescribing aspirin alternatives.

Cox enzyme is involved in the formation of certain kinds of tumors, such as colorectal, prostate, and breast cancers. According to a recent study, taking adult-strength aspirin (325 mg or more) daily for at least 5 years is associated with a 50% lower risk of colorectal cancer, a 20% lower risk of prostate cancer, and a 15% less risk of breast cancer. But another study has shown that women who take an aspirin a day may raise their risk of getting pancreatic cancer. There is a need for clinical trials to look at aspirin's benefits at high doses and also to determine Cox activity in different tumors.

The PGI synthetase is inhibited by tranylcypromine, a clinically used antidepressant and monoamine oxidase inhibitor in vitro. Nicotine is also a potent inhibitor of this enzyme in vascular tissues of humans, and it may be an important factor in the association of smoking with the development of cardiovascular disease.

Aspirin and other NSAIDs do not inhibit 5-lipoxygenase and may facilitate LT formation by making more of the ArA available for metabolism via this pathway. One classic disease situation in which this occurs is aspirin-induced asthma symptoms. By the inhibition of Cox pathway ArA is available for the lipoxygenase pathway and formation of LTs, which are well known to enhance the inflammatory process of the disease.

Efforts are being made to develop compounds that can inhibit the formation of LTs. Researchers are concentrating on four points in the pathway. The first two relate to the biosynthesis of LTs, and the goal is inhibition of 5-lipoxygenase or the membrane-bound protein (FLAP). The other two involve receptor antagonists directed against LTB_4 or D_4.[23] There are compounds (e.g., benoxaprofen, zileuton, and others) known to inhibit 5-lipoxygenase in vitro. Montelukast and zafirlukast are LTD_4 antagonists. Currently, available data indicate that the inhibition of LT formation or action has a salutary effect in the treatment of both induced and spontaneously occurring asthma.

5.7.1 CYCLOOXYGENASE 2: A TARGET FOR TREATMENT OF DISEASES

There are two Cox isoforms and are referred to as Cox-1 and Cox-2 for the order in which they were discovered. Each is encoded by a separate gene and exhibits a discrete pattern of tissue-specific expression. Cox-1 is predominantly expressed constitutively and functions as a physiological "housekeeping" enzyme in most tissues, including the gastric mucosa, kidneys, and platelets. Cox-2 activity is normally undetectable in most tissues and is primarily an inducible enzyme. In cells such as monocytes, macrophages, and synoviocytes, Cox-2 is expressed at higher levels after induction by inflammatory mediators (interleukin 1 and tumor necrosis factor) and growth factors. It is presumed to be the Cox of predominant importance in the generation of PGs of inflammation. However, it is constitutively expressed in the developing brain and kidneys, and therefore, may be involved in their development and proper maturation. Cox activity is inhibited by NSAIDs, which are most commonly administered for the relief of pain and inflammation. However, adverse side effects, including peptic ulcer disease, are associated with the use of such compounds, which are nonselective inhibitors of Cox-1 and Cox-2. PGE_2 is the predominant Cox-1 product of ArA formed in the gastric mucosa. It stimulates bicarbonate and mucus secretion, decreases acid secretion, and may regulate gastric blood flow, which most likely plays a role in limiting the effect of diverse physical and chemical insults to the gastric mucosa. This cytoprotective property is shared by PGI_2. Given the broad role of PGs in normal human physiology, it is not surprising that systemic suppression of PG synthesis through the inhibition of Cox can lead to unwanted side effects. Toxicity associated with the use of NSAIDs was the major stimulus to develop selective Cox-2 inhibitors. At position 523, Cox-1 has an isoleucine residue whereas Cox-2 has a valine residue. The presence of the less bulky valine in the Cox-2 provides an access for Cox-2–selective inhibitors. This led to the development of drugs that selectively inhibit Cox-2 without having adverse effects on the constitutive and maintenance pathway of Cox-1.[22,32] The selective Cox-2 inhibitors include rofecoxib (Vioxx), celecoxib (Celebrex), valdecoxib (Bextra), and others, which have dominated the market in the United States.

Recently, some Cox-2–selective inhibitors have shown adverse cardiovascular side effects resulting in withdrawal of Vioxx from the market.[18] Selective inhibition of Cox-2 without reducing Cox-1–mediated TX production could alter the balance between PGIs and TX and promote prothrombotic state, which explains the observed Cox-2 inhibitors' cardiovascular risk.

In 2006, an analysis of 138 randomized trials and almost 150,000 participants showed that selective Cox-2–inhibitors are associated with a moderately increased risk of cardiovascular events mainly due to a twofold increased risk of myocardial infarction. Also, high doses of some traditional NSAIDs such as ibuprofen are associated with similar increase in risk of vascular event. Other selective Cox-2 inhibitors are still in the market.

Cox-2 inhibitors originally designed as anti-inflammatory agents against arthritis may have broader utility. The relationship between NSAIDs and other diseases was suggested epidemiologically before Cox-2 inhibitors were tested. The interest in NSAIDs as potential cancer-fighting agents was fueled a decade ago by a major study linking the regular use of aspirin to an unexpectedly low incidence of colon cancer.[2] Since then, several population-based studies have detected a 40%–50% decrease in the relative risk of colorectal cancer in persons who regularly use aspirin and NSAIDs. The NSAID sulindac caused a decrease in the number and size of polyps in patients with familial adenomatous polyposis, a rare inherited disease that develops in colon cancer. An increased expression of Cox-2 and an increased PG formation are found in polyps and colon cancer. Based on these findings, the U.S. Food and Drug Administration approved Celebrex to treat familial adenomatous polyposis. The majority of both human and animal colorectal tumors express high levels of Cox-2,

TABLE 5.1
Possible Roles of Cox-2 in Carcinogenesis

1. Appears in excessive amounts in a wide range of tumors, including lung, breast, pancreas, and colon tumors—causes an excessive formation of PGs.
2. Interrupts the life cycle of cells, preventing their natural cell death—inhibits apoptosis, leading to carcinogenesis.
3. Promotes the formation of new capillaries—stimulates angiogenesis.
4. Compromises the immune system.

whereas the surrounding tissues have low to undetectable Cox-2 expression. Levels of Cox-1 are not increased. Elevated Cox-2 expression has been reported in human cancers of the breasts, lungs, and head and neck. Although Cox-2 appears to play a role in carcinogenesis, the exact mechanism(s) by which it acts is only partially understood.[15] The possible roles are listed in Table 5.1.

There is compelling evidence that the inhibition of Cox-2 (and thereby the blocking of the formation of PGs) protects against colon, mammary, esophageal, lung, and oral cancers.

Angiogenesis, the formation of new capillaries, is essential not only for the growth and metastasis of solid tumors but also for wound and ulcer healing.[11] Blood flow for oxygen and nutrient delivery to the healing site cannot be restored without angiogenesis. Angiogenesis and suppressed cell-mediated immunity are central to the development and progression of malignant diseases. Recent work indicates that Cox-2 may play a very important role in the regulation of angiogenesis associated with neoplastic tumor cells. NSAIDs such as aspirin have antiangiogenic and immunomodulatory properties.

Experimental studies have shown that overabundant Cox-2 can interfere with the normal life cycle of cells by preventing their normal, natural cell death (apoptosis). Experimental studies have also linked Cox-2 with compromising the immune system. Based on animal studies, the benefits of NSAIDs may be, as a combination with other medications, delivering a one–two punch to tumors to control their growth rather than getting rid of them. Further studies are continuing in this exciting field.

Other potential use for Cox-inhibitors (in particular Cox-2–selective inhibitors) may include the treatment of Alzheimer's disease (AD). AD is characterized by a progressive dementia and the extracellular deposition of β-amyloid fibrils within the brain. It is thought that an inflammatory component may be involved in this process. Several epidemiological studies have indicated that patients taking NSAIDs for other diseases (e.g., rheumatoid arthritis) have a 50% lower risk of developing AD than those not taking NSAIDs. Other studies have shown no benefits. Transgenic mice overexpressing Cox-2 have neurons that are more susceptible to damage. The inflammatory cytokines may play a part in the disease's pathogenesis. They may contribute to the precursor plaques. Clinical trials are underway to measure the ability of celecoxib to prevent AD and to slow the disease's progression.

Recent studies suggest the involvement of Cox-2 in amyotrophic lateral sclerosis (ALS), a neurodegenerative process. Cox-2 inhibitors may have some promise as therapy for the treatment of ALS.

5.7.2 CYCLOOXYGENASE 3

A new variant of Cox has been identified recently and is named Cox-3. Like the other Cox enzymes, Cox-3 is involved in the synthesis of PGs and plays a role in pain and fever.[8] However, unlike Cox-1 and Cox-2, Cox-3 appears to have no role in inflammation. Therefore, it is not classified as NSAID.

The activity of Cox-3 is inhibited by acetaminophen, which has little effect on the other two Cox enzymes. If this is the target of acetaminophen, the same thing can be done with Cox-3 that was done for Cox-2—try to develop better inhibitors.

5.8   EICOSANOIDS AND CHRONIC DISEASES

Many of today's chronic diseases are related to the impact of an imbalance in the ω_6- and ω_3–based eicosanoids. Having higher levels of eicosanoids formed from ArA tend to increase the risk of many inflammatory and autoimmune diseases.

Eicosanoids help regulate the balance between osteoclasts, which are involved in bone resorption and osteoblasts that rebuild the bone. PGE_2 favors osteoclast-induced resorption at the expense of osteoblast-induced bone formation and may contribute to osteoporosis. ArA may adversely affect cystic fibrosis (CF) patients by contributing to a proinflammatory effect in lung tissue through an increase in LTB_4. A diet low in ArA appears to ameliorate inflammation in patients with rheumatoid arthritis possibly because of reduction in proinflammatory eicosanoids. ArA has been implicated as a risk factor for asthma possibly due to its being a precursor of LTs with bronchoconstrictive effects. Eicosanoids derived from ArA are present at much higher concentrations in mucosa of patients with inflammatory bowel disease. An increase in the formation of PGE_2 triggers proliferation of tumor cells and regular use of Cox inhibitors has been associated with reduced risk of some types of cancer such as breast and colon cancers.

Inhibiting eicosanoid synthesis by modern drugs is effective for many people in reducing inflammation and the accompanying pain of many diseases, particularly arthritis. Even though a drug therapy can successfully block Cox and lipoxygenase pathways ArA can still be converted into other damaging molecules such as epoxy derivatives. So another approach to treat diseases is to prevent eicosanoid formation by dietary modification.

5.9   EFFECTS OF DIET ON EICOSANOIDS

The precursors of eicosanoids are DHGL, ArA, and EPA. The type and amount of PUFAs consumed (ω_6 vs. ω_3) are important considerations. In most individuals subsisting on a Western diet, there is an abundant intake of preformed ArA from meat products. This product is also formed from dietary linoleic acid present in commonly used vegetable oils. Therefore, ArA is the predominant constituent of membrane phospholipids, and most eicosanoids generated are derived from ArA.[28] These include prothrombotic TXA_2, immunosuppressive prostaglandin (PGE_2) and proinflammatory leukotriene (LTB_4), which have deleterious effects. In general, eicosanoids derived from the other two precursors have a more favorable spectrum of biological activities.[1,3]

Dietary intake determines to a great extent the type of precursor present on membrane phospholipids, and some of the dietary constituents can affect the biosynthesis of eicosanoids. Reducing the intake of ω_6 fatty acids (particularly ArA from animal products) while proportionately increasing the intake of ω_3 fatty acids results in the production of eicosanoids with reduced potential to do harm (e.g., TXA_3, PGE_3, and LTB_5).

5.9.1   Factors Affecting the Formation of 20-Carbon PUFAs

Linoleic, linolenic, and oleic acids are metabolized in the body by the same sequence of enzymes with alternating desaturases and elongases. The affinity of these fatty acids, assuming that they are present at equal concentration, for the enzyme system is as follows: linolenic acid > linoleic acid > oleic acid.

Our diet normally contains a very small amount of linolenic acid in relation to linoleic acid. Oleic acid, when present in amounts several times greater than linoleic acid, suppresses the conversion of linoleic acid to ArA. Supplementing the diet of healthy individuals with oleic acid results in diminished ArA content in their platelet phospholipids and a reduction in TXA_2 formation. This may explain the low incidence of myocardial infarction in countries with a high consumption of olive oil, a rich source of oleic acid. A diet rich in saturated and monounsaturated fatty acids at the expense of PUFAs and the avoidance of meat products decrease ArA content and increase Mead acid in membrane phospholipids. Alcohol inhibits Δ_6 desaturase, which converts linoleic acid to γ-linolenic acid (GLA), the initial step in the formation of ArA.

The tissue level of DHGL, which is normally very low, can be increased by taking GLA. Rich sources of GLA are the oils of borage, black currant, and evening primrose. The advantage of taking GLA is that it bypasses the Δ_6 desaturase step.

The EPA content of membrane phospholipid can increase by consuming oils that are relatively good sources of linolenic acid such as rapeseed (canola) and soybean oils and green leafy vegetables, which contain significant amounts of linolenic acid. Canola oil is considered valuable because it has low saturated fat, relatively favorable ω_6 to ω_3 ratio (the best of the available vegetable sources) and is easy to get and inexpensive. Conversion of linolenic acid to EPA and further to DHA in humans is limited but varies with individuals. Women have higher conversion efficiency than men. Preformed EPA is abundant in fats and oils of cold-water fish. Clinical studies have shown that the exchange of marine fish oil for vegetable oil in an otherwise typical Western diet leads to a decrease in platelet TXA_2 formation and an increase in those of TXA_3 and PGI_3. The replacement of proaggregatory and vasoconstrictive TXA_2 with TXA_3, which is much less potent in both respects, leads to a shift in the TX/PGI balance and produces the antithrombotic state. EPA competitively inhibits the formation of prostanoids (including TXA_2) from ArA. Also, LTB_5 (from EPA) is far less active than LTB_4 (from ArA).

In areas where fish consumption is high, such as Japan, Greenland, and the areas bordering the Mediterranean Sea, the population ingests a considerably higher proportion of ω_3 fatty acids than that in other areas where there is little fish consumption, and the measured risk of death by cardiovascular disease is decreased. This indicates that years of eating such a diet may reduce the vasoconstriction, platelet aggregation, and chronic arterial inflammation that lead to attacks and strokes. It is believed that such diets can reduce the incidence of some chronic diseases, including certain cancers by a similar mechanism of reducing adverse eicosanoid effects.

5.9.2 Factors Affecting Eicosanoid Synthesis

The effects of various factors[33] on eicosanoid formation are shown in Figure 5.6. The antioxidants vitamin E and vitamin C protect the precursor fatty acids in phospholipids from lipid peroxidation and thereby maintain the levels of precursors for the formation of eicosanoids. In relatively higher concentrations, vitamin E inhibits phospholipase A_2 and decreases the Cox and lipoxygenase products.[17] Vitamin C at concentrations of 3 mg/dL inhibits TX synthetase. Garlic, onion, and ginger contain a substance named "ajoune," which inhibits platelet aggregation by blocking TX synthetase and thus reducing TXA_2 generation from ArA. Epidemiological data have shown that those who consume liberal quantities of garlic and onion have a lower incidence of cardiovascular disease. The active component in garlic and onion also inhibits 5-lipoxygenase pathway and provides relief in rheumatoid arthritis by reducing pain and improving the movement of joints in patients with arthritis.

Alcohol in concentrations as low as 10 mg inhibits platelet TXA_2 synthetase and potentiates vascular PGI_2 synthesis. These observations, together with the effect of alcohol on Δ_6 desaturase, are of interest because moderate alcohol ingestion is thought to offer some protection against cardiovascular disease. The antioxidants present in wine also have an inhibitory effect on 5-lipoxygenase.

5.10 ALTERNATIVE MEDICINE FOR PAIN

One of the most common inflammatory diseases associated with pain is arthritis. It is characterized by the slow progressive deterioration of articular cartilage. Current therapeutic regimens address mainly pain but not degeneration. More than 40% of arthritis sufferers in the United States report using alternative medicine including dietary supplements and the use of all remedies have increased since the FDA issued a health warning about Cox-2 inhibitors. However, the effectiveness of many

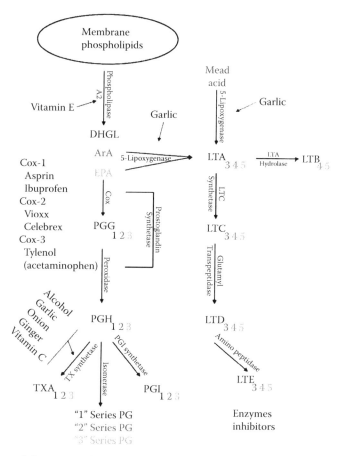

FIGURE 5.6 Effects of dietary constituents on eicosanoid formation.

ingredients in supplements has not been adequately studied. Also, the over-the-counter supplements are not regulated in the same way as drugs and their composition can vary widely.

5.10.1 Turmeric

Turmeric has been used for centuries by practitioners of Ayurvedic medicine to treat inflammatory disorders.[20] It has been accepted that curcumin, a yellow-colored compound, is the active anti-inflammatory ingredient in turmeric. It is marketed widely in the Western world as a dietary supplement for the treatment of a variety of disorders.

Curcumin has been shown to inhibit Cox-2 and lipoxygenase. Patients with arthritis taking turmeric over a period of time have reported an increase in mobility, flexibility, less stiffness, less pain, and swelling in their joints. Results from a pilot study indicated that turmeric may help alleviate symptoms of irritable bowel syndrome. No significant adverse events have been reported.

In animal models of rheumatoid arthritis, curcumin was found to be a significant inhibitor of joint inflammation and peri-articular joint destruction in a dose-dependent manner.[12] Curcumin inhibited the transcriptional factor nuclear factor-kappa B (NF-κB) and subsequent expression of key inflammatory genes mediating joint inflammation and destruction. These findings suggest that NF-κB inhibition may be an important mechanism of turmeric's protective effect against arthritis. There is a need to determine the most effective dose in preclinical and clinical trials to explore the potential benefit of turmeric in the prevention or treatment of arthritis.

5.10.2 AVOCADO SOY UNSAPONIFIABLE

Avocado soybean unsaponifiable (ASU) is an extract made from avocado and soybean oils. It increases the synthesis of aggrecan, a protein expressed in chondrocytes. It is a major proteoglycan in the articular cartilage and is important for its proper functioning. Aggrecan has been shown to have beneficial effects on osteoarthritis. Patients who took 300 mg/day of ASU did not have to take as much medication as was required without ASU.[16] There was no significant difference on increasing the dose from 300 to 600 mg/day.

5.10.3 GLUCOSAMINE AND CHONDROITIN

Glucosamine, an amino sugar, is thought to promote the formation and repair of cartilage. Chondroitin is a cartilage component that is thought to promote water retention and elasticity and to inhibit the enzymes that break down the cartilage. Both compounds are made in the body. Glucosamine and chondroitin have been widely promoted as a treatment for osteoarthritis. Some human studies have found benefits such as relief from pain and stiffness with fewer side effects than conventional arthritis drugs. Other studies have shown no benefits. It does take 2–3 months to get the benefits, and pills containing in addition calcium and vitamin D are found to be more effective.

Defects in Eicosanoid Metabolism

Deficiency of Cyclooxygenase—A Case

A 25-year-old woman was admitted to the hospital because of mild bleeding tendency. Since childhood, she has had repeated episodes of bruisability after slight injuries. Dental extraction on three occasions was not followed by prolonged bleeding. Tonsillectomy at the age of 3 years, however, was accompanied by a prolonged postoperative bleeding. Appendectomy at the age of 18 years was uneventful.

On admission, the patient had normal blood pressure, pulse rate, and temperature. Platelet count and prothrombin time were normal. The skin bleeding time was 8 minutes (normal: 4 minutes). TXA_2 was less than 0.5 pmol/10^8 platelets (normal: 300–500 pmol/10^8 platelets). When incubated with ArA, platelets did not form TXA_2. The metabolite, $PGF_{1\alpha}$, from PGI was less than 3 pmol/mL blood (normal: 11–17 pmol/mL). Platelets failed to aggregate with ArA but did so in the presence of PGH_2, which bypasses Cox. PGI_2 formation could not be detected but the lipoxygenase pathway was functional.[35]

This is a very interesting case of congenital Cox deficiency[34] associated with mild vascular defect expressed as a prolonged bleeding time. Although PGs and other prostanoids have a physiological role, this case suggests that their absence results in no dramatic consequences. This patient had normal blood pressure probably because both TXA_2, a vasoconstrictor, and PGI_2, a vasodilator, were absent. It is interesting that without these eicosanoids, she had normal menses, normal growth and development, and—other than mild bleeding tendency—appeared to be in good health. She resembled patients on low-dose aspirin therapy or those who subsist on fish rich in ω_3 fatty acids.

Deficiency of LTC$_4$ Synthase—A Case

A girl was born after an uncomplicated pregnancy. Her birth weight, length, and head circumference were all in the third percentile. At 2 months of age, muscular hypotonia was recorded and psychomotor retardation became apparent. She had microcephaly, deep-seated eyes, wide nasal root, and epicanthal folds. Over the next 4 months, muscular hypotonia progressed rapidly. Deep tendon reflexes were reduced. There was poor visual contact and no head control.

The blood cell count, protein, glucose, and several other plasma components were normal. Urinary components, including organic acids, were normal. Lysosomal storage disorders and defects in mitochondrial respiratory chain were ruled out. She failed to thrive and died at the age of 6 months. No permission was given for necropsy.

Further studies were performed on samples that were saved. In the cerebrospinal fluid, LTC_4 was below detectable levels.[36] Stimulated monocytes in the presence of a precursor could not form LTC_4, but LTB_4 synthesis was increased. Based on these results, this patient had LTC_4 synthase deficiency. This is a new inborn error of eicosanoid metabolism and may be associated with the clinical disorder of this patient.

The pathological roles of cysteinyl LTs in allergic and inflammatory disorders are well established. This case illustrates that these eicosanoids may also have an important physiological role as messengers or neuromodulators in the central nervous system. The clinical features of deficiency include muscular hypotonia, psychomotor retardation, failure to thrive, and a fatal outcome. This is the only case reported on this disorder. Therefore, the essentiality of LTC_4 synthase in humans at this time is suggestive.

REFERENCES

1. Balik, E. M., A. H. Lichtenstein, M. Cheng et al. 2006. Effects of omega-3 fatty acids on serum markers of cardiovascular disease risk: A systematic review. *Atherosclerosis* 189:19.
2. Baron, J. A., and R. S. Sandier. 2000. Non-steroidal anti-inflammatory drugs and cancer prevention. *Annu Rev Med* 51:511.
3. Bays, H. E. 2007. Safety considerations with omega-3 fatty acid therapy. *Amer J Cardiol* 99:535.
4. Boyce, J. 2005. Eicosanoid mediators of mast cells: Receptors, regulation of synthesis and pathologic implications. *Chem Immunol Allergy* 87:59.
5. Capdevila, J. H., J. R. Falck, and R. W. Estabrook. 1992. Cytochrome P-450 and the arachidonate cascade. *FASEB J* 6:731.
6. Catella-Lawson, F., M. P. Reilly, S. C. Kapoor et al. 2001. Cyclooxygenase inhibitors and the antiplatelet effects of aspirin. *N Engl J Med* 345:1809.
7. Cawood, A. L., M. P. Carrol, S. A. Wootton et al. 2005. Is there a case for n-3 fatty acid supplementation in cystic fibrosis? *Curr Opin Clin Nutr Metab Care* 8:153.
8. Chandrasekharan, N. V., H. Lamar Turepu Roos, N. K. Evanson et al. 2002. Cox-3, a cyclooxygenase-1 variant inhibited by acetaminophen and other analgesic/antipyretic drugs: Cloning, structure, and expression. *Proc Nat Acad Sci* 99:13926.
9. Clegg, D. O., D. J. Reda, C. E. Harris et al. 2006. Glucosamine, chondroitin sulfate, and the two in combination for painful knee osteoarthritis. *New Engl J Med* 354:795.
10. Drazen, J. M., E. Israel, and P. M. O'Byrne. 1997. Treatment of asthma with drugs modifying the leukotriene pathway. *N Engl J Med* 340:197.
11. Farooqui, M., Y. Li, T. Rogers et al. 2007. Cox-2 inhibitor celecoxib prevents chronic morphine-induced promotion on angiogenesis, tumor growth, metastasis and mortality, without compromising analgesia. *Brit J Cancer* 97:1523.
12. Funk, J. L., J. B. Frye, J. N. Oyarzo et al. 2006. Efficacy and mechanism of action of turmeric supplements in the treatment of experimental arthritis. *Arthritis Rheum* 54:3452.
13. Garcia Rodrigues, L. A., and A. Gonzalez-Perez. 2004. Risk of breast cancer among users of aspirin and other anti-inflammatory drugs. *Brit J Cancer* 91:525.
14. Giardiello, F. M., V. W. Yang, L. M. Hylind et al. 2002. Primary chemoprevention of familial adenomatous polyposis with sulindac. *N Engl J Med* 346:1054.
15. Harizi, H., J. Corcuff, and N. Gualde. 2008. Arachidonic acid–derived eicosanoids: Roles in biology and immunopathology. *Trends in Mol Med* 14:461.
16. Henrotin, Y. E., C. Sanchez, M. A. Deberg et al. 2003. Avocado/soybean unsaponifiable increase aggrecan synthesis and reduce catabolic and proinflammatory mediator production by human osteoarthritic chondrocytes. *J Rheumatol* 30:1825.

17. Jiang, O., and B. N. Ames. 2003. Gamma tocopherol, but not alpha tocopherol, decreases proinflammotry eicosanoids and inflammation damage in rats. *FASEB J* 17:816.
18. Kearney, P. M., C. Baigent, J. Godwin et al. 2006. Do selective cyclic-oxygenase-2 inhibitors and traditional non-steroidal anti-inflammatory drugs increase the risk of atherothrombosis? Meta analysis of randomized trials. *Brit Med J* 332:1302.
19. Khanapore, S. P., D. S. Garvey, D. R. Janero, and L. G. Letts. 2007. Eicosanoids in inflammation, biosynthesis, pharmacology, and therapeutic frontiers. *Curr Top Med Chem* 7:311.
20. Kohli, K., J. Ali, M. J. Ansari, and Z. Raheman. 2005. Curcumin: A natural anti-inflammatory agent. *Ind J Pharmacol* 37:141.
21. Leaf, A., and P. C. Weber. 1988. Cardiovascular effects of *n*–3 fatty acids. *N Engl J Med* 318:549.
22. Lichtenstein, D. R., and M. M. Wolfe. 2000. Cox-2 selective NSAIDs. New and improved? *J Am Med Assoc* 284:1297.
23. Lipworth, B. T. 1999. Leukotriene receptor antagonists. *Lancet* 353:57.
24. Naramiya, S., Y. Sugimoto, and F. Ushikubi. 1999. Prostanoid receptors: Structures, properties, and functions. *Physiol Rev* 79:1193.
25. Requirand, R., P. Gibart, P. Tramini et al. 2000. Serum fatty acid imbalance in bone loss: Example with periodontal disease. *Clin Nutr* 19:271.
26. Sardesai, V. M. 1992a. The essential fatty acids. *Nutr Clin Pract* 7:179.
27. Sardesai, V. M. 1992b. Biochemical and nutritional aspects of eicosanoids. *J Nutr Biochem* 3:562.
28. Simopoulos, A. P. 2001. Evolutionary aspects of diet and essential fatty acids. *World Rev Nutr* 21:323.
29. Srivastava, K. C. 1986. Onion exerts antiaggregatory effects by altering arachidonic acid metabolism in platelets. *Prostaglandins Leukot Med* 24:43.
30. Stenson, W. F. 1990. Role of eicosanoids as mediators of inflammation in inflammatory bowel disease. *Scand J Gastroent* 25(supple 172):13.
31. Subbaramaiah, K., D. Zakim, B. B. Weksler, and A. J. Dannenberg. 1997. Inhibition of cyclooxygenase: A novel approach in cancer prevention. *Proc Soc Exp Biol Med* 216:201.
32. Turini, M. F., and R. N. Dubois. 2002. Cyclooxygenase-2: A therapeutic target. *Annu Rev Med* 53:35.
33. Willis, A. L. 1981. Nutritional and pharmacological factors in eicosanoid biology. *Nutr Rev* 39:289.

CASE BIBLIOGRAPHY

34. Boda, Z., E. Tamas, I. Altorjay et al. 1981. Congenital deficiency of cyclooxygenase in a woman with generalized atherosclerosis. *Scand J Hematol* 27:65.
35. Mayateper, E., and B. Flock. 1998. Leukotriene C$_4$—synthase deficiency: A new born error of metabolism linked to a fatal developmental syndrome. *Lancet* 352:1514.
36. Pareti, F. I., P. M. Mannucci, A. D. D'Angelo, J. B. Smith, L. Sautebin, and G. Galli. 1980. Congenital deficiency of thromboxane and prostacyclin. *Lancet* 1:898.

6 Inorganic Elements (Minerals)

At least 35 chemical elements occur in human tissues, although some are present in extremely small amounts. Four elements (i.e., oxygen, hydrogen, carbon, and nitrogen) form and make up 96% of the weight of the human body. The remaining 4% of the body weight is composed of essential and nonessential elements. Over 50% of the weight of the body is oxygen, and oxygen and hydrogen together constitute 75% of the body weight (mostly as body water).

The term most commonly used is *mineral* to represent each of the elements found in biological material, although some elements such as iodine and fluorine are not minerals; however, custom has established this terminology. Some minerals occur in the body tissues in relatively large amounts (100 milligrams to gram quantities) and are designated as macrominerals, while others are present in much smaller concentrations (milligrams or micrograms). Such small concentrations were not easily quantified by early analytical methods and were called "trace minerals" or elements. The development of instruments with increased sensitivity has enabled investigators to study the role of these trace elements more carefully.

An element is considered to be essential when a diet adequate in all respects except the mineral under study consistently results in altered or diminished physiological function and when a diet supplemented with physiological levels of the element, but not of others, prevents or cures this impairment. Essentiality must be demonstrated by more than one independent investigator and in more than one species before the trace element is generally accepted as essential. Deficiency is correlated with lower-than-normal levels of the mineral in the blood and tissues of the body. Like other essential nutrients, increasing amounts of essential minerals evoke an increasing biological response until a plateau is reached. Larger intakes of minerals may produce pharmacological actions and still larger intakes may produce toxic effects.

The inorganic elements or minerals can be divided into essential macrominerals (i.e., those required in the diet at levels of 100 mg or more per day), essential trace minerals (i.e., those needed in amounts not more than a few milligrams per day), ultratrace minerals (i.e., those that may be essential for animal metabolism but for which human requirements have not been established), and trace contaminants for which there is no evidence of requirement for either animal or man. Essential macrominerals include calcium, phosphorous, magnesium, potassium, sodium, chloride, and sulfur (Table 6.1). Essential microminerals include iron, copper, zinc, cobalt, molybdenum, selenium, manganese, iodine, chromium, and fluorine (Table 6.2). The ultratrace elements are silicon, nickel, vanadium, tin, arsenic, boron, lithium, rubidium, silver, antimony, and others.[22,23]

6.1 ESSENTIAL MACROMINERALS

6.1.1 CALCIUM

Calcium is the most abundant cation in the human body and comprises about 1.5%–2% of the total body weight. The body of healthy humans contains about 1250 g of calcium, about 99% of which is present in bones and teeth as deposits of calcium phosphate and calcium hydroxide. The remaining 1% is found in extracellular fluid, soft tissues, and as a component of various membrane structures.

6.1.1.1 Food Sources

Calcium is present in significant amounts in only a few foods, with milk and dairy products as the best sources. A quart of milk supplies about 1200 mg of calcium in a readily assimilable form.

TABLE 6.1
Essential Macrominerals in the Adult Human Body and Their Major Functions

Mineral	Body Weight (%)	Total[a] (g)	Function
Calcium	1.78	1250	Structural component of bones and teeth; regulation of excitable tissues (nerve and muscle excitability); blood clotting; activation of some enzymes; mediates action of some hormones.
Phosphorus	0.96	670	Structural component of bones and teeth; component of nucleic acids, nucleotide coenzymes, ATP, GTP, etc.; essential in intermediary metabolism, enzyme systems; maintenance of osmotic and acid–base balance.
Magnesium	0.04	25	Constituent of bones and teeth; nerve impulse transmission; activator of some enzymes; structural integrity of mitochondrial membranes.
Potassium	0.19	130	Regulation of nerve and muscle excitability; regulation of osmotic pressure; acid–base balance, water balance.
Sodium	0.14	100	Excitability of nerves, muscles, active transport of glucose, regulation of osmotic pressure, acid–base balance, water balance.
Chloride	0.15	105	Component of gastric juice, regulation of osmotic pressure, acid–base balance, water balance.
Sulfur	0.25	175	Component of thiamin, biotin, pantothenic acid, lipoic acid, methionine, cysteine, taurine; stabilizes structures of several proteins.

[a] Average amount in adults weighing 70 kg.

Broccoli and leafy, green vegetables such as turnip greens and kale have appreciable amounts of calcium. Other foods relatively high in calcium salts are beans, shellfish, and fish of the sardine type in which bones are eaten. Some vegetables such as spinach contain appreciable quantities of oxalic acid, which forms insoluble calcium oxalate in the intestinal tract and lessens the absorption and utilization of calcium present.

6.1.1.2   Absorption

The absorption of calcium is quite variable and depends on a number of factors including various ions, acid–base status, lactose, and vitamin D.[1] Calcium can be precipitated as phosphate, carbonate, oxalate, phytate, sulfate, or calcium soap in the presence of excess fatty acids. All of these are insoluble and therefore poorly absorbed. Calcium salts are more soluble in acid than in basic solutions. Lactose exerts a favorable effect on calcium absorption. The beneficial effect is the result of chelation of calcium by lactose, which forms a soluble complex of low molecular weight. Vitamin D is important in facilitating the absorption of calcium. The active form of vitamin D induces the synthesis of a transport protein for calcium that increases calcium absorption. Calcium from the intestine is absorbed by active transport (i.e., against the concentration gradient by a process requiring energy). The average person has a high degree of adaptability to high or

TABLE 6.2
Essential Trace Minerals in the Human Body and Their Major Functions

Mineral	Body Weight (%)	Total[a]	Functions
Iron	0.006	4	Structural component of hemoglobin, myoglobin, cytochromes, some enzymes.
Copper	0.0001	80 mg	Component of ceruloplasmin (iron mobilization), cytochrome oxidase (energy metabolism), superoxide dismutase (free radical inactivation), lysyl oxidase (cross-linking of elastin), tyrosinase, dopamine hydroxylase.
Zinc	0.003	2 g	Component of several enzymes (e.g., alcohol dehydrogenase, carbonic anhydrase, alkaline phosphatase, carboxypeptidase, thymidine kinase); role in wound healing.
Cobalt	trace	1.1 mg	Component of vitamin B_{12}.
Molybdenum	0.00001	9 mg	Component of xanthine oxidase, aldehyde oxidase, sulfite oxidase.
Selenium	0.00002	15 mg	Component of glutathione peroxidase, iodothyronine 5-deiodinase.
Manganese	0.00002	20 mg	Component of pyruvate carboxylase; activation of many enzymes; necessary for normal skeletal and connective tissue development.
Iodine	0.00004	30 mg	Constituent of thyroxine, triiodothyronine.
Chromium	0.00001	8 mg	Component of glucose tolerance factor; potentiates insulin action; involved in glucose transport into the cell.
Fluorine	0.0015	1 g	Structural component of calcium hydroxyapatite of bones and teeth.
Silicon[b]	0.001	700 mg	Apparent role in the formation of connective tissue and bone matrix.

[a] Average amount in adults weighing 70 kg.
[b] Human requirement for this mineral is not known.

low amounts of calcium in the diet. Those eating a low-calcium diet appear to have more efficient calcium absorption than those consuming a diet high in calcium. Thus, if the intake of calcium is lowered, intestinal efficiency and the ability to absorb and retain calcium increase, whereas raising the intake reduces the efficiency of absorption. Under normal conditions, approximately 33% of the ingested calcium is absorbed.

Once calcium is absorbed through the walls of the intestine it is transported in the plasma and released to fluids bathing the tissues of the body. From there, the cells absorb whatever calcium is needed for their normal functioning and growth.

The level of calcium in plasma is maintained at about 10 mg/dL and is regulated by the endocrine system involving parathyroid hormone (PTH), calcitonin, and the active form of vitamin D. Plasma calcium exists in three forms. About 50% of the calcium in the plasma is ionized; it is the only fraction that is physiologically active and is assumed to be the fraction under hormonal control. The other 50% is nonionized and physiologically inert: 40%–45% is bound to plasma protein, primarily to albumin, and 5%–10% is complexed with ions such as citrate, bicarbonate, and phosphate. As the blood plasma is filtered in the kidney, about 99% of the calcium (10 g/day) is reabsorbed and the remaining 1% (usually about 100–175 mg/day) is excreted in the urine.

6.1.1.3   Functions

Calcium serves as the principal component of the skeleton and provides the strength and rigidity of the skeleton and teeth.[2,7] It is deposited in bone as calcium phosphate and calcium hydroxide, which make up a physiologically stable compound called hydroxyapatite, $Ca_{10}(PO_4)_6(OH)_2$. Because calcium and phosphorus are the predominant elements in these compounds, an adequate supply of both must be present before they can be precipitated from fluids surrounding the bone matrix. Calcification apparently occurs when the product of the level of calcium and phosphorus in the blood and extracellular fluid exceeds 30 (e.g., mg of calcium × mg of phosphorus in 100 mL of blood >30). The skeleton serves as a vital physiological tissue, providing a readily available source of calcium and phosphorus for homeostatic control when the absorbance of these nutrients from the intestine is insufficient or when their excretion from the body is excessive. The bone tissue is constantly being reshaped (or remodeled) according to various body needs and stresses, with as much as 700 mg of calcium entering and leaving the bones each day.

Cells use their internal calcium ion concentration to regulate a variety of processes.[3] The calcium ion level is kept low by an ATP-dependent calcium pump; in nerves and muscles, an additional pumping system is also present. In most cells, calcium release from the endoplasmic reticulum by inositol triphosphate triggers the actions, which differ according to cell type. In nerve cells, calcium-gated ion channels are used to start neurotransmitter release. Glycogen breakdown, muscle contraction, and the secretion of small molecules such as insulin by the pancreas or histamine by mast cells are calcium-regulated processes. Calcium is required to initiate the blood clotting process. The ionized calcium stimulates the blood platelet to release thromboplastin, which is a necessary cofactor for the conversion of prothrombin to thrombin. In addition, it mediates the intracellular action of many hormones.

To carry out these various roles, calcium must be available to the appropriate tissue in the proper concentrations.[6] This is accomplished by PTH, calcitonin, and the active form of vitamin D by controlling the site of entry of calcium in the circulation (intestinal absorption) and the site of exit (the kidney). In addition, the large store of calcium in bone is available for deposits or withdrawals depending upon peripheral demands. When the blood calcium level falls, PTH is secreted, which restores calcium to its normal concentration range. PTH stimulates renal tubular calcium absorption and inhibits phosphate reabsorption. This leads to decreased excretion of calcium and increased excretion of phosphate in urine. PTH mobilizes bone calcium by direct stimulation of osteoclasts. It also stimulates the conversion of vitamin D to its active form by the kidney. The active form of vitamin D acts on intestinal cells to induce the synthesis of a specific calcium-binding protein that facilitates intestinal calcium absorption. All these actions of PTH increase blood calcium. Calcitonin is secreted when blood calcium levels are elevated.[4] It acts to lower both calcium and phosphorus by inhibiting bone resorption. Thus, it aids in counterbalancing the action of PTH and maintaining blood calcium at normal level. The active form of vitamin D not only increases intestinal absorption but also promotes bone resorption directly, an apparently paradoxical situation because it is also required for adequate calcification of cartilage and osteoid.

6.1.1.4   Disorders of Calcium

Calcium deficiency in children can lead to rickets, and in adults to osteomalacia. These two diseases are associated with vitamin D deficiency or, rarely, with alterations in vitamin D metabolism or action. In osteoporosis, the amount of bone is reduced without a change in its chemical composition. This disorder is associated with a variety of factors and a negative calcium balance. Whether deficient dietary intake of calcium is the cause of the disease is not clear. Calcium supplementation and hormones are frequently used in treatment. Potassium bicarbonate to balance the metabolic production of acid is beneficial. Plasma calcium level is closely regulated within a fairly limited range. Hypocalcemia is a total plasma calcium concentration less than 8.8 mg/dL in the presence of normal plasma protein concentration or plasma ionized calcium level less than 4.7 mg/dL. Hypoproteinemia can reduce the protein-bound fraction of calcium but the ionized calcium level is unchanged. The causes of hypocalcemia include hypoparathyroidism, vitamin D deficiency, and renal disease.

A decrease in ionic plasma calcium is a cause of tetany, a condition marked by severe, intermittent spastic contraction of muscles and by muscular pain. Tetany occurs occasionally in newborn infants and sometimes in infants affected by rickets and in fat malabsorption. In the last instance, a loss of vitamin D accounts for diminished calcium absorption, resulting in a plasma calcium level too low to be compensated by the PTH. Treatment is administration of calcium preferably with vitamin D. Hypercalcemia is a plasma total calcium concentration above 10.4 mg/dL or plasma ionized calcium above 5.2 mg/dL.

Malignancy and primary hyperparathyroidism are the most common causes for hypercalcemia. Hematological malignancies, such as multiple myeloma, tend to be responsible for hypercalcemia in patients with solid tumors. Because calcium is an important regulator of many cellular functions, hypercalcemia can produce abnormalities in the neurologic, cardiovascular, pulmonary, renal, gastrointestinal, and musculoskeletal systems. The clinical manifestations include muscle weakness, anorexia, thirst, polyuria, and dehydration.

The role that calcium might have in reducing the rates of colorectal cancer, the nation's second leading killer, has been the subject of many studies. Higher intakes of calcium are associated with lower risk for colorectal cancer.[8,9] Higher calcium intake also reduces the occurrence of polyps that can turn cancerous. The protective ability of calcium to reduce the risk of this disease may be due to calcium's effect on proliferation, differentiation, and binding of bile acids that may act as mutagens in the colon. Recently, scientists analyzed 10 studies that together traced nutrient consumption of more than half a million people, nearly 5000 of whom eventually got colorectal cancer. People who consumed 6–8 ounces of milk a day had a 12% lower risk of developing colorectal cancer than those who drank less than two glasses a week. With more than a glass a day, the risk reduction was 15%. A total calcium intake—from diet plus calcium supplements—of 1000 mg a day was protective too. It is estimated that if all study participants had consumed that much, the women may have suffered 15% fewer cases, and the men 10% fewer.

Vitamin D, which is commonly added to milk, is thought to also decrease the risk of colorectal cancer. It is not clear whether the vitamin acts directly or indirectly on increased intestinal calcium absorption, but the study has found the largest protective effect with the highest doses of both calcium and vitamin D. The study could not determine vitamin D's role but found the biggest protective effect with the highest doses of both nutrients.

Some studies have shown an increase in prostate cancer risk among the highest consumers of dairy products. The association between calcium and prostate cancer may be related to calcium's tendency to suppress the conversion of vitamin D to its active form.[10,11] One of the roles of vitamin D is maintenance of cellular differentiation within the prostate. Therefore, men should avoid taking more than 1000 mg calcium per day.

6.1.1.5 Requirements

The amount of calcium retained by the body depends not only on the amount in the diet but also on the efficiency of absorption and on excretion; hence, it is difficult to set an absolute standard for the calcium requirement. Moreover, the need for calcium appears to be flexible. In certain parts of the world, the adult population gets along well with a diet containing low amounts of calcium.

The calcium requirements are based on balance studies that measure the intake and output of calcium over time. The Food and Nutrition Board of the National Academy of Science in its 1989 revision recommends 800 mg/day of calcium for adults. This amount covers the basic needs and allows for a margin of safety. This allowance is on the basis that calcium losses are approximately 320 mg/day. Because only a portion of the dietary calcium is absorbed, 800 mg is suggested for maintaining balance. The Recommended Dietary Allowance (RDA) for infants up to 1 year old is between 400 and 600 mg. For children 1–10 years old, the allowance is set at 800 mg, and for those between the ages of 11 and 18 years, the recommended amount is 1200 mg per day. To meet the needs of the growing fetus and the mother during pregnancy, the RDA for calcium during gestation is 1200 mg/day compared with 800 mg for nonpregnant women. Human milk contains 25–35 mg calcium/100 mL. For lactating women, this represents an additional 150–200 mg depending on the amount of milk produced, so to meet this demand the RDA during lactation is set at 1200 mg/day.

6.1.1.6 Toxicity

A number of conditions involving increased bone breakdown or calcium absorption can increase the blood calcium. A very high intake of calcium and a high intake of vitamin D are a potential cause of hypercalcemia. This may lead to excessive calcification not only in the bone but also in the soft tissues such as the kidneys.

6.1.2 PHOSPHORUS

Phosphorus as a primary, secondary, or tertiary ion is present in the body fluids (about 16% of the total) and as a constituent of bones and teeth (about 84% of the total). Phosphorus constitutes 1% of the human body weight. It is estimated that the adult body contains 12 g of phosphorus per kilogram of fat-free tissue or about 670 g in men and 630 g in women.

6.1.2.1 Food Sources

Phosphorus is a major constituent of all plant and animal cells and therefore is present in all natural foods. In general, foods rich in protein are also rich in phosphorus. Meat, poultry, fish, eggs, milk, and cereal products are good sources of phosphorus as they are for calcium.

6.1.2.2 Absorption

Most of the dietary phosphorus is absorbed as free phosphate, and about 60%–70% of our normal intake is absorbed. The most favorable absorption of inorganic phosphate takes place when calcium and phosphorus are ingested in approximately equal amounts. Because milk has calcium and phosphorus in equal amounts, it is a good source of phosphorus. Organic phosphate esters of phytic acid in cereals and seeds are not a source of phosphorus because the human intestinal tract lacks phytase. Phytic acid forms insoluble calcium salts in the intestinal lumen and interferes with calcium absorption. Available evidence indicates that phytic acid also interferes with the absorption of iron and zinc. The transport of phosphate from the small intestine is an active, energy-dependent process. Like calcium, phosphorus absorption is regulated by the active form of vitamin D. In general, in adults, about two-thirds of the ingested phosphate is absorbed and what is absorbed from the intestine is almost entirely excreted in the urine. However, in growing children, there is a positive balance of phosphate. The serum inorganic phosphate level is maintained closely in the range of 3–4 mg/100 mL in adults. Levels are higher in infants (6 mg/dL) and young children (4.5 mg/dL). The kidneys provide the main excretory route for the regulation of serum phosphate level.

6.1.2.3 Functions

The addition or removal of phosphate groups of proteins is the main method of regulating metabolism, cell division, and differentiation. Along with calcium, phosphorus has a major role in the formation of bones and teeth. Phosphorus has several other very important functions. It has a critical role as part of nucleic acids (i.e., DNA and RNA), which are essential for cell protein synthesis. Phosphorus is present in phospholipids, the key components in the structure of cell membranes. It is essential in carbohydrate metabolism as the phosphate esters of several compounds. Phosphorylation to glucose-6-phosphate initiates glucose catabolism. Many high-energy phosphate bonds involve phosphoryl groups. Phosphate is part of some conjugated proteins such as casein of milk. Some of the water-soluble vitamins function as coenzymes only when combined with phosphate. The phosphate buffer system is of importance in the regulation of pH.

6.1.2.4 Deficiency

A primary deficiency of phosphorus is not known to occur in humans. Despite a relatively low intake of phosphorus, a deficiency is rarely seen because it is efficiently recycled by the kidney; about 90% of the filtered phosphate is reabsorbed by the proximal tubule. Phosphorus metabolism may be disturbed in many types of diseases, notably those involving the kidney and the bone. Hypophosphatemia is observed in 0.25%–2.15% of general hospital admissions.[5] Alcohol abuse is the most common cause of severe hypophosphatemia, possibly due to poor food intake and vomiting. Hypophosphatemia is associated with the administration of glucose or total parenteral nutrition (TPN) without sufficient phosphate, excessive use of antacids that bind phosphate, hyperparathyroidism, recovery from diabetic acidosis, alcoholism, and some other conditions. Hypophosphatemia is induced by a number of mechanisms, including urinary excretion, decreased intestinal absorption, or a combination of these abnormalities. Increased urinary excretion is usually secondary to hyperparathyroidism, renal tubular defects, X-linked vitamin D–resistant rickets, aldosteronism, and diuretic therapy. Hypophosphatemia due to urinary losses is observed in up to 30% of patients with malignant neoplasms such as certain leukemias and lymphomas and osmotic diuresis. Low serum phosphate level causes muscle weakness because the muscle cells are deprived of phosphorus essential for energy metabolism. Hypophosphatemia may also have profound, deleterious effects on the viability of human red blood cells. It may cause a decrease of red cell 2,3-bisphosphoglycerate (BPG) and ATP. BPG promotes oxygen release from oxygenated hemoglobin.[12] A reduction of concentration of this phosphoric acid ester lowers tissue oxygen by shifting the oxygenated hemoglobin dissociation curve to the left. Tissue hypoxia can result despite a pO_2 tension in the normal range. Parenteral phosphate is given for critically depleted patients. Because the kidney is capable of excreting 600–900 mg of phosphorus daily, hyperphosphatemia is rare in the absence of chronic renal disease.

6.1.2.5 Requirements

The Food and Nutrition Board recommends that the daily intake of phosphorus be at least 800 mg/day and approximately equal to the calcium intake. Because phosphorus is widely distributed in foods, there is little possibility of a dietary inadequacy if the food contains sufficient protein and calcium.

6.1.3 Magnesium

Magnesium is the fourth most abundant cation in the body and quantitatively it is second to potassium as the intracellular cation. An adult human weighing 70 kg contains 20–28 g of magnesium, with about 60%–65% of the total present in bone, 27% in muscle, 6%–7% in other cells, and approximately 1% in extracellular fluid. The erythrocyte content varies from 4.3 to 6.2 mEq/L (1 mEq/L = 12 mg) depending on the age of the cells. As the red blood cells age, the magnesium content falls slowly. Magnesium ion in erythrocytes and plasma exists in free, complexed, and protein-bound forms. In plasma, the approximate percentages are 55% free, 13% complexed with citrate, phosphate, and other ions, and 32% protein bound. Plasma magnesium concentrations range from 1.4 to 2.4 mg/dL.

6.1.3.1 Food Sources

Magnesium is widely distributed in foods. Because it is present in chlorophyll, green vegetables are important sources. Whole grains, beans, peas, and some seafoods are rich in magnesium.

6.1.3.2 Absorption

Absorption occurs largely in the upper part of the small intestine, where about 33% of the ingested magnesium is absorbed.[14] It is excreted primarily by the kidney and is regulated in response to magnesium levels in blood. In healthy adults, the serum magnesium is 1.4–1.75 mEq/L, with approximately 20% of the magnesium bound to proteins. When magnesium intake is low, the kidney reabsorbs almost all of the magnesium so that practically none is lost by the body. As a result, variation in dietary intake seldom affects blood levels. Urinary losses increase with the use of diuretics and with the consumption of alcohol.

6.1.3.3   Functions

Just as calcium is responsible for the integrity of the cell membrane, magnesium is responsible for the structural integrity of the mitochondrial membrane.[15] It is an essential constituent of all soft tissues and bones. The soluble, ionic form participates as a cofactor for countless enzymatic reactions, especially where MgATP is involved. The magnesium-dependent and magnesium-activated enzymes include those of mitochondrial oxidative phosphorylation and of intermediary metabolism of glucose and fatty acids. It plays an important role in neurochemical transmission and muscle excitability. Magnesium plays a vital role in the reversible association of intracellular particles and in the binding of macromolecules to subcellular organelles; for example, the binding of RNA to ribosomes is magnesium dependent.

6.1.3.4   Deficiency

Because of the wide distribution of magnesium in plant and animal products, primary deficiency of magnesium is rare in individuals with normal organ function. The fall in circulating magnesium concentration is seen only with extreme depletion. Hypomagnesemia can occur in gastrointestinal disorders such as malabsorption syndromes, diarrhea, and steatorrhea; chronic alcoholism; diabetes mellitus, with prolonged intravenous feeding with magnesium-free solutions; during hemodialysis; and some other conditions.[13] Deficits are accompanied by a variety of structural and functional disturbances. Hypomagnesemia is clinically manifested by anorexia, increased irritability, disorientation, convulsions, and psychotic behavior.

In magnesium deficiency, especially if severe, hypocalcemia can occur that persists despite increased calcium intake until the deficit of magnesium is corrected. Apparently, magnesium is required for the mobilization of calcium from the bone.

6.1.3.5   Requirements

The estimates of requirements are based on a large number of balance studies and range from 200 to 700 mg/day. The present RDA for magnesium is 350 mg/day for men and 300 mg/day for women. The magnesium content of the average American diet is about 250 mg/day. Therefore, there is some potential for deficiency, but this has not been identified.

6.1.3.6   Toxicity

Hypermagnesemia is usually a result of renal insufficiency; however, magnesium toxicity is not uncommon. Many antacids and laxative preparations have magnesium salts as the active ingredients. The use of magnesium sulfate as a cathartic in patients with impaired renal function can lead to severe toxicity.

An elevated serum concentration of magnesium alters the normal function of the neurologic, neuromuscular, and cardiovascular systems. In mild magnesemia, the patient may experience nausea and vomiting. At higher serum magnesium concentrations, drowsiness, lethargy, and altered consciousness may be present. At serum concentrations of magnesium between 8 and 10 mEq/L, respiratory paralysis, hypertension, and difficulty in talking and swallowing may also be present.

6.1.4   Potassium

Potassium constitutes 5% of the total mineral content of the body. The average man weighing 150 pounds has about 130 g of potassium, most of which is found inside the cells; it is the major cation of the intracellular fluid. The total body potassium content expressed per body weight increases with age and is greater in men than in women. The concentration of potassium in the lean body tissues is fairly constant and is about 440 mg/100 g. This relationship has become the basis for determining the lean body mass. The normal range of potassium in plasma is between 14 and 20 mg/100 mL. The cellular elements of the blood contain about 20 times as much as the plasma.

6.1.4.1   Food Sources

Potassium is widely distributed in natural foods. Whole grain, legumes, leafy vegetables, broccoli, potatoes, fruits, and meat are rich sources. A large banana or a cup of citrus fruit juice provides about 0.5 g of potassium.

6.1.4.2   Absorption

The potassium present in food is readily absorbed from the small intestine. It is excreted primarily in the urine. The kidney maintains normal plasma levels through its ability to filter, reabsorb, and excrete. The normal obligatory loss of potassium amounts to about 160 mg/day. The adrenal cortex hormone, aldosterone, influences potassium excretion; it conserves sodium in exchange for potassium, which is excreted. Alterations in acid–base balance are also reflected in compensatory changes in the amount of potassium excreted in the urine.

6.1.4.3   Functions

Along with sodium, potassium is involved in the maintenance of normal water balance, osmotic equilibrium, and acid–base balance.[21] It has a very important role in extracellular fluid in that it influences muscle activity, notably cardiac muscle. The normal level of potassium in extracellular fluid is 4–6 mEq/L, and it is critical that the concentration remains within this range. The myocardium is exquisitely sensitive to slight changes in the potassium concentration of plasma. Hyperkalemia, an increase above 8 mEq/L, can cause myocardial arrest in diastole, whereas a decrease in plasma potassium to 2 mEq/L can provoke systolic arrest. Characteristic changes in the electrocardiogram accompany the development of these conditions. Potassium functions within the cell as a cation for neutrality regulation, a regulator of osmotic pressure, and a catalyst in many biological reactions. The intracellular concentrations of both potassium and hydrogen ions are higher than those of extracellular fluid. When the extracellular concentration of hydrogen ion is increased, as in acidosis, there is a shift of potassium from cells to extracellular fluid. When the extracellular concentration of hydrogen ion is decreased, potassium moves into cells. Thus, extracellular acidosis produces hyperkalemia and extracellular alkalosis causes hypokalemia. A change of 0.1 unit of plasma pH can be accompanied by a change of opposite sign of 0.6 mM in the plasma concentration of potassium.

6.1.4.4   Deficiency

Because of the widespread distribution of potassium in foods, deficiency is unlikely under normal circumstances. Hypokalemia, plasma potassium concentration less than 3.5 mEq/L, occurs in less than 1% of normal healthy people. However, it is common in ambulatory practice, often as a consequence of drug therapy or disease. Hypokalemia frequently results from commonly used diuretics, corticosteroids, and insulin. Experimental deficiency in rats results in a slow growth rate, thinning of hair, renal hypertrophy, necrosis of the myocardium, and death. In man, serious loss of both potassium and sodium can result from diseases of the gastrointestinal tract involving loss of secretions by vomiting or diarrhea. Trauma, surgery, anoxia, diabetic acidosis, shock, and any damage to or wasting away of tissues may result in the transfer of potassium to the extracellular fluid and plasma and loss from the body through urinary excretion. Recovery with rapid uptake of potassium by tissues may result in low plasma potassium levels. Low extracellular potassium concentration causes muscular weakness, increases nervous irritability, mental disorientation, and cardiac irregularities. Because sodium is antagonistic to potassium, excessive intake of sodium may have the same effects as a low potassium intake.

Other effects of hypokalemia and potassium depletion include decreased insulin secretion resulting in carbohydrate intolerance, metabolic alkalosis, and increased renal ammoniagenesis.

6.1.4.5   Toxicity

Hyperkalemia may be caused by several factors. Increased potassium levels may be due to excessive intake, either therapeutically or nutritionally. It may also result from the failure of the kidneys to excrete potassium. Addison's disease (hypoaldosteronism), diuretics, and renal glomerular failure may also cause this problem. Redistribution of potassium in the body, causing hyperkalemia, may be due to acidosis, severe acute starvation (as in anorexia nervosa), and severe tissue damage. Blood transfusion may lead to hyperkalemia because of the leaching of potassium from the erythrocytes in the transfused unit of blood. The cardiac toxicity of hyperkalemia is a major cause of morbidity and mortality, with electrocardiographic changes paralleling the degree of hyperkalemia.

6.1.4.6   Requirements

Although it is a dietary essential, there is no information on its minimal requirements. The normal dietary intake is about 3–5 g/day. It is assumed that the amount of potassium in the diet is adequate.

6.1.5   Sodium

Sodium constitutes 2% of the total mineral content of the body. The body of a healthy adult contains about 256 g of sodium chloride or 100 g of sodium. Of this, a little more than half is in the extracellular fluid, about 34.5 g is in the bone as inorganic bound material, and less than 14.5 g is in the cells. It is the major cation of the extracellular fluid. Normal serum values range from 310 to 340 mg/dL.

6.1.5.1   Food Sources

Foods of both animal and plant origin contain sodium and, as a general rule, animal foods contain more sodium than plant foods. However, the main dietary source of sodium is common salt used in cooking and for seasoning, the sodium salts such as monosodium glutamate and sodium nitrite, and other preservatives that are used in processed foods.

6.1.5.2   Absorption

Most of the ingested sodium is mainly absorbed from the small intestine. The absorption of sodium is an active (energy-dependent) process. It enters the bloodstream and is filtered by the kidney and reabsorbed to maintain the blood levels within the narrow range required by the body. Normal serum sodium is 134–146 mEq/L. Any excess, which with a normal diet amounts to 90%–95% of the ingested sodium, is excreted in the urine; this is controlled by aldosterone. There is a limit to the amount of sodium that can be excreted by the kidney in a certain volume of urine. If the dietary intake exceeds the kidney's ability to excrete sodium, the volume of blood and extracellular fluid will rise. Sodium is also lost through perspiration. Normally, sodium losses are minimal, but environmental conditions such as exercise or fever leading to excessive perspiration can lead to substantial loss of sodium and water by this route. An altered proportion of sodium to water in extracellular fluid indicates an abnormality in sodium balance, water balance, or both.

6.1.5.3   Functions

Sodium is the principal cation of the extracellular fluid.[16] In combination with potassium, the principal cation of the intracellular fluid, sodium regulates water balance. It contributes to the osmotic pressure, which keeps water from leaving the blood and going into the cells. Potassium acts to keep fluid within the cells. When the levels of either of these ions get out of balance, water shifts in or out of cells to keep the concentration of sodium or potassium at the correct level in their respective components.[18]

Sodium is essential for the absorption of glucose in the kidney and intestine and the transport of other nutrients across membranes. Through its association with chloride and bicarbonate, it is involved in the regulation of acid–base balance. As a component of the sodium pump, it is essential in the passage of metabolic materials across cell membranes. It plays a role in transmitting electrochemical impulses along nerve and muscle membranes and therefore maintains normal muscle irritability and excitability.

6.1.5.4 Deficiency

Hyponatremia, the most common electrolyte disorder, is defined as a reduced plasma sodium concentration (<134 mEq/L). Generally, clinical concern arises when the sodium concentration is less than 130 mEq/L. Although loss of fluid and loss of salt generally accompany each other, a defect of sodium alone may be encountered.[20] The main consequence of sodium depletion is a reduction in extracellular fluid volume with a decrease in cell and tissue perfusion. The most commonly encountered situations that cause sodium and chloride depletion are dehydration because of heavy sweating, severe diarrhea, or vomiting. Increased sodium losses in urine can occur in adrenal insufficiency when mineralocorticoids are not available to promote tubular reabsorption. The symptoms are weakness, fatigue, lack of appetite, nausea, a diminution of mental acuity, low blood pressure (BP), and rapid pulse rate. A thirst develops that cannot be alleviated by drinking fluid alone but is corrected by including salt. The specific serum concentration reflects the ratio of total body sodium to total body water and is not an accurate indicator of total body sodium. Both hyponatremia and hypernatremia can, therefore, occur in the presence of low, normal, and high total body sodium.

Hypernatremia is caused by loss of water, gain of sodium, or both. Loss of water could be due to increased loss or reduced intake, and a gain of sodium is due to either increased intake or reduced renal excretion. Increased loss of water can occur through the kidney (e.g., diabetes insipidus or osmotic diuresis), the gastrointestinal tract (osmotic diarrhea), or the skin. Reduced water intake occurs most commonly in comatose patients or in those with a defective thirst mechanism. If hypernatremia is due to water loss as a result of diarrhea or vomiting, the patient urinates very little. On the other hand, if the condition is due to kidney dysfunction, the patient urinates in large quantities. When the sodium concentration in the plasma is very high, it affects brain cells. The patient experiences muscle twitching and feels tired and confused. The role of sodium in hypertension is discussed in Section 6.1.8.

6.1.5.5 Requirements

Like potassium, there is no established dietary allowance for sodium. The usual daily intake of sodium chloride is about 10–15 g or 170–250 mEq of sodium. This is far greater than required, but the amount is used chiefly because of taste; most of it is excreted in the urine.

6.1.6 CHLORIDE

Chloride is present in the body to the extent of 0.15% of the body weight. It is widely distributed throughout the body but is present in higher concentration in extracellular fluids where it is closely associated with sodium. The normal chloride content of blood is 98–106 mM/L.

6.1.6.1 Food Sources and Absorption

Chloride is taken in the body largely as sodium chloride; therefore, when salt is restricted the chloride level drops. It is excreted in the urine, but the kidney is efficient in reabsorbing chloride when dietary intake is low. Its excretion in urine and sweat usually follows closely the excretion of sodium; however, chloride can also be excreted in association with ammonium or hydrogen ions.

6.1.6.2 Functions

As part of hydrochloric acid, it is used to maintain the normal acidity of the stomach contents required for initiating the digestion of proteins. It is essential in a number of vital body processes including water balance, osmotic pressure, and acid–base balance. It contributes to the ability of the blood to carry large amounts of carbon dioxide to the lungs. Abnormalities of chloride metabolism are generally accompanied by alterations in sodium metabolism. Recently, a number of cases of chloride deficiency were reported as a result of accidental omission of chloride in certain infant food formulas. The symptoms of chloride deficiency included alkalosis associated with hypovolemia and marked loss of potassium in the urine. Impaired growth, memory defects, and psychomotor disturbances also occurred. All the symptoms disappeared after administration of chloride.

Decreased concentrations of serum chloride occur in metabolic acidosis.[19] In uncontrolled diabetes, there is an overproduction of keto acids whose anions replace chloride; in renal disease, phosphate retention accompanies impaired glomerular filtration, with a concomitant decrease in serum chloride concentration. A deficit of body chloride and a decreased serum chloride accompany prolonged vomiting. High concentrations of serum chloride are usually found in dehydration, certain types of renal tubular acidosis, and respiratory alkalosis. Elevated sweat chloride values are of significance in diagnosing cystic fibrosis. The sweat glands appear morphologically unaffected, but the chloride content of the secretion is 2–5 times the normal level.

6.1.6.3 Requirements

Ordinary diets contain sufficient chloride in association with sodium and potassium, but when there is excessive excretion of any of them, more must be provided. Adrenal insufficiency and acidosis are examples. Persons working in industries in which they encounter intense heat and perspire freely must have salt supplies with their drinking water to make up for this loss of electrolytes.

6.1.7 SULFUR

Sulfur is present in every cell of the body and represents 0.25% of the body weight. It occurs primarily as a constituent of sulfur-containing amino acids: cystine, cysteine, methionine, and taurine. It is present in almost all proteins but is most prevalent in the keratin of skin and hair, which contain 4%–6% sulfur.

6.1.7.1 Food Sources and Absorption

In food it is found as inorganic sulfate and sulfur bound in organic form. Inorganic sulfur is absorbed from the intestine into the portal circulation. After digestion of proteins, the free sulfur-containing amino acids are absorbed into the portal circulation.

6.1.7.2 Functions

Sulfur has several metabolic functions.[17] It is necessary for collagen synthesis and the formation of many mucopolysaccharides. Disulfide linkages, S–S bonds, stabilize the structure of many proteins. Sulfur occurs in reduced form, –SH, in cysteine and is important in the activity of some enzymes. The sulfhydryl group is also able to form high-energy compounds that make it important in the transfer of energy. Sulfur participates in several important detoxification reactions by which toxic substances are conjugated with active sulfate and excreted in the urine. It is part of the vitamins thiamin, biotin, and pantothenic acid, and the cofactor lipoic acid.

6.1.7.3 Requirements

Although it is an essential macronutrient, no quantitative dietary requirement has been specified for sulfur. The major food sources are proteins containing methionine and cysteine. A diet containing 100 g of protein provides 0.6–1.6 g of sulfur, depending on the quality of the protein.

6.1.8 ROLE OF MACROMINERALS AND OTHER FACTORS IN HYPERTENSION

BP is a measure of the pressure of the blood against the walls of the blood vessels produced by the pumping action of the heart. When the BP is measured, two readings are generally taken: systolic and diastolic pressures. The systolic reading indicates the maximum pressure exerted on the arterial walls; this high point occurs when the left ventricle of the heart contracts, forcing blood through the arteries. Diastolic pressure is a measure of the lowest pressure in the blood vessel walls and happens when the left ventricle relaxes and refills with blood. Healthy BP is considered 120 mm Hg systolic and 80 mm Hg diastolic (usually presented as 120/80).

Hypertension is defined as an elevated systolic BP, elevated diastolic BP, or both. It is the most common chronic disorder in the United States, affecting 29% of the adult population. Many people can experience temporary increases in BP, particularly under stressful conditions. Some individuals experience "white coat" hypertension,[84] which refers to an elevated BP value measured in a clinical environment, which is higher than the one obtained outside of this environment. A clinical diagnosis of hypertension is made when the average of two or more readings taken on two or more occasions are consistently elevated above 140/90. For systolic BP, values between 120 and 129 mm Hg are considered normal and between 130 and 139 high normal. For diastolic BP, the corresponding value for normal is between 80 and 84 and high normal is between 85 and 90. BP values ranging from 120 to 139 mm Hg systolic or 80 to 89 mm Hg diastolic are considered prehypertensive.[88] Persons with BP in this range are at increased risk for the development of definite hypertension over time. Most people (90%–95%) suffering from high BP have no identifiable cause for the disorder. This type of high BP is called primary or essential hypertension. Patients have secondary hypertension when a specific cause for elevated BP has been identified; about 5%–10% of the people with hypertension have a secondary cause. Because hypertension is typically asymptomatic and therefore considered a "silent" disease, affected individuals often do not know they have the condition. In fact, about one-third of hypertensive persons are unaware of the disease and only about half of those who are aware achieve adequate BP control. So, hypertension is called a "silent" disease because unless BP is measured periodically, no one knows it is developing. The risk of hypertension increases with age and the prevalence is growing along with the aging population.

High BP is a major health problem throughout the industrialized world because of its high prevalence and association with increased risk of cardiovascular disease, stroke, and renal disease. It can also affect vision, increase mortality, and decrease longevity. Only 47% of adult Americans have optimal or healthy BP. Among adults 50 years of age or older, a much higher proportion have hypertension and a much lower proportion have optimal BP. Hypertension affects an estimated 65 million individuals in the United States and many more worldwide. After smoking, high BP is the leading cause of preventable illness and death. Hypertension is a key factor in heart attacks and strokes, which kill about 850,000 Americans a year.

An individual's BP is influenced by many factors including genetic predisposition, race, body weight, level of exercise, cigarette smoking, insulin resistance, psychological stress, and diet. Some of the factors are discussed below.

6.1.8.1 Genetics

Numerous family and population studies support a significant role for genetic factors. Hypertension in persons younger than 55 years is four times more common in individuals with a family history of hypertension than in those with no family history of it. Estimates of the genetic contribution to BP variation ranges from 30% to 50%. Multiple genes are likely involved, and although the effects of some genes may affect BP independently, most genetic effects involve gene-gene interaction and gene-environment interaction. Hypertension is more common in African Americans[78] than in whites. Compared to Caucasians, African Americans develop hypertension earlier in life and their average BP values become much higher. People who regularly eat foods high in salt are more susceptible to high BP.

6.1.8.2 Renin

Sodium is the main determinant of extracellular fluid volume. When the body contains too much extracellular fluid the arterial pressure rises. The elevated pressure in turn has a direct effect to cause kidneys to excrete the excess extracellular fluid, thus returning the pressure back to normal. Located throughout the vascular system are volume or pressure sensors that detect these changes and send either excitatory or inhibitory signals to the central nervous system and/or endocrine glands to effect appropriate responses by the kidneys.

The renin–angiotension–aldosterone system (RAAS) is a metabolic hormonal pathway that plays an important role in BP regulation and salt and water balance. Decreases in BP and renal blood flow, volume depletion or decreased sodium concentration, and an activation of the sympathetic nervous system can all trigger an increased secretion of the enzyme renin from the juxtaglomerular cells in the kidney. Renin acts on angiotensinogen, a plasma protein synthesized in the liver, and forms angiotensin I. Angiotensin I is converted to angiotensin II by the action of angiotensin-converting enzyme present in the lungs. Angiotensin II is a potent vasoconstrictor and causes a rise in BP. It also triggers the adrenal glands to secrete aldosterone, which causes an increase in the reuptake of sodium by the kidneys, and because water follows sodium, water retention increases as well. All of these processes work to restore BP and volume. The resultant increase in BP results in the suppression of renin release through negative feedback. With sodium restriction, adrenal responses are enhanced and renal vascular responses are reduced. Sodium loading has the opposite effect.

The range of plasma renin activities observed in hypertensive subjects is broader than that in normotensive individuals. Some patients have been defined as having low-renin essential hypertension and others as having high-renin essential hypertension. Approximately 20% of patients with hypertension have suppressed renin activity and higher plasma angiotensinogen levels. This situation is more common in individuals of African descent than White patients.

6.1.8.3 Sodium

There is historical basis for the assumption of a close relationship between salt intake and BP. In the early years of the last century, no measures were available to decrease BP other than a drastic reduction of dietary salt intake. The concept of dietary salt as a major factor in reducing BP gained support from the work of Dahl in the 1950s with a type of rat that was sensitive to salt. Since then an association between dietary sodium and hypertension has been inferred from epidemiological studies, animal experiments, and clinical trials. Data from population surveys are frequently cited as primary evidence for a link between sodium intake and mean arterial pressure. The highest incidence of hypertension occurs in northern Japan, where salt intake may be as high as 20 g/day. A low incidence of hypertension has been found in societies with low salt intake. However, there is substantial disagreement as to how strong this relationship is and whether the data support such an interpretation. This is because the response of BP depends on variables such as genetic susceptibility, body mass, mechanisms mediated by neuronal and hormonal systems, and the kidneys. The most comprehensive study on the role of sodium in hypertension was carried out by the Intersalt Cooperative Research Group, based on 10,079 volunteers in 52 participating centers in 32 countries.

The findings of this group showed a weak positive association between urinary sodium excretion, which reflects salt intake, and BP. Specifically, each 100 mmol sodium (6 g of salt or 2.4 g sodium) per day increase in habitual intake was associated with a 2.2 mm Hg increase in systolic BP. However, the association disappeared when four centers in Brazil, Kenya, and New Guinea were excluded. The population in these specific centers had unusually low salt intakes and BP and differed from the population of industrial countries in many respects.

Evidence from randomized clinical trials has shown that a 4.9 mm Hg reduction in systolic BP and a 2.6 mm Hg reduction in diastolic BP can be achieved with moderate sodium restriction. However, the efficacy of sodium reduction in hypertensive patients varies. Several clinical trials have shown significant BP lowering, but others have shown minimal or no reduction. A recent meta-analysis of 56 trials in hypertensive and normotensive individuals demonstrated only a 3.7 and 1.0 mm Hg reduction in systolic and diastolic BP, respectively, with sodium restriction. Compared with the overall population, diabetics, African Americans, and elderly persons respond best to sodium restriction. African Americans have a higher incidence of salt sensitivity that appears to be caused by racially determined differences in renal handling of sodium.

Although the association between sodium intake and BP is weak, the evidence suggests the general contention that habitual intake of salt is an important factor in the occurrence of hypertension. Taste for salt is acquired and can be modified. On average, Americans consume about 10–12 g of salt per day (2–2.5 teaspoons), about 20 times the requirement of less than 0.5 g/day. Since salt is about 40% sodium, 10–12 g of salt intake is equal to 4–4.8 g sodium per day. Susceptibility to salt-induced hypertension (i.e., salt-sensitive individual) cannot be identified easily for the entire population. Because there is no apparent risk to mild sodium restriction, the most practical approach is to advise mild dietary sodium restriction (up to 5 g salt/day), which can be achieved by eliminating all additions of salt to food that is prepared normally.

Many people are already aware that consuming too much salt has been linked to high BP and have reduced the amount they use in cooking and at the table (saltshaker). The real problem is not that people are overusing the saltshaker. Instead, high levels of sodium (about three quarters) come from processed foods and restaurant meals, and much of the sodium we consume is in foods that do not necessarily taste salty, like packaged bread and chicken dishes. Besides enhancing the taste, salt helps provide texture to many foods and acts as a preservative. Many people have become accustomed to the taste.

The American Medical Association (AMA) is calling for a public awareness campaign about lowering salt in the American diet. They want makers of packaged foods and restaurants nationwide to gradually lower sodium levels in foods by 50% over the next decade. They also have asked the Food and Drug Administration to review food-labeling rules related to sodium and have suggested that food labels start to carry warnings about high-sodium foods. The AMA recommends that any food that contains more than 480 mg of sodium per serving should be considered a high-sodium food. The Centers for Disease Control and Prevention (CDC) estimates that such a reduction in salt could save 150,000 lives and more than $10 billion in health-care expenditures a year. The CDC is urging anyone who has hypertension, is African American, or over age 40 years—nearly 70% of the U.S. population—to follow a stricter guideline of just 1500 mg of sodium a day. A new study shows that physical activity may diminish the negative impact of a high-sodium diet on BP. This is described in the section "Physical Activity."

6.1.8.4　Chloride

Most studies assessing the role of salt on the hypertensive process have assumed that it is the sodium ion that is important. However, some investigators have suggested that the chloride ion may be equally important. This suggestion is based on the observation that feeding chloride-free sodium salts to salt-sensitive hypertensive animals fails to increase arterial pressure. In humans, BP is not increased by high dietary sodium intake with anions other than chloride. These results suggest that chloride may also play a significant role in the hypertensive effects observed with sodium chloride.

6.1.8.5　Potassium

Potassium has been shown to be inversely related to BP.[86] A moderate lowering of BP is seen in humans by increasing potassium in the diet. Also, population surveys have suggested that lower BP values exist in societies where dietary potassium intake is relatively high. In some meta-analyses, dietary potassium supplementation of 50–120 mEq/day reduced BP by about the same amount as salt reduction (by 6 mm Hg systolic and 3.4 mm Hg diastolic). Hypertensive patients should maintain adequate potassium intake (50–90 mmol/day) by adding fresh fruits and vegetables.

6.1.8.6　Calcium

A number of observations in both experimental animals and humans suggest there is an inverse relationship between calcium intake and BP. In addition, analysis of the data collected in a U.S. national survey shows that, as a group, hypertensive adults consume less calcium per day than normotensive adults (573 vs. 897 mg). The association between calcium intake and BP is supported by the findings that in communities with hard water, there is lower cardiovascular mortality and BP. Calcium is the major determinant of water hardness. Evidence from clinical trials on the antihypertensive effect of calcium through dietary intake or supplements has been inconclusive. Although the effect of calcium on BP is still controversial, the fact that a moderately high calcium intake (1.5 g/day) probably also reduces the extent of age-related osteoporosis indicates that it is probably a useful adjunct.

6.1.8.7 Magnesium

Although an inverse association between magnesium intake and BP appears to exist, the role of magnesium in hypertension is not well established. There are no compelling data that recommend increased dietary intake of magnesium for lowering BP.

Preeclampsia is a pregnancy-specific condition, usually occurring after 20 weeks of gestation, consisting of hypertension associated with edema, proteinuria, or both. Women with preeclampsia may develop convulsions, a condition called eclampsia. Eclampsia has a high mortality rate. Women with preeclampsia may unpredictably progress rapidly from mild to severe preeclampsia and eclampsia within days and even hours. Magnesium sulfate has been used for several years as an anticonvulsant to treat preeclampsia and eclampsia, although its mode of action remains obscure. Magnesium sulfate is a potent cerebral vasodilator and increases the synthesis of prostacyclin, an endothelial vasodilator. It also causes a dose-dependent decrease in systemic vascular resistance, which may explain its transient hypotensive effect. Recently, in a large-scale clinical trial, which included 10,000 women in 33 countries, magnesium sulfate given to pregnant women with preeclampsia reduced the risk of eclampsia by 58% compared with a placebo. Magnesium sulfate appears to have an important role in preventing and controlling eclampsia, and the available evidence suggests that it is tolerably safe.

6.1.8.8 Folic Acid

Several studies have examined the role of folic acid in the prevention of high BP and found that it provides some benefit. In the Nurses' Health Study researchers analyzed diet and BP information from more than 150,000 women. None of the women had a history of high BP. Results showed that women aged 27–44 years who got at least 1000 µg a day of folic acid from their diet and supplement were 46% less likely to develop high BP than women who got less than 200 mg/day of folic acid.[82] Women aged 45–70 years who consumed more folic acid had an 18% lower risk of high BP. The beneficial effects of folic acid supplementation were greater among younger women. One possible explanation is that folate is an important cofactor for nitric oxide synthase and subsequent nitric oxide generation.

6.1.8.9 Vitamin D

A growing body of research suggests that vitamin D may also play a role in BP regulation and heart health.[82] It is known that cases of high BP increase during the winter and in places that are farther from the equator—both are situations where a decrease in available sunlight leads to lower vitamin D production. Some studies have found that plasma concentrations of 25-OH vitamin D are inversely associated with the risk for hypertension. Vitamin D supplementation reduces plasma renin activity and clinical as well as epidemiological evidence indicates that the vitamin may reduce BP in humans. More clinical trials are needed to establish whether this vitamin has BP-lowering effects.

6.1.8.10 Vitamin C

Studies show that BP rises as vitamin C depletion[84] occurs in humans and higher vitamin C intakes are associated with lower BP. One recent study of individuals with high BP found that a daily supplementation of 500 mg vitamin C resulted in an average drop of systolic BP of 9% after 4 weeks. One possible explanation: vitamin C helps support the body's production of nitric oxide, which is critical to normal functioning of blood vessels.

6.1.8.11 Chocolate

A study involving clinical trials has shown that eating cocoa-rich foods is associated with an average of 4.7 points lower systolic BP and 2.8 points lower diastolic BP.[87] Subjects were given 100 g/day of dark chocolate, estimated to contain 88 mg flavonols, or 90 g/day of flavonol-free white chocolate for 15 days. White chocolate had no effect on BP. Dark chocolate, but not white chocolate, was also associated with significant reduction in several measures of insulin resistance.

Also, some studies have shown that ω_3 fatty acids, especially docosahexaenoic acid, coenzyme Q10, garlic, celery, and a few others reduce BP. But more studies are needed to confirm the findings.

6.1.8.12 Other Factors

6.1.8.12.1 Calories

Cal intake may be the most important nutritional consideration in the pathogenesis of hypertension. Epidemiological studies demonstrate a clear direct relationship between an increase in body weight and BP. Overweight individuals have increased incidence of hypertension and increased cardiovascular risk. A weight loss as small as 10 pounds of body weight in overweight patients may significantly lower BP. Weight loss is found to decrease the activity of angiotensin-converting enzyme. In overweight hypertensive patients, the clinical data estimate that for every 1 kg of weight that is lost, systolic and diastolic BP is lowered by 2.5 and 1.5 mm Hg, respectively. Weight is potentially the most efficacious of all nonpharmacological measures to treat hypertension. Weight loss also enhances the efficiency of antihypertensive drugs.

6.1.8.12.2 Alcohol

Several large epidemiological studies have found that alcohol consumption may increase BP. Whereas findings at moderate levels of alcohol intake are inconsistent,[85] heavy drinkers consistently exhibit higher BP than nondrinkers. Patients who consume three to four drinks a day experience a 3–4 mm Hg increase in systolic BP and a 1–2 mm Hg increase in diastolic BP compared with those who do not consume alcohol. Alcohol consumption is not recommended for nondrinkers. For drinkers, intake should be limited to 1 ounce of alcohol (2 ounces of 100 proof whiskey, 8 ounces of wine, or 24 ounces of beer per day) in most men and half that amount in most women.

6.1.8.12.3 Physical Activity

Persons who are physically active have been shown to have lower BP than those who are less physically active. At least 30 minutes of moderate-intensity physical activity such as brisk walking, bicycling, or yard work 3 times a week (preferably once a day) can lower BP in both normotensive or hypertensive individuals. Regular exercise can also promote weight loss and overall cardiovascular[79] fitness.

Researchers recently found that the more people exercise the less likely it is that their BP will rise in response to a high-salt diet. The study was done on 1900 men and women (average age 38 years) living in a rural region in China. For one week all participants consumed 3000 mg sodium/day in their diet. The next week they were placed on a high-salt diet—18,000 mg/day. BP readings were taken each day. When switching from a low-sodium to a high-sodium diet, those who experienced a 5% or greater boost in systolic BP (the heart contraction measure represented by the top figure of a BP reading) were deemed "high-salt" sensitive.

Study results showed that compared to sedentary subjects, participants who exercised regularly were less likely to experience heightened BP after consuming a high-sodium diet for one week. The most active individuals had a 38% reduced risk of salt-sensitivity than the least active group. This group was the least likely to see a 5% or greater rise in their BP in response to a high-salt diet. Compared with the most sedentary group, those in the next-to-highest activity group had a 17% lower risk of salt sensitivity, and those in the next-to-lowest activity group had a 10% lower risk.

Engaging in physical activity has a "significant" independent and progressively healthful impact on the degree to which salt sensitivity relates to BP. So the take-home message is, first to encourage people to both lower their sodium intake and increase their physical activity. For those who cannot increase their physical activity because of age or disability, they should still be encouraged to follow a low-sodium diet because sodium has a marked effect on BP.

6.1.8.12.4 Smoking

Smoking is an independent risk factor for coronary heart disease. Although smoking may not be related to chronic alterations in BP, it may interfere with the response to certain antihypertensive drugs. In hypertensive patients, cigarette smoking cessation is probably the most significant and important modifiable risk factor.

6.1.8.12.5 DASH Combination Diet

A few years back, a number of dietary approaches were combined into a single intervention trial called Dietary Approaches to Stop Hypertension (DASH).[77,80] The participants were given a typical Western diet, a diet that was rich in fruits and vegetables (to increase potassium and fiber), or a fruit-and-vegetable diet combined with low-fat dairy products (to increase calcium) coupled with low saturated fat and total fat—DASH "combination" diet. The trial showed BP reduction of 11.4/5.5 mm Hg in hypertensive persons receiving the DASH diet compared with hypertensive patients ingesting a so-called usual American diet, with dietary sodium intake and body weight held constant. Furthermore, the DASH diet produced a reduction in BP of 3.5/2.1 mm Hg in subjects without hypertension. The follow-up study to DASH (DASH-sodium) was recently reported. In this study, the research group found that dietary sodium restriction on top of the DASH combination diet could be even more effective than the DASH diet alone. Results of the DASH-sodium trial confirm the earlier findings that the reduction of dietary sodium has a greater effect on BP in African Americans than in whites, in persons with hypertension than in those with high-normal BP, and in women than in men. The DASH-sodium investigators suggest that a reduction to about 3 g salt per day may be justified to all persons whether they have hypertension or not. This will require cooperation from the food industry because much of the salt in the U.S. diet comes from prepared food, rather than salt added in cooking.

The data from DASH studies provide strong support for a dietary approach to prevent and control mild hypertension. Thus, in well-motivated patients, modifying the lifestyle effectively lowers BP and may be more important than the initial choice of antihypertensive drugs. The same lifestyle-modification strategies that are effective in treating hypertensive patients may also be useful in the primary prevention of essential hypertension.

Lifestyle modifications for prevention and/or treatment of hypertension should include weight reduction, salt restriction, increased intake of fruits and vegetables (potassium), increased intake of low-fat dairy products (calcium), moderation of alcohol consumption, regular physical activity, and cessation of smoking. These are all appropriate measures shown to produce significant reduction in BP while reducing cardiovascular risks.

6.2 ESSENTIAL TRACE ELEMENTS

6.2.1 IRON

There is about 4 g of iron in the body of a healthy adult male and approximately 2.8 g in a female. The iron-containing compounds in the body are grouped into two categories. About 75% of body iron is considered functional. The majority of this is present in the hemoglobin of red blood cells whereas small portions occur in myoglobin, in certain respiratory enzymes that catalyze oxidation–reduction processes within the cell, and in other iron-containing enzymes. The remaining 25% of body iron is stored in the reticuloendothelial system chiefly in the liver, spleen, and bone marrow as storage or nonessential iron. The storage form is present as a soluble iron complex, ferritin, which contains about 20% iron, and as an insoluble iron protein complex, holding about 35% iron. Both forms can release iron as needed.

6.2.1.1 Food Sources

The best food sources of iron (>5 mg/100 g) include organ meats such as liver and heart, brewer's yeast, wheat germ, egg yolks, oysters, certain dried beans, dried fruits (e.g., figs and dates), and green vegetables. Iron, as ferrous sulfate, is added to some foods such as flour. Milk and milk products and most nongreen vegetables are low (<1 mg/100 g) in iron.

6.2.1.2   Absorption

Iron in foods is present as heme iron, which is found in animal products, and nonheme iron, present mainly in plant products. The efficiency of absorption of heme iron is much higher than nonheme iron.[25] Two substances, ascorbic acid and meat, facilitate the absorption of nonheme iron. Ascorbic acid forms complexes with and/or reduces ferric iron to ferrous iron. Meat facilitates the absorption of iron by stimulating the production of gastric acid, which helps reduce ferric iron to the ferrous state. Iron seems to be more readily absorbable in the ferrous state. Absorption takes place chiefly in the upper part of the small intestine. Some foods (e.g., bran, vegetable fiber, and those with phytates, polyphenols, oxalates, taurine, or phosphates) tie iron up so that it is absorbed poorly. Iron uptake is influenced by the amount of storage iron. As stores decrease the amount of iron absorbed increases, and as the stores increase the amount absorbed decreases. This regulatory mechanism in the intestinal mucosa helps maintain iron homeostasis and in large part protects against both iron deficiency and iron overload. It is estimated that in a normal healthy adult, only 5%–10% of the dietary iron is absorbed, but it increases to 10%–20% in iron-deficient individuals.

The regulation occurs primarily at the translational level where the amounts of transferrin, its receptor, ferritin, and the first enzyme of the heme synthesis pathway are regulated by an iron-responsive element (IRE), a stem loop structure 5′ to the coding region of the messenger RNAs for ferritin and transferrin, and in the 3′ untranslated region of the receptor.[27] Binding of a regulatory protein to the IRE in the presence of low intracellular iron decreases ferritin formation. By contrast, in the presence of high intracellular iron, protein binding increases ferritin formation and decreases transferrin synthesis. Increased ferritin formation decreases iron absorption because the incoming iron is sequestered and does not enter the circulation. The iron-containing mucosal cell is then sloughed into the intestine in the normal manner.

Some proteins involved in the regulation of body iron stores through control of iron absorption have been identified. One is HFE, the normal product of the gene *HFE*, which is mutated in most patients with hereditary hemochromatosis (HH; see Section 6.2.1.5). HFE is found in crypt cells in the duodenum, in tissue macrophages, and in Kupffer cells in the liver. Two functions have been suggested for HFE: decreasing iron uptake by binding to transferrin receptor (thereby competing with transferrin) and inhibiting iron release from macrophages. Hepcidin, a 25–amino acid peptide, is believed to be a central regulator of iron homeostasis through its effects on intestinal absorption, macrophage recycling of iron from senescent red blood cells, and iron mobilization from hepatic stores. It is produced in the liver. Its expression is inversely related to both iron absorption and macrophage iron release. But the mechanisms underlying the regulation of body iron absorption and storage are not clearly understood.

Plasma transferrin delivers iron to the cells where cell membrane receptors bind the iron–transferrin complex and carry it into the cells by receptor-mediated endocytosis. There the iron is released. The receptor then returns the apotransferrin to the cell surface for release into the extracellular environment to function once again. In humans, there is no way to excrete excess iron. Less than 1 mg is excreted per day, 67% of it from the gastrointestinal tract as extravasated cells, iron in the bile, and iron in exfoliated mucosal cells. The other 33% accounts for the small amount of iron in desquamated skin and urine.

6.2.1.3   Functions

Hemoglobin is the most abundant of the heme proteins and accounts for 62% of the body iron. It transports oxygen via the bloodstream from the lungs to the tissues. Hemoglobin is a tetramer made of four globin chains, each associated with a heme group that contains one iron atom. Hemoglobin makes up over 95% of the protein of the red cell and accounts for more than 10% of the weight of whole blood. Myoglobin, the red pigment of muscle, has a structure similar to the monomer unit of hemoglobin. It contains one globin chain, one heme group, and one atom of iron. It transports and stores oxygen for use during muscle contraction. Myoglobin accounts for about 8% of the body iron. The myoglobin content of human muscle is approximately 5 mg/g of tissue. Heme iron is also found in the cytochromes that are located in the mitochondria and other organelles. Cytochromes *a*, *b*, and *c* are present within the cristae of mitochondria in all aerobic cells and are essential for the oxidative production of cellular energy in the form of ATP. Cytochrome *c* is made up of one globin chain and one heme group containing one atom of iron. The cytochrome P450s are a family of proteins located primarily in the microsomal membrane and are involved in the oxidative degradation of drugs and endogenous substrates. Cytochrome *b*5 is a component of many membranes.

Other iron porphyrin enzymes include peroxidase, which, in conjunction with hydrogen peroxide, catalyzes the oxidation of certain organic compounds, and catalase, which is involved in the decomposition of hydrogen peroxide. There are also a group of iron-containing enzymes in which iron is not present in the form of heme. These enzymes contain iron–sulfur complexes and include reduced nicotinamide adenine dinucleotide dehydrogenase, succinate dehydrogenase, and other components of electron transport pathways. The enzymes that contain heme and nonheme iron account for about 3% of the body iron. In addition, there are enzymes such as aconitase and phosphoenolpyruvate carboxykinase, which require iron as a cofactor for enzymatic function.

6.2.1.4   Deficiency

Iron deficiency is the most common nutritional deficiency worldwide. Its prevalences are highest in developing countries where 30%–70% of the population may be affected. In comparison, the prevalence of iron deficiency is less than 20% in the industrialized countries of Europe and North America. In the United States, the CDC estimates that the prevalence of iron deficiency is greatest in toddlers 1–2 years of age (7%) and in adolescent girls and women 12–49 years of age (9%–16%).

The body is very efficient in conserving iron supplies. Simple iron deficiency occurs only during the growth period or when intake fails to meet needs after blood loss or in women who have experienced frequent pregnancies in rapid succession. During the deficiency, iron depletion occurs in three phases. In the first phase, there is depletion of iron stores (decrease in serum ferritin) and a compensatory increase in iron absorption, transferrin, and iron binding capacity. This is followed by a phase in which iron stores are exhausted and transferrin saturation is reduced. The amount of heme precursor, protoporphyrin, in erythrocytes increases, but the blood hemoglobin remains near normal level. In the third phase, anemia characterized by a low hemoglobin level develops. In the absence of adequate heme synthesis, there is failure of the cells to grow, and this leads to the production of small cells. Nutritional anemia is characterized by hypochromic and microcytic cells.

In addition to these changes, iron deficiency is associated with a drop in iron-containing enzymes, which play critical roles in cellular metabolism and in the functioning of enzymes that require iron as a cofactor. Evidence of these deficiencies shows up in decreased work capacity and altered behavior such as apathy and irritability.

Hypotransferrinemia, also called atransferrinemia, is a condition in which little or no transferrin is produced. This rare disorder leads to severe iron deficiency anemia that does not respond to iron therapy. Intravenous administration of transferrin normalizes iron kinetics. Individuals with this disorder are susceptible to infection (transferrin inhibits the growth of certain bacteria probably by binding iron required for the growth of these organisms). Patients with a rare congenital defect in the uptake of iron by red cell precursors have normal plasma iron and transferrin levels but have severe hypochromic anemia that does not respond to iron therapy.

6.2.1.5   Iron Overload

There are a number of conditions that cause excessive accumulation of iron in the body. The term *hemosiderosis* denotes an increase in iron storage without associated tissue damage. Hemochromatosis indicates that such damage is present, particularly in the liver, that the iron overload is generalized, and that the amount of iron is generally increased. The best defined is HH, an autosomal recessive disorder caused in most cases by mutation in the *HFE* gene.[26,28] It is characterized by an increase in the rate of dietary iron absorption by the small intestine. People with the disease absorb approximately 3–4 mg of iron per day—compared to the normal rate of 1–2 mg of iron per day. Because the body has no mechanism to increase the excretion of iron beyond that which occurs by normal daily skin desquamation and gastrointestinal and genitourinary tract sloughing, the excess absorbed iron accumulates at a rate of approximately 0.5–1 g per year. During adulthood, total body iron stores in HH patients can reach 20–40 g, compared to a normal value of 3–4 g. The capacity of cells to sequester iron through complexing with ferritin, the major intracellular iron storage protein, is eventually exceeded. This leads to excess intracellular "free" iron.

The onset of clinical signs and symptoms of HH usually occurs in mid to late adulthood and commonly consists of fatigue, malaise, and vague abdominal pain. As the disease progresses, more serious clinical sequelae develop and include gonadal and cardiac failure, diabetes mellitus, cirrhosis of the liver, and arthritis. There is an increased incidence of hepatocellular carcinoma after substantial damage to the liver has occurred.

HH is one of the most common genetic disorders, clinically presenting in men twice as frequently as in women. The reduced clinical presentation in women is thought to be a result of menstrual iron loss and extra iron demands from pregnancy. HH is predominantly a disorder of Caucasians, with a prevalence of 1 in 200–400. The treatment of hemochromatosis involves the removal of excess iron as quickly as possible. Iron is most readily removed by weekly phlebotomy of 500 mL until body stores return to normal as indicated by serum ferritin level. Thereafter, one phlebotomy every 3 months usually suffices to maintain normal iron stores. Patients are advised to restrict intake of vitamin C because it facilitates iron absorption; red meat, a rich source of heme iron; and alcohol.

Repeated transfusion leads to rapid iron loading because each unit of blood contains 200–250 mg of iron and can cause what is known as transfusional siderosis. Reticulendothelial macrophages become iron loaded and, ultimately, iron is deposited in the same sites as in other iron-overload disorders (liver, heart, and endocrine tissues). Cardiomyopathy is more prevalent in patients with transfusional siderosis. Therapy consists of the administration of deferoxamine, an iron-chelating agent, by continuous infusion. The deferoxamine–iron complex is excreted in urine (iron is not normally excreted by this route).

Neonatal hemochromatosis is characterized by iron loading in the liver, heart, and pancreas, and liver failure in the perinatal period. The disease may be associated with metabolic disorders such as hypermethioninemia, but the mechanism is poorly understood. Liver transplantation is the primary treatment but is often unsuccessful. In another disorder, termed *juvenile hemochromatosis*, patients at a young age present with cardiomyopathy and endocrinopathy but not severe liver disease. Patients usually die of heart failure before the age of 30. The genetic basis of this disorder is unknown.

Aceruloplasminemia is a rare autosomal recessive condition caused by mutations in the ceruloplasmin gene. This disorder is distinct from Wilson's disease, in which low serum ceruloplasmin levels result from a copper transport defect. Patients with aceruloplasminemia have low serum iron but have massive accumulation of iron in neural and glial cells of the brain, hepatocytes, and pancreatic islet cells. Treatment with plasma or ceruloplasmin concentrate may be helpful.

Hemosiderosis results when iron is present in excessive quantities in a diet that permits its maximum absorption. A distinct iron-loading disorder is prevalent in Africa, affecting up to 10% of some rural populations. Formerly termed *Bantu siderosis*, iron overload results from ingestion over many years of large amounts of highly bioavailable iron derived from cooking pots and from drinking beer brewed in nongalvanized steel drums. In men, the intake may exceed 100 mg iron per day. The condition frequently becomes manifest in early adulthood and reaches severity after the age of 40. The pathological pattern of the iron overload is one of hepatic and reticuloendothelial involvement. Hemosiderosis can progress to hemochromatosis, cirrhosis, and diabetes. Serious iron overload does not develop in all beer drinkers, and not all patients with iron overload consume excessive amounts of beer. Some investigators have suggested that there is also a genetic predisposition, but the defective gene has not yet been identified.

The production of tissue-damaging free radicals is an essential component of the pathogenesis of chronic diseases, and iron may help form free radicals, resulting in lipid peroxidation, low-density lipoprotein (LDL) oxidation, and DNA damage. Iron overload is associated with a greater incidence of cancer. Patients with HH have 200 times greater risk of hepatocellular carcinoma than those with around normal iron stores. Several studies have suggested that even a modest increase in iron status may be a risk factor for the development of heart disease.[29] Serum ferritin concentration is considered the best measure of body iron stores and is the most feasible to use in epidemiological studies. In a cohort study of over 1900 Finnish men, from 40 to 64 years of age, men with serum ferritin greater than 200 μg/L had a 2.2 times greater risk of myocardial infarction compared to men with lower ferritin levels. Furthermore, serum ferritin was observed to be one of the strongest indicators of the presence and prognosis of carotid artery disease. Blood donations, which deplete iron stores in the donors, were associated with reduced risk of myocardial infarction and cardiovascular disease. In premenopausal women, the incidence of cardiovascular disease is less than half that of age-matched men. Depletion of iron stores by regular menstrual blood loss may be a source of protection in premenopausal subjects.

Excess iron is quite toxic, even to healthy individuals.[30] Ferrous sulfate tablets are a cause of infant morbidity and mortality. Human clinical data support the concept that high iron stores impose additional risk of many types of diseases. Diseases such as Alzheimer's, Parkinson's, and Huntington's have also been associated with the defective regulation of iron in the brain. Iron accumulates in the brain with aging, and evidence suggests that iron contributes to amyloid protein and free radicals that characterize Alzheimer's disease. Elevated body iron stores are associated with insulin resistance, and reductions in iron stores increase insulin sensitivity.

6.2.1.6 Requirements

The RDA for adults is based on the assumption that an adult male must obtain about 1 mg of iron per day to replace body losses, and an adult female must obtain about 1.2–2 mg of iron per day. Because the average amount of absorption is about 10% of ingested iron, it is recommended that men obtain 10 mg and women obtain 18 mg from dietary sources. Iron needs for women are higher than that for men because of menstrual loss and the demands of pregnancy and lactation. During pregnancy, about 300 mg are needed for the growth of the fetus, 70 mg for the placenta, and 500 mg for the synthesis of hemoglobin associated with increase in blood volume that occurs at this time. As a result, it is recommended that pregnant women take a supplement providing 30–60 mg of iron in addition to obtaining 18 mg from the diet. Human milk contains 0.2 μg/mL of iron. Because only 0.5–1 mg is transferred to milk, the recommended intake during lactation is the same as that for women.

6.2.2 Copper

The adult human being weighing about 150 pounds has on average about 80 mg of copper (70–120 mg), with about a third of it evenly divided between the liver and the brain, a third in the muscle, and the rest dispersed in other tissues.

6.2.2.1 Food Sources

The amount of copper in foods of plant origin varies according to the soil in which they are grown, but green leafy vegetables, legumes, whole grain, and almonds are good sources. Raisins and other dried fruits rank fairly high in copper content. Meat, especially liver, and seafoods including shellfish such as oysters are rich in copper, whereas dairy products are low in copper.

6.2.2.2 Absorption

Copper is absorbed from the upper part of the small intestine and possibly from the stomach. Absorbed copper is transported in combination with albumin to the liver where it is incorporated into ceruloplasmin, an α_2-globulin, and released into the blood where it constitutes about 90% of the plasma copper pool. Ceruloplasmin delivers copper to target tissues in the body. One molecule of ceruloplasmin contains six atoms of copper. The major route of copper excretion is via the bile and ultimately the stools. Trace amounts are lost through the urine, hair, nails, sweat, and desquamation of skin. Absorption and excretory processes vary with the levels of dietary copper, providing a means of copper homeostasis.

6.2.2.3   Functions

Several cuproenzymes play critical metabolic roles, including ceruloplasmin, cytochrome c oxidase, lysyl oxidase, superoxide dismutase, tyrosinase, dopamine hydroxylase, and others. Ceruloplasmin is necessary for the oxidation of iron in the plasma for binding to transferrin, and thus it plays a role in the transport of iron to sites where hemoglobin synthesis can occur. Cytochrome c oxidase governs the terminal reaction in the electron transport chain and is essential for energy production. Lysyl oxidase catalyzes the deamination of lysine residues and is the key enzyme for cross-linking in collagen and elastin. When the activity of lysyl oxidase is low, pathological changes in connective tissue occur. This ultimately leads to vascular disease and spontaneous rupture of major vessels, as well as defective bone matrix and osteoporosis. Superoxide dismutase decomposes superoxide free radicals, which can cause membrane damage and cell death. Tyrosinase is important in the formation of melanin, and dopamine hydroxylase participates in the conversion of dopamine to norepinephrine.

6.2.2.4   Deficiency

Deficiency of copper is extremely rare in humans because the amount present in foods is more than adequate to provide the average needs. Copper deficiency has been demonstrated in malnourished infants, in those with prolonged diarrhea or malabsorption disorders, in individuals who have undergone intestinal bypass surgery, and in those who are receiving long-term TPN. Prolonged high doses of zinc can also induce copper deficiency because of the antagonistic relationship between zinc and copper. Excess zinc stimulates the synthesis of intestinal metallothionein, which chelates copper and inhibits its absorption.

The outstanding findings in copper deficiency are leukopenia, particularly neutropenia and granulocytopenia, and microcytic anemia that is unresponsive to iron therapy. Anemia arises from impaired utilization of iron and is, therefore, a conditioned form of iron deficiency anemia. Copper deficiency shortens the life span of erythrocytes. This may be related to the plasma membrane because of free radical accumulation when superoxide dismutase activity is low. Other changes seen in copper deficiency include a fall in serum copper and ceruloplasmin, failure of iron absorption and erythropoiesis, and bone demineralization. Neutropenia and leukopenia are early indications of copper deficiency in children.

There are two hereditary syndromes related to the disruption of copper homeostasis: Wilson's disease[30,31] and Menke's kinky hair syndrome. Wilson's disease is an autosomal recessive disorder of copper metabolism. It occurs in every ethnic and geographical population, with a worldwide prevalence of 1 in 30,000 live births. Patients with this disease have a defect in the ability to excrete copper via the bile. This appears to be a manifestation of a defective gene for ATPase copper transporter ATP7B in the chromosome 13 and results in the accumulation of abnormally high copper, especially in the liver, brain, kidney, and the cornea of the eye. There is a fall in serum copper and ceruloplasmin levels. This suggests that copper incorporation in ceruloplasmin and biliary excretion of copper are both mediated by the same ATPase copper transporter. The incorporation of copper in apoceruloplasmin is defective in Wilson's disease. Excess copper causes cirrhosis of the liver and brain disturbances. A defective metallothionein with an abnormally high affinity for copper may be the cause of the excessive storage of copper in tissues.[32] The extensive cellular damage seen in Wilson's disease may be because of the influence of copper on lipid peroxidation, which would cause damage to lysosomal membranes with the subsequent leakage of acid hydrolases. The disease is usually diagnosed during or after the third decade of life. Patients have a wide range of symptoms including hepatic, neurologic, and psychiatric disorders, as well as renal abnormalities, hematological disturbances, and endocrine dysfunctions. Early treatment with chelating agents such as penicillamine that promote copper excretion is essential to prevent severe tissue damage from copper toxicity. Pyridoxine (vitamin B_6) is usually prescribed concomitantly to counter the deficiency of this vitamin that tends to develop during long-term penicillamine administration. Some individuals are intolerant of penicillamine; side effects include neurotoxicity, hematologic abnormalities, and a distinctive rash on the neck. Other pharmaceutical agents are available. Triethylene tetramine hydrochloride is a suitable alternative chelating agent with somewhat less significant side-effect profile.

Oral zinc acetate has proved highly effective in Wilson's disease, the mechanism of which involves induction of metallothionein synthesis in intestinal epithelial cells. Increased metallothionein synthesis results in greater binding of dietary copper and decreased absorption. Zinc therapy has particular value in young presymptomatic patients, in patients who are pregnant, given the possible fetal teratogenic effects of other compounds, and as a maintenance therapy for patients after their initial "decoppering" is accomplished. Zinc acetate has minimal side effects. The only drawback to its use is the relatively long term (4–6 months) required for the maintenance of proper copper balance.

Tetrathiomolybdate forms a stable complex with protein and copper. It decreases copper absorption and reduces circulating free copper. It is fast acting and restores copper balance within weeks compared with several months required with other copper chelators or with zinc. Another consideration for patients with Wilson's disease is dietary restriction of shellfish and liver, both copper-rich foods.

Menke's kinky (steely) hair syndrome is an X-linked disease of male infants with onset in early infancy.[33] The prevalence of the disease is 1 in 300,000 live births. It is characterized by low serum copper and ceruloplasmin levels and low copper level in the liver and brain but markedly elevated cellular copper in the intestinal mucosa. The defect is a failure to transport copper to the fetus during development as well as a failure to absorb copper from the gastrointestinal tract. It is caused by mutations in the copper transporter ATP7A gene. The loss of protein activity blocks the export of dietary copper from the gastrointestinal tract and causes copper deficiency associated with Menke's disease. Infants have retarded growth and defective keratinization and pigmentation of the hair. Brain tissue is practically devoid of cytochrome c oxidase. The defect is in the transport of copper from the intestine into the blood. Intestinal cells absorb copper but are unable to release it into circulation. Parenteral administration of copper results in transient improvement, but a deficit in neurological tissue continues and infants experience cerebral degeneration and generally do not survive past infancy. The disease is usually recognized by the unusual (steely) texture of the hair and by a severe delay in development.

6.2.2.5 Requirements

There is no RDA for copper, but the 1989 revision established the estimated safe and adequate dietary intake for copper at 1.5–3 mg/day. This guideline represents a range of intake below which the copper in the diet might be considered inadequate and above which one would risk possible toxic accumulation. The recommendation for infants and children is 0.08 mg/kg/day. The actual amount in the adult diet is estimated to be about 1–1.5 mg/day.

6.2.2.6 Toxicity

Copper is toxic to humans only when it is ingested as the copper ion. It acts as an inhibitor of several enzymes. As little as 20–40 times the usual intake of copper causes mild to fatal signs of poisoning in experimental animals. In humans, 10–30 mg of orally ingested copper as ionic salts or from food stored in copper vessels has been reported to cause intestinal discomfort, nausea, vomiting, dizziness, and headaches. Copper toxicity occurs in Wilson's disease.

Copper Deficiency—A Case

A girl was born with the megacystis microcolon intestinal hypoperistalsis syndrome. She required TPN because of ineffective gastrointestinal function. On the second day after birth, a tube jejunostomy was created for drainage, and TPN was started. Her maintenance TPN contained only iron and zinc as trace elements. She had been well maintained until 9 months of age, when her legs became partially flexed in a frog-like position. Her right thigh was swollen, with limited range of motion because of pain. A radiograph revealed scurvy-like changes in the long bones. Her serum vitamin C was normal. Laboratory analysis showed that her serum copper level was 24 µg/dL (normal, 70–130 µg/dL) and ceruloplasmin level was 13 µg/dL (normal 20–45 mg/dL). Her white blood cell count was 1900/mm^3 (normal 6000) with neutropenia.

Intravenous copper was started at a dose of 410 µg/day. A significant elevation in the white blood cell count was observed on the fifth day of the treatment and she was relieved of pain on motion in the extremities and her serum copper and ceruloplasmin levels returned to near-normal levels. Several other cases of copper deficiency have been reported in children and adults. A 51-year-old nurse on TPN for 9 months developed neutropenia, anemia, and low levels of serum copper and ceruloplasmin. Another patient, a 68-year-old woman who was maintained on TPN developed severe anemia and neutropenia after receiving TPN for 2.5 years. Her serum copper and ceruloplasmin levels were low. The administration of copper led to a rapid improvement in anemia and neutropenia in both patients.

Copper deficiency has been demonstrated in infants and adults receiving prolonged TPN.[92,94] Anemia and leukopenia have been noticed in these patients. Copper deficiency in infants demonstrates an additional complication of severe bone demineralization (role of lysyl oxidase in cross-linking of collagen). Infants are more susceptible to severe copper deficiency than adults. Copper accumulates in the fetal liver late during gestation. Milk is very low in copper, so these liver stores are needed during the first months after birth. Because bile is a major excretory pathway for copper, the requirement of copper is increased in people with jejunostomies, or external biliary drainage. Supplemental copper is usually not required if TPN is limited to less than 4 weeks but should be considered for patients receiving long-term TPN.

6.2.3　ZINC

Zinc is a ubiquitous component of animal and plant tissues. The adult human body contains about 2–2.5 g of zinc with about 70% concentrated in the bone. The neonate contains up to 140 mg of zinc at birth. On average, most organs have zinc levels of 20–30 µg/g of wet tissue. Bone contains about 200 µg/g and muscle has about 50 µg/g. High zinc contents have been noted in ocular tissues, seminal vesicles, epididymis, prostate, and semen. Ocular tissues and the prostate gland have 600–800 µg/g. Human blood contains 7–8 µg/mL, of which 70%–85% occurs in red blood cells, 3% in white blood cells and platelets, and the remainder in the plasma. Zinc occurs in proteins and metalloenzymes in all three blood fractions.

6.2.3.1　Food Sources

Good dietary sources of zinc are meat, poultry, eggs, and seafood. Oysters are the richest sources of zinc. Cereals and legumes also contain significant amounts of zinc, but because of the presence of phytic acid in these foods, zinc is less available than that supplied by foods of animal origin.

6.2.3.2　Absorption

About 40% of dietary zinc is absorbed, primarily in the small intestine, although the segment where the absorption is optimal is not known. Intestinal absorption is enhanced by pregnancy and corticosteroids and is diminished in the presence of dietary phytates, phosphates, iron, and copper. Zinc is translocated across the cell membrane against a concentration gradient by a carrier-mediated system and enters the intracellular zinc pool. It is postulated that the absorption is facilitated by binding to a substance such as picolinic acid, citric acid, or an as yet unidentified compound. Prostaglandin E2 also binds zinc and may facilitate its absorption.

Homeostatic regulation of zinc appears to be related to the synthesis of intestinal metallothionein, a cysteine-rich protein that can bind zinc, copper, and other divalent cations. The release of zinc from the intestine to the portal circulation increases when the intestinal metallothionein concentration is low, as seen in zinc deficiency. On the other hand, metallothionein in the intestinal cell increases when zinc intake is high or during fasting. Dietary and hormonally induced factors may be responsible for regulating the amount of intestinal metallothionein and hence the zinc uptake or release by intestinal cells. This mechanism appears to allow for efficient regulation of zinc transfer to the circulation.

Metallothionein has more affinity for copper than zinc, and this is the reason for the copper deficiency in individuals ingesting excess zinc. Daily zinc supplements have been found to be of benefit in alleviating excess copper accumulation in patients with Wilson's disease. Copper absorption is inhibited because it remains bound to metallothionein.

Zinc is transported from the intestine into portal circulation, bound to albumin, and is concentrated in the liver. It is then distributed to the extrahepatic tissues via plasma. About 67% of the zinc in plasma is loosely bound to albumin and is considered to be the principal metabolically active fraction. A portion is bound to the α_2 macroglobulin, the transferrin, and the amino acids cysteine and histidine. The fraction bound to amino acids determines the amount that is filtered by the kidney. The normal route of excretion is via the gastrointestinal tract originating from the pancreatic, biliary, and mucosal secretions. A small fraction (about 400–600 µg) of zinc is normally excreted daily in the urine.

6.2.3.3   Functions

Zinc is essential in the composition or function of over 70 enzymes involved in digestion and major metabolic pathways. It is part of carbonic anhydrase, which is present in erythrocytes in very high concentration, and many other tissues also exhibit this enzyme activity. Without this enzyme, carbon dioxide elimination cannot take place with sufficient rapidity to sustain life; hence, this enzyme is as important to CO_2 transport as hemoglobin is to oxygen transport. As part of carboxypeptidase, zinc plays a role in protein digestion. As part of alkaline phosphatase, it is involved in bone, heart, kidney, and placental metabolism. Alcohol dehydrogenase, lactic dehydrogenase, glutamic dehydrogenase, and superoxide dismutase are zinc metalloenzymes. Zinc is also required for the proper activity of DNA and RNA polymerases and thymidine kinase. Zinc functions as a cofactor in the synthesis of collagen. Another possible role of zinc is to maintain membrane integrity and function.

It has a role in the synthesis, storage, and secretion of insulin by the pancreatic islet β cells. It is absolutely important for normal spermatogenesis, embryonic development, and fetal growth. Zinc is necessary for the binding of steroid hormone receptors and several other transcription factors to DNA, and thereby plays an extremely important role in the regulation of gene transcription. Zinc binding to certain transcription factors results in the formation of a loop or "finger" in the protein that permits the folded region of genes. Zinc finger motifs require four amino acid residues as ligands (4 cysteinyl or 2 cysteinyl and 2 histidyl residues) per mole of zinc. Several transcription factors have been reported to contain "zinc finger" regions.

Zinc is vital to the proper development and maintenance of the immune system. It performs important functions in basic cellular processes such as DNA replication, RNA transcription, cell division, and cell activation that are indispensable for immunological mechanisms. Without zinc, the body cannot fight off invading viruses and bacteria. Even mild deficiency may increase the risk of infections. Zinc lozenges (13 mg elemental zinc every 2 hours while awake) have significantly reduced the development of colds in some studies but not in others, and meta-analysis of controlled trials has not confirmed the effectiveness of this treatment.[37,38] These discrepancies may be due to formulations of zinc lozenges that seem to influence their effectiveness. Formulations such as zinc aspartate and zinc glycinates bind zinc tightly and do not release zinc ions needed for the beneficial effect. Other forms such as zinc gluconate are found to be effective. But zinc gluconate also may cause nausea and bad taste. Potential for zinc toxicity exists with prolonged use of zinc lozenges.

Pneumonia is a leading cause of morbidity and mortality in children younger than 5 years. In a recent study researchers investigated whether zinc, which is known to boost the body's immune system to infection, would help children aged 2–23 months with severe pneumonia.[35] In Bangladesh 220 children were randomly assigned to receive either 20 mg zinc per day or placebo in addition to standard hospital antibiotics. Those given zinc recovered an average of 1 day earlier, and their average stay in hospital was 1 day shorter. In another study, zinc administered as a therapeutic agent to young children with acute or persistent diarrhea reduced the direction of the diarrhea and was associated with a lower rate of treatment failure or death.

These results suggest that zinc treatment could reduce antimicrobial resistance by decreasing multiple antibiotic exposures and lessening complications and deaths where second-line drugs may not be available.

6.2.3.4 Deficiency

Zinc deficiency can occur as a result of malnutrition or because of gastrointestinal disorders,[39,40,41] renal disease, diabetes, cirrhosis, acquired immunodeficiency syndrome, sickle cell disease, alcoholism, or chronic infection. Zinc deficiency is characterized by low levels of zinc in plasma and hair. Prolonged zinc deficiency in children can result in hypogonadism and dwarfism. This has been described in the Middle East and probably occurs in other parts of the world (including the United States) where the intake of zinc is low and/or the intake of dietary fiber is high. In both children and adults, zinc deficiency results in poor wound healing. Zinc is present in gustin, a salivary polypeptide that appears to be necessary for the normal development of taste buds; thus, zinc deficiency also leads to decreased taste acuity. Other signs of zinc deficiency include depressed immune function, anorexia, dermatitis, alopecia, and altered reproductive performance manifested by congenital abnormalities, poor pregnancy outcome, and gonadal dysfunction. Cornea, the tissue with the highest zinc concentration in the body, is affected by zinc deficiency. Corneal edema occurs and may progress to corneal clouding and opacities.

The decreased acuity of taste and smell and the depressed immune function seen in some elderly populations have been attributed to zinc deficiency. The concentration of zinc in plasma is lower in elderly individuals than in younger subjects; this may be related to a drop in food consumption and a concomitant reduction in zinc intake.

Zinc deficiency has been reported in infants fed formula diets low in zinc content. Premature infants are especially at risk of zinc deficiency because of their rapid growth. The high zinc content of colostrum helps satisfy this need. Infants fed human milk have higher levels of plasma zinc than do infants fed cow's milk despite the fact that human and cow's milk contain similar amounts of zinc. This suggests that zinc in human milk is more available than the zinc in cow's milk. A similar situation exists with iron from the two milks. A more severe zinc deficiency occurs in infants with the rare genetic disease acrodermatitis enteropathica. This disease is transmitted by an autosomal recessive gene and the symptoms usually appear after the infants have been weaned from breast milk. Infants with this disease have a characteristic dermatitis in an acral distribution (face, hands, anogenital areas, and feet), diarrhea, failure to thrive, infection, and, if not treated, death. The disease is due to an abnormality in zinc absorption. The syndrome can be rapidly reversed by simple oral supplementation with zinc in doses 3–4 times the daily RDA.

Patients with major burns suffer acute trace element deficiencies at least partly because of large exudative losses through the burned areas.[36] A deficiency of zinc can exacerbate poor immunity, and burns are the second-leading cause of immune deficiency (after HIV infection). Addition of zinc into a standard enteral formula is associated with a significant decrease in the number of bronchopneumonia infections and with a shorter hospital stay.

Reduced intake of zinc plus inability to store it in the body can lead to prolonged abnormal eating behaviors.[40] Many hospitalized anorexic and bulimic patients are zinc deficient. Zinc is found to enhance the rate of recovery in anorexics by increasing weight gain and improving anxiety and depression.

6.2.3.5   Requirements

Studies in human subjects have demonstrated that normal adults require about 12.5 mg of zinc daily when ingesting a mixed diet. The turnover of body zinc is estimated to be about 6 mg/day. Based on these and other data and the assumption that about 40% of dietary zinc is absorbed, an RDA is established at 15 mg/day for males over 10 years of age and 12 mg for females over 10 years of age (with an additional 3 mg during pregnancy and 7 mg during lactation). The RDA for infants is about 3–5 mg and for the preadolescent it is 10 mg.

6.2.3.6   Toxicity

Zinc is relatively less toxic than other microminerals. Doses up to 200 mg have produced no ill effects. The ingestion of excess zinc resulting from the storage of food in galvanized containers has resulted in fever, nausea, vomiting, and diarrhea. Zinc and copper are mutually antagonistic, and prolonged ingestion of excess zinc may produce evidence of copper deficiency if the copper intake is marginal. To avoid this complication, chronic use of zinc supplements should be limited to 40 mg/day.

6.2.4   COBALT

Cobalt is essential for some species of animals but not for others. For example, cattle and sheep in certain regions develop a peculiar disease characterized by emaciation and anemia while horses grazing on the same land remain healthy. This disease is due to cobalt deficiency and is corrected by the administration of cobalt.

The whole body of a normal adult human contains about 1.1 mg of cobalt. It is not known to concentrate in any organ or tissue, although the liver, kidney, and bones are normally higher in cobalt content than other tissues. Human liver contains about 0.034 μg/g wet weight.

6.2.4.1   Food Sources

The richest food source of cobalt is seafood, which contains 1.56 μg/g wet weight. Other good sources include buckwheat, figs, cabbage, lettuce, spinach, beet greens, and watercress. Dairy products and cereals contain much less. The average intake of cobalt in humans is about 0.3 mg/day. It is well absorbed but most of it, about 0.26 mg/day, is excreted in the urine. It does not accumulate in tissues.

6.2.4.2   Functions

Cobalt is utilized primarily as a component of vitamin B_{12}.[42] Synthesis of vitamin B_{12} by bacteria requires cobalt. In ruminants, this occurs in the proximal part of the intestine from which the vitamin is then absorbed. In other animals and men, however, where the bacterial formation of vitamin B_{12} takes place only in the colon, absorption is minimal. Therefore, to be of nutritional value for humans, cobalt must be ingested as vitamin B_{12}. Humans obtain their requirement of this nutrient largely from animal tissues. If humans have a need for cobalt other than vitamin B_{12}, the requirement is not known. The Food and Nutrition Board has not yet established an RDA for cobalt or presented an estimated safe and adequate daily intake range for humans. Administration of a pharmacological dose (10–15 mg/day) of cobalt, either orally or parenterally, causes polycythemia in animals and humans; other signs include reticulocytosis, elevated number of erythrocytes, and increased hemoglobin levels. This effect is not mediated by vitamin B_{12}. Cobalt may exert this effect by increasing the formation or inhibiting the destruction of erythropoietin secreted by the kidney. It does this in pharmacological but not physiological doses.

6.2.4.3   Toxicity

Several instances of severe cardiomyopathy in heavy beer drinkers have been attributed to cobalt. At one time, 1.2 ppm of cobalt were used to improve the foaming properties of beer; however, the amount of cobalt that would be ingested by someone who drank 12 quarts of beer daily would be 8–10 mg, which is less than the amount of cobalt used in the treatment of anemia. It seems that high cobalt and high alcohol intakes are necessary to induce the distinctive cardiomyopathy, beer drinker's cardiomyopathy, and perhaps a low protein intake or a thiamin deficiency.

6.2.5   Molybdenum

Molybdenum occurs in low concentrations, comparable with those of manganese, in all tissues and fluids of the body. The liver, kidney, adrenal gland, and bone contain the most molybdenum. The adult body contains about 9 mg of the element.

6.2.5.1   Food Sources

The molybdenum content of foods varies greatly within and among the different classes of foods, particularly in relation to the soil type from which they are derived. Foods rich in this nutrient are dairy products, dried legumes, organ meats (liver, kidney), grain products, and some green leafy vegetables. Fruits, berries, and most root or stem vegetables are poor sources.

6.2.5.2   Absorption

Inorganic molybdenum is readily and rapidly absorbed from diets; the hexavalent water-soluble forms, sodium and ammonium molybdates, are particularly well absorbed. After absorption, it is rapidly eliminated via the kidney, which is the major homeostatic mechanism for this element. It exists in blood and urine as the molybdate ion.

6.2.5.3   Functions

Evidence that molybdenum is an essential trace element for humans is based on the fact that it is part of the molecular structure of the flavoproteins, xanthine oxidase and aldehyde oxidase, and the heme protein sulfite oxidase. Aldehyde oxidase oxidizes and detoxifies various purines, pyrimidines, pteridines, and related compounds.[45] The flavoprotein enzyme xanthine oxidase catalyzes the transformation of hypoxanthine to xanthine and of xanthine to uric acid. Sulfite oxidase catalyzes the conversion of sulfite to sulfate. The sulfite is the penultimate product in the pathway of metabolism of sulfur moieties of methionine and cysteine. Molybdenum may possess cariostatic properties because children living in areas where the soil content of this mineral is high have less than average dental decay.

6.2.5.4   Deficiency

There has been no deficiency of molybdenum reported in humans under natural conditions. The only observations in humans have been from patients with an inborn error, sulfite oxidase deficiency, and a patient on TPN. The patients described with the inborn error were newborns who showed congenital abnormalities, feeding difficulties, and failure to thrive; also, urinary excretion of sulfite and thiosulfate excretion was radically increased. The clinical manifestations included neurological disease that caused brain damage and mental retardation; these were accompanied by an abnormal pattern of sulfur excretion in the urine. The pathology of the disease could be either due to the toxicity of sulfite itself or from the abnormal development of the neurological system in the absence of sulfate, a component of sulfolipids and sulfoproteins in the brain and other tissues in the early stages of development.

A 24-year-old patient with Crohn's disease was on TPN for a prolonged period. He developed headache, irritability, lethargy, and coma. A metabolic study on urinary metabolites showed high

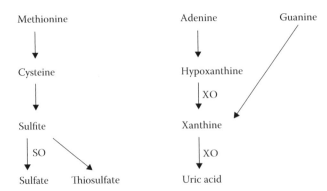

FIGURE 6.1 Catabolism of sulfur-containing amino acids and purines. SO, sulfite oxide; XO, xanthine oxidase.

levels of sulfite and thiosulfate and a low level of sulfate, symptoms of sulfite oxidase deficiency, high levels of hypoxanthine and xanthine, and low uric acid, indicative of xanthine oxidase deficiency (Figure 6.1). Supplementing the TPN with ammonium molybdate (300 μg molybdenum/day) led to a dramatic decrease in the urinary content of abnormal metabolites and improved the clinical condition.

There is a tiny region in northern China called Limxian, which has very low quality soil that is lacking in a number of essential minerals including molybdenum. People living there suffer from a number of deficiencies, one of which is molybdenum deficiency. Symptoms of molybdenum deficiency at that place are mainly cancer related, especially stomach and esophagus cancer.[43] The incidence of cancer is 10 times higher than the average in China and 100 times higher than the average in the United States. It is not clear whether dietary molybdenum supplementation is beneficial in decreasing the risk of cancer.

A study was conducted to see if molybdenum supplementation could correct the high cancer rate. Molybdenum (30 μg/day) and vitamin C (120 mg/day) were given over a 5-year period. There was no decrease in the incidence of gastroesophageal cancer or other cancers.

It is believed that people in that region have increased intake of nitrosamine, which is a known carcinogen. This may be one of a number of dietary and environmental factors that contribute to the development of gastroesophageal cancer in this population. Plants require nitrate reductase, a molybdoenzyme necessary for the conversion of nitrate from soil to amino acids. When molybdenum content of soil is low, plants preferentially convert nitrate to nitrosamine instead of amino acids. This causes increased nitrosamine exposure for those who consume the plants. Adding molybdenum to the soil in the form of ammonium molybdate may help decrease the risk of gastroesophageal cancer by limiting nitrosamine exposure.

6.2.5.5 Requirements

The minimum dietary requirements compatible with satisfactory growth and health cannot be given, and molybdenum deficiency has not been observed under natural conditions. Based on balance studies, the Food and Nutrition Board established that a safe and adequate intake is 75–250 μg/day; the usual daily intake of molybdenum is about 50–350 μg.

6.2.5.6 Toxicity

Molybdenum is relatively nontoxic. More than 500 mg/kg of food or water is required to produce signs of toxicity, which include diarrhea, anemia associated with the failure of red blood cells to mature, and high blood uric acid. There can be a significant increase in xanthine oxidase activity in the blood of some individuals living in high-molybdenum geochemical areas. In this population, uric acid in blood and urine is elevated and the incidence of gout is high. There is physiological antagonism between molybdenum and copper. Studies in humans have shown that urinary copper excretion increases as the dietary intake of molybdenum is increased. High doses of molybdenum have been found to inhibit the metabolism of acetaminophen in rats;[44] however, it is not known whether this occurs in clinically relevant doses in humans.

Molybdenum Deficiency—A Case

A 24-year-old man with Crohn's disease underwent multiple small bowel resections with a resultant small bowel syndrome. He was started on TPN as the sole method of nutritional support. A year later he developed a syndrome characterized by tachycardia, tachypnea, severe headache, nausea, and night blindness, which then progressed to severe generalized edema, disorientation, and coma. Laboratory analysis showed that his plasma methionine was 250 mmol (normal, <55 mmol/L) and uric acid 0.5 mg (normal, 5 mg/dL); his urinary excretion of thiosulfate was high and inorganic sulfate and uric acid was low.

Because the two enzymes involved in the metabolism of sulfur-containing amino acids and purines are both molybdenum-containing proteins, the possibility of molybdenum deficiency was considered. Ammonium molybdate (300 mg/day) was started intravenously. The patient showed improvement in clinical signs. Plasma methionine and uric acid and the excretion of sulfate and uric acid in the urine returned toward normal. This is a classic case of molybdenum deficiency induced by molybdenum-free TPN. Individuals genetically deficient in xanthine oxidase suffer from only mild myopathy secondary to deposition of purine crystals in muscle.

Patients with inborn errors of sulfite oxidase deficiency exhibit severe neurological abnormalities. The main biochemical feature of this disorder is very low to virtual absence of inorganic sulfate in the urine.[89] The mental disturbances and occasional coma observed in this case appear to be related to sulfite oxidase deficiency. It is conceivable that excess sulfite accumulating in the plasma could lead to symptoms by a direct action on the central nervous system. Sulfite may also be converted to hydrogen sulfite, which is extremely toxic (Figure 6.1).

6.2.6 SELENIUM

Selenium occurs in all cells and tissues of the body in concentrations that vary with the tissue and the level and chemical form of selenium in the diet. The liver and kidney usually have the highest concentration with much lower levels in other tissues. Cardiac muscle has consistently higher selenium than skeletal muscle. On the average, the normal adult has about 15 mg of selenium.

6.2.6.1 Food Sources

The level of selenium in individual foods of plant origin is highly variable and depends mainly on the soil conditions under which they are grown. The average selenium content in soil is 1 ppm, but the geographical distribution is uneven. Most areas have an adequate supply, while in some areas the supply is deficient. The northeastern parts of the United States, parts of Canada, China, New Zealand, and Scandinavia are deficient in selenium, whereas Venezuela and parts of Colombia have a high selenium concentration. Fruits and vegetables are generally low in selenium (<0.01 ppm). Grains and cereals reflect the varying selenium concentrations of the soil in which they were grown. Organ meats (e.g., liver, kidney) are good sources (>0.1 ppm). Fish, especially tuna and shellfish, are rich in selenium (5.1–6.2 ppm).

6.2.6.2   Absorption

Selenium is incorporated in foods through proteins containing the selenoamino acids, seleno-methionine and selenocysteine. Selenium supplements are added as inorganic selenium such as sodium selenite. All forms of the mineral are generally absorbed well from the small intestine. After absorption, selenium is bound to a protein and transported in the circulation for distribution to the tissues. The excretion of selenium is largely by way of the kidney, although small amounts can be eliminated in the feces. It is excreted in the urine as trimethyl selenite and in the breath as dimethyl selenide, a volatile compound with a garlic-like odor. The latter appears in the breath only when selenium intake is high and is a sign of selenium intoxication.

6.2.6.3   Functions

Four selenoproteins are known and all contain selenocysteine.[51,52] Glutathione peroxidase prevents oxidative damage by destroying hydrogen peroxide and a variety of other peroxides by using reducing equivalents from glutathione. The other selenoproteins are type I iodothyronine 5'-deiodinase, which is responsible for the production of biologically active triiodothyronine, and selenoproteins[47] P and W. The latter is found in white skeletal muscles and is presumably involved in a selenium-sensitive myopathy of lambs and calves that is associated with skeletal muscle calcification. Selenoprotein P is the major selenoprotein in rat serum and contains about eight selenium atoms per molecule. Selenocysteine is made by way of a phosphoserine tRNA intermediate. The selenocysteine is carried by a specific tRNA, which has an anticodon complimentary to UGA. The secondary structure of the mRNA determines whether the UGA will act as a stop codon or a code for selenocysteine. Selenium also influences the metabolism and toxicity of certain drugs and chemicals. The toxicity of some compounds is enhanced in selenium deficiency. It also appears that this mineral somehow binds with toxic minerals such as arsenic, mercury, and cadmium and renders them less harmful.

Selenium is reported to mimic the action of insulin.[53] Studies have shown that selenium mediates a number of insulin-like actions such as stimulating glucose uptake and regulating metabolic processes including glycolysis, gluconeogenesis, the pentose phosphate pathway, and fatty acid synthesis. Although the exact mechanism of the insulin-mimicking action of selenium has yet to be determined, it is reported that those actions are mediated through the activities of key proteins involved in the insulin-signal cascade. Selenium is also reported to play a role in reducing the oxidative stress associated with diabetes, thereby retarding the progression of secondary complications of diabetes such as neuropathy, retinopathy, and cataracts.

6.2.6.4   Deficiency

There are no clear-cut signs or symptoms of mild-to-moderate deficiency of this essential nutrient in humans, and clear deficiencies have not been seen in the Western population even in low-selenium areas of the United States; however, special diets formulated without selenium have caused deficiency. Several cases of deficiencies have occurred in patients on TPN. The symptoms of deficiencies included chronic muscle pain, elevated plasma enzymes from tissue damage, and abnormal nail beds. Cardiomyopathy and skeletal muscle weakness have been observed in a few patients. Children with inborn errors of amino acid metabolism, who received synthetic diets that were low in selenium, had low plasma selenium and low erythrocyte glutathione peroxidase activity.

Selenium deficiency can be the cause of Keshan disease, an endemic and often fatal cardiomyopathy that affects mainly young children and women of childbearing age. It occurs in a broad zone from northeast to southwest China, known to be very low in this mineral. Although other etiological factors may also be involved, selenium supplementation controls this disease. Epidemiological studies in the low-selenium region of China show that Kashin–Beck Syndrome, a painful inflammatory disease related to arthritis, is also probably caused by selenium deficiency. It seems to be responsive to selenium, but the relationship is less clear than in Keshan disease. Numerous studies suggest that deficiency of selenium is accompanied by the loss of immunocompetence; both cell-mediated immunity and B-cell function can be impaired.

Low plasma selenium levels are associated with lymphocyte infiltration of the thyroid, suggesting a link between selenium and autoimmune thyroid disease. Selenium supplementation offers benefits in patients with autoimmune thyroiditis receiving thyroxine (T4).[54] Controlled clinical trials using selenium (200 µg/day) for several weeks have shown 25%–50% reduction in thyroid peroxidase (an enzyme involved in the iodination of T4 and triiodothyronine) antibody concentration.

Selenium deficiency reduces the activity of the selenium-dependent antioxidant enzyme, leading to a number of functional disorders, including skeletal muscle dysfunction, and increased capillary permeability. Low selenium status has been associated with arthritis. It has also been linked with senility and Alzheimer's disease. Low levels of plasma selenium in HIV/AIDS sufferers have been linked with higher mortality.

Numerous studies[49] have shown an association between high cancer rates and low geographical selenium concentrations in the soil and between low cancer rates and diet rich in selenium. The plasma selenium content of cancer patients is significantly lower than that in healthy persons. Studies have also shown that individuals with the highest plasma selenium levels had a 40% lower risk of colorectal adenoma and 30% lower risk for adenoma recurrence, compared with individuals having the lowest plasma selenium levels.[50] Men who consume high levels of selenium or have high levels of selenium in the body tissues are about half as likely to develop prostate cancer compared with those who have the lowest selenium intake. Data also suggest that selenium supplementation (200 µg/day) may reduce prostate cancer risk.[47]

In one study, a woman receiving chemotherapy for ovarian cancer and selenium supplementation (200 µg/day) had significantly increased white blood cell count, decreased hair loss, abdominal pain, weakness, malaise, and loss of appetite.[52]

A number of epidemiological studies suggest that selenium deficiency is associated with increased risk of developing heart disease. Research has shown that lower antioxidant status is linked to higher incidence of cardiovascular disease due to increased levels of LDL oxidation. Selenium as part of one of the antioxidant enzymes may help inhibit LDL oxidation. There is an inverse correlation between the plasma selenium and severity of atherosclerosis.

6.2.6.5   Requirements

Researchers in China determined the dietary selenium intake needed to prevent Keshan disease; they found that the disease was absent in areas where the dietary intake averaged 19 and 14 µg/day for a man and a woman, respectively. They also estimated what they called the "physiological selenium requirement" based on saturation of plasma glutathione peroxidase activity. Individuals ingesting 40 µg/day or more of this nutrient were found to have similar enzyme values. In 1989, the Food and Nutrition Board adjusted the physiological requirement values obtained in China to account for differences in body weight and incorporated an appropriate safety factor. The RDAs for selenium of 70 and 55 µg/day were suggested for men and women, respectively. The RDA values for younger age groups were extrapolated downward on the basis of metabolic body size.

6.2.6.6   Toxicity

Supplementation with selenium must be done carefully. The element is toxic in large doses, and the range between deficiency and toxicity is small. The mechanism of toxicity is not known, but it may interfere with sulfur metabolism. The upper limit of the safe intake is 200 µg/day. Excessive selenium produces cirrhosis of the liver, enlargement of the spleen, gastrointestinal bleeding, and depression.

Fatal Cardiomyopathy—A Case

A 42-year-old man with Crohn's disease who was receiving home parenteral nutrition (HPN) as the only nutritional support for about 10 years was admitted to the hospital with severe chest pain and dyspnea. During the 3 days following admission, his symptoms of congestive heart failure and compensated metabolic acidosis persisted despite aggressive treatment. A normal serum albumin, calcium, magnesium, potassium, phosphorus, and other tests excluded the common nutritional cardiomyopathy. On day 6, the patient developed increased ventricular irritability and refractory ventricular fibrillation and died.

At autopsy, all chambers of the heart were dilated and the myocardium was grossly flabby. Samples of the liver, heart, and kidney were obtained. These tissues along with plasma taken on the day of admission were analyzed for several parameters, including selenium. Extremely low concentrations of selenium (5%–12% of normal) were found in all samples.

This is a case of fatal cardiomyopathy, secondary[90,93] to selenium deficiency, developed on a long-term HPN program. Similar complications have been described in other patients on TPN for 2–8 years. It is not possible to predict the onset of cardiomyopathy or other less severe adverse effects of selenium deficiency. Therefore, it is recommended that patients on long-term HPN and hospitalized patients receiving extended TPN be monitored for selenium deficiency and given supplements if necessary.

6.2.7 MANGANESE

A normal 70-kg adult contains about 12–20 mg of manganese. This relatively small amount is distributed throughout the tissues and body fluids. The highest concentration occurs in the bones, liver, and pituitary gland (2.5–3.3 µg/g) and the lowest in muscle (0.04–0.18 µg/g). Manganese levels in plasma are very low, ranging from 0.4 to 1 ng/mL. The concentration of manganese is greater in tissues rich in mitochondria because manganese is more concentrated in mitochondria than in the cytoplasm. There is little variation in the content of manganese with age. In contrast to several other essential trace metals, the fetus does not accumulate manganese in the liver and fetal concentrations are significantly lower than in adults.

6.2.7.1 Food Sources

Grains, cereals, fruits, and vegetables are good sources of manganese whereas dairy products, meat, poultry, and fish contain very little. Tea is the richest source of manganese.

6.2.7.2 Absorption

Manganese is poorly absorbed from the gastrointestinal tract. Only about 3% is absorbed in healthy individuals. Factors that have been reported to have detrimental effects on absorption include iron, calcium, fiber, phytates, and sugar. After absorption, it is transported to the liver where a small portion is bound to a specific carrier protein, transmagnamin. The primary route of excretion is in the bile and a little appears in the urine. In spite of the small amount of manganese in tissues, its concentration is accurately controlled primarily by promoting the elimination of the excess metal from the body by a dose-dependent biliary excretion.

6.2.7.3 Functions

Manganese is a component of pyruvate carboxylase, which contains four moles of manganese per mole of enzyme, and superoxide dismutase in mitochondria, the cellular organelle that contains the highest concentration of manganese.[55] Superoxide dismutase is one of the body's main defenses against free radicals. Manganese is required for the activation of glycosyl transferases that catalyze the synthesis of glycosaminoglycans and glycoproteins; it is also a cofactor for a number of enzymes such as arginase. Manganese is necessary for normal skeletal and connective tissue development. A relationship with stress and mood alteration has been suggested because the manganese concentration in tears is 30 times greater than that found in plasma.

6.2.7.4 Deficiency

Although manganese is essential, a deficiency has not been reported in the free-living human population. One possible and unsubstantiated case of human deficiency may have occurred when manganese was inadvertently omitted from the vitamin K–deficient, purified diet that a patient received as a volunteer. The clinical signs in this patient included weight loss, transient dermatitis, nausea and vomiting, slight reddening of the hair, and slow growth of hair. These symptoms responded to manganese supplementation. More recently, young adults fed a manganese-deficient diet for 5 weeks developed a finely scaling, minimally erythematous rash. The rash was diagnosed as miliaria crystallina, a condition in which sweat cannot be excreted through the superficial epidermis because the sweat gland openings are occluded by alterations in the stratum corneum. This results in small, clear blisters filled with fluid. The dermatitis observed in these experimentally induced deficiencies suggests a requirement of manganese for the activity of enzymes necessary for the maintenance of skin integrity. Manganese-dependent glycosyltransferases function in the synthesis of mucopolysaccharides of collagen in the skin and other tissues.

Other findings in this study were a decline in total and high-density lipoprotein and serum cholesterol and an increase in serum calcium, phosphorus, and alkaline phosphatase. The increase in plasma calcium and phosphorus suggests that stores of manganese in the bone are mobilized as a consequence of manganese deficiency. Dissolution of bone to release manganese would also release calcium and phosphorus in blood. Similar increases of plasma calcium and phosphorus are seen in manganese-deficient rats. This suggests that manganese deficiency can be a contributing factor for osteoporosis.

Women suffering from osteoporosis have low levels of plasma manganese. In one study, researchers gave women with osteoporosis a supplement that included manganese, along with a number of other minerals. The women given this supplement experienced less bone deterioration than the women who received just a calcium supplement. The researchers could not definitely say, however, that manganese was responsible for this positive effect.

Those who suffer from epileptic seizures typically have lower levels of manganese in their blood and brain than those without epileptic seizures. However, it is not known whether there is a direct relationship between epileptic seizures and manganese deficiency. There is a need to determine whether correcting manganese deficiency can be of benefit to patients with seizures.

6.2.7.5 Requirements

The exact human requirement for manganese is not known. Balance studies have shown that 1–2 mg is required to maintain equilibrium. The estimated safe and adequate range recommended by the Food and Nutrition Board is 2–5 mg/day for adults; infants and children require 0.3–3 mg, depending on age. Various dietary components affect the bioavailability of manganese. Factors that have been reported to have a detrimental effect on either the absorption or retention include iron, calcium, fiber, phytate, and sugar. For example, the consumption of three bran muffins per day produced a negative manganese balance despite the dietary intake of about 13.9 mg/day.

6.2.7.6 Toxicity

In contrast to other trace elements, manganese has a low toxicity. Intakes of greater than 1 mg/g of food are needed to produce toxic signs. The few cases of poisoning reported have been the result of ingesting megadoses of vitamin/mineral supplements for several years or the result of industrial exposure to dust. Chronic poisoning appears mainly in miners working either in manganese mines or in ore-crushing mills. The mineral enters the body by inhalation of the dust in the air. Toxicity produces dementia and a psychiatric disorder resembling schizophrenia, followed by neurological changes similar to those of Parkinson's and Wilson's diseases. Manganese has been shown to interfere with iron absorption. On the other hand, iron deficiency leads to an increase in manganese absorption. Thus, iron deficiency can make an individual vulnerable to manganese toxicity, whereas manganese exposure might induce anemia by inhibiting iron absorption.

Manganese Deficiency and Osteoporosis—A Case

A professional basketball player decided to go on a "bizarre" macrobiotic diet. Several months later, he was having problems with broken bones that would not heal. Extensive laboratory tests showed that his serum manganese level was zero, and calcium and phosphorus levels were elevated. This young man had an osteoporosis-like disease.[91] Fortunately, diet changes and mineral supplements brought speedy improvement.

Interest in this case led to experimental studies in rats. It was found that the rate of bone resorption in manganese-deficient animals was slowed and the rate of bone rebuilding was slowed even more. The net result was loss of bone mass. Meanwhile, data accumulated in Belgium revealed that the average serum manganese level of postmenopausal osteoporotic women was 25% as much as that of age-matched normal women. These two studies provide concrete evidence that manganese plays a key role in bone development.

Surveys suggest that U.S. women consume on average less manganese than the 2–5 mg/day considered safe and adequate. People who are dieting to lose weight or who are vegetarians should consider taking a vitamin–mineral supplement that includes trace amounts of manganese.

6.2.8 Iodine

The total amount of iodine in the body of an average adult is about 20–50 mg distributed as follows: muscle, 10%; skin, 10%; skeletal structures, 7%; thyroid, 20%; and the remaining 13% is scattered in other endocrine organs and the central nervous system. The concentration of iodine in the thyroid gland is more than 100 times that in the muscle and 10,000 times that in the blood.

6.2.8.1 Food Sources

Generally, vegetable products are low in iodine because the iodine content of a given plant food depends on the type of soil, and the soil usually contains little of this element. Seawater contains iodine, and when the sea spray is deposited on coastal regions, it enriches the soil and the drinking water with this element. Vegetables grown in these regions take up iodine from the soil, and the inhabitants of coastal areas get this element from drinking water and vegetables as well as from seafood, which is the only rich source of iodine. The amount of iodine in dairy products, meat, and eggs is generally good but depends on the composition of animal feed.

6.2.8.2 Absorption and Metabolism

Iodine occurs in foods primarily as iodide, but also in lower amounts as inorganic iodine or as an organically bound complex. Most, but not all, organically bound iodine is freed and reduced to iodide prior to absorption. Thyroxine and triiodothyronine are largely absorbed without degradation. The iodide is rapidly absorbed by the stomach and the upper part of the small intestine. Once absorbed, the iodide appears immediately in the bloodstream where it constitutes the major part of the iodide pool, all in the extracellular space. About 33% of the absorbed iodide is selectively taken up by the thyroid gland. The remaining 67% is usually taken up by the kidney for excretion in the urine, and this provides protection against the accumulation of toxic levels of this element in other tissues.

The uptake of iodide from the plasma across the thyroid cell membrane is an active process against electrical and concentration gradients. The normal concentration of iodide in the thyroid cell is several times higher than that of the plasma. Thyroid-stimulating hormone (TSH) of the pituitary gland stimulates the uptake of iodide into the thyroid, in direct response to the plasma levels of thyroid hormone.

Once in the thyroid, the iodide ion is oxidized to free iodine, the reaction being catalyzed by a specific peroxidase in the presence of hydrogen peroxide. The free iodine rapidly iodinates position three of the tyrosyl group of the protein thyroglobulin to form monoiodotyrosine (MIT) and subsequently iodinates position five to form diiodotyrosine (DIT). The coupling of two forms of iodinated tyrosines then takes place. Two DITs couple to form T4 with the release of alanine, and one MIT and one DIT couple to form triiodothyronine (T3). The two forms of the hormone, T3 and T4, still bound to thyroglobulin, are stored in the bound form, and the thyroid may contain 2 weeks' supply of the hormone.

Secretion of the hormone follows proteolytic degradation of the thyroglobulin. The hormones T3 and T4 are secreted into the bloodstream and largely bound to a carrier protein. Iodine metabolism is controlled primarily by a biofeedback system, which includes the thyroid itself and the pituitary through TSH.

6.2.8.3   Functions

Iodine is an integral component of the thyroid hormones T3 and T4. These hormones stimulate cell oxidation and play a major role in regulating the basal metabolic rate of the adult and the growth and development of the child. Iodine is present in high concentrations in the ovary and some other tissues, but so far as is known the entire functional significance of iodine is accounted for by its presence in the thyroid hormone.

6.2.8.4   Deficiency

Worldwide, the soil in large geographic areas is deficient in iodine. Twenty-nine percent of the world's population, living in approximately 130 countries, is estimated to live in areas of deficiency.[57] Those who consume only locally produced foods in these areas are at risk for deficiency. In the United States and in a number of other nations iodine consumption is mainly through iodized salt.

Over the last decade salt consumption in the United States has significantly decreased due to concerns over high BP. About 45% of American households buy salt without iodine, which grocery stores also sell. Most of the ingested salt (approximately 70%) in the United States comes from processed food that is typically not iodized in the United States and Canada.

Another source of iodine used to be commercially baked bread. Iodine was used as a dough conditioner in making bread, and each slice of bread contained 140 μg of iodine. In the early 1980s, bread makers started using bromide as a conditioner instead of iodine. Iodine was also more widely used in the dairy industry 30 years ago than it is now. These small changes caused Americans to consume less iodine.

The U.S. National Health and Nutrition Examination surveys (NHANES) have demonstrated that the median urinary iodine (UI) excretion fell from 320 μg/L to 145 μg/L, a decrease of more than 50%, between the early 1970s and the early 1990s.[58] The NHANES of 2001–2002 and 2003–2004 showed that the median UI excretion has stabilized.

The majority (>90%) of dietary iodine absorbed in the body appears in the urine. The UI concentration is an indicator of the adequacy of iodine intake. Thus, UI is recommended for assessing recent dietary iodine intake worldwide. The criteria for iodine deficiency has been established by the World Health Organization (WHO) stating that the median UI concentration in a population should be >100 μL/L (corresponding to daily intake of 150 μg/day) and ≤20% of the population should have UI concentration of <50 μg/L. Median levels of UI of 0–19 μg/L, 20–49 μg/L, and 50–99 μg/L indicate severe, moderate, and mild iodine-deficient populations, respectively. Table 6.3 shows the relationship between UI, iodine intake, and iodine status. A minimum of approximately 70 µg of iodine is needed to produce T3 and T4 in the thyroid gland each day. But more than that is required because iodine—whether ingested or released from T3 and T4—is rapidly excreted in the urine.

The WHO estimates that approximately 2 billion people, including 285 million school-age children, still have iodine deficiency.

If there is iodine deficiency or the availability of iodine is low for a prolonged period of time, the thyroid gland attempts to compensate for the deficiency by increasing its secretory activity. This causes the thyroid to enlarge (hypertrophy) to the point where a large nodule is visible in the neck, a condition known as simple or endemic goiter (Figure 6.2). The deficiency of the hormone causes accumulation of mucinous material under the skin, which presents a coarseness of features giving the characteristic appearance of myxedema. Goiter is one of the most frequent diseases of the endocrine system throughout the world, and it can be prevented by an intake of iodide. This may be accomplished by adding inorganic iodides to table salt (in ratios of about 1:5000 to 1:200,000).

Iodine deficiency in infants and children is associated with an endemic goiter[60] called cretinism. It is characterized by a wide range of clinical abnormalities including mental retardation and biochemical signs related to the impairment of the central nervous system and thyroid function. Clinical signs observed in infants include large birth size, subnormal temperature, lethargy, thick, dry skin, and an enlarged tongue. Recognition of the syndrome in the first weeks of life is essential

TABLE 6.3
Relationship between Iodine Intake, Urinary Excretion, and Iodine Nutritional Status

Urinary Iodine Excretion (µg/L)	Iodine Intake (µg/day)	Iodine Status
<20	<30, insufficient	Severe deficiency
20–49	30–74, insufficient	Moderate deficiency
50–99	75–49, insufficient	Mild deficiency
100–199	150–299, adequate	Optimal
200–299	300–449[a], more than adequate	More than adequate
>299	>499[b], excessive	Possibly excessive

[a] Risk of iodine-induced hyperthyroidism within 5–10 years following introduction of iodized salt in susceptible individuals.

[b] Risk of adverse health consequences; iodine-induced hyperthyroidism and autoimmune thyroid disease.

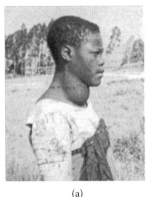 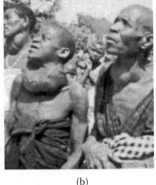

(a)   (b)

FIGURE 6.2   (a) A simple goiter in a young woman. (b) Advanced modular goiter in an endemic area in Tanzania. (Courtesy of Shari Roehl, Pharmacia & Upjohn Co.)

to minimize mental retardation. The cause of the deficiency in the fetus and the newborn is low iodine intake during pregnancy by the mother.[62]

Iodine deficiency is the most preventable cause of mental retardation in the world,[61,62] Some researchers estimate that 15% of women in the United States have moderate iodine deficiency that may be linked to breast cancer. Now, nearly 1 in 7 women will develop breast cancer. That number was 1 in 20 30 years ago, when iodine consumption was high. Women with goiter due to iodine deficiency have a three times greater incidence of breast cancer. The incidence of breast cancer is high in the United States and low in Japan. The diet in Japan is rich in iodine. Japan has the lowest incidence of iodine deficiency, goiter, hypothyroidism, and breast cancer. Iceland, another high iodine intake country, has low rates of goiter and breast cancer. It has been suggested that iodine impacts breast health by making estrogen receptors in the breast less sensitive to estrogens. Systematic studies are needed to determine the beneficial effects of iodine against breast cancer.

Iodine deficiency can also occur despite adequate intake. Some foods contain substances that block the transport and utilization of iodine by the thyroid. These substances are known as goitrogens. Cabbage and similar species of the Cruciferae family contain glucosinolates, which are degraded to thiocyanate, a goitrogen, during digestion. Cassava, a staple source of carbohydrates for many people in tropical countries, contains cyanogenic glycosides that release cyanide, which is subsequently converted in the body to thiocyanate. Phenolic derivatives present in peanuts are also active goitrogens.

6.2.8.5   Requirements

The 1989 RDA is 40–120 μg for infants and children up to the age of 10 years old, and 150 μg for older children and adults. An additional 25 and 50 μg are recommended during pregnancy and lactation, respectively. To ensure adequate dietary intake, it is advisable to use iodized salt. The current level of enrichment of iodine in table salt is 76 μg/g of salt. The average use of 3.4 g of enriched salt per person per day would supply a daily intake of approximately 200 μg of iodine.

6.2.8.6   Toxicity

Iodine in large amounts (more than 50 mg/day) disturbs all thyroid functions, starting from the transport of iodine and continuing to the synthesis and secretion of thyroid hormone; thus, iodine in excess works like a goitrogen and can cause "iodine goiter." Excess amounts of iodine can also cause acne-like skin lesions or can worsen preexisting acne of preadolescents or young adults. Lododerma is the term used for nodular, ulcerating, pustular, or fungating lesions that occur on the skin of some individuals after long-term ingestion of iodides (usually from expectorants). Similar signs are also seen in those who eat kelp (seaweed), sold in health food stores as a dietary supplement. The iodine content of kelp is high.

6.2.9   CHROMIUM

Chromium is widely distributed throughout the human body in low amounts without special concentration in any known tissue or organ. There is a progressive decline in the tissue levels of this metal with age, at least in the United States, as measured in the liver and other organs (except lungs). Chromium is the only heavy metal to show a continuing decrease in tissue levels throughout life. The total body content of this mineral in the adult at the age of 30 is estimated to be 6–10 mg. The tissues of human infants contain higher amounts of chromium than adults. These levels decline rapidly in the first decade of life. The hepatic chromium in children less than 10 years of age is about 10 times that of adults 30 years old.

6.2.9.1   Food Sources

The best food sources of chromium include brewer's yeast (but not torula yeast), some spices (e.g., black pepper), shellfish (especially oysters), eggs, meat products, cheeses, whole grain, and unrefined brown sugar. Vegetables are poor sources of available chromium.

6.2.9.2 Absorption

Chromium in diets is available in two forms: a highly absorbable organic form and an inorganic form that is poorly absorbed (i.e., <1%) regardless of the chromium status of the individual. After absorption from the intestine, trivalent chromium binds to transferrin, which is involved in the transport of chromium to body tissues. It is excreted primarily in the urine, with small amounts lost in hair, perspiration, and bile.

6.2.9.3 Functions

The primary role of chromium appears to be in the maintenance of normal glucose tolerance.[64] In its biologically active trivalent state, it forms complexes with organic compounds that are important for biological activity. One such complex, glucose tolerance factor (GTF), has been identified in brewer's yeast as a complex of trivalent chromium, nicotinic acid, glutamic acid, glycine, and a sulfur-containing amino acid. GTF is believed to be the compound through which the effects of chromium are mediated. It may be involved in the binding of insulin to insulin receptors. It is hypothesized that chromium is mobilized into plasma from body stores in response to a glucose challenge and acts along with insulin in glucose metabolism. It appears that chromium in the form of GTF forms a complex between insulin and insulin receptors and facilitates the interaction of insulin with tissues; thus, it may potentiate insulin action.[65,66]

Recently, studies have begun to reveal the mechanism of chromium's actions. Research has suggested that after chromium is released from transferrin, it binds to an oligopeptide in order to become biologically active. The chromium peptide complex binds to the insulin receptor and increases the activity of the insulin receptor tyrosine kinase, thereby amplifying insulin action. Recent reports also indicate that chromium works by increasing the presence of insulin-responsive glucose transporter (GLUT4) to the plasma membrane.[65]

Chromium has a possible role in regulating lipoprotein metabolism. Chromium supplementation in normal and hyperlipidemic individuals decreases plasma triglycerides and cholesterol and increases high-density lipoprotein cholesterol. Epidemiological evidence points to low serum chromium as a risk factor for the development of coronary heart disease.

Analysis of the chromium content of adult male aortas indicates that Americans have 35% as much of this element as Africans, 17% as much as that of Near East Asians, and only 13% as much as the residents of the Far East. The three populations with which Americans are compared exhibit a far lower incidence of coronary heart disease. It is possible that these populations take a higher amount of chromium in their daily diet than Americans.

6.2.9.4 Deficiency

Plasma chromium decreases during pregnancy, with increasing age, in insulin-dependent diabetes, and in protein Cal malnutrition. The most common situation in which a deficiency can appear is in patients receiving TPN. The deficiency signs in a patient on TPN for 3 years were glucose intolerance, peripheral neuropathy, and metabolic encephalopathy. The symptoms were not improved with increased caloric intake or with the administration of 45 units of insulin per day. Supplementation with 250 μg/day of chromium for 2 weeks led to lowering of plasma glucose, weight gain, and reversal of the diabetes-like symptoms. The 45 units of exogenous insulin were no longer needed. Similar symptoms were reported in another patient on TPN for months. In this case, 150 μg/day of chromium chloride (trivalent chromium) was administered intravenously and within 4 days the blood glucose levels were normal, the encephalopathy cleared, and the patient began to gain weight. The AMA has recommended supplementation of TPN with 10–15 μg of chromium per day for stable adults.

Chromium supplementation appears to improve glucose utilization and to decrease exogenous insulin requirements in some diabetics. In some cases, it also leads to improved glucose tolerance in normal subjects, children with protein-Cal malnutrition, the elderly, and subjects with marginally elevated blood glucose.

6.2.9.5 Requirements

The amount of chromium ingested daily by adults is about 0.05–0.12 mg. An RDA intake for chromium has not been established, partly because there is not sufficient information on which to base a recommendation. A normal, healthy adult loses about 1 μg of chromium daily in the urine; the dietary intake of chromium needed to replace this loss ranges from 4 μg of GTF chromium in brewer's yeast (as much as 25% of this form may be absorbed) to 200 μg of chromium from inorganic salt (less than 1% of this form is absorbed). In the 1989 revision, the Food and Nutrition Board established a safe and adequate intake of 50–200 μg/day for healthy adults.

6.2.9.6 Toxicity

It is unlikely that individuals will get too much chromium in their diets because only minute amounts of the element are present in most foods, and trivalent chromium, the form found in foods, is poorly absorbed. Toxicity is almost exclusively from the hexavalent form of chromium. Poisoning is limited to accidental ingestion of chromic acid or chromates. Toxicity to the kidney, liver, nervous system, and blood are major causes of skin allergies, ulceration, and bronchial asthma.

6.2.10 FLUORIDE

Fluoride has been detected in trace amounts in all organs and tissues of humans, but studies have demonstrated that where diets are high in fluoride, its concentration in the body increases. On average, the adult human contains less than 1 g of fluorine, approximately 99% of which is in the bones and teeth. The concentration in soft tissues is normally low and does not increase with age.

The understanding of fluoride's role in tooth decay prevention got its start in 1901, when a young dental school graduate named Frederick S. McKay decided to open a practice in Colorado Springs, Colorado. When he arrived, McKay was astounded to find scores of townspeople with brown stains on their teeth. At the same time, he later learned, the mottled teeth were surprisingly resistant to decay. McKay's quest to determine the cause of staining ended three decades later with the discovery that the town's drinking water had high levels of naturally occurring fluoride.[68,71]

Subsequent research determined that water fluoride levels below 1 ppm prevent decay without the attendant staining. In a trial launched in 1945, Grand Rapids, Michigan, became the first city to fluoridate its water; 11 years later, the benefits of the practice were clear and widespread fluoridation began. Knowledge about the benefits of water fluoridation led to the development of other modalities for delivery of fluoride, such as toothpastes, gels, mouth rinses, tablets, and drops. Several communities in Europe and Latin America have added fluoride to table salts.

6.2.10.1 Food Sources

Fluoride is ubiquitous, occurring in minute amounts in all foodstuffs and water supplies. The content of foods varies widely and is affected by the fluorine content of the air, soil, and/or water in the environment in the areas in which they are produced. The fluoride content of vegetables grown in areas with water fluoridation is often 3 or 4 times higher than that in areas where fluoride is not added. Nevertheless, some foods contain more fluoride than others. Vegetables, meat, cereals, and fruits contain about 0.2–1.5 ppm; seafood has about 5–15 ppm, and tea has about 75–100 ppm. A cup of tea supplies approximately 0.1 mg of fluoride.

6.2.10.2 Absorption

The availability of fluoride in foods is generally lower than in water. Soluble fluoride is rapidly and almost completely absorbed through the stomach and the small intestine, even at higher intakes. The less-soluble sources of fluoride (e.g., bone meal) are poorly absorbed. Absorption is considered to occur by passive diffusion. The second most common route of absorption is by way of the lung. Pulmonary inhalation of fluoride present in dusts and gases constitutes the major route of industrial exposure. It enters the circulation and is rapidly distributed throughout the body as fluoride ion.

About 50% of the absorbed fluoride is taken up readily by bones and teeth where it becomes an integral and important component. The other 50% is excreted in the urine within 24 hours. Regardless of the amount ingested, blood levels of fluoride remain amazingly constant because of the ability of the kidneys to excrete amounts in excess of the body's needs.

6.2.10.3 Functions

Fluoride may not be, in the strictest sense, an essential trace element. It does, however, produce documented positive effects on skeletal and dental health, and it is certainly biologically active. Fluoride ions at a proper level assist in the prevention of dental caries (tooth decay; Figure 6.3). When children under 9 years old consume drinking water containing 1 ppm of fluoride, there is less dental caries in childhood, adolescence, and throughout life. This has led to the fluoridation of water supplies in many countries. Thus, it is reasonable to classify fluoride as an important ingredient in the diet on the basis of its proven beneficial effect on dental caries.[68]

The mechanism by which fluoride increases the resistance of the teeth to decay is not fully understood, but it appears that crystals of fluoroapatite can replace the crystals of hydroxyapatite normally deposited during tooth formation. Fluoroapatite in tooth enamel is apparently less soluble in acid and more resistant to the cariogenic action of acids in the oral environment. The fluorine content of the outer layer of the enamel may be more than 20 times that found in the inner layers where caries activity is less likely to be initiated. The levels of fluorine in both the outer and inner layers of the enamel are considerably lower when fluoridated water is not available. Fluoride may

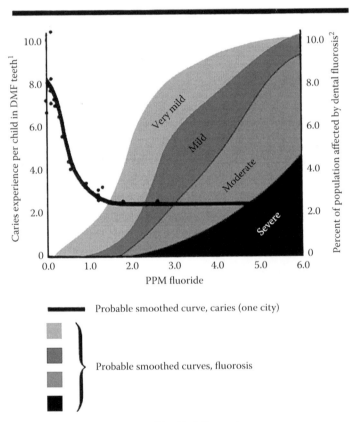

Probable smoothed curve, caries (one city)

Probable smoothed curves, fluorosis

1. Data from Dean, H. T. 1945. New York Symposium.
2. Data from Dean, H. T. 1954. *Int Den J* 4:311–37.

FIGURE 6.3   Dental caries and dental fluorosis in relation to fluoride in public water supplies. DMF, decayed, missing, and filled. (Courtesy of Shari Roehl, Pharmacia & Upjohn Co.)

exert a protective effect on teeth by inhibiting the formation of acid by bacterial enzymes in the plaque on the teeth of persons receiving fluoridated water. A proper intake of fluoride is essential for maximum resistance to dental caries, a beneficial effect that is particularly evident during infancy and early childhood and which persists through adult life.

Laboratory and epidemiological research suggests that fluoride prevents dental caries predominately after eruption of the tooth into the mouth, and its actions primarily are topical for both adults and children. These mechanisms include inhibition of demineralization, enhancement of remineralization, and inhibition of bacterial activity in dental plaque. Fluoride enhances remineralization by adsorbing on the tooth surface and attracting calcium ions present in saliva. Fluoride also acts to bring the calcium and phosphate ions together and is included in the chemical reaction that takes place, producing a crystal surface that is much less soluble in acid than the original tooth mineral. Fluoride from topical sources such as fluoridated drinking water is taken up by cariogenic bacteria when they produce acid. Once inside the cells, fluoride interferes with enzyme activity of the bacteria and the control of intracellular pH. This reduces bacterial acid production, which directly reduces the dissolution rate of tooth mineral.

The prevalence of dental caries declined in the United States during the second half of the last century even in communities without fluoridated water. This trend has been attributed to the availability of fluoride through foods and beverages processed in areas with fluoridated water and the widespread use of fluoride toothpaste. Despite the beneficial role of fluoride, 8 of the 50 largest cities in United States and several smaller cities have not instituted fluoridation. This may be because the voters in these places rejected fluoridation in their public water supplies. There are persons who make unsubstantiated claims about the adverse health effects of fluoride. Therefore, fluoridation can become a political issue. There is also expense for fluoridation, and the per capita cost may increase especially in smaller communities.

There is evidence that the ingestion of fluoride at the relatively high level of up to 8 ppm during adult life gives protection against osteoporosis in later life with no adverse effects. Fluoride stimulates osteoblast activity and can replace hydroxyl ions in the hydroxyapatite structure of bone. This substitution results in bone with increased crystalline size but decreased elasticity and quality. Increased retention of calcium accompanied by a reduction in bone demineralization has been observed in patients receiving fluoride salts. This suggests that dietary fluoride is essential for optimal bone structure and prevention of osteoporosis in men. Fluoride alone or in combination with vitamin D and calcium currently is used therapeutically in the treatment of metabolic bone disease on the premise that fluoride promotes positive calcium balance and causes remineralization of the skeleton.

6.2.10.4 Water Fluoridation

Water fluoridation is the controlled addition of fluoride to a public water supply to reduce tooth decay. The deliberate addition of fluoride into drinking water has been a controversial topic for decades. Some claim it does little or nothing to prevent tooth decay and is dangerous for health.[70] Others, including most dentists and public health officials, say it significantly lowers rates of tooth decay and presents no health risks. Fluoride has both beneficial and adverse effects on dental health. While the prevalence of dental caries is inversely related to a range of concentrations of fluoride in drinking water consumed, the prevalence of dental fluorosis has been shown to be positively related to fluoride intake from many sources.

Epidemiological investigation of patterns of water consumption and the prevalence of dental caries across various U.S. regions with different water fluoride concentrations led to the development of a recommended optimum range of fluoride concentration of 0.7–1.2 mg/L; the lower concentration was recommended for warm climates where the water consumption is higher, and the higher concentration was recommended for colder climates. The safe upper limit was set at 4 mg/L.

About 171 million people in the United States (61.5% of the U.S. population) drink fluoridated water. In addition, 200,000 people live in places where water has fluoride levels of at least 4 mg/L and an additional 1.4 million live where the concentration is about 2 mg/L. Most are in South

Carolina, but there are thousands in Texas, Oklahoma, and Virginia as well. Fluoride levels of as high as 4 mg/L are caused by natural rock and soil formations, not by the addition of fluoride to water. Water fluoridation has been listed as one of the 10 great public health achievements in the twentieth century in the United States.

Between 1950 and 1980, clinical studies in 20 different countries demonstrated that the addition of fluoride to community water supplies reduces caries by 40%–50% in primary (baby) teeth and 50%–60% in permanent teeth. Health and dental organizations worldwide have endorsed fluoride safety and effectiveness. An estimated 12 million in Western Europe and 355 million worldwide (5.7% of world population) receive artificially fluoridated water. In addition, at least 50 million people worldwide drink water that is nationally fluoridated to optimum levels. In some locations, notably parts of Africa, China, and India, natural fluoridation exceeds recommended levels.

Bottled water can have fluoride. U.S. regulations for bottled water do not require declaring fluoride content, so the effect of always using bottled water is not known.

Some organizations and individuals are opposed to water fluoridation. They are concerned that the fluoride intake cannot be easily controlled and that children may be more susceptible to health problems. As with other drugs fluoride carries side effects and risks beyond the proclaimed benefits. For this reason consumers should have the right to choose whether to undergo treatment. They feel that fluoridation of public drinking water constitutes nonconsensual mass medication of the populace and therefore presents an ethical as well as public health issue. They feel that there is no need for fluoride to be ingested since other alternatives are available for its delivery to the teeth. Tooth decay rates have dropped at the same rate in countries with or without water fluoridation. Studies indicate fluoride's potential to cause a wide range of adverse systemic effects. In recent years, when towns and cities across the country have held voter referenda on fluoridation, its use has been rejected more than half the time.

In 2006, a 12-member panel of the U.S. National Research Council (NRC) reviewed the health risks associated with fluoride in water. They unanimously concluded that the maximum amount of fluoride the Environmental Protection Agency allows in nation's drinking water (4 mg/L) can cause health problems and "should be lowered." The limit was previously 1.4–2.4 mg/L, but it was raised to 4 mg/L in 1985.

On average, about 10% of children exposed to 4 mg/L level develop severe dental fluorosis. Children who drink water at a level of 2 mg/L are at risk of a less severe form of dental fluorosis. At the level used in fluoridated water, decreased bone fractures are expected, but the NRC found the overall evidence suggestive but inadequate for drawing firm conclusions about the risk or safety of exposure at 2 mg/L. But the report states that fractures do seem to increase as fluoride is increased from 1 mg/L to 4 mg/L, suggesting a dose-related adverse effect of lifetime exposure. The report discusses a number of other adverse health effects that may be associated with excessive fluoride exposure.

Fluoride has a suppressive effect on the thyroid gland. Doses of 0.03–0.14 mg/kg/day are known to relieve hyperthyroidism. The effect of fluoride is more severe when iodine is deficient and fluoride is associated with lower levels of iodine. Thyroid effects in humans are associated with fluoride levels 0.05–0.13 mg/kg/day when iodine intake is adequate and 0.01–0.03 mg/kg/day when iodine intake is inadequate. Its mechanism and effects on the endocrine system remains unclear.

Epidemiologic studies have noted a correlation between increased fluoride and low IQ.[69] The most rigorous of these studies compared an area with mean fluoride water concentration of 0.36 mg/L to an area with 2–47 mg/L. The NRC speculates that effects on the thyroid could lead to poor test results. The committee expressed concern about the effect of fluoride on IQ, noting that the "consistency of study results appears significant enough to warrant additional research" on the question of IQ. IQ deficits, the committee noted, have been strongly associated with dental fluorosis. But the existing data are "not adequate" to say for sure whether fluoride can impair IQ.

Kidney patients and diabetics are at special risk from fluoridated water because they tend to drink more liquid than healthy individuals. Chronic ingestion in excess of 12 mg/day is expected to cause adverse effects and an intake that high is possible when fluoride levels are around 4 mg/L.

A separate study concludes that fluoride raises the risk of osteosarcoma, a rare bone cancer, especially in boys. The risk of osteosarcoma among boys drinking water with 0.5 mg per liter fluoride was estimated to be five times as great as among boys drinking nonfluoridated water. At 1 mg or more, the risk was an estimated seven times as high. But because only about 400 cases of the disease are diagnosed annually in the United States, the absolute risk of the disease remains very low.

In 1997, the Institute of Medicine set a safe upper limit of 0.7 mg of fluoride per day for children under 6 months of age. According to the Environmental Working Group in 25 of the 28 largest cities in the United States, at least 15% of formula-fed infants are exposed to excess levels of fluoride, mostly from tap water used to make infant formula.

A study was done in Canada that measured the fluoride content of bones in Toronto, where drinking water is fluoridated, and Montreal, where it is not. The study found that the average level of fluoride in bone is 1033 ppm in Toronto and 645 ppm in Montreal. The Toronto bone samples had altered architecture, which decreased their resistance to compression, and higher density but less mineral that increased their brittleness. In Toronto, moderate dental fluorosis was seen occurring at rates as high as 30% in some fluoridated communities.

Dental fluorosis[72] is the first visible sign of fluoride overdose. During the years 1999–2002, CDC conducted the NHANES, which found a 9% higher prevalence of dental fluorosis in American children than was found in a similar survey 20 years ago. The 1999–2002 survey found an overall rate of 32% among U.S. school children aged 6–19 years. This compares to an incidence of 22.4% reported in the 1985 survey. According to the latest information reported by CDC, March 2007, 41% of children aged 10–15 now have some form of fluorosis, whereas 36% of children 16–19 years old have fluorosis. Moderate and severe fluorosis was observed in less than 4% of both age groups.

A 35-year-old woman who drank water with 1.9 mg/L level fluoride developed a subtle form of skeletal fluorosis that doctors initially suspected to be a form of "seronegative" arthritis. Seronegative arthritis refers to a form of arthritis that mimics the symptoms of rheumatoid arthritis (RA) but lacks autoantibodies diagnostic of RA. In this case, the woman presented with joint pain involving the lower back, both heels, and the knee, for the past 3 years. In addition to these symptoms she suffered from gastrointestinal disturbances prompting the doctors to suspect the possibility of enteropathic arthritis—a form of arthritis associated with inflammatory bowel disease.

The doctors finally began to suspect the role of fluoride after X-rays revealed increased bone density in the pelvic area and calcification of some ligaments. There was slight elevation of fluoride in blood. The patient was diagnosed to have skeletal fluorosis.

Another study at Mayo Clinic suggested similar cases of fluorosis may be occurring in the United States among habitual tea drinkers. A woman was diagnosed to have fluorosis. She was taking several cups of tea every day. She took steps to reduce tea intake, which led to improvement of symptoms.

Fluoride intake at moderate levels is known to strengthen teeth, but views have changed on how best to get it. Scientists used to believe that the benefits occurred mostly when people ingested fluoride and it circulated in blood. New studies suggest that topical exposure (through toothpaste, gels, and fluoride applications at a dental office) is equally good. Some countries that were using fluoridated water have discontinued. These countries include Finland, Germany, Japan, the Netherlands, Sweden, Switzerland, Czechoslovakia, and Russia. The change was probably motivated by public opposition to water fluoridation and/or because the need for water fluoridation was met by alternative strategies. Some use fluoridated salt, milk, toothpaste, gel, and mouthwash. A rough estimate is that an adult in a temperate climate consumes 0.6 mg/day of fluoride in places where water is not fluoridated and 2 mg/day with water fluoridation.

6.2.10.5 Deficiency

Fluoride has not yet been proved to be an essential trace element for humans, but areas with low fluoride content of water supplies have high rates of dental caries. Also, there is an indication that a deficiency of fluoride results in increased incidence of osteoporosis in the aged.

6.2.10.6   Requirements

There is insufficient data to establish an RDA for fluoride, but the Food and Nutrition Board established a safe and adequate daily intake of fluoride for seven age categories. These range from 0.1–0.5 mg/day for infants up to 6 months old to 1.5–4 mg/day for adults. A water supply containing 1 ppm fluoride can provide 1–2 mg/day depending on the amount of water and liquids (e.g., coffee, juices) consumed. Fluoridation of the water supply is the simplest and most effective method of providing dietary fluoride. Different forms of fluoride (e.g., sodium fluoride, sodium silicofluoride, and fluorosilicic acid) have all been used effectively to provide fluoride ions in the water supply. For persons who do not have access to a community water supply that is fluoridated, 2-mg tablets of sodium fluoride are available, which release 1 mg of fluorine. The well-documented protective effect of fluoride against dental caries occurs only at a daily dietary intake of 1.5 mg/day or more. Intakes above 2.5 mg/day in children cause some mottling of the teeth. Adults living in areas where the drinking water contains more than 4 mg/L enjoy some protection against osteoporosis.

6.2.10.7   Toxicity

Fluoride has a small range of safety, yet the range is wide enough that the normal fluctuation in the fluoride content of foods poses no risk of excessive intake. Acute toxicity can occur following the ingestion of larger quantities of soluble fluoride compounds such as sodium fluoride. Intakes in the range of 1–5 mg/kg body weight produce gastrointestinal distress lasting for a few hours. A lethal dose is approximately 2–5 g of soluble fluoride. Fluoride inhibits a large number of enzymes and diminishes tissue respiration and anaerobic glycolysis. The latter effect is due to the inhibition of enolase, which catalyzes the conversion of 2-phosphoglycerate to phosphoenolpyruvate.

The major manifestation of chronic ingestion of excessive amounts of fluoride is dental fluorosis and osteosclerosis. In those localities where the fluoride concentration is relatively high, it usually has deleterious effects on the teeth. This is most evident in permanent teeth that develop during high fluoride intake. If fluoride is ingested in toxic quantities during childhood while the teeth are undergoing calcification, characteristic signs appear. Instead of the normal glistening translucent appearance, patches or even the entire surface of the teeth may look dull and chalky. This is called dental fluorosis (Figure 6.4). Pitting—the result of the breaking off of the ends of the enamel prisms—is a common occurrence. The teeth may also have brown mottling. The problem occurs only when a high amount of fluoride is ingested during tooth development and cannot occur afterward; however, even severely mottled teeth are resistant to dental caries. As the level of fluoride content increases, the severity and extent of mottled enamel increase until at levels of 8–10 ppm in community water almost all individuals who grow up in the area have disfiguring mottled enamel. In some countries (e.g., India) where, in certain regions, unusually large amounts of fluoride are consumed, the mineral can cause endemic skeletal fluorosis (i.e., the density and calcification of bone are increased). This type of fluoride intoxication results from the ingestion of 10–25 mg fluoride per day for 10–20 years.

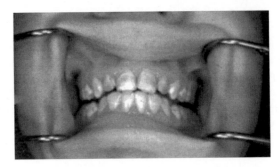

FIGURE 6.4   Moderate fluorosis shown as mottling of the permanent teeth. This 14-year-old drank well water containing 5.5 ppm of fluoride from birth (5.5 × optimal level). (Courtesy of Shari Roehl, Pharmacia & Upjohn Co.)

It is thought to represent the replacement of hydroxyapatite by the denser fluoroapatite, but the mechanism of its development is not known. The degree of skeletal involvement varies from changes that are barely detectable radiologically to marked thickening of the cortex of large bones and calcification of ligaments and tendons. In its severest form, it is a disabling disease and is designated as crippling skeletal fluorosis.

6.3 ULTRATRACE MINERALS

6.3.1 SILICON

Silicon is present in all cells of the body in varying amounts, the concentration being between 3 and 60 μg/g wet weight. Higher concentrations are found in the connective tissues such as aorta, trachea, tendon, bone, skin, and its appendages. Among the foods, barley and oats have high contents with 2610 μg and 4310 μg/g, respectively, whereas fruits, meat, fish, and dairy products contain considerably less. Silicon enters the alimentary tract from the foods as monosilicic acid, as solid silica, and in organically bound forms with pectin and mucopolysaccharides. It appears to be well absorbed. Even over a wide range of intake, the concentration in blood remains relatively constant at not more than 1 mg/dL. It is excreted easily in both stools and urine.

6.3.1.1 Functions

Silicon appears to be necessary for calcification, growth, and in mucopolysaccharide formation as a cross-linking agent.[73] It accumulates in high concentration in the line of ossification of new bone together with increasing calcium content. There is also high silicon content within the mitochondria of the bone-forming osteoblasts. In whole cells the calcium to silicon ratio is approximately 5:1, whereas the concentration of silicon within the mitochondria exceeds that of calcium. It is present in high concentration in mucopolysaccharides and collagen and a portion is bound so tightly that it can be hydrolyzed only by strong acid or alkali treatment. This lends support to the postulate of a strong, possibly regulatory role of silicon in the formation of connective tissue matrix and subsequent calcification.

6.3.1.2 Deficiency

In experimental animals deficient in silicon, there is reduction of glycosaminoglycans in cartilage and the collagen concentration in the bone is decreased. Deficiency of this nutrient has not been produced in humans; however, the silicon content of aorta decreases from a high of about 205 μg/100 mg tissue nitrogen in infants to 86 μg/100 mg in persons aged 40 years. The atherosclerotic process itself is associated with a decline in the silicon content of the vessels; normal arteries contain 180 μg/100 mg nitrogen, whereas those with moderate pathology have 105 μg/100 mg and severely sclerotic arteries have 63 μg/100 mg.[76] The human requirement for this trace mineral is not known.

6.3.1.3 Toxicity

A common nondietary form of silicon toxicity is a lung condition known as silicosis because of the inhalation of airborne silicon oxide dust. The amount of silicon in blood and urine increases in silicosis. Silicon does not appear to be toxic in the levels usually found in foods.

6.3.2 NICKEL

Nickel is distributed throughout the body without particular concentration in any tissue and does not accumulate with age in a particular tissue or organ other than the lungs. The total amount of nickel in an adult body is estimated to be about 10 mg.

6.3.2.1 Food Sources and Absorption

Nickel occurs mainly in foods of plant origin. Cereal grains (especially buckwheat, oats, and rye) and vegetables are good sources, whereas foods of animal origin contain little of this element. The average daily intake in the American diet is 0.3–0.6 mg of which 5%–10% is absorbed by the small intestine. The level of nickel in human serum is about 2.6 (1.4–4.6) μg/L. A small amount of nickel is ultrafilterable, with the remainder present in nearly equal proportions bound to albumin and to the α_2 macroglobulin, nickeloplasmin. The nickel content of sweat is surprisingly high, 49 μg/L, which is about 20 times the nickel concentration in blood serum.

6.3.2.2 Functions

The physiological function of nickel is not quite clear. There is some evidence that it plays a role as an activator of arginase and DNAase and helps maintain the conformation of membranes. It is firmly associated with DNA and RNA and may help maintain their structure. Clear signs of deficiency of this element have been described in at least six different species. These signs include impaired growth and hematopoiesis and changes in the levels of iron, copper, and zinc in the liver.

Little is known about the role, if any, of nickel in human metabolism, but based on animal data, it is reasonable to postulate that this element is required by humans. Abnormal serum concentrations occur in several diseases in man. Serum nickel is elevated to about twice the normal in the 12–36 hours after the onset of symptoms in patients with myocardial infarction (5.2 μg/L). The source of this increase and its cause are unknown. Nickel in cardiac muscle, even if completely released and distributed solely in the serum, is insufficient to account for the hypernickelemia. It could possibly come from other organs such as the liver and lungs. It rises also following acute stroke and severe burns. Significantly diminished mean concentrations are found in patients with hepatic cirrhosis (1.6 μg/L) and chronic uremia (1.7 μg/L). Patients with acute myocardial ischemia without infarction and acute trauma exhibit normal levels. During pregnancy, especially in the third trimester, the serum level of this element is significantly less. A greater than 15-fold increase occurs 5 minutes after delivery and returns to normal level within an hour. The transient hypernickelemia may be important to the separation of the placenta.

6.3.2.3 Requirements

A dietary requirement for adults, extrapolated from animal data, is about 30 μg/day, and a good mixed diet should supply these needs. No nickel-deficiency state has been observed, but it could become a concern in malabsorption disease. Nickel is generally nontoxic.

6.3.3 BORON

Boron is of nutritional interest because there is evidence of its essentiality for higher plants. It is inevitably a constituent of the tissues of animals and men that consume plants. It is distributed throughout the tissues and organs of humans at concentrations of about 0.5–1.5 ppm (dry basis) in soft tissues and several times these levels in bone. Approximately 48 mg is present in the human body.

Foods of plant origin, especially fruits, leafy vegetables, nuts, and legumes, are rich sources of this element. Wine, cider, and beer also have a high content of boron. The boron in food, sodium borate, and boric acid is rapidly and almost completely absorbed and is distributed in tissues and organs. It is then excreted largely in the urine.

Several experiments have been performed to produce boron deficiency in rats but without much success. One group has reported that chicks with a deficiency of this element show depressed growth; eventually, boron may be found essential for animals and men.

The precise biochemical role, if any, of boron is not known at the present time. Some human studies suggest that this element influences mineral metabolism via a regulatory role involving a hormone at the cell membrane[75] level. Supplementation with 3 mg boron in postmenopausal women causes a marked increase in their serum levels of 17-β-estradiol and testosterone and a decrease in their urinary excretion of calcium and magnesium. The increase in the steroid concentration in serum is of significance because 17-β-estradiol is the most biologically active form of human estrogen, and testosterone is its precursor.

Estrogen administration is an effective way to slow down the loss of calcium from bone that occurs after menopause. Boron may be one of the important nutritional factors that can prevent or slow down osteoporosis by maintaining a relatively high serum estrogen level.

The deficiency of boron has not been reported in humans, but based on the studies that show positive effects of this element on mineral metabolism, a requirement of at least 1 mg/day may be appropriate. A limited number of surveys indicate that daily boron intake is about 0.5–3 mg depending on the proportion of various food groups in the diet. Boron is only mildly toxic; a concentration exceeding 100 μg/g is required to produce typical signs of toxicity. These include nausea, vomiting, diarrhea, dermatitis, and lethargy.

6.3.4 ARSENIC

Arsenic is widely distributed throughout the tissues and fluids of the body. In humans, the concentration in most tissues is about 0.04–0.09 ppm (dry basis), with skin, nails, and hair having higher levels (0.65 ppm). Adult humans may contain as much as 20 mg of arsenic.

Arsenic occurs in the air in areas where coal is burned, particularly near smelters and refineries, in sea water at levels of 3–6 ppb, and in normal soil at levels of 1–40 ppm. Most foods contain less than 0.5 ppm and rarely exceed 1 ppm. This applies to fruits, vegetables, grains, meats, and dairy products. Seafood (2–8 ppm), oysters (3–10 ppm), and mussels (as high as 120 ppm) are much richer in arsenic than other foods. Arsenic from food is well absorbed and rapidly excreted, primarily in the urine. Small amounts are also excreted by way of bile, sweat, hair, and skin losses. Urinary excretion is a satisfactory homeostatic mechanism that prevents arsenic accumulation.

No specific mode or site of action of arsenic has been found. It can activate and inhibit several enzymes, but these actions are not specific. It may affect zinc and/or arginine metabolism. Recent studies in rats and chicks suggest that it may have a function as a methylated compound and can affect labile methyl metabolism.

Signs of deficiency (e.g., depressed growth) are seen in several species of animals, but there is no evidence that arsenic is of nutritional importance in humans. If it is needed by humans, based on experiments in animals the requirement may be 12–15 μg/day, which is usually present in a normal diet.

The organic forms of arsenic that occur naturally in foods are easily excreted after absorption and toxicity from food is not likely. The signs of acute poisoning are nausea, vomiting, diarrhea, a burning sensation in the mouth, and abdominal pain. Normal hair always contains arsenic in small amounts, but this is greatly increased by excessive intakes of the element in certain forms. The level remains high for some days after cessation of intake and then rapidly returns to normal level. The diagnosis of arsenic poisoning is usually done by hair analysis.

In some places, ground water is contaminated with arsenic and can be toxic if present in high amounts. Arsenic enters groundwater from the weathering of minerals in rocks and soils. Drinking arsenic-contaminated groundwater is linked to health problems including diabetes and cardiovascular disease. Arsenic attacks certain proteins that have sulfur–sulfur bonds such as keratin, found in hair and skin. This results in skin lesions and hair loss. It also interferes with energy metabolism. In the United States, the upper safe limit is 10 ppb.

There are several wells in Bangladesh with arsenic content near 500 ppb. Researchers are exploring ways to remove arsenic from ground water.

6.3.5 TIN

Tin is found in most tissues, except brain, and approximately 14 mg is present in adult humans. The exact nature of this element in tissues is not known at this time. Various organic tin compounds are lipid soluble, and a substantial proportion of tin is found in tissue lipids.

A diet composed largely of fresh meat, cereals, and vegetables (which usually contain less than 1 ppm tin) can supply tin at about 1 mg/day, whereas a diet that includes substantial amounts of canned vegetables, fruit juices, and fish can provide as much as 38 mg/day. Tin is poorly absorbed and retained by man.

The biological function of this element is unknown, but it has a number of properties that offer possibilities for a role. Tetravalent tin has a strong tendency to form coordination complexes with 4, 5, 6, and possibly 8 ligands. It could participate in oxidation–reduction reactions in biological systems because the Sn^{2+}/Sn^{4+} oxidation–reduction potential of 0.13 V is within the physiological range and is near the potential of flavin enzymes.

Naturally occurring tin deficiency is not known in animals or men; however, rats raised on an experimental diet deficient in tin do not grow normally. Supplements of various tin compounds produced significant growth responses in tin-deficient rats maintained on purified diets inside trace-element-controlled isolators. At 0.5, 1.0, and 2.0 ppm of tin the growth increased by 24%, 53%, and 59%, respectively. Tin may be a necessary trace element in human nutrition; because it is poorly absorbed and poorly retained in the tissues, tin has a low toxicity.

6.3.6 Vanadium

Vanadium is widely distributed in tissues of animals and human beings in low concentrations in the range of 0.01–0.6 μg/g wet weight. Adult humans contain about 25 mg of vanadium in their bodies, most of which is present in the fatty tissues, blood serum, and bones and teeth. Environmental factors may influence mineral concentration.

Foods rich in vanadium include shellfish, mushrooms, dill seed, black pepper, and parsley; fresh fruits and vegetables contain little of this mineral. It is poorly absorbed, and the main route of excretion is by way of the kidney.

The biochemical function of vanadium is not known; however, it may have a role in the regulation of Na^+, K^+, ATPase, adenyl cyclase, and protein kinase. Vanadium may affect iodine metabolism and thyroid function. The hepatic synthesis of cholesterol and fatty acids in rats and rabbits decreases in the presence of trace amounts of vanadium. The site of inhibition of cholesterol biosynthesis is localized at the enzyme squalene synthetase.

Vanadium is essential for both the chick and the rat. Chicks fed low-vanadium diets demonstrated reduced growth and rats fed low-vanadium diets responded to dietary mineral supplementation with increased weight gain; however, some believe that these results are the consequences of high-vanadium supplements (10–100 times the amount normally found in the diet) that caused pharmacological changes. The final proof of its essentiality as a trace metal in humans is still lacking.[74] Some of the experimental low-vanadium diets contained 4–25 ng/g, which did not affect the animals, so if humans need vanadium, the requirement may be very small. The amount in an average daily diet is estimated to be about 6–20 μg. The toxicity of oral vanadium is low because it is poorly absorbed. Those exposed to vanadium via the respiratory system show signs of toxicity. These include depressed growth, diarrhea, and decreased appetite.

REFERENCES

Calcium and Phosphorus

1. Allen, L. H. 1982. Calcium bioavailability and absorption. A review. *Am J Clin Nutr* 35:783.
2. Anderson, J. B. 1990. Dietary calcium and bone mass throughout the life cycle. *Nutr Today* 25(2):9.
3. Arnaud, C. D. 1978. Calcium homeostasis: Regulatory elements and their integration. *Fed Proc* 37:2557.
4. Austin, L. A., and H. Heath. 1981. Calcitonin: Physiology and pathophysiology. *N Engl J Med* 304:269.
5. Berner, Y. N., and M. Shike. 1988. Consequences of phosphate imbalance. *Annu Rev Nutr* 8:121.
6. Bronner, F., ed. 1990. *Intracellular Calcium Regulation*. New York: Wiley-Liss.
7. Eaton, S. B., and D. A. Nelsen. 1991. Calcium in evolutionary perspective. *Am J Clin Nutr* 54:281s.

8. Gorham, E. D., C. F. Garland, F. C. Garland et al. 2007. Optional vitamin D status for colorectal cancer prevention: A quantitative meta analysis. *Amer J Prev Med* 32:210.

9. Hartman, T. J., P. S. Albert, K. Snyder et al. 2005. The association of calcium and vitamin D with risk of colorectal adenomas. *J Nutr* 135:252.

10. Lappe, J. M., D. Travers-Gustafson, K. Michael Davies et al. 2007. Vitamin D and calcium supplementation reduces cancer risk: Results of a randomized trial. *Amer J Clin Nutr* 85:1586.

11. Larsson, S. C., L. Bergkvist, J. Rutegard et al. 2006. Calcium and dairy food intakes are inversely associated with colorectal cancer risk in the Cohort of Swedish Man. *Amer J Clin Nutr* 83:663.

12. Lichtman, M. A., D. R. Miller, and R. B. Freeman. 1969. Erythrocyte adenosine triphosphate depletion during hypophosphatemia in a uremic subject. *N Engl J Med* 280:240.

MAGNESIUM

13. Flink, E. B. 1986. Magnesium deficiency in alcoholism. *Alcoholism* 10:590.

14. Hardwick, L. L., M. R. Jones, N. Brautbar, and D. B. Lee. 1991. Magnesium absorption. Mechanisms and the influence of vitamin D, calcium and phosphate. *J Nutr* 121:13.

15. Shils, M. E. 1988. Magnesium in health and disease. *Annu Rev Nutr* 8:429.

POTASSIUM, SODIUM CHLORIDE, SULFUR

16. Blaustein, M. P. 1985. Sodium chloride, extracellular fluid volume, and hypertension. *Hypertension* 7:834.

17. Huxtable, R. J. 1986. *Biochemistry of Sulfur*. New York: Plenum.

18. Maxwell, M. H., C. R. Kleman, and R. G. Narins. 1987. *Clinical Disorders of Fluid and Electrolyte Metabolism*. New York: McGraw-Hill.

19. Simopoulos, A. P., and F. C. Bartter. 1980. The metabolic consequences of chloride deficiency. *Nutr Rev* 38:201.

20. Simpson, F. O. 1988. Sodium intake, body sodium, and sodium excretion. *Lancet* 2:25.

21. Whang, R., ed. 1983. *Potassium: Its Biologic Significance*. Boca Raton, FL: CRC Press.

TRACE AND ULTRATRACE ELEMENTS/GENERAL

22. Mertz, W., ed. 1988. *Essential and Toxic Trace Elements in Human Health and Disease*. New York: Alan R. Liss.

IRON

23. Andrews, N. C. 1999. Disorders of iron metabolism. *N Engl J Med* 341:1986.

24. Beard, J. L., H. Dawson, and D. J. Pinero. 1996. Iron metabolism: A comprehensive review. *Nutr Rev* 54:295.

25. Beutler, E. 2003. The HFE Cys 282 Tyr mutation as a necessary but not sufficient cause of clinical hereditary hemochromatosis. *Toxicology* 180:169.

26. Donovan, A., C. N. Roy, and N. C. Andrews. 2006. The ins and outs of iron homeostasis. *Physiology* 21:115.

27. Fleming, R. E., and W. S. Sly. 2002. Mechanisms of iron accumulation in hereditary hemochromatosis. *Annu Rev Physiol* 64:663.

28. Klipstein-Grobusch, K., J. F. Koster, D. E. Grobbee, J. Lindemans, H. Boeing, A. Hofman, and J. C. M. Witteman. 1999. Serum ferritin and risk of myocardial infarction in the elderly: The Rotterdam study. *Am J Clin Nutr* 69:1231.

29. Thompson, K. J., S. Shoham, and J. R. Connor. 2001. Iron and neurodegenerative disorder. *Brain Res Bull* 55:155.

COPPER

30. Ala, A., A. P. Walker, K. Ashkan et al. 2007. Wilson's disease. *Lancet* 369:397.

31. Bingham, M. J., T. Ong, K. H. Summer, R. B. Middleton, and H. J. McArdle. 1998. Physiologic function of the Wilson disease gene product, ATP7B. *Am J Clin Nutr* 67:982S.

32. Brewer, G. J., and F. K. Askari. 2005. Wilson's disease: Clinical management and therapy. *J Hepatol* 42 (supple 1):S13.

33. Mercer, J. F. B. 1998. Menkes syndrome and animal models. *Am J Clin Nutr* 67:1022S.

ZINC

34. Bhutta, Z. A., S. M. Bird, R. E. Black et al. 2000. Therapeutic effects of oral zinc in acute and persistent diarrhea in children in developing countries: Pooled analysis of randomized controlled trials. *Amer J Clin Nutr* 72:1516.
35. Bose, A., C. L. Coles, Gunavathi et al. 2006. Efficiency of zinc in the treatment of severe pneumonia in hospitalized children <2 year old. *Amer J Clin Nutr* 83:1089.
36. Herndon, D. N., and R. G. Tomkins. 2005. The pharmacologic modulation of the hypermetabolic response to burns. *Adv Surg* 39:245.
37. Hulisz, D. 2004. Efficacy of zinc against common cold viruses: An overview. *J. Amer Pharm Assoc* 44:594.
38. Kurugol, Z., M. Akilli, N. Bayram, and G. Koturoglu. 2006. The prophylactic and therapeutic effectiveness of zinc sulphate on common cold in children. *Acta Pediatr* 95:1125.
39. Prasad, A. S. 2002. Zinc deficiency in patients with sickle cell disease. *Am J Clin Nutr* 75:181.
40. Su, J. C., and C. L. Birmingham. 2002. Zinc supplementation in the treatment of anorexia nervosa. *Eat Weight Disord* 7:20.
41. Zemel, B. S., D. A. Kawchak, E. B. Fung, K. Ohene–Frempong, and V. A. Stallings. 2002. Effect of zinc supplementation on growth and body composition in children with sickle cell disease. *Am J Clin Nutr* 75:300.

COBALT

42. Underwood, E. J. 1977. Cobalt. *Nutr Rev* 33:65.

MOLYBDENUM

43. Blot, W. J., J. Y. Li, P. R. Taylor et al. 1993. Nutrition intervention trials in Limxian, China: Supplementation with specific vitamin/mineral combinations, cancer incidence, and disease specific mortality in the general population. *J Nat Cancer Inst* 85:1483.
44. Boles, W., and C. D. Klaassen. 2000. Effects of molybdate and pentachlorophenol on the sulfation of acetaminophen. *Toxicology* 146:23.
45. Kones, R. 1990. Molybdenum in human nutrition. *J Natl Med Assoc* 82(1):11.

SELENIUM

46. Berry, M. J., and R. Larsen. 1992. The role of selenium in thyroid hormone action. *Endocr Rev* 19:207.
47. Duffield-Lillico, A. J., B. L. Dalkin, M. E. Reid et al. 2003. Selenium supplementation, baseline plasma selenium status and incidence of prostate cancer: an analysis of the complete treatment period of the Nutritional Prevention of Cancer Trial. *BJU Int* 91:608.
48. Hurwitz, B. E., J. R. Klaus, M. M. Llabre et al. 2007. Suppression of human immunodeficiency virus type 1 viral load with selenium supplementation: A randomized controlled trial. *Arch Intern Med* 167:148.
49. Jacobs, E. T., R. Jiang, D. S. Alberts et al. 2004. Selenium and colorectal adenoma: Results of a pooled analysis. *J Natl Cancer Inst* 96:1669.
50. Oldfield, J. E. 2001. Historical perspectives on selenium. *Nutr Today* 36(2):100.
51. Rayman, M. P. 2000. The importance of selenium in human health. *Lancet* 356:233.
52. Sieja, K., and M. Talerczyk. 2004. Selenium as an element in the treatment of ovarian cancer in woman receiving chemotherapy. *Gynecol Oncol* 93:320.
53. Stapleton, S. R. 2000. Selenium: An insulin-mimetic. *Cell Mol Life Sci* 57:1874.
54. Turker, O., K. Kumanlioglu, I. Korapolat, and I. Dogan. 2006. Selenium treatment in autoimmune thyroiditis: 9 month follow-up with variable doses. *J Endocrinol* 190:151.

MANGANESE

55. Freelan-Graves, J. H. 1988. Manganese: An essential nutrient for humans. *Nutr Today* 23(6):13.

IODINE

56. Anderson, M., B. Takkouche, I. Egli et al. 2005. Current global iodine status and progress over the last decade towards the elimination of iodine deficiency. *Bull World Health Organ* 83:518.

57. Borak, J. 2005. Adequacy of iodine nutrition in the United States. *Conn Med* 69:73.

58. Caldwell, K. L., R. Jones, and J. G. Hollowell. 2005. Urinary iodine concentration: United States National Health and Nutrition Examination Survey 2001–2002. *Thyroid* 15:692.

59. Kotwal, A., and P. R. Quadeer. 2006. Goiter and other iodine deficiency disorders: A systematic review of epidemiologic studies to deconstruct the complex web. *Arch Med Res* 38:1.

60. Pierce, E. N. 2008. U.S. Iodine nutrition: Where do we stand? *Thyroid* 18:1143.

61. Utiger, R. D. 2006. Iodine nutrition—more is better. *New Engl J Med* 354:2819.

62. Zimmerman, M. B. 2007. The adverse effects of mild-to-moderate iodine deficiency during pregnancy and childhood: A review. *Thyroid* 17:829.

CHROMIUM

63. Cefalu, W. T., and F. B. Hu. 2004. Role of chromium in human health and in diabetes. *Diabetes Care* 27:2741.

64. Chen, G., P. Lin, R. Guruprasad et al. 2006. Chromium activates glucose transporter 4 trafficking and enhances insulin-stimulated glucose transport in 3T3-L2 adipocytes via a cholesterol-dependent mechanism. *Mol Endocrinol* 20:857.

65. Mertz, W. 1998. Interaction of chromium with insulin: A progress report. *Nutr Rev* 56:174.

66. Vincent, J. B. 2000. The biochemistry of chromium. *J Nutr* 130:715.

FLUORIDE

67. Dean, H. T., F. A. Arnold, P. Jay, and J. W. Knutson. 1950. Studies on mass control of dental caries through fluoridation of the public water supply. *Public Health Rep* 65(43):1403.

68. Featherstone, J. D. 1999. Prevention and reversal of dental caries: Rate of low level fluoride. *Community Dent Oral Epidemiol* 27:31.

69. Hileman, B. 2006. Fluoride risks are still a challenge. *Chem Eng New* 84(38):34.

70. Lennon, M. A. 2006. One in a million: The first community trial of water fluoridation. *Bull World Health Organ* 84:759.

71. Marshall, T. A., S. M. Levy, J. J. Warren et al. 2004. Association between intake of fluoride from beverages during infancy and dental fluorosis of primary teeth. *J Amer Coll Nutr* 23:108.

72. McCoy, M. 2001. What is that stuff? Fluoride. *Chem Eng News* 79(16):42.

ULTRATRACE ELEMENTS

73. Carlisle, E. M. 1982. The nutritional essentiality of silicon. *Nutr Rev* 40:193.

74. Hopkins, L. L., and M. E. Mohr. 1974. Vanadium as an essential nutrient. *Fed Proc* 33:1773.

75. Nielsen, F. H. 1988. Boron: An overlooked element of potential nutritional importance. *Nutr Today* 23(1):4.

76. Schwartz, K. 1977. Silicon, fiber and atherosclerosis. *Lancet* 1:454.

MINERALS AND HYPERTENSION

77. Appel, L. J., T. J. Moore, E. Obarzanek, W. M. Vollmer, L. P. Svetkey, F. M. Sacks, G. A. Bray, T. M. Vogt, J. A. Cutler, M. M. Windhauser, P. Lin et al. 1997. A clinical trial of the effect of dietary patterns on blood pressure. DASH Collaborative Research Group. *N Engl J Med* 336:1117.

78. Cooper, R. S., C. N. Rotimi, and R. Ward. 1999. The puzzle of hypertension in African Americans. *Sci Am* 280 (2):56.

79. Dickinson, H. O., J. M. Mason, D. J. Nicolson et al. 2006. Lifestyle interventions to reduce raised blood pressure: A systematic review of randomized controlled trials. *J Hypertens* 24:215.

80. Fleet, J. C. 2001. DASH without the DASH (of salt) can lower blood pressure. *Nutr Rev* 59:291.

81. Forman, J. P., E. Giovannucci, M. D. Holmes et al. 2007. Plasma 25-hydroxy vitamin D levels and risk of incident hypertension. *Hypertension* 491:1063.

82. Forman, J. P., E. B. Rim, M. J. Stamper and G. C. Curhan. 2005. Folate intake and the risk of hypertension among U.S. Women. *J Amer Med Ass* 293:320.

83. Glen, S. K., H. L. Elliott, J. L. Curzio, K. R. Lees and J. L. Reid. 1996. White-coat hypertension as a cause of cardiovascular dysfunction. *Lancet* 348:654.

84. Hajjar, I. M., V. George, E. A. Sasse, and M. S. Kochar. 2002. A randomized double-blind, controlled trial of vitamin C in the management of hypertension and lipids. *Amer J. Ther* 9(4):289.
85. Renaud, S. C., R. Gueguen, P. Conard et al. 2004. Moderate wine drinkers have lower hypertension-related mortality, a prospective cohort study in French men. *Amer J Clin Nutr* 80:621.
86. Suter, P. M. 1998. Potassium and hypertension. *Nutr Rev* 56:151.
87. Taubert, D., R. Roesen, and E. Schomig. 2007. Effect of cocoa and tea intake on blood pressure: A meta analysis. *Arch Int Med* 167:626.
88. Wang, Y., and Q. J. Wang. 2004. The prevalence of prehypertension and hypertension among U.S. adults according to the new Joint National Committee Guidelines. *Arch Int Med* 164:2126.

CASE BIBLIOGRAPHY

89. Abumrad, N. N., A. J. Schneider, D. Steel, and L. S. Rogers. 1981. Amino acid intolerance during prolonged total parenteral nutrition reversed by molybdate therapy. *Am J Clin Nutr* 34:2251.
90. Bluhm, G. 1990. Selenium and cardiovascular disease. *Trace Elem Med* 7:139.
91. News of the week. 1986. Manganese lack may lead to osteoporosis. *Chem Eng News* 64(37):5.
92. Percival, S. S. 1995. Neutropenia caused by copper deficiency: Possible mechanism of action. *Nutr Rev* 53:59.
93. Quercia, R. A., S. Kom, D. O'Neill, J. E. Dougherty, M. Ludwig, R. Schweizer, and R. Sigman. 1984. Selenium deficiency and fatal cardiomyopathy in a patient receiving long-term home parenteral nutrition. *Clin Pharm* 3:531.
94. Tokuda, Y., S. Yokoyama, M. Tsuji, T. Sugita, T. Tajina, and T. Mitomi. 1986. Copper deficiency in an infant on prolonged total parenteral nutrition. *JPEN J Parenter Enteral Nutr* 10:242.

7 Vitamins—An Overview

7.1 HISTORICAL PERSPECTIVE

In earlier times, it was thought that illness was always caused by eating something and not by the absence of some factors in the diet. The absence of certain nutrients from the diet leads to what we now know as deficiency diseases. Although individual vitamins were not actually discovered until the early part of the 1900s, a considerable amount of evidence had accumulated long before that time that substances, in addition to carbohydrates, proteins, fats, inorganic elements, and water, were required by animals and men. The connections among dietary habits, specific diseases, and the special curative effects of certain foods have been recorded throughout history. In the 1500s, explorers on long voyages vividly described "scurvy" in their sailors and speculated that it was caused by a lack of something in food. The successful treatment of this condition with citrus fruits and fresh vegetables was reported in 1753 by James Lind, a physician in the British Navy, and a half century later, the British Navy made routine the provision of lime juice for its seamen. In 1810, Marzari from Italy first made a connection between maize diets and pellagra, and stated that the disease resulted from some form of dietary inadequacy. People unable to see properly at night were asked to eat roasted ox liver or the liver of a black cock. As early as 1825, people in India recognized that night blindness was caused by bad and insufficient food.

In 1911, the first successful preparation of an essential food factor was obtained by Casimir Funk, a Polish biochemist working in the Lister Institute in London. He obtained a crystalline compound from rice polishings that was effective in curing and preventing a dietary deficiency called polyneuritis in pigeons,[1] and beriberi in humans. The name "vitamine" was proposed for the compound because of its vital need for life and because chemically it was an amine. It was also called water-soluble factor B because of its ability to cure beriberi. As work by several investigators progressed and other "vitamins" were discovered, it was found that only a few were amine in nature, and so the final "e" was dropped to give the presently used general term "vitamin."

7.2 DEFINITION

Vitamins[2] are organic compounds that the body requires in small amounts for its metabolism, yet cannot make for itself, at least in sufficient quantity. For the most part, they are not related chemically and differ in their physiological role.[5] They are not used primarily to supply energy, or as a source of structural tissue components. The primary function of vitamins is to promote a wide variety of biochemical and physiological processes necessary for life. The basic reason that vitamins are essential constituents of an adequate diet is the lack (in humans) of the enzymatic machinery necessary to achieve rates of synthesis in accordance with the body's need.

7.3 NAMES

During 1913–1914, McCollum and Davis extracted a factor from butter fat, which they called "fat-soluble A" to distinguish it from the water-soluble factor B. These two essentials became known as vitamin A and vitamin B respectively. As more and more vitamins were discovered, each was assigned a letter. Thus, antiscorbutic factor became known as vitamin C, antirachitic factor as vitamin D, antihemorrhagic factor as vitamin K, and so on, because their chemical nature was unknown. Later, vitamin B was shown to consist of several substances and subscripts were added

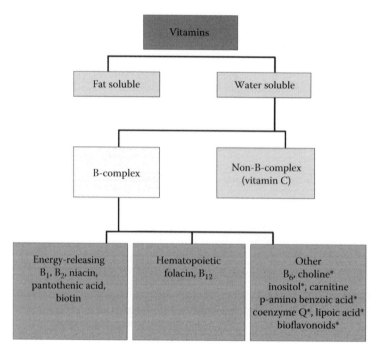

FIGURE 7.1 Classification of vitamins. *Indicates the dietary substances that are given vitamin status but are not established as vitamins.

(i.e., B_1, B_2, etc.). These terms continue to be used although they are being replaced by the chemical names.[12] After the vitamins were identified chemically, they were given specific names. It is entirely correct to use the specific names; however, there are advantages in certain circumstances for retaining some of the original letters. Vitamins such as A, D, E, K, and B_{12} each consist of several closely related compounds with similar physiological properties.

7.4 CLASSIFICATION

Vitamins are divided into groups on the basis of their solubility (Figure 7.1). Fat-soluble vitamins A, D, E, and K are found in foods associated with lipids. They are absorbed from the intestine with dietary fats, so conditions unfavorable to normal fat uptake also impair their absorption. Because they are lipid-soluble, significant quantities of the fat-soluble vitamins can be stored in the body, so they do not have to be consumed every day.

Water-soluble vitamins are not associated with dietary lipids, and the derangement of fat absorption does not interfere with their own absorption. They are normally excreted in the urine in small quantities. With the exception of vitamin B_{12}, they are not stored in appreciable quantity; therefore, these vitamins have to be supplied frequently to avoid their depletion.

The water-soluble vitamins are divided into B-complex (all the B vitamins) and non-B-complex (C). The B-complex group is further separated into the energy-releasing vitamins, the hematopoietic group (concerned with blood cell formation), and others with miscellaneous functions.

7.5 FUNCTIONS

Vitamins participate in a wide variety of biochemical and physiological functions,[3,5,6] including the expression of genetic information (vitamin A, differentiation of epithelial cells), the transcription of specific mRNA that codes for the synthesis of the protein responsible for calcium absorption (vitamin D), the posttranslational modification of proteins involving carboxylation of glutamate residues (vitamin K), the protection of cellular lipids from free radical attack (vitamin E), the reduction of metals, so that the associated enzyme systems can act on the transport of molecular oxygen (vitamin C), and as components of coenzymes that play vital roles in the metabolism of all cells (B vitamins, vitamin K).

Each coenzyme participates in the catalysis of a specific enzyme reaction associated with the metabolism of carbohydrates, fats, proteins, and nucleic acids. The utilization of many substrates for energy, the formation of cellular constituents such as protein, the deposition of energy reserves (e.g., glycogen, triglycerides), and the integrity of the repair and defense mechanisms require the participation of vitamins.[2,8,9]

Historically, nutritionists have been concerned with vitamins for their role in preventing and treating nutritional deficiency diseases.[7] The absence of one or more vitamins in the diet leads to characteristic disorders known as deficiency diseases, corrected by specific vitamins. Pieces of evidence accumulated during the last few years suggest that some of the vitamins may also provide health effects beyond preventing deficiency diseases. For example, increased intakes of vitamin D may offer protection against diabetes; vitamins C and E may reduce the risk of coronary heart disease and cataracts; vitamin K may reduce the risk of osteoporosis; and vitamin C may prevent the formation of nitrosamines, which are potent carcinogens. Increased intakes of folic acid, vitamin B_{12}, and vitamin B_6 during pregnancy may protect against delivery of infants with neural tube defects. These findings make it necessary to examine the criteria used to establish the recommended levels of vitamins for consumption.

7.6 DEFICIENCY

Hypovitaminosis or avitaminosis is a deficiency disease resulting from an inadequate supply of one or more vitamins in the diet. Dietary vitamin deficiencies in economically developed countries are rare, but are still common in some developing countries. The deficiencies usually coincide with a lack of basic nutrients. A lack of one or more vitamins produces rather characteristic symptoms. The vitamin deficiency can be classified as primary or secondary. Primary deficiency is caused by consuming an inadequate diet, which can be evaluated by dietary history. People who eat a varied diet are unlikely to develop a severe primary vitamin deficiency. In secondary deficiency, the recommended amount may be consumed, but because of some problems (conditioning factors) such as gastrointestinal disorders, malabsorption,[15] medication, allergies, metabolic defects, and so on, the nutrient is not efficiently absorbed and/or metabolized. The secondary deficiency can be assessed from clinical history. Regardless of the etiology, the deficiency, if prolonged, leads to a stepwise loss of body reserves of the vitamin(s).

Because most vitamins are not stored in the body, humans must consume them regularly to avoid deficiency. The body stores of different vitamins vary widely; vitamins A, D, and B_{12} are stored in significant amounts in the human body, mainly in the liver and an adult human's diet may be deficient in vitamins A and B_{12} for many months before developing a deficiency condition. Thiamin is not stored in significant amounts, so stores may be left only for a couple of weeks.

A full-blown deficiency of vitamin does not develop overnight. One of the earliest consequences of a deficiency is the reduction in the level of excretion of the vitamin or its metabolite in the urine and/or a lowering of the level in plasma.[17] Thus, determining the level of the vitamin in the plasma or urine is one way of assessing the vitamin status of the individual. If the deficiency continues, tissue levels become gradually depleted and the enzymes (or functions) dependent on vitamins will be less active and result in a biochemical lesion. Also, the substrate for the enzyme (and/or if the substrate is diverted to another pathway, its products) accumulates in the tissues and in the blood, and appears in the urine in greater quantities. The measurement of enzyme activity in the blood and substrate and other products in plasma and urine can be

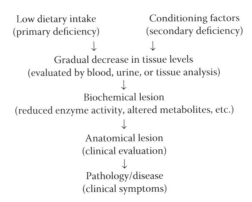

FIGURE 7.2   Sequence of events occurring in vitamin deficiency.

used to assess the extent of deficiency. Further, the continuation of the deficiency can lead to anatomical lesion and finally to cellular disease. This sequence of events is shown schematically in Figure 7.2.

7.7   NEED FOR SUPPLEMENTS

Minimum daily requirements (MDR) have been established for vitamins and other nutrients to protect normal, healthy individuals from deficiency syndromes. The MDR is set for each vitamin at a level below which signs of deficiency appear. In many countries throughout the world, scientific committees periodically assess the evidence about the requirements of the population for individual nutrients. The scientific group charged with setting nutrient allowances in the United States is the Food and Nutrition Board of the National Academy of Sciences. This group reviews research findings on each nutrient and establishes values for the nutrient requirement of the average individual in specific age and sex groups. The average requirement is then turned into an allowance by providing for individual variation and the body's inefficient use of the nutrient. This is generally two to six times the MDR. The resulting recommended daily allowances (RDA) are the levels of intake of essential nutrients that are considered adequate to meet the known nutritional needs of practically all healthy individuals. Dietary supplements often containing vitamins are used to ensure that adequate amounts of these nutrients are obtained on a daily basis if optimal amounts of the nutrients cannot be obtained through a varied diet. It is estimated that about 37% of the general adult population takes vitamin supplements, and there is little argument against supplements in reasonable amounts. There is, however, a concern with the use at unproven pharmacological levels as opposed to nutritional levels. A well-balanced diet contains adequate amounts of all nutrients including vitamins, but marginal intakes do occur within some segments of the population. While these problems can and should be solved by dietary improvements, there are instances where supplementation is justified. Examples of those who may have increased requirements include women who are pregnant or breast-feeding; people consuming a very low-calorie diet; strict vegetarians who eliminate all meat and dairy foods from their diet; and individuals whose nutrient needs are altered by illness,[10,11] medication, or other factors (Table 7.1).

A meta-analysis in 2006 suggested that vitamin A and E supplements provide no tangible health benefits for generally healthy individuals.[4] Another study found that vitamins E and C may actually curb some benefits of exercise. Tobacco smoking alters the metabolism of several vitamins. Smokers have lower levels of plasma vitamin C, E, folic acid, and carotenoids than nonsmokers, even after adjustment for dietary intake. Furthermore, cigarette smokers have increased turnover of the whole body vitamin C pool. Smoking is also associated with diminished levels of folate in the cells of the oral mucosa, diminished vitamin C levels in leukocytes, and decreased concentrations of vitamin E

TABLE 7.1
Conditions That Increase the Need for Vitamin Supplements

Women who are pregnant or breast feeding

Women with excessive menstrual bleeding

People on very low-calorie diets

Strict vegetarians

Elderly people

Individuals with diseases of the gastrointestinal tract

Patients on some medications

Tobacco smokers

Individuals with vitamin-responsive inborn errors of metabolism

in the alveolar fluid. The mechanisms responsible for these effects have not been identified, but when human plasma is exposed in vitro to the gas phase of cigarette smoke, there is degradation of vitamin C, vitamin E, and carotenoids. Because of extensive exposure of plasma constituents to cigarette smoke during passage through the lung vasculature, these in vitro findings may have physiologic significance for heavy smokers. The safest course is to quit smoking. For those who continue to smoke, two different dietary recommendations have been advocated: (1) increase the consumption of fruits and vegetables and (2) recommend supplements of β-carotene, and vitamins A, C, and E. However, recent findings raise serious questions about the safety of high-dose supplements of some of these vitamins in smokers.

Some enzymes are dependent on vitamins of the B group and vitamin K as components of the coenzymes. Because the body can synthesize apoenzyme the limiting factor affecting enzyme activity is the availability of coenzymes derived from vitamins, which must be consumed in the diet. Some of the classical deficiency symptoms are the result of inadequate coenzyme levels. Once the apoenzyme associated with the coenzyme is saturated, a further increase in the level of coenzyme (by ingesting supplements) does not increase enzyme activity. Therefore, higher intakes of vitamins with coenzyme functions serve no useful purpose; however, there are individuals with vitamin-responsive errors of metabolism. These genetically determined disorders result in increases in individual vitamin requirements by 10–1000 times the RDA. This can be due to a defect in the absorption or transport of the vitamin, impairment in the formation of the coenzyme, a defect in the binding of the coenzyme to the genetically abnormal apoenzyme, and the short half-life of the enzyme. Inborn errors of metabolism involving eight water-soluble vitamins and two fat-soluble vitamins are known. Although these disorders are rare, their clinical response to pharmacological doses of appropriate vitamins is well documented.

7.8 HYPERVITAMINOSIS

The likelihood of consuming too much of any vitamin from food is remote, but overdosing from vitamin supplements does occur. At high doses, some vitamins cause side effects such as nausea, vomiting, and diarrhea.[14] Some other vitamins, especially the fat-soluble vitamins A and D, can be toxic. Vitamin A at intakes five times or more of the RDA can result in toxic signs such as headache, vomiting, and so on. Although water-soluble vitamins are generally less toxic than similar amounts of fat-soluble vitamins, they, too, can have adverse effects. A high level of the metabolite of the vitamin or the vitamin itself can interfere with the action of other nutrients. The toxicity varies widely among individuals, depending on the dose of the supplement and the individual's body size, health, and use of medication. For example, some people may tolerate 5 g of vitamin C without adverse effects, whereas others may exhibit toxic symptoms with 1 g. Unfortunately, there is no way to predict the exact level at which a particular nutrient will be toxic in a particular individual.

7.9 ANTIVITAMINS

There are naturally occurring substances, as well as synthetic ones, that interfere with biological functions of vitamins.[8,9] They are sometimes consumed as natural components of foods or medications. These substances—antivitamins—can cause deficiency symptoms similar to those observed when the corresponding vitamin is absent, and the administration of the specific vitamin reverses the deficiency symptoms. Isonicotinic acid hydrazide, also called isoniazid, is used to treat tuberculosis. Isoniazid can cause the deficiency of niacin and vitamin B_6, and the deficiency symptoms are reversed after giving supplements of these two vitamins.

The metabolic antagonism by these substances is accomplished in one of three ways:

1. The antagonist can cleave the vitamin and render it inactive. Some foods (e.g., raw fresh water fish) contain the enzyme thiaminase, which cleaves vitamin B_1 molecule. People have acquired vitamin B_1 deficiency by eating raw clams and raw fish as a major part of their diet. This antagonist is easily destroyed by cooking.
2. The substance can complex with the vitamin as what happens between avidin, which is present in raw egg white, and biotin. Like thiaminase, avidin is inactivated by cooking.
3. Substances that have structural similarity to vitamins occupy the vitamin's receptor sites and thereby deny them to the vitamins; an example is dicoumarol, an antagonist to vitamin K.

Although these substances are known to provoke problems in the normal, orderly process of metabolism, they can perform some useful functions. They serve as research tools in animal experiments to generate defined vitamin deficiency states with minimal disturbances of other components of the diet. Some of them have clinical uses. Dicoumarol, a structural antagonist to vitamin K, has found application in postsurgical therapy to prevent the formation of potentially obstructive blood clots. Methotrexate, an antagonist to folic acid, has been used to treat leukemia.

7.10 ENRICHMENT OF FOODS

A common practice in recent years is the enrichment of food products with respect to certain vitamins. Some foods are supplemented to make up for the losses that occur during processing, and others to enrich foods with low-vitamin content. Flour is an example of a staple that is supplemented with vitamins. Wheat is rich in vitamins, but during processing to white flour, a considerable amount of these micronutrients is lost because they are contained in the outer layer of the cereal. The amount added is generally of the same order as that lost in the course of processing. Milk may contain added vitamin D and breakfast cereals often have supplements of the B-complex constituents.

A Boy with a Limp—A Case

A 6-year-old boy was referred to a hospital for evaluation of hip pain and a limp for 6 weeks. There was no history of trauma, fever, or weight loss. The pain had worsened progressively until a day earlier when he had become unable to walk. The boy's parents reported that he had intermittent bleeding from his gums during the past month.

On physical examination, he was apprehensive, but did not speak. His weight was 16.7 kg (less than 5th centile), and his height was 113 cm (10th centile). His gums were swollen and one of his upper incisors was loose. Proximal leg muscles were tender bilaterally. Skin and joint examinations were normal. Routine laboratory tests and coagulation tests were normal. Radiographs of his legs showed diffuse osteopenia. A bone scan showed hyperactivity in the right tibiofibular joint. The first diagnosis considered was acute leukemia, but a bone marrow smear and biopsy specimen did not support the diagnosis. Therefore, clinical and radiographic findings were reassessed. A further history from the boy's parents revealed that the boy's diet consisted of cookies, yogurt, whole milk, biscuits, and water for the past 1 year. He did not eat any fruit, vegetable, meat, or fish. Scurvy was suspected. A leukocyte ascorbic acid concentration of less than 0.6 mg/dL (normal: 0.6–2 mg/dL) confirmed the diagnosis of scurvy. The patient was treated with vitamin C (200 mg/day orally) for 10 days and a balanced diet. There was rapid resolution of gingival bleeding and resumption of weight bearing within 2 weeks. He was recommended a balanced diet. When examined after 6 months, he was well.

Primary vitamin deficiencies are rare in developed countries. Vitamins are present in adequate amounts in a balanced diet. If the diet is deficient in a particular vitamin, a deficiency disease can develop, which can be treated by the administration of that particular vitamin. A diagnosis of deficiency can be made by the presence of characteristic clinical findings. In the case of scurvy, some symptoms can mimic other disorders such as deep vein thrombosis, arthritis, and leukemia, and the disease may be misdiagnosed. In this case, leukemia was first considered, but after getting a dietary history, further tests were done and scurvy was confirmed. This patient's diet was deficient in vitamin C. This vitamin has an important role in the formation of collagen, which serves as a matrix on which bones and teeth are formed. Vitamin C[19] and its functions are discussed in Chapter 10, "Water-Soluble Vitamins II." The same author earlier reported scurvy in an adult who was following a fad "natural" diet that avoided "acidic" foods. This case makes the point that for diagnosis, it is important to note not only the clinical findings but also the dietary history of the patient.

A Man Who Lost Weight and Sight—A Case

A 55-year-old man was referred to a hospital because of poor vision in both eyes. For about 10 years he had weighed 150 kg and had tried several diets to lose weight but without success. A year earlier, he weighed 170 kg and agreed to surgical procedure to treat obesity. A gastroplasty was done and after 6 months he lost 90 kg, but at this time, he started having visual problems. He waited another 6 months before entering the hospital. Ophthalmological examination showed bilateral optic atrophy. His visual acuity was reduced to 5/60 in his right eye and 3/60 in his left eye. The color-determination test was defective. He had normal electroretinogram, but visual-evoked responses were abnormal. He weighed 80 kg, his general physical condition was good, and neurological examination was normal.

Blood analysis showed that this patient had mild macrocytic anemia and marginal deficiency of vitamin B_{12}. He was treated with 1000 µg of vitamin B_{12} in combination with other B vitamins daily for 2 weeks, then with 250 µg of vitamins weekly for 1 month and then with 250 µg monthly. The hematological findings returned to normal but visual acuity remained unchanged. After 6 months of treatment, visual acuity was the same, and visual-evoked responses were still abnormal.

The cause of vitamin B_{12} deficiency in gastropathy may be a disturbance in the secretion of intrinsic factor required for vitamin B_{12} absorption (Chapter 10). Also, this patient had been on several weight-reducing diets for 10 years prior to surgery, which might have been responsible for the deficiency of vitamin B_{12} and other B-complex vitamins. The status of other B-complex vitamins in this case was not made.

Optic nerve involvement may be part of the pathologic findings attributed to pernicious anemia. This nerve involvement may be similar to other neurologic lesions of pernicious anemia.[18]

Optic neuropathy because of vitamin B_{12} deficiency is rare. In most cases, no single vitamin deficiency alone has been implicated. In the case presented here, the deficiencies of other vitamins cannot be ruled out. Vision problems were reported in some World War II prisoners who had been malnourished. Dietary supplementation with vitamin B_{12}, niacin, and other B vitamins restored some vision in these patients. Thiamin and multiple B vitamin treatment also resulted in visual improvement in Korean War prisoners.

The patient described is 55 years old. In some elderly patients impairment of secretion of intrinsic factor may exist. If optic neuropathy is observed, prognosis for recovery of vision may be good if vitamin treatment is started at an early stage.

REFERENCES

1. American Diabetes Association. 1967. *Essays in the History of Nutrition and Diabetes.* Chicago: American Diabetes Association.
2. Bender, D. A. 1992. *Nutritional Biochemistry of the Vitamins.* New York: Cambridge University Press.
3. Combs, G. F. 1992. *The Vitamins, Fundamental Aspects in Nutrition and Health.* San Diego, CA: Academic Press.
4. Bjelakovic, G., D. Nikolova, L. L. Gluud et al. 2007. Mortality in randomized trials of antioxidant supplements for primary and secondary prevention: A systematic review and meta-analysis. *J Amer Med Assoc* 297:842.
5. Bolander, F. F. 2006. Vitamins not just for enzymes. *Curr Opin Investig Drugs* 7:912.
6. Friedrich, W. 1988. *Vitamins.* New York: Walter de Gruyter.
7. Gaby, S. K., A. Bendich, V. N. Singh, and L. J. Machlin. 1991. *Vitamin Intake and Health.* New York: Marcel Dekker.
8. Harris, L. J. 1955. *Vitamins in Theory and Practice.* Cambridge: Cambridge University Press.
9. Machlin, L. J., ed. 1984. *Handbook of Vitamins: Nutritional, Biochemical and Clinical Aspects.* New York: Marcel Dekker.
10. Maqbool, A., and V. A. Stallings. 2008. Update of fat-soluble vitamins in cystic fibrosis. *Curr Opin Pulm Med* 14:574.
11. McCollum, E. V. 1957. *A History of Nutrition.* Boston: Houghton-Miffin Co.
12. 1987. Nomenclature policy: Generic descriptors and trivial names for vitamins and related compounds. *J Nutr* 120:12.
13. Ristow, M., K. Zarse, A. Oberbach et al. 2009. Antioxidants prevent health-promoting effects of physical exercise in humans. *Proc Natl Acad Sci* 106:8665.
14. Rudman, D., and P. J. Williams. 1983. Megadose vitamins: Use and misuse. *N Engl J Med* 309:488.
15. Sahid, H. M., and Z. M. Mohammed. 2006. Intestinal absorption of water-soluble vitamins: An update. *Curr Opin Gastroenterol* 27:140.
16. Scriver, C. R. 1973. Vitamin-responsive inborn error of metabolism. *Metabolism* 22:1319.
17. Thrunham, D. I. 1981. Red cell enzyme tests of vitamin status: Do marginal deficiencies have any physiological significance? *Proc Nutr Soc* 40:155.

CASE BIBLIOGRAPHY

18. Moschos, M., and D. Droutsas. 1998. A man who lost weight and his sight. *Lancet* 351:1174.
19. Shetty, A. K., R. W. Steele, V. Silas, and R. Dehne. 1998. A boy with a limp. *Lancet* 351:182.

8 Fat-Soluble Vitamins

8.1 VITAMIN A

Vitamin A was the first fat-soluble vitamin to be discovered and has been known chemically since 1927, when its structure was determined.

8.1.1 CHEMISTRY

The term "vitamin A" is reserved to designate any substance or mixture of substances that possesses activity similar to vitamin A. Retinol (also known as vitamin A alcohol and vitamin A_1) is the most commonly known and the most abundant of all naturally occurring vitamin A compounds. Other compounds of biological interest include retinal (also called retinaldehyde) and retinoic acid. The more general term, retinoids, includes both naturally occurring compounds with vitamin A activity and synthetic analogs of retinol, irrespective of whether they have biological activity.

Retinol is a primary alcohol containing a β-ionone ring with an unsaturated side chain that terminates in an alcohol group (Figure 8.1). The β-ionone ring is essential for activity, and when it is absent or altered structurally, the compound loses its biological activity. Vitamin A has been isolated in pure form as pale yellow crystals and has been synthesized chemically. It is sensitive to oxidation, isomerization, and/or polymerization when dissolved in a dilute solution under light and in the presence of oxygen, especially at high temperature; however, at ordinary cooking temperature, it is stable. When retinol is oxidized (the alcohol group is changed to aldehyde), it is converted to retinal. Further oxidation results in the formation of retinoic acid. In food, the alcohol is usually esterified with fatty acids (retinyl esters), especially palmitic acid. Vitamin E, if present, protects it from oxidation. Vitamin A_2 is 3-dehydroretinol and is found in the eyes of fresh water fish.

8.1.2 FOOD SOURCES

Preformed vitamin A is available only in foods of animal origin in which the animal has converted the precursor into the active vitamin.[5] Rich sources of the vitamin include the liver, kidneys, and animal fats including those found in milk, cream, butter, egg yolk, and some fatty fish. Liver is the richest source of dietary retinol in the U.S. diet. A 3-ounce portion of liver contains 100 times the retinol present in one glass of whole milk, 116 times that in one whole egg, and 200 times that in a pat of butter. Because milk and butter are important sources of retinol, the U.S. Food and Drug Administration (FDA) defined the identity of low-fat and nonfat milk as well as margarines to contain 624 μg/L and 55 μg/pat of all-*trans* retinol, respectively, to preserve the nutritional quality of these dietary substitutes. In the United States, approximately two-thirds of the recommended daily intake of vitamin A is met by direct intake of retinol. The remaining one-third is obtained by consuming carotenoids.

Plant foods are rich in carotenoids, which are chemically related to vitamin A. They are known as the precursors (or provitamin A) that are converted in the body by an enzyme-catalyzed reaction to active vitamin A. There are more than 400 carotenoids, but only 60 of those can be converted to vitamin A, the most important of which are α-carotene, β-carotene, and γ-carotene. The major dietary sources of provitamin A are the yellow and green vegetables and fruits (e.g., carrots, sweet potatoes, apricots, spinach). The carotenes are useful nutritionally only in so far as they may be converted to

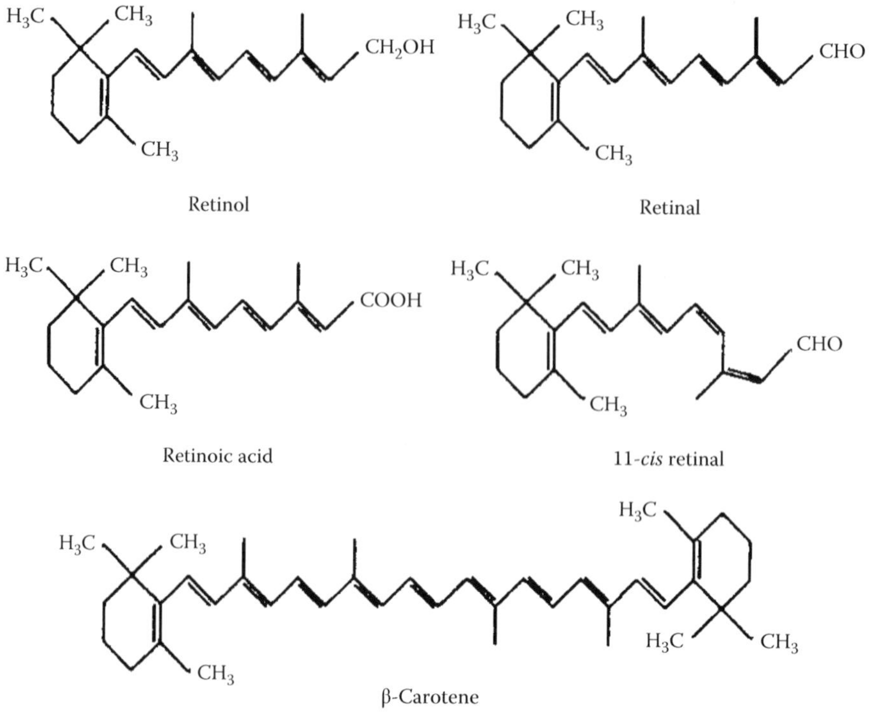

FIGURE 8.1 Structures of retinol, retinal, retinoic acid, 11-*cis* retinal, and β-carotene.

retinol. One β-carotene molecule can theoretically give rise to two molecules of retinol. In α-carotene and γ-carotene as well as cryptoxanthin (the yellow pigment of corn), one of the rings differs from that of retinol, so these carotenes are half as active as β-carotene in the formation of retinol.

8.1.3 ABSORPTION

Vitamin A in the diet is present in the form of provitamin, particularly β-carotene from plant sources, or as preformed retinol or retinol derivatives (retinol esters, retinal) from foods of animal origin.

8.1.3.1 Absorption of Carotenes and Their Conversion to Retinol

Those carotenes that possess at least one β-ionone ring (e.g., α-carotene, β-carotene, and γ-carotene and cryptoxanthin) can be converted to retinol. Carotenes must first be absorbed at least as far as the cells of the intestine because the principal site of cleavage is the intestine. As carotenes are hydrocarbons, they are not readily soluble in aqueous medium and are better absorbed in the presence of fat. After the carotene enters the intestinal cell, it is cleaved into two molecules (in the case of β-carotene) of retinal by the enzyme 15,15-dioxygenase (Figure 8.2), which is located in the cytosol of the intestinal cell. In the presence of reduced nicotinamide adenine dinucleotide (NADH), alcohol dehydrogenase[4] (retinal reductase) converts retinal to retinol. The cleavage enzyme is also present in the liver, and intravenously administered carotene is converted to vitamin A even after the removal of the intestine; however, the rate of conversion in the liver is about one-eighth of that in the intestine.

8.1.3.2 Absorption of Preformed Vitamin A

Retinol, if present as an ester, is first hydrolyzed to free retinol by hydrolysis in the lumen of the small intestine. The free retinol is then absorbed in the intestinal cell. The free retinol, whether formed from carotenes or coming preformed from the diet, is esterified by esterases in the intestinal cell microsomes to form retinyl ester. Palmitic acid is the major fatty acid for this esterification.

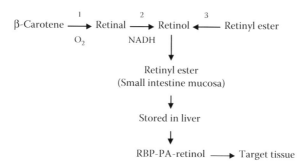

FIGURE 8.2 Absorption and transport of dietary carotenes and vitamin A. (1) 15,15-dioxygenase (small intestine) splits β-carotene into two moles of retinal. (2) Alcohol dehydrogenase (retinal reductase). (3) Dietary preformed vitamin A as retinyl ester is hydrolyzed by pancreatic esterase and converted to retinol. This, along with retinol derived from carotenes, is reesterified immediately after passage through the gut wall. The esters are conveyed to the liver where they are stored in ester form. From the liver, vitamin A is distributed to various organs by way of the plasma in the form of a protein complex.

8.1.4 TRANSPORT

After absorption in the intestinal cell, retinyl ester is transported to the liver via the intestinal lymphatic system and thoracic duct in the low-density lipoprotein (LDL) fraction of the blood, mainly in association with lymph chylomicrons. It is stored in the liver in combination with LDL. Approximately 80%–90% of the total body retinol is stored in the liver when vitamin A status is adequate. When there is a demand for vitamin A in tissues, the retinyl ester is hydrolyzed to free retinol and combines with its specific transport protein, called retinol-binding protein (RBP), while still in the liver. The retinol–RBP then combines with another protein, prealbumin (PA), in a protein–protein complex. This complex then leaves the liver and enters the circulation to be carried to the target tissue. Both RBP and PA are synthesized in the liver. In protein deficiency, RBP and PA cannot be synthesized in adequate quantities, and vitamin A is not released into circulation. Alternately, if there is vitamin A deficiency, RBP accumulates in the liver. If vitamin A is then administered, RBP immediately combines with retinol and is released in a protein–protein complex.

Zinc has a role in vitamin A metabolism. Deficiency of zinc results in decreased synthesis of RBP and decreased activity of the enzyme that releases retinol from its storage form, retinyl palmitate, in the liver. And zinc is part of the enzyme alcohol dehydrogenase, which converts retinol to retinal.

8.1.5 BIOCHEMICAL ROLE

There are three active forms of vitamin A: retinol (alcohol), retinal (aldehyde), and retinoic acid (acid). Retinal has a role in vision, retinol is required for reproductive activity, and retinoic acid is used for other vitamin A functions. Retinol and retinal are intercovertible, but once retinoic acid is formed, it cannot be reconverted and it cannot be stored in the body.

$$\text{retinol} \leftrightarrow \text{retinal} \rightarrow \text{retinoic acid}$$

Vitamin A, in the form of retinoic acid, plays an important role in gene transcription. Retinoic acid is a ligand for certain nuclear receptors that act as transcription factors. The retinoid receptors belong to two subfamilies: retinoic acid receptors (RARs) and retinoid X receptors (RXRs). These are active in retinoid-mediated gene transcription. Retinoid receptors regulate transcription by binding to specific DNA sites—the retinoic acid response elements (RAREs)—in target genes. RAR and RXR must dimerize before they can bind to the DNA. RAR will form a heterodimer with

RXR (RAR–RXR) but does not readily form a homodimer (RAR–RAR). RXR, on the other hand, readily forms a homodimer (RXR–RXR) and will form heterodimers with many other nuclear receptors, including the thyroid hormone receptor, TR, (RXR–TR), the vitamin D receptor, VDR, (RXR–VDR) and others. The RAR–RXR heterodimer recognizes RAREs on the DNA whereas the RXR–RXR homodimer recognizes retinoid "X" response elements on the DNA. The other RXR heterodimers will bind to various other response elements on the DNA. Once retinoic acid binds to the receptors and dimerization has occurred, the receptors undergo a conformational change that causes corepressors to dissociate from the receptors. Coactivators can then bind to the receptor complex, which may help to loosen the chromatin structure from the histones or may interact with the transcriptional machinery. The receptors can then bind to the response elements on the DNA and upregulate (or downregulate) the expression of target genes. Retinoic acid is a powerful mediator of cell function. Through the stimulation and inhibition of transcription of specific genes, retinoic acid plays an important role in controlling cell proliferation, differentiation, and apoptosis during normal cell development. Too much or too little retinoic acid creates a disruption of these highly regulated processes.

8.1.5.1 Vision

The light receptors of the eye are the rod and cone cells of the retina. The outer segments of both kinds of receptors contain light-sensitive pigments that require vitamin A for their formation and proper functioning. The rod and cone outer segments are surrounded by pigmented epithelium cells that store vitamin A. The light-sensitive pigment of the rods is rhodopsin (visual purple), which consists of a glycoprotein, opsin, that is linked to 11-*cis* retinal. The cone cells contain one of three possible iodopsins. In each case, 11-*cis* retinal is bound (via the formation of a Schiff's base) to a specific lysyl residue of the respective protein (collectively referred to as opsins).

Retinol and retinal have four double bonds in their chain and can exist in a number of stereo-isomers. The most stable form is the all-*trans* form; this form does not combine with opsin and must be isomerized to the 11-*cis* form. During the light reaction, rhodopsin is split into opsin and all-*trans* retinal. As light strikes the retina, visual purple is bleached, and the reaction causes a light stimulus to excite the optic nerve which, in turn, transfers the stimulus to the brain (Figure 8.3). The bleaching of rhodopsin is a means whereby the human eye can see at night. To regenerate the pigment, the all-*trans* retinal has to be isomerized by an isomerase in the rod outer segments. The whole process is a cycle of events in light and dark. Small amounts of retinol are continually lost in the visual process and must be replaced from the body's supply of vitamin A. Concurrent zinc deficiency can interfere with the mobilization of vitamin A from liver stores as well as the synthesis of rhodopsin. Thus, vitamin A deficiency is exacerbated by concurrent zinc deficiency.

The visual cycle uses a panel of proteins whose roles in enzymatic processing and trafficking enable regeneration of 11-*cis* retinal. One of these proteins, retinal pigment epithelium (RPE) 65, is essential and functions as a chaperone for all-*trans* retinal delivering it to the enzyme, which converts it to 11-*cis* retinal. Isotretinoin (Accutane), discussed in Section 8.1.5.6, competitively binds to RBP65, and this competition inhibits visual cycle function and induces night blindness.

8.1.5.2 Maintenance of Epithelial Cells

Retinol deficiency has a deleterious effect on epithelial structures, in general. Epithelial cells are found in the linings of all openings in the interior part of the body (e.g., alimentary tract, respiratory tract) as well as in glands and ducts. They also form the outer protective layer of the skin. Most epithelial cells secrete mucus, but in vitamin A deficiency, there is a reduction in mucus-secreting cells; these cells are replaced by keratin-producing cells in many tissues of the body, particularly in the conjunctiva and cornea of the eye, the trachea, the skin, and other ectodermal tissues. The production of glycoprotein in mucus secretion is reduced. The administration of vitamin A induces a shift to the mucus-producing cells, but the mechanism by which this occurs is not understood.

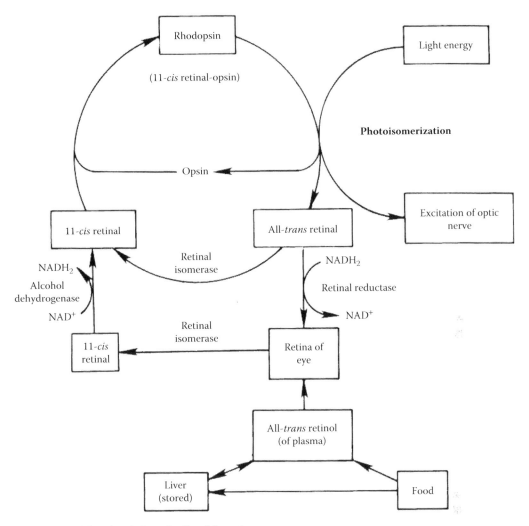

FIGURE 8.3   Visual cycle in rod cells of the retina.

8.1.5.3   Bone Development

Vitamin A is required for normal bone growth.[7] In vitamin A deficiency, the bones fail to grow in length, probably because the remodeling process that is an essential phase of bone growth is poorly controlled. The skull and spinal column do not continue to enlarge to accommodate the growing nervous system. Children lacking vitamin A fail to grow. When given vitamin supplements, these children gain weight and grow taller. Vitamin A is also necessary for enamel-forming epithelial cells in the development of teeth. There is evidence that retinoic acid performs the vitamin A function in the development of bone and epithelial tissue.

8.1.5.4   Reproduction

In vitamin A-deficient rats, there is a failure of spermatogenesis in the male and a decrease in estrogen synthesis in the female. Deficiency also interferes with placental development and other aspects of female reproduction in the rats and chicks. Vitamin A is necessary for embryogenesis and tissue differentiation. In women, vitamin A supports fetal development during pregnancy. There is a significant transfer of vitamin A between the mother and the fetus, and fetal vitamin A needs can be met by mobilizing as little as 10% of the typical stores of a well-nourished mother. A lower maternal status of vitamin A is associated with fetal malformation and intrauterine growth retardation. An excessive consumption of vitamin A or its analog, isotretinoin (13-*cis* retinoic acid), which is used for the treatment of acne, in the early months of pregnancy can lead to spontaneous abortion. Excessive vitamin A poses teratogenic risks. Among women who took more than 10,000 IU of supplemental vitamin A daily, approximately one out of every 57 infants was born with a malformation attributable to vitamin A toxicity. Higher intakes before the seventh month of pregnancy appear to be most damaging. Because 13-*cis* retinoic acid is known to be teratogenic in humans, it is marketed in the United States as contraindicated during pregnancy.

8.1.5.5 Immunity

Vitamin A is commonly known as the anti-infective vitamin.[17] It plays an important role in immune response. The skin and mucosal cells (cells that line the airways, digestive tract, and urinary tract) function as a barrier and form the body's first line of defense against infection. Retinol is required to maintain the integrity and function of these cells. Retinol and retinoic acid play a central role in the development and differentiation of white blood cells, such as lymphocytes, which play critical roles in the immune response. Activation of T-lymphocytes, the major regulatory cells of the immune system, appears to require the binding of retinoic acid to RARs.

There is evidence that vitamin A is protective against measles.[18] High doses of vitamin A supplements improve recovery from measles; and decrease mortality, duration of disease, and risk of complications. Controlled trials suggest clinical benefits from a high dose of vitamin A in severe and potentially severe measles, especially in children under the age of 2 years. A dose of 50,000 IU is used for infants 1–6 months of age, 100,000 IU for infants 7–12 months of age, and 200,000 IU for children over 1 year of age.

Vitamin A supplementation reduces mortality in children with human immunodeficiency virus. Vitamin A supplementation also protects against the complications of other life-threatening infections including malaria and lung disease. One well-controlled study has shown that vitamin A supplements decrease the severity of malaria infection in children 6 months to 5 years of age. Supplementation reduced the number of febrile episodes, the parasite density, and the proportion of subjects with spleen enlargement.[15]

8.1.5.6 Dermatology

Vitamin A appears to function in maintaining normal skin health. Natural and synthetic retinoids influence epithelial cell proliferation and epidermal differentiation and have been used increasingly as systemic or topical agents in the treatment of dermatological disorders. 13-*cis* retinoic acid (isotretinoin) inhibits sebum production and is the drug of choice for the treatment of severe cystic acne, and is useful in the treatment of other forms of acne. Acitretin normalizes hyperproliferative states and induces the differentiation of basal cells in the dermis toward a less keratinized, more epithelial phenotype. Etretinate is used in Europe for the treatment of psoriasis and related disorders.

Acne vulgaris is the most common dermatologic problem of the adolescent years. Age of onset and severity of disease are affected by sex, genetics, and external factors such as cosmetics and medications. It is stimulated by androgens, primarily testosterone in males and testosterone and dehydroepiandrosterone in females. It generally resolves as androgen levels decline; but some cases persist in adulthood. It has been suggested that chocolate, fried foods, soda, and iodine in milk may be linked to acne. A group of investigators have proposed that diets rich in refined sugar and the Western diet may be involved. They have examined indigenous populations that eat plant-based diets composed mainly of unprocessed or minimally processed foods high in carbohydrate and fiber and low in saturated fat. They are largely free of acne. But the role of nutritional factors in the prevalence of acne remains unclear. Acne is not due to vitamin A deficiency, but some derivatives of the vitamin do improve the condition. Isotretinoin (Accutane) appears to be extremely effective at clearing up the scarring, inflamed, and pus-filled cysts that cover the face, neck, and back of severe acne sufferers. However, it can cause severe birth defects if used during pregnancy.[16] Other adverse effects include dry skin, lips, nose and eyes, reduced night vision, modest elevation of blood triglycerides and cholesterol, depression and, in rare cases, suicide.

Each year roughly one million prescriptions for Accutane are written and the Food and Drug Administration (FDA) estimates at least 120 women take the drug while pregnant. Since March 2006, the dispensing of Accutane in the United States has been controlled by an FDA-mandated website called iPLEDGE. It is designed for doctors, patients, and pharmacists to control the distribution of this drug because it causes severe birth defects.[2] Doctors must pledge that they know how to treat acne, know about Accutane's birth defect risk, and know how patients can avoid pregnancies. They must also pledge to register every patient, enter the primary and secondary methods of birth control of all females of child-bearing potential (unless they swear to abstinence), and record the results of regular pregnancy tests, which must be performed by federally certified laboratories, not with at-home kits. Patients must sign iPLEDGE as well, getting a personal identification number in order to fill their prescriptions. They must verify online or by phone that their doctors counseled them and obtained pregnancy tests, and every month patients must repledge the two forms of birth control they are using.

On June 29, 2009, Roche Pharmaceuticals, the original creator and distributer of the Accutane brand in the United States, officially discontinued both the manufacture and distribution of Accutane in this country. Generic isotretinoin will remain available in the United States through various manufacturers. Hoffman LaRoche will continue to manufacture and distribute Accutane outside of the United States.

8.1.5.7   Other Functions

Retinol appears to be involved in mucopolysaccharide biosynthesis at the enzymatic level. The glycoprotein content in the mucus secretion is reduced in deficiency. There is a loss of appetite, which is attributed to a change in the taste buds, perhaps as a result of a decrease in mucopolysaccharide synthesis or due to the clogging of taste bud pores with keratinized cells. Vitamin A may also have a role in the stability of membranes of lysosomes, mitochondria, and outer cell membranes.

Epidemiological and experimental data support a role for vitamin A and retinoids in decreasing the risk of certain cancers, especially those of epithelial origin. Studies in cell culture and animal models have shown the ability of retinoids to reduce carcinogenesis. It has been suggested that physiologic retinoids may act as endogenous chemoprotective factors, suppressing the expression of early aberrant clones, thus preventing the formation of premalignant lesions. Intracellular retinoid bioavailability is regulated by the presence of specific receptors, the cellular retinol binding proteins (CRBPs). In humans, three CRBPs have been described: CRBP1 is distributed throughout the body, whereas CRBP2 is mainly restricted to the small intestine, and CRBP3 is present in the cardiac and skeletal muscle. In normal human breast epithelium, CRBP1 is uniformly expressed but appears to be downregulated in breast cancer. A loss of CRBP1 gene is also reported in human ovarian cancer cell lines. These findings suggest that a reduction of CRBP1 expression causes local vitamin A deficiency and contributes to oncogenetic processes.

Some case-controlled epidemiologic studies have implicated vitamin A as a beneficial dietary factor in reducing cancer risk. But there is no difference in blood levels of vitamin A between cancer patients and matched controls. There is insufficient evidence in humans that vitamin A is effective in treating or preventing cancer.

8.1.6   Deficiency

Vitamin A deficiency is rarely seen in the United States and other developed countries, but a subgroup of patients suffering from malabsorption, cholestasis, or inflammatory bowel disease, or those who have undergone small-bowel bypass surgery may have subclinical deficiency. Vitamin A deficiency is common in underdeveloped countries. In addition to dietary problems, iron deficiency can affect vitamin A uptake, and excess alcohol consumption can deplete vitamin A in the liver. About 127 million preschool children and 7 million pregnant women around the world are vitamin A deficient. For children, lack of vitamin A causes severe visual impairment and blindness and significantly increases the risk of severe illness and even death from common childhood infections such as diarrheal disease and measles. Vitamin A deficiency diminishes the ability to fight infection. For pregnant women in high-risk areas, vitamin A deficiency occurs especially during the last trimester when the demand by both the unborn child and the mother is the highest. The mother's deficiency is demonstrated by the high prevalence of night blindness during this period.

Night blindness is an inability to see in dim light (nyctalopia) and is usually the first sign of vitamin A deficiency (Figure 8.4). The rod cells are particularly sensitive to vitamin A deficiency. Xerophthalmia (Figure 8.5b) is an eye disease characterized by drying of the eyes. The cells of the

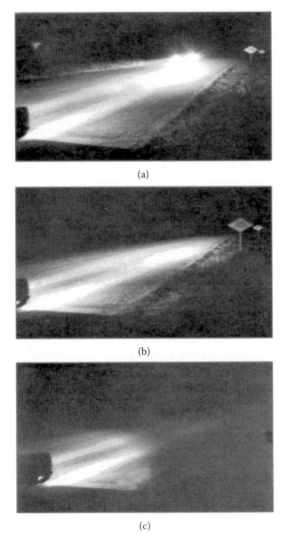

(a)

(b)

(c)

FIGURE 8.4 (a) Headlights of an approaching car as seen by a normal individual or one with vitamin A deficiency. (b) Wide stretch of road as seen by a normal individual after the approaching car has passed. (c) View of the road as seen by a vitamin A-deficient subject after the approaching car has passed. Only a few feet in front of the car are visible and one cannot see the road sign at all. (Courtesy of Shari Roehl, Pharmacia & Upjohn Co.)

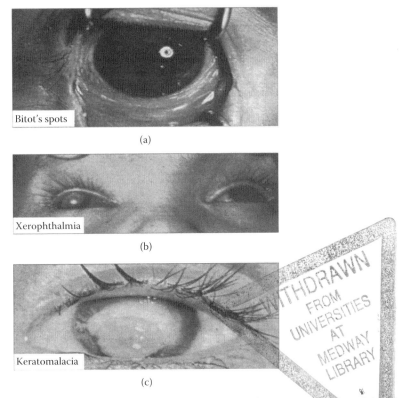

FIGURE 8.5 (a) Bitot's spots—white foamy plaques on the temporal side of the cornea. (b) Xerophthalmia in an Indonesian child with severe involvement of one eye. (c) Keratomalacia in a young child. (Courtesy of Shari Roehl, Pharmacia & Upjohn Co.)

lacrimal gland become keratinized (Figure 8.5c) and stop secreting tears, possibly as a result of a decreased ability to synthesize mucopolysaccharides or because the lacrimal duct is blocked. This condition is called keratomalacia. If the condition is untreated, an infection can cause ulceration and the loss of intraocular fluid. Pus is exuded and the eye hemorrhages; this condition is known as Bitot's spots (Figure 8.5a).

Vitamin A deficiency has been recognized as the leading cause of preventable pediatric blindness in developing countries. Approximately 250,000–500,000 children become blind each year due to vitamin A deficiency, with the highest prevalence in the Southeast Asia and Africa. During the past 25 years, combating vitamin A deficiency has emerged as one of the most cost-effective interventions for saving the sight and lives of children. The United Nations Special Session on Children in 2002 set the goal to eliminate vitamin A deficiency and its tragic consequences including blindness, disease, and premature death. The World Health Organization (WHO) and the United Nations International Children Emergency Fund (UNICEF) have issued a joint statement recommending that vitamin A be administered to all children, especially those younger than 2 years who are diagnosed with measles. Coexistent vitamin A deficiency in young children increases the risk of death.

Several studies indicate that vitamin A deficiency enhances susceptibility to carcinogenesis both in experimental animals and in humans. The vitamin seems to have a role in promoting a normal differentiation of epithelial cells and in maintaining the controls that prevent the development of malignancy in these cells.

There are no specific deficiency signs or symptoms that result from carotene deficiency. However, dietary carotenoids have been suggested to protect against cataract formation, LDL oxidation, and certain cancers. It was hoped that β-carotene would be an effective chemopreventive agent for cancer because numerous epidemiological studies had shown that diets high in β-carotene were associated with lower incidences of cancers of the respiratory and digestive systems. However, intervention studies using high doses of β-carotene actually resulted in more lung cancer than in the placebo-treated groups.

8.1.7 Units

The units are presently expressed as retinol equivalents (RE). It takes into account the variations in absorption and conversion of different precursors into vitamin A. One RE is equal to 1 μg of retinol, 6 μg of β-carotene, and 12 μg of other carotene precursors. When vitamin A is expressed in international units, 1 RE = 3.3 IU of retinol = 10 IU of β-carotene.

The Institute of Medicine's recently released recommended daily intake guideline has reduced by half the amount of provitamin A carotenoids expected to be converted into retinol. Renamed "retinol activity equivalents," 12 mg of β-carotene or 24 mg of other provitamin A carotenoids is now considered to be equivalent to 1 mg of all-*trans* retinol. The poor conversion of carotenoids into vitamin A is due to the interference of vegetable matrix with absorption.

8.1.8 Recommended Dietary Allowance

The requirement of vitamin A is proportional to body weight. The 1990 Recommended Dietary Allowance (RDA) for adult males is 1000 RE; the RDA for women is lower (800 RE) to allow for lesser body weight. These are about twice the amount to meet the minimal needs. During pregnancy, 1000 RE is recommended, and during lactation, 1200 RE is prescribed; children need 600–1000 RE daily, with the amount increasing from infancy to 14 years of age.

8.1.9 Assessment of Vitamin A Status

The diagnosis of vitamin A deficiency is made through the measurement of retinol in plasma. A retinol concentration in plasma of less than 10 μg/dL indicates deficiency, and a concentration higher than 100 μg/dL is considered toxic. In the latter case, the presence of a significant amount (>70%) of circulating retinyl ester in fasting plasma is a confirmation of a hypervitaminosis state.

The relative dose response (RDR) method indirectly assesses the adequacy of liver vitamin A stores. When vitamin A stores in the liver are low, apo-RBP accumulates in the hepatocytes. After the oral administration of a small dose (450–1000 RE) of vitamin A in oil, the apo-RBP concentration in the plasma rapidly rises to a plateau at approximately 5 hours. The increments in plasma retinol levels between 0 and 5 hours (after vitamin A administration) divided by the retinol value at 5 hours and then multiplied by 100 yields the RDR value as a percentage. Values above 20% have been found in adult subjects with night blindness or liver reserve stores below 20 mg/g. Average values of liver vitamin A concentrations in well-nourished adult individuals are approximately 100 mg/g. A suggested adequate reserve for both adults and children is 20 mg/g.

Quantitative measures of dark adaptation for night vision and electroretinograms are useful functional tests.

8.1.10 Toxicity

Excessive doses of vitamin A are toxic and can destroy cell membranes and membranes of subcellular organelles of tissues by penetration into and expansion within the lipid portion of these membranes.[3] Membranes of lysosomes are more sensitive. The toxicity occurs when the amount of vitamin ingested is so much that the liver storage and serum transport capacities are exceeded. Symptoms of vitamin A toxicity include drowsiness, headaches, double vision, vomiting, loss of appetite, coarsening and loss of hair, scaly skin eruption, bone fragility, and weakness.

An acute toxicity of vitamin A was first noted in arctic explorers who had consumed polar bear liver; vitamin A toxicity has been seen after the administration of 150 mg in adults and 100 mg in children. The long-term ingestion of high amounts of vitamin A can lead to hypercalcemia and bone abnormalities. In addition, lower bone mass and decreased biochemical markers for bone turnover have been observed in patients treated with retinoids for skin diseases. Vitamin A stimulates bone resorption and inhibits bone formation.[6] This combination would be expected to produce bone loss and to contribute to osteoporosis development and may occur with relatively low levels of vitamin A intake. It is possible that unappreciated hypervitaminosis A contributes to osteoporosis pathogenesis. In the most recent prospective cohort study of postmenopausal women, the risk of hip fracture was almost doubled among women with retinol intakes of about 2000 μg/day or more compared with those who consumed less than about 500 μg/day. In contrast to retinol, higher intakes of β-carotene did not significantly increase the risk of hip fracture, presumably because of a limitation on the conversion of β-carotene to retinol. The amounts of retinol in fortified foods and vitamin supplements may need to be reassessed because these add significantly to total retinol consumption in the United States.

Several water-soluble sugar derivatives of vitamin A have been synthesized by attaching glucose or glucuronic acid to retinol and retinoic acid. These compounds are as efficiently absorbed by the body as the fat-soluble forms. They promote growth and alleviate vitamin A deficiency in rats and are less toxic. The reduced toxicity of these water-soluble compounds may make them clinically useful in people suffering from defects in lipid absorption, such as cystic fibrosis or cholestasis, as well as in treating retinoid-responsive skin disorders such as acne, psoriasis, and wrinkling and possibly some forms of skin cancer. However, some studies have found that children given water-soluble vitamin A suffer asthma twice as much as a control group supplementing with the fat-soluble vitamin.

Hypercarotenemia, also called hypercarotenosis, is caused by the ingestion of large quantities of foods containing carotene. It results merely in the deposition of carotene in tissues, particularly the skin and plasma, which then can become distinctly orange–yellow. It gives the person the appearance of having jaundice, but the eyes do not become yellow. It is a benign condition and the removal of carotenes from the diet for some days causes the disappearance of the orange skin color of the individual.

Hypervitaminosis A has been observed in adults taking more than 5000 IU/day for several years. If the toxicity is detected in time and vitamin A intake is stopped, the symptoms disappear in a few days, although it may take longer depending on the amount of vitamin A that has been ingested and the extent of liver storage of vitamin A.

8.2 VITAMIN D

Since the Middle Ages, cod liver oil has been used as a remedy for rickets, but it was not until 1922 that the cause of rickets and the scientific basis for its cure were established. Rickets can be counteracted by a fat-soluble factor, and the antirachitic activity is produced in some foods and other biological materials after ultraviolet irradiation. This discovery provided the basic information for the isolation and identification of vitamin D in the 1930s; later, it was discovered that the vitamin has to be converted in the body to the metabolically active form for it to have a biological function.

8.2.1 CHEMISTRY

Vitamin D is a generic name for a family of distinct, closely related compounds that have rickets-preventing properties. The two major forms of nutritional significance for humans are cholecalciferol, which is also known as vitamin D_3 (Figure 8.6), and ergocalciferol or vitamin D_2 (Figure 8.7). Vitamin D has a structure similar to steroids except that the B-ring is absent. Therefore, it is technically a secosteroid, a term used for a steroid that has one of the rings open. The structural differences between vitamin D_2 and vitamin D_3 are in their side chains. The side chain of vitamin D_2 contains a double bond between carbons 22 and 23 and a methyl group on carbon 24. Vitamin D_3 is produced by the action of sunlight or ultraviolet irradiation from the precursor,

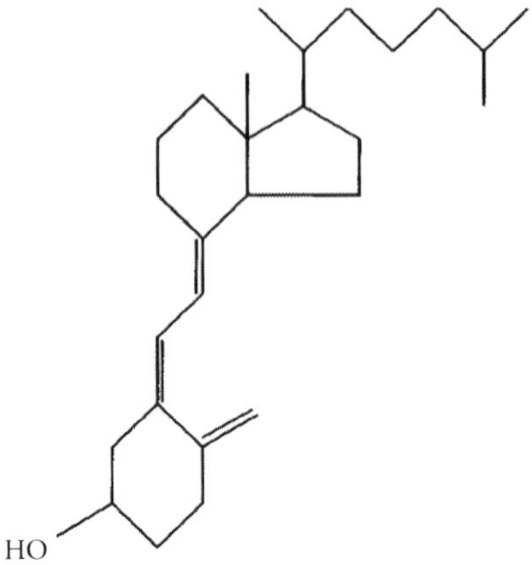

FIGURE 8.6 Cholecalciferol, vitamin D_3, formed by ultraviolet irradiation of 7-dehydrocholesterol.

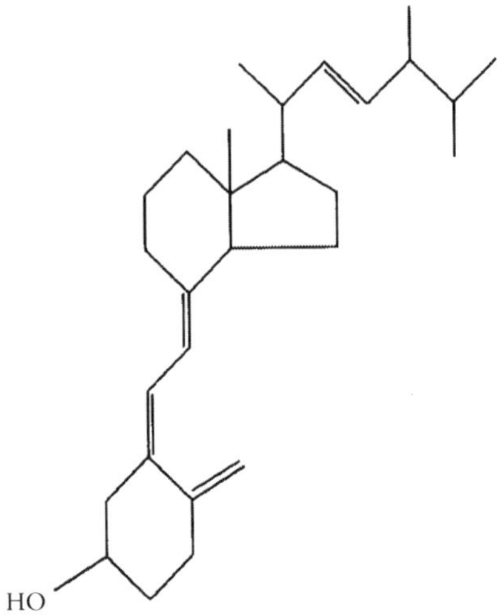

FIGURE 8.7 Ergocalciferol, vitamin D_2, formed by ultraviolet irradiation of ergosterol.

7-dehydrocholesterol (7-DC), that is synthesized in the skin of animals and humans. Vitamin D_2 is made synthetically by irradiation of the plant steroid, ergosterol. Vitamin D is fairly stable and is soluble in a wide range of organic solvents.

During exposure to sunlight, the solar ultraviolet B photons (290–315 nm) penetrate into the skin where they cause photolysis of 7-DC to precholecalciferol (PC). Once formed, PC undergoes a thermally induced rearrangement of its double bonds to form cholecalciferol over a period of few hours. Double bonds present in the fifth and sixth carbons in the B-ring structure are necessary for this conversion, which in essence opens the B-ring. The vitamin formed diffuses gradually through the basal layers of the skin into the circulation. In adult skin, approximately 60% of the cutaneous stores of 7-DC are found in the epidermis and the other 40% resides in the dermis. The average concentration of 7-DC in 1 cm^2 of young adult skin is approximately 0.8 μg for the epidermis and 0.15–0.5 μg for the dermis. The concentration of 7-DC in the epidermis decreases with increasing age: at the age of 70, there is a 75% decrease of 7-DC compared with that in young adults.

Latitude, season of the year, and time of day as well as ozone pollutants in the atmosphere influence the number of solar ultraviolet B photons that reach the Earth's surface, and thereby affect the cutaneous production of cholecalciferol. More ultraviolet B photons are able to penetrate the ozone layers in the spring, summer, and fall months because the sun is directly overhead. As winter approaches, the solar zenith angle of the sun becomes more oblique. This configuration causes ultra-violet B photons to be absorbed more efficiently by the atmospheric ozone layer, thereby decreasing the number of photons that reach the Earth's surface. At latitude 42°N (Boston), exposure to sun-light during the month of November through February will not produce any significant amounts of cholecalciferol in the skin. Ten degrees north of Boston (52°N, Edmonton, Canada), this period is extended to include October and March. Because windowpane glass absorbs ultraviolet radiation, exposure to sunlight through glass windows will not result in any production of cholecalciferol. The topical application of sunscreen diminishes the cutaneous production of the vitamin.

Excessive exposure to solar radiation causes conversion of 7-DC to tachysterol and lumisterol, which are biologically inactive. Melanin is an excellent sunscreen that can reduce the formation of the vitamin by absorbing part of the solar radiation. Those with dark skin pigmentation require as much as tenfold longer exposure to sunlight to make the same amount of vitamin D in their skin as does a light-skinned individual. This effect may partly explain the greater susceptibility of dark-skinned children to rickets.

8.2.2 FOOD SOURCES

Vitamin D is found in only small amounts in butter, cream, egg yolk, and liver. Plant foods are extremely poor sources of this nutrient. Fish liver oils and saltwater fish (e.g., herring, salmon, and sardines) are the only rich sources of dietary vitamin D. In the United States, the major sources of dietary vitamin are fortified foods such as milk, to which is added 400 IU of vitamin D per quart. The fortification has greatly improved the vitamin D content of milk from approximately 0.03–0.13 to 1 μg/100 g. Although milk is fortified with vitamin D, dairy products made from milk, such as cheese and ice cream, are generally not fortified with vitamin D and contain only small amounts of the vitamin. Some ready-to-eat breakfast cereals and juices may be fortified with vitamin D often at the level of 10%–15% of the daily values. Margarine also has been fortified to contain approximately 11 μg/100 g. A 3-oz serving of salmon, sardines, tuna, or shrimp contains 3.5–4.5 μg of vitamin D. One egg contains about 0.8 μg.

This nutrient is unique in the sense that it is not required in the diet when the individual is exposed to a sufficient amount of ultraviolet light; therefore, it has been called the sunshine vitamin. The 7-DC in the skin, when exposed to ultraviolet rays, is converted to vitamin D_3 (Figure 8.8). However, because adequate exposure to sunlight is not possible in some geographical regions and in conjunction with recommendations to reduce exposure to sunlight to decrease the risk of skin cancer, dietary vitamin D is deemed essential. The amount of vitamin produced is influenced more by the amount of ultraviolet light to which the individual is exposed than by the amount of the precursor present. The pigment on the skin acts as a protection against the over-production of the vitamin in the dark-skinned individuals in the tropics. It reduces the benefits for the much smaller amount of irradiation available to these individuals when living in temperate zones. Substantial vitamin D is required in the diet of this population. Because of the very small amount of the nutrient present in most foods, milk and some other foods have been fortified with this vitamin.

8.2.3 ABSORPTION

Dietary vitamin D is absorbed with the aid of bile salts from the small intestine. Being lipid-soluble, it is primarily absorbed with fat through the lacteal system; once absorbed, it is incorporated into the chylomicrons and transported in the lymphatic system. The vitamin is removed from the chylomicrons and attached to a carrier protein α_2-globulin, vitamin D–binding protein (DBP). Vitamin D formed from 7-DC by irradiation also is bound to the same transport protein and, from then on, it is indistinguishable from vitamin D obtained from food sources. The vitamin is stored

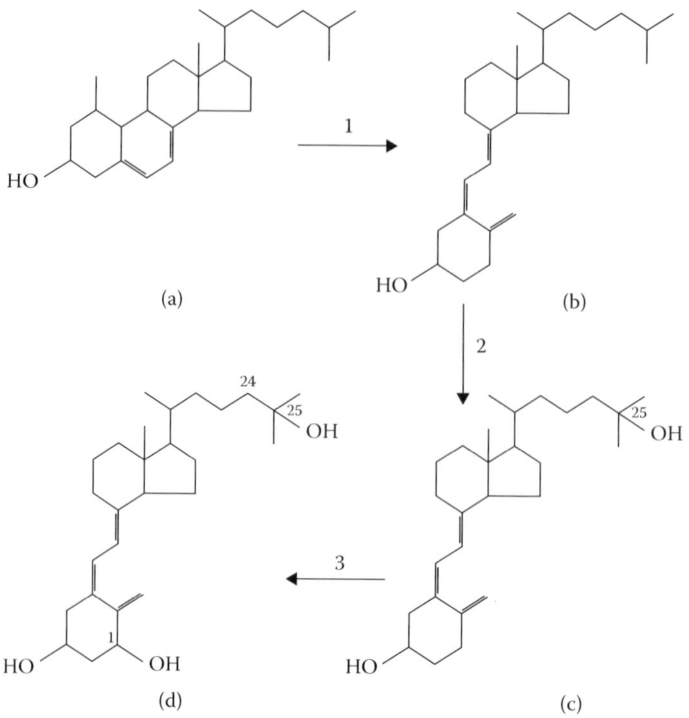

FIGURE 8.8 Step 1 is the formation of cholecalciferol (b) by irradiation of 7-dehydrocholesterol (a) in the skin by ultraviolet light. Step 2 is the conversion of cholecalciferol to 25-hydroxycholecalciferol (c) in the liver. Step 3 is the formation of 1,25-dihydroxycholecalciferol (d) in the kidney from compound (c).

in adipose tissues and muscles or metabolized to the active form. Obesity, age, and conditions that lead to malabsorption can affect the availability of the vitamin. Vitamin D, being fat-soluble, is deposited in adipose tissue, and people who are overweight cannot access it as readily as others. By age 65, changes in the skin may reduce vitamin production by as much as 60%. Malabsorption conditions like Crohn's disease, pancreatic enzyme deficiency, and celiac disease may cause less vitamin D absorption.

8.2.4 METABOLISM

Following the intestinal absorption of the dietary vitamin or synthesis in the skin, vitamin D has to be metabolically altered in order for it to be biologically active (Figure 8.8). In the liver, the vitamin undergoes its initial transformation, which involves the addition of a hydroxyl group to C_{25}. This reaction is catalyzed by microsomal vitamin D–25-hydroxylase to yield 25-OH–vitamin D. This metabolite is the predominant form of vitamin D in the blood, where it is transported attached to DBP. It undergoes further hydroxylation in the kidney by mitochondrial 1-hydroxylase. The enzyme is found in the inner mitochondrial membrane of the cells lining the proximal convoluted renal tubules. The 1-hydroxylase is part of the enzyme system associated with cytochrome P450. The product 1,25-dihydroxycholecalciferol (or 1,25-dihydroxyergocalciferol) is also called calcitriol, and it functions as a hormone which, along with calcitonin and parathyroid hormone (PTH), regulates calcium and phosphorus metabolism. The calcitriol is transported via a transport protein to the intestines, bones, kidneys, and perhaps other sites where it carries out its known actions of the vitamin.

25-OH–vitamin D also undergoes other metabolic conversions, the most important of which is 24-hydroxylation in the kidney mitochondria to form 24,25-dihydroxy vitamin D. It appears to have no biological function and represents an alternate hydroxylation for the removal of 25-OH–vitamin D.

Dietary calcium suppresses the synthesis of calcitriol and stimulates the synthesis of 24,25-dihydroxy vitamin D. On the other hand, a low level of dietary calcium increases the synthesis of calcitriol. In vitamin D deficiency, the kidney has high 1-hydroxylase and low 24-hydroxylase activity; with the administration of vitamin D, 1-hydroxylase activity declines while that of 24-hydroxylase increases. Hence, it has been suggested that there is some reciprocal regulation of these two enzyme systems. A low serum calcium results in an increased production of 1,25-dihydroxy vitamin D and the result-ing hypercalcemic effect and a decreased formation of 24,25-dihydroxy vitamin D. When the serum calcium approaches a normal level, the synthesis of 1,25-dihydroxy vitamin D stops and that of 24,25-dihydroxy vitamin D is stimulated. It appears that PTH (which is released in response to low serum calcium) is the mediator that stimulates the production of 1,25-dihydroxy vitamin D. The major excretory route for vitamin D is bile. Vitamin D metabolites may undergo conjugation in the liver prior to secretion. An enterohepatic circulation of vitamin D metabolites has been demonstrated in humans.

Although the kidneys are the major site for calcitriol production, the placenta has the capacity to synthesize it. This may be important during the third trimester of pregnancy. Elevated circulating calcitriol levels can enhance the efficiency of the mother's intestinal calcium absorption to meet an increased need of the fetus for calcium to mineralize the skeleton. Prostate also can synthesize calcitriol.

8.2.5   Functions

The major target tissues for calcitriol are the intestines, bones, and kidneys. It functions like a steroid hormone. Upon entry into target cells, calcitriol (ligand) migrates into the nuclei where it binds to the VDR, a member of the superfamily of nuclear receptors that regulate gene expression. The bind-ing of the ligand to VDR brings about conformational changes so that the RXR can combine with it, forming a heterodimer complex. The ligand–VDR–RXR complex recruits additional coactivators and binds to vitamin D response elements (VDREs) in target genes. The VDREs are short sequences of DNA and are found in DNA regions associated with calcitriol-activated genes such as those for osteocalcin (expressed in osteoblasts). The target genes can either be upregulated or downregulated. The example of upregulation is calcium-binding protein, which facilitates intestinal calcium absorp-tion. The inhibition of PTH gene in the parathyroid gland is an example of downregulation.

The most important function of calcitriol (together with PTH and calcitonin) is to maintain calcium and phosphorus hemostasis. In response to low blood calcium levels, calcitriol mediates important biological actions in the intestines, bones, and kidneys. The normal calcium concentra-tion in the blood is about 10 mg/dL. A drop in blood calcium below the normal level stimulates the release of PTH from parathyroid glands. One of the actions of this hormone is the activation of renal-1-hydroxylase, which results in the formation of calcitriol.

In the small intestine, the biological action of calcitriol is analogous to other steroid hormones. Calcitriol binds to a receptor on the intestinal cell and is transferred to the nucleus, where it stimulates a series of events that results in the biosynthesis of both a calcium-binding protein and a phosphorus-binding protein. These are then transferred to the cell surface where they facilitate the intes-tinal absorption of both calcium and phosphorus, thus increasing blood calcium and phosphorus levels.

In the bones, calcitriol, together with PTH, stimulates the release of calcium into the blood, prob-ably by increasing the production of the enzyme that accelerates the breakdown of bone matrix. This response of calcitriol is also thought to represent an initial event in the bone remodeling pro-cess. By activating bone resorption (which is a precursor for bone formation in the bone remodeling system), calcitriol may have a role in the synthesis of new bones.

In the kidneys, about 10 g of calcium is filtered daily, but only about 100 mg is actually lost in the urine; the difference is actively reabsorbed by the distal tubule cells and restored to the bloodstream. This reabsorption is controlled by the concerted action of calcitriol and PTH.

All these effects of calcitriol on the intestines, bones, and kidneys result in raising the blood cal-cium to the level optimal for the calcification of bone and the promotion of normal neuromuscular activity. The response to low plasma calcium levels is characterized by an elevation of PTH and hence of calcitriol; calcitriol acts to enhance the intestinal absorption of calcium. Calcitriol and PTH increase bone resorption and inhibit urinary calcium excretion. High plasma calcium levels cause the production of calcitonin, which inhibits bone resorption and enhances calcium excretion. Furthermore, the high levels of calcium and phosphorus in plasma increase the rate of bone mineralization. Thus, the bones serve as an important reservoir of the calcium and phosphorus needed to maintain homeostasis of plasma levels. When vitamin D and dietary calcium are adequate, no net loss of bone calcium occurs, but when dietary calcium is low, PTH and calcitriol cause a net demineralization of bones to maintain normal plasma calcium level. Hence, vitamin D deficiency causes a net demineralization of bones due to an elevation of PTH.

The active form of vitamin D is considered to be a hormone because it is produced exclusively in the kidneys and has specific target organs—the intestine and bone. Also, its formation is regulated either by direct or indirect feedback by plasma calcium, PTH, and vitamin D itself. Thus, vitamin D is a nutrient and a prohormone. It is needed in the diet as a nutrient only when exposure to sunlight is insufficient to internally produce enough vitamin D_3 from the irradiation of 7-DC.

In addition to its well-known function in calcium metabolism, vitamin D appears to have a role in several noncalcemic tissues. There is evidence that vitamin D may offer protection against such diverse chronic diseases as hypertension, certain cancers, type 2 diabetes, and autoimmune disorders including multiple sclerosis (MS). Several recent European studies suggest that supplementing infants with vitamin D during their first year might offer protection against type 1 diabetes. One large prospective study has shown that the relative risk of developing type 1 diabetes by the age of 30 among children who were given vitamin D in their first year (at least 50 μg/day) was only 0.12 compared with children who were not given supplements—a substantial reduction.

The VDR is present in the small intestine, colon, osteoblasts, most cells of the immune system including activated T and B lymphocytes, β-islet cells, and most organs in the body, including brain, heart, skin, gonads, prostate, and breast. Vitamin D is a potent immune system modulator. Autoimmune diseases occur when the body mounts an immune response against its own tissues. In type 1 diabetes, the targets are the β-cells of the pancreas; in MS the targets are the myelin-producing cells of the central nervous system; and in rheumatoid arthritis (RA), the targets are the collagen-producing cells of the joints. Autoimmune responses are mediated by T cells. The active form of vitamin D has been found to modulate T cell responses, and diminish autoimmune responses in animal models of type 2 diabetes, MS, and RA. MS causes the disintegration of the protective myelin sheath surrounding nerve cells in the brain and spinal cord, leading to the gradual loss of function and disability. It affects 350,000 people in the United States and 2 million around the world. A study based on stored blood samples from more than 7 million U.S. military personnel found that young people who had the highest levels of vitamin D had a 62% lower risk of developing MS than people with the lowest level. Scientists first linked vitamin D's role in MS more than 30 years ago when they noticed the disease was more prevalent in northern latitudes where sunlight is sparse during winter months. People living in cities like Detroit, Boston, and New York synthesize no vitamin D from sunlight between December and February. More recent studies have shown that vitamin D injections prevent MS from developing in mice that can be induced in a laboratory setting to develop myelin destruction as in MS. In two large cohorts of U.S. women followed for at least 10 years, vitamin D supplement use was associated with a significant reduction in the risk of developing MS. Postmenopausal women with the highest total vitamin D intakes were at significantly lower risk of developing RA after 11 years of follow-up than those with the lowest intakes. Thus, the evidence from experimental and human epidemiological studies suggest that maintaining adequate vitamin D levels may help decrease the risk of several autoimmune diseases.

Calcitriol can inhibit the proliferation and induce the terminal differentiation of a variety of normal and tumor cells by directly or indirectly altering the transcription of cell growth regulatory genes. Epidermal cells possess a VDR, and calcitriol and its analogs have been used successfully for treating hyperproliferative skin disorder (psoriasis). An analog calcipotriene (Dovonex) suppresses keratinocyte proliferation and has anti-inflammatory effects. The analog is highly effective for the treatment of psoriasis when applied locally twice daily as an ointment.

Thus, the functions of vitamin D include regulation, proliferation, differentiation, and immunomodulation.

Several studies suggest that vitamin D may have a role in blood pressure regulation and heart health. Both the blood vessels and the heart have VDR, which means that vitamin D is providing some function in regulating these tissues. Research indicates that vitamin D may play a role in preventing or reversing coronary disease. Low levels of vitamin D have been implicated in hypertension, elevated triglycerides, and impaired insulin metabolism. The Nurses' Health Study and the National Health and Nutrition Examination Surveys (NHANES) have shown that serum concentrations of 25-hydroxy vitamin D are inversely associated with blood pressure. Research in mice lacking the gene encoding the VDR indicates that the biologically active form of vitamin D decreases the expression of the gene encoding renin through its interaction with the VDR. Because inappropriate activation of the renin–angiotensin system is thought to play a role in some form of hypertension, adequate vitamin D levels may be important for decreasing the risk of high blood pressure. The results of animal studies suggest that vitamin D plays a role in insulin secretion under conditions of increased insulin demand. A report on a clinical trial conducted in men with congestive heart failure (CHF) suggests that vitamin D has a protective effect on the heart itself and on atherosclerosis that may precipitate CHF.

Two characteristics of cancer cells are lack of differentiation and rapid growth and proliferation. The biologically active form of vitamin D induces cell differentiation and inhibits proliferation of a number of cancerous and noncancerous cell types maintained in cell culture. These effects may be mediated through VDR expressed in cancer cells. A 2006 study using data of more than 4 million cancer patients from 13 different countries showed a marked difference in cancer risk between countries classified as sunny and countries classified as less sunny, for a number of different cancers.

Research suggests that vitamin D can improve mood and may help reduce depression. There is an association between low serum vitamin D levels and Parkinson's disease. Whether Parkinson's disease causes low vitamin D levels or whether vitamin D levels play a role in the pathogenesis of Parkinson's disease has not been established. Vitamin D alone or together with curcumin, a component in turmeric, may help stimulate the immune system to clear the brain of amyloid β, which forms the plaque considered the hallmark of Alzheimer's disease.

Vitamin D might be a factor in longer life. A study of more than 57,000 participants has shown that those who took supplemental vitamin D had a 7% lower risk of death from all causes than those who did not.

The mechanism of how vitamin D plays a role in the prevention of various diseases involving noncalcemic tissues has not been well established. So far, there is very little information on whether taking vitamin D supplements can avoid or reduce the risks of these diseases. Vigorous scientific studies are needed to clarify the relationship between vitamin D and cardiovascular disease, cancer, and other chronic diseases. The findings are based on 25-hydroxy vitamin D levels in serum and disease incidence and epidemiologic studies that have pointed to a connection between sunlight exposure, a surrogate for vitamin D levels, and various diseases.

In general, people who live closer to the equator have a lower incidence of these diseases. Researchers have been able to establish a dose–response relationship between sunlight and serum 25-hydroxy vitamin D levels. Each degree of latitude corresponds to 0.8–1 ng/mL of 25-hydroxy vitamin D. A person living near the 0° latitude (equator) is expected to have a level of about 60 ng/mL. In an individual living at 60° latitude such as Southern Alaska or Sweden, it may be 2–10 ng/mL. Researchers in this field consider a level of 55–60 ng/mL as optimal for cancer prevention. Using a new WHO database of cancer incidence, mortality, and prevalence in 177 countries, it is estimated that about 250,000 cases of colorectal cancer and 350,000 cases of breast cancer could be prevented worldwide by boosting the serum level of 25-hydroxy vitamin D to 55–60 ng/mL.

8.2.6 Deficiency

Vitamin D deficiency can result from inadequate intake coupled with inadequate sunlight exposure, disorders of the gastrointestinal tract that can affect absorption, conditions such as liver and kidney disorders, and body characteristics such as skin color and body[28] fat.

Vitamin D deficiency is much more common than previously thought, affecting up to half of adults and apparently healthy children in the United States. It is estimated that >50% of African Americans in the United States are either chronically or seasonally at risk of developing vitamin D deficiency. In the third NHANES, 42% of African American women 15–65 years of age are found to be vitamin D deficient at the end of the winter and 84% of African Americans over 65 years old are vitamin D deficient. It is estimated that one billion people in the world are currently vitamin D deficient. Data from supplementation studies indicate that vitamin D intakes of at least 800–1000 IU/day are required to achieve serum 25-OH vitamin D of at least 32 ng/mL, a value considered in the optimum range (see Section 8.2.8).

The deficiency of vitamin D tends to increase the risk of infections such as influenza. People with low serum levels of vitamin D are more likely to acquire a cold and flu than those with adequate amounts. The effect of the vitamin appears to be strongest in people with asthma and other lung diseases who are predisposed to respiratory infections. People with the worst deficiency are 36% more likely to suffer respiratory infections than those with adequate levels, according to new research findings. Among asthmatics those who are vitamin D deficient are 5 times more likely to get sick than their counterparts with healthy vitamin levels.

Vitamin D deficiency may be an underlying factor in musculoskeletal pain and is a potentially treatable cause. Recently, doctors have come across adults who were disabled by severe pain, sometimes for years, until they were treated for undiagnosed vitamin D deficiency. In a cross-sectional study of 150 consecutive patients referred to a clinic in Minnesota for the evaluation of persistent nonspecific musculoskeletal pain, 93% were found to have levels of 25-hydroxy vitamin D indicative of deficiency. Physicians may be wise to suspect hypovitaminosis D in patients with persistent nonspecific musculoskeletal pain. This is especially true for patients from areas with a prolonged winter.

There is a lot of data that suggests that adults with low vitamin D levels are at risk of diabetes,[40] high blood pressure, cardiovascular disease, and cancer. Two recent studies have reported that 70% of American children are not getting enough vitamin D. In one study researchers looked at the serum levels of vitamin D of more than 6000 people who were between 1 to 21 years old. They checked vitamin D deficiency defined as <15 ng/mL of 25-hydroxy vitamin D and insufficiency, which is defined as 15–29.5 ng/mL. Overall 7.5 million or 9% of U.S. children were found to be vitamin D deficient and another 50.8 million or 60% had insufficient vitamin D level in their blood. Children with low levels of vitamin D were more likely to have high blood pressure and lower levels of good cholesterol—two factors that are considered major risk factors for heart disease later in life. Children with lower vitamin D levels also had higher PTH than their counterparts with adequate vitamin D in their blood. PTH is a measure of bone health. High levels of PTH suggest that bones need more calcium to grow. Overall, those most at risk for vitamin D deficiency were older, female, obese, drank milk less than once a day, and spent more than 4 hours a day watching TV, playing video games, or working at a computer. They were also more likely to be children with darker skin, including non-Hispanic blacks and Mexican-Americans.

In a second study, researchers looked at 3577 adolescents, 12–19 years of age. Those with low vitamin D levels were more likely to have high blood pressure, high blood sugar, and other risk factors for heart disease than their counterparts with ample vitamin D in their blood, regardless of how much they weighed.

Vitamin D deficiency leads to rickets in children,[19] which usually develops in infancy or early childhood (Figure 8.9) and is among the most frequent childhood diseases in many developing countries. It is caused by defective bone formation as a result of inadequate deposition of calcium

Bowlegs—Rickets

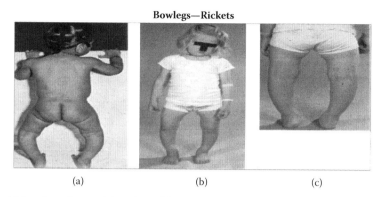

(a)   (b)   (c)

FIGURE 8.9   (a) Bowlegs due to rickets in a child from a moderately affluent family. (b) Close-up of front standing. (c) Close-up from back standing; note the angle of the feet. (Courtesy of Shari Roehl, Pharmacia & Upjohn Co.)

and phosphorus in the bone. The bones become soft and pliable, and a number of different deformities may ensue: bow legs, knock knees, enlargement of the ends of bones, and so on. When the poorly calcified bones are called upon to perform weight-bearing functions for which they are not properly prepared, they yield, and a bowing of legs occurs when a vitamin D–deficient child slowly starts to walk or supports weight of any kind on the incompletely mineralized bone. Other signs include bone pain or tenderness, muscle weakness, increased tendency to fracture, and growth disturbances. Unless effective measures are employed early in the disease, permanent malformation of bone may persist. There is commonly a delay in dentition as the appearance of the first tooth in rachitic babies is delayed.

While the predominant cause of rickets is vitamin D deficiency, the lack of adequate calcium in the diet may also lead to rickets. Those at high risk for developing rickets include breast-fed infants whose mothers are not exposed to sunlight, breast-fed infants themselves who are not exposed to sunlight, and individuals not consuming fortified milk, such as those who are lactose intolerant.

In the United States and other developed countries rickets was common in the 19th and early 20th centuries. With the introduction of vitamin D–fortified foods the disease was largely eliminated by the 1950s. In recent years, however, despite the better understanding and wide choice of preventive and therapeutic strategies, the crippling bone disease is reappearing, not only in temperate zones with limited sunshine but also in sunny climates. Indeed, rickets is more common in some sunny countries than in temperate ones. An old problem of nutritional child health, once eliminated, has resurfaced. One of the reasons appears to be due to the greatly increased rate of exclusive breast-feeding in this and other countries. Baby formula is fortified with vitamin D.

Vitamin D content of breast milk from a mother with adequate vitamin D status is approximately 22 IU/L, and this cannot provide by itself the intake of 200 IU/day recommended for infants. Most breast-fed infants may obtain vitamin D through sunlight exposure. However, the amount of vitamin D synthesized through sunlight exposure is affected by the amount of time exposed to sun, the amount of skin exposed, air pollution, time of day, latitude, and skin pigmentation. It is estimated that light-skinned infants require about 30 minutes of sunlight per week to get adequate vitamin D if they are wearing only diapers, and 2 hours per week if they are fully clothed with no hat. Infants with dark skin need to spend much more time in the sunlight to synthesize the same amount of vitamin D. Breast-fed infants should be given vitamin D supplements beginning in the early days of life.

Osteomalacia in adults, a condition that might be called adult rickets, occurs after skeletal development is complete. It affects primarily women of childbearing age who become calcium-deficient after repeated pregnancies. As in rickets and even though bone mineralization has ceased, collagen formation continues. This results in the formation of uncalcified bone matrix, causing the bone to become softer and susceptible to fracture. The main symptoms of osteomalacia are muscular weakness and bone pain. Osteomalacia is easily distinguishable from the more common osteoporosis by the fact that the osteoid matrix remains intact in the former but not in the latter.

Vitamin D deficiency is rare in America and Europe because of fortification of dairy products with the vitamin. The deficiency cases that do occur are most often seen in low-income groups with poor dietary habits, the elderly with minimal exposure to sunlight, strict vegetarians, those with fat malabsorption or severe liver and kidney disease, and those taking some drugs that interfere with vitamin D metabolism. The use of anticonvulsant drugs for epilepsy has caused rickets in infants and osteomalacia in adults. These drugs stimulate the hepatic cytochrome P450 microsomal enzyme systems, leading to degradation of the vitamin and its metabolite.

Classical rickets and osteomalacia can be cured by vitamin D supplementation; however, there are occasional cases of rickets that are not due to inadequate dietary intake of the vitamin and/or exposure to sunlight. These cases of rickets can be due to any number of unrelated causes. Vitamin D–dependent rickets, type 1, is an autosomal recessive disorder in which serum calcitriol levels are very low and 25-hydroxy vitamin D levels are normal. This disease is caused by a mutation in the gene encoding the 1-α hydroxylase, leading to a clinical syndrome of vitamin D deficiency. It is characterized by hypocalcemia and elevated serum alkaline phosphatase. PTH levels in the serum are elevated; consequently, urinary excretion of phosphate is increased and urinary calcium excretion is decreased. Symptoms usually appear before the age of 2 years, including rickets and growth retardation. Treatment with calcitriol (0.5–1 µg/day) leads to a rapid correction of abnormalities and the resolution of the bone disease. Calcium and phosphorus supplements are usually not required.

Hereditary vitamin D–resistant rickets, also called vitamin D–dependent rickets, type 2, is a rare autosomal recessive disease that results from target organ resistance to the action of calcitriol. Mutations in the gene from VDR result in an inability of VDR to bind to calcitriol, or an inability of the VDR–RXR complex to bind to the VDRE in DNA. Affected patients usually present with severe rickets during their early childhood, although some may have a mild form of the disease not recognized until adulthood. Alopecia is common especially in severe childhood forms and may be due to defective VDR in the hair follicles. Serum calcium and phosphorus are low. Secondary hypoparathyroidism is present. Circulating calcitriol levels are elevated (unlike rickets, type 1). Pharmacological doses (5–30 µg/day) of calcitriol, along with mineral supplements, improve the biochemical disorder and bone disease, although some patients may not respond to massive doses of calcitriol.

X-linked hypophosphatemic rickets, also called vitamin D–resistant rickets, is an X-linked dominant disorder characterized by hypophophatemia with renal phosphate wasting, rickets, and short stature. Hypophosphatemia is present soon after birth and rachitic bowing of the legs develops when the child begins to walk. Children have growth retardation. Serum levels of calcium and 25-hydroxy vitamin D are normal and levels of calcitriol are low normal. As hypophosphatemia is a potent inducer of 1-α hydroxylase, calcitriol levels should be high but they are not. This suggests the existence of a functional defect in the 1-α hydroxylase, most likely caused by the abnormal phosphate transport. Oral neutral phosphates combined with calcitriol is an effective therapy for this disorder.

Severe burn injury is associated with vitamin D deficiency. The conversion of 7-DC to vitamin D is reduced in these patients. Therefore, vitamin D supplementation is necessary in these patients.

Patients who are suffering from chronic renal failure have a defect in vitamin D metabolism. They generally have low levels of calcitriol in their blood because the kidney enzyme responsible for the biogenesis of the active metabolite of vitamin D is inoperable. This condition appears to be responsible for renal osteodystrophy—bone degeneration—in patients with kidney failure. It can be treated successfully in most cases by calcitriol.

Individuals without functional parathyroid glands do not secrete PTH when needed; this affects the activity of 1-hydroxylase, which is dependent on the hormone, and the synthesis of calcitriol. Calcium is not mobilized and the sensitive neuromuscular junction reacts in a convulsive or tetanic state. This condition is treated with calcitriol and calcium.

There is an age-dependent loss of calcium absorption and bone mass associated with low blood levels of calcitriol. This is attributed to the low activity of 1-hydroxylase, and calcitriol may help in preventing bone loss in old age.

8.2.7 UNITS

The international unit of vitamin D recommended for adoption by the WHO is the vitamin D activity of 0.025 µg of crystalline vitamin D. The dietary requirement depends on the amount synthesized by the individual that, in turn, depends on skin pigmentation and exposure to sunlight. It has been estimated that depending on skin pigmentation, exposing the hands, face, and arms on a clear summer day for 10–15 minutes two to three times a week is sufficient to meet requirements. An intake of 2.5 µg/day vitamin D (100 IU) prevents rickets and ensures adequate calcium absorption, satisfactory growth, and normal mineralization of the bone in infants; however, the RDA is considered to be 400 IU to promote calcium absorption and some increase in growth. The requirements for older children and adults have not been precisely determined, but the current RDA takes account of adverse conditions and provides for 7.5 µg/day for those aged 19–22 years.

For adults, the RDA for vitamin D is set at 5 µg/day. Prevalence rates of low plasma vitamin D levels in older adults range from 5% to 15% in the Framingham cohort to over 50% of hospitalized and institutionalized elderly patients. Reasons for these high prevalence rates include poor dietary intake, inadequate exposure to the sun, chronic liver and renal diseases, and therapy with drugs that can impair vitamin D activity. A recent U.S. trial involving healthy older men and women demonstrated that supplemental vitamin D and calcium (700 IU and 500 mg, respectively) can reduce bone loss and decrease fracture rates. The Institute of Medicine recently recommended the doubling of the previous RDA for vitamin D to 10 µg/day (400 IU) for adults aged 51–70 years, and a tripling to 15 µg/day (600 IU) for adults over age 70 years. Because mean intake in community-dwelling elderly individuals is approximately 2.5 µg/day, a low-dose supplement (10 µg/day) should be considered for all older adults. Multivitamin pills typically contain at least 400 IU.

8.2.8 ASSESSMENT OF VITAMIN D STATUS

The serum concentrations of 25-hydroxy vitamin D are several times greater than that of calcitriol and have a much longer biological half life, around two to three weeks compared with 4–6 hours for calcitriol. Because of this relative stability, the principal biomarker used to assess vitamin D status is serum 25-hydroxy vitamin D. But the cutoff values have not been clearly defined. Generally, a value of 0–14.9 ng/mL indicates severe deficiency, 15–31.9 ng/mL mild deficiency, and 32–100 ng/mL is optimal. In patients with chronic renal failure, there is impairment in renal 1-hydroxylase, which results in disassociation between 25-hydroxy vitamin D and calcitriol concentrations. Measuring serum calcitriol is then necessary. Vitamin D intoxication is usually associated with a 25-hydroxy vitamin D concentration above 150 ng/mL, with attendant hypercalcemia and hyperphosphatemia. Calcitriol concentrations are not substantially altered.

8.2.9 TOXICITY

During exposure to sunlight, some fraction of the precursor, 7-DC, is converted to vitamin D_3 and only short exposures are necessary for sufficient cutaneous production of the vitamin. With continued exposure to sunlight, the remaining vitamin is rapidly isomerized to biologically inert products (mainly lumisterol and tachysterol), which do not enter the circulation. Therefore, excess exposure to sunlight does not result in an overproduction or toxic amounts of the vitamin. Ingestion of vitamin D in excess of the recommended amount provides no added benefit and large doses can be harmful. There is a narrow gap between the nutrient requirement and the toxic dose. An intake of five times the RDA over a prolonged period has led to toxic effects. Normal dietary sources do not contain excessive amounts of vitamin D; however, there is great concern among individuals who take large amounts of supplemental vitamins and those who are treated with vitamin D or its analogs for various clinical conditions.

Excessive vitamin D can cause irreversible calcification of the heart, lungs, kidneys, and other soft tissues. Therefore, care should be taken to detect early signs of intoxication in patients receiving pharmacological doses of the vitamin. Symptoms of intoxication include hypercalcemia, nausea, vomiting, loss of appetite, muscular weakness, and joint pains. The intoxication is thought to be caused as a result of 25-OH–vitamin D levels in the blood rather than calcitriol because large doses of 25-OH vitamin D can mimic the action of calcitriol. The treatment includes the withdrawal of vitamin D and the reduction of dietary calcium intake until the serum calcium falls to near-normal level. In more severe cases, glucocorticoids are administered, which are thought to antagonize the action of vitamin D. As calcitonin can also bring serum calcium levels down, it may also be used.

8.3   VITAMIN E

Vitamin E was discovered during investigations on the influence of nutrition on reproduction in rats.[41] Rats fed a diet of casein, corn starch, and rancid lard failed to reproduce unless lettuce or whole wheat was included in the diet. Subsequently, it was found that wheat germ oil contained all the "vitamin" properties of wheat. The letter E was adopted to designate the factor following the then recognized vitamin D. In the 1930s, vitamin E was isolated from wheat germ oil, and its structure was established. It was given the name tocopherol, which is derived from the Greek words "tokos" (child birth) and "pherein" (to bear). The suffix "–ol" indicates that the factor is an alcohol.

8.3.1   CHEMISTRY

Eight compounds with characteristic vitamin E-like biological activity have been isolated from plant sources. They all have a 6-chromanol ring structure and a side chain. There are four tocopherols (α, β, γ, and δ) with a fully saturated side chain, and four tocotrienols that have a similar structure but with double bonds at the 3′, 7′, and 11′ positions of the side chain. The individual tocopherols and tocotrienols differ within the group only with respect to the number and the position of the methyl groups in the aromatic ring of the molecule (Figure 8.10). α-tocopherol is the most abundant and the most biologically active isomer of vitamin E. β-tocopherol and γ-tocopherol are 50% and 10% as potent, respectively, as α-tocopherol. α-tocotrienol is about 30% as active as α-tocopherol, and the other isomers of vitamin E have very little activity. The vitamin E isomers are light yellow substances, which are oils at room temperature. They are insoluble in water and soluble in nonpolar solvents. They are fairly stable to heat and acid and unstable to alkali, ultraviolet light, and oxygen. They are destroyed when in contact with rancid fats. Freezing and deep-frying of fat destroys most

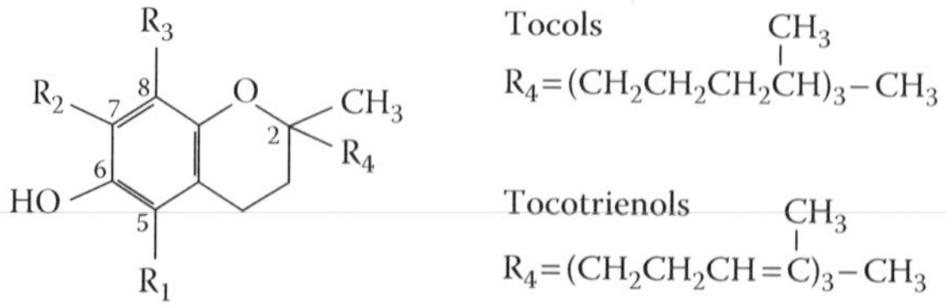

Tocopherol	Methyl positions
	5, 7, 8
	5, 8
	7, 8
	8

FIGURE 8.10   Structures of naturally occurring tocopherols.

of the tocopherol present in food. Tocopherols protect vitamin A, carotene, and vitamin C in foods from oxidative destruction. Their most important chemical characteristic is their antioxidant properties. In addition to the naturally occurring isomers, several types of synthetic vitamin E are available commercially. Synthetic vitamin E consists of a mixture of all eight isomers. The naturally occurring α-tocopherol is designated RRR α-tocopherol to distinguish it from the synthetic form, which is known as all-racemic α-tocopherol. RRR is used to explain molecular configuration. The natural form is 100% and is the most biologically active. Synthetic vitamin E has 12.5% of RRR.

8.3.2 FOOD SOURCES

All eight isomers are widely distributed in nature. Vegetable oils are the richest sources. Tocopherols are found in conjunction with plant oils, especially with polyunsaturated fatty acids (PUFAs). Grains and other seeds have these substances mostly in their germ. As if by design, there appears to be a relationship between the concentration of linoleic acid in various plant oils and the concentration of tocopherols. The latter are able to preserve and prevent the oxidation of the relatively unstable fatty acid. The processing of wheat in the preparation of white flour removes most of the vitamins through separation of their germ, and some are destroyed by bleaching.

With the possible exception of the liver, foods of animal origin contain little vitamin E activity, and all of it is accounted for by α-tocopherol. In vegetable seed oils, other isomers occur in substantial amounts. Coconut oil and fish oils are low in tocopherols.

8.3.3 ABSORPTION AND TRANSPORT

Tocopherol occurring naturally in food is in the free form, but in vitamin supplements, it is mostly as ester, which is readily hydrolyzed in the intestine. Over 20%–40% of the ingested vitamin is absorbed. As with other fat-soluble vitamins, the efficiency of absorption is enhanced by the simultaneous digestion and absorption of fats. Studies in animals and humans have shown that bile and pancreatic juices are necessary for maximum absorption of vitamin E.

After absorption from the intestine, vitamin E is transported to the circulation by lipoproteins primarily in the β-lipoprotein fraction. There is no evidence for the existence of a specific transport protein. Some vitamin E can translocate into circulating high-density lipoprotein. However, the majority of absorbed vitamin E remains in chylomicron remnants and is released in hepatocytes as remnants are removed and catabolized. A tocopherol transfer protein (TTP) in the liver binds with vitamin E and enhances its transfer into very low-density lipoprotein (VLDL) particles, which then enter the circulation. The TPP preferentially interacts with the RRR isomeric form of α-tocopherol; thus, the natural isomer has the most biological activity. α-tocopherol remains in VLDL during transformation to LDL and then circulates within LDL. It is accumulated in tissues in proportion to the fatty acid content, especially in the structures of the cells that contain phospholipid membranes such as the mitochondria, microsomes, and plasma membranes. The adrenal glands, pituitary glands, testes, and platelets have high concentrations. Vitamin E is found in tissues unmodified only in unesterified form. It undergoes very little metabolism, and the major route of excretion is via the bile. When the intake is large, it is converted to a lactone of tocopherol quinone and then is excreted in the urine as glucuronide.

8.3.4 FUNCTIONS

Being fat soluble, vitamin E is found in all cell membranes.[42,46] It is readily oxidized, and this characteristic is the basis for what is probably its prime biological function—serving as a lipid antioxidant. Antioxidants are reducing substances that help maintain a low oxidation–reduction potential in tissues. Vitamin E seems to prevent the oxidation of unsaturated and PUFAs. It appears to protect cellular and subcellular membranes from deterioration caused by free radicals—highly reactive compounds that (in the body) arise most frequently from PUFAs that have been oxidized in various physiological processes. Vitamin E can react with these free radicals to convert them to a less reactive, nontoxic form. When insufficient vitamin E is present, free radicals are able to catalyze the lipid peroxidation of membranes and their destruction. Vitamin E deficiency is accelerated by the ingestion of large amounts of PUFAs, and cell damage occurs from the deposition of lipofuscin pigment. Individuals whose diets regularly contain large amounts of unsaturated fats may gain protection against the formation of free radicals by the use of a supplemental vitamin. Aside from maintaining the integrity of cell membranes throughout the body, vitamin E protects the fat in LDL from oxidation. Oxidized LDL has been implicated in the development of cardiovascular disease.

Products of oxidative deterioration occur in tissues of aged patients. As vitamin E therapy can prevent or slow down such reactions, it may also slow the aging process. Other substances, such as selenium (as part of glutathione peroxidase) and vitamin C (ascorbic acid), also participate in inhibiting tissue-damaging oxidations. Some, but not all, of the signs of the vitamin deficiency are alleviated by these nutrients. Therefore, it is possible that the vitamin has other functions apart from scavenging of free radicals and reacting with active forms of oxygen. Animal research suggests possibilities for the role of tocopherols in human nutrition, but the many claims for the vitamin in relieving or preventing ischemic heart disease, muscular dystrophy, menstrual disorders, toxemias of pregnancy, spontaneous abortion, and sterility have not been substantiated.

Increasing evidence suggests a role of vitamin E in the prevention of cancer. Dietary supplementation of vitamin E has been reported to reduce the incidence of various cancers,[44] including colon, esophageal, and prostate cancers, although not all studies showed a beneficial effect. The proposed mechanism for this anticarcinogenic effect is thought to involve at least two theories: (1) the inhibition of lipid peroxidation and its formation of reactive products and (2) the inhibition of the formation of powerful mutagenic nitric oxide species such as peroxynitrite and nitrosamines known to react with DNA and other biological molecules. The androgen receptor is required for the development of the normal prostate gland and prostate cancer. In the early stages of prostate cancer, almost all cancer cells are androgen dependent and highly sensitive to anti-androgens. Recent work has shown that vitamin E suppresses the expression of androgen receptor in prostate cancer cells. This mechanism may explain how vitamin E inhibits the growth of prostate cancer cells and help establish new therapeutic concepts for the prevention and treatment of prostate cancer. There have been theories that vitamin E, especially when coupled with selenium, may reduce the risk of prostate cancer by 30%. However, a large placebo-controlled intervention study using α-tocopherol and selenium supplementation (the SELECT, or Selenium and Vitamin E Cancer Prevention Trial) alone or in combination was recently halted because there was no evidence of benefit in preventing prostate cancer. Several other functions of vitamin E have been identified that are not likely related to its antioxidant capacity. It is known to inhibit the activity of protein kinase C, an important cell-signaling molecule. α-tocopherol also appears to affect the expression and activities of enzymes in immune and inflammatory cells. It has been shown to inhibit platelet aggregation and to enhance vasodilation.

High doses (60–800 mg/day) of vitamin E have been shown in controlled trials to improve parameters of immune function. Two intervention studies have shown that vitamin E supplementation at 400–800 mg/day may protect against cardiovascular diseases possibly by inhibiting LDL oxidation. Other randomized trials indicate that vitamin E supplements (2000 mg/day) may slow the progression of Alzheimer's disease. Also supplemental intake of vitamin E (100–200 mg/day) has been associated with a decreased risk of cataracts.

Although both tocopherols and tocotrienols possess excellent antioxidant activity tocotrienols suppress reactive oxygen species more efficiently. In addition, tocotrienols show promising non-antioxidant activities in various in vitro and in vivo models. Most notable are the interactions of tocotrienol with the cholesterol biosynthetic pathway leading to the lowering of plasma cholesterol levels, the prevention of cell adhesion to endothelial cells, and the suppression of tumor cell growth. They also possess powerful neuroprotective and anticancer properties. Tocotrienols are found in abundance in plant foods such as rice bran or palm oil.

8.3.5 DEFICIENCY

In experimental animals, vitamin E deficiency signs are observed in the reproductive, muscular, nervous, glandular, vascular, and hemopoietic systems. Male rats on a vitamin E-deficient diet produce immotile sperm and exhibit degeneration of the germinal epithelium. Pregnant rats fed vitamin E-deficient diets either abort, or have prolonged gestational periods or resorption of the fetuses; a vascular lesion of the placenta apparently is the common denominator of these conditions. Muscle paralysis and creatinuria indicative of muscle lesions can be seen. Skeletal muscle as well as the myocardium become ischemic and suffer from calcium and lipofuscin deposits. These effects are magnified when PUFAs are added to the vitamin E-deficient diet.

Vitamin E is present in a wide variety of foods; because it is stored in the body and turns over very slowly, its deficiency is rarely seen in humans. Several years may be necessary for a previously healthy adult to deplete endogenous vitamin E stores. Persons suffering from a variety of disorders associated with fat malabsorption, such as celiac disease, pancreatitis, sprue, and biliary cirrhosis, have been found to have low plasma tocopherol levels. Common manifestations of what appears to be a vitamin E deficiency are muscle weakness, creatinuria, and an increased susceptibility of the membranes of the erythrocytes to hemolysis. Ataxia, weakness, reflex change, impaired vision, and retinopathy are associated with chronic advanced deficiency. The outer rod segments of the retina contain an exceptionally high concentration of PUFAs in an oxygen environment and hence particularly need antioxidant protection; this probably accounts for the retinal dysfunction in vitamin E deficiency.

The NHANES III examined the dietary intake and blood levels of vitamin E in 16,295 adults. Twenty-seven percent of white participants, 41% of African Americans, 28% of Mexican Americans, and 32% of the other participants were found to have blood levels of α-tocopherol less than 20 μmol/L. This cutoff value was chosen because of the reports that suggest an increased risk for cardiovascular disease below this level. Recent data from NHANES indicate that mean dietary intake of vitamin E is 7.8 mg/day for men and 6.3 mg/day for women, both well below the current intake recommendations of 15 mg/day. It is estimated that more than 90% of Americans do not meet daily dietary recommendations for vitamin E.

The developing nervous system appears to be vulnerable to vitamin E deficiency. Infants who have severe vitamin E deficiency at birth and are not treated with the vitamin rapidly develop neurological symptoms. In contrast, adults who develop serious vitamin E deficiency as a result of malabsorption syndromes may not develop neurological symptoms.

Infants, particularly premature ones, are born with low vitamin E levels (0.25 mg/dL) because most of the vitamin is transferred to the fetus in the last 2 months of fetal life. As these infants also have impaired fat absorption, they need an oral supplement preferably of water-soluble α-tocopherol in addition to that present in either breast milk or infant formula. Human milk provides 1.3–3.3 mg/L α-tocopherol, about four times as much as is present in cow's milk, and results in a faster increase in serum tocopherol levels of breast-fed infants. All milk formulas for infants now contain added vitamin E to provide 5 mg/100 Cal or 7 mg/g linoleic acid.

Infants with low plasma α-tocopherol develop hemolytic anemia and thrombocytopenia. In adults with a vitamin E–deficient diet, there is a decrease in red blood cell survival time with less than 0.5 mg/dL α-tocopherol. There is no clear consensus as to the optimal level of α-tocopherol in plasma below which is considered the vitamin deficiency. When the level of plasma tocopherol falls below 0.5 mg/dL, peroxide hemolysis tests in vitro become positive and most probably in vivo hemolysis occurs when tocopherol reaches a level equal to or below 0.2 mg/dL in plasma.

Children with abetalipoproteinemia cannot absorb or transport vitamin E and become deficient quite rapidly. Patients with a familial form of isolated vitamin E deficiency have extremely low plasma vitamin E because of a defect in the TTP. In these individuals, the absorption and transport of vitamin E to the liver are normal, but hepatic incorporation of α-tocopherol into nascent VLDL is impaired. Patients with TTP deficiency exhibit peripheral neuropathy and ataxia. High doses of vitamin E can prevent or mitigate the neurological course of the disease. Serum vitamin E concentrations in patients increase when they are treated with large doses of vitamin E, presumably because of the direct transfer of tocopherol from chylomicrons to other circulating lipoproteins.

8.3.6 UNITS

The vitamin E requirements are expressed as tocopherol equivalents (TE). One milligram of α-tocopherol equals 1 mg of TE. The RDA for infants is 4–5 TE; for children and adolescents, the range is 6–15 TE; and for adult males and females, it is 15 and 8 mg TE, respectively. During pregnancy and lactation, an additional 2–3 mg TE is recommended.

In establishing the RDA, it is recognized that the need for vitamin E is directly related to the PUFA content of the diet. When the dietary PUFA is low, the need for the vitamin is lower, and when PUFA is increased in the diet, the need for vitamin E also increases. In general, the increase in PUFA is the result of an increased use of vegetable oils, which are the best sources of vitamin E. In the United States, the average dietary intake of vitamin E is estimated to be in the range of 7.5–9 mg TE and 21 g of PUFA; a ratio of α-tocopherol to PUFA of approximately 0.4 is considered to be adequate in preventing the deficiency. It has been suggested that a ratio of 0.6 mg TE per gram of PUFA be present in the diet in persons who consume large amounts of fish and fish oils, which have elevated peroxidative potential and low vitamin E content.

8.3.7 ASSESSMENT OF VITAMIN E STATUS

The laboratory diagnosis of vitamin E deficiency is made on the basis of low plasma levels of α-tocopherol (5 μg/mL) or < 0.8 mg of α-tocopherol per gram of total plasma lipids. The red blood cell peroxide hemolysis test is not entirely specific but is a useful functional measure of the antioxidant potential of cell membranes.

8.3.8 TOXICITY

Because tocopherol deficiency is associated with pathological changes in some species of animals, there has been a temptation to use vitamin E in the treatment of several different conditions in humans. The vitamin has been prescribed in large doses (and hence used essentially as a drug) in the treatment of diseases of the circulatory, reproductive, and nervous systems, and as a protection against the effects of aging and air pollution. The extent of self-medication also has given rise to concerns for its possible toxicity. Fortunately, this vitamin is the least toxic among the fat-soluble vitamins. Some individuals have experienced gastrointestinal distress with daily intakes of up to 300 mg. The only well-known pharmacological action of vitamin E is that it interferes with vitamin K metabolism, thus increasing prothrombin time and predisposing the individual to bleeding. For most people, α-tocopherol doses up to 600 mg/day appear to be safe, but the long-term effect of the large amounts needs to be determined.

The Food and Nutrition Board of the Institute of Medicine established 1000 mg/day as a tolerable upper intake level for α-tocopherol supplements based on the prevention of hemorrhage. Some physicians recommend discontinuing high-dose vitamin E supplementation 1 month before elective surgery to decrease the risk of hemorrhage. Premature infants are vulnerable to adverse effects of vitamin E supplementation, which should be used only under supervision of a pediatrician.

8.4 VITAMIN K

The discovery of vitamin K resulted from the observation that some chicks ingesting diets that had been extracted with nonpolar solvents to remove the sterols developed hemorrhages under the skin, in muscle, in other tissues, and that the blood taken from these animals clotted more slowly. Furthermore, this hemorrhagic disease could not be cured by the administration of any of the known vitamins or other physiologically active lipids. In 1935, it was proposed that the antihemorrhagic factor was a new fat-soluble vitamin; it was given the name K, the first letter of German word "koagulation." It was isolated in 1939 from alfalfa and was synthesized in the same year.

8.4.1 CHEMISTRY

Vitamin K is a generic term for a group of naphthaquinone derivatives with characteristic antihemorrhagic effects in animals fed a vitamin K-deficient diet.[54] The vitamin exists in nature in two forms (Figure 8.11). Vitamin K_1, originally isolated from lucerne (alfalfa), is the only form that occurs in green plants. It is called phylloquinone, phytylmenaquinone, or phytomenadione. It has a 20-carbon phytyl side chain attached to 2-methyl-1,4-naphthaquinone. Chemically, it is 2-methyl-3-phytyl-1,4-naphthaquinone. The compound isolated from putrefied fish meal is called vitamin K_2 and is one of a family of vitamin K_2 homologs produced by bacteria; these have 4–13 isoprenyl units in the side chain attached to the basic 2-methyl-1,4-naphthaquinone. They are called menaquinone-4 (MK-4) to menaquinone-13 (MK-13), depending on the number of isoprenyl units.

Vitamin K_3 is produced synthetically and has no isoprenyl side chain; it is known as menadione. In addition to these three groups of fat-soluble compounds with vitamin K activity, several water-soluble and water-miscible preparations are available that make them especially suited for the treatment of vitamin K deficiency when fat absorption is impaired. Menadione sodium bisulfite

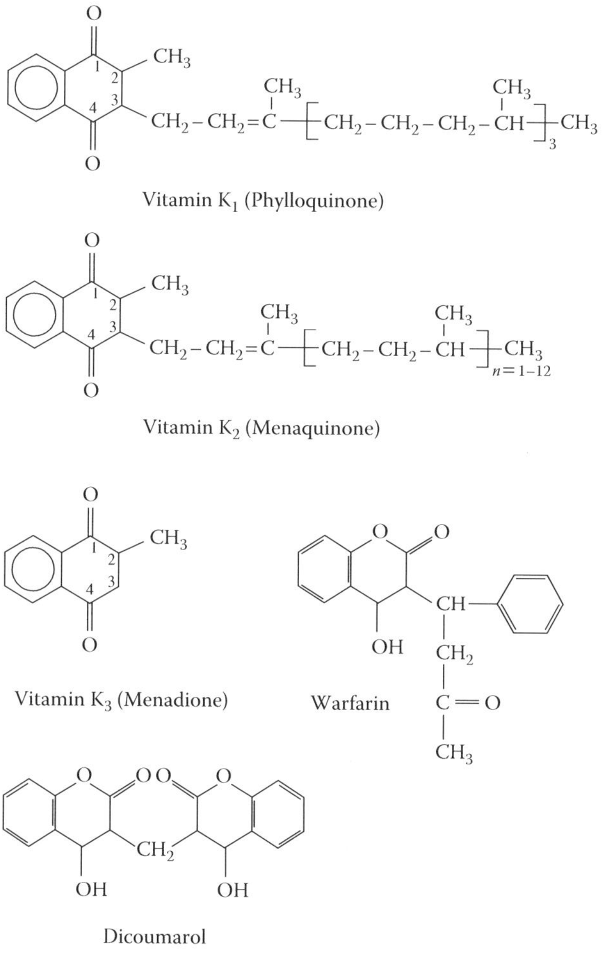

FIGURE 8.11 Structures for vitamin K and the two antagonists.

(Hykinone) and sodium menadiol diphosphate (Synkevite) are water-soluble; Mephyton, Konakin, and Mono-Kay are water-miscible.

Phylloquinone is yellow oil at room temperature. Various menaquinones can be crystallized and have melting points of 35–60°C, depending on the length of the isoprenoid chain. The naturally occurring vitamin K compounds are unstable in ultraviolet light and are destroyed by oxidation. The vitamins are stable at ordinary cooking temperatures.

8.4.2 Food Sources

Vitamin K is present in fresh, green, leafy vegetables such as spinach, cabbage, lettuce, broccoli, kale, and cauliflower; peas, carrots, and cereal are poor sources. Many species of bacteria (including *Escherichia coli*), which are present in the large intestine of humans, synthesize this vitamin and in part provide for the needs of the body. This explains why healthy human beings (with the exception of newborn infants) appear to be not dependent on the supply of vitamin K in their diet.

8.4.3 Absorption

Vitamin K is absorbed in micellar form with dietary fats and requires a normal supply of bile and pancreatic juice. It enters the lymph ducts as chylomicrons and is released by the liver; it then goes into the general circulation associated with β-lipoproteins. An obstruction of the bile duct (e.g., in obstructive jaundice and liver failure) will reduce absorption.

8.4.4 Functions

Vitamin K functions as an essential cofactor for the enzyme carboxylase that converts specific glutamic acid residues of precursor proteins to γ-carboxyglutamic acid (GLA) residues in the new proteins[64] (Figure 8.12). The active form of the vitamin is the hydroquinone (the reduced form); this is an electron donor for a microsomal electron transport system for which oxygen is the terminal acceptor. This electron transport system is coupled to a carbon dioxide fixation reaction that converts peptide-bound glutamate to GLA (Figure 8.13).

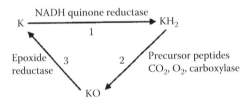

FIGURE 8.12 Vitamin K is converted to its reduced form, KH_2, catalyzed by nicotinamide adenine dinucleotide and thiol-dependent quinone reductase (reaction 1); KH_2-dependent carboxylase (in the presence of CO_2 and O_2) catalyzes the γ carboxylation of peptide-bound glutamic acid residues (reaction 2), and KH_2 is converted to the epoxide (KO); in reaction 3, vitamin K is regenerated from the epoxide, catalyzed by dithiol-dependent epoxide reductase. Reactions 1 and 3 are inhibited by warfarin and dicoumarol.

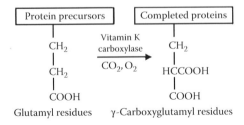

FIGURE 8.13 The vitamin K–dependent carboxylation reaction.

The carboxylation reaction will only proceed if the carboxylase enzyme is able to oxidize vitamin K hydroquinone to vitamin K epoxide at the same time; the carboxylation and epoxidation reactions are said to be coupled reactions. Vitamin K epoxide is then reconverted to vitamin K by vitamin K epoxide reductase. These two enzymes comprise the vitamin K cycle. Vitamin K is continually recycled in our cells. Vitamin K–dependent carboxylase activity[58] is present in most tissues, and a large number of proteins are subject to posttranslational modification. The presence of GLA residues is critical to the calcium-binding function of these proteins. At this time, 14 human proteins containing GLA residues have been discovered, and they play key roles in the regulation of physiological processes.

Vitamin K is required to maintain normal levels of blood clotting factors: prothrombin; factors VII, IX, and X; protein C and protein S; and protein Z. Prothrombin and factors VII, IX, and X possess procoagulant activity, and they make up the core of the coagulation cascade. The term coagulation cascade refers to a series of events, each dependent on the other, that stop bleeding through clot formation. Protein C and protein S act as anticoagulants that provide control and balance in the coagulation cascade. Protein Z appears to enhance the action of thrombin by promoting its association with phospholipids and cell membranes. It also has an anticoagulatory function. Control mechanisms for the coagulation cascade exist because uncontrolled clotting may be as life threatening as uncontrolled bleeding. Each of these specific factors is a protein synthesized by the liver as an inactive precursor at the ribosomal level. The vitamin participates in the posttranslational carboxylation of specific glutamic acid residues of precursor proteins to GLA residues in completed proteins. Severe liver disease results in lower blood levels of these clotting factors and an increased risk of uncontrolled bleeding (hemorrhage). Vitamin K–dependent carboxylase activity is present in most tissues, and a large number of proteins are subjected to posttranslational modification.

Of the known vitamin K–dependent proteins, prothrombin has been the most extensively studied. In the NH_2 terminal region of this protein, there are 10 tightly clustered GLA residues, which occur at positions 7, 8, 15, 17, 20, 21, 26, 27, 30, and 33.

GLA is an amino acid with a dicarboxylic acid side chain. The carboxyl groups are adjacent and thereby impart unique calcium-binding characteristics to proteins in which they reside. The six proteins involved in the coagulation system are required for normal blood clotting by facilitating protein–calcium–phospholipid interactions. The administration of vitamin K antagonists such as coumadin and warfarin (Figure 8.11) inhibits the conversion of vitamin K to its active form (hydroquinone); this, in turn, prevents the carboxylation of GLA precursors to GLA and results in blood clotting abnormalities.

The soft tissues that transport calcium have been found to have either GLA-containing proteins (e.g., kidney, chorioallantoic membrane) or the vitamin K–dependent carboxylating system (e.g., intestine, placenta). The GLA-containing proteins have also been found in various pathological calcifications (e.g., renal calculi, atherosclerotic plaque). Osteocalcin, which is present in the bone matrix, is the most abundant GLA-containing protein. It contains 49 amino acids, including three GLAs. After collagen, it is the major protein component of bone matrix and is the seventh most abundant protein in the body. It constitutes 1% of the total proteins and 10%–20% of the noncollagen proteins. Osteocalcin is synthesized in osteoblasts and is expressed under the influence of vitamin D and retinoic acid. Osteocalcin is thought to play a role in bone metabolism. It is often used as a biochemical marker for bone formation. Some studies have shown that a lack of osteocalcin leads to increased bone formation suggesting that it may also function as a negative regulator of bone formation. However, this does not explain other recent findings in which increased serum undercarboxylated osteocalcin was found to be a strong predictor of hip fracture risk in both institutional and free-living elderly women.

Recently, it was reported that osteocalcin acts like a hormone in the body, causing β-cells of the pancreas to produce more insulin and at the same time directing fat cells to release a hormone called adiponectin, which increases insulin sensitivity. It also reduces fat stores in the body. Mice with high levels of osteocalcin activity do not gain weight or become diabetic even when they eat a high-fat diet. Mice lacking osteocalcin have type 2 diabetes, increased fat mass, decreased insulin and adiponectin expression, and decreased β-cell proliferation. People with type 2 diabetes have been shown to have low osteocalcin levels, suggesting that altering the activity of osteocalcin could be an effective therapeutic strategy. Additional studies are needed to see whether osteocalcin works the same way in humans as it does in mice.

Matrix GLA protein (MGP) contains 84 amino acids, including five GLAs. MGP is found in bone, cartilage, and many soft tissues, including blood vessels. Animal studies suggest that MGP prevents the calcification of soft tissues and cartilage while facilitating normal bone growth and development. A lack of MGP results in arterial calcification, suggesting that this protein acts as an inhibitor of soft tissue calcification. The metabolic alterations responsible for these observations are not yet known. The anticoagulant protein S is also formed by osteoblasts, but its role in bone metabolism is not clear. Children with inherited deficiency of protein S suffer complications related to increased blood clotting as well as decreased bone density.

Gas6 is a vitamin K–dependent protein found throughout the nervous system, as well as the heart, lungs, stomach, kidneys, and cartilage. Gas6 appears to be a cellular growth-regulating factor with cell-signaling activities, but its exact mechanism of action has not been determined. It appears to be important in cell adhesion, cell proliferation, and protection against apoptosis. There are four transmembrane GLA proteins, but the specifics of the role of these apparent cell-surface receptors are not yet known.

Vitamin K has been shown to protect against nerve cell damage due to oxidation. It may be of benefit in the treatment of Alzheimer's disease. A study in Japan on the prevention of bone loss in females with liver disease has shown that those receiving vitamin K supplementation were 90% less likely to get liver cancer. A German study in men found a significant inverse relationship between vitamin K consumption and prostate cancer.

Vitamin K appears to have a role in maintaining strong, healthy bones. An analysis of data from more than 72,000 women in the Nurses' Health Study showed that women in quintiles 2–5 of vitamin K intake had a significantly lower age-adjusted risk of hip fractures than women in the last quintile (< 109 µg/day). More recently, studies from 888 elderly men and women participating in the Framingham Heart Study also showed similar results. There were significantly more incidences of hip fractures among elderly in the lowest reported quartiles of vitamin K intake than in those in the highest quartile of intake. In contrast, there was no significant association between vitamin K intake and bone mineral density in this cohort. The lowest intake in this study averaged 56 µg/day; the highest averaged 254 µg/day. This work suggests that people may need more vitamin K than the current RDA of about 65–80 µg/day. One serving of spinach or two servings of broccoli provide four to five times the RDA. The presence of GLA residues in proteins other than vitamin K–dependent clotting factors suggests that vitamin K may have functions in addition to its role in blood clotting, such as calcium transport and calcium deposition in the bone matrix.

8.4.5 DEFICIENCY

A prolonged blood coagulation time and an increased incidence of hemorrhage are the only known symptoms of vitamin K deficiency. The deficiency is marked by a diminished plasma prothrombin concentration. The hypoprothrombinemia is readily corrected by the administration of 2–5 mg/day vitamin K orally. A primary deficiency is uncommon in healthy individuals because of the widespread distribution of vitamin K in plants and because the microbiological flora of the gut can synthesize a significant part of the daily requirement of vitamin K. The most common causes of the deficiency are thus largely secondary due to impaired fat absorption, severe liver disease, or drug therapy. Among the first type of disorders are biliary obstruction or fistula, pancreatic insufficiency, celiac disease, and regional enteritis. In the absence of functioning liver tissue, vitamin K cannot be converted to its active form, and there will also be a carboxylase deficiency. When liver damage is the cause of hypoprothrombinemia, vitamin K is ineffective as a therapeutic agent. Anticoagulant drugs such as coumarin act as antimetabolites by inhibiting the conversion of vitamin K to its active form. Sulfa drugs and certain broad-spectrum antibiotics that cause sterilization of the gut can produce vitamin K deficiency.

In contrast to healthy adults, newborn breast-fed infants sometimes have a prolonged prothrombin time due to vitamin K deficiency. This is usually true in the first week of life. Very little vitamin K passes the placental barrier from the maternal circulation for storage in the fetal tissues. Also, newborns have a relatively sterile intestinal tract (i.e., it does not contain the organisms that synthesize vitamin K), and they are generally fed foods that are relatively free of bacterial contamination.

Infants whose mothers are on anticonvulsive medication to prevent seizures are also at risk of vitamin K deficiency. Human milk is a poor source of vitamin K. It contains 1–4 μg/L of the vitamin. Therefore, young infants are likely to suffer from a subnormal synthesis of active prothrombin. If prothrombin concentrations fall below 10% of the normal level, hemorrhagic disease of the newborn will appear 1–7 days postpartum. Premature infants are more susceptible than full-term infants. The prevalence of vitamin K deficiency in infants without bleeding can occur in as many as 50% of infants younger than 5 days. The classic disease occurs in 0.25%–1.7% of infants. The American Academy of Pediatrics and a number of similar international organizations recommended that a prophylactic dose of 0.5–1 mg of vitamin K be administered to all newborns shortly after birth. The deficiency signs persist only until a bacterial flora is established in the infant's intestine.

In the early 1990s, there was controversy regarding the practice of administering vitamin K injections to newborns. Two studies showed a relationship between administration of vitamin K and childhood leukemia and other forms of childhood cancer. But studies in the United States and Sweden that reviewed the medical records of 54,000 and 1.3 million children, respectively, found no evidence of a relationship between childhood cancer and vitamin K injections at birth.

8.4.6 Requirements

Vitamin K is a dietary essential but no specific estimate of vitamin requirement has been made. Requirements are met by a combination of dietary intake and microbiologic synthesis in the intestine. In humans, about 50% of vitamin K in the liver is vitamin K_1 (from plant food) and the remainder is vitamin K_2 (from bacterial origin). The American Academy of Pediatrics estimates that newborn infants require 1.5–2.5 μg/kg body weight per day. Assuming the efficiency of absorption of the orally fed vitamin K to be about 10% for that age, a daily intake of 20 μg appears to be adequate for the neonate (assuming no intestinal synthesis). Adult requirements are estimated to be about 2 μg/kg body weight with 1 μg/kg from food or 70–140 μg/day, an amount easily supplied in the diet.

8.4.7 Assessment of Vitamin K Status

Prothrombin time is typically used as a measure of functional vitamin K status. When the prothrombin concentration declines to below 30% of normal, prothrombin time rises above 30 seconds. A deficiency of vitamin K can be distinguished from hypoprothrombinemia of liver disease by a measurement of nongammacarboxylated prothrombin precursor (i.e., abnormal prothrombin) that accumulates in plasma when the vitamin is deficient. In persons with vitamin K deficiency, liver disease, or both, the values can rise to 30% of the total prothrombin. In addition, low gammacarboxyglutamate levels in the urine indicate vitamin K deficiency.

8.4.8 Toxicity

Although vitamin K is fat soluble, there are no known causes of human toxicity related to the natural vitamins K_1 and K_2. Excessive doses of the synthetic vitamin menadione and its derivatives have been reported to produce hemolytic anemia in rats and hyperbilirubinemia and kernicterus in some low birth weight infants. These water-soluble compounds are known to react with free sulfhydryl groups of proteins and cause the breakdown of red blood cells and increase bilirubin in the blood.

To prevent neonatal hemorrhage, it became the practice to give menadione orally to the mother in the last few weeks of pregnancy, or by injection during labor to prevent hemorrhage; however, because of the adverse effects of the synthetic vitamin, if the vitamin is to be given, it should be in a controlled dose sufficient to prevent hemorrhage but low enough to prevent adverse reactions.

Megavitamin Therapy—A Case

A 20-year-old girl was admitted to a hospital for evaluation of a possible brain tumor. On admission, she appeared chronically ill, complained of severe headache, and preferred to be left without motion. Flexion of her neck increased her discomfort. Her vital signs were normal. Two days before admission, she experienced emesis, diplopia, and severe headache. Two months before admission, she became anorectic with increasingly severe headache and diffuse scaling erythematous dermatitis. Eight months earlier, she went on a reducing diet and gradually decreased her weight from 56 to 41 kg. Two years before admission, a dermatologist recommended a daily supplement (50,000 IU) of vitamin A for acne. The patient had taken this vitamin, faithfully increasing her intake sometimes to amounts of 200,000 IU/day.

The patient had bilateral abducens nerve palsies. A liver scan showed hepatomegaly and portal hypertension. Laboratory data revealed that she had total plasma vitamin A of 128 µg/dL (normal: 50 µg/dL), retinyl esters of 41 µg/dL (normal: 1.6 µg/dL), and elevated levels of plasma alkaline phosphatase and glutamic oxaloacetic transaminase. She was placed on a diet low in vitamin A and carotenes. Her appetite improved, her weight increased to 46 kg, and her vitamin A and retinyl esters levels were reduced by the time she was discharged 22 days after admission.

This is a classical case of vitamin A toxicity.[68,69] Several cases have been reported, many traceable to high intake of the vitamin prescribed as a therapy for dermatological disorders or to self-medication by individuals. Headache, nausea, stiff neck, anorexia, lip fissuring, and elevated blood vitamin A are all common to hypervitaminosis A. Rarely, hepatic inflammation with hepatomegaly, abnormal results of liver function tests, and pathological evidence of hepatocellular damage are found. A daily consumption of 50,000 IU of vitamin A for a few days would generally be considered safe. Vitamin A toxicity occurs when the capacity of RBP to transport the vitamin in plasma is exceeded. Substantial amounts of vitamin A are then transported in plasma in a manner other than bound to the carrier protein. It may manifest nonspecific toxicity to cell membranes. RBP functions not only to regulate the supply of retinol to tissues but also to protect from the surface-active properties of the vitamin.

The noncurative nature of many chronic diseases often spawns a host of quasimedical therapies including megavitamin therapy. These may not only be ineffective but potentially dangerous.

REFERENCES

Vitamin A

1. Bates, C. J. 1995. Vitamin A. *Lancet* 345:31.
2. Berard, A., L. Azoulay, G. Koren et al. 2007. Isotretinoin, pregnancies, abortions and birth defects: A population-based perspective. *Brit J Clin Pharmacol* 63:196.
3. Binkley, N., and D. Krueger. 2000. Hypervitaminosis A and bone. *Nutr Rev* 58:138.
4. Christian, P., and K. P. West Jr. 1998. Interactions between zinc and vitamin A: An update. *Am J Clin Nutr* 68:435S.
5. Denke, M. A. 2002. Dietary retinol—a double-edged sword. *J Am Med Assoc* 287:102.

6. Feskanich, D., V. Singh, W. C. Willett, and G. A. Colditz. 2002. Vitamin A intake and hip fractures among postmenopausal women. *J Am Med Assoc* 287:47.

7. Hadi, H., R. J. Stoltzfus, M. J. Dibley et al. 2000. Vitamin A supplementation selectively improves the linear growth of Indonesian preschool children. Results from a randomized controlled trial. *Am J Clin Nutr* 71:507.

8. Jang, J. T., J. B. Green, J. L. Beard, and M. H. Green. 2000. Kinetic analysis shows that iron deficiency decreases liver vitamin A mobilization in rats. *J Nutr* 130:1291.

9. Kim, S. R., N. Fishkin, J. Kong et al. 2004. Rpe 65 Len 450 Met variant is associated with reduced levels of the retinal pigment epithelium lipofuscin fluorophores, A2E and iso-A2E. *Proc Natl Acad Sci U S A* 101:11668.

10. Kull, I., A. Bergstrom, E. Melen et al. 2006. Early-life supplementation of vitamins A and D in water-soluable form or in peanut oil, and allergic diseases during childhood. *J Allergy Clin Immunol* 113:1299.

11. Lotan, R. 2005. A crucial role for cellular retinol-binding protein-1 in retinoid signaling. *J Natl Cancer Inst* 97:3.

12. Orlandi, A., A. Ferlosio, A. Alessandro et al. 2006. Cellular retinol binding protein-1 expression in endometrial hyperplasia and carcinoma: Diagnostic and possible thereapeutic implications. *Mod Pathol* 19:797.

13. Pryor, W. A., W. Stahl, and C. L. Rock. 2000. β carotene: From biochemistry to clinical trials. *Nutr Rev* 58:39.

14. Semba, R. D. 1998. The role of vitamin A and related retinoids in immune function. *Nutr Rev* 56:538.

15. Shankar, A. H., B. Genton, R. D. Semba et al. 1999. Effect of vitamin A supplementation on morbidity due to *Plasmodium falciparum* in young children in Papua New Guinea: A randomized trial. *Lancet* 354:203.

16. Soprano, D. R., and K. J. Soprano. 1995. Retinoids as teratogens. *Annu Rev Nutr* 15:111.

17. Stephenson, C. B. 2001. Vitamin A, infection, and immune function. *Annu Rev Nutr* 21:167.

18. West, C. E. 2000. Vitamin A and measles. *Nutr Rev* 58:46.

Vitamin D

19. Abrams, S. A. 2002. Nutritional rickets: An old disease returns. *Nutr Rev* 60:111.

20. Autier, P., and S. Gandini. 2007. Vitamin D supplementation and total mortality: A meta-analysis of randomized controlled trials. *Arch Int Med* 167:1730.

21. Evatt, M. L., M. R. Delong, N. Khazai et al. 2008. Prevalence of vitamin D insufficiency in patients with Parkinson disease and Alzheimer's disease. *Arch Neurol* 65:1348.

22. Ford, E. S., W. H. Giles, and A. H. Mokdad. 2004. Increasing prevalence of the metabolic syndrome among U.S. adults. *Diabetes Care* 27:2444.

23. Garland, C. F., W. B. Grant, S. B. Mohr et al. 2007. What is the dose-response relationship between vitamin D and cancer risk? *Nutr Rev* 65:591.

24. Grant, W. B. 2009. Does vitamin D reduce the risk of dementia? *J Alzheimer's Dis* 17:151.

25. Griffin, M. D., N. Xing, and R. Kumar. 2003. Vitamin D and its analogues as regulators of immune activation and antigen presentation. *Annu Rev Nutr* 23:117.

26. Guyton, K. Z., T. W. Kenslir, and G. H. Posner. 2001. Cancer chemotherapy using natural vitamin D analogs. *Annu Rev Pharmacol Ther* 41:421.

27. Harris, S. 2002. Can vitamin D supplementation in infancy prevent type 1 diabetes? *Nutr Rev* 60:118.

28. Holick, M. F. 2007. Vitamin D deficiency. *New Engl J Med* 357:266.

29. Hollis, B. W., and R. L. Horst. 2007. The assessment of circulating 25(OH) D and 1,25(OH)2D: Where we are and where we are going. *J Steroid Biochem Mol Biol* 103:473.

30. Ingraham, B. A., B. Brangdon, and A. Nohe. 2007. Molecular basis of the potential of vitamin D to prevent cancer. *Curr Med Res Opin* 24:139.

31. Klein, G. L., T. C. Chen, M. F. Holick et al. 2004. Synthesis of vitamin D in skin after burns. *Lancet* 363:291.

32. Liewellyn, D. J., K. Langa, and J. Lang. 2009. Serum 25-hydroxy vitamin D concentration and cognitive impairment. *J Geriatr Psychiatry Neurol* 22(3):188.

33. Mascarenhas, R., and S. Mobarhan. 2004. Hypovitaminosis D–induced pain. *Nutr Rev* 62:354.

34. Masoumi, A., B. Goldenson, S. Ghirmai et al. 2009. 1 α, 25-dihydroxyvitamin D interacts with curcuminoids to stimulate amyloid-β clearance by macrophages of Alzheimer's disease patients. *J Alzheimer's Dis* 17:703.

35. Norman, A. W. 1998. Sunlight, season, skin pigmentation, vitamin D and 25-hydroxy vitamin D integral components of the vitamin D endocrine system. *Am J Clin Nutr* 67:1108.

36. Posner, G. H. 2002. Low-calcemic vitamin D analogs (deltanoids) for human cancer prevention. *J Nutr* 132:3802S.

37. Vieth, R., and S. Kimball. 2006. Vitamin D in congestive heart failure. *Am J Clin Nutr* 83:731.

38. Wang, T. J., M. J. Pencina, S. L. Booth et al. 2008. Vitamin D deficiency and risk of cardiovascular disease. *Circulation* 117:503.

39. Weng, R. L., J. Shults, M. B. Leonard et al. 2007. Risk factors for low serum 25-hydroxyvitamin D concentrations in otherwise healthy children and adolescents. *Am J Clin Nutr* 86:150.

40. Zeitz, U., K. Weber, D. W. Soegiarto et al. 2003. Impaired insulin secretory capacity in mice lacking a functional vitamin D receptor. *FASEB J* 17:509.

VITAMIN E

41. Ahuja, J. K., J. D. Goldman, and A. J. Moshfegh. 2004. Current status of vitamin E nutriture. *Ann N Y Acad Sci* 1031:307.

42. Brigelius-Flohe, R., and M. G. Traber. 1999. Vitamin E: Function and metabolism. *FASEB J* 13:1145.

43. Gotoda, T., M. Arita, H. Arai et al. 1995. Adult-onset spinocerebellar dysfunction caused by a mutation in the gene for the α-tocopherol-transfer-protein. *N Engl J Med* 333:1313.

44. Lippman, S. M., E. A. Klein, P. J. Goodman et al. 2009. Effect of selenium and vitamin E on risk of prostate cancer and other cancers: The Selenium and Vitamin E Cancer Prevention Trial (SELECT). *J Am Med Assoc* 301:39.

45. Maras, J. E., O. I. Bermudez, N. Qiao et al. 2004. Intake of α-tocopherol is limited among U.S. adults. *J Am Diet Assoc* 104:567.

46. Meydani, M. 1995. Vitamin E. *Lancet* 345:170.

47. Müller, D. P. R. 1986. Vitamin E—Its role in neurological function. *Postgrad Med J* 62:107.

48. Theriault, A., J. Chao, Q. Wang et al. 1999. Tocotrienol: A review of its therapeutic potential. *Clin Biochem* 32:309.

49. Traber, M. G., and H. Arai. 1999. Molecular mechanisms of vitamin E transport. *Annu Rev Nutr* 19:343.

50. Traber, M. G. 2007. Vitamin E regulatory mechanisms. *Annu Rev Nutr* 27:347.

51. Traber, M. G., B. Frei, and J. S. Beckman. 2008. Vitamin E revisited: Do new data validate benefits for chronic disease prevention? *Curr Opin Lipidol* 19:30.

52. Zhang, Y., J. Ni, E. M. Messing et al. 2002. Vitamin E succinate inhibits the function of androgen receptor and the expression of prostate specific antigen in prostate cancer cells. *Proc Natl Acad Sci U S A* 99:7408.

VITAMIN K

53. Allison, A. C. 2001. The possible role of vitamin K deficiency in the pathogenesis of Alzheimer's disease, and in augmenting brain damage associated with cardiovascular disease. *Med Hypothesis* 57:151.

54. Berkner, K. L., and K. W. Runge. 2004. The physiology of vitamin K nutriture and vitamin K-dependent protein function in atherosclerosis. *J Thromb Haemost* 2:2118.

55. Booth, S. L., G. Dallal, M. K. Shea et al. 2008. Effect of vitamin K supplementation on bone loss in elderly men and women. *J Clin Endocrinol Metab* 93:1257.

56. Dowd, P., S. W. Ham, S. Naganathan, and R. Hershline. 1995. The mechanism of action of vitamin K. *Annu Rev Nutr* 15:419.

57. Ducy, P., C. Desbois, B. Boyce et al. 1996. Increased bone formation in osteocalcin-deficient mice. *Nature* 382:448.

58. Ferland, G. 1998. The vitamin K-dependent proteins: An update. *Nutr Rev* 56:223.

59. Feskanich, D., P. Weber, W. C. Willett et al. 1999. Vitamin K intake and hip fractures in women: A prospective study. *Am J Clin Nutr* 69:74.

60. Lee, N. K., H. Sowa, E. Hinoi et al. 2007. Endocrine regulation of energy metabolism by the skeleton. *Cell* 130:456.

61. Luo, G., P. Ducy, M. D. McKee et al. 1997. Spontaneous calcification of arteries and cartilage in mice lacking matrix GLA protein. *Nature* 386:78.

62. Nimptsch, K., S. Rohrmann, and J. Linseisen. 2008. Dietary intake of vitamin K and risk of prostate cancer on the Heidelberg Cohort of the European Prospective Investigation into Cancer and Nutrition (EPIC-Heidelberg). *Am J Clin Nutr* 87:985.

63. Saxena, S. P., E. D. Israels, and L. G. Israels. 2001. Vitamin K-dependent pathway regulating cell survival. *Apoptosis* 6:57.
64. Shearer, M. J. 1995. Vitamin K. *Lancet* 345:229.
65. Sokoll, L. J., and J. A. Sadowski. 1996. Comparison of biochemical indexes for assessing vitamin K nutritional status in healthy adult population. *Am J Clin Nutr* 63:566.
66. Suttie, J. W. 1995. The importance of menaquinones in human nutrition. *Annu Rev Nutr* 15:399.
67. Yoshida, M., P. F. Jacques, J. B. Meigs et al. 2008. Effect of vitamin K supplementation on insulin resistance in older men and women. *Diabetes Care* 31:2092.

CASE BIBLIOGRAPHY

68. Clinical Nutrition Cases. 1982. The pathological basis of vitamin A toxicity. *Nutr Rev* 40:272.
69. Smith, F. R., and D. S. Goodman. 1976. Vitamin A transport in human vitamin A toxicity. *N Engl J Med* 294:805.

9 Water-Soluble Vitamins I

9.1 THIAMIN—B$_1$

The paralyzing disease beriberi, prevalent in many countries of the world, particularly in Asia where polished rice is a staple food in the diet, has been known for generations. The first real breakthrough in the treatment came during the study by Takai, a Japanese medical officer, on the high incidence of the disease among men in the Navy during 1878–1883. He reported that he cured the strange sickness in his sailors by giving them less polished rice and more vegetables, barley, meat, and canned milk. He believed that the beneficial effect was due to the higher protein content of the diet. In 1897, Dutch physician Eijkman found that a disease resembling beriberi could be produced in chickens fed on polished rice and that the disease could be prevented or cured by feeding rice bran. He also showed that he could cure the disease in humans by a similar treatment.

In 1911, Casimir Funk, a chemist at the Lister Institute in London, obtained a substance from rice bran extracts and gave the name "vitamine" to the antiberiberi principle because it was vital for life and it also had an amine function. In 1926, the vitamin was isolated in crystalline form from rice bran. The identification of the structure and the chemical synthesis of the vitamin were accomplished in 1936 by Williams in the United States. The name thiamin was given to this compound because of the presence of sulfur (thio) and amine.

9.1.1 FOOD SOURCES

All foods of animal origin and plant tissues contain thiamin, and it is, therefore, present in all whole natural foods, but the only important source in the biological world is the seeds of plants. In cereals, the vitamin is present mainly in the germ and outer coat of the seed. Much of the vitamin is lost when cereals are milled and refined. For example, 100 g of whole wheat flour contains 0.56 mg thiamin, while 100 g of white flour contains only 0.06 mg thiamin. In the United States, processed foods must be enriched with thiamin mononitrate (along with niacin, riboflavin, folic acid, and iron) to replace the amount lost in processing. All green vegetables, fruits, roots, meat, and dairy produce (except butter) contain significant amounts of the vitamin, but none is a rich source. Pork contains substantial amounts of the vitamin.

9.1.2 CHEMISTRY

Thiamin consists of a pyrimidine ring joined by a methylene bridge to a sulfur-containing thiazole nucleus (Figure 9.1). It is stable to heat at temperatures up to 100°C in solutions that are somewhat acidic.[1] In alkaline solution and in the presence of mild oxidants such as potassium ferricyanide, thiamin is converted to thiochrome, a blue fluorescent compound. This reaction serves as a basis for the detection and the quantitation of thiamin. Pure thiamin hydrochloride is a crystalline, colorless, water-soluble compound with a very characteristic odor and a slightly bitter taste.

9.1.3 ABSORPTION AND TRANSPORT

In most animal products, thiamin occurs in a phosphorylated form (thiamin monophosphate, pyrophosphate, and triphosphate), with about 80%–85% as pyrophosphate. In plant products, most of the vitamin occurs in the nonphosphorylated form. The phosphorylated form cannot penetrate

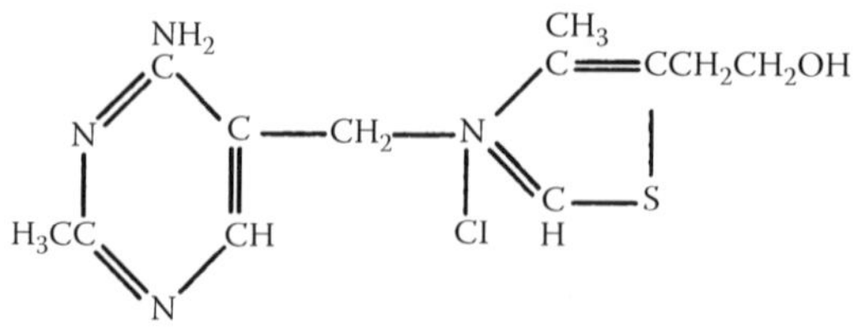

FIGURE 9.1   Thiamin.

cell membranes and is hydrolyzed in the intestinal lumen prior to its uptake into the mucosa. The absorption of the vitamin occurs primarily in the duodenum. At high concentrations, it is passively absorbed (passive diffusion), and at low concentrations, it is absorbed by an active process requiring energy and sodium. Active transport is inhibited by alcohol consumption and by folic acid deficiency. In the serum, thiamin is mostly bound to albumin. Approximately 90% of the total thiamin in blood is in erythrocytes. A specific protein called thiamin-binding protein has been identified in rat serum and is believed to be a hormonally regulated carrier protein that is important to tissue distribution of the vitamin.

As with most of the water-soluble vitamins, the body is unable to store thiamin to any great extent.[2] The liver, the heart, and the brain have higher concentrations of the vitamin than other tissues or organs. The amount of thiamin present in the body is not great, accounting to only about 50 mg. Of the total vitamin in the body, about 80% is thiamin pyrophosphate (TPP), 10% is triphosphate, and the remainder is monophosphate and free thiamin.

Excess thiamin is rapidly excreted in the urine. When intake is low, urinary excretion decreases, and when intake is high, a proportionate increase in urinary excretion is observed, which provides a measure of adequacy of thiamin stores. At least 20 metabolites of thiamin have been identified in the urine of rats and humans; pyridine acetic acid and thiazole acetic acid are the major ones.

9.1.4   FUNCTIONS

Thiamin was the first vitamin whose precise activity in the body was stated in biochemical terms.[4] The known biochemical functions of thiamin require its conversion to TPP, which serves as a coenzyme in a number of metabolic processes. The reaction is catalyzed by TPP kinase that is found in all cells in which TPP functions as a coenzyme. TPP is also known as cocarboxylase because of its major role in the oxidative decarboxylation of α-ketoacids:

$$\text{Thiamin} + \text{ATP} \xrightarrow{\text{Thiamin pyrophosphate kinase}} \text{TPP} + \text{AMP}$$

In animal cells, TPP plays a critical role in the generation of energy. The decarboxylation of pyruvate to acetyl coenzyme A (CoA) is a key reaction for the further oxidation of carbohydrate and some amino acid substrates in the citric acid cycle, and for the storage of excess carbohydrate as fat in adipose tissues. Similarly, the decarboxylation of α-ketoglutarate to succinyl CoA is a key step in the energy-producing citric acid cycle itself. Oxidative decarboxylation is a complex reaction with many steps, which, in addition, requires lipoic acid and coenzymes of three other B vitamins (e.g., pantothenic acid [in CoA], niacin [in nicotinamide adenine dinucleotide, NAD], and riboflavin [in flavin adenine dinucleotide, FAD]), thereby demonstrating the interdependent roles of several of the B vitamins in energy metabolism. The multienzyme complex is called pyruvate dehydrogenase (in the case of pyruvate decarboxylation). It consists of three enzymes: TPP-dependent pyruvate decarboxylase, a lipoic acid-bound dihydrolipoyl transacetylase, and a dihydrolipoyl dehydrogenase; the last is a FAD-dependent enzyme that oxidizes reduced lipoic acid (Figure 9.2). The oxidative

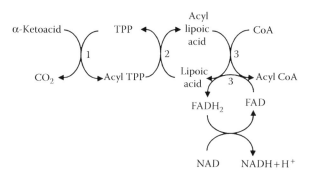

FIGURE 9.2 Thiamin pyrophosphate-dependent α-ketoacid dehydrogenases. (1) Pyruvate decarboxylase in pyruvate dehydrogenase converts pyruvate to acetyl CoA; α-ketoglutarate decarboxylase in α-ketoglutarate dehydrogenase converts α-ketoglutarate to succinyl CoA and succinyl replaces the acetyl group throughout the reaction; branched-chain α-ketoacid decarboxylase in branched-chain α-ketoacid dehydrogenase converts branched-chain α-ketoacids (formed from leucine, isoleucine, and valine) to their corresponding acyl CoA. (2) Dihydrolipoate transacetylase. (3) Dihydrolipoyl dehydrogenase.

decarboxylation of α-ketoglutarate to succinyl CoA involves an analogous series of reactions catalyzed by α-ketoglutarate dehydrogenase.

Another important function of thiamin is to serve as a coenzyme in the process of transketolation in the phosphogluconate pathway, which generates glyceraldehyde-3-phosphate and sedoheptulose-7-phosphate from two pentoses. Transketolase is active in erythrocytes, kidneys, and other tissues, and it is important in providing five-carbon sugars for the synthesis of various ribonucleotides including those found in DNA and RNA. A normal function of the phosphogluconate pathway also produces the reduced form of nicotinamide adenine dinucleotide phosphate (NADP), which is needed for several synthetic reactions such as fatty acid synthesis, cholesterol, and steroid synthesis.

TPP is thus an important coenzyme in carbohydrate metabolism and in the normal operation of the citric acid cycle. This explains why vitamin B_1 deficiency can be accelerated by a high-carbohydrate diet and the onset of deficiency is delayed by a diet rich in fats. The three branched-chain α-ketoacids derived from the deamination of leucine, isoleucine, and valine (i.e., α-ketoisocaproic, α-keto-β-methyl valeric, and α-ketoisovaleric acids) are also oxidatively decarboxylated by a multienzyme complex branched chain keto acid (BCKA) dehydrogenase analogous to that of pyruvate.

Benfotiamine is a synthetic fat-soluble form of thiamin. It has been found to prevent the most common form of diabetes-related eye disease in rats. A clinical trial is being considered to assess whether a similar result would occur in humans.

9.1.5 Deficiency

The classical disease resulting from vitamin B_1 deficiency in humans is called beriberi (derived from Singhalese, "beri-weakness" or "I can't"). All cells of the body require thiamin in the coenzyme form for energy metabolism; thus, it would seem to affect all the organ systems. But the most prominent symptoms include the gastrointestinal disorders (anorexia, indigestion, and the accompanying weight loss), neurological disorders, and cardiovascular disorders.

When the cells of the smooth muscle and secretory glands do not receive energy from glucose, they cannot do their functions in digestion to provide still more glucose and other substrates. The secretion of hydrochloric acid in the stomach and the digestive enzymes in the gastrointestinal tract are dependent on the supply of energy. A vicious cycle then ensues as the deficiency continues.

The central nervous system is dependent on glucose for energy to do its work, so without thiamin, neuronal activity is impaired. The failure of energy metabolism affects neurons and their functions in selected areas of the central nervous system. Alertness and reflex responses are diminished and general apathy and fatigue result. Depending on the extent of deficiency, lipid synthesis is impaired, and damage or degeneration of the myelin sheath (lipid tissue) covering nerve fibers follows and causes increased nerve irritation and pain. Paralysis results if the deficiency continues.

Heart muscle weakness causes cardiac failure; smooth muscles of the vascular system may be involved, causing dilation of peripheral blood vessels and—as a result of cardiac failure—edema in the extremities.

Clinically, beriberi, like many other diseases, presents a spectrum of manifestations depending on the severity of the deficiency and stress factors. Individuals on a diet containing 0.2–0.3 mg of thiamin per 1000 Cal (which is slightly less than the requirement of 0.25–0.5 mg/1000 Cal) may slowly become depleted of the vitamin and may develop peripheral neuropathy including numbness of the feet, heaviness of the legs, anesthesia, and fatigue. Edema is not a feature at this stage and, therefore, it is called dry beriberi. If the patient is subsisting on a diet containing less than 0.2 mg of the vitamin per 1000 Cal (4200 kJ), the deficiency is more severe. In addition to the manifestations for marginal deficiency, the heart enlarges and there is an accumulation of edema fluid in the legs, face, and trunk. This is called wet beriberi and is known as shoshin in Japan. In spite of the edema, albumin does not appear in the urine, which is an important diagnostical feature. Beriberi heart disease is treated with 100 mg of thiamin administered intravenously once a day for 1 week followed by 10–15 mg per day orally.

Infantile beriberi occurs most frequently in breast-fed infants between the ages of 2 and 6 months. The nursing mother may have no clinical signs of thiamin deficiency, but she will have a history of poor diet and the milk is undoubtedly low in vitamin B_1. The infant with beriberi very rapidly develops such symptoms as cyanosis, tachycardia, and a thin cry. The condition has a rapid onset and can progress suddenly to death (usually from heart failure) unless the deficiency is corrected. Once thiamin is administered, symptoms are dramatically relieved within a matter of hours.

The most acute type of deficiency frequently encountered in western countries and particularly the United States is associated with alcohol abuse or alcoholism and is the well-known Wernicke–Korsakoff syndrome or Wernicke encephalopathy. This is generally thought to result from a high intake of empty calories in the form of alcohol, coupled with a low intake of nutritionally adequate food. It is also encountered in patients who suffer from severe nutritional depletion unrelated to drinking. In order of frequency, the most common presenting symptoms are mental confusion that soon gives way to a characteristic disorder of memory (faulty immediate recall and recent memory) and confabulation, abnormal ocular mobility, and peripheral neuropathy. As the disturbances of immediate recall and recent memory associated with Korsakoff syndrome may become irreversible, this condition requires prompt recognition and therapeutic intervention. Usually 100 mg of thiamin is administered intramuscularly followed by 10–15 mg of oral dose daily. The response is complete recovery if the treatment is started early in the course of the disease.

Approximately 10%–15% of chronic alcoholics develop cirrhosis of the liver. Alcohol-induced cirrhosis of the liver may impair hepatic uptake or storage of the vitamin. This may be due to the failure of binding sites within the damaged liver cells or the failure of the liver to elaborate the enzymes required for converting the vitamin to its coenzyme form.

The heart may undergo pathological changes as a result of alcohol and its associated thiamin deficiency. Specific nutritional heart disease in the alcoholic may occur in a form similar to that of beriberi, but in contrast to beriberi heart disease, alcoholic cardiomyopathy manifests with symptoms of heart failure, low cardiac output, and peripheral vasoconstriction.

Many people with type 1 and type 2 diabetes have low plasma concentrations of thiamin, and this may be linked to some of the complications seen in diabetics.[10] Because thiamin deficiency can result in a form of dementia (Wernicke–Korsakoff syndrome), its relationship to Alzheimer's disease and other forms of dementia have been investigated. A case-control study in 38 elderly women found that blood levels of thiamin were lower in those with dementia of Alzheimer's type compared to those in the control group. Some investigators have reported that the activities of transketolase and α-ketoglutarate dehydrogenase were decreased in the brains of patients who died of Alzheimer's disease.[3]

All diuretics lead to increased urinary thiamin excretion, depending on the urinary flow rate. In a subject at risk, such as an elderly patient, chronic diuretic treatment may lead to a subclinical thiamin deficiency. Whether subclinical thiamin nutrition is a modulator of the prevalence and/or severity of heart failure is not known. Thiamin supplementation should be considered in all patients expected to undergo a period of sustained diuresis when inadequate dietary intake is possible.

Malarial infection leads to a large increase in metabolic demands for glucose as well as a requirement for increased disposal of lactate.[6] This can cause severe thiamin deficiency and can contribute to a dysfunction of the central nervous system. Routine administration of thiamin as an adjunct to antimalarial therapy is necessary to meet the increased demands for this vitamin.

Patients with thiamin deficiency can be treated with physiological doses of this vitamin. However, there are several thiamin-responsive disorders that require pharmacological doses of the vitamin. These disorders include branched-chain ketoacidurias (maple syrup urine disease), subacute necrotizing encephalopathy due to thiamin disphosphate deficiency in the brain (Leigh syndrome), thiamin-responsive lactic acidosis (deficiency of pyruvate decarboxylase), and thiamin-responsive megaloblastic anemia (TRMA) associated with diabetes mellitus and deafness. TRMA is presumably secondary to reduced thiamin cellular transport and absorption (caused by lack of a membrane-specific carrier) and impaired intracellular pyrophosphorylation. TRMA is inherited in an autosomal recessive manner. Megaloblastic anemia occurs between infancy and adolescence. The anemia is corrected with life-long use of pharmacologic doses (25–75 mg/day) of thiamin because anemia can recur if thiamin is withdrawn. The progressive sensorineural hearing loss is generally early and can be detected in toddlers, is irreversible, and may not be prevented by thiamin treatment. The diabetes mellitus is non-type 1 in nature, with age of onset from infancy to adolescence. For maple syrup urine disease, many patients respond to a pharmacological excess of thiamin supplementation (8 mg/kg/day). For other disorders, therapeutic doses of 10–50 mg/day have proved beneficial in some cases.

9.1.6 REQUIREMENTS

Thiamin is water soluble and because the body cannot store it to any appreciable extent, a daily intake of this vitamin is essential. The requirement varies with the composition of the diet. As the vitamin participates in the metabolism of energy-yielding nutrients, the requirement is based on the energy content and more particularly on the amount of carbohydrate in the diet. The substitution of fat for carbohydrate exerts a thiamin-sparing effect and such diet requires less thiamin than a carbohydrate diet of the same caloric value. This is because the oxidation of fatty acid requires TPP in one reaction while for carbohydrate this coenzyme participates in at least three sites of metabolism. The minimum daily adult thiamin needs are 0.23–0.35 mg/1000 Cal. The recommended daily allowances (RDA) standard is 0.5 mg/1000 Cal to provide a margin of safety for individual variation and to afford some protection during periods of stress. The daily allowance for men between the ages of 20 and 50 is 1.4 mg, and for women of the same age group is 1 mg. An additional 0.4 mg over the allowance is suggested for pregnant women and 0.5 mg for nursing mothers. The recommendations for infants and children are the same as for adults (i.e., 0.5 mg/1000 Cal). The elderly utilize vitamin B_1 somewhat less efficiently and, therefore, an allowance of at least 1 mg is recommended even though their caloric intake may be below 2000 Cal (8400 kJ). To maintain optimal stores, a minimum intake of 1 mg is also recommended for all adults when energy intakes are restricted.

The need for the vitamin increases with the amount of alcohol consumed; this accounts for the increased incidence of beriberi among chronic alcoholics. Thiamin deficiency in alcoholics can be due to an inadequate intake from decreased consumption of balanced diet, decreased absorption, and decreased utilization. Fever and infection increase cellular energy requirements and hence thiamin needs.

It has been claimed that megadoses of thiamin improve central nervous system disorders, prevent senility, and cure mental illnesses. The clinical benefits have not been documented.

9.1.7 ASSESSMENT OF THIAMIN STATUS

One of the commonly used procedures for assessment of thiamin status is determining the urinary excretion of the vitamin by oxidizing it to thiochrome and measuring the latter by means of the intensity of its fluorescence in ultraviolet light. The excretion of the vitamin decreases with decreased intake.

Biochemical tests based on the functional level of TPP are a more accurate assessment of the vitamin B_1 status of the individual. During thiamin deficiency, the pyruvate decarboxylase activity in the pyruvate dehydrogenase complex is reduced, and pyruvate accumulates in the tissues and the blood. The measurement of blood pyruvic acid after administration of glucose and standard exercise has been used to assess the thiamin status of the individual; however, thiamin deficiency may not be the only cause for an elevated blood pyruvic acid. A more specific test in the diagnosis of thiamin deficiency is the measurement of transketolase activity in erythrocytes with and without the addition of TPP. Thiamin deficiency is indicated when TPP addition increases the enzyme activity by more than 25%. This test correlates closely with thiamin nutrition and is believed to be useful in detecting marginal deficiency before clinical symptoms become apparent.

9.1.8 ANTITHIAMIN SUBSTANCES

Several thiamin analogs rapidly induce symptoms of vitamin B_1 deficiency. These include pyrithiamin, in which a pyridine group is substituted for the thiazole ring, and oxythiamin, in which a hydroxyl group is substituted for the free amino group on the pyrimidine ring. Pyrithiamin inhibits the formation of TPP and oxythiamin appears to displace thiamin in tissues.

Thiamin-destroying or thiamin-inactivating factors have been found in fish, shellfish, and a variety of vegetables. Thiaminase I, which is thermolabile, is found in some fresh water fish; it decomposes thiamin at the methylene bridge. Thiaminase II, which is also thermolabile, is present in some microorganisms and can hydrolyze the vitamin; it is found in raw clams and seafood. In addition to these thermolabile thiaminases, thermostable factors that inactivate thiamin have been found in fern, tea, betel nuts, and a large number of other plants and vegetables. These foods have a variety of substances such as tannic acid, caffeic acid, and polyphenols, which are powerful inhibitors of thiamin. Tannic acid is most likely the substance in tea that inactivates thiamin by forming a tannin–thiamin complex. An acute syndrome (seasonal ataxia) has been associated with thiamin deficiency caused by thiaminase in African silkworms, a traditional, high-protein food for some Nigerians. Sulfites that are added to foods, usually as preservatives, will attack thiamin at the methylene bridge in the structure, cleaving the pyrimidine ring. The rate of this reaction is increased under acidic conditions.

9.1.9 TOXICITY

As vitamin B_1 is water soluble and the body has limited capacity to store it, any excess amount is excreted in the urine. There is no indication of toxicity from an excess use of the vitamin. The kidney has no known threshold, and intolerance to thiamin is rare. Daily doses of 500 mg have been administered in humans for as long as a month without ill effects, but a few cases of sensitization have been described following repeated parenteral injections.

9.2 RIBOFLAVIN—B₂

The existence of a yellow–green fluorescent pigment in milk whey was recognized in 1879, but the biological role of this substance was understood only after 1932. The water-soluble B vitamin was first shown to have two components: a beriberi-preventive material, which was destroyed by heat, and a heat-stable component, which was effective in promoting growth in rats. To differentiate the heat-labile component from the heat-stable fraction, the two components were designated vitamin B_1 and vitamin B_2, respectively. In 1925, there were reports from four different laboratories on the isolation of four substances necessary for growth that were called heptaflavin, lactoflavin, ovoflavin, and verdoflavin. These names were based on the sources of isolation (e.g., liver, milk, eggs, and grass, respectively) and because they were flavin compounds, which gave an intense yellow–green fluorescence in water. In 1932, Warburg and Christian isolated "Warburg's yellow enzyme" from yeast and demonstrated that it was capable of acting as a hydrogen carrier. They also showed that it had a protein component combined with a yellow pigment, neither of which alone was enzymatically active, but were effective in combination. In 1933, Kuhn and his group isolated about a gram of the active principle (yellow pigment) from 5400 L of milk and showed that it was related to Warburg's yellow enzyme. The vitamin was synthesized in 1935. It got its name riboflavin from its color and its component ribose derivative.

9.2.1 CHEMISTRY

Riboflavin is orange–yellow in color and has an intense greenish yellow fluorescence. Its solubility in water is relatively slight. It is stable to heat in acidic and neutral solution, but not in an alkaline medium. In an aqueous solution, it decomposes in the presence of light. Reduced riboflavin is insoluble in water and advantage is taken of this property to get the vitamin in crystalline form. Riboflavin is composed of an isoalloxazine ring structure linked to an alcohol derived from the pentose sugar ribose (Figure 9.3).

9.2.2 FOOD SOURCES

Riboflavin is widely distributed in both plants and animal tissues. The most important food source is milk. One of the pigments in milk, lactoflavin, is the milk form of the vitamin. Other good sources include eggs, liver, kidneys, and green leafy vegetables. The best natural source of riboflavin is yeast, but this is not normally part of a dietary regimen. Fruits and vegetables are moderately good sources of the vitamin, but they are not consumed in sufficient quantities to meet the daily requirements. It has been estimated that in the American diet, milk and milk products provide about 50% of daily needs; meat, eggs, and legumes contribute about 25%; and fruits, vegetables, and cereals about 10% each of the daily requirement of the vitamin. Riboflavin is obtained commercially from a culture medium of several molds, which produce the vitamin in abundance.

9.2.3 ABSORPTION AND TRANSPORT

Riboflavin occurs in foods as flavin mononucleotide (FMN), FAD, and as free riboflavin; all three forms can fulfill the vitamin requirement of the human body. Both FMN and FAD are hydrolyzed in the upper gastrointestinal tract to free riboflavin, which then enters the mucosal cells of the small

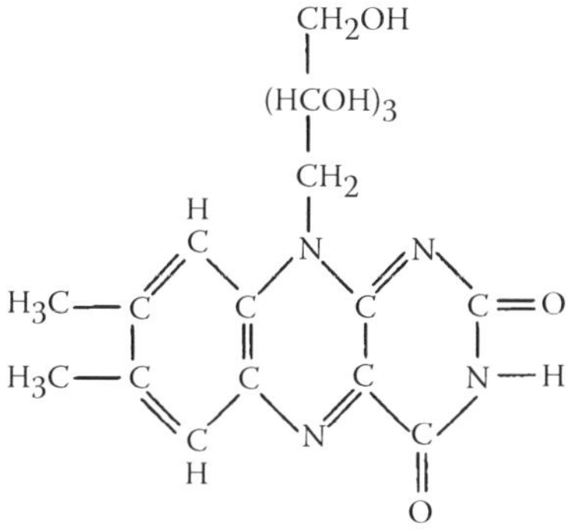

FIGURE 9.3 Riboflavin.

intestine by a saturable transport system. In the mucosal cells, it is phosphorylated to FMN by the enzyme flavokinase in the presence of ATP. It then enters the portal system and is bound to plasma albumin. FMN is readily released from the blood to the tissues, principally in the liver, where it is converted to FAD. In the tissues, it is stored as FMN and FAD rather than as free riboflavin. The liver is the major site of storage and contains about one-third of the total body flavins; other organs with high content of flavins are the heart and kidneys. In tissues, FAD can be hydrolyzed to FMN and free riboflavin by phosphatases. It is excreted primarily in the urine after the kidneys have allowed the reabsorption of sufficient vitamin to maintain tissue saturation within established limits. A small fraction is eliminated via the bile.

9.2.4 BIOCHEMICAL ROLE

Riboflavin combines with phosphoric acid in tissues to become part of the coenzyme FMN.[12,15] The latter, with the addition of adenosine monophosphate, forms FAD (Figure 9.4). The degradation of FAD to FMN is catalyzed by FAD pyrophosphatase and the further degradation of FMN to riboflavin by FMN phosphatase. In a strict sense, the mononucleotide and dinucleotide designations given to the riboflavin coenzymes are not chemically correct because the carbohydrate attached to the flavin is a polyhydric alcohol (reduced sugar) and not ribose. These coenzymes are the prosthetic groups of the flavoprotein enzymes, which catalyze oxidation–reduction reactions in numerous metabolic pathways and in energy production via the respiratory chain. These enzymes include amino acid oxidases, xanthine oxidase, cytochrome c reductase, succinic dehydrogenase complex, glutathione reductase, and many others. They use the alloxazine ring moiety of FMN or FAD as the acceptor or donor of two hydrogen atoms.

Large amounts of free riboflavin are present in the retina, but its function[13] there is not understood. The vitamin is essential for growth and is believed to participate in multiple functions, including the synthesis of corticosteroids in the adrenal glands, the formation of red blood cells in the bone marrow, the synthesis of glycogen, the metabolism of fatty acids, and the effectiveness of thyroid hormone in regulating enzyme activity. Riboflavin has been used as a part of the phototherapy treatment for neonatal jaundice. A randomized placebo-controlled trial examined the effect of 400 mg/day of riboflavin for 3 months on migraine prevention[19] in 54 men and women with a history of recurrent headaches. The vitamin was found to result in significant reductions in headache frequencies and headache days. Another study also showed the beneficial effect of riboflavin in the prevention of migraines.[11]

9.2.5 DEFICIENCY

Riboflavin deficiency is not known to be a primary etiological factor in a major human disease, although patients with beriberi and protein deficiency are generally also deficient in vitamin B_2.[17] The deficiency may produce severe systemic symptoms in experimental animals, but in humans, the manifestations appear to be limited primarily to the skin and mucus membranes. The symptoms are usually not severe. It is not a specific deficiency disease comparable to beriberi. Early signs include soreness and burning of the lips, mouth, and tongue. Some of the signs of the deficiency include swollen and reddened (magenta) tongue (a condition called glossitis), fissuring at the corners of the mouth and lips (a condition called cheilosis; Figure 9.5), seborrheic dermatitis especially at the nasal–labial folds, and corneal vascularization. These signs have generally been accepted as the clinical picture of vitamin B_2 deficiency. In addition, ocular symptoms and signs that respond to

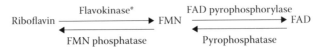

FIGURE 9.4   The conversion of riboflavin to FAD. * Flavokinase is stimulated by thyroxine.

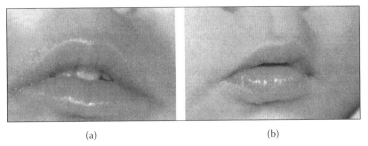

(a)   (b)

FIGURE 9.5   (a) Close-up of a young child with cheilosis, or, as it is sometimes called, cheilitis. It is usually the first and most characteristic sign of riboflavin deficiency. The lesion begins as areas of pallor at the angles of the mouth, with hyperkeratosis of the epidermis and with dermal inflammatory infiltrate. Cracks or fissures radiate from the corners of the mouth. These tend to become secondary, get infected, and produce a macerated, bleeding, inflammatory fissure lesion. (b) The same child but fully recovered after 4 weeks of therapy with 2 mg of riboflavin daily. (Courtesy of Shari Roehl, Pharmacia & Upjohn Co.)

administration of vitamin B_2 have been reported. A case-control study found that men and women in the highest quintile of dietary riboflavin intake (1.6–2.2 mg/day) had significantly decreased risk (33%–51%) of cataracts compared to those in the lowest quintile (0.08 mg/day). Another case-control study reported that individuals in the highest quintile of riboflavin nutritional status, as measured by red cell gluthathione reductase activity, had about 50% reduction in the occurrence of age-related cataracts as those in the lowest quintile of riboflavin nutritional status. Also a recent study in 408 women found that higher dietary riboflavin intake was inversely associated with 5-year change in lens opacification.

Preeclampsia is hypertension that develops during pregnancy accompanied by proteinuria. Its cause is not known. A study in 154 pregnant women at increased risk of preeclampsia found that those who were deficient in riboflavin were 4.7 times more likely to develop preeclampsia than those who had adequate riboflavin nutritional status. However, another small randomized, placebo-controlled, double-blind trial in 450 pregnant women with prior preeclampsia found that supplementation with 15 mg of riboflavin did not prevent the condition.[16]

In view of the importance of the vitamin in cell respiration, it seems surprising that the clinical changes attributed to the deficiency are minor.

Thyroid disease has profound effects upon vitamin B_2 physiology and metabolism. Thyroxine stimulates intestinal motility and, as a result, the absorption of the vitamin is decreased in hyperthyroidism and is increased in hypothyroidism. Thyroxine regulates flavokinase, the enzyme that converts riboflavin to FMN. In hypothyroidism,[14] the enzyme activity results in a diminished formation of FMN from riboflavin and hepatic levels of FMN and FAD are decreased, similar to the condition in vitamin B_2 deficiency. On the other hand, there is increased formation of FMN in hyperthyroidism, and this may increase turnover and thereby impose a strain on vitamin reserves; however, the level of FAD remains near normal.

Riboflavin is sensitive to light and is rapidly inactivated. Therefore, phototherapy of neonatal jaundice and of certain skin disorders may promote riboflavin deficiency.

In contrast to thiamin, riboflavin deficiency is recognized as protective against malaria both in experimental animals and in humans.[18] With dietary riboflavin deficiency, parasitemia is decreased dramatically. In a study with human infants suffering from malaria, normal riboflavin nutritional status was associated with higher parasitemia. The mechanism by which riboflavin deficiency inhibits parasitemia is not known. Hypothyroidism, which inhibits the formation of FAD, is associated with diminished parasitemia. Also a number of antimalarial drugs inhibit the biosynthesis of FAD. Based on these observations, it has been suggested that the requirements of the parasites for riboflavin are higher than that of human cells. Therefore, marginal riboflavin deficiency is selectively detrimental to the parasites.

9.2.6   REQUIREMENTS

The minimal requirement for riboflavin is defined as the level that prevents clinical signs of deficiency and allows for normal urinary excretion of the vitamin. In adults, the consumption of no more than 0.55 mg/day results in clinical signs of deficiency and reduces urinary excretion. Levels of 0.8–0.9 mg/day prevent the appearance of clinical signs, but urinary excretion is still below normal; this suggests that the minimal requirement is more than 0.9 mg/day. The RDA is based on energy allowances and is 0.6 mg/1000 Cal for all ages. For men, it is 1.3–1.7 mg/day and for women, it is 1.1–1.3 mg/day, depending on age. An additional 0.3 mg is recommended in pregnancy, and for lactating mothers, an additional 0.5 mg is recommended (based on the content of riboflavin in milk and assuming 70% utilization efficiency). Some pieces of evidence show that the vitamin B_2 need is increased among women using oral contraceptives.

9.2.7   ASSESSMENT OF NUTRITIONAL STATUS

One of the methods used to assess riboflavin deficiency is the measurement of urinary excretion of the vitamin. Normal adults excrete 120 µg or more of the vitamin every 24 hours; excretion of less than 50 µg/day is characteristic of deficiency. Results are often expressed in terms of micrograms of riboflavin per gram of creatinine, and the excretion of less than 27 µg of vitamin B_2 per gram of creatinine has been suggested as an indicator of deficiency. The vitamin can be measured fluorometrically. The measurement of the activity of the erythrocyte glutathione reductase, a FAD-containing enzyme, is a more specific and sensitive indicator of vitamin B_2 status.

9.2.8   ANTAGONISTS

Several antagonists have been identified and used for experimental studies to produce vitamin B_2 deficiency. The antagonist D-galactoflavin has been used experimentally in animals and humans to hasten the development of riboflavin deficiency. A few foods such as Jamaican ackee nut are known to contain riboflavin antagonists.

9.2.9   TOXICITY

The vitamin appears to be relatively nontoxic, and no cases of toxicity from ingestion of excess vitamin B_2 by experimental animals and humans have been reported. The transport system necessary for absorption of riboflavin across the intestine becomes saturated, limiting the amount of vitamin that can be absorbed. The capacity of the human gastrointestinal tract to absorb orally administered vitamin B_2 may be less than 20 mg in a single dose. After absorption, riboflavin is rapidly excreted in the urine; therefore, it is unlikely to cause a health risk, even with the ingestion of large doses. Oral doses of 10 g/kg body weight in rats and 2 g/kg body weight in dogs produced no toxic effects. Mice receiving 340 mg/kg body weight intraperitoneally (5000 times the therapeutic dose, or an equivalent of 20 g/day for humans) showed no apparent effect.

The vitamin is excreted primarily as free riboflavin in the urine, to which it imparts a yellow fluorescent color; it is sometimes prescribed with drugs so that it can act as a marker to determine whether a patient took the medication.

9.3   NIACIN

Nicotinic acid has been known to organic chemists since 1867 when it was discovered and isolated as an oxidation product of nicotine; however, its role as a vitamin was not recognized until 1937. In 1913, Funk isolated it from yeast and rice polishings in the course of an attempt to identify the water-soluble antiberiberi vitamin, but the interest in this compound was lost when it was found to be ineffective in curing pigeons of beriberi. Nicotinic acid was recognized as the component of the coenzymes NAD and NADP by Warburg and Von Euler in 1935. Thus, its metabolic role was known before its nutritional significance was established.

The disease pellagra was first reported in 1735 by Casal, a Spanish physician.[30] It appeared in Europe when corn became the major staple food stuff around the Mediterranean in Spain, France, Italy, and eastward. The disease was unknown in the United States until the beginning of the last century, when cultivation of corn increased, especially in the southern states. From 1910 to 1935, as many as 170,000 cases of pellagra per year were reported. The association of the disease with corn led to the theory that it was caused by a toxic substance present in spoiled corn. Goldburger, a physician working with the United States Public Health Service, was assigned the task of identifying the cause of the disease. In 1917, he conducted experiments with a group of prisoners who were either given the regular prison diet or the one typical of the villages in which pellagra was prevalent. After about 5 months, the prisoners on the village-type diet showed symptoms of pellagra while those on a regular prison diet were healthy. These studies established the theory that a dietary factor was involved in the disease. About the same time, Spencer, a veterinarian in North Carolina, first called attention to the similarity between the symptoms of a spontaneous canine disease "black tongue" and those of human pellagra. He cured the disease in dogs by giving them milk, eggs, and meat, and concluded that the cause of the disease was a diet low in nitrogen.

The link between pellagra and nicotinic acid was established in 1937, when Elvehjem and his group working at the University of Wisconsin found that nicotinic acid was effective in curing black tongue in dogs and pellagra in humans. The use of nicotinic acid in treating pellagra brought dramatic results, and the number of pellagra victims in southern hospitals dropped precipitously. The disease was once a common worldwide problem, but the fortification of wheat flour with niacin and the ready availability of multivitamins have virtually eradicated the disease except in some chronic alcoholics and in some maize-eating populations that eat few green vegetables and red meat.

The term niacin is used for nicotinic acid and derivatives that exhibit the qualitative nutritional activity of nicotinic acid. Nicotinamide or niacinamide is the amide of nicotinic acid.

9.3.1 FOOD SOURCES

Niacin is present in small amounts in most foods; particularly rich sources are cereal grains (e.g., whole wheat, rye) and enriched bread, legumes, meat, poultry, and peanuts. Tea and coffee also can contribute significantly to niacin intake. Vegetables and fruits are poor sources. The main source in the diet is the cereal staple consumed. Whole grains or lightly milled cereals contain more nicotinic acid than refined cereal grain and flours because as much as 90% of the vitamin is in the outer husks and is removed in the milling process. Niacin is added in enriched cereal products to compensate for the loss.

9.3.2 TRYPTOPHAN–NIACIN RELATIONSHIP

Some foods such as milk and eggs have a low content of the vitamin, but are effective in curing or preventing pellagra; also, diets low in niacin are not always pellagragenic. This discrepancy was explained in 1945 by Krehl and his associates at the University of Wisconsin. They showed that tryptophan and niacin were both effective in treating pellagra; subsequently, it was established that tryptophan is a precursor of niacin. The human body, therefore, is not entirely dependent on dietary sources of nicotinic acid as it may be synthesized from tryptophan. On average, 60 mg of tryptophan is converted to 1 mg of niacin, and the efficiency of conversion to niacin depends on nutritional and hormonal factors.[25,29] Of special interest are data showing that women in the third trimester of pregnancy and those who are on oral contraceptive steroids can convert tryptophan to niacin three times as effectively as nonpregnant females. This is because estrogens stimulate tryptophan oxygenase, the first and rate-limiting enzyme of the tryptophan–niacin pathway.

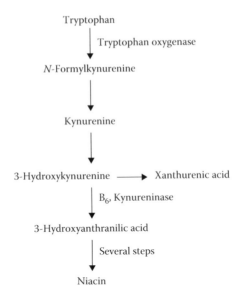

FIGURE 9.6 Pathway for the synthesis of niacin from tryptophan.

The synthesis of niacin begins with the oxidation of tryptophan to *N*-formylkynurenine (FK) catalyzed by the liver enzyme tryptophan oxygenase (Figure 9.6). FK is converted to kynurenine by the enzyme formamidase. Kynurenine is metabolized to produce 3-hydroxykynurenine, which, by the action of kynureninase, a vitamin B_6-dependent enzyme, forms 3-hydroxyanthranilic acid (HA). HA is then converted by a series of reactions to niacin. In deficiency of vitamin B_6, niacin is not formed. HA is shunted toward the alternate pathway and produces xanthurenic acid, which is excreted in the urine. Thus, vitamin B_6 deficiency can be diagnosed by a measurement of urinary xanthurenic acid after administration of oral tryptophan (tryptophan load test).

9.3.3 BOUND FORMS OF NIACIN

Corn is poor in niacin and its principle protein, zein, is very low in tryptophan, a biosynthetic source of the vitamin. In several Central and South American countries, there is an absence of pellagra among those whose staple food is maize. There is evidence that some niacin in corn is present in a carbohydrate-bound form, called niacytin, and a peptide-bound form, niacinogen, which may not be available. It can be liberated from the bound form by treatment with alkali. In Mexico, tortillas are made from maize treated with lime water; this practice may account for a low incidence of pellagra in Mexico. It may also be due to the liberal consumption of coffee, which is rich in niacin. The Hopi Indians of Arizona roast sweet corn in hot ashes. This is another traditional practice that liberates the nicotinic acid, but the ways of food preparation used in most countries do not have this favorable effect.

9.3.4 CHEMISTRY

Nicotinic acid is a simple derivative of pyridine. It is 3-pyridine carboxylic acid (Figure 9.7).[32] It is an odorless, nonhygroscopic, white crystalline compound, which is stable in air and resistant to autoclaving, and is in fact one of the most stable water-soluble vitamins. It is soluble in water, dilute acids, and alkaline solutions. It is active both as acid or amide (nicotinamide). The amide is preferred for therapeutic purposes because the acid acts as a vasodilator.

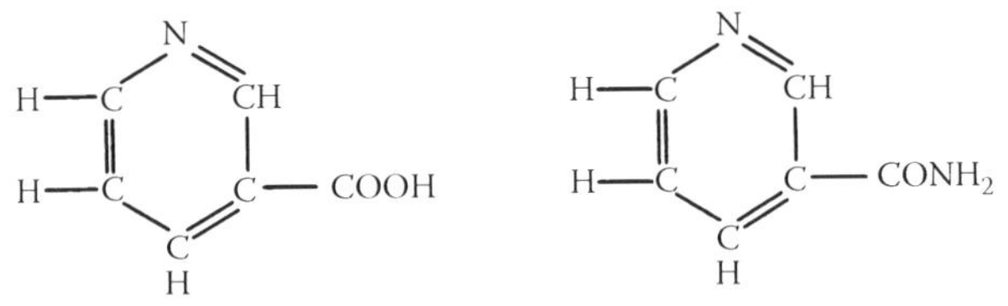

FIGURE 9.7   Niacin and niacinamide.

9.3.5   ABSORPTION AND TRANSPORT

Niacin is rapidly absorbed from the upper small intestine by simple diffusion, and it enters the circulatory system and reaches all the cells where it is incorporated into its coenzymes. Excess niacin is methylated and excreted in the urine either as *N*-methyl nicotinamide or as a pyridone of *N*-methyl nicotinamide. Little free nicotinic acid or nicotinamide is excreted. About two-thirds of the niacin metabolized by adults may come from tryptophan.

9.3.6   FUNCTIONS

Niacin is required by all living cells as part of the two coenzymes NAD and NADP.[22,24] They can accept or release hydrogen atoms readily and are effective in assisting several dehydrogenases in removing hydrogen in many biological reactions.[26] They are essential in the metabolism of carbohydrates, fats, proteins, and alcohol. NADP is required in the hexose monophosphate shunt of glucose metabolism, and its reduced form, NADPH, has important roles in the synthesis of fats and steroids. Niacin is part of the "glucose tolerance factor" of yeast, which enhances the response to insulin.

Niacin has been used for almost 50 years as a lipid-lowering drug.[20,28] The pharmacologic effect requires doses (1–3 g) that are much higher than those provided by a normal diet. It has potent triglyceride-lowering and high-density lipoprotein (HDL) cholesterol-elevating effect and a modest low-density lipoprotein (LDL) cholesterol-lowering effect. The most common side effect is flushing of the skin, which frequently diminishes over time. The precise mechanism of action of niacin's therapeutic effect has not been fully elucidated. Recent evidence indicates that niacin mediates its action through its G-protein receptor called GPR109A (HM74A) in adipocytes.[33] By binding to its receptor niacin reduces intracellular cyclic adenosine monophosphate (cAMP), thereby inhibiting hormone-sensitive lipase. It blocks the breakdown of adipose tissue fat, decreases free fatty acids in blood and as a result decreases secretion of very low density lipoprotein (VLDL) and cholesterol by the liver. Niacin also modulates the metabolism of HDL by inhibiting its catabolic pathway. However, it modestly increases insulin resistance and may worsen glycemic control in individuals with type 2 diabetes. It may also elevate liver enzymes in some individuals.

One popular supplement is inositol hexanicotinate, usually sold as "flush-free" or "no flush" niacin in units of 250, 500, or 1000 mg tablets or capsules. In the body, it is broken down into its components, releasing niacin. It is claimed to be as effective as niacin and does not cause flushing. But the evidence that it has lipid-modifying functions is contradictory. The American Heart Association and the National Cholesterol Education Program suggest that only prescription niacin should be used to treat dyslipidemia and only under the management of a physician. This is because niacin may have adverse effects including elevation of liver enzymes.

Nicotinamide has been shown to be a cure in some cases of type 1 diabetes. In some studies, newly diagnosed type 1 diabetics have experienced complete resolution of their diabetes with nicotinamide supplementation. In vitro and animal studies have indicated that high levels of nictinamide protect β-cells from damage caused by toxic chemicals and white blood cells. Several studies done on high-risk groups led to a large population-based study in New Zealand to see if supplements can prevent diabetes from developing in high-risk groups. The results of screening 32,000 5–7-year-old children for islet cell antibodies and treating those at risk have proved impressive. But some studies have reported that high doses of nicotinamide decrease insulin sensitivity. Unlike nicotinamide, niacin has not been found effective in the prevention of type 1 diabetes. Niacinamide is used currently to treat Hartnup disease.

9.3.7 DEFICIENCY

A deficiency of niacin causes pellagra (Figures 9.8 and 9.8A). The word is derived from the Italian words "pelle" (skin) and "agra" (rough). The disease is classically characterized by the three Ds—dermatitis, diarrhea, and dementia—but these are actually the symptoms of the advanced condition. Mild and early cases may lack any of the three components of the syndrome. Early symptoms of deficiency often are burning pain throughout the oral cavity and the tongue becomes red and swollen. The most common finding is a scarlet glossitis in the acute stages, somewhat similar to riboflavin deficiency, and a smooth atrophic tongue if the condition is chronic. Erythematous (acute) or pigmented and scaly (chronic) skin lesions are often seen on those parts of the body that are either subject to pressure and irritation, or exposed to sunlight. The hands and forearms up to the elbow and the skin around the neck and upper thorax are affected (Casal's necklace).

The gastrointestinal membrane is inflamed and atrophied, and the symptoms include anorexia, nausea, vomiting, constipation, and abdominal pain; but the most important in the advanced stages of the disease is intractable diarrhea. The latter induces malabsorption of most nutrients, causing the picture of chronic general malnutrition.

The neurological symptoms are associated with the degeneration of nervous tissues and include insomnia, irritability, vertigo, headache, delusion, and hallucination (in chronic cases). Some of the mental symptoms seen in chronic alcoholics have been ascribed to niacin deficiency, at least in part, because the diet of many alcoholics is deficient in several of the B vitamins.

Although the cause of pellagra has been attributed to the deficiency of niacin (and tryptophan), there are other complicating factors that can alter the availability of the vitamin. Some steps in the pathway from tryptophan to niacin are dependent on the coenzyme derived from vitamin B_6. The chronic administration of drugs such as isoniazid and 3-mercaptopurine, used in the treatment of tuberculosis and leukemia, respectively, can cause niacin deficiency. These drugs interfere with vitamin B_6 metabolism. Pellagra has also been shown to be associated with the consumption of millet jowar (*Sorgum vulgarae*). Unlike corn, jowar has niacin in the free form and also has adequate tryptophan content. The cause of the disease in a jowar-eating population has been attributed to the

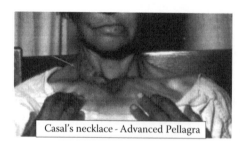
Casal's necklace - Advanced Pellagra

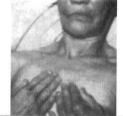
Same patient after niacin therapy

FIGURE 9.8 Casal's necklace—advanced pellagra. Dermatitis outlining the exposed area of the neck is pathognomonic of pellagra, as are the characteristic lesions on the backs of the hands. Either sunlight or heat from a stove may have been a precipitating factor. The same patient after nicotinamide therapy. (Courtesy of Shari Roehl, Pharmacia & Upjohn Co.)

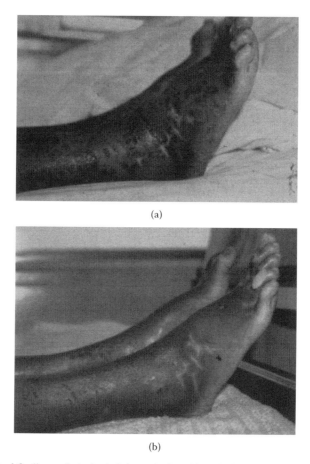

(a)

(b)

FIGURE 9.8A Clinical findings of niacin deficiency before (a) and after (b) therapy in an alcoholic patient.

presence of a relative excess concentration of leucine in jowar.[21] Experimental studies have shown that excess leucine in the diet inhibits the conversion of tryptophan to niacin. This effect of leucine can be counteracted by supplementing the diet with isoleucine.

Hartnup disease, a rare disorder, is characterized by skin lesions that mimic pellagra in all respects.[23] It is caused by an inborn error of tryptophan metabolism due, at least in part, to an absorption defect. The name of the disease comes from the first family in which it was recognized. In general, patients with this disease respond to the administration of niacin.

9.3.8 REQUIREMENTS

As dietary tryptophan also contributes to niacin nutrition, the term niacin equivalent (NE) is introduced, which is equal to 1 mg of niacin or 60 mg of dietary tryptophan. Niacin is intimately involved in the release of energy from food and, therefore, the requirement is based (as for thiamin) on caloric intake. Various studies suggest that 4.4 NE/1000 Cal protects all persons from pellagra, and this is considered to be the minimum need. To this, a 50% margin of safety is added in the recommended allowances of 6.6 NE/1000 Cal. It is also suggested that a minimum of 13 NE be maintained regardless of caloric intake. The RDA for infants, children, and adults is 6–9 NE/day, 11–18 NE/day, and 13–19 NE/day, respectively. During pregnancy, an increase of 2 NE is recommended, and during lactation an additional 5 NE over normal needs is indicated.

The average content of tryptophan in animal and vegetable proteins is 1.4% and 1%, respectively. If the daily diet contains 60 g of protein, it should provide about 600 mg of tryptophan, which can yield 10 mg of niacin. Most diets in the United States contain 500–1000 mg of tryptophan to provide 8–14 mg of niacin. In addition, the average diet also contains about 10 mg of preformed niacin, giving a total daily intake of 18–24 mg NE—an amount sufficient for all adult needs.

9.3.9 EVALUATION OF NIACIN STATUS

There is little storage of niacin in the body, and the excess is excreted as its metabolites in urine. The excretion of metabolites falls to low levels in deficiency, usually less than 3 mg/day. Normally, about one-fourth of the vitamin is excreted as methyl nicotinamide and the balance as its derivative pyridone, but the latter disappears before clinical signs appear. A measurement of excretion of methyl nicotinamide in a random sample of urine in relation to creatinine output gives the information on niacin status. An excretion of 0.5 mg of methyl nicotinamide per gram of creatinine is suggestive of deficiency.

9.3.10 TOXICITY

Niacin is essentially nontoxic. Nicotinic acid acts as a vasodilator and, therefore, may cause flushing of the skin with intakes as low as 50–100 mg. This reaction is not adverse and lasts only about 20 min. About half of those taking the vitamin will develop a tolerance to this effect. The niacinamide form that is usually found in vitamin supplements does not cause this reaction.

Niacin and its amide are used in megadoses (excess of 3 g/day) for the treatment of schizophrenia, but the evidence seems to question this use, and there are no data to support its effectiveness. Doses of 1–2 g of nicotinic acid (but not nicotinamide) three times a day lower both plasma triglycerides and cholesterol with corresponding decreases in LDL and VLDL. It also causes unpleasant flushing, skin rashes, and a variety of potentially unfavorable biochemical lesions. It should, therefore, be used as a lipid-lowering agent only under close supervision. Niacin increases blood glucose, and this may be a problem for diabetic patients. But it can cause decreased insulin sensitivity at doses of 2 g/day in adults at high risk for type 1 diabetes.

9.4 PANTOTHENIC ACID

Pantothenic acid, also called vitamin B_5, was recognized by Roger Williams in 1933 as an acidic substance required as a growth factor for yeast. The substance was also known to other investigators as a "liver filtrate factor" required for normal growth of rats and as "chick antidermatitis factor," which prevented and cured dermatitis in chicks. It was isolated and identified in 1939 and was synthesized in 1940. Tissue extracts from a variety of biological materials were found to contain the growth factor for yeast and it was named pantothenic acid, which is derived from the Greek word "pantos" (from everywhere). It was found to be an essential nutrient for a wide range of animals and birds.

9.4.1 FOOD SOURCES

In general, the distribution of pantothenic acid resembles that of the other B vitamins. Yeast, liver, and eggs are among the richest sources. Milk and meat are important sources because of the concentration of the vitamin and because of the quantities consumed. Cereal grains have a substantial amount, but about half of the vitamin may be lost when the whole grain is milled for the manufacture of flour. Moderate amounts of the vitamin are present in avocados, broccoli, molasses, and sweet potatoes.

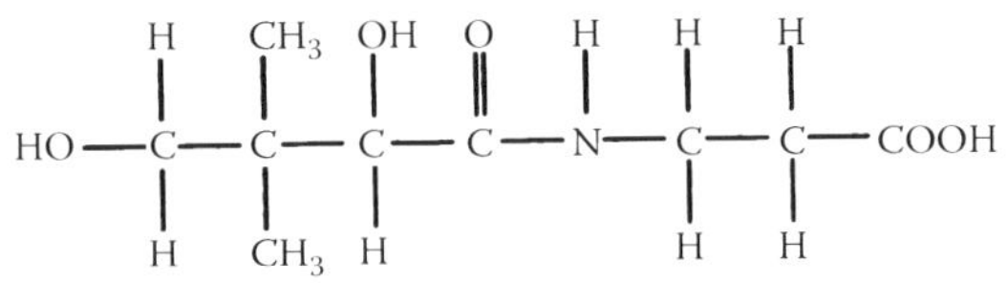

FIGURE 9.9   Pantothenic acid.

9.4.2   CHEMISTRY

Pantothenic acid is composed of pantoic acid and β-alanine, which are joined together by a peptide-like linkage (Figure 9.9). It is a pale yellow viscous oil that is easily destroyed by alkali and acid, but is stable in neutral solution. Pantothenic acid produced commercially is a synthetic, white, crystalline calcium salt, calcium pantothenate. It has a bitter taste. The derivative of pantothenic acid, pantothenol, is a more stable form of the vitamin and is often used in multivitamin supplements. It is rapidly converted to pantothenic acid in humans. Calcium and sodium pantothenate are also available as supplements. Various other derivatives of pantothenic acid have been synthesized, and their antagonistic action studied. W-methyl pantothenic acid is the most common derivative used to produce a deficiency of the vitamin in humans.

9.4.3   ABSORPTION AND TRANSPORT

Pantothenic acid in food is present in free form and also as a coenzyme in a bound form. The bound form is hydrolyzed by intestinal pyrophosphatase and phosphatase to release the vitamin. Free pantothenic acid is then absorbed from the small intestinal mucosa by a specific transport system that is saturable and sodium-dependent. After absorption, it enters the portal circulation and is transported to various tissues from which it is taken up by most cells and where it is probably incorporated into the coenzyme form. The serum contains only free pantothenic acid while most of the vitamin in the erythrocytes is present as a coenzyme. The concentration of the vitamin is higher in the liver, adrenals, kidneys, brain, and heart, all of which are organs characterized by high metabolic activity. Pantothenic acid is excreted in the urine as free vitamin, and the amount excreted reflects the dietary intake.

9.4.4   FUNCTIONS

Pantothenic acid is an essential component of CoA and the acyl carrier protein (ACP).[35,39] CoA is an atypical dinucleotide with the usual mononucleotide being replaced by phosphopantetheine. Pantetheine is pantothenic acid that is joined to β-mercaptoethylamine through a peptide linkage. At the other end, pantothenic acid is joined by a pyrophosphate to an adenylic acid group. This adenylic acid consists of adenine, D-ribose, and phosphate, but the phosphate is linked onto the 3-carbon of the ribose.

The activation of CoA involves the addition of the two-carbon acetate compound to form acetyl CoA. These acetate molecules are readily accepted by and transferred from the CoA molecule. CoA is present within the cell but not in the blood, suggesting that it is synthesized intracellularly and can pass through the cell membrane with difficulty, if at all. In red blood cells, it exists bound to protein.

CoA occupies a central and basic role in the metabolism of carbohydrates, fats, and proteins (Figure 9.10). The acetyl CoA that is formed from these three major nutrients combines with oxaloacetate to form citrate, which initiates the citric acid cycle. The oxidation of pyruvate and α-ketoglutarate requires CoA. It provides an acetyl group for the formation of acetyl choline needed in the transmission of nerve impulses and for the detoxification of sulfonamides and some other

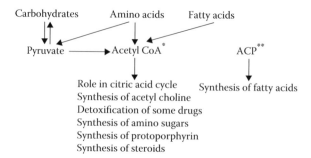

FIGURE 9.10 Metabolic functions of pantothenic acid. * Pantothenic acid is an essential component of coenzyme A. ** 4-Phosphopantetheine is the prosthetic group of ACP, which has a role in fatty acid synthesis.

drugs that are acetylated prior to excretion. It is essential for the synthesis of cholesterol, steroid hormones, and protoporphyrin (a part of hemoglobin), and for the stimulation of antibody response. In essence, because of its role in energy metabolism, CoA can be considered vital to all energy-requiring processes within the body. Proteins are acetylated by the addition of acetate group donated by CoA. Protein acetylation affects the three-dimensional structure of proteins, potentially affecting their functions. For example, acetylation of peptide hormones can alter the activities of these hormones. Protein acetylation plays a role in cell division and DNA replication and also affects gene expression by facilitating transcription of mRNA. A number of proteins can be acylated by the attachment of fatty acids donated by CoA. The acylated proteins play a role in cell signaling.

Fatty acid synthesis in the cytoplasm and mitochondria involves an additional role of pantothenic acid in the form of the cofactor 4-phosphopantetheine. This factor is bound to a protein commonly called the ACP. The acyl intermediates are esterified to the sulfhydryl groups of 4-phosphopantetheine linked to the acyl protein. The ACP appears to be involved in all fatty acid synthesis systems.

Pantothenic acid may have a role in wound healing. Treatment with oral pantothenic acid and application with oral pantothenol ointment have been shown to accelerate the closure of skin wounds and increase the strength of scar tissue in animals. But there are fewer studies to support accelerated wound healing in humans. A preliminary study has indicated that pantothenol ointment can help cure the foot ulceration commonly associated with diabetes.[34]

9.4.5 DEFICIENCY

Experimental deficiency in rats produces growth failure, impaired reproduction, adrenal cortical hypofunction, and graying of black hair. These pathological effects are accompanied by a reduction in plasma and urinary concentration of pantothenic acid and a decrease in the concentration of CoA in most tissues. Severe pantothenic acid deficiency has also caused loss of hair in mice. The cosmetic industry has used these observations to add pantothenic acid in various products such as shampoo. These products, however, showed no benefits in human trials. Pantothenic acid deficiency has also been induced in calves, pigs, guinea pigs, mice, monkeys, and rabbits when fed natural diets containing low levels of the vitamin. The deficient animals had a functional impairment of the gastrointestinal, reproductive, and hormonal systems as well as the neuromuscular system. These symptoms were reversed by supplementing the diet with the vitamin.

There seems to be no evidence of pantothenic acid deficiency disease in free human populations. In view of the importance of reactions dependent on this vitamin, one would expect the deficiency to be of serious concern in humans; however, this does not appear true, probably because the vitamin is present in most natural foods and most symptoms of pantothenic acid deficiency are vague and mimic those of other B vitamins. A deficiency has been produced experimentally. Human subjects were given a synthetic diet to which was added every known essential vitamin and mineral except pantothenic acid. This resulted in lowered blood cholesterol and altered response to corticotropin, but no clinical signs of deficiency were evident. It was, however, possible to produce a deficiency in human volunteers by the use of a metabolic antagonist (w-methyl pantothenic acid, 1–4 g/day) with a pantothenate-deficient diet. In 8–10 weeks, signs of deficiency appeared in these individuals, including depression, vomiting, malaise, abdominal distress, burning cramps, sleep disturbances, and paresthesia of the hands and feet. This list of symptoms probably reflects an impaired health of cells in many tissues. Biochemical abnormalities included decreased acetylation of p-aminobenzoic acid, abnormal glucose tolerance, and lowered blood cholesterol. All the symptoms were cured by the administration of the vitamin.

During World War II, a group of Americans imprisoned in a Japanese prison camp developed a neurological disorder characterized as "the burning foot syndrome." The symptoms consisted of numbness and tingling in the toes and burning pain in the feet and were associated with neurological and mental disturbances. After these men were liberated, some of them were administered, one at a time, each of the water-soluble vitamins in an effort to determine what accounted for this disease. Therapy with thiamin and niacin relieved some of the symptoms, but pantothenic acid relieved the burning foot syndrome. These subjects also had reduced ability to acetylate p-aminobenzoic acid, suggestive of pantothenic acid deficiency.

9.4.6 REQUIREMENTS

It is established that humans need pantothenic acid, but we know very little about the adequacy of intake or the effect of marginal deficiency on human health. It is generally assumed that pantothenic acid deficiency does not occur in humans because dietary intake is adequate and/or the vitamin is synthesized by the intestinal microflora, which contributes to the needs; however, recent studies suggest that the synthesis of vitamin by intestinal microorganisms does not contribute significantly to the maintenance of adequate pantothenate nutrition. Although no official value has yet been established as a recommended dietary allowance for humans, the 1989 report of the Food and Nutrition Board has recommended a safe and adequate estimated daily dietary intake for normal healthy individuals of different ages. The recommended intakes of pantothenic acid per day are as follows: infants up to 1 year of age, 2–3 mg; children and adolescents, 2–5 mg; and adults, 4–7 mg. These recommendations are based on studies on healthy persons whose intakes, blood levels, and urinary excretion were measured. A slightly higher intake may be warranted for pregnant and lactating women. Human milk contains approximately 2 mg of pantothenic acid per liter.

9.4.7 ASSESSMENT OF PANTOTHENIC ACID STATUS

As urinary output of pantothenic acid is directly proportional to dietary intake, the present assessment relies mainly on this index. Urinary excretion of less than 1 mg/day is considered abnormally low.

9.4.8 EFFECT OF EXCESS PANTOTHENIC ACID

Pantothenic acid as a calcium salt has been used successfully in treating the paralysis of the gastrointestinal tract after surgery, which causes the accumulation of gas and severe abdominal pain. It appears to stimulate gastrointestinal motility. Although the vitamin has been prescribed for neurotoxicity, salicylate toxicity, alopecia, osteoarthritis, diabetic neuropathy, psychiatric state, and some other ailments, it has not been proven to have any therapeutic use. Pantothenic acid neither prevents nor cures the graying of hair in humans despite the claims to the contrary by vendors of food supplements.

Pantothenic acid derivatives, pantothenol and pantethine, have been used to improve lipid profile in the blood. These derivatives can lower LDL cholesterol and triglycerides in mice. Doses of 900 mg of pantethine (300 mg three times daily) are effective in lowering total cholesterol and triglycerides in humans. Pantothenic acid (2 g/day) may reduce the duration of morning stiffness and pain sensitivity in arthritis patients.

There is no evidence that therapeutic doses of 10–100 mg of pantothenic acid chronically administered cause any harmful effects. Even with amounts as high as 10–20 g of calcium salt, the only reported problem was occasional diarrhea. However, there is one case of serious toxic reaction in an elderly woman who took a combination of 10 mg/day of biotin and 300 mg/day of pantothenic acid for 2 months. Therefore, as is true for all micronutrients, the use of pantothenic acid and its derivatives for the treatment of various diseases should be made under the guidance of a qualified healthcare provider.

9.5   BIOTIN

In 1901, Wildiers reported on a substance present in extracts of meat and some natural food materials, which permitted the rapid growth of yeast when added to a sugar and salt medium. He called this substance "bios," a Greek term meaning "life." Subsequent investigators recognized the complex nature of bios and were able to fractionate and identify its different components. Bios I was later shown to be inositol, and bios II was shown to be a mixture of pantothenic acid and another substance that was necessary for the growth and respiration of Rhizobium. This substance was called coenzyme R. In 1927, Boas reported that a toxic condition was produced on feeding raw egg whites to animals and the toxicity was prevented by giving a "protective factor x" found in liver. It was later named vitamin H (from "haut," which is German for skin). In 1936, two Dutch chemists Kogl and Tonnis succeeded in isolating a substance in crystalline form from the bios fraction of egg yolk. They obtained 1.1 mg of the substance from 250 kg of dried egg yolks and gave the name biotin for this material required for the growth of yeast. In 1940, du Vigneaud and his group proved that coenzyme R and vitamin H were identical to biotin. Its structure was then determined, and it was synthesized in 1945.

9.5.1   FOOD SOURCES

Biotin is widely distributed in natural foods. Those containing the greatest concentrations of the vitamin include yeast, liver, kidneys, soybeans and rice bran, cow's milk, egg yolk, peanuts, and molasses. Some vegetables such as cauliflower, tomatoes, and legumes are good sources. Most meats, grains, fruits, and vegetables contain lower quantities. Biotin occurs in food partly in a free form as well as partly bound to protein as part of the enzyme system.

9.5.2   CHEMISTRY

Biotin is a relatively simple compound, a cyclic urea derivative that contains sulfur. It has a bicyclical structure consisting of a ureido ring fused with a tetrahydrothiophene ring bearing a valeric acid side chain[42,46] (Figure 9.11). It is synthesized biochemically by a variety of microorganisms from pimelic acid, a seven-carbon dicarboxylic acid, alanine, and cysteine. In its free form, it is a crystalline substance, and is very stable to heat in cooking, processing, and storage. It is somewhat labile to alkali and oxidizing agents.

The substance in raw egg white, which causes the toxic manifestations that are reversed by biotin, is the glycoprotein called avidin. Avidin has a high affinity to biotin, and it combines with the vitamin in a firm linkage to form a complex that cannot be hydrolyzed and/or absorbed and, therefore, is excreted. Thus, the ingestion of large amounts of avidin results in an induced biotin deficiency (or egg white injury). The heating of egg white denatures avidin and destroys its ability to bind with biotin.

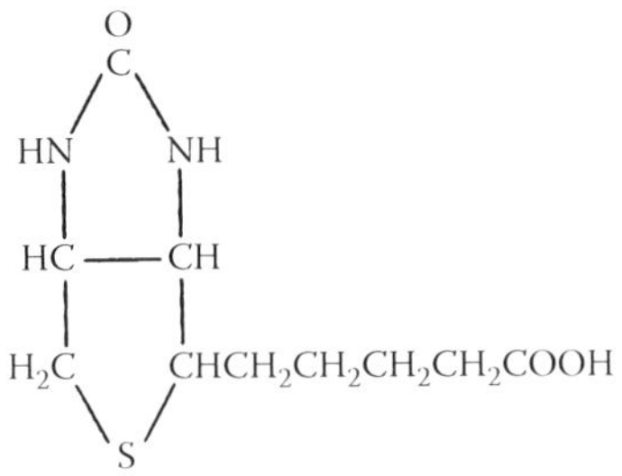

FIGURE 9.11   Biotin.

9.5.3   ABSORPTION AND TRANSPORT

Food contains biotin in its free form and bound to protein. The digestion of dietary proteins containing bound biotin yields considerable biocytin (biotinyl lysine). The enzyme biotinidase is present in pancreatic juice and in the intestinal mucosa; it cleaves biotin from biocytin. Only free biotin can be absorbed. The proximal part of the small intestine is the site of maximum absorption of biotin, and the transport occurs by a carrier-mediated process that is sodium-dependent, electroneutral, and capable of accumulating biotin against a concentration gradient. Free biotin is taken up by cells via active transport and is incorporated into biotin-dependent enzymes.

The ring system is not degraded by humans and animals to any appreciable extent. Mammals do convert a small fraction of the vitamin into sulfoxides. Partial degradation of the valeric acid side chain takes place by β-oxidation to form bisnorbiotin, which is two carbons shorter in length. These compounds and unchanged biotin are excreted in the urine.

9.5.4   FUNCTIONS

Biotin serves as a prosthetic group of five enzymes in human and animal tissues,[41] namely, pyruvate carboxylase (PC), acetyl CoA carboxylase 1 (ACC1), acetyl CoA carboxylase 2 (ACC2), propionyl CoA carboxylase (PCC), and β-methyl crotonyl CoA carboxylase[41] (MCCC; Table 9.1). Acetyl CoA carboxylase 1 (ACC1) is a cytosolic enzyme while the other four are mitochondrial enzymes. Biotin is covalently linked by an amide bond that involves the e-amino group of a lysyl residue of these carboxylases. The linkage is established by holoenzyme synthetase. Biotinidase catalyzes the cleavage of biotin from biocytin (biotinyl lysine) or biotinyl peptides.

Biotin-containing enzymes catalyze an ATP-dependent, carbon dioxide–fixation reaction utilizing bicarbonate as the carbon dioxide donor. The vitamin functions as a carbon dioxide carrier on the surface of the enzyme. The catalysis involves two steps: first, the binding of carbon dioxide to the ureido-1-nitrogen of biotin in combination with apoenzyme, and second, the transfer of the carbon dioxide moiety to an acceptor compound. These reactions occupy key roles in vitally important metabolic pathways such as the biosynthesis and utilization of glucose, fatty acids, and amino acids.

PC converts pyruvate to oxaloacetate, a critical reaction in gluconeogenesis. The formation of oxaloacetate also permits the continuous feeding of acetyl CoA into the citric acid cycle; when not needed for energy production, the citrate formed from oxaloacetate and acetyl CoA transfers two carbons of acetyl CoA to the cytosol for fatty acid synthesis (acetyl CoA cannot penetrate the mitochondrial membrane and is regenerated from citrate in the cytosol). ACC1 catalyzes the carboxylation of acetyl CoA, leading to the formation of malonyl CoA. This represents the first committed step in fatty acid synthesis. ACC2 catalyzes the formation of malonyl CoA in mitochondria. Malonyl CoA is an inhibitor of carnitine palmitoyl transferase J, the enzyme that regulates the transfer of long chain fatty acyl CoA into mitochondria. By virtue of this effect, it is thought to play a key role in regulating fatty acid oxidation.

TABLE 9.1
Biotin-Dependent Enzymes and Their Functions

Enzyme	Location	Function
Acetyl CoA carboxylase 1	Cytosol	Formation of malonyl CoA from acetyl CoA for fatty acid synthesis
Acetyl CoA carboxylase 2	Mitochondria	Formation of malonyl CoA from acetyl CoA for regulation of fatty acid oxidation
Pyruvate carboxylase	Mitochondria	Formation of oxaloacetate from pyruvate; role in citric acid cycle and gluconeogenesis
Propionyl CoA carboxylase	Mitochondria	Formation of methylmalonyl CoA from propionyl CoA (produced by catabolism of odd-chain fatty acids, valine, isoleucine)
Methyl crotonyl CoA carboxylase	Mitochondria	Role in leucine catabolism

PCC is the key enzyme that catalyzes the formation of methyl malonyl CoA from propionyl CoA. Methyl malonyl CoA then can enter the citric acid cycle via succinyl CoA and, through a series of reactions, form oxaloacetate. The latter can either form glucose (gluconeogenesis) or can oxidize to provide energy. Thus, propionyl CoA, which is produced as a result of the oxidation of odd carbon-numbered fatty acids (and metabolism of isoleucine and valine), can be used for energy derivation and glucose production. MCCC plays an essential role in the degradation of the branched-chain amino acid leucine. The conversion of methyl crotonyl CoA, an intermediate formed in leucine catabolism, to methyl glutaconyl CoA is catalyzed by MCCC. Methyl glutaconyl CoA is then degraded to acetyl CoA.

9.5.5 DEFICIENCY

The deficiency of biotin does not occur frequently in the human and animal species. The small amounts required are usually readily supplied in the diet and are further augmented in most species by microfloral synthesis. For this reason, it is only after the feeding of raw egg whites as a source of avidin that the deficiency symptoms appear. If rats are fed such a diet, they develop a characteristic group of symptoms, which include loss of appetite and growth rate, hair loss (alopecia), change in fatty acid composition, extensive dermatitis, hair loss in the region of the eye (which is sometimes called "spectacled eye"), and neural disorders.

Biotin deficiency has been produced in humans by a low-biotin diet containing large amounts of raw egg white for 10 weeks. This was done experimentally in four volunteers. Beginning with the third or fourth week, symptoms appeared in this order: scaly desquamation, lassitude, muscle pain, hyperesthesia, pallor of skin and mucous membranes, anemia, anorexia, and nausea. In addition, the blood cholesterol level increased significantly and urinary excretion of biotin decreased to about 10% of the normal level. All these abnormalities were cured within 5 days when 150 µg/day of biotin was given orally. Similar deficiency symptoms were also seen in one patient who had for years subsisted on a diet that included four to six dozen raw eggs a week.

Although no evidence exists of a natural biotin deficiency in human adults, two types of dermatitis that occur in young infants, Leiner's disease and seborrheic dermatitis, appear to be due to a lack of the vitamin. The deficiency can result because of a low content of biotin in milk or possibly defective digestion or persistent diarrhea. Dermatitis resolves completely after biotin therapy.

Significantly lower blood levels and urinary excretion of the vitamin are found in pregnant women, some alcoholics, and among the elderly.

Biotin deficiency has also been reported or inferred in sudden infant death syndrome (SIDS). Autopsy studies suggest that hepatic biotin was significantly lower in SIDS infants than in infants dying from other causes. Additional studies are needed to confirm or refute this hypothesis.

Biotin deficiency has been reported in some patients on total parenteral nutrition without biotin supplementation for a long time. The symptoms in these patients included an erythematous rash that is exfoliative in nature, alopecia, waxy pallor, irritability, lethargy, depression, hallucination, numbness and tingling of extremities, mild hypotonia (low muscle tone), and organic acidosis. The excretion of propionic acid in urine was increased. These patients responded to the administration of 10 mg/day biotin; after 1 week, the organic aciduria was eliminated and the rash improved.

Biotin deficiency is a potent teratogenic event in some animal species, and the resulting malformations are similar to certain human birth defects. Recent studies have shown that marginal asymptomatic biotin deficiency is a common occurrence in normal human pregnancy. However, a link between biotin deficiency and deleterious effects on the fetus and mother has not been established.

Children with phenylketonuria often develop skin conditions such as eczema and seborrheic dermatitis in areas of the body other than the scalp. The changes may be related to poor ability to use biotin. Increasing dietary biotin is known to improve seborrheic dermatitis in these cases.

Individuals on long-term anticonvulsants may have reduced blood levels of biotin as well as increased urinary excretion of organic acids indicating decreased activities of carboxylases. Some anticonvulsants inhibit intestinal absorption of biotin. People on long-term sulfa drugs or other antibiotics may have decreased intestinal bacterial synthesis of biotin, theoretically increasing the requirement for dietary biotin.

There is increased interest in biotin metabolism as a result of the discovery of infants and children with inherited defects in the utilization of biotin and by the fact that some of them can be treated successfully with pharmacological doses of the vitamin. Inborn errors of biotin metabolism include abnormal holocarboxylase synthetase, defects in individual carboxylases, and biotinidase deficiency. Common clinical features associated with these disorders are hypotonia, skin rash (dermatitis), developmental delay or regression, and alopecia. Some of the biochemical abnormalities include lactic acidemia, metabolic acidosis, and hyperammonemia.

Abnormal holocarboxylase synthetase is characterized by an abnormally high K_m value for biotin and leads to deficiencies in the mitochondrial PC, PCC, and MCCC; this is known as multiple carboxylase deficiency. The disease manifests itself in the first week of life and is characterized as a neonatal form. In this disorder, patients respond dramatically to biotin administration. At a dose of 10 mg/day of biotin (200 times normal intake), plasma biotin concentration rises above the K_m value, which allows the effective conversion of the mitochondrial apocarboxylases to the holoenzymes. The clinical symptoms and biochemical abnormalities disappear.

Defects in the individual mitochondrial biotin-containing carboxylases are due to abnormal apoenzyme structures, and the patients generally do not respond to biotin therapy. A deficiency of PCC causes propionic aciduria. Patients with this disorder typically have episodes of vomiting, severe ketosis, and acidosis.

Isolated deficiency of MCCC[44,47] has been reported in three patients. Two of them were asymptomatic on a low-protein diet, but increasing the dietary protein in one patient caused vomiting, aciduria, and excretion of the metabolites of methyl crotonyl CoA. They did not respond to biotin therapy, but were clinically well after treatment with a diet low in protein.

Isolated PC deficiency causes an elevation of pyruvate and lactate in blood. These patients usually have severe neurological problems and early death. They do not respond to biotin therapy.

Biotinidase is the enzyme necessary for the normal recycling of biotin that has been incorporated into the carboxylases. In patients with a deficiency of this enzyme, the recycling of biotin is blocked and, therefore, additional biotin must be ingested to prevent deficiency. Patients with this type of disorder also show multiple carboxylase deficiency, but the symptoms appear at 2 or 3 months of age, and this deficiency is characterized as the juvenile form. Patients deficient in biotinidase usually respond to 10 mg of biotin/day with the reversion to normal of all the biochemical and clinical features of the disease.

Patients with biotin-responsive multiple carboxylase deficiency due to abnormal holocarboxylase synthetase and those with biotinidase deficiency can be identified as follows. In the case of multiple carboxylase deficiency, fibroblasts cultivated in a medium containing biotin only in amounts provided by fetal calf serum show low activities of carboxylases. The activities increase when the medium is supplemented with high concentrations of biotin. In the case of biotinidase deficiency, the fibroblasts from patients with this disease show normal activities of carboxylases in both types of media.

9.5.6 ASSESSMENT OF BIOTIN STATUS

In order to assess biotin nutrition in humans, the plasma level of vitamin and urinary excretion is measured. Biotin levels in plasma of over 250 mg/L, and urine biotin levels of 20 μg/l or 25 μg/24 hours seem to indicate an adequate supply of biotin in humans. The deficiency of the vitamin can be established by demonstrating a decreased urinary excretion of biotin, an increase in characteristic organic acids, and an alleviation of symptoms in response to biotin supplementation.

Methyl crotonyl CoA, an intermediate of leucine metabolism, is converted to glutaconyl CoA catalyzed by MCCC. In biotin deficiency, methyl crotonyl CoA is shunted to an alternate metabolic pathway, producing 3-hydroxyisovaleric acid (3-HIA), which is then excreted in increased amounts in the urine. Thus, an increased urinary excretion of 3-HIA is an early and sensitive indicator of reduced biotin status.[45]

9.5.7 REQUIREMENTS

The dietary requirement for biotin in man is not known with certainty. This is partly due to the uncertainty of the amount of vitamin in food. It is also synthesized by the normal human intestinal flora in amounts that make a significant but precisely undetermined contribution to the body pool of the vitamin. Based on studies of usual intakes and urinary excretion of the nutrient, the Food and Nutrition Board has recommended a safe and adequate daily dietary intake range of biotin for normal individuals of various age groups. The values may be summarized as follows: infants up to 1 year of age, 25–35 μg/day; children and adolescents, 40–50 μg/day; older children and adults, 50–100 μg/day. The average American diet supplies an estimated 100–200 μg of the vitamin per day. This amount plus that uncertain quantity synthesized by the intestinal flora is more than adequate to supply the recommended allowance under normal conditions.

9.5.8 EFFECT OF PHARMACOLOGICAL DOSES

Biotin in amounts of 500 μg daily administered either orally or intramuscularly has been used successfully to treat seborrheic dermatitis and Leiner's disease. In amounts of 1 mg/day orally for 8–12 weeks or 1.5 mg daily for 6–8 weeks, biotin is beneficial in the treatment of seborrheic eczema and acne. The use of a topical cream once daily and a shampoo three times weekly containing 0.25%–1% biotin is effective in reducing and controlling hair loss in male pattern alopecia. Injected doses of 150–300 μg have been administered for acute biotin deficiency and higher amounts (e.g., 4–10 mg/day) are given to patients with inborn errors of biotin metabolism.

Biotin is generally accepted to be well tolerated by humans without any side effects, even at high doses.

Thiamin-Responsive Disorder—A Case

A 3-week-old baby girl, the second child of healthy parents, became breathless and had difficulty feeding. Two weeks later, she had heart failure and was admitted to a hospital. Echocardiography showed normal cardiac anatomy but a greatly enlarged left ventricle, severely impaired left ventricular function, and mild mitral insufficiency. Plasma amino acids, pyruvate, and lactate and urinary organic acids were normal. Treatment with diuretics was started. Over the next few days, severe hypotonia appeared and the infant was unable to suck. Cardiac biopsy done at 2 months of age showed myofibrillar degeneration and fibrosis. Histochemical and ultrastructural studies did not reveal any specific disease. Cardiomyopathy was classified as the one of unknown origin. Total parenteral nutrition was started. At 4 months of age, the patient developed glucose intolerance and lactic acidosis. Cardiac transplantation was recommended but the baby's parents did not consent. At the age of 6 months, the baby was considered terminally ill.

The medical team treating this baby came across a case of cardiomyopathy, reported about 8 years earlier, that responded to pharmacological doses of thiamin. Because of the poor clinical condition of this patient and the possibility that this case may also be a thiamin-responsive disorder, treatment with thiamin (50 mg/day, i.m.) was started. Within 2 days, the baby regained control of her head and could suck. Her cardiac function started improving slowly. Diuretic treatment was stopped when she was 9 months old. However, her erythrocyte thiamin content and TPP kinase were low. She was started on a lipophilic form of thiamin, benfotiamin, 600 mg/day by mouth. At the age of 20 months, her body weight, height, and psychomotor development were normal, and she had no signs of heart failure.

It is not known why plasma lactate was not elevated when the baby was 5 weeks old and had cardiac failure. Perhaps she had marginal deficiency. Diuretics could have accelerated the deficiency to the point that there was glucose intolerance and lactic acidemia. Another case of a patient with neonatal thiamin-dependent cardiomyopathy was described in 1991. Studies on fresh muscle homogenates showed a deficiency of pyruvate oxidation. Freezing and thawing of the homogenate and the addition of TPP brought the rate of pyruvate oxidation to normal. Based on these studies, it was suggested that the abnormality was due to a defect in the cellular uptake of thiamin. It is possible that the case described above involves a similar defect. Formation of the coenzyme may also be defective.

Benfotiamin[5,7] is absorbed from the small intestine by passive diffusion, in contrast to thiamin, which is absorbed by active process. At high doses, a small fraction is passively absorbed. Benfotiamin is similar to thiamin except that its thiazole ring is open. During absorption, the ring is closed, and the resulting thiamin is converted to the coenzyme form. The high dose of benfotiamin is expected to substantially increase the plasma level of thiamin. And even if a small fraction of plasma thiamin is passively transported into the cell, it should be adequate. It would be helpful to determine the plasma and erythrocyte levels of thiamin and erythrocyte TPP kinase activity in the patient receiving such a high dose of benfotiamin.

This case illustrates that a simple nutritional treatment was able to save a baby who was terminally ill. Transplantation would not have helped her.[50,51] Dilated cardiomyopathy, although not common in children, accounts for several deaths and is the most common reason for cardiac transplantation in children. The measurement of plasma thiamin levels and the treatment with parenteral thiamin in neonatal patients with cardiomyopathy should be considered. This may prevent unnecessary transplantations as this case has clearly demonstrated.

REFERENCES

THIAMIN—B$_1$

1. Brown, M. L. 1990. Thiamin. In Present Knowledge in Nutrition, ed. M. L. Brown, 142–145. Washington, DC: Nutrition Foundation.
2. Combs, G. F., Jr. 2008. *The Vitamins: Fundamental Aspects in Nutrition and Health*. 3rd ed. Ithaca, NY: Elsevier Academic.
3. Glaso, M., G. Nordbo, L. Diep, and T. Bohmer. 2004. Reduced concentrations of several vitamins in normal weight patients with late-onset dementia of the Alzheimer type without vascular disease. *J Nutr Health Aging* 8:407.
4. Gubler, C. J. 1991. Thiamin. In Handbook of Vitamins, 2nd ed., ed. L. J. Machlin, 233–281. New York: Marcel Dekker.
5. Hammes, H., X. Du, D. Edelstein et al. 2003. Benfotiamine blocks three major pathways of hyperglycemia damage and prevents experimental diabetic retinopathy. *Nat Med* 9:294.
6. Krishna, S., A. M. Taylor, W. Supanaranond, S. Pukrittayakamee, F. ter Kuile, K. M. Tawfiq, P. A. H. Holloway, and N. J. White. 1999. Thiamin deficiency and Malaria in adults from Southeast Asia. *Lancet* 353:546.
7. Loew, D. 1996. Pharmacokinetics of thiamin derivatives especially of benfotiamin. *Int J Clin Pharmacol Ther* 34:47.
8. Rieck, J., H. Halkin, S. Almog, H. Seligman, A. Lubetsky, D. Olchovsky, and D. Ezra. 1999. Urinary loss of thiamin is increased by low doses of furosemide in healthy volunteers. *J Lab Clin Med* 134:238.
9. Rindi, G., C. Patrini, U. Laforenza, H. Mandel, M. Berant, M. B. Viana, V. Poggi, and A. N. F. Zarra. 1994. Further studies on erythrocyte thiamin transport and phosphorylation in seven patients with thiamin-responsive megaloblastic anemia. *J Inherit Metab Dis* 17:667.
10. Thomalley, P. J. 2005. The potential role of thiamin (vitamin B$_1$) in diabetic complications. *Curr Diabetes Rev* 1:287.

RIBOFLAVIN—B$_2$

11. Boehnke, C., U. Reuter, U. Flach et al. 2004. High-dose riboflavin treatment is efficacious in migraine prophylaxis: an open study in a tertiary care center. *Eur J Neurol* 11:475.
12. Cooperman, J. M., and R. Lopez. 1991. Riboflavin. In *Handbook of Vitamins*, 2nd ed., ed. L. J. Machlin, 283–310. New York: Marcel Dekker.
13. Jacques, P. F., A. Taylor, S. Moeller et al. 2005. Long-term nutrient intake and 5-year change in nuclear lens opacities. *Arch Opthalmol* 123:517.
14. Lee, S. S., and D. B. McCormick. 1985. Thyroid hormone regulation of flavocoenzyme biosynthesis. *Arch Biochem Biophys* 237:197.
15. McCormick, D. B. 1994. Riboflavin. In *Modern Nutrition in Health and Disease*, ed. M. E. Shils, J. A. Olson, and M. Shike, 366–375. Malvern, PA: Lea and Febiger.
16. Neugebauer, J., Y. Zahre, and J. Wacker. 2006. Riboflavin supplementation and preeclampcia. *Int J Gynecol Obstet* 93:136.
17. Powers, H. 2003. Riboflavin (vitamin B$_2$) and health. Review article. *Amer J Clin Nutr* 77:1352.
18. Rivlin, R. S., and P. Dutta. 1995. Vitamin B$_6$ (Riboflavin). Relevance to malaria and antioxidant activity. *Nutr Today* 30(2):62.
19. Sandor, P. S., J. Afra, A. Ambrosini, and J. Schoenen. 2000. Prophylactic treatment of migraine with β blockers and riboflavin: differential effects on the intensity dependence of auditory evoked cortical potentials. *Headache* 40:30.

NIACIN

20. Benjo, A. M., R. C. Maranhao, S. R. Coimbra et al. 2006. Accumulation of chylomicron remnants and impaired vascular reactivity occur in subjects with isolated low HDL cholesterol: Effects of niacin treatment. *Atheroscler* 187:116.
21. Cook, N. E., and K. J. Carpenter. 1987. Leucine excess and niacin status in rats. *J Nutr* 117:519.
22. Friedrich, W. 1988. *Vitamins*. New York: W. de Gruyter.
23. Halverson, K., and S. Halverson. 1963. Hartnup disease. *Pediatr* 31:29.
24. Henderson, L. M. 1983. Niacin. *Annu Rev Nutr* 3:289.

25. Horwitt, M. K., A. E. Harper, and L. M. Henderson. 1981. Niacin–tryptophan relationships for evaluating niacin equivalents. *Am J Clin Nutr* 34:423.
26. Kamanna, V. S., and M. L. Kashyap. 2008. Mechanism of action of niacin. *Am J Cardiol* 101:20B.
27. Mrocheck, J. E., R. L. Jolley, D. S. Young, and W. J. Turner. 1976. Metabolic response of humans to ingestion of nicotinic acid and nicotinamide. *Clin Chem* 22:1821.
28. Richman, J. G., M. Kanemitsu-Parks, I. Gaidarov et al. 2007. Nicotinic acid receptor agonists differentially activate downstream effectors. *J Biol Chem* 282:18028.
29. Satyanarayana, V., and B. S. Narasinga Rao. 1980. Dietary tryptophan level and the enzymes of tryptophan–NAD pathway. *Br J Nut* 43:107.
30. Sebrell, W. H., Jr. 1981. History of pellagra. Fed Proc 40:1520.
31. Walters, R. W., A. K. Shukla, J. J. Kovacs et al. 2009. β-Arrestin 1 mediates nicotinic acid-induced flushing, but not its antilipolytic effect in mice. J Clin Invest 119:1312.
32. Weiner, M., ed. 1983. Nicotinic Acid: Nutrient–Cofactor Drug. New York: Marcel Dekker.
33. Zhang, Y., R. J. Schmidt, P. Foxworthy et al. 2005. Niacin mediates lipolysis in adipose tissue through its G-protein coupled receptor HM74A. *Biochem Biophys Res Commun* 334:729.

Pantothenic Acid

34. Abdelatif, M., M. Yakoot, and M. Elemaan. 2008. Safety and efficacy of a new honey ointment on diabetic foot ulcers: A prospective pilot study. *J Wound Care* 17:3.
35. Combs, G. F. 2008. *The Vitamins: Fundamental Aspects in Nutrition and Health.* 3rd ed. Boston: Elsevier.
36. Eissenstat, B. R., B. W. Wyse, and R. G. Hansen. 1984. Effect of pantothenic acid status on the content of the vitamin in human milk. *Am J Clin Nutr* 40:317.
37. Naruta, E., and V. Buko. 2001. Hyperlipidemic effect of pantothenic acid derivatives in mice with hypothalamic obesity induced by aurothioglucose. *Exp Toxicol Pathol* 53:313.
38. Plesofsky-Vig, N., and R. Brambl. 1986. Pantothenic acid and coenzyme A in cellular modification of proteins. *Annu Rev Nutr* 6:41.
39. Song, W. O. 1990. Pantothenic acid: how much do we know about this B-complex vitamin? *Nutr Today* 25(2):19.

Biotin

40. Corbett, J. W., and J. H. Harwood. 2007. Inhibitors of mammalian acetyl-CoA carboxylase. *Recent Pat Cardiovasc Drug Discov* 2:162.
41. Dakshinamurty, K., and J. Chauhan. 1988. Regulation of biotin enzymes. *Annu Rev Nutr* 8:211.
42. Hommes, F. A. 1986. Biotin. *World Rev Nutr Diet* 48:35.
43. Mock, D. M., N. I. Mock, and S. Weintraub. 1988. Abnormal organic aciduria in biotin deficiency: rat is similar to man. *J Clin Lab Med* 12:240.
44. Mock, D. M., J. G. Quirk, and N. I. Mock. 2002. Marginal biotin deficiency during normal pregnancy. *Am J Clin Nutr* 75:295.
45. Mock, N. I., M. I. Malik, P. J. Stumbo, W. P. Bishop, and D. M. Mock. 1997. Increased urinary excretion of 3-hydroxyisovaleric acid and decreased urinary excretion of biotin are sensitive early indicators of decreased biotin status in experimental biotin deficiency. *Am J Clin Nutr* 65:951.
46. Said, H. M. 2002. Biotin: The forgotten vitamin. *Am J Clin Nutr* 75:179.
47. Sweetman, L., and W. L. Nyhan. 1986. Inheritable biotin-treatable disorders and associated phenomena. *Annu Rev Nutr* 6:317.
48. Tong, L. 2005. Acetyl-Coenzyme A carboxylase: crucial metabolic-enzyme and attractive target for drug discovery. *Cell Mol Life Sci* 62:1784.
49. Wolf, B., R. E. Grier, J. R. Secor McVoy, and G. S. Heard. 1985. Biotinidase deficiency, a novel vitamin recycling defect. *J Inherit Metab Dis* 8(Suppl. 1):53.

CASE BIBLIOGRAPHY

50. Baker, H. D., H. R. Scholte, J. E. M. Luyt-Houwen, A. H. Van Gennip, N. G. Abeling, and J. Lam. 1991. Neonatal cardiomyopathy and lactic acidosis responsive to thiamin. *J Inherit Metab Dis* 14:75.
51. Rocco, M. D., C. Patrini, A. Rimini, and G. Rindi. 1997. A 6-month old girl with cardiomyopathy who nearly died. *Lancet* 349:616.

10 Water-Soluble Vitamins II

10.1 FOLIC ACID

The discovery of folic acid began in 1930 with the work of Lucy Wills in Bombay, India, on pernicious anemia of pregnancy. Her patients were pregnant women who had been living for a long period on poor diets that consisted of polished rice and white bread and lacked foods of animal origin and vegetables. Wills produced anemia in monkeys by feeding them a diet similar to that eaten by her patients. She then tried all of the vitamins known at that time for the possible favorable effect, but she was unable to cure the disease; however, good responses were obtained by feeding them a commercial preparation of autolyzed yeast called marmot or crude liver extract. Thus, she had discovered a previously unrecognized factor (Wills' factor), which was subsequently called vitamin M (for monkeys). A number of other investigators were also working on the seemingly unrelated problems of purification of a growth factor for certain strains of bacteria and an antianemic factor for chicks. The antianemic factor of the chick was obtained in 1940 by extraction of liver autolysates with 95% alcohol. It was called vitamin B_c. The same year, a factor was identified in yeast and liver, which was essential for the growth of *Lactobacillus casei*. These studies turned out to be decisive for the isolation of the antianemic factor. In 1941, Snell and his group reported the isolation of an acid that supported the growth of *L. casei*. This factor was named folic acid because of its abundance in green leaves (from the Latin *folium*, meaning leaf). These scientists recognized that folic acid or one with similar chemical and physiological properties also occurred in a number of animal tissues of which liver and kidney are the best sources.

Interest in the constituents of yeast that cured the anemia of pregnancy stimulated the scientists at Parke, Davis, and Company to isolate and characterize the active principle. These investigators used both the *L. casei* growth-stimulation activity and the chick antianemic activity to monitor their purification attempts. The active principle in liver and yeast extracts that cured pernicious anemia of pregnancy described by Wills had many properties in common with bacterial growth factors present in liver and spinach leaves and with a dietary factor required to prevent the development of anemia in chicks and monkeys. The purification of folic acid from natural sources was accomplished in the 1940s, and its structure was determined by degradation in 1948. The same year, it was synthesized and established as a dietary essential for humans, many animals, and microorganisms.

10.1.1 FOOD SOURCES

Folic acid is present in almost all natural foods, but the highest concentrations are found in yeast, liver, fresh green leafy vegetables, asparagus, and lettuce. Fair sources include beef, veal, and wheat whereas root vegetables, tomatoes, bananas, rice, corn, and sweet potatoes contain little folic acid.

10.1.2 CHEMISTRY

Folic acid (also called folacin) consists of three main parts: a two-ring nitrogenous compound called pteridine, a yellow pigment first isolated from butterflies' wings; *p*-amino-benzoic acid; and glutamic acid. Pteridine is linked through a methylene bridge to a molecule of *p*-aminobenzoic acid to form pteroic acid. This combines with a molecule of glutamic acid to form pteryl glutamic acid or folic acid (Figure 10.1). Folic acid is a yellow crystalline substance that is slightly soluble in water and stable in acid solution. When heated in neutral or alkaline solution, however, it undergoes

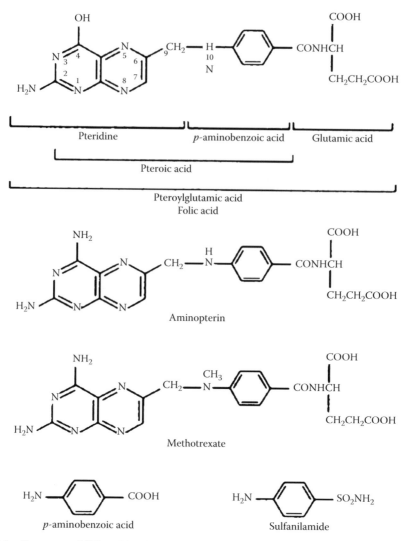

FIGURE 10.1 Structures of folic acid and related compounds.

rapid destruction, so it may be destroyed by some methods of cooking. We now know that the vitamin occurs in food mostly as pteryl polyglutamates (i.e., compounds containing more than one glutamic acid residue). The term folate is used for the broader group of substances that give rise to folic acid in the body.

10.1.3 ABSORPTION

Most of the folic acid in foods is present as a polyglutamate that contains three to seven gluta-mate residues. Polyglutamates cannot be absorbed as such; however, human mucosal cells of the duodenum and jejunum contain an enzyme called conjugase that splits off the extra glutamate residues. In vivo hydrolysis probably occurs at the intestinal cell surface. The vitamin is absorbed predominantly in the jejunum by an active process that is stimulated by glucose and exhibits satu-ration kinetics. After folic acid enters the circulation from the gut, it is reduced and methylated to methyl tetrahydrofolate (THF), which is the major form of the vitamin in circulation. Methyl THF is taken up by cells and is metabolized intracellularly to the polyglutamate form, which is retained by cells. The normal serum folate level is maintained by dietary intake and by an efficient enterohepatic circulation. After cellular uptake, methyl THF must first be converted to THF via methionine synthase catalyzed reaction. Only then can the THF be polyglutamated by folate polyglutamate synthase, which allows it to play a central role in 1-carbon metabolism. Also, only polyglutamate form can be retained by cells. Normal body stores in humans have been estimated at 5–10 mg of which half is in the liver. Folic acid is excreted in the urine and in the bile.

10.1.4 Functions

Folic acid as such is not active biologically. It must go through two reduction steps, first to dihydrofolic acid (FH_2) and then to 5,6,7,8 tetrahydrofolic acid (FH_4 or THF), which is the active coenzyme form; the enzyme dihydrofolate reductase (in the presence of NADPH) catalyzes both reduction steps. FH_4 carries 1-carbon units on the N-5 and N-10 nitrogen atoms of the pteridine ring in the form of formyl, methyl, methenyl, and methylene groups for the biosynthesis of a variety of biomolecules.

The biochemical role of folate coenzymes in mammalian tissues is to serve as an acceptor and a donor of 1-carbon units in a variety of reactions that are involved in purine and thymidine biosynthesis and in the interconversions of histidine–glutamate, serine–glycine, and homocysteine[5]–methionine.[1] The coenzyme is essential in the insertion of methyl groups in deoxyuridylic acid to form thymidylic acid, which is catalyzed by thymidylate synthetase. Thus, folate is essential for DNA synthesis, repair, and methylation.

Methylene THF is formed from THF by the addition of methylene group from one of three carbon donors: formaldehyde, serine, or glycine.[14] In addition to its use as a coenzyme for thymidylate synthase, methylene THF has a central role in the cycle of 1-carbon utilization. It involves the reduction of methylene THF to methyl THF followed by the transfer of methyl group to homocysteine and the regeneration of THF as given below

1. THF → Methylene THF
2. Methylene THF → Methyl THF
3. Methyl THF + homocysteine → THF + methionine

Reaction 2 is catalyzed by methylene THF reductase (MTHFR). It contains a bound flavin cofactor and uses NADPH as the reducing agent. Reaction 3 is catalyzed by methionine synthase, which is a vitamin B_{12}–dependent enzyme. Inactivation of methionine synthase during vitamin B_{12} deficiency results in accumulation of methyl THF, which cannot be polyglutamylated and thus leaks out of the cell, thereby resulting in an intracellular THF deficiency and reduction in 1-carbon metabolism. Deficiency of MTHFR can limit the availability of methyl THF for reaction 3 and can also result in intracellular THF deficiency. Vitamin B_{12} deficiency responds to replacement with folic acid, which can be converted to THF via dihydrofolate reductase, or to replacement with 5-formyl THF (folinic acid), which bypasses methionine synthase and can be converted to methylene THF or to 10 formyl THF via intermediates.

10.1.5 Deficiency

Folic acid deficiency may be the most common hypovitaminosis of humans, affecting the indigent of the world. Since the vitamin is present in almost all foods, the occurrence of a deficiency state because of inadequate intake is rare in western countries; however, the deficiency secondary to malabsorption frequently occurs in patients with disease involving the upper small intestine (e.g., celiac disease or tropical sprue, a disease characterized by intestinal lesions) or following proximal bowel resection. Other factors that can lead to folate deficiency include the increased demands during pregnancy, infancy, and adolescence that are associated with growth and related needs for DNA, alcoholism, and so on. Oral contraceptives may lower serum or erythrocyte folate levels, perhaps because of decreased absorption of the vitamin because of impairment in the action of the conjugase on polyglutamate, or perhaps because of increased excretion or transfer to the tissues from plasma.

Folic acid is necessary for the production and maintenance of new cells. It is especially important during periods of rapid cell division and growth such as infancy and pregnancy. Folic acid is needed to synthesize components of nucleic acids (most notably thymine, but also purine bases). Thus, folate deficiency slows DNA synthesis and cell division, affecting hematopoietic cells the most because of rapid cell division. Erythropoiesis is slowed and leads to megaloblastic anemia, which is characterized by large immature red blood cells.

In humans, the deficiency of folate is characterized by macrocytic anemia,* glossitis, and gastrointestinal disturbances involving impaired digestion and absorption. Experimental human folate deficiency was produced by Herbert who observed the following signs of vitamin deficiency: in 3 weeks on a low-vitamin diet, serum folate falls below 3 ng/mL; in 7–10 weeks, white cell hyperpigmentation is evident; in 12–16 weeks, the urinary excretion of formiminoglutamic acid (FGA) is increased (this demonstrates a block in the conversion of histidine to glutamic acid); and in 18–20 weeks, megaloblastic anemia appears. Administration of folic acid brings about dramatic reversal of these changes. The interrelationship of folic acid and vitamin B_{12} as it pertains to megaloblastic anemia is discussed in Section 10.2.4.

Folate deficiency is associated with forgetfulness, irritability, and often hostile and paranoid behavior. This may be related to the high level of plasma homocysteine, which is seen in folate and/ or vitamin B_{12} deficiency. Several studies have shown that plasma homocysteine levels correlate with cognitive decline and depression in the general population. Low blood folate concentrations are associated with significantly greater risk for relapse in persons with antidepressant therapy, and folate status predicts response to antidepressant treatment in the elderly. Also, adding folic acid to an antidepressant regimen further reduces depressive symptoms.

A recent epidemiologic study suggests that folate could help prevent Alzheimer's disease.[5,11] The researchers found that people who reported getting at or above 400 µg of folate per day had a 50% lower risk than people who were consuming less than that amount. The findings, if confirmed by other studies, could lead to a relatively simple way to avoid Alzheimer's disease that afflicts 4.5 million Americans.

Epidemiological studies have suggested that folate deficiency is associated with increased risk for certain types of cancer. Several studies indicate that dietary folate intake is inversely associated with the risk of developing colorectal neoplasms[4] in a dose-dependent fashion. Approximately 40% reduction in the risk of colorectal neoplasms is observed in individuals taking the highest amount of folate compared with those taking the lowest amount of the vitamin. Two recently published large, prospective epidemiological studies suggest that maintaining adequate levels of serum folate or moderately increasing folate intake from dietary sources and vitamin supplements can significantly reduce the risk of pancreatic cancer[15] in male smokers and breast cancer in women[6] regularly consuming moderate amounts of alcohol. Interactions appear to exist between folate status, mutations in MTHFR, plasma homocysteine, and cervical cancer. Supplementation with folate may reduce cancer risk.

The mechanism by which folate provides protection against cancer is not clearly understood. Epidemiologic studies on whether folate intake affects breast cancer risk have reported mixed results. Most studies suggest that diets high in folate are associated with decreased risk of breast cancer. One broad cancer screening trial has reported a potential harmful effect of folate intake on breast cancer risk, suggesting that routine folate supplementation should not be recommended as a breast cancer preventive measure. A more recent study has shown no significant effect of folic acid on overall risk of breast cancer among women. It has been suggested that folate may help prevent cancer as it is involved in the synthesis and functions of DNA, and a deficiency of folate may result in damage to DNA that may lead to cancer.

---

* Anemias definitions are given in Section 10.5.

Evidence from animal studies suggests that folate deficiency is associated with DNA damage, abnormal DNA methylation, and impaired DNA repair. Folate-deficient humans have markedly elevated levels of uracil in DNA and chromosome breaks. Such breaks could contribute to the increased risk of cancer associated with folate deficiency. Folate status can be a key determinant of DNA strand breaks, leading to genetic instability and thus to increased cancer risk. Folate appears to be an ideal candidate for chemoprevention.

Folate deficiency during pregnancy is a risk factor for delivering infants with neural tube defects[3,8] (NTDs). The defects occur between the 21st and 27th day after conception. An abnormality in folate metabolism can be caused by mutation in the gene that expresses MTHFR. Two common alleles, the C677T (thermolabile) allele and the A1298 allele, have been described. Women who are homozygous for C677T are predisposed to mild hyperhomocysteinemia because they have less active MTHFR available to produce methyl THF (which is required to decrease homocysteine).[7] Women who are homozygous for this defect are thought to be at higher risk for pregnancies affected by NTDs. About 5%–25% of individuals may have inherited 2 copies of the defective gene. When folate intake is low, the individuals with the defective gene have lower levels of MTHFR enzyme and high levels of homocysteime in their blood. Improved folate nutritional status appears to stabilize the enzyme, resulting in improved enzyme levels and lower homocysteine levels in their blood.

Several studies have shown that preconceptional supplementation with folic acid reduces the incidence of these defects by about 70%. In 1996, the U.S. Food and Drug Administration issued a regulation, to be effective by January 1998, requiring that all enriched flour, rice, pasta, cornmeal, and other grain products contain 140 mg of folic acid per 100 g in addition to the B_1, B_2, niacin, and iron already present in such products. The goal of this fortification was to increase the intake of folate by women of childbearing age in response to a recommendation by Public Health Service that at least 0.4 mg of folic acid should be consumed daily to prevent NTDs.[9] Many pregnancies are unplanned, and adequate folate must be present early in pregnancy when the fetal nervous system is developing—a time before most women are aware they are pregnant. Folic acid supplementation has had substantial effect on plasma folate and homocysteine levels in a population sample of middle aged and older adults.

The Centers for Disease Control and Prevention (CDC) reported in 2004 that severe brain and spinal birth defects dropped 27% in the United States since the folic acid fortification mandate. Before fortification, about 4130 babies had such neural defects each year in the United States, and nearly 1200 died. After fortification, the yearly average dropped to about 3000, with 840 deaths. According to the CDC, only 30%–35% of women of childbearing age get at least 400 µg of folic acid daily, whether through enriched foods or supplements. It is estimated that we could avert another 1000 NTDs if all women in this age group consumed at least 400 µg of folic acid daily. Studies in Canada, where food fortification is nearly identical to that of the United States, have reported a decrease of about 50% in the incidence of NTDs.

Folic acid is now viewed not only as a nutrient needed to prevent megaloblastic anemia in pregnancy but also as a vitamin essential for reproductive health. Low plasma levels of folic acid during pregnancy may also lead to preeclampsia. It affects 3%–5% of pregnant women and is a common cause of premature births. It typically occurs very late in pregnancy. Besides inducing high blood pressure, it can cause kidney failure, swelling of hands, seizures, and death. In the United States, only a few hundred women die from pregnancy-related causes each year, but preeclampsia kills thousands in developing countries. Black women have higher incidents of preeclampsia, and when they experience this disorder, they are more likely to have a more severe form that shows up as early as 6 months into pregnancy.

In a recent study, researchers examined 85 white women and 78 black women. Thirty-four white women and twenty-six black women had preeclampsia. Blood samples were taken from each woman near delivery time and were used to measure the levels of folic acid and homocysteine. Homocysteine was higher in all the women with preeclampsia. But black women with the condition had the highest levels. Folic acid levels were lower in women with preeclampsia, and black women had lower levels of this vitamin compared to white women.[12] These findings strongly suggest that black women might need to take more folic acid.

10.1.6 ANTAGONISTS

Several compounds have been synthesized to serve as inhibitors of folic acid metabolism. These are important in cancer chemotherapy and in fighting bacterial and protozoan infections. Among the most important antagonists of folic acid are aminopterin (Figure 10.1), amethopterin (methotrexate), trimethoprim, and pyrimethamine. These are structural analogs of folic acid and compete with dihydrofolate reductase. Methotrexate binds with the enzyme 1000 times better than folic acid and is a powerful competitive inhibitor of the enzyme and thus prevents the formation of THF. This, in turn, inhibits purine nucleotide synthesis and the formation of thymidylate. Since cell division is dependent on thymidine as well as other nucleotides, fast-growing cancer cells (e.g., leukemic cells) cannot multiply. One problem is that rapidly dividing cells of bone marrow are also sensitive to this drug for the same reason. Methotrexate has been used successfully for many years in cancer chemotherapy.

Dihydrofolate reductase from different organisms differs in structure, and thus it is possible to choose drugs that can selectively inhibit bacterial and protozoal enzymes while not affecting the mammalian enzyme; therapeutic concentrations of the drug in the body are not hazardous to the cells of mammalian host. Trimethoprim, in conjunction with sulfonamide, is used extensively in treating some forms of bacterial infections in man. Sulfonamides, although not folate analogs, are analogs of an intermediate in folate biosynthesis, p-aminobenzoic acid. Sulfanilamide is the simplest member of the class of sulfa drugs (Figure 10.1).

Bacteria cannot absorb folic acid from a host but must synthesize it. The enzyme that incorporates p-aminobenzoic acid into a folic acid moiety can be tricked into making a compound that has sulfanilamide in place of p-aminobenzoic acid. This is not folic acid and thus cannot form the coenzyme THF. The bacteria are starved of the required coenzyme and thus cannot grow and divide. Since man requires dietary folate, the sulfanilamide is not harmful at the dose that will kill bacteria.

10.1.7 ASSESSMENT OF FOLIC ACID STATUS

The most useful procedure is the direct determination of folic acid levels in serum and red blood cells. This provides a sensitive indicator of vitamin status long before clinical symptoms of deficiency appear. Normal values in blood serum are 6–20 ng/mL, but drops to less than 3 ng/mL in just 1 week on a low-folate diet. It takes about 15–20 weeks of deficient diet for the level of folate to decrease in red blood cells.

An abnormal amount of FGA, an intermediate in the conversion of histidine to glutamic acid, accumulates in blood and is excreted in the urine in folate deficiency. The normal excretion of FGA is 0–6 µg/mL of urine or less than 4 mg/24 hr. In order to determine the folate nutrition, the patient is given three doses of histidine (5 g each) during a 24-hour period. Normal FGA in urine is less than 25 µg/mL (25 mg/24 hr). In folate deficiency, however, the excretion is greater than 30 µg/mL (35 mg/24 hr).

10.1.8 REQUIREMENTS

The minimum daily requirement of folic acid for adults is about 50 µg/day as determined by the amount of folic acid needed to maintain serum folate levels in normal range. In calculating the recommendation, it is assumed that 25%–50% of the vitamin present in food is available for absorption. Allowing a margin of safety for differences in availability from various foods, the current Recommended Dietary

Allowances (RDA) for folates is set at 200 µg/day for adult males and 180 µg/day for adult females. During pregnancy and lactation, folate requirements clearly increase, and the RDA is set at 400 µg/day during pregnancy and 280 µg/day during the first 6 months of lactation. The allowances for infants and children vary with age and body weight and are set at 3.6 µg/kg/day.

In general, only half the folate in food is nutritionally available (bioavailable), whereas over 85% of folic acid that is added to food or ingested as a supplement is bioavailable. Because of the differences in bioavailability between supplemental folic acid and different forms of folic acid (polyglutamates) found in food, the Food and Nutrition Board of the Institute of Medicine introduced a new unit, the Dietary Folate Equivalent (DFE); 1 µg of food folate provides 1 µg of DFE; 1 µg of folic acid taken with meals provides 1.7 µg of DFE; and 1 µg of folic acid supplement taken on an empty stomach provides 2 µg of DFE.

Folate deficiency occurs most often in dialyzed patients because folic acid is removed by dialysis. Therefore, the daily prophylactic administration of the water-soluble vitamins, including 1 mg of folic acid, is recommended.

10.1.9 Excess Folate

Large doses of folate have been useful in the treatment of few rare diseases (i.e., homocysteinuria, defect in absorption of the vitamin, deficiency of dihydrofolate reductase). Large doses of folic acid (10–30 mg/day) have been used to reverse hematological signs of folate deficiency. Deficiency of vitamin B_{12}, though often undiagnosed, may affect a significant number of people, especially older adults. One symptom of vitamin B_{12} deficiency is megaloblastic anemia, which is indistinguishable from that associated with folate deficiency. Large doses of folic acid given to an individual with an undiagnosed vitamin B_{12} deficiency could correct megaloblastic anemia without correcting vitamin B_{12} deficiency. This can make the individual at risk of developing irreversible neurologic damage. Such cases of neurologic damage due to vitamin B_{12} deficiency have been seen at folic acid doses of 5 mg and above. To prevent such problems in vitamin B_{12}–deficient individuals, the Food and Nutrition Board of the Institute of Medicine advises all adults to limit their intake of folic acid to 1 mg/day. Doses as high as 100 mg/day for 10 days have been used to treat patients with tropical sprue without toxic effects; however, there are few reports that have shown deleterious effects of the ingestion of 15 mg folate/day for 1 month. The signs included sleeplessness, irritability, and gastrointestinal symptoms, but these claims have not been confirmed. There appears to be no toxic reaction to folic acid taken at 10 mg/day. Large doses may, however, interfere with the action of other drugs such as anticonvulsants. Parenteral administration of massive doses of folic acid will induce convulsions in individuals receiving anticonvulsant drugs because of epilepsy. Folic acid may reverse the anticonvulsant drug effects.

10.2 VITAMIN B_{12}

A severe anemia that was due to "some disorder of the digestive and assimilative organs" was first reported by Combe in 1822. In 1855, Addison, an English physician, gave a description of an anemia that occurred mostly in the middle-aged and the elderly that led to the death of the patients in 2–5 years. There was no known treatment available, and the disease was inevitably fatal and became known as pernicious anemia. Following the observation by Whipple that the liver is a source of potent hematopoietic substance for iron-deficient dogs, Minot and Murphy in 1926 showed that feeding large quantities (at least 0.3 kg) of beef liver cured this type of anemia. That same year, Castle reported abnormal gastric secretion in patients with pernicious anemia and concluded that the causative mechanism of the disease was "an inability to carry out some essential steps in the process of gastric digestion." He postulated that the antipernicious substance was formed by a combination of an extrinsic factor in food (e.g., liver) with an intrinsic factor (IF) in the normal gastric secretion and that both factors were necessary for the prevention or cure of the disease. Biochemists then began a long series of experiments to isolate the active component present in liver, which was then called antipernicious anemia factor or Castle's extrinsic factor.

Protein-free liver extracts were prepared and concentrated, which could be injected in patients. The injected dose of the liver extract was much more effective than the same amount ingested; this observation cast doubt on Castle's theory that the active antipernicious anemia factor was a combination of an extrinsic factor and an IF. Attempts to identify the active factor took several years because no animals other than humans were known to exhibit a need for this substance, and there were no easy methods to detect the factor. All experimental work of the evaluation of liver extracts had to be done on human subjects suffering from pernicious anemia. It was then discovered that the microorganism *Lactobacillus lactis* also needed the antipernicious anemia factor for growth. The availability of this microbiological method led to more extensive experimental work for the isolation of the pure active factor.

In 1948, two groups of investigators working independently (one in England and the other in the United States) isolated the active substance in a crystalline form. Positive hematological responses were obtained with doses as low as 3 μg of the substance. On the basis of water solubility, the substance was classified as a "B vitamin" and was named vitamin B_{12}. This was the last vitamin to be discovered. About 1 ton of fresh beef liver was needed to isolate 20 mg of the vitamin. The substance was identified chemically as one containing about 4% of its weight as the mineral cobalt. The structure was established by degradation and by x-ray crystallography.

10.2.1 Food Sources

Naturally occurring vitamin B_{12} is synthesized by microorganisms; higher plants and animals cannot synthesize it. Thus, this vitamin is unique among the B group in that it is not present in fruits, vegetables, and grains. Animals get their vitamin by ingesting microorganisms containing vitamin B_{12} and/or the B_{12} activity of microorganisms high enough in the alimentary tract for absorption and storage in tissues (especially the liver). Shellfish concentrates the vitamin from plankton and bacteria-rich seaweeds. The best sources of vitamin B_{12} include meats, clams, oysters, seafood, eggs, and milk. An average nonvegetarian Western diet contains 5–7 μg/day of vitamin B_{12}, which adequately sustains normal vitamin B_{12} equilibrium. Strict vegetarians do not get vitamin B_{12} except in seaweed and water or foods of nonanimal origin that have been contaminated by bacteria from soil. The reliable sources are foods fortified with vitamin B_{12} such as fortified breakfast cereals, fortified soy-based products, fortified energy bars, and fortified energy and soft drinks.

10.2.2 Chemistry

Vitamin B_{12} is a red crystalline substance that is a neutral, odorless, and tasteless compound and is soluble in water. It is resistant to boiling in neutral solution but unstable in the presence of alkali. The molecule consists of two major portions; a porphyrin-like "corrin ring" that is linked to a central cobalt atom (the ring is designated "corrin" because it is the core of the vitamin B_{12} molecule; all of the compounds containing this ring are designated corrinoids), and an odd ribonucleotide that has the base 5,6-dimethylbenzimidazole linked to ribose in an α-N glucosidic linkage (rather than a β-linkage found in other nucleotides). The ribonucleotide is covalently bound to the corrin ring by an ester linkage and coordinately bonded to cobalt (Figure 10.2).

Because of the presence of cobalt, the biologically important forms of vitamin B_{12} are also known by the generic term cobalamins. Vitamin B_{12} is present in the body in several forms differing only in the ligand attached to cobalt. They include cyanocobalamin (CN), hydroxocobalamin (OH), deoxyadenosylcobalamin (5-deoxyadenosyl), and methylcobalamin (CH_3). The last two are the coenzyme forms known to be metabolically active in mammalian tissues. In the original isolation procedure, cyanide was added to promote crystallization and the substance isolated was cyanocobalamin. This form has not been found in natural materials. Hydroxocobalamin appears to be the

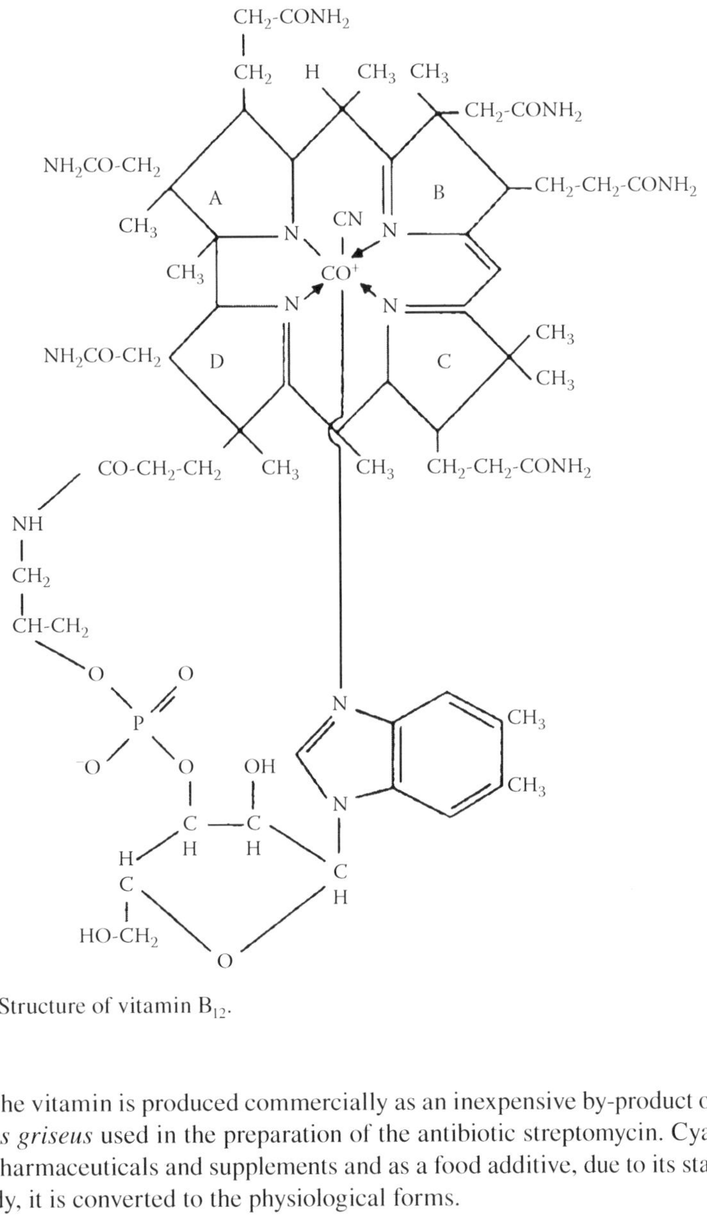

FIGURE 10.2 Structure of vitamin B_{12}.

natural form. The vitamin is produced commercially as an inexpensive by-product of the cultivation of *Streptomyces griseus* used in the preparation of the antibiotic streptomycin. Cyanocobalamin is used in many pharmaceuticals and supplements and as a food additive, due to its stability and lower cost. In the body, it is converted to the physiological forms.

10.2.3 ABSORPTION AND TRANSPORT

Vitamin B_{12} in food is mostly bound to protein; it is released by cooking, acidification (in the stomach), or proteolysis (specifically by pepsin). Two mechanisms are known for the absorption of the vitamin. Active absorption of physiological amounts (1–2 µg) is dependent on the presence of an IF and is highly specific; there is also a passive, nonspecific, IF-independent absorption mechanism, which has an efficiency of only about 1% of the ingested vitamin.

After the release of the free vitamin from food in the stomach, it is bound to a glycoprotein, IF, which is secreted by gastric parietal cells. Normal stomach cells secrete IF greatly in excess of that required to form complex with the amount of the vitamin present in a daily diet; however, in the gastric juice there are other proteins known as rapid (R) binders, a family of cobalamin-binding proteins of unknown function. At a low pH in the stomach, cobalamins have a much greater affinity for R binders than for IF. Even at a pH of 8, the affinity of cobalamin is 2 to 3 times as much for R binders than for IF. Thus, in the stomach cobalamin binds to R binders and then passes as a cobalamin–R binder complex into the intestine. The change in pH that occurs when the gastric contents pass into the duodenum and the action of proteolytic enzymes secreted by the pancreas, which partially degrade R binders, causes cobalamin to shift from R binders to IF. The R binders are digested, but cobalamin–IF complex remains intact because IF is resistant to proteolysis. The complex passes through the small intestine until it reaches the ileum. There it attaches to a specific receptor and is taken up into ileal mucosal cells. After 1–2 hours, vitamin B_{12} is released from its complex with IF and then finds its way across the enterocyte into the portal venous blood at which point it is attached to transcobalamin (TC) II, a transport protein for cobalamin produced by the liver and possibly by other tissues. The newly absorbed cobalamin circulates as cobalamin–TC II complex. It is as this complex that cobalamin is absorbed by cells that contain specific receptors that bind this complex. Once bound, the complex along with the receptor is carried into the cell by pinocytosis, and the vitamin is released from TC II, which is degraded by lysosomal enzymes. The vitamin is then converted to its coenzyme form. There are two other cobalamin-binding proteins, TCI and TC III, in the serum, which are synthesized by granulocytes and possibly also in the salivary gland, gastric mucosa, and some hepatoma cells; they appear to have largely a storage function. TC II is a pure protein while TC I and TC III are glycoproteins. Cobalamin is excreted via bile although a small amount less than 0.25 μg/day may be eliminated in the urine.

10.2.4 Biochemical Functions

There are two coenzyme forms of cobalamin: methylcobalamin and adenosylcobalamin[26] (also called coenzyme B_{12}).

10.2.4.1 Interrelationship between Folic Acid and Vitamin B_{12}

Methylcobalamin is necessary for the conversion of methyl THF to THF. In this reaction, the methyl group from methyl THF is transferred to homocysteine to produce methionine (methyl THF + homocysteine → THF + methionine). The reaction is catalyzed by cobalamin-dependent methionine synthase (Figure 10.3). The significance of this reaction appears to be the conversion of the circulating form of folate (methyl THF) to THF; the THF then can be conjugated to a polyglutamate chain and stored in the cell, and it can also be converted to methylene THF, the form necessary for thymidylate synthesis. In cobalamin deficiency, conjugation is compromised because of impairment in the conversion of poorly conjugable methyl THF to the readily conjugable THF. This results in leakage of folate out of the cells and leads to a deficiency of tissue folate. There is a buildup of methyl THF (i.e., methyl folate trap)[33] and a deficiency of THF and its derivatives needed

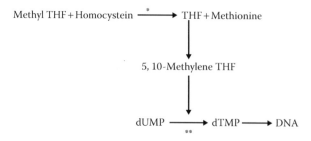

FIGURE 10.3 Reactions requiring both folic acid and cobalamin. * Methionine synthase, a methylcobalamin-dependent enzyme converts homocysteine to methionine and methyl THF to THF, which is used to generate methylene THF. ** Thymidylate synthase reaction utilizes methylene THF as 1-carbon donor in the methylation of dUMP to dTMP, a rate-limiting step in DNA synthesis. dUMP = deoxyuridine monophosphate; dTMP = deoxythymidine monophosphate.

for purine and thymidylate synthesis; this leads to megaloblastic anemia. The deficiency of either folate or vitamin B_{12} causes hematologically indistinguishable anemia. Cobalamin deficiency also leads to signs such as stomatitis and gastrointestinal mucosal alterations that are similar to those seen in folate deficiency; this is probably based on the defect[22] in the conversion of methyl THF to THF. The anemia due to cobalamin deficiency cannot be corrected by the administration of high doses of folic acid.

The inefficient conversion of homocysteine to methionine may indirectly cause neurologic disorder. Methionine is required to form *S*-adenosylmethionine (SAMe), which is necessary for methylation of myelin sheath phospholipids. SAMe is also involved in the synthesis of certain neurotransmitters, catecholamines, and in brain metabolism. These neurotransmitters are important for maintaining mood, possibly explaining why depression is associated with vitamin B_{12} deficiency. Methylation of myelin sheath phospholipids may also depend on adequate folate, which in turn is dependent on vitamin B_{12}–dependent methionine synthase recycling.

10.2.4.2 Homocysteine

Homocysteine is an amino acid not found in proteins·and is not a normal dietary constituent. The sole source of homocysteine is methionine. Methionine is activated by adenosine triphosphate to form SAMe, which serves as a convenient methyl donor to a variety of acceptors. The by-product of these methylation reactions is homocysteine.

Homocysteine is metabolized by one of two pathways: remethylation and transsulfuration. In the remethylation pathway (Figure 10.3) homocysteine receives a methyl group from methyl THF to form methionine in a reaction catalyzed by cobalamin-requiring methionine synthase. This reaction occurs in all tissues. Methyl THF is formed from methylene THF in a reaction catalyzed by MTHFR, a flavin adenine dinucleotide (FAD)–dependent enzyme. Homocysteine can also accept a methyl group from betaine, but this reaction is confined mainly to the liver and is B_{12} independent. In the transsulfuration pathway, homocysteine condenses with serine to form cystathionine in a reaction (Figure 10.4) catalyzed by vitamin B_6—pyridoxal phosphate (PLP)—requiring cystathionine β synthase (CS). Cystathionine is subsequently hydrolyzed by a second PLP–requiring enzyme γ cystathionase to form cysteine and α-ketobutyrate. Thus, the metabolism of homocysteine involves four water-soluble vitamins: riboflavin, folic acid, B_{12}, and B_6.

Because of the existence of efficient pathways for the removal of homocysteine, its concentration in plasma normally is low, averaging 10 μM/L. The levels are higher in men than in women up to menopause and increase with age, especially after the age of 60. The levels also go up in patients with renal failure, hypothyroidism, and during therapy with drugs such as methotrexate,[30] nitrous oxide, isoniazid, and some antiepileptic agents. Homocysteine level in plasma is considered a sensitive index of folate or B_{12} deficiency. Hyperhomocysteinemia is defined as a plasma level of >15 μM/l and is denoted as moderate (15–30 μM/L), intermediate (30–100 μM/L), and severe (>100 μM/L) hyperhomocysteinemia.

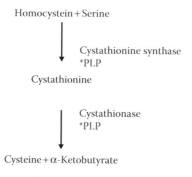

FIGURE 10.4   Conversion of homocysteine to cysteine. * PLP = Pyridoxal phosphate.

Elevations in plasma homocysteine are typically caused either by deficiencies or impairment in the conversion of required vitamins to their coenzyme forms or genetic defects in the enzymes involved in homocysteine metabolism. CS deficiency is the most common genetic cause of severe hyperhomocysteinemia. The homozygous form of this disease—congenital homocystinuria—can be associated with plasma homocysteine levels of up to 400 μM/L. It is rare, occurring in 1 in 200,000 births. Heterozygotes have much less marked hyperhomocysteinemia with plasma levels in the range of 20–40 μM/L. A common thermolabile variant of the enzyme MTHFR is homozygous in 5%–7% of the population. Such individuals tend to have slightly elevated plasma homocysteine levels, particularly in the presence of suboptimal folate nutrition. Other abnormalities of the remethylation cycle are also associated with an increase in plasma homocysteine.

Hyperhomocysteinemia is now recognized as a strong, independent risk factor for cardiovascular disease[18] and venous and arterial thrombosis. Many studies have shown that elevated plasma homocysteine levels are frequently found in patients with arteriosclerosis affecting coronary, cerebral, and peripheral arteries. At any given time, from 25% to 45% of patients with coronary heart disease (CHD) have high plasma homocysteine levels. A 1 μM/L rise in homocysteine level is associated with a 10% increase in CHD risk. The mechanism of this association is unknown. The homocysteine-induced adverse vascular changes appear to result from endothelial and smooth muscle cell effects and increased thrombogenesis. Although plasma homocysteine levels have been correlated with CHD risk, neither a cause–effect relationship nor a treatment outcome benefit has been established in clinical trials. Elevated plasma homocysteine levels are associated with heightened stroke risk. Because dietary supplementation with folic acid, vitamin B_{12}, and pyridoxine reduces homocysteine levels, two large supplementation trials were carried out with these vitamins. There was no observable decrease in stroke risk. Hyperhomocysteinemia during pregnancy is associated with increased risk for delivery of infants with NTD. This presumably indicates impaired homocysteine remethylation, resulting in a possible methionine shortage at a crucial stage of fetal development. Increasing evidence indicates that the homocysteine-lowering effect of folic acid plays a critical role in lowering the risk of NTD. Homocysteine may accumulate in the blood when there is less folate and/or vitamin B_{12} for methionine synthase to function effectively. Decreased vitamin B_{12} levels in the blood of pregnant women have been associated with an increased risk of NTD. Adequate vitamin B_{12} intake, in addition to folate, is likely to be beneficial in the prevention of NTD.

Mild homocysteinemia is very common, occurring in >20% of the elderly. Elevated homocysteine in elderly patients is an independent risk factor for dementia in general, including both vascular dementia and Alzheimer's disease. Plasma homocysteine levels are known to increase proportionately to the number of cigarettes smoked per day. The dose–response relationship is found to be the strongest in the oldest age group and in women. Increased homocysteine level per cigarette smoked per day is about 1% in women and 0.6% in men. The reason why plasma homocysteine level is increased in smokers is not known. It is possible that the intake of vitamins in smokers is reduced. Plasma homocysteine level is inversely related to physical activity. The most pronounced difference is found in the older age group between the physically inactive and the physically active subjects. Many individuals with inflammatory bowel disease (IBD) have elevated levels of plasma homocysteine, and recent evidence indicates that homocysteine plays a pathogenic proinflammatory role in IBD. Several studies have reported that high homocysteine levels significantly increase the risk of osteoporotic fractures. Elevated plasma homocysteine levels also seem to be associated with glaucoma.

The relations between elevated homocysteine and diseases are obtained through epidemiological studies. The question of causality remains to be determined. Most elevated levels of homocysteine can be lowered by folate supplementation alone or in combination with other B vitamins. There are concerns about the large amount of folate intake because it can mask the hematological abnormalities and allow neurologic complication to progress or accelerate. Homocysteine levels can be reduced by increasing the intake of folic acid, B_{12}, and B_6 and reducing the intake of methionine[24,28] (principally from animal protein). It is not known whether lowering homocysteine level diminishes the vascular occlusive risk that accompanies hyperhomocysteinemia. Large prospective trials are underway in the United States and Europe to answer this critical question but will require several years. Positive trial results would indicate an inexpensive relatively safe intervention for patients at risk of CHD.

10.2.4.3   Role of Coenzyme B_{12}

Coenzyme B_{12} is required for the conversion of methylmalonyl CoA to succinyl CoA, a reaction catalyzed by the adenosylcobalamin-dependent enzyme methylmalonyl CoA mutase (Figure 10.5). Methylmalonyl CoA is generated by the carboxylation of propionyl CoA, which is the product of the catabolism of isoleucine, valine, and odd-chain fatty acids. In the deficiency of vitamin B_{12}, the further metabolism of methylmalonyl CoA is impaired and methylmalonyl CoA accumulates and is excreted in the urine. The neurological disorders seen in B_{12} deficiency are due to the progressive demyelination of nervous tissue. Accumulation of methylmalonyl CoA interferes with the myelin sheath in two ways. First, methylmalonyl CoA is a competitive inhibitor of malonyl CoA in fatty acid biosynthesis; because the myelin sheath is turning over continually, a decrease in fatty acid synthesis can lead to its eventual degeneration. Second, the accumulated methylmalonyl CoA is converted to propionyl CoA (a three-carbon compound) that can substitute for acetyl CoA (a two-carbon compound) as a primer for fatty acid synthesis. The resulting odd-chain fatty acids are incorporated into membrane lipids where they disrupt membrane function possibly because of their unusual physical properties.

10.2.5   Deficiency

The deficiency of vitamin B_{12} can occur because of inadequate dietary intake, such as in strict vegetarians living in highly hygienic conditions,[22] but in most cases the deficiency is secondary to a defect in absorption that can result from disorders affecting the stomach, the intestine, and the pancreas. The most common cause of cobalamin deficiency is a failure of IF secretion that is caused by atrophy of gastric mucosa. This is thought to be caused by autoimmune destruction and leads to the disease known as pernicious anemia. Diseases such as regional enteritis (Crohn's disease) and tropical sprue can impair the ability of the ileum to absorb cobalamin. Normally, the small intestine is free of bacteria, but conditions such as intestinal diverticula and surgically created blind loops favor bacterial growth. Microorganisms can compete with IF for the vitamin, making it unavailable for absorption. A normally functioning pancreas is also important because it secretes pancreatic juice that is rich in bicarbonate and that has the enzymes required for degradation of R binders.

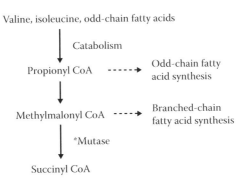

FIGURE 10.5   The role of adenosylcobalamin. * Methylmalonyl-CoA mutase is an adenosylcobalamin-dependent enzyme. Cobalamin deficiency in humans results in decreased conversion of methylmalonyl CoA to succinyl CoA and increased excretion of methylmalonic acid in the urine.

This facilitates the combination of IF with cobalamin, a key step for cobalamin absorption. Defects in the transport and metabolism of the vitamin may also cause a deficiency. Patients with inborn errors of TC II deficiency as well as deficiencies in other proteins involved in vitamin B_{12} metabolism have been reported.

There are two major symptoms of vitamin B_{12} deficiency in humans: hematological and neurological. Methylcobalamin, one of the coenzyme forms of vitamin B_{12}, is required to generate THF and methylene THF, which is essential for the conversion of uridylic acid to thymidylic acid. In the deficiency of B_{12}, methylene THF is not available for normal production of thymidylic acid and, as a result, of DNA. Cell duplication and differentiation are impaired, and megaloblastosis develops in tissues that depend on continuous cell duplication. The sensitivity of the hematopoietic system is due to its high rate of turnover of cells. Maturing cells are unable to complete nuclear division while cytoplasmic maturation continues at a relatively normal rate. This results in the production of morphologically abnormal cells or the death of cells during maturation, a phenomenon referred to as ineffective hemopoiesis. Other tissues with high rates of cell turnover (e.g., mucosal cells) have similar high requirements of vitamin B_{12}.

The hematological manifestations of vitamin B_{12} deficiency anemia can be relieved by the administration of high doses of folate, but a treatment with B_{12} itself is essential because folate cannot replace cobalamin in reactions involving other coenzyme forms of vitamin B_{12}.

Deficiency of vitamin B_{12} causes a macrocytic, megaloblastic anemia that is marked by a progressive decrease in the number and increase in size of red blood cells and physical symptoms of pallor and weakness; there is also leukopenia and thrombocytopenia. The individual appears pale, has glossitis and irritated mucosa, and may present with either diarrhea or constipation. Appetite loss, constipation, and tongue soreness are associated with vitamin B_{12} deficiency. These symptoms may be related to the increased vulnerability of rapidly dividing gastrointestinal cells to impaired DNA synthesis.

Vitamin B_{12} deficiency can cause disorders of the nervous system. Damage to the myelin sheath is the obvious organic lesion in neuropathy associated with cobalamin deficiency. This causes a wide variety of neurological signs and symptoms, including paresthesias of the hands and feet, loss of memory, and dementia. Although the progression of neurologic complications is generally gradual, such symptoms are not always reversible with the treatment of vitamin B_{12} deficiency, especially if they have been present for a long time.

Vitamin B_{12} deficiency was recently shown to be associated with elevated levels of tumor necrosis factor and decreased levels of epidermal growth factor in both rats and humans. It has been proposed that these changes may have a positive relationship between B_{12} deficiency and certain disorders including Alzheimer's disease and rheumatoid arthritis.[21] A recent prospective study has found that B_{12} deficiency may be associated with breast cancer. Among postmenopausal women, the risk of breast cancer more than doubled with plasma vitamin B_{12} levels in the lowest quintile compared to women in the four highest quintiles.

10.2.5.1   Acquired Vitamin B_{12} Deficiency

Nitrous oxide constitutes a major component of the anesthesia procedures practiced all over the world. Each year approximately 45 million people in North America undergo anesthesia. Nitrous oxide irreversibly oxidizes the cobalt atom of vitamin B_{12}, leading to inactivation of the vitamin and functional intracellular vitamin B_{12} deficiency.[34] An 80-minute period of anesthesia with nitrous oxide has been shown to cause hyperhomocysteinemia and neurological deterioration about 6 days after the anesthetic administration in people with subclinical vitamin B_{12} deficiency. Symptoms are treated with high doses of vitamin B_{12}, but recovery can be slow and incomplete. People with normal vitamin B_{12} levels have significant vitamin stores to make the effect of nitrous oxide insignificant.

The inactivation of methionine synthase by nitrous oxide has been demonstrated with purified enzyme, in cultured cells, in animal models, and in humans. The mean half-time of inactivation is

46 minutes. Residual methionine synthase more than 200 minutes after the start of nitrous oxide approaches zero. To restore the activity, the de novo synthesis of enzyme is required, which may take days. This can cause hyperhomocysteinemia and extreme deficiency of methionine in the blood and brain. Individuals with severe MTHFR deficiency exhibit high homocysteine and low methionine concentrations in plasma. These individuals may be more susceptible to nitrous oxide. For example, an infant boy was anesthetized twice before he was diagnosed to have severe MTHFR deficiency and subsequently died because of neurologic deterioration, perhaps due to extreme deficiency of methionine in the brain. Hence, patients with diagnosis of severe MTHFR deficiency should not receive nitrous oxide anesthesia.

10.2.6 REQUIREMENTS

The average mixed diet in the United States supplies between 5 and 10 μg of vitamin B_{12}/day. It is assumed that at this level of intake, approximately 15%–25% is absorbed and available for tissue use. The average amount of the vitamin in the tissue stores of normal adults is 5 mg, and the liver is the principal storage site. The half-life of B_{12} is more than a year, and daily losses are of the order of 1.3 μg. Therefore, day-to-day needs constitute a tiny fraction of the total storage supply, and several years are required for the development of significant B_{12} deficiency. Using these data together with the amounts of B_{12} required to initiate hematological response and to maintain health in patients with pernicious anemia, the RDA for adolescents and adults is set at 2 μg/day; for infants, the RDA is 0.5–1 μg/day, and for children, it is 1–1.5 μg/day. During pregnancy and lactation, the RDA is increased to 4 μg/day.

10.2.7 ASSESSMENT OF B_{12} STATUS

Serum levels of the vitamin in normal individuals range from 200 to 900 pg/mL, and deficiency should be suspected when the value is less than 100 pg/mL. The size and appearance of red blood cells can also be used initially to differentiate the anemia from that caused by the lack of iron. Vitamin deficiency is associated with megaloblastic anemia, along with low white blood cell and platelet counts. There is increased excretion of methylmalonic acid in the urine. Normal excretion in 24 hours is about 3 mg; an amount greater than 5 mg is considered a sign of cobalamin deficiency.

If pernicious anemia is suspected, either an absence of IF or an ileal defect may be the cause. The simplest means of sorting out the possible cause of malabsorption is the Schilling test. The patient is given a small oral dose of radioactive cobalamin (0.5–2 μg), followed immediately by a 1000-μg parenteral dose of nonradioactive vitamin. The nonradioactive vitamin binds to most available receptor sites in the liver and other body tissues, and any radioactive cobalamin that is absorbed does not have binding sites and is excreted in the urine. The amount of radioactivity in the patient's 24-hour urine collection provides an index of the degree of malabsorption. If this test shows malabsorption, it is repeated, but this time the patient is given a dose of IF concentrate in addition to cobalamin. If the absorption then becomes normal, the patient is deficient in IF. If the added IF does not correct the malabsorption, the defect lies in the ileum or pancreas. The test can be repeated by giving the vitamin along with bicarbonate and/or pancreatic enzymes. If the malabsorption is not corrected, the malfunction of ileum can be suspected by exclusion.

10.2.8 TOXICITY

The only established use of vitamin B_{12} is the treatment of its deficiency. It is administered orally or intramuscularly in doses of 1–1000 μg. The only need for excessive vitamin administration is in very rare cases of patients with a congenital defect such as B_{12}-responsive methylmalonic aciduria. Large doses of hydroxocobalamin hydroxide (5–10 g intramuscularly) have been used as an antidote to acute cyanide poisoning. The hydroxocobalamin hydroxide ligand is displaced by cyamide ion, and the resulting vitamin B_{12} complex is excreted in urine. In 2006, the Food and Drug Administration approved the use of hydroxocobalamin for acute treatment of cyanide poisoning. Aside from this use, the vitamin has been promoted for a number of conditions including multiple sclerosis and other neuropathies, but has no known value. There have been no reported health problems associated with intakes of vitamin B_{12} in excess of 1000 times the RDA level except in rare cases of allergic reaction. The vitamin has a very low toxicity.

10.3   PYRIDOXINE

By the late 1920s, it became clear that there was more than one water-soluble B vitamin. To investigate the pellagra-preventive factor, rats were fed a diet deficient in what was considered to be this factor. The animals developed dermatitis (rat acrodynia), which was thought to be an experimental model for pellagra in humans. After the antiberiberi (B_1) vitamin was separated from the crude preparation, riboflavin was isolated and found to be ineffective in curing rat dermatitis. After the identification of the real antipellagra factor, it was observed that this factor also could not cure the disease in rats. In 1936, Gyorgi distinguished the water-soluble factor whose deficiency was responsible for dermatitis from vitamin B_2 and named it vitamin B_6.[41,42]

Rapid progress was made in the study of this new vitamin, and it was isolated from rice bran and yeast in 1938 by five different research groups. The structure was quickly established and confirmed by synthesis, and the name pyridoxine (PN) was proposed for this substance because of its structural resemblance to the pyridine ring.

10.3.1   CHEMISTRY

The three naturally occurring forms of vitamin B_6 are PN, pyridoxal (PL), and pyridoxamine (PM). The compounds differ in the nature of the substitution on the carbon atom in position four of the pyridine nucleus. PN is primary alcohol, PL is the corresponding aldehyde, and PM has the aminomethyl group in this position (Figure 10.6). These three forms have equal biological activity. The commonly available synthetic form is pyridoxine hydrochloride, which is a white, crystalline, and odorless substance. It is light sensitive, especially in alkaline pH, and substantial loss occurs during cooking. Freezing of vegetables causes about 25% reduction in the amount of vitamin present.

10.3.2   FOOD SOURCES

The vitamin is widely distributed in plant and animal tissues. In the animal kingdom, it is present as PL and PM; in foods of plant origin, it is found primarily as PN. Beef, chicken, pork, and fish are rich in vitamin B_6. Among vegetable foods, bananas, nuts, peanuts, and soybeans are good sources; other fruits and vegetables have moderate amounts of the vitamin.

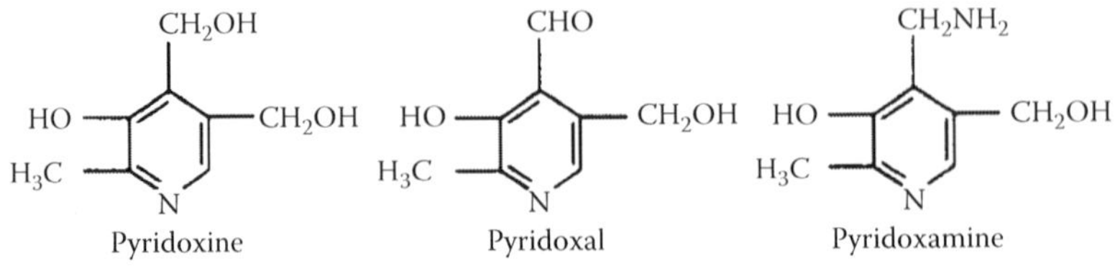

FIGURE 10.6   Structures of pyridoxine, pyridoxal, and pyridoxamine.

10.3.3 ABSORPTION AND TRANSPORT

The three forms of the vitamin are present in food in free forms as well as their phosphorylated derivatives (these require hydrolysis prior to absorption by the nonspecific phosphatases of the gastrointestinal tract). The free forms of the vitamin are absorbed by passive diffusion in the jejunum. PN, PL, and PM are then transported to the liver where they are phosphorylated by a single kinase to form, respectively, pyridoxine 5-phosphate (PNP), pyridoxal 5-phosphate (PLP), and pyridoxamine 5-phosphate (PMP). PNP and PMP can then be oxidized to PLP by a flavin-dependent oxidase. PNP can be converted to PLP and PMP, but neither of them can be converted back to PNP. All three phosphorylated derivatives can be dephosphorylated to the free vitamin by the action of phosphatases. Any excess of vitamin B_6 in the liver is metabolized via PL in an irreversible reaction catalyzed by aldehyde oxidase (or aldehyde dehydrogenase) to 4-pyridoxic acid (Figure 10.7). This is the primary metabolite of the vitamin excreted in the urine and accounts for 40%–60% of the ingested vitamin consumed by the individual in an adequate diet.

The free forms of the vitamin (mostly PL) and their phosphorylated derivatives (primarily PLP) are bound to albumin and enter the circulation where they are available for uptake by other tissues. The phosphorylated compounds do not readily penetrate the cell membrane and are hydrolyzed by phosphatases prior to entry into the cell.

The enzymes required for the interconversion of PNP, PLP, and PMP are not found in all tissues, but pyridoxal kinase is present in all cells. This may be the reason for the findings that circulating PLP accounts for 60%–70% of the total vitamin B_6, with PL as the next abundant form of the vitamin. The concentrations of PM, PN, and their phosphorylated derivatives in circulation are very low.

10.3.4 FUNCTIONS

PLP represents the coenzyme form of the vitamin although PMP can also activate a number of vitamin B_6–dependent enzymes. PLP is the coenzyme for over 60 different enzymes, most of which are on the pathways of amino acid and protein metabolism, including aminotransferases[45] and decarboxylases. In one way or another, PLP is involved in the metabolism of all the amino acids. In the case of transamination, enzyme-bound PLP is aminated to PMP by the donor amino acid, and the bound PMP is then deaminated to PLP by the acceptor α-keto acid. PLP is necessary for the normal metabolism of tryptophan. A notable reaction is the conversion of tryptophan to 5-hydroxytryptamine. In vitamin B_6 deficiency, a number of metabolites of tryptophan, particularly xanthurenic acid in the niacin biosynthetic pathway, are excreted in the urine in abnormally large quantities. The conversion of methionine to cysteine is also dependent on the vitamin.

Vitamin B_6 plays a role in the formation of neurotransmitters serotonin, epinephrine, norepinephrine, dopamine, and γ-aminobutyric acid. It is also involved in the formation of histamine

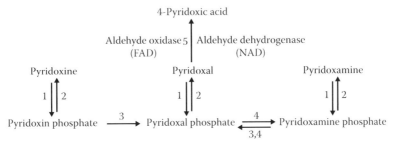

FIGURE 10.7 Metabolism of vitamin B_6. 1. Pyridoxal kinase. 2. Phosphatase. 3. Pyridoxine phosphate oxidase (FMN dependent). 4. Aminotransferase. 5. FAD-dependent aldehyde oxidase or NAD-dependent aldehyde dehydrogenase.

from histidine. The vitamin may increase the ability to recall dreams. It is thought that this effect may be due to the role PLP plays in the conversion of tryptophan to serotonin. PLP participates in the biosynthesis of protoporphyrin as a coenzyme for δ-aminolevulinic acid synthetase. This enzyme is the first and rate-limiting enzyme in the porphyrin biosynthesis. The enzymatic activity of glycogen phosphorylase is dependent on PLP. The catabolism of glycogen is initiated by phosphorylase, and PLP affects the enzyme's conformation. Vitamin B_6 has a role in gluconeogenesis. PLP catalyzes transamination reactions that are essential for providing substrates derived from amino acids for the formation of glucose.

In addition to its classical cofactor functions, PLP seems to modulate actions of steroid hormones in vivo by interacting with steroid receptor complexes. Steroid receptors are proteins and contain lysine residues that can interact with PLP and, as a result, less steroid binds to the receptor. In addition, PLP also binds to another site on the receptor that binds to DNA; thus, PLP can decrease the expression of the steroid. The binding of PLP to steroid hormone receptors suggests that the vitamin B_6 status of an individual may have implications for diseases affected by steroid hormones including breast cancer and prostate cancer. PN has been implicated in increasing or decreasing the expression of certain genes by interaction with transcription factors.

10.3.5 Deficiency

Because vitamin B_6 is required for several enzymes, its deficiency can have a significant effect on health, but primary deficiency in humans is rare because of the widespread distribution of the vitamin in foods. Even on a deficient diet, long periods of deprivation are required before the effects are noted. By the use of structural antagonists, however, it is possible to produce symptoms of deficiency. These include hypochromic microcytic anemia and seborrheic-like skin lesions around the eyes, nose, and mouth accompanied by glossitis and stomatitis. These lesions clear rapidly after administration of PN. Convulsive seizures, depression, and confusion may occur in individuals on a vitamin-deficient diet. Anticonvulsants may not be effective in treating these seizures. Low vitamin B_6 intake and nutritional status have been associated with impaired immune function, especially in the elderly. Decreased production of lymphocytes and interleukin-2 has been reported in vitamin B_6–deficient individuals. Bringing the vitamin B_6 status to normal resolves the immune function. According to a prospective study from the Netherlands, the intake of vitamin B_6, especially in smokers, could cut the risk of Parkinson's disease by half. Because the synthesis of the neurotransmitters serotonin and norepinephrine is dependent on PLP, it has been suggested that vitamin B_6 deficiency may lead to depression. Supplementation with this vitamin may be a treatment for depression.

Convincing evidence of the essential nature of the vitamin in humans came several years ago from reports of a curious syndrome in infants in various parts of the United States. They presented a picture of inadequate growth, nervousness, irritability, and seizures and had abnormal electro-encephalographic patterns. All the infants showing these signs were receiving the same proprietary canned liquid formula that lacked vitamin B_6. Evidently, the sterilization process used in the preparation had accidentally destroyed the vitamin. Rapid recovery followed injection of PN, thus proving conclusively that the symptoms were the result of the deficiency of vitamin B_6. The seizures associated with vitamin deficiency may be because of the lower activity of PLP-dependent glutamate decarboxylase, resulting in depressed levels of the neurotransmitter γ-amino-butyric acid. The formation of norepinephrine from tyrosine also requires PLP-dependent carboxylase.

Vitamin B_6 deficiency increases urinary excretion of oxalate and is implicated in renal calculus formation; this is attributed to an inability to convert glyoxylate to glycine and serine.

10.3.6 Effect of Drugs

Some chronic alcoholics develop sideroblastic anemia, which is similar to that seen in iron deficiency except that the bone marrow is filled with sideroblasts (iron-loaded red blood cell precursors).

Serum PLP concentrations are reduced in such patients. The experimental chronic administration of alcohol to human volunteers (when given with an inadequate diet) leads to sideroblastic anemia, but this is prevented when adequate PN is supplied. Acetaldehyde, the first intermediate of alcohol oxidation, inhibits pyridoxal kinase and accelerates the destruction of PLP in erythrocytes. Alcohol may thus cause anemia by inducing a depletion of PLP; however, this can be overcome if the intake of the vitamin is abundant.

Isonicotinic acid hydrazide, a chemical relative of PN, acts as its antagonist. Patients treated with this drug for tuberculosis experience neuritic symptoms apparently because of the imposed B_6 deficiency. The condition is corrected when a PN supplement is prescribed. Penicillamine, a drug used as a copper chelator in the treatment of Wilson's disease and cystinuria, is also a vitamin B_6 antagonist, so a PN supplement is usually prescribed for these patients. Some women who use oral contraceptives show biochemical evidence of vitamin deficiency such as low activity of PLP-dependent transaminase in erythrocytes and an increased excretion of xanthurenic acid in urine. These effects may be because estrogens induce increased activity of the enzyme system that converts tryptophan to niacin in the liver, and this may increase the requirement for PN. These women may also show signs of depression. There is evidence that depression is sometimes associated with the disturbance of amine metabolism in the brain, particularly serotonin, a product of tryptophan metabolism. These changes can be corrected by increased intake of PN.

10.3.7 GENETIC DEFECTS

There are several genetic B_6-dependency syndromes in which defective enzyme proteins are unable to function under physiologic levels of PLP. In these disorders, the characteristic lesions of vitamin B_6 deficiency are not present, but instead there are specific symptoms related to one particular enzyme. The conditions improve markedly and the symptoms disappear after the administration of pharmacological doses of the vitamin (i.e., 10–1000 mg/day), in contrast to the normal requirement of approximately 2 mg. These conditions are vitamin B_6-responsive syndromes and are not due to PN deficiency. Prominent among these is PN-responsive sideroblastic anemia. This condition is due to a defective PLP-dependent enzyme, δ-aminolevulinic acid (ALA) synthetase, which catalyzes the formation of ALA from glycine and succinyl CoA. ALA is the precursor of heme, and ALA synthetase is the first and rate-limiting enzyme of the heme biosynthetic pathway. In this condition, there is impairment of heme synthesis; it responds to about 2 g/day of PN. Other disorders in this category include xanthurenic aciduria, homocystinuria, and cystathionuria.

A second disorder is seen in children who have a defective PLP-dependent glutamate decarboxylase; this causes a reduction in brain γ-aminobutyric acid. These children develop convulsions and brain damage unless they are treated with large doses of PN starting at birth.

10.3.8 REQUIREMENTS

The human requirement of vitamin B_6 is closely related to the amount of protein intake and is satisfied at the level of 0.02 mg/g of protein; hence, the RDA for adult men and women is set at 2.2 and 2 mg/day, respectively, to provide a reasonable margin of safety. These levels permit a daily protein intake of 100 g for women and 110 g for men. The RDA for infants begins at 0.3 mg/day, increases to 0.6 mg/day for older infants who consume mixed diets, and increases to 1–2 mg from childhood through adolescence. The requirement is high in pregnancy because of the increased catabolism of tryptophan as a result of hormonal effects and the active transfer of the vitamin to the fetus; therefore, during pregnancy and lactation, 2.6 and 2.5 mg/day, respectively, are recommended.

The amount of vitamin B_6 in human milk is directly related to the amount in mother's diet. To assure at least 0.5 mg of vitamin B_6 per liter of milk, it may be necessary to increase the supplement to about 10 mg/day.

10.3.9 ASSESSMENT OF VITAMIN B$_6$ STATUS

In vitamin B$_6$ deficiency, the rate of conversion of tryptophan to niacin is decreased and more trypto-phan is diverted toward an alternate pathway that is normally insignificant. If a large dose of trypto-phan is administered (e.g., as in the tryptophan load test) to an individual who is vitamin B$_6$ deficient, there will not be adequate supply of PLP to allow for the normal conversion of tryptophan to niacin. Instead, various metabolites of the alternate pathway accumulate, including xanthurenic acid, which is not utilized in the body and is excreted in the urine. Excretion of high amounts of xanthurenic acid in urine after the tryptophan load test is, therefore, an indirect measure of B$_6$ status.

Normally, about 60% of ingested vitamin B$_6$ is converted to its major metabolite, 4-pyridoxic acid, and is excreted in the urine. In deficiency, however, the amount of this metabolite excreted is reduced, and in severe deficiency, it disappears from the urine. The measurement of 4-pyridoxic acid in urine can give an index of the vitamin B$_6$ intake. The excretion of less than 1 mg of the metabolite in 24 hours suggests an inadequate intake of the vitamin.

The activity of the PLP-dependent enzymes, alanine aminotransferase and aspartate amino-transferase, in red blood cells is considered a sensitive indicator of vitamin B$_6$ status; however, the direct measure of total vitamin B$_6$ and PLP is the most sensitive index of vitamin B$_6$ nutrition.

10.3.10 EFFECT OF PHARMACOLOGICAL DOSES

Large doses of vitamin B$_6$ are used in the prophylaxis and treatment of deficiency diseases,[43] as well as in the treatment of dermatological, neuromuscular, neurological, and various other conditions,[46] including certain anemias, hyperoxaluria, nausea, and vomiting of pregnancy, undesirable lacta-tion, depression associated with oral contraceptive use, schizophrenia, atherosclerosis-associated thrombosis, and kidney stones. Doses in the 100–400 mg/day range are generally used, but the efficacy of the vitamin for some of these ailments is certainly not proven. Carpal tunnel syndrome is a disease in which nerves that travel to the wrist are pinched as they pass through a narrow opening in a bone in the wrist. It causes pain or numbness in the hand. The symptoms are aggravated by use of the hands for work. Vitamin B$_6$ has been shown in at least small-scale clinical studies to have a beneficial effect on carpal tunnel syndrome. Vitamin B$_6$ has been used to treat nausea during preg-nancy. The administration of 25 mg of PN every 8 hours for 3 days or 10 mg of PN every 8 hours for 5 days have been found to be beneficial in alleviating morning sickness. The study found a slight but significant reduction in nausea and vomiting. Premenstrual syndrome is an ill-defined group of symptoms affecting a certain proportion of women between the middle and the end of the men-strual cycle. Decreased synthesis of neurotransmitters has been postulated to cause mood changes and water retention. Since the metabolism and the availability of the vitamin in the body appear to be normal, perhaps the entry of the vitamin into cells may be affected because of its interaction with steroid hormones. Administration of 50–500 mg/day of PN is of benefit for some individuals. One of the popular alternative medicine choices for autism[37] is a combination of vitamin B$_6$ and magnesium.[44] Higher doses of vitamin B$_6$ confer benefits to about half of all autistic children and adults on whom it has been tried. The dose used was 6 mg/kg body weight and magnesium 0.6 mg/kg body weight per day. Some studies have shown that this treatment can help attention deficit dis-order. Vitamin B$_6$ ingestion can alleviate some of the symptoms of alcoholism hangover. Limited data have shown that supplementation of vitamin B$_6$ at levels higher than the tolerable upper intake (100 mg/day) decreases elevated urinary oxalate level, an important determinant of calcium oxalate stone formation in some individuals.

The effects of megadoses of the vitamin were studied in normal adults.[39] They were given 200 mg of PN daily for 33 days. When these large doses were withdrawn, these individuals required greater than normal intakes of vitamin B$_6$ to maintain normal biochemical levels. Thus, there is the possibility of inducing B$_6$ dependence as a result of high intake of the vitamin. Large doses of PN may be undesirable or potentially hazardous to certain individuals. PN can reverse the therapeutic effect of levodopa used in Parkinson's disease. Very high doses (e.g., 2–5 g) of PN cause sensory nervous system dysfunction.

The acute toxicity of vitamin B_6 is quite low; daily doses of under 500 mg (i.e., 250 times RDA) for up to 6 months appear to be safe, but prolonged consumption of the vitamin in amounts considerably above RDA may increase the individual's daily requirement because of dependency and can also result in neurotoxicity. In most cases, the individuals recover normal functions after they stop taking the megadoses. Large doses of vitamin B_6 should not be taken unless the individual has been proven to have a deficiency and the use of such doses is warranted.

10.4   VITAMIN C—ASCORBIC ACID

Scurvy was one of the earliest recognized deficiency syndromes. It was described about 1500 BC in Egyptian literature and later in the Greek and Roman literature, and it was known for about 400 years that the disease could be controlled by dietary means. It is said that scurvy literally reshaped the course of history because many military and naval rations were grossly deficient in the necessary food factor. Military campaigns and voyages of discovery were cut short if the ration of the participants contained little antiscorbutic factor.

In the seventeenth century, sailors developed the disease if they were at sea for long periods of time without an opportunity to replenish supplies. A large portion of the crew died or was incapacitated by scurvy. For instance, Vasco da Gama lost 100 of 150 men on his way to India, and Magellan lost many of the 196 men who started around Cape Horn in 1520. When Jacque Cartier was exploring North America in 1535, many of his men suffered from scurvy; friendly American Indians gave his men pine needle broth, which cured them. At that time, the disease was thought to be caused by the cold, damp condition on board the ship.

British naval rations were devoid of antiscorbutic factor, but it was present to some extent in the rations of French, Spanish, and Portuguese navies who included pickled peppers, cider, vinegar, and so on. Analysis of the records kept by many of the early British sailors revealed that seamen consumed a diet that was basically composed of dried beans, cheese, and some salted dried beef. There were no fruits and vegetables for the common sailors, but the officers had a supply of these foods and they were less prone to the disease until much later. In the middle of the eighteenth century, James Lind, a British medical officer and one of the first to study scurvy, was interested in the difference between the diet of officers on board the ship and the common sailors. He ran an experiment where he fed the sailors different diets including cider vinegar, garlic, salt, alcohol, oranges, and other foods. From his results, he concluded that the disease was caused because of the lack of fresh fruits and vegetables in the diet. Furthermore, he established that lemon juice was an excellent remedy for the disease. Upon his return to London, Lind went before the Royal Medical Society and presented the results of his experiments; however, he was criticized for the simplicity of the results. No one believed that a disease could so easily be cured by a change in diet. At that time, of course, nothing was known of the accessory food factors or vitamins. The British navy did not allow him to continue his experiments on other ships.

In 1772, Captain James Cook was the first person to show that a long voyage could be undertaken without the crew developing scurvy, provided that they were supplied with fresh fruits and vegetables (including oranges and lemons) whenever they touched land. At that point, the British navy finally concluded that the results of Lind's experiments were meaningful, and in 1805, it adopted the use of lemon juice rations for all crews. At that time, lemons were called limes, and the routine use of lime juice led to the term *limey* to refer to a British seaman, a term now extended to all British.

By the beginning of this century, it was widely known that there was an antiscorbutic factor present in certain fruits and vegetables. The step toward the final isolation of this factor was the discovery in 1907 by Hoist and Frohlich in Norway that guinea pigs, like men, were susceptible to scurvy. They found that guinea pigs remained healthy on a diet of cereal grains and cabbage, but when restricted to cereal grains alone, they developed scorbutic lesions. Supplements of fruits, fresh vegetables, and juices protected the animals. An important aspect of this work was that it provided an experimental animal, the guinea pig, which led to the development of an assay for the biological determination of the antiscorbutic potency of foods. Thereafter, the search for the active factor was directed toward isolating it from citrus juices and trying its effect in curing scorbutic guinea pigs. It was clear that the antiscorbutic factor was a water-soluble, organic substance, which did not contain nitrogen and had extremely strong reducing properties. Since the terms "fat-soluble A" and "water-soluble B" had already been chosen, the antiscorbutic substance was logically named "Vitamin C."

The first isolation of the factor in pure form came in 1928 from an unrelated field of biochemistry, that of tissue oxidation. Szent-Györgi, in investigating the oxidation–reduction system in plants and animals, succeeded in isolating from adrenal glands, oranges, and cabbage a reducing agent in crystalline form but did not recognize its properties as a vitamin. The substance was acidic in nature, exhibited very strong reducing properties, gave color tests characteristic of sugars, and had an empirical formula $C_6H_8O_6$. For these reasons, he named it "hexuronic acid." About the same time, King and Waugh from the University of Pittsburgh also isolated an antiscorbutic substance in pure form from lemon juice. Later Szent-Györgi and King and Waugh independently demonstrated that hexuronic acid was identical with the antiscorbutic substance. The trivial chemical name ascorbic acid was assigned to designate its function in preventing scurvy. In 1933, Hirst and Haworth determined its structure and accomplished its synthesis.

10.4.1 Food Sources

Vitamin C is widely distributed in the vegetable kingdom where it is easily synthesized. Fruits, especially citrus fruits and berries, tomatoes, green vegetables, parsley, lettuce, and green peppers are excellent sources. A 4-ounce serving of orange juice contains about 45 mg of ascorbic acid. Cabbage, cauliflower, papayas, spinach, and other green vegetables are good sources. Although low in vitamin C, potatoes and the root vegetables are consumed in such quantities that they become a good source. Dormant plant foods such as cereal grain, seeds, and nuts are relatively poor sources of vitamin C. Most animals can synthesize their own supply of vitamin C, but relatively little is stored in their tissues and, as a result, animal products are poor sources of ascorbic acid.

10.4.2 Chemistry

L-ascorbic acid is a white, crystalline, water-soluble compound that is stable in dry form. It is very sensitive to oxidation, especially on exposure to heat and particularly in the presence of copper (but not of aluminum). Therefore, foods prepared in copper vessels lose ascorbic acid quickly. It is also rapidly destroyed in alkaline solution but is fairly stable in weakly acidic solution. Consequently, baking soda has a harmful effect, but cooking in steam has little destructive action on the vitamin C content of food. It is the least stable of all the vitamins.

Ascorbic acid is a hexose derivative and is classified as a carbohydrate, one closely related to monosaccharides (Figure 10.8). It is a very powerful reducing agent, and its biological function is linked to this important property both in plants and in animals. It is readily oxidized to form dehydroascorbic acid (DHA). The DHA may be reduced back to the original form (i.e., there is a reversible oxidation–reduction reaction); both forms are biologically active. The synthetic form is derived from the monosaccharides glucose or galactose and is used to enrich food products and in nutrient supplements.

D-ascorbic acid is structurally related to L-ascorbic acid but has a weak antiscorbutic action; however, it has a similar redox potential. Both compounds have been used to prevent nitrosamine formation from nitrites in cured meats such as bacon. The weak antiscorbutic action of D-ascorbic acid may be because it is not retained in tissues in sufficient concentration to be effective. It may be effective if given in small doses throughout the day. To avoid possible confusion and any implications that it is a vitamin, the term erythrobic acid is used for the D-isomer.

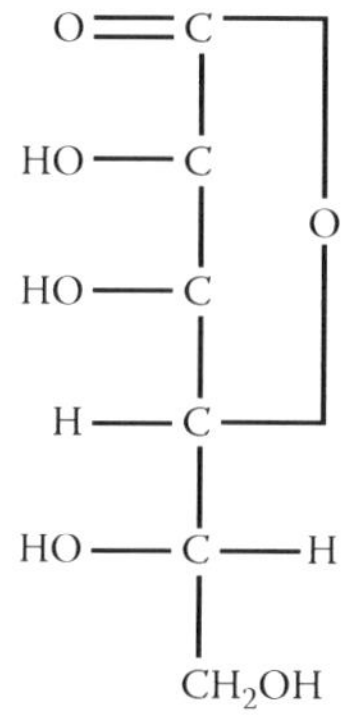

FIGURE 10.8 Structure of ascorbic acid.

10.4.3 ABSORPTION AND METABOLISM

Vitamin C is readily and almost completely absorbed from the upper part of the small intestine when ingested in physiological amounts. The process of facilitated diffusion and active transport similar to those operating in the absorption of simple hexoses are involved in the absorption of vitamin C in the intestinal cell. When progressively large doses of ascorbic acid are ingested, the absorption efficiency falls. Thus, doses of 100 mg, 180 mg, 1.5 g, and 5 g will be absorbed at rates of 100%, 70%, 50%, and 20%, respectively. The portion of ascorbic acid that is not absorbed and remains in the lumen exerts the same osmotic effect as other sugars and can cause watery diarrhea. After absorption, it is distributed throughout the water component of the body. There is no extensive storage of vitamin C, but certain tissues such as adrenal cortex, pituitary, thymus, corpus luteum, and retina have relatively large amounts of the vitamin. The metabolically active pool has been estimated to be approximately 1500 mg in a healthy adult and about 3% of it (45 mg) is catabolized per day. Thus, an intake of 45 mg/day should be sufficient to maintain an adequate body pool. Ascorbic acid is reversibly oxidized to DHA and then irreversibly oxidized further to diketogulonic acid and then to oxalic acid. These are the main metabolites of ascorbic acid and are excreted in the urine.

10.4.4 BIOCHEMICAL FUNCTIONS

Ascorbic acid appears to be essential for normal functions of plant and animal cells. In contrast to most water-soluble vitamins, it has no clear-cut role as a catalyst nor is it a part of an enzyme or structure. Its specific functions[49] at the biochemical level are not fully understood. It appears to protect, regulate, and facilitate the biological processes of other enzyme systems. It serves as a reducing agent in a number of hydroxylation reactions in the body. A major function of ascorbic acid is in the formation of collagen, a fibrous protein made up of three polypeptide chains coiled together to form a helix. These polypeptides have an unusual amino acid composition consisting of glycine (about 33% of the amino acids present), hydroxyproline, and hydroxylysine. The hydroxylation of proline and lysine takes place after they are incorporated into the polypeptide, and this step is essential for the normal physical structure of the completed protein molecule. The hydroxylation reactions are catalyzed by proline hydroxylase for proline and lysyl hydroxylase for lysine; ascorbic acid serves as a specific nonreplaceable reducing agent to generate iron in the reduced form (Fe^{2+}). The tissue levels of collagen proline hydroxylase are lower in scorbutic guinea pigs than in normal animals. Higher concentrations of enzyme and ascorbic acid are found in injured tissues in which wound healing and scar tissue formation are occurring.

Collagen fibers give rigidity to the amorphous ground substance of connective tissue that fills the space between the cellular and circulatory components of tissues and aids in holding them together. Collagen is also a major component in organic matrix of bone and teeth and in the scar tissue formed during healing of wounds and bone fractures. In the absence of vitamin C, the hydroxylation step is impaired and defective collagen cannot form fibers. This results in the skin lesions and blood vessel fragility that is prominent in scurvy. Vitamin C is essential for healing of wounds and for the repair and maintenance of cartilage, bones, and teeth.

Ascorbic acid also appears to have a role in other hydroxylation reactions such as the hydroxylation of tryptophan, which leads to the formation of serotonin, and in the conversion of tyrosine to norepinephrine. The abnormalities in vascular and neurologic activity seen in scorbutic patients may be because of impaired synthesis of these biologically active substances. Ascorbic acid is apparently required for the metabolism of tyrosine. Alkaptonuria in guinea pigs results when they are fed a diet deficient in vitamin C and containing excess tyrosine. The vitamin seems to protect the enzyme that oxidizes p-hydroxyphenyl pyruvic acid (PHPPA), a metabolite of tyrosine. The subsequent administration of vitamin C reduces or abolishes the output of PHPPA. Vitamin C participates in the hydroxylation of trimethyllysine in carnitine biosynthesis. It has been postulated that vitamin C is required for the hydroxylation reactions involved in the synthesis of corticosteriods.

As a reducing agent, ascorbic acid aids in the absorption of iron by reducing it to the ferrous state in the stomach. It protects vitamin A and vitamin E from oxidation and also helps maintain THF in the reduced state; it also appears to regulate cholesterol metabolism. Recent studies suggest that vitamin C is involved in the conversion of cholesterol to bile acids, which may have implications for blood cholesterol level and the incidence of gall stones. Ascorbic acid is considered to have cancer prevention properties; it inhibits the formation of nitrosamine from nitrite in foods and induces the activity of some enzymes involved in the metabolism of xenobiotics such as the cytochrome P-450 system. Vitamin C has been shown to reduce the risk of colon cancer in case–control studies and to induce detoxifying enzymes in human colon cancer cells. Individuals consuming the highest amount of vitamin C appear to have about half the risk for pancreatic cancer as those with the least vitamin C in their diets.

In spite of the foregoing information on the biological effects of vitamin C, no precise biochemical reaction for this vitamin has been established.

10.4.5 DEFICIENCY

Vitamin C is unique in the sense that it is a vitamin only for humans, monkeys, guinea pigs, fruit-eating bats, red-vented bulbul birds, trout, and carp; most other species do not require dietary vitamin C for the prevention of scurvy. They synthesize it from glucose through the intermediate formation of D-glucuronic acid, L-gulonic acid, and L-gulonolactone. Humans, monkeys, and guinea pigs have lost L-gulonolactone oxidase, an enzyme that normally catalyzes the conversion of L-gulonolactone to L-ascorbic acid.

D-glucose → D-glucuronic acid → L-gulonic acid → L-gulonolactone $\overset{*}{\rightarrow}$ L-ascorbic acid
*gulonolactone oxidase

An adult goat, an example of an ascorbic acid–producing animal, synthesizes about 13 g of vitamin C per day in normal health, and the synthesis increases manyfold under stress. Trauma and injury also cause humans to use more vitamin C. The loss of ability to synthesis ascorbic acid in humans strikingly parallels the evolutionary loss of the ability to break down uric acid. It has been suggested that in humans uric acid has taken over some functions of ascorbate. More recently it has been reported that a glucose transport protein on the surface of human red blood cells is altered by another protein called stomatin so that the vitamin C's oxidized form, DHA, is preferentially imported into red blood cells instead of glucose. DHA is then quickly reduced to vitamin C inside the red blood cell. In fact, humans express three orders of magnitude more of these glucose-turned-DHA transporters on their red blood cells than do mammals that produce their own vitamin C. Because of this efficient vitamin C cycling (and the role of uric acid), humans need only consume 1 mg vitamin C per kg of body weight per day, whereas goats have to synthesize 200 times that amount.

In humans, the deficiency in vitamin C results in scurvy. The signs of the disease in adults include aching joints, bones, and muscle, impaired capillary integrity with subcutaneous hemorrhage (Figure 10.9), perifollicular hyperkeratosis (an accumulation of epithelial cells around the hair follicles), and bleeding gums (Figure 10.10). Impaired formation of collagen is the basis for all

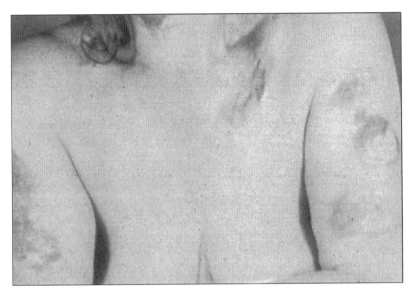

FIGURE 10.9 Ecchymoses of a patient with vitamin C deficiency. Capillary fragility, which is associated with vitamin C deficiency or scurvy, is illustrated by the appearance of the purple patches (bleeding in the tissue) on the arms and around the neck. (Courtesy of Shari Roehl, Pharmacia & Upjohn Co.)

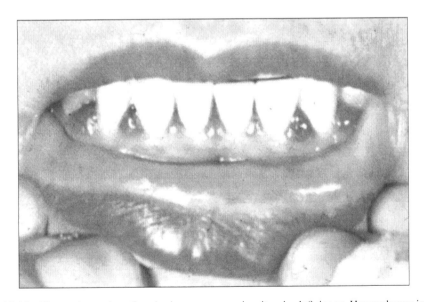

FIGURE 10.10 Hemorrhages into the gingiva may occur in vitamin deficiency. Hemorrhages into a number of other areas include the conjunctivae, eyeballs, brain, kidneys, and joints. Nosebleeds, hematuria, and melena may also occur on the basis of capillary fragility. It should be noted that other conditions such as leukemia and certain other bleeding diathesis may produce similar capillary bleeding. (Courtesy of Shari Roehl, Pharmacia & Upjohn Co.)

these changes. Other symptoms of scurvy[54] are weakness, anorexia, mental depression, hysteria, and anemia. The anemia is related to the action of vitamin C in facilitating the absorption of iron. Weakness may be attributed to the role of vitamin C in the biosynthesis of carnitine, which is involved in the transport of fatty acids into mitochondria, where they are oxidized and provide energy.

Pain, tenderness, swelling of thighs and legs, hemorrhage of the costochondral cartilages, and irritability are frequent symptoms of infantile scurvy. Because of the pain, the infant does not want to move and assumes a position with legs flexed (Figure 10.11). The infant is generally pale and irritable and cries when handled. A transient tyrosinemia may occur in some patients.

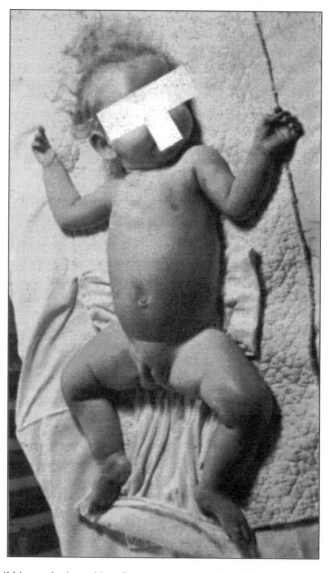

FIGURE 10.11   Child in scorbutic position. Because movement is painful, the scorbutic infant usually lies on its back and makes little attempt to lift the afflicted leg or arm. Both legs may be tender and sometimes both arms as well. This "pithed frog position" is usually the first sign of scurvy. (Courtesy of Shari Roehl, Pharmacia & Upjohn Co.)

Scurvy is considered to be rare in developed countries. However, vitamin C deficiency or depletion was found in 5%–17% of participants in the Third National Health and Nutrition Examination Survey, in 30% of samples of hospice patients, in 68% of a population of hospitalized elderly patients, and in individuals who eat meat-based diets and avoid fruits and vegetables. In smokers, this risk of vitamin C deficiency is roughly four times greater than in nonsmokers.

Oral contraceptives are known to decrease vitamin C levels in plasma and white blood cells. Aspirin can lower vitamin C levels if taken frequently. Taking 2 aspirin tablets every 6 hours for a week has been reported to lower vitamin C in white blood cells by 50% primarily by increasing urinary excretion of vitamin C.

10.4.6 Requirements

The allowances are derived from the amount of vitamin C that will cure or prevent scurvy, the amount that is metabolized in the body, and the amount necessary to maintain adequate body reserves. A dietary intake of 10 mg/day ascorbic acid will cure the clinical signs of scurvy, which is associated with levels of 0.13–0.24 mg/dL plasma and a body pool of 300 mg. The normal body pool of ascorbic acid is about 1500 mg, and approximately 3%–4% of it is metabolized daily. On the basis of this information, the RDA for adults of both sexes is set at 60 mg/day.[49] Human milk contains 35–55 mg/L of ascorbic acid, depending on the mother's dietary intake. Consequently, the infant consuming 850 ml/day of milk receives about 35 mg/day of ascorbic acid. For adolescents, the recommended allowance is 50 mg. An increase of 40 mg/day during pregnancy and lactation is recommended.

Plasma concentration of ascorbic acid is lowered by the use of cigarettes and oral contraceptive agents; in these cases, additional intake of vitamin C is recommended although the significance of the decrease in plasma ascorbic acid level in these circumstances is unclear. Conditions that may require a large quantity of vitamin C are thyrotoxicosis, infection, physical trauma, and surgery. In such instances, 200 mg/day or more of ascorbic acid may be administered, and even larger amounts have been suggested for use in the prevention of the common cold. Evaluation of such claims for the common cold by carefully controlled double-blind studies has demonstrated that any benefits derived from such large doses are too insignificant to justify routine use.

10.4.7 Assessment of Vitamin C Status

The measurement of plasma or serum concentration of ascorbic acid is the most commonly used and practical procedure for evaluation of vitamin C nutriture. The normal range of ascorbic acid in plasma is 0.6–2.5 mg/dL, and subnormal values are seen in deficiency, some cases of pregnancy and lactation, infectious diseases, congenital heart failure, and kidney and liver diseases. Ascorbic acid concentration of less than 0.2 mg/dL is considered indicative of inadequate vitamin intake.

The concentration of ascorbic acid in white blood cells may more closely reflect the level of vitamin C in tissues than does the amount in plasma, but the procedure is somewhat more tedious and more prone to analytical errors. The white blood cells of healthy adults have a concentration of about 27 μg of ascorbic acid per 10^8 cells. Vitamin C is a threshold substance (i.e., it is not excreted by the kidneys until the ascorbic acid level in the blood exceeds a certain value that depends on the degree of saturation of body tissues). The saturation test depends on the amount of ascorbic acid excreted in the urine after a test dose of the vitamin (about 500 mg) has been administered. If the tissues are well supplied with vitamin C, a large amount of it is eliminated, but if the tissues are not saturated, it will be retained and little will be excreted. Normal individuals excrete at least 50% of the dose within 24 hours, whereas severely deficient subjects may excrete very little of the administered vitamin.

10.4.8 EFFECTS OF HIGH DOSES OF VITAMIN C

Several placebo-controlled trials have examined the effect of vitamin C supplementation on the prevention and treatment of common colds.[51,55] It was found that vitamin C supplementation in doses of 2 g/day did not decrease the incidence of cold. However, in individuals under significant physical or environmental stress, such as marathon runners, skiers, soldiers, and people exposed to severe cold, doses ranging from 250 mg to 1 g/day decreased the incidence of colds by 50% compared with the risk in individuals not using supplements. Among the same group, taking vitamin C had 80%–100% reduction in pneumonia incidence, compared with persons given placebo.

Higher dietary intakes of vitamin C are associated with lower cardiovascular disease risk, but randomized-controlled trials have not found supplementation to reduce the risk of cardiovascular disease in diabetics or other high risk individuals. People who take large quantities of vitamin C that exceed U.S. RDA have a lower incidence of cataracts than those ingesting the amount within the RDA, suggesting a potential preventive role for high doses of vitamin C. Nevertheless, insufficient interventional data exist to assume conclusively a preventive role of the vitamin in cataract and macular degeneration.

High blood levels of vitamin C are independently associated with lower prevalence of elevated blood lead concentrations. Vitamin C may inhibit intestinal absorption or urinary excretion of lead.

There is some evidence that vitamin C interacts with anticoagulant medications such as warfarin. Large doses of vitamin C may block the action of warfarin, requiring an increase in anticoagulant dose to maintain its effectiveness.

Vitamin C is perhaps the most controversial vitamin in terms of views on the benefits and risks of high doses. The use of megadoses (e.g., 1 g or more) of ascorbic acid became popular shortly after Linus Pauling advocated it for prevention of the common cold. Since then, this vitamin has been cited as beneficial against other respiratory infections, cardiovascular defects, cancer, schizophrenia, and a variety of other diseases. The efficacy of pharmacological levels of the vitamin remains controversial because many of the claims have not been substantiated.

For most individuals, ascorbic acid has a very low toxicity and excessive intakes are tolerated; however, adverse effects of megadoses of vitamin C have been reported in some individuals, including induced uricosuria, hypoglycemia, hemolysis in patients with erythrocyte glucose-6-phosphate dehydrogenase deficiency, impaired bactericidal activity of leukocytes, and excessive absorption of iron.

Vitamin C is a powerful reducing agent and antioxidant and, therefore, can raise the oxygen required for cells and tissues. A significant loss of high-altitude resistance has been observed following high doses of vitamin C. This may increase the risk of hypoxia in individuals working under limited oxygen conditions. Ascorbic acid is partially converted to oxalic acid, the excretion of which increases after ingestion of vitamin C in megadose quantities. The hyperoxaluria can increase the risk of urinary tract stones, especially in populations with a predisposing metabolic abnormality.

Since the efficiency of intestinal absorption of vitamin C decreases with increased intake, it can cause gastrointestinal disturbances such as diarrhea, nausea, and abdominal pain. These are the most common adverse reactions due to megadoses of vitamin C. The unabsorbed portion of vitamin C leads to its high concentration in the feces, which may interfere with some tests for occult blood in the stool. As a strong reducing agent, it may also interfere with several laboratory procedures including urinary glucose determination.

Ascorbic acid dependency may be induced through high intakes of vitamin C. Ascorbate conditioning was observed in human infants whose mothers ingested more than 400 mg/day of ascorbic acid during pregnancy. The deficiency disease is believed to result from the induction of vitamin catabolism from prenatal conditioning. The induction of neonatal scurvy by prenatal conditioning has been confirmed in guinea pigs. Individuals taking megadoses of ascorbic acid for long periods of time, therefore, should reduce their daily intake gradually when they decide to discontinue the supplement.

Massive doses of ascorbic acid do not produce toxicity. This may be because of its rapid excretion in the urine and limited storage in the human body, but in view of the potential to cause adverse reactions described above, the routine intake of large amounts of vitamin C should be avoided.

Sensory Neuropathy from PN Abuse—A Case

A 27-year-old woman came to a doctor's office because of increased difficulty in walking. Approximately 2 years before, she had been told by a friend that vitamin B$_6$[59,60] provided a natural way to get rid of body water, and she had begun to take 500 mg/day for premenstrual edema. One year before presentation, she had started to increase her intake, until she reached a daily consumption of 5 g/day. During this period of increase in dosage, she initially noticed that flexing her neck produced a tingling sensation down the neck and into the legs and soles of her feet. In the 4 months immediately preceding her examination, she became progressively unsteady when walking, particularly in the dark, and noticed difficulty handling small objects. She also noticed some change in the feeling in her lips and tongue, but she had no other positive sensory symptoms and was not aware of any limb weakness.

Examination showed that the patient could walk only with the assistance of a cane and that she was unable to walk with her eyes closed. Physical examination was consistent with peripheral sensory polyneuropathy.[61] However, motor strength was normal. The sensations of touch, temperature, pinprick, vibration, and joint position were severely impaired in both the upper and lower limbs. There was a mild subjective alteration of touch-pressure and pinprick sensation over the cheeks and lips but not over the forehead. Motor nerve conduction was normal. The results of spinal fluid examination were normal, as were those of other clinical laboratory investigations.

Two months after the patient stopped taking PN her symptoms improved noticeably. Seven months after withdrawal she felt much improved; she could walk without a cane, could stand with her eyes closed, and had returned to work. Electrophysiological sensory nerve status remained abnormal but was very much improved. Clinical evaluation disclosed no likely cause for the sensory neuropathy other than the vitamin B$_6$ ingestion. This implicated PN megavitaminosis as the sole cause of her illness.

Interestingly, in both the syndrome of PN toxicity described above and the syndromes of genetic and acquired PN deficiency, the nervous system is affected. A deficiency of PN causes convulsions (low level of γ-aminobutyric acid) and peripheral neuropathy, which illustrates the role of B$_6$ in the formation of sphingomyelin at the level of serine palmitoyltransferase, which requires PLP. The mechanism for the toxic effects of PN in large doses is not understood. It is possible that excessive PN may occupy binding sites on the appropriate apoenzymes and act as a competitive inhibitor for the PLP resulting in neuropathy. PN is a substituted pyridine. As a family, pyridines are neurotoxic with the minimal toxic dose depending on structure.

Water-soluble vitamins are for the most part extremely safe because it is assumed that they are rapidly cleared from the body. "Vitamin megadosing" has been a favorite subject in the popular press. Because these substances can be obtained over the counter, the practice of megadosing is extensive. The case described above illustrates that even water-soluble vitamins do have their own profile of risk and can cause harmful effects. Vitamin intake should be routinely included in a patient's medication history to allow the identification of potentially hazardous self-medication. Individuals who take nutritional supplements at levels substantially greater than the RDA should be informed of the possible risks.

10.5   ANEMIAS

The various anemias mentioned in this chapter are defined as follows:

1. *Anemia* is any condition in which the number of red blood cells per cubic millimeter, the amount of hemoglobin per 100 ml of blood, or the volume of packed cells per 100 ml of blood are less than normal.
2. *Hypochromic anemia* is the one in which the erythrocytes contain less hemoglobin than normal.
3. *Microcytic anemia* is the one in which red cell size or mean corpuscular volume is smaller than normal.
4. *Macrocytic anemia* is the one in which red cell size or mean cell volume is above normal.
5. *Megaloblastic anemia* is a condition in which the erythroblasts in the bone marrow show a characteristic abnormal maturation of the nucleus being delayed relative to the maturaion of the cytoplasm.
6. *Sideroblastic anemia* is a refractory anemia in which the marrow shows increased iron present as granules arranged in a ring around the nucleus in developing erythroblasts. A defect in heme synthesis is present.
7. *Pernicious anemia* is caused by autoimmune attack on the gastric mucosa leading to atrophy of the stomach. The wall of the stomach becomes thin. There is achlorhydria (absence of hydrochloric acid), and the secretion of intruinsic factor is absent or almost absent.
8. *Megaloblast* is a large nucleated, embryonic type of cell that is a precursor of erythrocyte, in an abnormal erythropoietic process observed almost exclusively in pernicious anemia.
9. *Normoblast* is a nucleated red blood cell, the immediate precursor of normal erythrocyte in man.

REFERENCES

Folic Acid

1. Bailey, L. B., ed. 1995. *Folate in Health and Disease*. New York: Marcel Dekker.
2. Blount, B. C., M. M. Mack, C. M. Wehr et al. 1997. Folate deficiency causes uracil mis-incorporation into human DNA chromosome breakage. Implications for cancer and neuronal damage. *Proc Natl Acad Sci USA* 94:3290.
3. Cherian, A., S. Seena, R. K. Bullock et al. 2005. Incidence of neural tube defects in the least-developed area of India: A population-based study. *Lancet* 366:930.
4. Cole, B. F., J. A. Baron, R. S. Sandler et al. 2007. Folic acid for the prevention of colorectal adenomas: A randomized clinical trial. *J Am Med Assoc* 297:2351.
5. Corrada, M. M., C. H. Kawas, J. Hallfrisch et al. 2005. Reduced risk of Alzheimer's disease with high folate intake: The Baltimore Longitudinal Study of Aging. *Alzheimer's Dement* 1:11.
6. Ericson, U., E. Sonestedt, B. Gullberg et al. 2007. High folate intake is associated with lower breast cancer incidence in postmenopausal women in the Malmo Diet and Cancer cohort. *Am J Clin Nutr* 86:434.
7. Eskes, T. K. 1998. Open or closed? A world of difference: A history of homocysteine research. *Nutr Res* 56:236.
8. Goh, Y. I., and G. Koren. 2008. Folic acid in pregnancy and fetal outcomes. *J Obstet Gynaecol* 28:3.
9. Jacques, P. F., J. Selhub, A. G. Bostom, P. W. F. Wilson, and L. H. Rosenberg. 1999. The effect of folic acid fortification on plasma folate and total homocysteine concentrations. *N Engl J Med* 340:1449.
10. Kim, Y. I. 2006. Does a high folate intake increase the risk of breast cancer? *Nutr Rev* 64:468.
11. Luchsinger, J. A., M. K. Tang, J. Miller et al. 2007. Relation of higher folate intake to lower risk of Alzheimer's disease in the elderly. *Arch Neurol* 64:86.
12. Parick, T. E., R. W. Powers, A. R. Daftari et al. 2004. Homocysteine and folic acid are inversely related in black women with pre-eclampsia. *Hypertension* 43:1279.
13. Refsum, H., P. M. Ueland, O. Nygard, and S. E. Vollset. 1998. Homocysteine and cardiovascular disease. *Annu Rev Med* 49:31.

14. Selhub, J. 1999. Homocysteine metabolism. *Annu Rev Nutr* 19:217.

15. Stolzenberg-Solomon, R. Z., D. Albanes, F. Javier-Nieto, T. J. Hartman, J. A. Tangrea, M. Rautalahti, J. Schlub, J. Virtamo, and P. R. Taylor. 1999. Pancreatic cancer risk and nutrition-related methyl group availability indicators in male smokers. *J Natl Cancer Inst* 91:535.

16. Tamura, T., and M. F. Picciano. 2006. Folate and human reproduction. *Am J Clin Nutr* 83:993.

17. Van Guelpen, B. 2007. Folate in colorectal cancer, prostate cancer and cardiovascular disease. *Scand J Clin Lab Invest* 67:459.

18. Welch, G. N., and J. Lscalzo. 1998. Homocysteine and atherothrombosis. *N Engl J Med* 338:1042.

19. Zhang, S. M., N. R. Cook, C. M. Albert et al. 2008. Effect of combined folic acid, vitamin B_6 and vitamin B_{12} on cancer risk in a women: A randomized trial. *J Am Med Assoc* 300:2012.

20. Zhang, S., D. J. Hunter, S. E. Hankinson, E. L. Giovannucci, B. A. Rosner, G. A. Colditz, F. E. Speizer, and W. C. Willett. 1999. A prospective study of folate intake and the risk of breast cancer. *J Am Med Assoc* 281:1632.

Vitamin B_{12}

21. Andres, A., N. H. Loukill, E. Noel et al. 2004. Vitamin B12 (cobalamin) deficiency in elderly patients. *J Can Med Assoc* 171:251.

22. Carmel, R. 2001. Current concepts in cobalamin deficiency. *Annu Rev Med* 51:357.

23. Cashman, K. D. 2005. Homocysteine and osteoporotic fracture risk: A potential role for B vitamins. *Nutr Rev* 63:29.

24. Clarke, R., S. Lewington, P. Sherliker et al. 2007. Effects of B Vitamins on plasma homocysteine concentrations and on risk of cardiovascular disease and dementia. *Curr Opin Clin Nutr Metab Care* 10:32.

25. Cooper, B. A., and D. S. Rosenblatt. 1987. Inherited defects of vitamin B_{12} metabolism. *Annu Rev Nutr* 7:291.

26. Glusker, J. P. 1995. Vitamin B_{12} and the B_{12} coenzymes. *Vitam Horm* 50:1.

27. Leibovitch, J., S. Kurtz, G. Shemesh et al. 2003. Hyperhomocysteinemia in pseudoexfoliation glaucoma. *J Glaucoma* 12:36.

28. Lonn, E., S. Yusul, M. J. Arnold et al. 2006. Homocysteine-lowering with folic acid and B vitamins in vascular disease. *N Engl J Med* 354:1567.

29. Loscalzo, J. 2006. Homocysteine trials: Clear outcomes for complex reasons. *N Engl J Med* 354:1627.

30. Malinow, M. R. 1996. Plasma homocyst(e)ine: A risk factor for arterial occlusive diseases. *J Nutr* 126:1238S.

31. Metz, J. 1992. Cobalamin deficiency and the pathogenesis of nervous system disease. *Annu Rev Nutr* 12:59.

32. Miller, J. W. 1998. Vitamin B_{12} deficiency, tumor necrosis factor-α and epidermal growth factor: A novel function for vitamin B_{12}. *Nutr Rev* 56:236.

33. Scott, J. M., J. J. Dinn, P. Wilson, and D. G. Weir. 1981. The methyl-folate trap and the supply of *S*-adenosyl methionine. *Lancet* 2:755.

34. Selzer, R. R., D. S. Rosenblatt, R. Laxova, and K. Hogan. 2003. Adverse effect of nitrous oxide in a child with 5, 10-methylenetetrahydrofolate reductase deficiency. *N Engl J Med* 349:45.

35. Woodson, R. D., ed. 1990. Symposium on new frontiers in vitamin B_{12} metabolism. *Am J Hematol* 34:81.

36. Wu, K., K. J. Helzlsouer, G. W. Comstock, S. C. Hoffman, M. R. Nadeau, and J. A. Selhub. 1999. A prospective study on folate, B_{12}, and pyridoxal 5-phosphate (B_6) and breast cancer. *Cancer Epidemiol Biomarkers Prev* 8:209.

Pyridoxine

37. Angley, S., S. Semple, C. Hewton et al. 2007. Children and autism—part 2—management with complementary medicines and dietary interventions. *Aust Fam Physician* 36:827.

38. Balk, E. M., G. Raman, A. Tatsioni et al. 2007. Vitamin B_6, B_{12} and folic acid supplementation and cognitive function: A systematic review of randomized trials. *Arch Int Med* 167:21.

39. Bossier, K. H. 1988. Megavitamin therapy with pyridoxine. *Int J Vitam Nutr Res* 58:105.

40. Combs, G. F. 2008. *The Vitamins: Fundamental Aspects in Nutrition and Health*. San Diego: Elsevier.

41. Dakshinamurti, K., ed. 1990. Vitamin B6. *Ann N Y Acad Sci* 585:1.

42. Leklem, J. E. 1990. Vitamin B6: A status report. *J Nutr* 120:1503.

43. Leklem, J. E., and R. D. Reynolds, eds. 1988. *Clinical and Physiological Applications of Vitamin B6*. New York: Alan R. Liss.

44. Mausain-Bosc, M., M. Roche, A. Polge et al. 2006. Improvements of neurobehavioral disorders in children supplemented with magnesium-vitamin B$_6$: Attention deficit hyperactivity disorders. *Magnes Res* 19:46.
45. Vanderlind, R. E. 1986. Review of pyridoxal phosphate and the transaminases in liver disease. *Ann Clin Lab Sci* 16:79.
46. Williams, A. L., A. Cotter, A. Sabina et al. 2005. The role for vitamin B$_6$ as treatment for depression: A systematic review. *Fam Pract* 22:532.

Vitamin C—Ascorbic Acid

47. Block, G. 1991. Vitamin C and cancer prevention: The epidemiological evidence. *Am J Clin Nutr* 53:270S.
48. Feiz, H. R., and S. Mobarhan. 2002. Does vitamin C intake slow the progression of gastric cancer in *Helicobacter pylori*-infected populations? *Nutr Rev* 60:34.
49. Gershoff, S. N. 1993. Vitamin C (ascorbic acid): New roles, new requirements? *Nutr Rev* 51:313.
50. Hampl, J. S., C. A. Taylor, and C. S. Johnston. 2004. Vitamin C deficiency and depletion in the United States: The Third National Health and Nutrition Examination Survey, 1988 to 1994. *Amer J Public Health* 94(5):870.
51. Hemila, H. 1992. Vitamin C and the common cold. *Br J Nutr* 67:3.
52. Levi, F., C. Pache, F. Lucchini, and C. L. Vecchia. 2000. Selected micronutrients and colorectal cancer: A case control study from the Canton of Vand, Switzerland. *Eur J Cancer* 36:2115.
53. Montel-Hagen, A., S. Kinet, N. Manel et al. 2008. Erythrocyte glut1 triggers dehydroascorbic acid uptake in mammals unable to synthesize vitamin C. *Cell* 132:921.
54. Olmedo, J. M., J. A. Yiannias, E. B. Windgassen, and M. K. Gomet. 2006. Scurvy: A disease almost forgotten. *Int J Dermatol* 45:909.
55. Sasazuki, S., S. Sasaki, Y. Tsubono et al. 2006. Effect of vitamin C on common cold: randomized controlled trial. *Eur J Clin Nutr* 60:9.
56. Sauberlich, H. E. 1995. Pharmacology of vitamin C. *Annu Rev Nutr* 14:37.
57. Velandia, B., R. M. Centor, V. McDonnell, and M. Shah. 2008. Scurvy is still present in developed countries. *J Gen Intern Med* 23:1281.
58. Wittes, R. E. 1985. Vitamin C and cancer. *N Engl J Med* 312:178.

CASE BIBLIOGRAPHY

59. Podell, R. N. 1985. Nutritional supplementation with megadoses of vitamin B$_6$. Effective therapy, placebo, or potentiator of neuropathy? *Postgrad Med* 77(3):113.
60. Rudman, D., and P. J. Williams. 1983. Megadose vitamins. Use and misuse. *N Engl J Med* 309:488.
61. Schaumburg, H., J. Kaplan, A. Windebank, N. Vick, S. Rasmus, D. Pleasure, and M. J. Brown. 1983. Sensory neuropathy from pyridoxine abuse: A new megavitamin syndrome. *N Engl J Med* 309:445.

11 Vitamin-Like Substances

In addition to the nutrients that have been definitely established as vitamins, there are several other substances that have some properties of vitamins but do not meet all the criteria to be classified as vitamins. Some are present in much larger amounts than the vitamins, some are synthesized endogenously in adequate amounts to meet the needs of the body, and for some it has not been possible to determine any essential biological role in humans. These substances may be considered "conditional" vitamins in that they may be required by humans under special conditions, they may be taken by some individuals in supplemental or pharmacological form, or they may be essential to other animals. These vitamin-like substances include choline, carnitine, bioflavonoids, lipoic acid, coenzyme Q, inositol, and *p*-aminobenzoic acid (PABA). A brief description of each of these substances follows.

11.1 CHOLINE

In 1849, Strecker, a German chemist, isolated a compound from hog bile to which he subsequently gave the name choline (from the Greek word "chole," meaning bile). It was synthesized in 1867, and its structure was established, but the compound did not attract the attention of nutritionists and biochemists at that time. In 1932, Best and his associates in Toronto observed that pancreatectomized dogs that were maintained on insulin developed fatty livers. Feeding fresh beef pancreas or egg yolk, however, cured the fatty liver, and the effective agent (or one of the effective agents) was choline present in the pancreas and egg yolk. Subsequently, other investigators reported that choline was essential for the growth of young rats, thereby indicating its vitamin-like nature.

Choline is a relatively simple molecule containing three methyl groups. It has the following structure:

$$H_3C - \underset{\underset{CH_3}{|}}{\overset{\overset{CH_3}{|}}{N}} - CH_2CH_2OH$$

It is a colorless, bitter-tasting, water-soluble substance that absorbs water rapidly and reacts with acids to form stable crystalline salts such as choline chloride and choline bitartarate. Choline is widely distributed in foods and is present in relatively large amounts in most foods. The richest sources are egg yolk and liver; other good sources include soybeans, potatoes, cabbage, wheat and rice bran, and whole grains (e.g., barley, com, oats, rice, wheat, sorghum). Fruits and fruit juices have negligible amounts of choline.

The most abundant choline-containing compound in the diet is lecithin. Less than 10% of choline is present either as a free base or as sphingomyelin. Both pancreatic secretions and intestinal mucosal cells are capable of hydrolyzing lecithin to glycerophosphoryl choline or lysolecithin, which, after absorption, passes to the liver to liberate choline or goes to peripheral tissues via the intestinal lymphatics. Only about 33% of free choline, especially in large doses, is fully absorbed. About 67% is metabolized to trimethylamine by the intestinal microorganisms and is either eliminated in the stool, or, after absorption, is excreted in the urine. Trimethylamine has a fishy odor. When large amounts of choline are consumed, the individual may suffer from a fishy body odor. Plasma choline increases after the ingestion of lecithin. Choline is stored as lecithin and sphingomyelin in organs such as the liver, kidneys, and brain.

Choline has several functions in the body. As a component of phospholipids (primarily lecithin), it affects the mobilization of fat from the liver (lipotropic action). In the liver, choline is incorporated into lecithin, and during this process fatty acids are removed from the glycerides of the liver, resulting in a decrease of triglyceride content. Choline is a constituent of the abundant plasmalogens in the mitochondria and in the sphingomyelin of the brain. Choline thus provides an essential structural component of many biological membranes and also of plasma lipoproteins. It has a role in nerve transmission as a constituent of acetyl choline. It is part of a platelet-activating factor, which functions in inflammatory and other processes. Choline via its metabolite, betaine, can donate methyl groups that are necessary for the synthesis of other biologically important compounds. As part of phospholipids, it participates in signal transduction—an essential process for cell growth, regulation, and function. Betaine is the source of methyl groups required for methylating reactions. Methyl groups from betaine may be used to convert homocysteine to methionine. Betaine cannot be converted back to choline. Thus, the oxidation of choline to betaine diminishes the availability of choline to tissues. In the liver, fat and cholesterol are packaged into very low-density lipoprotein (VLDL) for transport through the blood to tissues. Phosphatidyl choline is a required component of VLDL particles; without adequate phosphatidyl choline, fat and cholesterol accumulate in the liver.

Fatty liver, hemorrhagic kidneys, and poor growth are the common deficiency symptoms in animals. Because low-density lipoprotein (LDL) is formed from VLDL, choline-deficient individuals also have reduced levels of LDL cholesterol. A recent study has shown that a newborn's risk for neural tube defects (NTDs) rises if the mother has low blood level of choline during pregnancy. NTDs have become less common since the 1996 decision in the United States to fortify the food supply with folic acid, which is known to prevent the defect; but NTDs have not disappeared.[22] About 500 pregnancies per year are affected by NTDs in California alone. The study targeted a group of nutrients suspected to promote brain and spinal-cord development. In early pregnancy, a sealed tube forms along the embryo's back that later grows into the brain and spinal cord. NTDs occur if the tube does not seal correctly. Researchers measured blood levels of 13 nutrients in two groups of women who participated in California's prenatal birth-defect screening program.

Of 18,000 pregnant women screened between 2003 and 2006, the researchers identified 80 whose pregnancies were affected by NTDs. Their blood samples were compared to 405 samples randomly selected from among the women whose infants had no structural birth defects. Choline was the only nutrient whose blood levels were linked to the risk of NTDs.[23] As blood choline levels went up, risk of NTDs went down. The risk for NTDs was 2.4 times higher in women with the lowest blood choline levels compared to women with average blood choline levels. The highest blood choline levels were associated with the lowest risk. The blood samples were obtained between the 15th and 18th week of pregnancy well after the formation of the neural tube, which seals around the sixth week of pregnancy. More studies are needed to examine blood samples in early pregnancy. There is also a need to test whether choline supplements given in early pregnancy reduce the rates of NTDs. At this time, multivitamin supplements contain no choline. In humans, the need for choline is met from dietary sources as well as endogenous synthesis. It is biosynthesized from serine, provided that methionine is present to supply the methyl groups, or by a series of reactions requiring vitamin B_{12} and folic acid as cofactors. Thus, an adequate supply of methyl group donors in the diet is required to protect against the accumulation of lipid in the liver. Premenopausal women may be resistant to choline deficiency because estrogen induces endogenous synthesis of choline. There are a small number of genetic polymorphisms that predict the risk for developing symptoms of liver dysfunction when deprived of dietary choline.

Studies in patients receiving long-term total parenteral nutrition have shown that low levels of choline are common and can be associated with hepatic steatosis. The treatment of these patients with an oral administration of choline improved plasma levels and decreased hepatic fat content. Recent evidence suggests a link among choline deficit and lecithin availability, neural membrane defects, and amyloid deposition associated with the progression of Alzheimer's disease. Choline appears to be a "conditionally essential" nutrient.

Choline is used in the treatment of alcohol-related or protein deficiency–induced fatty liver but without demonstrable benefits, whereas pharmacological doses seem to alleviate symptoms of tardive dyskinesia, Huntington's disease, and other neurological disorders. There is little evidence to suggest that the administration of choline cures fatty liver, cirrhosis, or other defects that resemble those associated with choline deficiency.

Due to its role in lipid metabolism, choline has also found its way into nutritional supplements which claim to reduce body fat, but there is no evidence to prove that it has any effect on reducing excess body fat or that taking high amounts of choline will increase the rate at which fat is metabolized. A supplement is often taken as a form of smart drug due to the role that neurotransmitter acetylcholine plays in various cognitive systems with the brain.

Consumption of a high dose (10–15 g/day) of choline is associated with a fishy body odor, vomiting, salivation, and increased sweating. Taking large doses of choline in the form of phosphotidyl choline does not generally result in fishy body odor because its metabolism results in little trimethylamine. A dose of 3.5 g choline per day can have a slight blood pressure–lowering effect.

There is a genetic disorder in which the body is unable to metabolize trimethylamine, which is produced from choline in foods. It is an autosomal recessive disorder involving a trimethylamine oxidase deficiency. Persons with this disorder may suffer from strong fishy or otherwise unpleasant odor. They are advised to restrict intake of foods high in choline.

Food provides 600–900 mg of choline per day as a constituent of lecithin. Because of the large amount present in a variety of foods, it is difficult to consume a diet deficient in choline, and deficiency syndrome in humans has not yet been identified. Based on the limited human data that is currently available, the Food and Nutrition Board of the Institute of Medicine set an adequate intake level for choline at 550 mg/day for men and 425 mg/day for women. The tolerable upper limit level for choline is set at 3.5 g/day for adults. This recommendation is based primarily on preventing hypotension and secondarily for preventing fishy body odor. The Food and Drug Administration requires that infant formulas not made from cow's milk be supplemented with choline. The amount of choline utilized by humans is much larger than the catalytic amounts of vitamins required in metabolic reactions. Therefore, choline is not considered to be a vitamin for men.

11.2 CARNITINE

Carnitine was discovered in 1905 as a minor nitrogenous constituent of muscle, and its structure was established in 1927, but it received little attention for the next several years. Frankel, in 1947, while investigating the role of folic acid in the nutrition of insects found that the meal worm (*Tenebrio molitor*) required a growth factor that was present in yeast, thus implying that it had an important physiological function. This factor was named vitamin B_T—"vitamin B" because of its water solubility and "T" for *Tenebrio*; however, because it was not recognized as a vitamin, the name was changed to carnitine. Subsequent studies showed that carnitine-deficient larvae died "fat" when they were starved; that is, they were unable to utilize their fat stores in order to survive. The interest in the role of carnitine increased in 1955 when Friedman and Frankel discovered that it can be reversibly acetylated by acetyl coenzyme A (CoA) and when Fritz showed that it stimulated fatty acid oxidation in liver homogenates.

Carnitine has the following structural formula:

$$(H_3C)_3N - CH_2 \underset{\underset{OH}{|}}{-} CH - CH_2 - COOH$$

It is a very hygroscopic compound that is easily soluble in water and alcohol. In general, carnitine content is high in foods of animal origin and low in plant foods. Meat and dairy products are the major sources of carnitine in the diet; other good sources include asparagus and wheat germ. Cereals, fruits, and other vegetables contain little carnitine.

Like the water-soluble vitamins, carnitine is easily and almost completely absorbed from the intestine. It is transported into most cells by an active mechanism. There is little metabolism of carnitine. Renal handling is highly conserved in humans; at normal physiological concentrations in blood plasma, more than 90% of filtered carnitine is reabsorbed by the kidneys and what is excreted in the urine is mostly as acyl carnitines.

Carnitine has an important role in the β-oxidation of long-chain fatty acids.[14] The first step in the oxidation of a fatty acid is its activation to fatty acyl CoA. This reaction occurs in the endoplasmic reticulum on the outer mitochondrial membrane. The oxidation site for fatty acids is inside the inner membrane of the mitochondria, which is impermeable both to fatty acyl CoA and long-chain fatty acids. Carnitine acts as a carrier of acyl groups across the membrane (Figure 11.1).

The transport system is believed to consist of carnitine acyl transferase I (CPT1), located on the outer side of the membrane, and carnitine acyl transferase II (CPT2), located in the mitochondrial matrix and connected by a translocase. First, CPT1 catalyzes the transacylation reaction:

$$acyl\ CoA + carnitine \rightarrow acyl\ carnitine + CoA$$

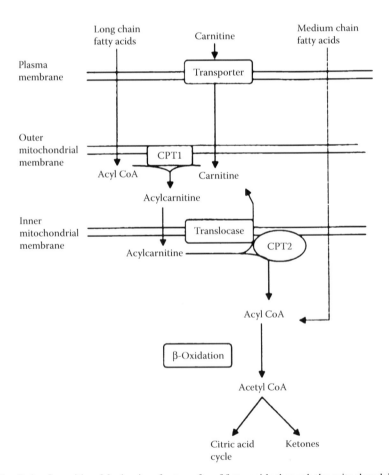

FIGURE 11.1   Role of carnitine. Mechanism for transfer of fatty acids through the mitochondrial membranes for oxidation.

Translocase transports the acyl carnitine across the inner mitochondrial membrane into the matrix and simultaneously transports free carnitine from the matrix to the cytosol. In the matrix, CPT2 resynthesizes the acyl CoA and releases carnitine:

$$\text{acyl carnitine } + \text{ CoA } \rightarrow \text{ acyl CoA } + \text{ carnitine}$$

Acyl CoA is then oxidized by β-oxidation to release energy. Medium-chain and short-chain fatty acids are activated in the mitochondrial matrix, and the oxidation of these fatty acids is independent of carnitine.

Carnitine exerts antioxidant activity, thereby providing a protective effect against lipid peroxidation of membrane phospholipids and against oxidative stress induced at the myocardial and endothelial cell level.[12]

Carnitine is an essential growth factor for some insects such as the meal worm; however, higher animals and humans appear to be able to synthesize carnitine to meet their total needs within their bodies. It is synthesized endogenously from two essential amino acids: lysine and methionine. Four micronutrients are required for the various enzymatic steps: ascorbic acid, niacin, pyridoxine, and iron. The lower level of carnitine in plant foods in comparison to animal foods can be explained on the basis that plant materials are most likely to be deficient in lysine and methionine—the precursors of carnitine. Thus, a vegetarian diet is likely to be low in both preformed carnitine and its precursor amino acids. Carnitine deficiency from inadequate dietary intake has not been reported. Patients suffering from severe protein malnutrition have been found to have significantly lowered blood levels of carnitine. As to what extent these depressed levels have significant clinical implications needs further study.

Glucose is the major fuel for the fetus. Newborn infants use glycogen stores within the first 24 hours and then must turn to fatty acids from their diet and from body fat stores. These are the preferred sources of energy for the heart through the suckling period. Newborn infants do not have the full biosynthetic capacity for carnitine, and they may be at risk for carnitine deficiency if they do not receive adequate amounts of this substance in their diet. The carnitine content of breast milk is appreciably higher than that of cow's milk; most milk formulas contain comparable levels of carnitine, except those based on soybean protein and casein hydrolysates. In general, the plasma concentration of carnitine is lower in preterm infants than normal term infants, but it is increased by feeding on milk-based formulas.

Carnitine deficiency symptoms have been reported in rare cases of inborn errors of metabolism. Primary deficiency syndromes are classified either as myopathic or systemic. Primary muscle carnitine deficiency is associated with generalized muscle weakness (usually beginning in childhood) and excess lipids in skeletal muscle fibers. The clinical features overlap with muscular dystrophy. Muscle carnitine level is low while serum carnitine level is normal. Primary systemic deficiency is associated with multiple episodes of metabolic encephalopathy, nausea, vomiting, confusion, hypoglycemia, hyperammonemia, and excess of lipids in hepatocytes during acute attacks. In this respect, it resembles Rye's syndrome. The low carnitine level in serum distinguishes it from the myopathic form. Systemic deficiency can arise from a defect in the endogenous synthesis of carnitine, absorption and/or transport, uptake by tissues, or increased excretion.

Clinical deficiency has also been recognized secondary to a variety of defects of intermediary metabolism and other disorders. Patients with inborn errors of metabolism associated with increased circulating organic acids become deficient in carnitine. This is attributed to the role of carnitine in promoting the excretion of organic acids as acyl carnitines. Some patients on long-term enteral or parenteral nutrition lacking in carnitine exhibit lower plasma carnitine levels and show symptomatic evidence of carnitine deficiency. Renal tubular disorders that involve an excessive excretion of carnitine and patients with chronic renal failure, in which hemodialysis may promote excessive loss, show signs of deficiency. Recently, levocarnitine has received approval for use in patients undergoing hemodialysis.

The administration of carnitine is beneficial in some cases of myopathic and systemic deficiency. It may also be useful in the treatment of secondary deficiencies. About 1–2 g/day appears to be adequate for most therapeutic purposes. The treatment also includes a high-carbohydrate and low-fat diet. Because the oxidation of short-chain and medium-chain fatty acids is not dependent on carnitine, these can be substituted for the long-chain triglycerides. Carnitine supplementation has been hypothesized to improve exercise performance in humans through various mechanisms.[9,10] However, experimental data suggest that carnitine supplementation does not modify performance in healthy humans. Carnitine is concentrated within the epididymis and contributes directly to the energy supply required by sperm for maturation and motility. Treatment with carnitine or acyl carnitine (1–2 g/day) increases the number and motility of sperm and the number of spontaneous pregnancies.

A decline in mitochondrial function is thought to contribute to the aging process.[2] Carnitine may be involved since its concentration in tissues declines with age and thereby reduces the integrity of mitochondrial membrane. Particularly adversely affected are bones which require the continuous reconstructive and metabolic function of osteoblasts for maintenance of bone mass. There is a close correlation between changes in plasma levels of osteocalcin and osteoblast activity, and a reduction in plasma osteocalcin level is an indicator of reduced osteoblast activity, which appears to underlie osteoporosis in elderly subjects and in postmenopausal women. Administration of carnitine increases plasma osteocalcin concentrations in animals thus treated, whereas plasma osteocalcin levels decrease with age in controlled animals.

Carnitine supplements may cause mild gastrointestinal symptoms, including nausea, vomiting, abdominal cramps, and diarrhea. But in general, carnitine appears to be well tolerated; toxic effects related to carnitine overdose have not been reported.

For normal healthy individuals, the need for carnitine is met from dietary sources and endogenous synthesis. Therefore, its deficiency is unlikely, and it should not be considered a vitamin; however, it may be a dietary essential in individuals with specific metabolic disorders.

11.3 BIOFLAVONOIDS

In 1936, Szent-Györgyi and his associates reported that extracts of red pepper and lemon juice were effective in the treatment of patients with certain pathological conditions characterized by an increased permeability and fragility of capillary walls. The crystalline material was isolated from lemon juice and was named citrin. This compound decreased tissue hemorrhages and prolonged the life of scorbutic guinea pigs; it was later found that citrin was a mixture of flavonoids. The name vitamin P was proposed for these flavone substances because of their presumed action on vascular permeability. Subsequent work showed that these substances were nonessential food factors, and the term "bioflavonoids" was given to these flavonoids exhibiting biological activity. Bioflavonoids are a large group of phenolic substances that are found in all higher plants. These include anthocyanidins (purple and dark-red pigments), flavanols such as catechin and epicatechin, flavanones, flavones, and isoflavones. They are largely responsible for the colors of many fruits and flowers.

The basic flavone structure consists of 1,4-benzopyrene with a phenyl substitution at the 2-position (Figure 11.2). The presence of a hydroxyl group in the molecule enables flavonoids to

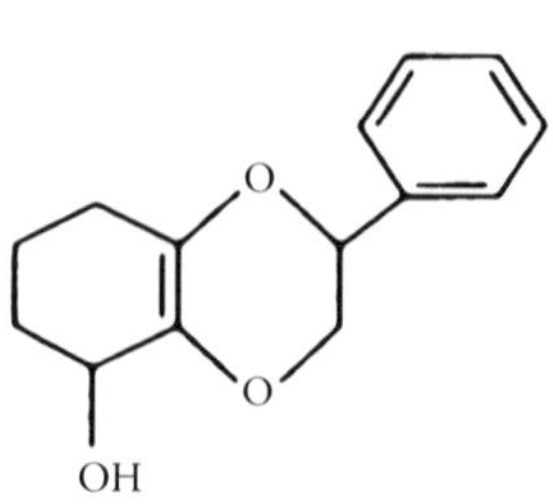

FIGURE 11.2 Bioflavonoid.

form glycosides by binding with sugars. Most naturally occurring flavonoids are present as glycosides; they can also form chelates with metals. They are brightly colored, water-soluble substances that are relatively stable and resistant to heat and—to a moderate degree—to acidity.

Bioflavonoids are present in foods of plant origin, with higher concentrations found in colored exterior tissues such as peels, skin, and the outer layer of fruits and vegetables.[4] A significant amount enters the human body in the form of beverages such as tea, coffee, cocoa, wine, and beer. Citrus fruits contain about 50–100 mg. It is estimated that our daily diet contains, on the average, about 1 g of flavonoids.

The absorption, storage, and excretion of the flavonoids are very similar to vitamin C. They are readily absorbed from the upper part of the small intestine and excess amounts are excreted in the urine.

The mechanism by which flavonoids exert their claimed influence on capillary permeability and fragility is not clear. They are active antioxidants and their biological activity may be related to their ability to protect ascorbate by functioning as antioxidants[17] by chelating divalent metal cations. Their effect on the maintenance of capillary permeability would thus be indirect via ascorbic acid. Flavonoids have been referred to as "nature's biological response modifiers" because of strong experimental evidence of their inherent ability to modify the body's reaction to allergens, viruses, and carcinogens. They show antiallergic, anti-inflammatory, antimicrobial, and anticancer activity. The beneficial effects of fruits, vegetables, tea, and wine have been attributed to flavonoid compounds, rather than to their known content of nutrients.[19] Some flavonoids inhibit aldose reductase, the enzyme involved in the formation of cataracts in diabetes and galactosemia, but there is no evidence that they actually inhibit cataract formation in humans.

Bioflavonoid deficiency has been produced in animals; it results in a syndrome characterized by increased capillary permeability and fragility. Although the deficiency syndrome has not been seen in humans, these compounds have been used clinically in the treatment of diseases in which vascular abnormality is a factor; however, there is no evidence for a requirement of flavonoids in human nutrition.

11.4 LIPOIC ACID

The continuing study of vitamin B_1 as a coenzyme in carbohydrate metabolism revealed that this metabolic system required other coenzyme factors in addition to thiamin. In a work with lactic acid bacteria, Reed discovered in 1951 that one of these factors is a fat-soluble acid, which he named "lipoic acid" (from the Greek word "lipos," meaning fat). He showed that this substance was a growth factor and that it was a requirement for pyruvate oxidation by certain microorganisms. In the same year, it was isolated in crystalline form from the water-insoluble residue of beef liver. Lipoic acid is an eight-carbon, disulfide-containing carboxylic acid and is also known as thioctic acid. Its formula is shown in Figure 11.3. It occurs in minute amounts, usually in a protein-bound form in a wide variety of foods. Yeast, liver, kidney, spinach, broccoli, brussel sprouts, and rice bran are rich sources. It is synthesized endogenously in humans from octanoic acid in mitochondria.

Lipoic acid functions in the same manner as some of the B-complex vitamins. It serves as a coenzyme for pyruvate dehydrogenase and α-ketoglutarate dehydrogenase. In these multienzyme complexes, lipoic acid is linked to the enzyme dihydrolipoyl transacetylase by an amide bond (to the e-amino group of lysine). It functions as a carrier of acyl groups, which are transferred

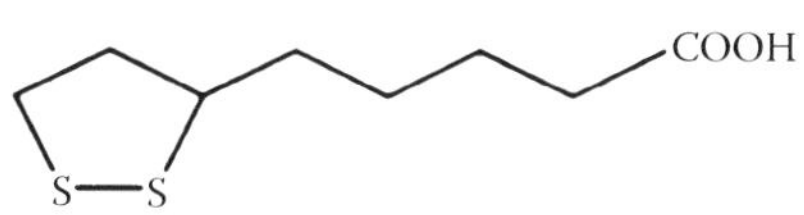

FIGURE 11.3 Lipoic acid.

from thiamin pyrophosphate derivatives. The disulfide bond is reduced and an acyl thioester linkage is formed. The lipoic acid then transfers the acyl group to the final acceptor molecule (coenzyme A). Lipoic acid also is an effective antioxidant. Lipoic acid has been shown in cell culture experiments to increase the cellular uptake of glucose by recruiting the glucose transporter GLUT 4 to the cell membrane, suggesting its use in diabetes. There is limited evidence that high doses of lipoic acid can improve glucose utilization in individuals with type 2 diabetes, but these findings are controversial because lipoic acid is found to worsen the condition in type 1 diabetes–induced[18] rats. Aging studies in rats suggest that the use of lipoic acid and acetyl carnitine results in improved memory performance and delayed structural mitochondrial decay. Thus, it may be helpful for people with Alzheimer's disease or Parkinson's disease. It reduces plasma triglyceride levels in mice.

Since the early 1990s, lipoic acid has been consumed as a dietary supplement and is available in the United States without a prescription; typical doses[11] are 100–200 mg/day. In Germany, lipoic acid is approved for the treatment of diabetic neuropathies and is available by prescription. Oral administration of lipoic acid at doses as high as 1800 mg/day for 6 months and 1200 mg/day for 2 years have resulted in no serious adverse effects when used to treat diabetic peripheral neuropathy. The most frequently reported side effects to oral lipoic acid supplementation are allergic reactions affecting the skin, including rashes.

Lipoic acid and biotin have structural similarities, and there is some evidence that high concentration of lipoic acid can compete with biotin for transport across cell membranes. Administration of high doses of lipoic acid in rats is found to decrease the activities of two biotin-dependent enzymes by about 30%. But it is not known whether lipoic acid supplementation substantially increases the requirement for biotin in humans.

Lipoic acid can be called vitamin-like for two reasons. First, it functions as a coenzyme in the oxidative decarboxylation of pyruvate and α-ketoglutarate. Second, it occurs in extraordinarily small amounts in the tissues. Unfortunately, no attempt to induce a deficiency of lipoic acid has been successful, and it has never been demonstrated to be required in the diet of humans. Humans can apparently synthesize this compound in adequate quantities.

11.5   COENZYME Q

In 1957, coenzyme Q was discovered independently by two groups of investigators. One group detected it in lipid extracts of mitochondria and gave it the name coenzyme Q when it was found to undergo reduction and reoxidation in the mitochondria. A second group found coenzyme Q in the unsaponifiable portion of tissues from vitamin A–deficient rats; they gave it the name ubiquinone because of its ubiquitous (widely distributed) appearance. The structure of coenzyme Q was determined first, and on the basis of similar properties, ubiquinone was considered to be closely related or identical (Figure 11.4).

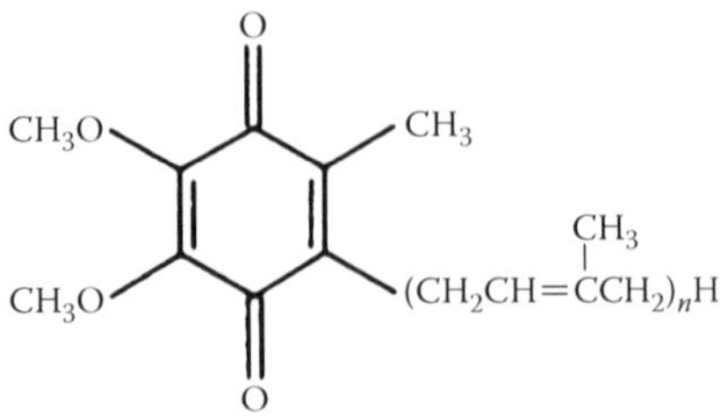

FIGURE 11.4   Coenzyme Q.

Coenzyme Q (ubiquinone) is a collective name for a group of lipid-like compounds that are chemically somewhat similar to vitamin E. These compounds have a basic quinone ring structure to which 30–50 carbon atoms are attached as isoprenoid units in the side chain in the 6-position. The number of isoprenoid units in the side chain varies from 6 to 10. The different members of the group are designated by a subscript following the letter Q to denote the number of isoprenoid units in the side chain. Human mitochondria have coenzyme Q with 10 isoprenoid units in the side chain, and it is called coenzyme Q_{10}. If the compound is expressed as ubiquinone, the number of carbon atoms in the side chain is indicated in parenthesis. Ubiquinone (30) is the same as coenzyme Q_6.

The rich food sources of coenzyme Q_{10} include meat, poultry, and fish. Other relatively rich sources are soybean and canola oils and nuts. Fruits, vegetables, eggs, and dairy products are moderate sources of coenzyme Q_{10}. The daily dietary intake is about 5–8 mg. The absorption follows the same process as that of lipids and the uptake mechanisms appear to be similar to vitamin E.

Coenzyme Q_{10} is formed in most human tissues. The quinone portion is synthesized from tyrosine, and the isoprene side chain is formed from CoA via the mevalonate pathway, and then the two structures are joined.

Coenzyme Q_{10} functions in the mitochondria as a link between various flavin-containing dehydrogenases (e.g., reduced nicotinamide adenine dinucleotide [NADH] dehydrogenase, succinate dehydrogenase, or fatty acyl CoA dehydrogenase) and cytochrome b of the electron transport chain. The quinone portion of coenzyme Q is alternately oxidized and reduced by the addition of two oxidizing/reducing equivalents (e.g., two protons, H^+, and two electrons, e^-). The isoprenoid side chains render coenzyme Q lipid-soluble and facilitate the accessibility of this electron carrier to the lipophilic portion of the inner mitochondrial membrane where the enzymatic aspects of the mitochondrial electron transport chain are localized. Coenzyme Q_{10} is a central player in the electron transport chain that delivers the electrons needed to convert the oxygen we breathe into water. It is also a powerful antioxidant.

Coenzyme Q_{10} is available as a dietary supplement. Doses for adults range from 30 to 100 mg/day, which are considerably higher than the normal dietary intake. It is recommended that the supplement be taken with a meal that contains fat to improve absorption. Coenzyme Q_{10} supplementation has garnered considerable attention in the medical community as a potential treatment for aging, heart disease, and neurodegenerative disorders such as Parkinson's disease. It has gained popularity for the prevention and treatment of various cardiac disorders. The findings that myocardial coenzyme Q_{10} levels were lower in patients with more severe versus moderate heart failure led to several clinical trials of coenzyme Q_{10} supplementation in heart failure patients. A meta-analysis of controlled clinical trials with coenzyme Q_{10} has found significant improvements in stroke volume, cardiac output, cardiac index, and end-diastolic volume in patients with heart failure, regardless of etiology (e.g., idiopathic, dilated, ischemic, hypertension, and congestive heart failure). As a supplement to conventional treatment, dosage typically used ranged from 150 to 300 mg/day. Other studies, however, have failed to show positive results. Large intervention studies are needed to determine whether coenzyme Q_{10} supplementation has value as an adjunct to conventional medical therapy in the treatment of congestive heart failure.

A 16-month, randomized controlled trial evaluated the safety and efficacy of 300, 600, and 1200 mg/day of coenzyme Q_{10} in 80 people with early Parkinson's disease. Coenzyme Q_{10} supplementation was well tolerated at all doses and was associated with slower deterioration of function in Parkinson's disease patients compared to placebo. However, the difference was statistically significant only in the group taking 1200 mg/day. The neuroprotective effects of coenzyme Q_{10} (300, 600, or 1200 mg/day) are under further investigation for a potential role in Parkinson's disease treatment, but significant benefits have not yet been demonstrated, and it is premature to make definitive recommendations.

Coenzyme Q_{10} is also being used for a variety of other conditions, including hypertension, human immunodeficiency virus, and migraine headaches. There is very little evidence to support its use for these conditions. Supplementation of coenzyme Q_{10} is a treatment for some of the very rare and serious mitochondrial disorders and other metabolic disorders where patients are not capable of producing enough coenzyme Q_{10} because of their disorders.

Coenzyme Q_{10} shares a common biosynthetic pathway with cholesterol. The synthesis of an intermediary precursor of coenzyme Q_{10}, mevalonate, is inhibited by some β blockers, blood pressure–lowering medications, and statins.[8,20] Statins that are prescribed to reduce plasma cholesterol suppress the biosynthesis of coenzyme Q_{10}. Some of the side effects of statins such as myopathies suggest generalized mitochondrial injury as a result of coenzyme Q_{10} deficiency. It is logical to consider complementing extended statins therapy with coenzyme Q_{10} to support the deficient cellular biogenetic state and ameliorate oxidative stress.

In certain laboratory animals, coenzyme Q can alleviate some symptoms of vitamin E deficiency. It appears to have beneficial effects in certain disease states such as muscular dystrophy, periodontal disease, hypertension, and congestive heart failure.[7] There have been no reports of significant adverse effects of oral coenzyme Q_{10} supplementation at doses as high as 1200 mg/day for up to 16 months. Some individuals have experienced gastrointestinal symptoms such as nausea and diarrhea and loss of appetite. Concomitant use of warfarin and coenzyme Q_{10} has been reported to decrease the anticoagulant effect of warfarin in at least 4 cases. An individual on warfarin should not take coenzyme Q_{10} supplements without consulting the health care provider that is managing the individual's anticoagulant therapy.

Coenzyme Q is found in most living cells, and it seems to be concentrated in the mitochondria. It can be synthesized in mammalian cells and, therefore, is not a true vitamin; however, the aromatic ring moiety must presumably be supplied from dietary sources.

11.6   INOSITOL

Inositol was discovered in 1850 and 75 years later, it was found to be a component of bios I, a yeast concentrate that promotes the growth of various bacteria. In 1940, Wooley, at the University of Wisconsin, described a deficiency syndrome in mice characterized by inadequate growth and alopecia that could be prevented by inositol. It was classified as a member of B complex (often referred to as vitamin B_8) but was found to be synthesized by the human body in adequate amounts (thus declassifying it as a vitamin).

Inositol is a cyclic, six-carbon compound with six hydroxyl groups; it is closely related to glucose (Figure 11.5). There are nine isomers of inositol (seven that are optically inactive and two that are optically active), but only one—designated as myo-inositol—is biologically active and of importance in animal and plant metabolism. It is an optically inactive, sweet crystalline substance that is water soluble. It is found in nature as free inositol, phytin (a mixed calcium and magnesium salt of insoluble hexaphosphate phytic acid), phosphatidyl inositol, and a water-soluble nondialyzable complex. It is widely distributed in plant and animal cells. Cereal grains are the richest sources and contain inositol as phytic acid; this can adversely affect the absorption of minerals such as calcium,

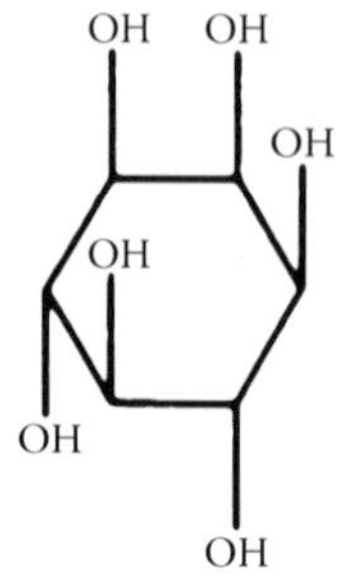

FIGURE 11.5   Inositol.

zinc, and iron by binding these metals to form salts. Other rich sources include nuts, red beans, and fruits, especially citrus fruits and cantaloupes.

D-chiro-inositol (DCI) is a member of a family of related substances often collectively referred to as "inositol." Inositol is known to be an important second messenger in insulin signal transduction.[16] It is possible that it is made in humans from myo-inositol by the action of epimerase. It is not abundant in most diets. It is found in significant quantities in buckwheat and in some other foods. It is available as a dietary supplement in the United States.

Inositol is absorbed from the small intestine, is readily metabolized to glucose, and is about 33% as effective as glucose in alleviating ketosis of starvation. In addition to food sources, it is synthesized in the cells from glucose.

The physiological role of inositol resembles to some extent that of choline.[6] It is present in the form of phosphatidyl inositol in the phospholipids of cell membranes and plasma lipoproteins. It has a lipotropic effect in preventing certain types of fatty livers from developing in experimental animals. This may be associated with the requirement of inositol to complete the assembly of fat-carrying lipoproteins in plasma.

In mice, the dietary deficiency of inositol causes a failure of growth and alopecia. There is no evidence of its requirement in humans; however, studies on the nutrient requirements of cells in tissue culture have shown that 18 different human cell lines all need myo-inositol for growth, probably because of its structural role in the formation of cell membranes. Inositol concentrations in the male and female reproductive organs are several times higher than in serum. This suggests that inositol has a certain role in reproduction.[5] It affects overall embryogenesis in several animal species and may prevent NTDs and stimulate the production of lung surfactant. Infants of diabetic mothers have an increased risk of congenital malformation, especially in the central nervous system and the heart. In vitro studies have shown that high glucose concentrations in the medium lower the inositol content in the embryo of the cultured rat conceptus and increase the sorbitol content. This may be explained by the fact that glucose competitively inhibits inositol transport into the cell, resulting in intracellular inositol depletion. A low inositol level may be a factor in diabetic pregnancy that leads to an increased incidence of dysmorphogenesis caused by the increase of sorbitol, the decrease in inositol, or both.

People suffering from clinical depression generally have decreased levels of inositol in their cerebrospinal fluid. Inositol participates in the action of serotonin, a neurotransmitter known to be a factor in depression. Neurotransmitters are chemicals that transmit messages between nerve cells. For this reason, inositol has been proposed as a treatment for depression, and preliminary evidence suggests that it may be helpful. Limited studies suggest that at doses of 12–18 g/day inositol reduces anxiety symptoms as effectively as selective serotonin reuptake inhibitors with a low incidence of side effects. Some preliminary studies on high dose supplements show promising results for people suffering from problems such as bulimia, panic disorder, obsessive-compulsive disorder, and unipolar and bipolar disorder. Other potential uses include Alzheimer's disease and attention deficit disorder.

Inositol is proposed as a treatment for diabetic neuropathy,[21] but there has been no double-blind, placebo-controlled studies on this subject, and two uncontrolled studies had mixed results. Inositol has also been investigated for potential cancer-preventive properties. DCI has been shown to influence the action of insulin in women who have insulin resistance and hyperinsulinemia due to DCI deficiency. The amount of DCI in muscle has been found to be lower in subjects with type 2 diabetes than in normal subjects. Inositol has been found in clinical trials to be an effective treatment for many of the clinical hallmarks of polycystic ovarian syndrome (PCOS) in both lean and obese women, including insulin resistance, hyperandrogenism, and oligo-amenorrhea.[15] The benefits of the drug metformin in PCOS appear at least partly due to increasing inositol[3] availability. According to some reports, inositol strengthens the cells of the hair by helping it to retain moisture. It is available as an ingredient in some shampoo formulas.

No serious adverse effects have been reported for inositol even with a dosage of 18 g/day. However, no long-term safety studies have been performed. Safety has not been established for young children, women who are pregnant or nursing, and those with severe liver or kidney disease.

There has been no deficiency of inositol reported in humans. This is probably due to the availability of inositol in the diet and its endogenous synthesis. In view of the need for inositol for growth by some human cell strains, it is possible that inositol is synthesized only by certain organs and is then made available for all cells.

11.7   *p*-AMINOBENZOIC ACID

PABA was identified as an essential nutrient for certain microorganisms; later, it was shown to be an antigray factor in rats and mice and a growth-promoting factor for chicks. In 1941, it was found that a failure of lactation occurred in rats whose diet contained all the then known B vitamins, including riboflavin, niacin, pyridoxine, pantothenic acid, and choline; this effect was reversed after the administration of PABA. It has been referred to as vitamin B_x because it serves as a provitamin for some bacteria in the intestinal tract such as *Escherichia coli*. The chemical structure of PABA is shown in Figure 11.6. It is a yellow, crystalline substance that is slightly soluble in cold water, but quite soluble in hot water. It is widely distributed in nature but is more concentrated in the liver, yeast, rice bran, whole wheat, molasses, and yogurt.

For humans and other higher animals, PABA functions as an essential part of the folic acid molecule. The suggested role is to provide this chemical for the synthesis of folic acid by those organisms that do not require a preformed source of folic acid. PABA resembles sulfanilamide and can reverse the bacteriostatic effects of sulfa drugs; this antimetabolite action is explainable on the basis of similarity of structure. Sulfonamides suppress bacterial growth by replacing PABA in the bacterial enzyme system; in excess, PABA reverses the effect. In view of the antagonism between PABA and the sulfa drugs, the continuous ingestion of extremely large doses of PABA is to be avoided. By itself, PABA is nontoxic, but the presence of a high PABA level in the blood and tissues might render sulfonamide therapy of little value. PABA is occasionally used in pill form by sufferers of irritable bowel syndrome to treat its associated gastrointestinal symptoms and for nutritional epidemiological studies to assess the completeness of the 24-hour urine collection for the determination of urinary sodium, potassium, and nitrogen levels. Despite the lack of any recognized PABA deficiency in humans, many claims are made by commercial suppliers of PABA as a nutritional supplement. Benefit is claimed for fatigue, eczema, scleroderma, and premature gray hair.

PABA is sometimes included in multivitamin preparations and adverse effects from oral doses have not been reported. It has also gained acceptance as a sunscreen, and topical preparations containing PABA are widely used. Other than being an essential component of the folic acid molecule, this compound appears to have no other function in human metabolism. It has no vitamin activity in humans who need a preformed folic acid, and thus it is not required in the diet. It is not accepted as a true vitamin, contrary to the listing in many vitamin preparations in the market.

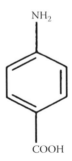

FIGURE 11.6   *p*-Aminobenzoic acid.

Jamaican Vomiting Sickness—A Case

Role of Carnitine

A 37-year-old woman of Jamaican descent was in normal health 4 hours before presenting to the hospital emergency department with excruciating headache and intractable vomiting. Earlier that day, she cooked canned ackee on low heat for 10 minutes and consumed a large portion of the fruit. About 20 minutes later, she experienced an acute onset of severe bitemporal and occipital headache and profuse vomiting. Thinking this would go away, and not associating her symptoms with ackee, she took two tablets of aspirin but had no relief. Because her symptoms persisted, she went to the hospital.

Upon arrival at the hospital, she complained of having headache, nausea, vomiting, and weakness. She also experienced slight paresthesia with numbness and tingling over her entire trunk and extremities. Her medical history was unremarkable with no medications or drug allergies. On examination, her blood pressure was 135/70 mm Hg, pulse was 85/minute and regular, and temperature was 98 F; she was alert and oriented to person, place, and time. Laboratory studies revealed low blood glucose and electrolyte imbalance, especially hypokalemia. She was lavaged with 3 L of saline and received 50 g of activated charcoal; there was an immediate relief of her vomiting. Intervention for the patient included an initiation of an intravenous line and correction of hypokalemia and glucose. The patient was discharged in 2 days.

Ackee fruit is indigenous to West Africa and Jamaica. The fruit is pear-shaped and yellowish–red in color. When ripe, the fruit splits open longitudinally and only then is it potentially edible. Unripe ackee contains hypoglycin, which is converted in the body to methylenecyclopropyl acetic acid (MCPA). Both hypoglycin and MCPA exert toxic effects. In unripe ackee, hypoglycin is found in the arillus that surrounds the seeds of the fruit. During ripening, most of the hypoglycin is translocated into the seeds. Toxicity may occur when unripe ackee is consumed because it is the arillus that is cooked and eaten.

MCPA inactivates several enzymes involved in catabolism (e.g., general acyl CoA dehydrogenase and butyryl CoA dehydrogenase, valeryl CoA dehydrogenase, and glutaryl CoA dehydrogenase). The inhibition of acyl CoA derivatives results in an accumulation of these carboxylic acids and the diagnosis of Jamaican Vomiting Sickness.[26]

Isovaleryl CoA is formed from leucine catabolism (Figure 11.7), and glutaric acid is an intermediate in the catabolism of lysine and tryptophan. Isovaleric acid is neurotoxic and causes depression, vomiting, and ataxia. Isovaleric acid and other organic acids have an affinity

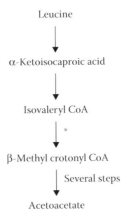

FIGURE 11.7 Leucine catabolism. * Isovaleryl CoA dehydrogenase. This enzyme is inhibited by methylene-cyclopropyl acetic acid.

for carnitine and are excreted in the urine as acyl carnitine. In the liver, hypoglycin forms nonmetabolizable esters with CoA and carnitine, depleting CoA and carnitine, thereby inhibiting fatty acid oxidation. The transport of long-chain fatty acids into the mitochondrial matrix for β-oxidations requires carnitine. A deficiency of carnitine causes an inhibition of fatty acid oxidation. There is a corresponding decrease in adenosine triphosphate (ATP) production and an inhibition of gluconeogenesis.

Normally, β-oxidation of fatty acids stimulates gluconeogenesis by providing ATP, NADH, and acetyl CoA, the latter functioning as an allosteric effector of pyruvate carboxylase. The competitive inhibition of the activation of pyruvate carboxylase by the increased concentrations of isovaleryl CoA and glutaryl CoA appears to be the principal mechanism by which toxicity is exerted.

Recently, there was an outbreak of endemic fatal encephalopathy in preschool children at Burkina Faso, West Africa, as a result of the consumption of unripe ackee fruit.[27] Fatal ackee poisoning occurs more often in children than in adults, who more commonly present with a chronic disease characterized by a self-revolving cholestatic jaundice. Pathologically, liver damage in Jamaican Vomiting Sickness and hypoglycemic syndrome is indistinguishable from that of Rye's syndrome. Experimental studies in rats show resistance to hypoglycin toxicity if animals are coadministered glycine, suggesting a possible directed therapy. As yet, no direct evidence exists for the use of glycine for Jamaican vomiting sickness in human beings.

REFERENCES

1. Agarwal, A., K. P. Nallella, S. S. Allamaneni, and T. M. Said. 2004. Role of antioxidants in treatment of male infertility: An overview of the literature. *Reprod Biomed Online* 8:616.
2. Ames, B. N., and J. Liu. 2004. Delaying the mitochondrial decay of aging with acylcarnitine. *Ann N Y Acad Sci* 1033:108.
3. Baillargeon, J. P., D. J. Jakubovicz, and M. J. Iuorno. 2004. Effects of metformin and rosiglitazone, alone and in combination, in nonobese women with polycystic ovary syndrome and normal indices of insulin sensitivity. *Fertil Steril* 82:893.
4. Beecher, G. R. 2003. Overview of dietary flavonoids: Nomenclature, occurrence and intake. *J Nutr* 133:324s.
5. Beemster, P., P. Groenen, and R. Steegers-Theunissen. 2002. Involvement of inositol in reproduction. *Nutr Rev* 60:80.
6. Berdanier, C. D. 1992. Is inositol an essential nutrient? *Nutr Today* 27(2):22.
7. Bhagavan, H. N., and R. K. Chopra. 2005. Potential role of ubiquinone (coenzyme Q_{10}) in pediatric cardiomyopathy. *Clin Nutr* 24:331.
8. Bliznakov, E. G. 2002. Coenzyme Q_{10}, lipid-lowering drugs (statins) and cholesterol: A present day pandora's box. *J Am Nutr Assoc* 5:32.
9. Brass, E. P. 2000. Supplemental carnitine and exercise. *Am J Clin Nutr* 72:618S.
10. Brass, E. P., and W. R. Hiatt. 1998. The role of carnitine and carnitine supplementation during exercise in man and individuals with special needs. *J Am Coll Nutr* 17(3):207.
11. Butler, J. A., T. M. Hagen, and R. Moreau. 2009. Lipoic acid improves hypertriglyceridemia clearance by stimulating triacylglycerol clearance and downregulating liver triacylglycerol secretion. *Arch Biochem Biophys* 485:63.
12. Calo, L. A., E. Pagnin, P. A. Davis et al. 2006. Antioxidant effect of L-carnitine and its short chain esters: Relevance for the protection from oxidative stress-related cardiovascular damage. *Int J Cardiol* 107:54.
13. Fischer, L. M., K. A. daCosta, L. Kwock et al. 2007. Sex and menopausal status influence human dietary requirements for the nutrient choline. *Am J Clin Nutr* 85:1275.
14. Foster, D. W. 2004. The role of the carnitine system in human metabolism. *Ann N Y Acad Sci* 1033:1.
15. Gerli, S., E. Papaleo, A. Ferrari et al. 2007. Randomized double-blind, placebo-controlled trial: Effects of myoinositol on ovarian function and metabolic factors in women with PCOS. *Eur Rev Med Pharmacol Sci* 11:347.

16. Lamar, J. 2002. D-chiro-inositol—its functional role in insulin action and its deficit in insulin resistance. *Int J Exp Diabetes Res* 3:47.
17. Lotito, S. B., and B. Frei. 2006. Consumption of flavonoid-rich foods and increased plasma antioxidant capacity in humans: Cause, consequence, or epiphenomenon? *Free Radic Biol Med* 41:1727.
18. Luz, J., J. C. Zemdegs, and L. S. Amaral. 2009. Chronic lipoic acid treatment worsens energy imbalance in streptozotocin-induced diabetic rats. *Diabetes Metab* 35(2):137.
19. Mink, P. J., C. G. Scrafford, L. M. Barraj et al. 2007. Dietary intakes of flavonols and flavones and coronary heart disease in U.S. women. *Am J Epidemiol* 165:1305.
20. Nawarskas, J. J. 2005. HMG-CoA reductase inhibitors and coenzyme Q_{10}. *Cardiol Rev* 13:76.
21. Packer, L., K. Kraemer, and G. Rimbach. 2001. Molecular aspects of lipoic acid in the prevention of diabetic complications. *Nutrition* 17:888.
22. Pitkin, R. M. 2007. Folate and neural tube defects. *Am J Clin Nutr* 85:285s.
23. Shaw, G. M., R. H. Finnell, H. J. Blom et al. 2009. Choline and risk of neural tube defects in a folate-fortified population. *Epidemiology* 20:714.
24. Sinclair, S. 2000. Male infertility: Nutritional and environmental considerations. *Alt Med Rev* 5:28.
25. Sucherowsky, O., G. Gronseth, J. Perlmutter et al. 2006. Practice parameter: Neuroprotective strategies and alternative therapies for Parkinson's disease (an evidence-based review): Report of the Quality Standards Subcommittee of the American Academy of Neurology. *Neurology* 66:976.
26. Zeisel, S. H., K. DaCosta, P. D. Franklin et al. 1991. Choline, an essential nutrient for humans. *FASEB J* 5:2093.

CASE BIBLIOGRAPHY

27. McTague, J. A., and R. Forney Jr. 1994. Jamaican vomiting sickness in Toledo, OH. *Ann Emerg Med* 63:1116.
28. Meda, H. A., B. Diallo, J. Buchet, D. Lison, H. Barennes, A. Ouangre, M. Sanou, S. Cousens, F. Tall, and P. Van de Perre. 1999. Epidemic of fatal encephalopathy in preschool children in Burkina Faso and consumption of unripe ackee (*Bligia Sápida*) fruit. *Lancet* 353:536.

Part II

Special Nutritional Needs

12 Nutritional Aspects of Pregnancy and Lactation

In adolescence, the human female experiences a surge in physical and physiological development that is more pronounced than in any other single period in her life. An optimal amount of body weight for height is apparently needed for normal ovulation and is therefore dependent on adequate nutrition. The growth of the fetus during pregnancy and the secretion of milk during lactation are nutrient-requiring processes. Thus, the mother's nutrition prior to pregnancy, during pregnancy, and during lactation has a strong impact on the pregnancy outcome and on the health of both the mother and the child.

12.1 NUTRITION PRIOR TO PREGNANCY

Malnutrition can impair the function of the human reproductive process. Pregnancy is possible when the normal process of ovulation and menstruation is functional. Recent observations suggest that body fat of at least 17% of body weight is required for menarche and about 22% of body weight as fat is necessary for maintaining a normal menstrual cycle. This minimal amount of fat is required apparently to maintain the normal levels of estrogen. The adipose tissue is known to convert androgen to estrogen, and it is estimated that this tissue provides roughly 33% of the estrogen that circulates in the blood of premenopausal women; it is also the main source of estrogen in postmenopausal women. Estrogen modulates the hormonal secretions of the pituitary, leading to a midcycle surge of luteinizing hormone and to ovulation (Figure 12.1). Gonadotropin-releasing hormone (GRH), which is secreted in pulses, controls the chain of events leading to ovulation. Its secretion depends on optimal estrogen level. In underweight or excessively lean women, the estrogen level is low. Therefore, the pattern of secretion of GRH is abnormal in amounts and timing and is similar to that of prepubertal girls. As a result, the cascade of events that normally leads to ovulation and prepares the uterus to support pregnancy is disrupted.

In mature women, GRH pulses stimulate the pituitary gland to release follicle-stimulating hormone. This hormone controls the growth of an ovarian follicle and luteinizing hormone, which controls the cyclical release of the egg from the follicle. When these hormones are low, ovulation cannot occur. The growing follicle normally releases estrogen, which modulates the hormonal secretions of the pituitary, and hence the ovulation. Estrogen also stimulates the growth of the uterine lining. After ovulation, the follicle becomes the corpus luteum (yellow body) and secretes progesterone, which increases the vascularity of the uterine lining in preparation for implantation of the fertilized egg. Progesterone also contributes to the development of the conceptus even before implantation because it specifically increases secretions of the fallopian tubes and uterus to provide appropriate nutritive matter for the developing conceptus. If no egg is implanted, the levels of progesterone and estrogen fall and the monthly flow of blood ensues. Thus, chronic dieting on very low–calorie diets may affect the level of hormones and may cause infertility in some women of reproductive age. In addition, other dietary factors can affect hormone levels. Some women who are infertile have a diet very high in carotenes or use tanning pills containing carotenes. Chronic exposure to low levels of lead appears to impair fertility by interfering with ovarian function. It suppresses the secretion of progesterone that is necessary for successful pregnancy and that is particularly crucial for implantation of the embryo in the uterus. New research[16] suggests that progesterone may also guide the

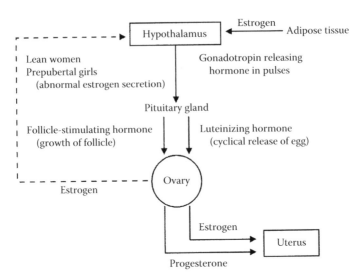

FIGURE 12.1 The role of estrogen in ovulation.

sperm toward the egg, as well as give it a final push to get there. The hormone makes calcium ions rush into human sperm by opening a pH-sensitive calcium channel called CatSper, which resides on sperm tail membranes. This finding could be used to design a new class of contraceptive drug. Body weight for men and women also matters for conception. One study has found that sperm count and sperm concentration are about 28.1% and 36.4% lower, respectively, in underweight men. The same measures are found to be 21.6% and 23.9% lower, respectively, in overweight men. Severe obese women show significantly reduced implantation and pregnancy rates. Women who are obese before pregnancy also face a higher risk of having babies with a variety of birth defects than do women with healthy weights, according to a study involving nearly 15,000 women from eight U.S. states. The abnormalities found were of the spine, heart, arms, legs, and abdomen. However, the absolute risk of having a birth defect is low, and the cause of the majority of birth defects is unknown. So, obese women should not be overly alarmed by these findings. Still the results underlie yet another reason for women to maintain a healthy weight.

Smoking is associated with a dose-related reduction in fertility and early menopause. Deficiency of nutrients such as vitamin B_6 and folic acid may develop as a result of the use of oral contraceptives.

New research suggests that a baby's sex is linked to his or her mother's diet at around the time of conception; a high-calorie diet at this time—and regular breakfast—might increase the odds of a boy. These findings might explain why the proportion of boys is lower in the developed countries.

A healthy pregnancy begins even before conception. The American College of Obstetricians and Gynecologists recommends educating patients about risk factors for bad pregnancy outcomes, such as use of alcohol or antiepileptic drugs. The Centers for Disease Control and Prevention (CDC) is attempting to standardize preconception care by more doctors, social workers, and nurses—and bring it more proactively into women's lives. CDC issued guidelines in April 2006 encouraging doctors of all specialties to ask women about their reproductive plans and consider all treatments, procedures, and medication in terms of what impact they would have on a possible pregnancy.

Many women and their doctors already work together to prepare for pregnancy. Women trying to have a baby often take precautions such as stopping smoking and drinking, losing weight, and ensuring that chronic problems such as asthma or diabetes are under control. Since studies showed that taking folic acid supplements before conception reduces the risk for having babies with neural tube defects (NTDs), some women who are trying to get pregnant do incorporate it into their routine.

Several doctors say that the most effective place to start would be a specific preconception visit to prepare for pregnancy a couple of months ahead. Preconception care is rarely covered by health insurance. But one major stumbling block is unplanned pregnancies. A study of 2001 birth data published in May 2006 in *Perspectives on Sexual and Reproductive Health* estimates that half of all pregnancies in the United States are unplanned, with about a quarter of pregnancies in college graduates coming as a surprise. These women may not see a doctor until 12 weeks or more after conceiving when the fetus's major organs have been formed, along with any birth defects.

12.2   NUTRITION DURING PREGNANCY

The fact that a woman's nutritional status can support fertility does not necessarily mean that it can support pregnancy. Many women conceive while consuming a nutritionally inadequate diet, but the incidence of low birth weight (LBW) and prematurity in their newborns is generally higher than those in normal-weight individuals. Underweight women also seem to have more pregnancy complications such as cardiovascular and respiratory problems.

12.2.1   LENGTH OF PREGNANCY AND BIRTH WEIGHT

The length of a normal pregnancy or gestation is considered to be 40 weeks (280 days) from the date of conception. Those born between 37 weeks and 41 weeks of pregnancy are called full-term babies. Infants born before 37 weeks of gestation are considered premature (preterm) babies. In the United States, about 12.8% of the babies (more than half a million a year) are born prematurely. This is an increase of 36% since the early 1980s.

Relatively little is known about the causes for the increase in preterm births. Variables such as an increase in the number of older women having babies and reproductive techniques that make multiple births more likely are probably contributing to the trend. Black women also have a 50% higher rate of preterm delivery than whites. More than 70% of premature babies are born between 34 and 37 weeks of gestation. These are called late preterm babies. About 12% of the premature babies are born between 32 and 33 weeks of gestation, 10% between 28 and 31 weeks, and 6% at less than 28 weeks of gestation. In many developed countries, the preterm birth rate is 5%–9%.

The majority of preterm children end up healthy. But many premature infants are at increased risk for short- and long-term health complications, including jaundice, respiratory problems, infections, disabilities, and impediments in growth and mental development. The earlier the babies are born, the greater their risk of health problems. Around the world, about 12.9 million babies are born too early each year, representing 9.6% of births. Of 4 million deaths that occur soon after birth, 28% are attributed to prematurity.

Typically, infant birth weight has been used as an indicator of a successful pregnancy. The average birth weight of a full-term baby is approximately 7.5 pounds but is typically in the range of 5.5–8.5 pounds. Babies weighing less than 5.5 pounds are considered LBW infants. About 8% of the babies born in the United States are LBW infants. The overall rate of these small babies is increasing in the United States. This may, in part, be due to the greater number of multiple births (twins, triplets, etc.) born early and weighing less. Birth weight generally correlates to gestational age; however, infants may be underweight for other reasons (malnutrition, other factors) than a preterm delivery. Very low birth weight (VLBW) is less than 1500 g, and extremely low birth weight (ELBW) is less than 1000 g. Almost all neonates in these two groups are born preterm.

12.2.2   PHYSIOLOGY

Conception begins with the fertilization of an ovum. The time after conception is the fertilization age. The gestational age is the time from the start of the last menstrual period and generally exceeds the developmental age by 2 weeks. The due date is typically calculated as 40 weeks from the date of the start of the last menstrual cycle (roughly 10–14 days before the date of conception). Pregnancy is divided into three trimesters, approximately 13–14 weeks each.

The newly fertilized ovum begins as a single cell with the combination of the nuclei of the sperm and egg and with the full human chromosome number 46. This new cell, called a zygote, can divide and grow into an individual. A series of divisions known as cleavage converts the zygote into a large number of cells. After four cleavages, the 16 cells appear as a solid ball or morula. The conceptus is slowly being transported into the uterine cavity as a result of the tubular muscular movements. With continued divisions, the cells form a hollow fluid-filled sphere—the blastocyst. The journey to the uterus takes about 3 days, and the developing blastocyst remains in the uterine cavity for an additional 1–3 days before it implants in the endometrium. Thus, implantation usually occurs on or about the fifth to seventh day after ovulation. Up until now, the developing conceptus is nourished by the secretions of the tube and the uterus, but its further growth requires more food and oxygen. The outer cell mass of the blastocyst differentiates into trophoblasts, while the inner cell mass gives rise to the embryo. Implantation results from the action of trophoblast cells. These cells secrete proteolytic enzymes that digest and liquefy the adjacent cells of the endometrium. The fluid and nutrients thus released are actively transported by the same trophoblast cells into the blastocyst, adding still further sustenance for growth. The blastocyst adheres to the endometrial epithelium where it undergoes implantation. The outer cell mass, or trophoblast, invades the endometrium, and the blastocyst becomes completely buried within the endometrium. Once implantation has taken place, the trophoblast cells and other adjacent cells both from the blastocyst and from the uterine endometrium proliferate rapidly, forming the placenta and the various membranes of pregnancy.

Progesterone secreted by the corpus luteum has a special effect on the endometrium to convert the endometrial stromal cells into large swollen cells that contain extra quantities of glycogen, proteins, lipids, and even some necessary minerals for the development of the conceptus. After implantation, the continued secretion of progesterone causes the endometrial cells to swell still more and store even more nutrients. These cells are now called decidual cells, and the total mass of cells is called decidua. Progesterone also decreases the ability of the uterine muscle to contract, thus preventing the embryo from being expelled from the body. As the trophoblast cells invade the decidua and imbibe it, the stored nutrients in the decidua are used by the embryo for growth and development. During the first week after implantation, this is the only means by which the embryo continues to obtain much of its nutrition. The decidual contribution to nutrition continues in this way for up to 8 weeks, although the placenta also begins to provide nutrition after the 16th day beyond fertilization (a little more than a week after implantation).

By the time the embryo is 8 weeks old, all the main internal organs have been formed, along with the major external body structure. During the embryonic development (weeks 2–8), the embryo is highly vulnerable to nutrient deficiencies and toxicities as well as harmful substances such as tobacco smoke. The term *fetus* is used for the developing individual from the beginning of the third month until birth.

There is no direct connection between a mother's circulation and that of the fetus; the placenta has evolved as part of the reproductive equipment, and the fetus is attached to it by means of the umbilical cord by which the transfer between the two circulatory systems occurs. The functions of the placenta are to transmit nutrients to the fetus, excrete fetal waste products into the maternal blood, and modify maternal metabolism at different stages of pregnancy by means of hormones.

In humans, the placental and fetal circulation forms during the early weeks of embryonic life. The placenta then continues to develop—growing in size, changing morphologically, and altering transport activity until its weight at term is about 15% that of the fetus. As in other organs, placental growth involves a period of active cell division (i.e., hyperplastic growth), which is reflected by an increase in DNA content and is followed by periods in which cell division is minimal but cell size may continue to increase. The phase of hypertrophic growth is reflected by increments in protein/DNA or weight/DNA ratio. In humans, the hyperplastic phase of growth is completed by the 34th to the 36th week of pregnancy. The size of the fetus varies directly with the size of the placenta, but placenta/fetal weight ratio changes considerably at different gestational ages.

The human placenta synthesizes two types of hormones: peptide and steroid. Early in pregnancy, the placenta secretes a peptide hormone, chorionic gonadotropin hormone (CGH), into the maternal circulation. It can be detected within a few days of implantation, and this provides the basis for early diagnostic tests for pregnancy. This hormone represses the pituitary secretion of the luteinizing hormone (the regulator of corpus luteum activity in the ovary) and arrests the normal menstrual cycle; at the same time, it also directly stimulates the corpus luteum to make progesterone. The level of CGH reaches maximum in about 50–70 days, after which there is a gradual decline throughout the remainder of pregnancy. From the seventh week of pregnancy, the placenta begins to take over the endocrine function of the ovary by producing large amounts of both estrogen and progesterone. CGH, in conjunction with a second peptide hormone, placental lactogen, promotes increased placental production of progesterone from maternal cholesterol (the placenta cannot synthesize cholesterol). Part of this placental progesterone passes into the maternal circulation to supplement progesterone made in the corpus luteum, and the remainder is exported to the fetus, which uses this steroid to form androstenedione and dehydroepiandrosterone—products that are then returned to the placenta to be chemically modified to estradiol and estriol. Thus, early pregnancy is marked by high blood levels of CGH along with a sharp rise in progesterone output, whereas in the latter part of pregnancy, there is a much lower level of CGH but increasing levels of estrogen and progesterone. In addition to its action on the corpus luteum, placental lactogen serves two other functions. It stimulates the growth of the mammary gland in preparation for lactation and makes glucose, amino acids, and fatty acids available to the fetus by diminishing maternal responsiveness to her own insulin. It causes these metabolites to be released from maternal tissues. As pregnancy progresses, maternal tissues show a decreased responsiveness to insulin. Progesterone and estrogen, as well as increased maternal weight, may also play roles in insulin resistance. In a sense, pregnancy has a slight diabetogenic effect in the mother.

The nutrients present in the maternal blood reach the fetal bloodstream via the placenta. Four major mechanisms are used for the maternal–fetal transfer of nutrients: passive diffusion (e.g., oxygen, carbon dioxide, fatty acids, steroids, nucleosides, electrolytes, and fat-soluble vitamins), facilitated diffusion (e.g., sugars), active transport (e.g., amino acids, some cations, and water-soluble vitamins), and endocytosis (e.g., proteins).

During pregnancy, the mother's body undergoes a series of adaptations that create an environment for optimal fetal growth and prepare the mother for the period of lactation. Changes in the maternal hormone secretions from the placenta lead to alterations in carbohydrate, fat, and protein utilization. In the first and second trimesters, increased serum concentrations of progesterone and estrogen lead to an increased sensitivity of maternal tissues to insulin. This results in a fundamental switch in energy balance so that pregnant women become strongly anabolic. They begin to store large quantities of energy above the immediate needs of the growing fetus. Breast enlargement and fat deposition prepare the mother for lactation. There is also an alteration in homeostatic control of almost all nutrients. Early in pregnancy while the placenta and fetus are still quite small, the size of the uterus begins to increase to accommodate the anticipated products of conception. The prepregnancy weight of the uterus is about 50 g but can increase up to 1000 g at term. After about the 10th week of pregnancy, the plasma and erythrocyte volumes begin to increase, reaching, at term, 50% and 25% (on the average), respectively, above the prepregnancy levels. With the increase in blood volume, more fluids carrying nutrients and oxygen are available to the placenta. At the same time, the larger blood volume facilitates the removal of CO_2 and metabolic waste products from the fetus.

In humans, a single fetus represents about 5% of maternal weight. Maternal genetic characteristics, including race, are known to influence the variance in birth weight. Both prepregnancy weight and weight gain during pregnancy are positively correlated with infant's birth weight. Weight of the term infant usually comprises at least 25% of the mother's total gestational weight gain. Women who are lean (prior to pregnancy) tend to have smaller newborns than those who are obese. Maternal diet and nutritional status are important factors that influence the course and the outcome of pregnancy. One manifestation of diminished support for the fetus in utero is the delivery of a full-term LBW infant (also called small for date, small for gestational age, fetal growth retarded, or intrauterine growth retarded). LBW is associated with increased mortality and morbidity, including a higher incidence of congenital abnormalities and poor postnatal growth. In 1990, the Institute of Medicine (IOM) evaluated the available scientific evidence and set guidelines for total gestational weight ranges that vary according to prepregnancy body mass index (BMI), a measure of obesity that takes into account a person's height and weight. Since then several studies have observed that infants of women with pregnancy weight gains within the IOM recommendations are relatively less likely to be at extremes of birth weight for a given gestational age. A total maternal weight gain, on average, of 24 pounds is considered optimal for adequate fetal development. Of greater importance than the total weight gain, however, is the gestational pattern of weight accumulation. The recommended pattern consists of a minimal weight gain of 2–4 pounds during the first trimester, with a linear rate of weight gain of 0.8 lb/week throughout the remaining two trimesters. Underweight women show the best pregnancy outcome with a weight gain of approximately 30 pounds. Obese women demonstrate satisfactory pregnancy course with weight gain of 16–20 pounds. Because the adolescent generally does not reach her full stature until 4 years after the onset of menstruation, and because pregnancy is also a period of rapid growth and development of the fetus and maternal tissues, a weight gain of about 35 pounds is recommended in adolescent pregnancy.

Excessive pregnancy weight gain is associated with increased risk of delivering an infant who is large for gestational age[3] and with serious neonatal complications such as hypoglycemia and hyperbilirubinemia.[21] Thin women who gain little weight during pregnancy and heavy women who put on too many pounds are at increased risk for preterm delivery compared to moderate weight women.[2] Premature birth is a major cause of illness and death among newborns, and hospital costs for premature infants are high. Thin women need to compensate for their low weight by making sure that they have a weight gain that will support a healthy fetus. Similarly, overweight women need to have adequate weight gain but should recognize that high weight gain is associated with increased risk.

A recent study has found that women who gain too much weight during pregnancy (>38 pounds) face an increased risk (40% increased risk) of breast cancer after menopause. The risk before menopause is no higher than usual. Researchers have not yet examined whether women who gain extra weight during pregnancy and then take it off have an increased risk of breast cancer. Fat cells produce estrogen, and it is believed that the extra hormone is what puts overweight women at risk of breast cancer. The message to women is to maintain their young adult weight throughout life.

If the maternal diet is inadequate, fetal growth is impaired and the birth weight of the infant is reduced. The fetus is unable to extract the necessary nutrients to maintain optimal growth. Evidence from both animals and humans suggests that inadequate nutrition, especially consumption of insufficient calories, can result in an incomplete maternal adaptation to pregnancy. The expected increase in maternal blood volume may not take place in undernourished animals and humans. This, in turn, leads to a reduction in uterine and placental blood flow. As a result, the placenta itself will not grow properly and will not transfer nutrients adequately. Thus, the process by which nutrients are actually passed to the fetus is impaired, and although these nutrients are available from maternal reserves, they cannot reach the fetus in normal quantities.

Maternal malnutrition in humans interferes with normal placental growth, as reflected by a lower weight and smaller placental size. The decrease in mean placental weight is in the range of 14%–50% of normal, depending on the severity of maternal malnutrition during pregnancy. Also, the urinary excretion of estriol and pregnanediol is less in malnourished pregnant women, and estriol excretion increases after the women receive food supplementation. Thus, maternal malnutrition apparently reduces the ability of the feto-placental unit to synthesize steroid hormones.

Evidence for an effect of maternal malnutrition on fetal development has been obtained from an examination of obstetrical records before, during, and after acute wartime starvation such as that which occurred during the 18-month famine in Leningrad in 1942–1943 and the 6-month famine in Holland during the winter of 1944–1945. In Leningrad, there was a reduction of the average birth weight of 600 g, while in Holland the birth weight fell by an average of 250 g. There was also a proportionate reduction in placental weights in the two regions. The difference between the Dutch and Russian experiences was probably related to the differing quality of nutritional status prior to the famine as well as to the severity of deprivation. For example, placental weights in poor Indian women are lower than those in Dutch women affected by famine during the second and third trimesters of pregnancy. As the famine condition is a more severe nutritional deprivation than the chronic moderate undernutrition of the low-income women in developing countries, the higher placental weight in the Dutch women as compared to women in Leningrad and India could be due to their better nutritional status at conception.

Further confirmatory evidence on the effect of nutrition on pregnancy outcome was provided by several nutritional intervention studies in various areas of the world. Protein–calorie supplementation during pregnancy to populations of known deficient nutritional status was associated with a significant maternal weight gain and an increase in birth weight. The weight gain was highest in those who were poorly nourished, so supplementation helped when it was needed. However, when the maternal diet was judged to be adequate, extra nutrition did not provide measurable changes in birth weight.

12.2.3 NUTRIENT REQUIREMENTS

A mother's nutritional status during pregnancy directly influences birth weight, which can have long-term effects on the health of her offspring. The rapid growth of the fetus and supporting maternal tissues necessitates an increase in the nutritional requirements of the pregnant woman above nonpregnant needs. Nearly all nutrients are required in greater amounts during pregnancy, but the magnitude of the increase is greater for some nutrients than for others. During a 40-week gestational period, the growing fetus accumulates about 400 g of protein, 475 g of fat, and 250 g of water containing minerals and other nutrients. These nutrients come from the mother via the placenta. During the same period, the mother expands her body fluids by 25%, or an average of 3 L, and accumulates 382 g of protein, and 3380 g of fat and minerals in her body tissues. The placenta grows with the fetus and contains 100 g of protein and 4 g of fat and minerals.

12.2.3.1 Energy

The energy requirement takes into consideration the placental, fetal, and maternal weight gain and the weight gain composition (i.e., the energy contained in all tissues gained during pregnancy). The progressive increase in the mass of the maternal and feto-placental tissues results in an increased basal metabolic rate, and the total gain of the mother's body mass means that any movement or activities she undertakes may require a larger expenditure of energy than in the prepregnant state. The energy required for normal pregnancy is estimated to be about 75,000 Cal (315,000 kJ; beyond the usual intake over the entire gestational period). An average of about an extra 150–200 Cal/day is recommended during the first trimester and 350 Cal/day thereafter. The National Research Council recommends an average of an additional 300 Cal/day for pregnant woman. For underweight or physically active pregnant women, more than an additional 300 Cal/day may be needed. In contrast, for obese women, pregnancy is viewed as an inappropriate time to limit energy intake or initiate weight loss. Women pregnant with boys consume about 10% more calories a day than those carrying girls but do not gain more weight. This appears to explain, at least in part, why newborn boys are heavier than girls and suggests that signals between the fetus and the mother drive appetite during pregnancy. Boys are on average 3.5 ounces heavier at birth than girls.

12.2.3.2 Protein

During the course of pregnancy, about 900 g of protein must be synthesized by the mother to support the development of the feto-placental unit and the maternal reproductive tissues. Considerable evidence suggests that protein deprivation during pregnancy has deleterious effects on the course of pregnancy and fetal development. Other clinical studies indicate that the level of certain maternal blood amino acids and proteins correlates significantly with infant birth weight, length, cranial volume, and motor and mental development. Amino acids derived from dietary protein are utilized for expanded maternal blood and other tissues and for fetal synthesis of its own proteins.

The optimal protein requirements during pregnancy have not been precisely determined and probably vary depending on the mother's age and nutritional status prior to pregnancy. The National Research Council recommends an additional 30 g/day protein from the second month of pregnancy to the end of gestation. This takes into account the lower efficiency of protein utilization and allows for maternal storage as well as fetal gain. A higher recommendation is made for adolescents to support their continued maturation.

12.2.3.3 Carbohydrates

Sufficient carbohydrate in the diet is required to prevent ketosis and excessive breakdown of proteins. Calories ingested early in pregnancy in any form may be stored in the maternal organism and used for subsequent fetal growth. A supply of sufficient calories in the form of carbohydrate can usually spare the metabolism of more important nutrients such as proteins during pregnancy. A minimum of 50–200 g/day of digestible carbohydrates should be provided.

12.2.3.4 Fats and Essential Fatty Acids

Maternal fat is accumulated primarily during the first and second trimesters as energy and essential fatty acid (EFA) reserves for lactation; fetal growth occurs mainly in the last 2 months of pregnancy. Dietary fat is important in fetal and early infant growth because this is the period of organogenesis, where there is a high demand for EFAs for the synthesis of cell structural lipids. This is true especially for the central nervous system in which the main period of cell division is prenatal. The approximate accumulation of EFAs during pregnancy is estimated to be about 620 g, which includes the demand for uterine, placental, mammary gland, and fetal growth, and the increased maternal blood volume. Most of the fats in fetal organs such as liver and brain are structural and contain a high proportion of phospholipids that require long-chain polyunsaturated fatty acids (PUFAs) that are derived from linoleic and linolenic acids (in the ratio of $\omega_6{:}\omega_3 = 5{-}7{:}1$). To meet these needs, 4.5% of the expected caloric intake in the form of EFAs is recommended during pregnancy.

Docosahexaenoic acid (DHA), an ω_3 fatty acid, had recently gained attention as a supplement for pregnant women, noting reports of improved attention and visual acuity. A study in the Netherlands has shown that the placenta pumps DHA from the mother to the fetus, thereby increasing the mother's susceptibility to depression. Postpartum depression strikes 15%–20% of women who give birth in the United States. It may be wise for mothers to increase their intake of DHA for both the benefit of the fetus and to help them avoid postpartum depression.

12.2.3.5 Minerals and Vitamins

Minerals and vitamins play a major role in regulating metabolic processes of living organisms. In pregnancy, there is an increased requirement for these nutrients to satisfy the needs of the growing fetus and to maintain the optimal nutritional status of the mother. Thus, an increased demand can only be met by available reserves or additional supply. Fortunately, these substances are found in abundance in the average diet; however, of particular concern are three minerals and one vitamin that might be lacking in the diets of pregnant woman: calcium, iron, zinc, and folic acid.

12.2.3.5.1 Calcium

At birth, the fetus contains about 28 g of calcium, which is mostly in the skeletal system. There are additional small quantities that are found in maternal supporting tissues and fluids that raise calcium deposition totals to about 30 g in pregnancy. A complex series of hormonal adjustments allows for increased calcium retention beginning early in pregnancy. The maternal body contains about 1120 g of calcium prior to pregnancy. To provide calcium for fetal development without depleting maternal tissues, an additional daily intake of 400 mg (or a total of 1200 mg)—the amount present in 1 quart of milk—is recommended during pregnancy.

12.2.3.5.2 Iron

Iron deficiency anemia is a common problem among nonpregnant women, and many women start their pregnancies with diminished iron stores. Normally, about 44 mL of blood is lost during each menstrual cycle; this amounts to the loss of 22 mg/month of iron or 0.7 mg/day. During pregnancy, this iron loss is saved, so during gestation (280 days), there is a total saving of 196 mg of iron. During pregnancy, expansion of hemoglobin mass requires about 480 mg of iron, and the formation of the placenta, umbilical cord, and fetus needs about 390 mg of iron; delivery blood loss (about 660 mL) amounts to 330 mg of iron. These add up to 1004 mg of iron to be supplied by the mother during pregnancy or about 3.6 mg/day. This is over and above her own normal requirements of 1 mg/day. The normal storage of iron in nonpregnant women is about 1000 mg. The fetus appears to be an effective parasite in extracting iron from its mother regardless of the state of maternal iron deficiency. Thus, the hemoglobin level of infants born to pregnant women with iron deficiency anemia is typically normal, and recent studies of plasma ferritin levels indicate that this index of storage iron in the newborn is unaffected by maternal iron status. Allowing for the increased efficiency of iron absorption during pregnancy, 30–45 mg/day supplemental iron is recommended during pregnancy.

12.2.3.5.3 Zinc

During pregnancy, blood zinc concentrations decrease by 30%–40% in many women and hair zinc levels also decline slightly. Zinc is an essential growth factor.[19] Although the fetal needs of this nutrient are highest in late pregnancy, it may also be critically important in very early pregnancy. Zinc concentrations in human embryos are seven times greater on the 35th day of gestation than on the 31st day. An additional 3–5 mg of zinc is recommended during pregnancy.

12.2.3.5.4 Vitamins

Adequate supplies of vitamins during pregnancy are necessary to ensure the normal development and viability of the offspring. The fat-soluble vitamins are principally stored in the liver and are readily available with increased demands; therefore, pregnancy-associated deficiency states of these nutrients are not known. As urinary excretion is limited, however, toxicity due to fat-soluble vitamins represents a potential danger with overdosage. In contrast to fat-soluble vitamins, water-soluble vitamins are not stored in the body in appreciable amounts. Because of an absence of reserves, deprivation is more likely to lead to deficiency states and toxicity, and overdosages are less likely. Recent studies have confirmed an association between low vitamin C and premature rupture of the membrane (PROM), causing premature delivery.[35] Vitamin C is specifically required for the synthesis and maintenance of collagen, a major component of the chorioamniotic membrane. Subjects with PROM were found to have weakened amniotic membranes associated with low levels of collagen, low amniotic fluid vitamin C levels, and low maternal plasma vitamin C levels in the third trimester. The incidence of weakened membranes is inversely correlated with smoking. Recently, scientists have discovered a possible link between reduced vitamin C availability during pregnancy and the devastating respiratory failure and massive cerebral bleeding that can occur immediately following premature birth. During pregnancy, there is a greater demand for folate for DNA synthesis in rapidly growing fetal, placental, and maternal tissues as well as for increased erythropoiesis, so pregnant women appear prone to develop folate deficiency. Even in well-nourished women, there is a predictable decrease in serum and red-cell folate during pregnancy, an increase in urinary folate excretion, and alterations in other laboratory findings suggestive of folic acid deficiency, although megaloblastic anemia is not common. Folic acid deficiency during pregnancy is a risk factor for delivering infants with NTDs in a minority of women. The frequency of maternal folate deficiency lends support to routine folate supplementation during pregnancy. A supplement of 400 µg/day folic acid is recommended during pregnancy.

NTDs are birth defects that involve an incomplete development of the brain, spinal cord, and/or their protective coverings. There are three types of NTDs: anencephaly, encephalocele, and spina bifida.[26] In anencephaly, infants are born with underdeveloped brains and incomplete skulls. These babies usually die within a few hours after birth. Encephalocele is a defect that results in a hole in the skull through which brain tissues protrude. Most of these babies do not live or have severe mental retardation. In spina bifida, the spinal column remains open. It can present as a mild defect that causes no problem or a serious defect involving muscle paralysis, loss of feeling, and loss of bowel control. Spina bifida is the most common disorder among babies born with NTDs occurring in about 60% of the cases, followed by anencephaly, which occurs in 35%, and encephalocele in 5% of the babies. NTDs are a worldwide problem affecting an estimated 300,000 or more fetuses or infants each year. Approximately 4000 pregnancies in the United States are affected by NTDs each year. NTDs occur within the first month of pregnancy, a time when many women do not know they are pregnant. The evidence that consumption of folic acid before conception and during early pregnancy can reduce the number of NTDs has been accumulating for many years.[6,11] One of the most rigorously conducted studies was the randomized controlled trial sponsored by the British Medical Research Council. The study showed that high-dose folic acid supplement (4 mg/day) used by women who had a previous NTD-affected pregnancy reduced the risk of having a subsequent NTD-affected pregnancy by 70%. In 1992, the United States Public Health Service recommended that all women with child-bearing potential should consume 0.4 mg of folic acid daily to reduce the risk of an NTD-affected pregnancy.[13] Because the effects of higher intakes are not well known and high doses of folate can mask vitamin B_{12} deficiency, care should be taken to keep total folate consumption to less than 1 mg/day, except under supervision of a physician.

Folate's exact role in preventing these birth defects remains unclear. Some women whose infants develop these defects are not deficient in folate, and others with severe folate deficiencies do not give birth to infants with birth defects. Other factors may also be involved. Folate participates in two metabolic pathways that, if disrupted, could have an adverse effect on the embryo. One of these pathways is important for nucleic acid synthesis, and the other for a range of methylation reactions. Disruptions in folate metabolism can also result in raised homocysteine concentrations that are teratogenic to the neural tube in some animal models. Individuals with low activity of methylene tetrahydrofolate reductase tend to have slightly elevated plasma homocysteine levels. Higher-than-average homocysteine levels in the blood been reported in women with NTD pregnancies and in patients with NTD. Moreover, several studies have shown a relationship between high plasma homocysteine and pregnancy complications or adverse neonatal outcomes that are associated with impaired folate status.

Folate and vitamin B_{12} are required for the conversion of homocysteine to methionine. Several researchers have shown an association between poor vitamin B_{12} status and the risk of NTD. Folic acid supplementation can overcome some of the metabolic effects of low vitamin B_{12} status. Animal studies have shown that the embryonic neural tube requires methionine for normal closure, and methionine (not folate) could prevent NTD. Some in vitro studies also suggest that homocysteine can cause embryonic malformations. In some individuals, the higher homocysteine level is due to a genetically inherited alteration in the activity of methionine synthase—the enzyme involved in the conversion of homocysteine to methionine. In about 6% of women, this enzyme occurs in a homozygous form. The body then requires more folate to keep homocysteine in the normal range (discussed in Chapter 10).

An alternative pathway for the removal of homocysteine involves its conversion to cysteine by reactions that require vitamin B_6. Thus, vitamin B_6 is involved indirectly in the regulation of homocysteine level. The most effective preconceptional prophylaxis to prevent NTDs may require vitamin B_6 and vitamin B_{12} as well as folic acid. Many of the epidemiological studies as well as the intervention studies of NTD prevention have yielded additional information, which suggests that other classes of major birth defects can also be reduced when women take folic acid containing multivitamins during the preconceptional periods. Folate metabolism is abnormal in mothers of children with Down syndrome, and this may be explained, in part, by a mutation in the methylene-tetrahydrofolate reductase gene.[23,28]

It has been reported recently that folic acid supplementation for a year prior to pregnancy reduced the risk of birth between 28 and 32 weeks of gestation by 50%.[10] The risk of birth between 20 and 28 weeks was reduced by 70%. The supplementation had no effect on the risk of preterm birth after 32 weeks. And beginning supplementation around the time of conception did little to reduce preterm births, even though such timing reduces the risk of NTDs. The finding reinforces the recommendation that all women of child-bearing age should take multivitamin supplements. Only 35%–40% of such women do take supplements, according to surveys conducted by the March of Dimes and other groups. Previous research had shown that women who deliver prematurely have lower than normal levels of folate in their blood. Preterm births—before 37 weeks of gestation—account for about 13% of U.S. deliveries and are associated with vision impairment and mental retardation in children and diabetes and cardiovascular disease as they grow older.

Although up to 70% of NTDs can be prevented by adequate folate consumption, some are unrelated to folate. More recently, it has been shown that a newborn's risk for NTD rises if the mother has low blood levels of choline. Inositol was found to reduce the incidence of spinal NTDs that were unrelated to folate in curly tail mice. Inositol is generally considered to be safe at doses as high as 12 g/day to treat depression and panic disorder. It is possible that inositol supplement could prevent more NTDs than with folic acid alone. However, further studies of the safety of high doses of inositol are needed before clinical trials can be initiated.

12.2.4 OTHER MATERNAL FACTORS

12.2.4.1 Age

One of the factors in the outcome of pregnancy is maternal age at the time of conception. There are greater risks of pregnancy complications at both ends of the age cycle in reproduction, specifically in very young adolescents 14 years of age and younger and in women 35 years and older. Complications for very young adolescents include an increased incidence of LBW infants and prenatal morbidity and mortality. In addition, there is a higher incidence of premature delivery and anemia. Conceiving at too early an age, smaller maternal size, and poor nutritional status of young adolescents have been given as explanations for poor pregnancy outcome. Young adolescents who become pregnant have not yet completed their own growth. Competition for nutrients between the mother's growth needs and those of her fetus may be one of the factors that contribute to unfavorable pregnancy outcome.

Women older than 35 years of age are at an increased risk of delivering LBW infants or infants with chromosomal abnormalities such as Down syndrome.

12.2.4.2 Diabetes

Women in their reproductive years with known diabetes of any kind should inform their physicians when they have decided to have a child. Conception when diabetes control is inadequate markedly increases the risk of major congenital abnormalities including NTDs and cardiac anomalies. Throughout pregnancy, normoglycemia (relative to normal pregnant state) is required to prevent intrauterine death and perinatal morbidity and mortality.

Maternal insulin requirements may fall slightly during the first 3 months of pregnancy when the fetus is actively removing rather large quantities of glucose and other metabolic fuels from the mother. As pregnancy progresses, maternal tissues show a decreased responsiveness to insulin. This resistance appears to be secondary to the effects of hormones secreted by the placenta such as lactogen. Increasing placental, fetal, and maternal weight may also play a role. Near the end of pregnancy, the woman's insulin requirement may double, but soon after delivery the insulin requirement falls abruptly. Thus, pregnancy per se has a mild diabetogenic effect.

In some women (estimated to be 1%–3% of all pregnancies), the increased need for insulin as pregnancy progresses may cause a temporary abnormality in glucose metabolism, termed *gestational diabetes*, which in the majority of cases disappears shortly after delivery.[1,24] The gestational diabetes occurs in women who may be genetically predisposed to the disease. It generally occurs between the 26th and 28th week of gestation. Some of these women may develop diabetes within the next 5–15 years.

Poorly controlled maternal diabetes (true or gestational) is associated with poor outcomes. Maternal hyperglycemia results in fetal hyperglycemia that, in turn, gives rise to insulinemia and contributes to increased triglyceride synthesis and deposition of subcutaneous fat. Therefore, the most common net result is fetal macrosomia (increased fetal body fat) and heavy birth weight. In some cases, the fetus may develop intrauterine growth retardation, which is apparently related to inadequate placental perfusion. Acetonuria occurring during pregnancy, regardless of etiology, appears to be associated with a demonstrable negative effect on intelligence quotient (IQ) in later childhood. The incidence of serious congenital malformations in diabetic women is approximately three times higher than that in nondiabetic women. Therefore, control of maternal blood glucose and acidosis can help lessen these risks, and good nutritional management is an essential part of this control.

New evidence is emerging for how important it is for pregnant mothers to eat good nutritious food. According to a recent study, expectant mothers who eat vegetables every day seem to have children who are less likely to develop type 1 diabetes. Compared to women who ate vegetables daily during pregnancy, those consuming only 3–5 times/week had a 71% increased risk of having a child with type 1 diabetes. Mothers-to-be should eat a vegetable-rich diet to protect their babies from type 1 diabetes.

12.2.4.3   Hypertension

Pregnancy-induced hypertension (PIH) or preeclampsia involves not only blood pressure elevation but also proteinuria and generalized edema.[34] It can progress to eclampsia, which produces seizures and often fatal complications of the liver, kidney, lungs, blood, and nervous system. More than 6 million women around the world and 70,000 in the United States suffer preeclampsia during pregnancy each year. It usually develops after the 24th week of gestation and about 67% of the cases are diagnosed after the 37th week of pregnancy. This disorder, once known as toxemia, occurs in about 6%–9% of pregnant women and most frequently in teenage girls, particularly blacks, during their first pregnancy. Pregnancy-induced hypertension is a peculiar form of high blood pressure because it occurs at a very specific time in pregnancy (22–24 weeks) and disappears almost as soon as the baby and placenta are delivered. In its severe form, it is a potentially life-threatening disease for both the mother and the infant. The maternal mortality attributed to hypertension is approximately 3–5/100,000 live births. It is also a factor in about 12.5% of all perinatal deaths because of its strong association with premature delivery and fetal growth retardation. How pregnancy sometimes causes dangerously high blood pressure is not known. Total weight gain during pregnancy and variation in sodium intake do not seem to influence its development. Some studies suggest that a low calcium intake during pregnancy is associated with preeclampsia. Urinary excretion of the prostacyclin I_2 metabolite is lower in pregnant mothers who later develop PIH. As the abnormality is detected early in pregnancy, long before the blood pressure becomes elevated, it may be a useful biochemical marker of PIH. Prostacyclin production is increased in normal pregnancy, and it may be an important regulator of blood pressure during those 9 months. Drug therapies, dietary moderation, inclusion of adequate foods rich in calcium, and rest are recommended for PIH.

One study has shown that taking multivitamin mineral supplements starting 3 months before pregnancy and through the first 3 months of pregnancy reduces the risk of developing preeclampsia by about 72%. Another study that involved taking high doses of vitamins C and E showed no benefit. Researchers have recently discovered biomarkers that could help diagnose and treat this disease.

Two antiangiogenic proteins secreted by placenta are identified: soluble forms, such as tyrosine kinase-1, and endoglin. These two proteins bind to vascular endothelial growth factors, disrupt the endothelium, and cause hypertension, proteinuria, and other systemic manifestations of preeclampsia. These proteins increase in their levels several weeks before the onset of clinical disease and thus may be useful to screen or identify patients at risk for the disease. Investigations are underway to counteract the effects of these proteins as a potential treatment for preeclampsia.[25]

Catechol-o-methyltransferase (COMT), which generates 2-methylestradiol (2-ME) in the human placenta, has recently been shown to have decreased activity in preeclampsia.[15] In experiments on the mouse model, researchers showed that decreased COMT activity and subsequent decreased 2-ME levels resulted in the clinical, histologic, and molecular changes characteristic of preeclampsia. Furthermore, both the preeclampsia-like characteristic features and angiogenic abnormalities completely resolved in rescue experiments with 2-ME. In addition, circulating levels of 2-ME were lower in 8 women with preeclampsia compared with 13 normotensive pregnant controls. The results may explain how the disease occurs and could point toward future therapies.

Ergothioneine, a compound made by fungi and found in unpasteurized food, has been detected in unusually high levels in the red blood cells of pregnant women with preeclampsia.[32] Ergothioneine is not synthesized by humans, and it finds its way into human cells exclusively through our diet.

The recent findings discussed above have profound implications for the diagnosis, treatment, and prevention of this devastating condition.

12.2.4.4 Alcohol

Alcohol is a known teratogen. It is estimated that at least 8% of all women of childbearing age are alcoholics; also, if one is a heavy drinker and is pregnant, the fetus is in danger. Roughly half of the infants born to alcoholic women have fetal alcohol syndrome (FAS); this refers to a series of effects seen in children of women who chronically drink alcohol to excess during pregnancy. Typical manifestations of FAS include prenatal and/or postnatal growth retardation with weight, length, and/or head circumference below the 10th percentile; central nervous system involvement with neurological abnormality, developmental delay, or intellectual impairment; and facial dysmorphology (birth defects) with at least two of the following three signs: microcephaly (small brain), microphthalmia (small eyes) and/or short palpebral fissures (the horizontal length of the eyes), and a poorly developed philtrum (the distance from the base of the nose to the upper lip) and thin upper lip. The data strongly suggest a causal association between maternal alcohol abuse and FAS, but how alcohol ingestion adversely affects the fetus is not clearly known. It freely crosses the placental barrier, and its concentration in the fetus can reach levels equivalent to that in the mother. Recently, scientists have studied the effects of alcohol administration on brain development in neonatal rats.[22] The animals were exposed to one episode of high blood alcohol level during the first 2 weeks after birth—a time when rat brains are going through developmental stages. In humans, this brain growth spurt starts in the sixth month of gestation and continues for 2 years after birth. In rat pups, exposure of the brain to alcohol caused the blockage of N-methyl-D-aspartate (NMDA) receptors and an excessive activation of γ-aminobutyric acid receptors. The disruption of signals of neurotransmitters resulted in massive apoptosis—a form of cell suicide—of developing brain cells. This study showed that it only requires one round of intoxication of about 4 hours for the damage to occur. The binge-drinking paradigm used in the study gave rats a blood alcohol level of 0.2 or 200 mg/dL blood. Such a level in people is twice the legal standard of drunkenness in many states.

A 1996 study by the IOM showed that about 20% of women who drink do not stop during pregnancy. About one in every 1000 babies born in the United States suffers from FAS, a disorder caused by exposure to alcohol in the womb. The disorder can cause stunted growth along with memory and learning problems. Thus, alcohol is the leading cause of preventable birth defects and mental retardation in the United States. Alcohol has secondary effects on nutrition: it may suppress appetite and replace food calories, and it may decrease absorption. Because the nutritional status of alcoholics tends to be poor, it is advisable to provide nutritional supplements to chronic alcohol users during pregnancy.

Mild-to-moderate alcohol use may not result in FAS but may result in infants being born with varying degrees of affliction or so-called fetal alcohol effects. A recent study has shown that children born to mothers who drink even small amounts of alcohol early in pregnancy are shorter and weigh less at age 14 than children born to mothers who abstain. Children born to women who are light drinkers (about 1½ drinks a week) in their first trimester weigh about 3 pounds less, and children born to heavy drinkers weigh up to 16 pounds less at age 14 than children born to abstainers.[14] Just one drink a day (12 ounces of beer or 4 ounces wine) during the first three months of pregnancy is associated with a two-point drop in overall IQ by the time the child is 10, according to one report. The effect shows up most clearly in certain visual tasks—such as fitting pieces of a puzzle into an empty space—and is strongest in African-American children. Federal health officials estimate that of the 4 million American women who get pregnant each year, more than half a million continue to drink: about 120,000 in the moderate-to-heavy range of seven or more drinks per week, and 400,000 in light-to-moderate range. A safe level of alcohol consumption during pregnancy has not been established; therefore, pregnant women are advised to avoid alcohol completely. All containers of beer, wine, and liquor carry the warning "women should not drink alcoholic beverages during pregnancy because of the risk of birth defects."

12.2.4.5 Phenylketonuria

Women with phenylketonuria (PKU) who are not on diet therapy just prior to and during pregnancy may face an increased risk of adversely affecting the development of their fetus. Congenital malformations, microcephaly, and retarded physical and mental growth are associated with in utero elevations of phenylalanine. The active transport of amino acids by the placenta to the fetus leads to a fetal blood phenylalanine concentration that is two to three times higher than that found in maternal blood. Therefore, even though the fetus may not carry PKU, pregnant mothers with PKU should be on diet therapy throughout the gestational period. Given that the damage is suspected to occur early in the first trimester, the ideal situation is to initiate diet therapy prior to conception to keep the maternal blood phenylalanine levels in the normal range. When the condition is well treated in the mother, pregnancy outcome for the children of women with PKU is generally good.

12.2.4.6 Smoking

The use of tobacco has a serious effect on the pregnant woman and the fetus. By smoking or using other forms of tobacco, the expectant mother absorbs thousands of chemical substances that reach the fetus through the placenta. Nicotine, tar, and carbon monoxide are thought to be the most dangerous to the fetus. Independent of most other variables (e.g., race, parity, maternal size, sex of the infant, gestational age, socioeconomic status), smoking is associated with reduced maternal weight gain and increased likelihood for LBW infants. In 1998, 12% of babies born to smokers in the United States were of LBW, compared to 7.2% of babies born to nonsmokers. Women who smoke also have a higher risk for spontaneous abortions than those who do not. The biochemical basis for these observations is not clear, but smoking may affect the endocrine status.

There is an increased risk of ectopic pregnancy. In ectopic pregnancy, the embryo becomes implanted in a fallopian tube or other abnormal site instead of the uterus. Cigarette smoking also appears to double a woman's risk of developing placental complications.

Using umbilical cord blood samples to assay for changes in HPRT (hypoxanthine-guanine phosphoribosyltransferase) gene researchers have found that smoking by the mother causes genetic mutations in the newborn. Also secondary maternal exposure produces quantitatively and qualitatively indistinguishable increases in fetal HPRT mutation. About one-third of attention-deficit hyperactivity disorder (ADHD) cases among U.S. children may be linked with tobacco smoke before birth, according to one study. ADHD is a brain disorder affecting between 4% and 12% of school-age children, or as many as 3.8 million U.S. youngsters. Affected children often have trouble sitting still and paying attention and act impulsively at home and at school. The findings highlight the need to strengthen public-health efforts to reduce prenatal tobacco smoke exposure. The take home message is "if one is planning a pregnancy, one should stop smoking and stay away from smokers."

12.2.4.7 Caffeine

During pregnancy, a woman consumes many foods and other substances that cross the placental barrier, enter the fetal circulation, and may possibly affect fetal development. Caffeine is present in high concentrations in coffee (45–155 mg/cup) and in tea (9–50 mg/cup), cola (30–65 mg/12 oz), cocoa (2–40 mg/12 oz), and milk chocolate (6 mg/oz). Caffeine rapidly crosses the human placenta and enters the fetal circulation. The fetus and neonate appear to lack the enzyme or enzymes necessary to demethylate caffeine.

The potential harmful effects of caffeine during pregnancy were shown in studies on small animals. A group from Harvard examined the effects of coffee consumption in more than 12,000 women interviewed at the time of hospitalization or delivery. After controlling for smoking, alcohol consumption, and demographic characteristics such as age, race, and medical history, their analysis showed no relation between LBW or short gestation and heavy coffee consumption (>4 cups/day); however, another group reported the cases of three women who gave birth to infants with missing fingers or toes and did not appear to have ingested other drugs or agents that might have such a teratogenic effect. These women consumed between 15–25 cups of coffee daily. Although studies in humans are inconsistent and generally have failed to demonstrate a negative effect of caffeine on pregnancy outcome, any substance that crosses the placenta may be regarded as potentially hazardous, especially during the first trimester. Therefore, pregnant woman who choose to use caffeine should do so in moderation.

12.2.4.8 Morning Sickness

Morning sickness (MS) refers to the nauseated feeling during pregnancy. The term is actually a complete misnomer. Symptoms occur throughout waking hours, not just in the morning, and "sickness" implies pathology. Healthy women experience the symptoms and bear healthy babies. For these reasons, the medical community uses the acronym NVP, short for "nausea and vomiting of pregnancy."

Nearly 80% of mothers experience nausea during pregnancy and about half actually vomit. A small number (0.3%–3%) of all pregnant women experience a more severe form of MS known as hyperemesis gravidarum.

The exact cause of MS is not known but may be due to physiologic changes that occur during pregnancy including increases in the levels of estrogen, progesterone, and CGH. Most likely, it may be related to CGH because the level of this hormone gradually increases up to the 12th week of pregnancy, at which point its levels start to decline. The symptoms of MS first appear about 5 weeks after the last menstrual period, peak during weeks 8–12, and gradually decline thereafter. Some scientists suggest that nausea and vomiting protect the embryo, expelling potentially dangerous foods that might contain harmful chemicals. Meat and dairy products, for example, are much more likely to harbor bacteria.

Thalidomide was prescribed in the 1950s and early 1960s as a cure for MS, but its use was discontinued when the drug's teratogenic effects came to light. Many medications are available for treatment of MS. However, concerns about the potential teratogenic effects of administered drugs during the critical embryogenic period of pregnancy drastically limit their use. Consequently, many pregnant women use complementary and alternative therapies. These include vitamins, herbal products, homeopathic preparations, acupuncture, and other natural modalities.

Ginger has been widely used as a spice to enhance the flavor in food and beverages and for medical purposes, particularly to treat ailments such as stomach ache, diarrhea, and nausea. In a recent randomized controlled trial of ginger to treat MS women took 1 g of ginger or 75 mg of vitamin B_6 daily for 3 weeks. Differences from baseline in nausea and vomiting scores were estimated for both groups at days 7, 14, and 21. The nausea scores and the number of vomiting episodes were significantly reduced following ginger and vitamin B_6 therapy. There was no significant difference between ginger and vitamin B_6 for the treatment of MS. Considering the largely positive results and the absence of adverse effects on pregnancy outcomes, ginger may be an effective treatment in managing nausea and vomiting symptoms during pregnancy.

12.2.4.9   Stress and Pregnancy Outcome

The notion that women must take it easy during pregnancy has long been dismissed as folklore. But now a growing body of research links high levels of stress or anxiety in some women to preterm—before 37 weeks' gestation—underweight (less than 5.5 pounds) babies and potential problems later, from respiratory ailments to developmental delays. Many women can work very hard in high-stress jobs and deliver healthy babies. But genetics and other environmental factors may predispose some women to higher risk. A study at Stony Brook University on 129 women showed that high-risk stress ranging from general anxiety to worries over specific events caused more preterm births and smaller babies. But the effect was erased when they took the women's attitudes into account. An optimistic outlook on life shielded women from risk.

A study on 335 women in India found preterm births and LBW were less common among women who practiced yoga[27] (stress reduction) one hour a day, compared with women who did no yoga. Other studies found that eating fewer than three meals and two snacks a day raised the risk of preterm delivery 30%. Therefore, one should not forget the basics. Pregnant women under stress must work especially hard to maintain good nutrition.

12.2.4.10   Other Factors

Infants born to women taking commonly prescribed antidepressants during the first trimester of their pregnancy have an increased risk of serious birth defects, though the danger remains tiny. Pregnant women taking aspirin increase the risk of miscarry but acetaminophen (Tylenol) appears safe. Studies have found that exposure to influenza in utero during the first half of pregnancy is tied to greater likelihood that an individual may someday develop schizophrenia. Pregnant women exposed to dental radiation are nearly four times as likely to have LBW infants. Direct exposure of a fetus to radiation is known to be harmful, but lead aprons and directional X-rays have virtually eliminated direct exposure. Thus, X-rays must be exerting an indirect effect on fetal development through the mother. Women should try to avoid elective dental and other X-rays during pregnancy, especially during the first trimester.

Mercury can seriously impair fertility and pregnancy outcome. Mercury passes readily through the placenta. Therefore, there is a risk to the fetus in chronically exposed pregnant women. High levels of mercury may harm the developing brain. Some types of fish should be avoided because of mercury contamination. These include shark, king mackerel, swordfish, tile fish, and tuna. Levels of air pollutants commonly found in many urban areas may cross the placenta and affect the fetus. More than a dozen studies worldwide have linked air pollution to LBW, still birth, and intrauterine growth retardation. According to the World Health Organization, air pollution can impair lung function in the womb.

Some common pesticides are thought to be so-called endocrine disrupters, chemicals that change hormone function in utero and can affect reproductive organ development and function later in life. A study has found that women who ate more than seven servings of beef a week during pregnancy had sons who were more likely to have poor sperm count and quality as adults,[4,30] possibly due to anabolic steroids used in the United States to fatten cattle. It could also be due to pesticides and other environmental contaminants. Phthalates are used in plastics and many products such as enteric coatings of some pharmaceutical pills, nutritional supplements, and personal care products, for example, perfumes, nail polishes, etc. One study has shown that exposure of women to phthalates during pregnancy can alter the reproductive organs of their male offspring.[29] Phthalate metabolites were measured in urine samples collected from pregnant women. After the birth of infants, the genital features and anogenital distances of baby boys born from these women were measured and correlated with the metabolite levels in the mothers' urine samples. Boys born to mothers with the highest levels of phthalates were seven times more likely to have shortest anogenital distance when adjusted for weight—the anogenital index (AGI).[31]

In rodents, the AGI is a sensitive measure of demasculinization of the male reproductive tract and of fetal exposure to endocrine disrupters; this parameter is rarely assessed in humans, and its significance is unknown. More human studies are needed to confirm that male reproductive development is affected by prenatal exposure to environmentally relevant levels of phthalates.

Recent studies[7] have linked prebirth exposure to organophosphates—pesticides widely used in food crops—and lower intelligence scores in children. Researchers looked at signs of exposure in urine samples taken from mothers during pregnancy and later from their children. For every 10-fold increase in organophosphates detected in urine during a mother's pregnancy corresponded to a 5.5-point drop in overall IQ scores in her children by age 7. The 20% of the children whose mothers appeared to be exposed to the least amount of pesticide had about a 7-point higher IQ level, on average, than those in the 20% born to mothers with the highest exposure of pesticides. The difference was equivalent to about 6 months of brain development in a typical child, according to the researchers. To avoid pesticide exposure, they suggested using organic produce and/or washing fruits and vegetables well.

12.2.4.11   Acquired Immunodeficiency Syndrome

Either in utero or during birth, 30%–50% of infants whose mothers are infected with the human immunodeficiency virus will also become infected.

12.3   FETAL ORIGINS OF ADULT DISEASE

Recently, attention has focused not only on the immediate health of the newborn but also his or her long-term health through childhood and into adulthood. Barker, an epidemiologist at the University of Southhampton in England, was the first to hypothesize that the major chronic diseases may have their origins in the womb and that a mother's nutritional intake may have a subsequent long-term impact on the health of her offspring.[18] He and his colleagues examined cardiovascular disease (CVD) in men born in Hertfordshire County, United Kingdom, in the early decades of the last century on whom good records were kept of birth size and growth in infancy. Studies showed a relationship between infant birth weight and CVD. It was proposed that the pathogenesis of CVD is programmed during the period of rapid growth in early life. The fetal origin hypothesis contends that undernutrition during critical periods of fetal development may permanently alter the body's structure, physiology, and metabolism, and thereby increase the susceptibility to disease in adult life. Subsequently, other similar studies have shown a relationship between infant birth size and stroke, hypertension, type 2 diabetes, renal failure, and metabolic syndrome. However, in most instances, epidemiologic studies have not actually measured nutritional intake of mothers, maternal undernutrition being inferred only indirectly from birth weight.

Data from the Dutch famine, a 5-month period of extreme food scarcity during World War II gave researchers a unique opportunity to study the effects of acute maternal undernutrition during early, mid-, and late gestation on the incidence of CVD. Researchers examined records of individuals born between November 1, 1943 and February 28, 1944. Famine exposure was defined as having experienced a period of >13 weeks of gestation during which the average adult's ration was <1000 calories. Eligible individuals were asked to participate in the study at the ages of 50 and 58 years. Overall, compared to individuals unexposed to famine, mothers who were exposed to the famine during early (conceived during the famine), mid-, or late gestation had twice the risk of CVD. Individuals exposed during early gestation developed CVD 3 years earlier than those not exposed. Exposure to famine during any of the three gestational periods was associated with decreased glucose tolerance and elevated blood cholesterol. These findings suggest that maternal nutrition, particularly during early gestation may have a significant impact on CVD risk later in life.

It appears that the developing fetus gathers clues from the womb about the world into which it will be born. For example, if the fetus receives only limited nutrients in the womb, its cells may react by becoming thrifty in the use of those nutrients, and that trait becomes engrained in the growing fetus. As a result, the body created by these cells may conserve fat after birth, an adaptation that would help the child survive if times outside are tough. But if times are not so tough, then the tendency to conserve fat, so valuable in the womb, may place that child at high risk for obesity as he or she grows into an adult. Indian babies are small with mean birth weight of 2700 g; 30% have a birth weight of 2650 or less. Their mothers are underweight. The economic conditions have improved considerably and with it the incidence of obesity,[33] heart disease, and type 2 diabetes are increasing, coinciding with increasing urbanization.

If during pregnancy the mother is diabetic, and it is not controlled, large amounts of glucose will be transferred to the fetus. This will cause the fetus to increase its levels of insulin, which may trigger permanent appetite changes in the brain. The result is an adult who is more likely to be obese and, if the individual is a female, may develop diabetes during pregnancy. Similar explanations are given for the relationship between LBW and heart disease, as well as hypertension and osteoporosis.

Evidence is also accumulating from animal experiments that environmental factors such as maternal nutrition, stress, and pollutants can change gene function epigenetically, that is, without altering the DNA sequence.[4]

Bispheriol A (BPA) is used to make hard polycarbonated plastic. It is found in a wide range of household items such as plastic water bottles, baby bottles, and food containers. Some animal studies have suggested that BPA has toxic health effects including reproduction and development. In a study to determine the effect of maternal BPA exposure on the fetus, researchers used a strain of mice (Agouti mice) that are usually brown in color and tend to be lean. When pregnant mothers of this strain were given BPA, a significantly higher number of their offspring was born with yellow fur. Mice that are yellow tend to have a higher risk of diabetes, obesity, and cancer compared to brown counterparts. In addition, the research team observed that when the pregnant females were given folic acid or genistein (an active ingredient in soy) in conjunction with BPA, it prevented the inherited changes. In another study, scientists have reported that they have changed the fur colors of baby mice simply by altering their mothers' diets. They fed pregnant mice (yellow) folic acid, vitamin B_{12}, choline, and betaine. Mice given the supplements gave birth to babies with predominantly brown coats. Pregnant mice not fed the supplements gave birth to babies with yellow coats.

The findings from human studies are largely based on epidemiological evidence. Attempts to confirm or refute the hypothesis using data from human pregnancies have only made limited progress because long-term experimental or intervention studies are difficult to undertake, or are ethically not possible. The National Children's Study that started recently will examine the effects of environmental influences on the health and development of 100,000 children across the United States following them from before birth until age 21. The study will help better understand how children's genes and their environments interact to affect their health and development.

Environmental Factors—A Case

Until around the 1940s, it was believed that the placental barrier protected the fetus from external harmful substances. Congenital defects were thought to be merely accidental, and no causal relationship was established between exogenous factors and these defects. Now we know that exposure to certain factors can affect the health of the expectant mother and her child. Birth defects in humans, especially in northern California and the Pacific Northwest, have been blamed on the exposure of pregnant women to herbicides used in forests in those regions; however, there may be other causes in addition to herbicides.

A deformity called crooked calf syndrome, characterized by bone defects in the calf's forelimbs, spine, and skull, is caused by the mother cow's eating lupine plants[36,37,38] in early pregnancy. These plants contain an alkaloid, anagyrine, that has been directly linked to the disease. In 1983, a baby boy born in the back country of northern California was brought to the University of California Medical Center at Davis. He had severe bone deformities in his arms and hands with a general appearance of crooked calf disease. The boy's mother revealed that her goats gave birth to stillborn or deformed kids during and after her own pregnancy and puppies born to her dog fed goat's milk during pregnancy also were deformed. The bone deformities were similar to those of "crooked" calves and the little boy. The mother also revealed that she regularly drank goat's milk during her pregnancy. It was then found that when lupine seeds were fed to lactating goats, anagyrine and other alkaloids appeared in their milk almost immediately. This suggests that anagyrine and other toxins from the lupine plant were present in goat's milk, which was regularly consumed by the boy's mother during her pregnancy. The presence of toxin(s) probably did adversely affect the development of the fetus and caused the bone deformities.

This case illustrates the significance of avoiding milk or milk products that are derived from foraging goats and cows. This case also makes the point that during pregnancy, mothers should be careful about what they take in their diet.

12.4 NUTRITION DURING LACTATION

During lactation, two important hormones, prolactin and oxytocin, are produced by the pituitary gland. Prolactin stimulates the production of milk in the breast tissue. Oxytocin allows milk to be released from the mammary gland to the nipples. The concentration of prolactin rises steadily during pregnancy, but high estrogen and progesterone levels inhibit milk secretion by blocking prolactin effect on the breast epithelium. The baby's delivery signals the end of the placenta's role by the sudden loss of both estrogen and progesterone secretions, which then lifts the block allowing the lactogenic effect of prolactin to assume its natural milk-promoting role. A few days after delivery, the prolactin level returns to nonpregnant levels. But each time the mother nurses her baby, nervous signals from the nipple to the hypothalamus causes a ten to twentyfold surge in prolactin secretion that lasts for about an hour. This keeps the mammary gland secreting milk for subsequent nursing. Infant suckling at the breast signals the pituitary gland to secrete oxytocin, which in turn stimulates the release of milk from the breast (milk letdown).

A new study reports that the neurotransmitter serotonin, which is produced in the brain and intestinal tract, is also produced in human mammary glands, where it controls milk production and secretion. Studies with human mammary cells and with mice show that the concentration of serotonin builds up in mammary glands as they fill with milk. The increase in serotonin inhibits further synthesis and secretion by suppressing expression of milk protein genes. After nursing, the cycle of milk and serotonin production begins again. The presence of so-called serotonin reuptake proteins in mammary cells "raises the possibility that selective serotonin reuptake inhibitors," which are used to treat depression, "could have effects on the breast milk production."

For the mother to produce sufficient milk to satisfy her infant's demands, she has to eat a well-balanced diet with special emphasis on critical nutrients such as calcium, iron, and water-soluble vitamins. This can be achieved with very little alteration in the normal diet. The energy, protein, carbohydrate, fat, and calcium remain relatively constant regardless of the mother's diet; however, if the dietary intake of these nutrients is severely restricted, the quantity of milk produced may be reduced. The volume of milk produced per day can be 550–850 mL/day, depending on several factors.

12.4.1 ENERGY

Human milk has a caloric content of approximately 70 Cal/100 mL. It is assumed that the caloric efficiency of milk formation and secretion is 80% and thus about 90 Cal is required for the production of 100 mL of milk or about 800 Cal for the daily production of milk. Following delivery, a woman ends up with about 9 pounds of extra weight over and above what she weighed before she became pregnant and about 250–300 Cal/day is available from mobilization of her body fat deposited during pregnancy. This, together with an extra 500 Cal/day (or an increase of 25% over and above the allowance for nonpregnant, nonlactating woman), should be sufficient to supply all the energy she needs to lactate properly.

12.4.2 PROTEIN

A mother's milk contains approximately 1 g protein per 100 mL, or 8.5 g/850 mL milk. It is assumed that the efficiency of milk protein synthesis is 70%; thus, about 12 g of extra protein is needed per day. It is suggested that an additional 30 g above the normal intake of 45 g of protein be consumed daily. This can be met solely by increasing meat intake by about 3 ounces or by increasing milk or fish intake.

12.4.3 ESSENTIAL FATTY ACIDS

Approximately 4%–5% of total energy in human milk is present as linoleic and linolenic acids and 1% as long-chain PUFAs derived from these acids; hence, about 6% of the total energy is supplied by EFAs and its metabolites. About 3–5 g/day EFA is secreted in milk. The efficiency of conversion of dietary EFAs into milk fatty acids is not known, but an additional 1%–2% of energy in the form of EFA is recommended during the first 3 months of lactation and an additional 2%–4% of the energy above the basic requirements is recommended thereafter.

12.4.4 CALCIUM

About 250–300 mg of calcium is present in a day's supply of milk. Although low maternal calcium intake is unlikely to affect the calcium content of human milk, it may decrease maternal bone density, especially if breast-feeding is prolonged. This can weaken the bones and may predispose a woman to osteoporosis in later life. This simply means that calcium intake of about 1200 mg daily is essential.

12.4.5 WATER-SOLUBLE VITAMINS

The vitamin content of human milk is dependent upon the mother's current vitamin intake and her vitamin stores. Because most water-soluble vitamins are not stored, the mother's diet should contain adequate amounts of these nutrients.

12.4.6 OTHER FACTORS

Alcohol consumption in excess of 0.5 g/kg body weight may result in decreased milk production. This corresponds to approximately 2–2.5 ounces of liquor, 8 ounces of table wine, or two cans of beer. Smoking, in addition to its harmful effects on the mother and her infant, can reduce milk volume. The use of illicit drugs should be discouraged and the use of certain legal substances by lactating women is also of concern because they may adversely influence the nutrient content of milk (e.g., excess coffee can influence the iron content of milk).

12.5 LACTATION EFFECTS

Lactation may be a good time for an overweight mother to lose weight. The energy expended by lactation is like performing vigorous exercise all day long. By moderate dietary restriction and by ensuring the availability of adequate amounts of essential nutrients, a nursing mother may lose significant weight and still provide adequate amounts of high-quality milk to her infant. Lactation minimizes postpartum blood loss and helps restore the uterus to its prepregnancy state sooner. Breast-feeding has been known to increase the length of time between delivery and the return of regular ovulation and to provide hormonal protection against conception, but the mechanism by which lactation exerts this effect on ovarian activity is not clear. It is suggested that suckling suppresses the pulsative release of GRH from the hypothalamus and also stimulates the release of prolactin. GRH is necessary for the pulsative release of luteinizing hormone from the pituitary.

Breast-feeding is a major factor that helps to reduce a woman's lifetime risk of developing breast cancer, according to a new analysis of research data from 30 countries. The relatively high risk of breast cancer found in developed countries is largely explained by the fact that women in those countries have chosen to have few children and to breast-feed them briefly or not at all according to the analysis of 47 studies recently published. It is the number of children and the duration of breast-feeding that is the key to the differences between developed and developing countries in breast cancer rates. Having a full-term pregnancy before the age of 30 lowers breast cancer risk, and having additional pregnancies further reduces the chance of developing the disease. A woman's relative risk of breast cancer declines by 7% with each birth and by an additional 4.5% for each year that she breast-feeds. Although these figures translate into modest risk reductions for an individual, the study concluded that if woman in developed countries had 2.5 children on average and breast-fed their infants for an extra 6 months, about 25,000 cases of breast cancer (or about 5% of cases) would be prevented each year. If each child were breast-fed for an additional 12 months, about 50,000 (11%) cases might be prevented annually. For the first time, the analysis confirms that breast-feeding itself can protect against breast cancer. In the United States and other developed countries, mothers of infants often find it difficult or impossible to keep breast-feeding once they return to work. In the United States, 70% of new mothers are working 30 hours or more per week by the time their infant is a year old. The majority of women do choose to start breast-feeding, but it does not last very long.

12.5.1 ROLE OF PROLACTIN OTHER THAN IN LACTATION

Multiple sclerosis (MS) involves the destruction of myelin sheath that protects nerve cells. Loss of this protective layer disrupts nerve signaling and leads to symptoms including loss of coordination. Women with MS suffer fewer symptoms during pregnancy. Recent studies in mice have shown that high prolactin levels reverse some of the damage associated with MS. Researchers have identified receptors of prolactin on the surface of myelin-producing cells and found that the hormone is able to boost the growth of these cells.

REFERENCES

1. Abrams, B., V. Newman, T. Key, and J. Parker. 1989. Maternal weight gain and preterm delivery. *Obstet Gynecol* 74:577.
2. Abrams, R. S., and D. R. Coustan. 1990. Gestational diabetes uptake. *Clin Diabetes* 8:19.
3. Armitage, J. A., L. Poston, and P. D. Taylor. 2006. Developmental origin of obesity and the metabolic syndrome: The role of maternal obesity. *Front Horm Res* 36:73.
4. Anway, M. D., A. S. Cupp, M. Uzumcu, and M. K. Skinner. 2005. Epitgenetic transgenerational actions of endocrine disrupters and male fertility. *Science* 308:1466.
5. Beemer, P., P. Groenen, and R. Stegers-Theunissen. 2002. Involvement of inositol in reproduction. *Nutr Rev* 60:80.
6. Berry, R. J., Z. Li, J. D. Erickson et al. 1999. Prevention of neural tube defects with folic acid in China. *N Engl J Med* 341:1485.
7. Bouchard, M. F., J. Chevrier, K. G. Harley et al. 2011. Prenatal exposure to organophosphate pesticides and IQ in 7-year old children. *Environ Health Perspect* doi:10.1289/ehp.1003185.
8. Brekke, H. K., and J. Ludvigsson. 2010. Daily vegetable intake during pregnancy negatively associated to islet autoimmunity in the offspring. The ABIS study. *Pediatr Diabetes* 11:244.

9. Brown, A. S., S. Gravenstein, C. A. Schaffer et al. 2004. Serologic evidence of prenatal influenza in the etiology of schizophrenia. *Arch Gen Psychiat* 61:774.

10. Bukowski, R., F. D. Malone, F. T. Porter et al. 2009. Preconceptional folate supplementation and the risk of spontaneous preterm birth: A cohort study. *PLos Med* 6(5):e1000061. doi:10.1371/journal .pmed.1000061.

11. Butterworth Jr., C. E., and A. Bendich. 1996. Folic acid and the prevention of birth defects. *Annu Rev Nutr* 16:73.

12. Callaghan, W. M., M. F. MacDorman, S. A. Rasmussen et al. 2006. The contribution of preterm birth to infant mortality rates in the United States. *Pediatrics* 118:1566.

13. Centers for Disease Control and Prevention. 1993. Recommendations for use of folic acid to reduce number of spina bifida cases and other neural tube defects. *J Am Med Assoc* 269:1233.

14. Day, N. L., S. L. Leach, G. A. Richardson et al. 2002. Prenatal alcohol exposure predicts continued deficits in offspring size. 14 years of age. *Alcohol: Clin Expl Res* 26:1584.

15. Dragun, D., and A. Hanse-Fielitz. 2009. Low catechol-o-methyltransferase and 2-methoxyestradiol in preeclampsia: More than a unifying hypothesis. *Nephrol Dial Transplant* 24:31.

16. Drahl, C. 2011. Sperm's come-hither channel. *Chem Eng* 89(12):12.

17. Frisch, R. E. 1990. Body fat, menarche, fitness and fertility. In *Adipose Tissue and Reproduction*, ed. R. E. Frisch, 1–26. Basel, Switzerland: Karger. (*Prog Reprod Biol Med* 14:1–26).

18. Godfrey, K. M., and D. J. P. Baker. 2000. Fetal nutrition and adult disease. *Amer J Clin Nutr* 71:1344 S.

19. Goldenberg, R. L., T. Tamura, Y. Neggers et al. 1995. The effect of zinc supplementation on pregnancy outcome. *J Am Med Assoc* 274:463.

20. Grant, S. G. 2005. Qualitatively and quantitatively similar effects of active and passive maternal tobacco smoke exposure on in utero mutagenesis at the HPRT locus. *BMC Pediatr* 5:20.

21. Hedderson, M. M., N. Weiss, D. A. Sacks et al. 2006. Pregnancy weight gain and risk of neonatal complications: Macrosomia, hypoglycemia and hyperbilirubinemia. *Obstet Gynecol* 108:1153.

22. Ikonomidou, C., P. Bittigau, M. J. Ishimaru et al. 2000. Ethanol-induced apoptotic neurodegeneration and fetal alcohol syndrome. *Science* 287:1056.

23. James, S. J., M. Pogribna, L. B. Pogribny et al. 1999. Abnormal folate metabolism and mutation in the methylenetetrahydrofolate reductase gene may be maternal risk factor for Down Syndrome. *Am J Clin Nutr* 70:495.

24. Jovanovic, L., and D. J. Pettitt. 2001. Gestational diabetes mellitus. *J Am Med Assoc* 286:2516.

25. Levine, R. J., and M. D. Lindheimer. 2009. First trimester prediction of early preeclampsia: A possibility at last. *Hypertension* 53:747.

26. Mitchell, L. E., N. Scott Adzick, J. Melchionne et al. 2004. Spina bifida. *Lancet* 364:1885.

27. Narendran, S., R. Nagarathna, V. Narendran et al. 2005. Efficacy of yoga on pregnancy outcome. *J Altern Complement Med* 11:237.

28. Rosenblatt, D. S. 1999. Folate and homocysteine metabolism and gene polymorphisms in the etiology of Down Syndrome. *Am J Clin Nutr* 70:429.

29. Stillerman, K. P., D. R. Mattison, L. Gludice, and T. G. Woodruff. 2008. Environmental exposure and adverse pregnancy outcomes. A review of science. *Reproductive Sci* 15:631.

30. Swan, S. H., F. Liu, J. W. Overstreet et al. 2007. Semen quality of fertile U.S. males in relation to their mothers' beef consumption during pregnancy. *Human Reprod* 22:1497.

31. Swan, S. H., K. M. Main, F. Liu et al. 2005. Decrease in anogenital distance among male infants with prenatal phthalate exposure. *Environ Perspect* 113:1056.

32. Turner, E., J. A. Brewster, N. A. Simpson et al. 2009. Imidazole-based erythrocyte markers of oxidative stress in preeclampsia—an NMR investigation. *Reproductive Sci* 18:1040.

33. Vickers, M. H., S. O. Krechower, and B. H. Breier. 2007. Is later obesity programmed in utero? *Curr Drug Targets* 8:923.

34. Witlin, A. G., and B. M. Sibai. 1997. Hypertension in pregnancy: Current concepts of preeclampsia. *Annu Rev Med* 48:115.

35. Woods Jr., J. R., M. A. Plessinger, and R. K. Miller. 2001. Vitamin C and E. Missing links in preventing preterm premature rupture of membranes? *Am J Obstet Gynecol* 185:5.

CASE BIBLIOGRAPHY

36. Cragmill, A., D. Crosby, and W. Kilgore. 1983. The transfer of teratogenic lupine alkaloids to human beings through milk. *J Am Vet Med Assoc* 183:351.

37. Crosby, D. G. 1983. Alkaloids in milk may cause birth defects. *Chem Eng News* 61(15):37.

13 Nutrition and Development

Human development generally denotes the series of changes that lead an embryo to become a mature organism. The first four stages of development in early life are fetal life, infancy, childhood, and adolescence. Nutrition is critical during all of the growth stages.

Nutrient intake is a major determinant of the health and vigor of infants and sets the pattern for the later stages of the lifespan. Newborn infants thrive because of complex physiological mechanisms of ingesting and digesting nutrients. Growth and development during infancy is a function of pre- and postnatal nutrition. Birth weight reflects prenatal growth, which is one of the most important clinical signs of fetal well-being.

The terms *low birth weight* (LBW) and *very low birth weight* (VLBW) describe infants with birth weights of less than 2500 and 1500 g, respectively, but these terms do not incorporate the concept of gestational age. Small-for-gestational age (SGA) or small-for-date (SFD) refers to those infants below the 10th percentile in growth adjusted for gestational age. Those between 10th and 90th percentiles in growth are termed appropriate-for-gestational age (AGA) and those above the 90th percentile adjusted for gestational age are referred to as large-for-gestational age (LGA). Insulin appears to play a significant role in fetal growth. The macrosomia of infants of diabetic mothers has been related to fetal hyperinsulinemia. Insulin can act as a fetal growth factor first by increasing nutrient uptake and utilization and second by exerting direct anabolic effect. Moreover, insulin can modulate the release of growth factors from the fetal tissues.

13.1 FETAL DEVELOPMENT

From conception to birth, the weight of human conceptus increases six billion times; cell number multiplies to 2000 billion, whereas the amounts of water, protein, fat, and minerals increase one to two billionfold. This rapid growth requires a continuous supply of energy and nutrients, which the fetus is unable to synthesize. The placenta transmits most of the elements essential for fetal growth and also removes metabolic waste from the fetus.

Several factors influence the birth weight. Maternal nutrition accounts for about 45%, and the mother's genetic characteristics, including race, are known to contribute about 25% of the variance in birth weight. Maternal height, age, prepregnancy weight, and a previous delivery of a LBW infant also contribute to the birth weight. Maternal malnutrition causes reduction in birth weight by interfering with the normal placental growth, size, and DNA content. It also causes reduction in the normal expansion of blood volume in pregnancy. This is associated with an inadequate increase in cardiac output and leads to decreased placental blood flow and therefore to reduced placental size. The consumption of coffee and alcohol and smoking also cause a reduction in birth weight.

Intrauterine life comprises two principal phases: embryonic and fetal.[25] The embryonic period is usually considered to be the first 8 weeks of growth, during which the ovum differentiates rapidly into an organism having most of the gross anatomic features of the human form. The fetal period spans from the end of the embryonic period through delivery. During early growth and differentiation, teratogenesis is a major consideration. Data accumulated recently suggest a relationship between maternal folic acid status and the frequency of neural tube defects. A variety of factors may impact on differentiation with an effect on fetal growth.

The human fetus requires nutrients to fuel the processes of cell growth and cell differentiation. The requirements depend on the current size of the fetus and the increment in fetal weight because of the synthesis of new tissues. In the earliest stages of development, growth is largely a matter of cell division, with little or no increase in cell size, so that first the embryo grows as fast as its cells divide. Only small amounts of nutrients are required to support this critical period of cell and system differentiation. As pregnancy proceeds, the fetal weight increases and the requirements for nutrients are progressively greater. The fetus grows at an accelerated rate during the first 37–38 weeks of gestation and gains approximately 5, 10, 20, and 35 g/day at 16, 21, 29, and 37 weeks, respectively (Table 13.1). After this period, the increase in weight drops considerably until term. The fetus that remains in utero postterm may experience weight loss because of the relative insufficiency of placenta, but height and head circumference are not affected. The fetus, which weighs approximately 500 g at 22 weeks, doubles its weight in another 5 weeks and doubles its body weight again in the next 5 weeks. At 32 weeks of intrauterine life, the fetus weighs about 2000 g. Over the next 8 weeks, it gains 1500 g to achieve body weight at term of 3300–3500 g.

Initially, the fetus contains a high amount of water (about 89%) and a very small amount of fat (1%–2%) and protein (8%–9%). With growth and maturation, at term the water content falls to about 74% of body weight while fat and protein increase to 15% and 12%, respectively. In early gestation, fat deposition takes place at a rate of about 28–35 mg/day and increases progressively throughout the gestation period. Fat content of the 12- to 20-week-old fetus is about 0.5% of the body weight; this increases to 2.1% at 24 weeks, 10% at 37 weeks, and 12%–15% at 40 weeks (Table 13.1). For up to about 26 weeks of gestation, fat is deposited in the fetal body mainly as phospholipids in the nervous tissue and cell membranes, and there is very little triglyceride in the adipose tissue. The fatty acids required by the phospholipids reach the fetus through the placenta, and this transfer goes on throughout gestation, but from 26 weeks, which is the time when β cells of the fetal pancreas begin to secrete insulin, the fetus synthesizes fat from glucose and the increment in body fat increases, so that during the last 4 weeks it amounts to over 9 g/day.

All through gestation, protein is synthesized by the fetus from amino acids reaching it from the mother's circulation. Fetal liver is capable of synthesizing all plasma proteins except γ-globulin, and this may be the only protein derived from the mother, because the placenta otherwise does not contribute significantly to the plasma proteins of the fetus. The total protein content of the human fetal body increases from the beginning of the perinatal period (e.g., the 20th week of gestation) from 22.5 g (7.5% of body weight) to 388 g (12.7%) at birth.

Analysis of the mineral content of the fetus shows retention of calcium, phosphorus, and magnesium with increasing gestational age consistent with skeletal growth. The calcification of the fetal skeleton begins at about 8 weeks. By week 22, the 1000-g fetus contains about 5 g of calcium, which increases to 30 g by 40 weeks with about 98% of it in the bones. Eighty percent of the total phosphorous is also in the bone with concentrations increasing along with calcium. The calcium:phosphorus ratio remains stable at 1.6:1 throughout gestation. The total magnesium

TABLE 13.1
Relationship of Gestational Age to Average Weight, Protein, and Fat of the Fetus

Gestational Age (Weeks)	Weight (kg)	Protein (g)	Fat (g)
12	0.02	1.1	0.1
16	0.10	6.3	0.6
20	0.30	22.5	2.7
24	0.75	65.0	13.1
28	1.35	123.0	47.2
32	2.00	189.0	130.0
36	2.70	277.0	250.0
40	3.50	446.0	525.0

content of the fetus at term is about 0.8 g with the accretion rate increasing exponentially during the third trimester of pregnancy. Zinc appears to be critically important in very early pregnancy. Its concentration in the human embryo is about 7 times greater on day 35 of gestation than on day 31. The term fetus contains about 300 mg iron, 140 mg zinc, and 15 mg copper. About 80% of these trace elements are accumulated at progressively increasing rates between 28 weeks of gestation and delivery.

The gastrointestinal tract is the interface between diet and metabolism across which all nutrients must pass. In the third week of gestation, the gut is formed from the endodermal layer of the embryo by the incorporation of the dorsal part of yolk sac during infolding by the embryonic disc. The intestine can be defined at week 6 as a tube extending from the mouth to the cloaca, divided according to its blood supply into fore-, mid-, and hindgut. A short esophagus, fusiform gastric and cecal swellings, pancreatic and hepatic buds, and a midgut loop in continuity with the yolk sac are recognizable. During the first few weeks of gestation, the small and large intestine grow in length at a rapid rate and loop into the umbilical cord. Villi, which provide the surface for absorption of nutrients and whose cells contain brush-border enzymes, begin to appear at about week 8 of gestation. By week 10, the abdominal cavity is large enough and reaccepts the small intestine followed by the colon. The cecum completes its descent to the right iliac fossa by 20 weeks when its mesenteric attachments are complete. The gastrointestinal tract appears anatomically prepared for oral feeding by the end of the second trimester. During the second and third trimesters of pregnancy, growth and maturation of the gastrointestinal tract occur in preparation for postnatal life. This is the period of maximal growth of the gut, which doubles in length between 25 and 40 weeks of gestation. At term, the volume of the stomach is about 30 mL and the lengths of the esophagus, small intestine, and large intestine are about 10, 250–350, and 40 cm, respectively.

Hepatic anlage appears during the fourth week of gestation as a solitary diverticulum from the duodenum growing within the ventral mesentery to reach the septum transversum where it proliferates to form anastomosing cords. Identifiable hepatic lobes are noted by the sixth week, and by the ninth week, it achieves its peak relative size, constituting 10% of the total fetal weight. The basic structure of the lungs is visible by 15 weeks of gestation, but they do not become fully operational before 34 weeks.

The development of the teeth begins in utero at 6 weeks of intrauterine life. Two weeks later tooth buds for all 20 primary teeth are present. By 40 weeks, tooth buds of the permanent first molars are present, and calcification of the primary teeth is in progress. Swallowing has been noted to occur at 16–17 weeks of gestation. At this time, the fetus is estimated to ingest approximately 2–7 mL of amniotic fluid every 24 hours; this increases to about 16–20 mL/day at 20 weeks. At term, the fetus ingests approximately 450 mL of amniotic fluid per day.

The parietal cells in the stomach are identifiable by 11 weeks of gestation, and the development of hydrochloric acid, pepsinogen, mucus, and gastric secretion occur throughout gestation. Functional hydrochloric acid production is present early in gestation and awaits appropriate environmental and hormonal stimuli. The disaccharidases sucrase, maltase, and isomaltase can be detected in the intestine by 10 weeks of gestation, and 70% of the adult level of these disaccharidases is reached between 26 and 34 weeks. Lactase activity, on the other hand, is detected at 12 weeks and by 26–34 weeks is only 30% of the term level, but from 35 weeks onward, there is a rapid rise to mature levels. The lactase level at term is 2 –4 times greater than that of infants 2–11 months of age. The cytosol and brush-border peptide hydrolases are present and increase in amount in relation to gestational age.

The pancreatic exocrine function is detectable in the second trimester. Lipase activity is found by 16 weeks of gestation and reaches term level by 28–30 weeks. Amylase can be detected by 22 weeks of gestation, but remains deficient (less than 10% of the adult level) in both term and preterm newborn infants. Trypsin is present by 16 weeks of gestation and is relatively high at term. Insulin is detected at 10–14 weeks of gestation and remains relatively constant throughout gestation. Its secretion in the fetal circulation starts around 26 weeks of gestation. Glucagon is present by the beginning of the second trimester, but normal fetal and maternal glucose concentrations do not appear to have significant regulatory function.

Bile secretion begins at approximately 12 weeks of gestation, but up to 32 weeks the bile acid pool is only 50% of that present at term due, in part, to inadequate hepatic synthesis and poor ileal reabsorption of bile acids. If the level of these acids in the gut falls below critical micellar concentration, it can lead to malabsorption of fat. The fetal intestine is developed for transport processes by 14 weeks of gestation. Absorption of lipids is detected as early as 10 weeks and the transport of glucose by 11–12 weeks; however, there is gestational maturation of the glucose transport mechanism and of other nutrients such as fatty acids, fat-soluble vitamins, calcium, and other minerals.

An adultlike pattern of distribution of most of the regulatory peptide hormones in the intestine is seen by 20–24 weeks of gestation. After this time, the peptide hormone concentrations increase so that by term adult levels are reached. It appears that substantial development of the gut neuro-endocrine system occurs by 25 weeks, the earliest time at which the fetus may first be able to be supported by oral feeding if born prematurely.

Glycogen appears in the liver at 8 weeks of gestation, and its concentration remains constant at 10–18 mg/g in fetal liver until 36 weeks of intrauterine life and then it begins to rise, reaching levels up to 50 mg/g by 40 weeks, and forms an important energy storage pool for the fetus and the newborn infant. The relatively high insulin:glucagon ratio present in the fetus preferentially stimulates glycogen synthesis and suppresses glycogenolysis by means of a multienzyme regulatory system. Similar increases are seen in skeletal and cardiac muscle. The efficient regulation of glycogen synthesis, storage, and degradation develops near term, and this may be a factor for altered glucose homeostasis in those born prematurely. Gluconeogenic enzymes are present in the fetus as early as 10 weeks of gestation, but when maternal glucose is available there is no significant hepatic glucose production. The ability to oxidize fatty acids is underdeveloped at birth.

Until term, the liver is a major erythropoietic organ, but under normal circumstances this function decreases sharply in the last month of intrauterine life. Renal function begins during 9 weeks and increases as a function of body mass rather than maturity, as does the tubular reabsorption of electrolytes. All nephrons are in place by 36 weeks, and no new nephrons are formed in postnatal life. The kidney, however, does not mature fully until about a year after birth. Fetal urine makes an increasingly larger contribution to the volume of amniotic fluid as gestation progresses. Although the fetal kidney is functional, the placenta acts as the major organ for the removal of fetal metabolic waste and the regulation of water and electrolyte homeostasis during fetal life. The fetal gastrointestinal tract is functional very early in gestation. The fetus ingests amniotic fluid beginning at 16 weeks of gestation and digests and absorbs the nutrients present in it. Unabsorbed nutrients and secretions accumulate in the intestine until birth in the form of meconium.

13.2   EXTRAUTERINE DEVELOPMENT

At birth, the gastrointestinal tract, the brain, kidney, and to some degree the liver are ready to function and have been functional in utero for some weeks. The transition from intrauterine to extrauterine life involves cardiopulmonary adaptation, thermoregulation, and enteral nutrition. Gastrointestinal tract and hepatic function must permit the interrelated events of absorption and metabolism to sustain growth and development.

Swallowing is an obligatory function for the survival of the neonate. After delivery, the infant may at first have an immature sucking pattern, but within 2 days a more mature pattern is established. A coordinated pattern of sucking and swallowing is absent in the neonate at less than 34 weeks of gestation, and 75% of the healthy preterm infants require tube feeding until this gestation. The newborn infant's gastrointestinal tract undergoes maturational changes during the first months of life. At delivery, the pH of the stomach is alkaline because of the presence of amniotic fluid. Gastric acid, a first line of defense against the ingestion of potentially pathogenic bacteria, is present within hours of birth, and the gastric pH falls to about 3. Thereafter, the acidity lessens until the age of 10 days when it again increases to reach the adult level by about 3 weeks.

Lingual lipase, which is secreted by glands at the base of the tongue, is acid stable and can function in an acidic environment in the stomach. It assumes a major role in newborn infants, especially the preterm infants whose pancreatic lipase and bile acid levels are low. The lingual lipase has a high activity level at birth. The pancreatic lipase level remains lower until the age of 4–6 months. Fat malabsorption in early life (physiological steatorrhea) is predominantly due to intraluminal bile acid deficiency, which leads to inadequate micelle formation and reduced solubilization of dietary triglycerides. The pancreatic amylase level, which is very low at birth, begins to increase slowly and reaches the adult level approximately at 2 years of age. After the first month of life, the amylase activity can be increased in response to increased starch intake. Salivary amylase may play a role in starch digestion in the first 6 months of life; its activity is about 33% of the adult level by 3 months of age.

At term, the microvillus membrane and mucosa of the intestinal epithelium may be immature in their barrier properties. Intestinal mucosal permeability is greatest during the neonatal period, particularly in preterm infants, and many large molecules including proteins, such as immunoglobulins, tend to be absorbed intact. This process provides a mechanism for the passive transfer of antibodies from the mother's milk and also permits the passage of whole protein with a potential to provoke allergic responses. The absorptive function of the intestine matures during the first year of life.

The ability of a newborn to oxidize fatty acids, which is low at birth, rapidly matures during the first few days of life. This is particularly important because milk, which is the major source of calories in this period of life, presents a large fat load. On a high-fat, low-carbohydrate diet, the newborn must generate active gluconeogenesis to maintain blood sugar concentration. The capacity to synthesize glucose from various precursors is acquired after birth. There is efficient utilization of dietary galactose for conversion to glucose, but there still remains a dependence on gluconeogenesis in early postnatal life. This is especially important if glycogen storage is limited.

The hepatic metabolic function is somewhat immature in the newborn. This is best reflected in bilirubin physiology and by the inefficiency of xenobiotic metabolism. The degree of hyperbilirubinemia is a measure of the functional immaturity of the infant's liver at the time of birth. There is decreased activity of UDP glucuronyl transferase, the rate-limiting enzyme involved in the excretion of bilirubin. Postnatal development of UDP glucuronyl transferase activity occurs in prematurely born infants irrespective of the gestational age, in contrast to slow development in utero, indicating that birth-related rather than age-related factors are important in the emergence of the enzyme. The absence of glucuronyl transferase may be a protection because conjugated bilirubin cannot leave the fetus through the placenta as effectively as unconjugated bilirubin.

The enzyme involved in the conversion of cystathionine to cysteine is absent in the fetus, and it appears only slowly after birth in preterm infants. As a result, the synthesis of cysteine is greatly reduced, and this amino acid must be considered essential in such infants. The absence of this enzyme limits the metabolism of methionine if given in excess. Taurine[1] is considered to be an essential nutrient for the neonate based on low concentrations observed in feeding studies. Carnitine also appears to be an essential nutrient in neonates and infants. This population has low body stores of carnitine and a decreased ability to synthesize it on their own. The premature infants have even lower stores of carnitine because they miss the carnitine accumulation that occurs during the third trimester.

The gastrointestinal tract is sterile in the fetus up to the time of birth. During delivery, the newborn infant picks up microbes from the birth canal and any other environmental source to which it is exposed.

13.3   NUTRITION AND DEVELOPMENT DURING INFANCY

Within 4–6 hours after birth, when the infant can safely tolerate enteral nutrition as judged by normal activity, alertness, and so on, feeding is necessary to maintain normal metabolism during transition from fetal to extrauterine life and to decrease the risk of hypoglycemia. In terms of body weight, the newborn infant's needs for all nutrients are more than that for adults because of the relatively high metabolic rate and special needs for growth and maturation. The development of the skeleton imposes special nutritive needs and the absence of teeth requires that the food be finely subdivided. Some nutrients were delivered to the fetus in surplus; these are stored in the liver to be used during the first few months of life. These include vitamin A, iron, and copper. Because vitamin K-dependent clotting factors do not pass the placenta, they are present in low concentrations in newborns. The current standard of practice in the United States is for newborn infants to receive 1 mg of vitamin K intramuscularly within a few hours of birth. The practice ensures that, at least for the short term, the infant will not become vitamin K deficient. When this practice is not routine, hemorrhage may occur in the newborn period. The amount of human milk ingested by the healthy infant from a well-nourished mother has been used as the primary basis for the recommended allowances during the first 6 months.

At birth, the human gastrointestinal tract is adapted for the consumption of a human-milk-based diet. Intestinal lactase is present and exhibits maximum activity during infancy. Pancreatic amylase secretion is low, and the bile salt pool is decreased relative to older persons, resulting in decreased fat absorption. Human milk provides nutrients in their most usable form for the development of the gastrointestinal tract.

13.3.1   NUTRITIONAL REQUIREMENTS

13.3.1.1   Energy

Except during the late gestational period, at no other period is the growth as intensive as the first 4 months after birth. The birth weight is doubled within 4 months' time with an average gain of 30 g/day, and the weight is tripled or quadrupled in 1 year. Such growth requires considerable nourishment. After the first year, the growth is slower and more steady. During the second year, the average gain in weight is about 2.5 kg. The length of the average healthy term infant increases 50% during the first year from a mean of 50 cm to 75 cm. The body fat content of the normal term infant at birth is 14%–15%, and it increases to about 25% at 4 months, the highest concentration during the first year of life. The gain in lipid is approximately 12 g/day. During the next 8 months, the gain is about 2.9 g/day, while during the second year it amounts to only 0.5 g/day. As a percent of body weight, the lipid content at 1 year of age decreases to 19%. The protein content of the body increases from 11% at birth to 14.6% at 1 year of age. It takes about 7.5 Cal to synthesize 1 g of protein and 11.6 Cal to synthesize 1 g of fat. In the infant, the brain occupies about 16% of the body weight and consumes in excess of 50% of the energy intake in the first few months, as compared to the brain of adults, which is about 2% of the body weight and consumes 20% of the energy utilized by the body.

Approximately 61,000 Cal are required to achieve the 3.5-kg growth between birth and 4 months of age, and 33% of these calories are utilized for growth during this period. This high proportion of calories used for growth drops to 7.4% of the 180,000 Cal consumed from 4 to 12 months of age. The energy requirement per day can vary considerably. A placid infant may thrive on as low as 70 Cal/kg body weight/day, whereas the one who cries a great deal may need 120 Cal or more. The recommended requirement per unit weight is about 2 times higher or 120 Cal/kg body weight/day during the first 6 months of life. These needs can be met through either breast-feeding or the use of formula. Most infant formulas provide 20 Cal/oz. After 6 months, the energy requirement as a function of body weight gradually decreases to approximately 105 Cal/kg/day.

13.3.1.2 Protein

Protein is required for maintenance (wear and tear), growth, and maturation of tissues. The postnatal period is characterized by further physiological and metabolic maturation, which involves changes in chemical composition of the body such as the increase in nitrogen content of cells and tissues. The protein content increases from approximately 338 g at birth to 469 g at the end of the perinatal period (28 days). Daily gain in protein is about 3.2 g during the first year but only 1.4 g during the second year. At birth, roughly about 12.5% of body weight is protein as contrasted with 18.75% for adults, and most of this change takes place during the first year. This increase makes the need for dietary protein both qualitative and quantitative. The protein requirement is 2–2.5 g/kg/day during the first year. As the infancy advances, the protein requirement drops off sharply because physical activity is then the major function for which calories are needed. About 15% of calories as protein is adequate during the first year.

13.3.1.3 Carbohydrates

The ability to hydrolyze maltose, sucrose, and lactose is adequate in newborn infants. Amylase, which is essential for digestion of starch, is very low during the first 4–6 months of age. Thereafter, the concentration begins to rise and reach the levels seen in adults. Therefore, foods containing starch are avoided during the first few months. The major carbohydrate source in early infancy is lactose (present in breast milk) and is the preferred sugar because it also enhances the absorption of dietary calcium and magnesium by lowering the pH of the intestinal contents. About half of the daily calories can be in the form of carbohydrates.

13.3.1.4 Lipids

Although no standards have been adapted for intakes of fat, the concentration of calories in fat is an asset during early infancy when the volume of milk voluntarily consumed by infants is limited. Fat also plays a role in the absorption of fat-soluble vitamins and is a source of essential fatty acids (EFAs). Normal growth of infants depends on an adequate supply of EFAs. Human gray matter and retinal membranes contain significant amounts of long-chain polyunsaturated fatty acids (PUFAs), especially docosahexaenoic acid (DHA). Rapid accretion of these fatty acids occurs in the central nervous system during the last trimester of pregnancy and first months of life. At present, there is insufficient information to determine whether term or preterm infants have sufficient enzymatic activities to synthesize their own long-chain PUFAs from dietary EFAs to meet their requirements for brain growth and development. Human milk provides both EFAs and their long-chain derivatives. Infants fed formula containing at least 2% of the total fatty acids as linoleic acid (0.95% of calories) and a ratio of linoleic:linolenic acid similar to that of human milk may permit incorporation of DHA and other PUFAs in infants.

13.3.1.5 Vitamins and Minerals

Adequate intakes of vitamins and minerals are required for normal growth and development of the infant. Many of these nutrients play important roles as cofactors and catalysts for cell function and replication. Increases in mineral content during growth result because of not only increase in size but also because of maturation of the structure as well. The mineral content of the body increases from 3% of body weight in the newborn to 4.3% in the adult.

The vitamin and mineral requirements of the normal infant are not as well defined as those of energy and protein. Vitamin K appears to be a concern only in newborn infants. It is routinely administered (0.5–1 mg intramuscularly or 1 mg orally) to protect them against hemorrhagic disease. This dose lasts until the infant's intestinal bacteria are established and begin to synthesize the vitamin. If the infant is exclusively breast-fed by a healthy, well-nourished mother and if it has adequate exposure to sunlight, then no vitamin supplementation is necessary after the first 6 months. Adequate exposure to sunlight means an area of body surface equivalent to the infant's head should be in the sun for 15 minutes. If the exposure to sunlight is limited, infants should receive 10 μg (400 IU) of vitamin D supplementation daily. Iron stores present at birth can last up to 6 months of age. Fluoride, important in the preeruptive as well as in the developing phase of tooth growth, may be a necessary supplement (0.25 mg daily) in the infant diet. This may not be necessary if the infant's water intake is adequate since much of the water in the United States is fluoridated.

13.3.1.6 Water

The infant is peculiarly susceptible to a lack of water because the obligatory water loss through the kidney and skin (in relation to body weight) is considerably greater than in the adult. The percentage of body water decreases from 75% at birth to 60% at 1 year of age. The water turnover in infants is approximately 15% of body water as compared to 6% in the adult. The renal capacity of the infant may be lower than that of the adult. It is suggested that water intake of 1.5 mL/Cal consumed is required daily. Under ordinary circumstances, human milk and properly prepared infant formulas supply sufficient water.

13.3.2 REQUIREMENTS FOR LOW BIRTH WEIGHT INFANTS

In recent years, the survival of LBW infants has greatly increased as a result of improvement in techniques for and the availability of high-risk perinatal care. Over 90% of LBW infants over 28 weeks of gestation and 40%–50% of those at 26 weeks of gestation now survive. These infants need early adequate nutrition because their stores of glycogen and some nutrients that normally accumulate during the last few weeks of gestation are limited. At the same time, they may be unable to maintain homeostasis. The generally accepted goal for nutritional management of LBW infants is to provide sufficient amounts of all nutrients to support continuation of the intrauterine growth rate. Depending on birth weight and weeks of gestation, they all need more calories, protein, and other nutrients in terms of body weight than the normal newborn infants. Hypoglycemia and jaundice are lessened in infants fed as early as 2 hours after birth as compared with those fed later. Small infants may have problems in their initial multiple-organ system adaptation, and parenteral nutrition may be needed as the sole nutrition or as a supplement during the period of slow adaptation of the infant's intestinal tract to enteral feedings. Parenteral nutrition is required particularly in infants with birth weight under 1500 g, but may be indicated in any infant facing a delay in reaching full oral feeding for any reason. Some small infants may require enteral tube feeding initially with small amounts (3–4 mL) of milk or formula.

Some manufacturers have devised formulas with types and amounts of nutrients designed specifically for small premature infants. LBW infants have a limited bile salt pool, and this appears to be a major factor in poor fat absorption. Also, because considerable accretion of long-chain PUFAs occurs in the central nervous system during the last trimester of gestation, these infants may have low storage of EFAs and PUFAs derived from them. Human infants, especially premature ones, probably have a low capacity for the synthesis of taurine and cysteine. Taurine has a role not only in the conjugation of bile acids, but also large amounts are found in the brain and retina. There is evidence from work with nonhuman primates and observations in humans that taurine deficiency in infancy can result in disturbances in retinal function.

It is generally agreed that for enteral feeding the milk from the premature infant's mother is higher in protein concentration during the first 4–6 weeks postpartum than is the milk of mothers of term infants. The protein concentration in the first month and its relation to the caloric value allows the milk from its mother to be sufficient to support good growth in many LBW infants. Milk from mothers of term infants is usually not adequate to support growth in premature infants under 1500 g because of its low protein content. The reason for the increased protein in milk of mothers of premature infants is not known, but may be due to the relatively low milk volume produced by these mothers.

13.3.3 Breast-Feeding

Although infants have been successfully breast-fed, attempts to develop breast-milk substitutes have included the use of easily available mammals (e.g., cows, goats) as well as the broths of some cereals. None of these substitutes were successful. As many as 95% of infants fed milk from animals died within the first 2 weeks of life. In the late nineteenth century, the major constituents of milk from different species were analyzed, and it was found that the milk of animals contained too much protein and electrolytes for infants. Protein and electrolyte intoxication caused diarrhea, fever, severe dehydration, hyperelectrolytemia, and death. Animal milk with a caloric density similar to that of human milk was diluted with water, and sugar was added in sufficient quantity to make the formula isocaloric with that of human milk. Infants grew when fed these formulas, and mortality was lowered to approximately 50%, which is similar to the present mortality of artificially fed infants in developing countries. With the development of refrigerators and less contaminated water, infant mortality has decreased to a level similar to that of breast-fed infants. Manufacturers have tried to make formulas containing nutrients in concentrations similar to those found in human milk; however, human milk is superior to any other kind of animal milk or formula and is the perfect food for the growth of infants. Breast milk provides the perfect infant nutrition. It is specifically targeted to meet the nutritional needs of a human baby and changes in composition as the baby grows to meet the infant's changing needs. A diet of breast milk for babies is correlated with benefits including less diarrhea as well as lower incidence of diabetes and asthma when compared to formula-fed babies. It provides not only optimum nutrition for infants but also protects against several diseases.[12] The benefits of human milk are related to its special biochemical, immunological, and psychosocial attributes.

13.3.3.1 Biochemical Benefits

The milk that is produced during the first few days after delivery is called colostrum, which is high in protein, minerals, and other substances (e.g., immunoglobulins) and low in fat in keeping with the needs and reserves of the newborn at birth. It also contains a number of substances that render the infant less susceptible to certain infections such as gastroenteritis. Colostrum causes the newborn infant's intestine to grow in size so as to be ready to receive an increased volume of food.[23] Beginning the third or fourth day after delivery, a slow transition occurs from colostrum to milk production, which contains a little more fat and lactose and less protein and salt concentrations. The infant formula cannot possibly duplicate this gradual change in milk composition, which continues for about 2–3 weeks; by the end of this period, the composition of milk is stable.

Human milk is dilute, and the infant's kidneys can easily handle its waste products even without taking any other fluid, including water. It has 1% protein (as opposed to 3%–4% in cow's milk). The protein when partly digested separates into two fractions: curd casein (about 30%) and the remainder is whey, which is soluble. In cow's milk, only 20% is whey and 80% is casein (Table 13.2). The casein of human milk is rich in cysteine, whereas that from cow's milk is low in this amino acid. This is of significance to some infants, especially LBW infants, who may not be able to convert methionine to cysteine and require the latter in the diet. Taurine is found in human milk in high amounts and is virtually absent in cow's milk. Taurine is an amino acid found free in almost every tissue in the body. It plays an important role in cardiovascular regulation and in the development of the central nervous system.[26] It improves fat absorption in preterm infants. Absence of taurine in the diet of infants is associated with abnormal electroretinograms. Because of the possible inability of some newborns to synthesize it, there is current interest in adding taurine to infant formulas and parenteral amino acid mixtures designed for use in neonates. Most infant formulas including soy protein-based formulas are now supplemented with taurine. Whereas α-lactoglobulin is the dominant whey protein in human milk, β-lactoglobulin is the major whey protein in cow's milk. β-lactoglobulin is the most common food allergen in infancy. The predominant carbohydrate of milk is lactose and it is present in high amounts (6.8 g/dL in human milk, 4.8 g/dL in cow's milk).

TABLE 13.2
Comparison between Human Milk and Cow's Milk

Constituent	Human Milk	Cow's Milk
Biochemical		
Total protein	1%	3.5%
Curd protein	0.30%	2.8%
Whey protein	0.77%	0.75%
Cysteine	↑	↓
Taurine	↑	↓
Lactose	6.8 g/dL	4.8 g/dL
Fat	3.8%	3.8%
Polyunsaturated fatty acids	++++	+
Bile-salt-stimulated lipase	++++	—
Immunological		
S-IgA (whey protein)	++++	—
Lactoferrin (whey protein)	++++	—
Lysozyme (whey protein)	↑ (300 × higher)	↓
Bifidus factor	++++	—

Lactose enhances calcium absorption and is a source of galactose for the biosynthesis of complex lipids of the brain and nervous system. The content of fat in human milk is about 3.8% (about the same as cow's milk) and provides 40%–50% of the energy. It contains more PUFAs derived from EFAs (over 10% of the total fatty acids), including DHA, than in cow's milk (2%). DHA is a major component of brain tissue, and its deficiency in the infant primate has been shown to cause neurological abnormalities.[14] Human milk also contains bile salt-stimulated lipase,[9] which helps digestion of fat. Therefore, nearly all milk fat is digested and absorbed, and very little is lost in the stool.

Several nucleotides are present in human milk, and their concentrations increase in the first few weeks of lactation. So, it seems likely that they are important for tissue development. Some of them have been linked to sleepiness.[11] Recently, researchers measured the levels of uridine monophosphate (UMP), adenosine monophoshate (AMP), and guanosine monophosphate (GMP)—the three nucleotides most strongly associated with sleep and sedation—in breast milk of 30 healthy mothers who had been breast-feeding for at least 3 months.[22] Samples of milk were collected before each feeding over a 24-hour period. The researchers found that the concentrations of AMP were highest at the beginning of the night, while levels of GMP and UMP increased as the night wore on. These sedatives were found at much lower concentrations in milk expressed during the day. AMP in milk might be fueling the release of the sleep-promoting neurotransmitter, γ-aminobutyric acid (GABA), while GMP might be involved in the secretion of melatonin, which helps regulate the natural body clock. UMP is known to promote the amount of both rapid eye movement (REM) and nonrapid eye movement (NREM)* sleep, which are two physiologically distinct states of normal sleep.

In another study, AMP and UMP were added to standard formula milk to make milk specifically for nighttime use. Infants receiving this particular night milk between 6 p.m. and 6 a.m., while relying on normal formula during the day, fell asleep faster and slept longer than when they drank standard formula milk all the time. Based on the above-mentioned findings, this would seem to indicate that mothers who use a breast pump to express milk during the day and then bottle-feed it to their babies at night may be inviting a sleepless night.

---

* Normal sleep includes two physiologically distinct states: rapid eye movement (REM) sleep and nonrapid eye movement (NREM) sleep.

Human milk is of such biological quality and bioavailability that adequate growth can be attained with a lower overall intake of protein than is provided by commercially prepared infant formulas,[5] which contain lower whey to casein ratios. The iron content of human milk is inadequate for term infants; however, supplementation generally is unnecessary in breast-fed infants because the iron present is better absorbed.

13.3.3.2 Immunological Benefits

Human milk contains about a dozen chemical substances that have complex and effective anti-infectious properties.[18,19] These substances neutralize, destroy, and eliminate viruses, bacteria, and parasites, which are known to cause enteritis, colitis, and some other diseases. Four of these substances are described in this section.

Secretory immunoglobulin A (S-IgA) contains most of the antibodies synthesized by the mother in response to the multiple stimuli she has experienced throughout her life. It is a whey protein and is resistant to the action of digestive enzymes. The concentration of S-IgA is very high in colostrum and decreases in mature milk, although its absolute amount remains high throughout lactation even 1 year postpartum.

Lactoferrin is part of the whey fraction of milk proteins. It has an extremely high affinity for iron, even greater than transferrin, and thus makes iron unavailable for the growth of certain iron-dependent bacteria in the gastrointestinal tract. It contributes to a large extent to the marked resistance against infectious gastroenteritis caused by *Escherichia coli*. Lactoferrin is present in human milk but not in cow's milk. Lactoferrin present in milk for the first 10 days of lactation is glycosylated, and then the sugar mostly disappears. Ten days is also the point at which bifidobacteria are generally well established in the intestine. It appears that the mother delivers glycosylated lactoferrin initially to play a protective role against pathogens while the infant builds up intestinal microbes. Once the bifidobacteria are well established, lactoferrin—easier to digest when not glycosylated—becomes a protein source. It also continues to deliver iron to the infant.

Lysozyme is an enzyme present in whey protein and has an antimicrobial action; it attacks bacterial cell walls. Its concentration in human milk is about 300 times more than in cow's milk. The enzyme is stable at acid pH and, therefore, remains active in the digestive tract. The stools of breast-fed infants have significantly greater amount of the enzyme than do bottle-fed infants.

The bifidus factor (methyl-*N*-acetyl D-glucosamine) is a specific factor that promotes the growth of *Lactobacillus bifidus*. The bifidus factor is present in human milk but not in cow's milk. The *L. bifidus* produces acetic acid and lactic acid, which result in a decreased stool pH, which, in turn, inhibits the growth of potential pathogens such as *E. coli*. Children who consume mother's milk in the early weeks of life have a significantly higher intelligence quotient (IQ) at 7–8 years of age than do those who receive no maternal milk. There are several other substances in human milk that provide an intrinsic immunological advantage to breast-fed infants. The incidences of acute infection, including otitis media, febrile upper respiratory tract infection, and acute diarrhea are significantly lower in breast-fed infants aged 3 months–1 year.

There are several other "bioactive" factors in human milk that provide infants with protection from infection by various microorganisms, hormones, and growth factors that affect development, agents that modulate immune function, and anti-inflammatory components. They tend to be present in highest amounts in early lactation. The concentrations of most of these compounds decline as lactation progresses while the infant's milk consumption increases. Many of these compounds are not present in formulas from protein hydrolysates and are present in very low or undetectable levels in formulas based on cow's milk. It is believed that there are several important ingredients in human milk that are not even discovered yet.

Macrophages and neutrophils in human milk may have direct phagocytic action. Oligosaccharides are found in large quantities (~1.5%) in human milk compared to cow's milk (~ 0.1%), which can intercept bacteria-forming complexes that can be excreted. Other substances such as hormones (e.g., cortisol) and smaller proteins including epidermal growth factor (EGF), nerve growth factor, and somatomedin C also protect against unwanted pathogens and other potentially harmful agents. Some of these factors also appear to play an important role in the maturation of the infant's intestinal mucosa. EGF accelerates wound healing. A portion of the low-density lipoprotein (LDL) receptor on human cells has an amino acid sequence very similar to that of the EGF precursor. It is possible that EGF provides a signal to appropriate cells for stimulation of the synthesis of LDL receptors. If so, mother's milk may have a role in the development of LDL receptors and cholesterol metabolism.

Some factors such as antioxidants, prostaglandins, and cytokine receptors may contribute resistance to inflammatory changes during gastrointestinal infections. Nucleotides in human milk enhance intestinal repair after injury and potentiate the immune response for some vaccines. Some nucleotides may promote the growth of *L. bifidus*, which suppresses the growth of enteropathogens in the newborn's intestine.

Other unknown compounds in human milk may stimulate the baby's own production of secretory IgA, lactoferrin, and lysozyme. These proteins are found in larger amounts in the urine of breast-fed babies than in that of bottle-fed infants. Because these proteins present in human milk cannot be directly absorbed by the infants it seems that these molecules must be produced in the mucosa of their urinary tract. It suggests that breast-feeding induces local immunity in the urinary tract. Recently, clinical studies have demonstrated that breast-fed infants have a lower risk of acquiring urinary tract infections.

13.3.3.3 Psychological Aspects

In addition to the biochemical and immunological benefits, one of the reasons for breast-feeding is to provide that special relationship and closeness that accompanies nursing.

13.3.3.4 Advantages

Breast-feeding is preferred as the first choice for most infants when available and appropriate. It is a natural food for full-term infants during the first months of life. It is readily available at the proper temperature and needs no time for preparation. It is fresh and free of contaminating bacteria and contains bacterial and viral antibodies; its allergic reactions are minimal, and it promotes sound feeding habits. The digestibility of human milk also confers an advantage for the breast-fed infant over cow's milk and commercial formula; however, commercial formulas that contain nearly all the known nutrients present in human milk are available, and they seem to work fine as far as the growth of the infant is concerned. Complications associated with breast-feeding are few; however, "breast milk" jaundice associated with hyperbilirubinemia can occur in the breast-fed infant during the first week of life and generally resolves by the fourth week of life. This is generally not a dangerous condition. Nevertheless, if the bilirubin level becomes high, the mother should temporarily stop breast-feeding and feed the infant formula until the jaundice starts to resolve. One important point that must be considered in breast-feeding is that the mother can concentrate chemicals to which she is exposed (e.g., DDT, PCBs), and they are presumed to be toxic to the offspring. Most of the drugs she may take appear in her own bloodstream and then in her milk in amounts that depend on pharmacological factors. There is disagreement as to whether milk can transfer the HIV virus to the infant, but until further studies are done women seropositive for HIV-1 should not breast-feed.

Breast-feeding has long been recognized as the ideal way to feed a newborn, with studies showing that breast-fed babies get fewer infections in infancy and gain long-term health advantages, including protection against adult obesity and diabetes. Breast milk plays a role in helping the baby's brain to develop. Breast-fed babies develop better vision and score higher on IQ tests,[16] results that are attributed to the long-chain fatty acids found in mother's milk. In addition to nutritional superiority, breast milk offers protection against several diseases, making *mother's milk the mother of all medicines for the infant*. Still, less than half of U.S. newborns leave the hospital on an exclusive diet of breast milk. Breast-feeding advocates say that it is in part because hospitals and doctors still accept formula as an alternative and fail to teach and support breast-feeding for new mothers.

According to 2004 statistics from hospitals and the U.S. Centers for Disease Control and Prevention (CDC), 64.7% of new mothers leave the hospital nursing their babies but some of those mothers already are supplementing with formula. Only 41.7% of mothers are exclusively breast-feeding when they leave the hospital.

Even for mothers who breast-feed exclusively in the early weeks and months, some debate exists over exactly how long babies should be breast-fed exclusively to achieve maximum benefit. The American Academy of Pediatrics (AAP) recommends that newborns be fed exclusively mother's milk for about the first 6 months, since this offers the best boost to the immune system and appears to help reduce infections among babies. The World Health Organization (WHO) recommends exclusive breast-feeding for the first 6 months of life, with solids gradually being introduced around this age when signs of readiness are shown. A new study from the Netherlands shows that at least 4 months of exclusive breast-feeding reduces the risk of respiratory and gastro-intestinal infections in babies by an average of 45%. Six months confers even better protection, lowering the infection rates an average of 65% below the rates for formula-fed babies. But a diet of mother's milk supplemented with formula during the first 6 months results in little protective effect. The results support AAP's and WHO's advice that all babies be breast-fed exclusively for 6 months. For some busy moms, the new findings suggest that even 4 months of breast-only feeding—but not less—can benefit babies' health. Supplemental breast-feeding is recommended until age 2.

Each year in the United States, there are hundreds of deaths and many more costly illnesses that breast-feeding may help prevent. These include stomach viruses, ear infections, asthma, juvenile diabetes, sudden infant death syndrome, and childhood leukemia. Researchers recently studied the prevalence of 10 common childhood diseases, costs of treating those diseases, including hospitaliz-ation, and the level of disease protection other studies have linked with breast-feeding. The report concludes that the lives of nearly 900 babies along with billions of dollars would be saved each year if 90% of U.S. women breast-fed their babies for the first 6 months. Breast-feeding is sometimes considered a lifestyle choice, but it is also a public health issue.

Benefits of breast-feeding also appear to stay with mothers for years to come, lowering risks of cardiovascular disease and cancer.

13.3.4 INFANT FORMULAS

The first commercially produced human milk substitute was introduced in the United States in 1869. Infant formulas were conceptualized as "dilutions" of cow's milk. Formulas were basically prepared by diluting cow's milk to the desired protein concentration and by adding sugar to restore energy density to, or close to, a desired level.

Formulas are based on several types of constituents: cow's milk base, soy protein, casein hyroly-sate, elemental amino acids, or meat base. Most regular ready-to-feed formulas have about 20 Cal/oz. Vitamins and minerals are added to meet the recommended intake for infants.

Infant formulas generally begin with cow's milk base. The predominant protein in cow's milk is casein, which is more difficult for infants to digest than the human milk protein, whey. Consequently, in infant formulas generally the casein content is reduced, although not to the level of human milk. In addition, the fat source in cow's milk is replaced by one of several vegetable oils allowing for easier digestion. The carbohydrate source in cow's-milk-based formula is supple-mented with lactose or sucrose because the lactose content of cow's milk is only 50%–70% of that in human milk.

Soy-based and protein-based hydrolysate formulas are available for infants who are intolerant of cow's-milk-based formulas.[2] Soy-based formulas use soybean as the protein source. Although nutrients such as methionine, zinc, and carnitine are still present, their concentrations are rela-tively low. Therefore, methionine is routinely added to all soy-based formulas. Zinc and carni-tine may not be added, and exogenous supplementation may be necessary. Soy-based formulas substitute sucrose, corn syrup, or a combination of the two for lactose as the carbohydrate source. Recently, soy-based formulas have come under scrutiny. Infants ingesting soy formulas grow as well as and absorb minerals at a rate equivalent to infants fed cow's-milk-based formulas. The concern about soy formulas stems from infants' exposure to phytoestrogens or isoflavones, which is several thousand times higher than the exposure from breast milk or cow's milk–based formulas, and whether this exposure poses a developmental hazard. It is estimated that a typical 4-month-old infant ingesting soy formula would be exposed to 29–47 mg of isoflavones per day. Plasma concentrations of isoflavones in infants receiving soy-based formula are found to be significantly greater than in infants fed breast milk or cow's-milk-based formulas. The biological impact of these elevated isoflavone levels on long-term infant development is not yet understood. The AAP recommends that the use of soy-based formula be limited to infants with primary lactase deficiency, galactosemia, secondary lactose intolerance from enteric infection or other causes, infants from vegetarian families who do not allow animal proteins, or infants who are potentially allergic to cow's milk protein but who have not demonstrated clinical manifestations of allergy.

Protein hydrolysate formulas are another option for infants who are intolerant of cow's-milk-based formulas. The milk proteins are heat treated and enzymatically hydrolyzed to enhance digestibility of protein hydrolysate formulas, which are fortified with additional amino acids that are lost during processing. Sucrose, tapioca, or corn syrup is substituted for lactose as the carbohydrate source. Protein hydrolysate formulas often include significant amounts of medium-chain triglycerides because they are better absorbed. Because proteins are hydrolyzed, these formulas are the least allergic of the infant formulas and therefore may be appropriate for infants with a true allergy to cow's milk protein.

The manufactures try to approximate the formulas as closely as possible to the function and composition of human milk, but many qualitative and functional properties of human milk have not yet been successfully reproduced. Human milk contains a number of components that provide benefits to the newborn infant. Some of these components are proteins such as lactoferrin, bile-salt-stimulated lipase, and others. These proteins aid the infant in the defense against infections, facilitate nutrient utilization, and create a beneficial intestinal microflora. Some of these proteins have been cloned and sequenced, and recombinant forms are now being produced. In the near future, it may be possible to add these recombinant milk proteins to infant formulas with the hope that their activities will provide benefits to formula-fed infants. However, several considerations need to be addressed before the addition of these recombinant proteins becomes a reality. These include the assessment of bioavailability and digestion, means of commercial production in an economically realistic manner, safety assessments, and ethical and consumer acceptance issues.

13.3.5 Solid Foods

For the past few decades, there has been a trend toward earlier introduction of solid foods, often after 4–6 weeks of life. The current recommendation is to delay it until 4–6 months of age. Starch digestion is not efficient during the early period of infancy, but improves as the infant grows. After 6 months, breast-feeding can continue, but the energy needs of the infant may exceed those that can be met by breast-feeding. The addition of semisolid foods is therefore desirable. This can also provide iron and other nutrients to supplement the basic intake from human milk.

The first solid foods to be given are usually iron-fortified cereals. It is important not to introduce mixed foods until each component has been given separately for about a week, for if an allergy or intolerance develops it will be difficult to identify the offending food component.[27] Rice is the best cereal to begin with because it is least likely to cause allergies. Strained fruits and vegetables are added next. Toward the end of the first year, tooth eruption and a greater ability to chew permit foods of coarser texture. Thus, a transition to family foods and self-feeding occurs.

13.3.6 Adverse Reactions to Food

Some infants may experience gastrointestinal symptoms or other metabolic derangement as a result of allergic reaction(s) to certain components of food, temporary deficiency of an enzyme because of some disease, or inborn errors of metabolism. Many of these adverse reactions can be readily avoided without compromising the nutritional adequacy of the diet.

13.3.6.1 Milk Allergy

The incidence of allergic reaction to cow's milk protein is probably 1%–3% in bottle-fed babies; cow's milk contains more than 25 distinct proteins, each of which potentially can act as an antigen to induce certain immunological responses. The most allergenic of the milk proteins is β-lactoglobulin, which primarily affects infants during the first few months of life and is attributed to the developmental immaturity of the infant's gastrointestinal tract. In most cases, milk protein allergy is a transient condition; it subsides within a few months and disappears by the third or fourth year of life. In infants prone to cow's milk protein allergy, breast-feeding may be ideal. Also, soy milk protein appears to be tolerated by most but not all infants with cow's milk allergy.

13.3.6.2 Wheat Allergy

Some infants experience reactions to wheat products. These reactions disappear after the removal of the offending substance. One specific syndrome associated with wheat ingestion is celiac disease. The children with this disease are asymptomatic until 6 months of age. They are sensitive to gluten, a protein that is present in wheat, barley, rye, and oats.

13.3.6.3 Lactose Intolerance

The disaccharide lactose is the primary sugar of mammalian milk. To be utilized, lactose must first be hydrolyzed into glucose and galactose by lactase, a membrane-bound enzyme of the brush-border of small intestinal epithelial cells. Lactose intolerance occurs in three forms. Congenital lactase deficiency is an extremely rare life-threatening condition because of a genetic enzyme defect that manifests itself at birth. As soon as the infant with this inborn error receives milk or milk-based formula, symptoms of flatulence, colic, diarrhea, and a lack of weight gain are observed. Acquired lactose intolerance occurs following diarrhea of any cause, including viral gastroenteritis as well as other malabsorption syndromes. This is a temporary state of low lactase activity in previously lactase-sufficient individuals following injury to small intestinal mucosa. This condition is reversible after temporary elimination of all lactose-containing foods from the diet. Developmental lactase deficiency occurs in 30%–70% of blacks and Asians and is present in about 15% of Caucasians, usually beginning at 2–3 years of age. These individuals can consume a moderate amount of lactose such as that provided by one cup of milk without symptoms.

13.3.7 Metabolic Disorders

There are several inborn errors of metabolism that are individually rare but collectively important because they cause significant morbidity and mortality that can in some cases be ameliorated or prevented by nutritional treatment. The basic principle in the management of inborn errors of metabolism is to manipulate the infant's biochemistry so that the metabolite(s) is as normal as possible in the tissue where the defect has its pathophysiological effect(s). The main strategies of nutritional support are dietary restriction of any compound or precursors or metabolites that accumulate as a result of the enzyme block, replenishing any deficient end product distal to the enzyme block, supplementing compounds that may combine with a toxic metabolite and facilitate its excretion, and providing a cofactor if it is deficient for the enzyme. Disorders of carbohydrate metabolism such as hereditary fructose intolerance (deficiency of fructose-1-phosphate aldolase) and galactosemia (deficiency of galactose-1-phosphate uridyl transferase) are treatable by simple dietary elimination of the offending carbohydrate, fructose, and galactose, respectively, and provision of alternate fuel sources to avoid hypoglycemia. Diseases such as phenylketonuria (deficiency of phenylalanine hydroxylase) and maple syrup urine disease (deficient activity of branched-chain keto acid decarboxylase) involve the metabolism of the essential amino acid phenylalanine and the branched-chain amino acids leucine, isoleucine, and valine, respectively. Treatment of these disorders is based on the principal of limiting the dietary intake of the offending amino acid(s) to the amount required for growth and maintenance. In the case of phenylketonuria, tyrosine becomes an essential amino acid and must be supplied in the diet.

13.4 NUTRITION AND DEVELOPMENT DURING CHILDHOOD

The time from 1 year of age until puberty is often referred to as the "latent" period of growth, in contrast to the dramatic changes that occur in infancy and adolescence. The growth during the first year and especially during the first 4 months of life is very rapid, but by the time the infants reach 12 months of age the speed of their growth decelerates. The gain in height decreases from about 25 cm the first year to about 12 cm the second year and 8 cm the third year. One half of the adult height is achieved by the age of 2.5–3 years. After 3 years, the amount of gain in height averages 5–6 cm/year and occurs evenly throughout the childhood years. Prior to adolescence, there is little difference in yearly height increments between the sexes. While the infant triples or quadruples its birth weight in 1 year, the gain in weight slows in the second year and is about 2.5–3 kg. Thereafter, the gains are relatively constant throughout childhood and average about 1.5–2 kg/year. At each age throughout childhood, boys weigh slightly more than girls until about 11–13 years when girls weigh somewhat more.

Body composition in preschool and school-age children remains relatively constant.[24] Fat gradually decreases during the early childhood years and reaches a minimum at approximately 6 years of age. After that it begins to increase slowly in preparation for pubertal growth. Generally, boys have more lean body mass per centimeter of height. Girls have a slightly higher percent of body weight as fat even in the early years, but these sex differences in lean body mass and fat are slight and do not become significant until adolescence.

Because children are growing and developing bones, teeth, muscle, and blood, they need more nutritious food in proportion to their weight than do adults.[7,8] An adequate intake of energy and other essential nutrients is critical to support normal growth and development. Prior to adolescence, there is little difference in yearly height increments between the sexes. As a result, differences in nutritional requirements for males and females have not been established for children under 11 years of age. The RDAs represent the current knowledge of nutritional intakes needed by children of different ages for optimal health. Most of the data for children of these ages are values interpolated from data on infants and adults.

13.4.1 ENERGY

The energy needs of children vary according to age, body size (height and weight), and physiological activity. Recommended energy intakes are given in Table 13.3 under three age groups: for 1–3 years, 102 Cal/kg body weight or 1300 Cal (5439 kJ) daily; for 4–6 years, 90 Cal/kg or 1800 Cal (7531 kJ) daily; and for 7–10 years, 70 Cal/kg or 2000 Cal (8368 kJ) daily.

About 15%–20% of school-age children are overweight. Both genetic and environmental factors contribute to obesity among school-age children. Obesity at this age is a significant risk factor for obesity in later years; therefore, it is important that school-age children be encouraged to keep their weight within normal range. Weight loss generally is not recommended as severe energy restriction could compromise children's growth and delay the onset of maturity. Generally, the goal in weight control for obese children is the maintenance of weight or reduction in the rate of weight gain.

TABLE 13.3
Daily Energy and Protein Intakes for Children

	Calories		Protein	
Age (Years)	Total	Per Kilogram Body Weight	Total	Per Centimeter Height
1–3	1300	102	16	1.2
4–6	1800	90	24	1.1
7–10	2000	70	28	1.0

Source: Food and Nutrition Board, National Research Council. 1989. *Recommended Dietary Allowances.* 10th ed. Washington, DC: National Academy Press.

13.4.2 PROTEIN

During the first year of life, body protein increases from 11% to 14.6%, and by 4 years of age it reaches the adult value of 18%–19%. This is accompanied by an increase in size and deposit of lean body mass. Protein requirements in childhood parallel an individual's caloric needs. Adequate growth and nitrogen retention will occur if the diet provides enough good-quality protein and other essential nutrients along with adequate calories. The average intake of total protein daily is 16, 24, and 28 g for the age groups 1–3, 4–6, and 7–10 years, respectively (Table 13.3).

13.4.3 VITAMINS AND MINERALS

Vitamin and mineral requirements for children have not been extensively studied. Most data are based on values for infants and adults. Because children are growing and developing bones, teeth, muscle, and blood, they need more nutritious food in proportion to their weight than do adults. Vitamins and minerals are necessary for normal growth and development.

Vitamin D is needed for calcium absorption and deposition in the bone. Calcium is needed for adequate mineralization and maintenance of growing bones. The greatest retention of calcium and phosphorus precedes the period of rapid growth by 2 years or more; therefore, liberal intakes of these minerals before age 10 are a distinct advantage. Zinc is essential for growth; its deficiency results in growth failure.

Vitamin and mineral requirements are covered in Chapters 6, 8, 9, and 10 on these topics.

13.5 NUTRITION AND DEVELOPMENT DURING ADOLESCENCE

Adolescence is the period between the onset of puberty and adulthood (i.e., 10–20 years of age). Puberty is an intensely anabolic period with increases in height and weight, alterations in body composition resulting from increased lean body mass, and changes in the quantity and distribution of fat. A growth spurt is experienced by every organ system in the body with the exception of the central nervous system, which remains stable, and the lymphoid system.[21] A rapid growth spurt begins in most girls between the ages of 10 and 13 years and in most boys between the ages of 12 and 15 years. This growth spurt lasts about 3 years. The annual peak for height and weight gain in girls averages about 9 cm and 8–9 kg, respectively. For boys, the annual peak rate is reached about 2 years later; they are 10 cm for height and 10 kg for weight gain. The growth spurt provides about 20% of the ultimate adult height and 50% of the ultimate adult weight. Girls attain their ultimate height by the age of 17–18 and boys by 18–20 years, but small increases in stature are often observed during the next decade.

The fat content of a girl's body increases from about 10% at 9–10 years to 20%–24% at the beginning of menarche. The fat content of a girl's body at age 20 years is about 1.5 times that of boys.

By 20 years of age, boys will have 1.5 times as much lean body mass as girls. The skeleton usually reaches its full size in girls by the age of 17 years and in boys at about the age of 20 years. The water content of the bones gradually diminishes as the mineralization increases. Provided the diet remains good, bone mineralization continues for several years after the attainment of full stature.

Nutrient needs are greatest during the pubescent growth spurt and gradually decrease as the individual achieves physical maturity. RDA values are extrapolated from infant data and/or adult values.

13.5.1 ENERGY

Caloric requirements for growing adolescents have not been studied enough to give an accurate expression of the energy needs of individual teenagers. Requirements increase with the metabolic demands of growth. Peak caloric intake closely tracks the peak growth spurt in both girls and boys. The peak energy intake for girls is at 11–14 years and is about 2200 Cal (9205 kJ). For boys, the peak energy intake is much later (15–18 years) and is of greater magnitude, about 3000 Cal (12,552 kJ). Intakes for three age groups are given in Table 13.4.

13.5.2 PROTEIN

The protein allowances, like those for energy and other nutrients, follow the growth pattern. The highest protein allowance for girls peaks at 11–18 years (46 g) and decreases to 44 g in adulthood. For boys, it is 56 g at 15 years and persists through adulthood.

13.5.3 VITAMINS AND MINERALS

Few data are available on which to base actual vitamin and mineral requirements, but like other nutrients they are all needed in increased amounts in proportion to energy requirements. Data on vitamin requirements for adolescents are more limited than for mineral requirements. Calcium, iron, and zinc may be in short supply, and all are needed during the growth spurt. Calcium is required for normal skeletal growth; during the growth spurt, about 45% of the adult skeletal mass is formed. Consequently, the RDA for calcium during adolescence is increased from 800 mg to 1200 mg/day. The need to consume good sources of calcium such as dairy foods is important for bone health during adolescence and beyond. Boys increase their muscle mass and blood volume faster than girls. Therefore, their need for iron increases during the adolescent growth spurt. Females

TABLE 13.4
Daily Energy and Protein Intakes for Adolescents

	Age (Years)	Calories		Protein	
		Total	Per Kilogram Body Weight	Total	Per Centimeter Height
Boys	11–14	2500	55	45	0.28
	15–18	3000	45	59	0.33
	19–24	2900	40	58	0.33
Girls	11–14	2200	47	46	0.29
	15–18	2200	40	44	0.26
	19–24	2200	38	46	0.28

Source: Food and Nutrition Board, National Research Council. 1989. *Recommended Dietary Allowances*. 10th ed. Washington, DC: National Academy Press.

require less iron for growth, but lose about 15 mg of iron per month as a result of menstruation, and this has to be replaced every month. The current RDA for iron is 18 mg/day for adolescents of both sexes. Zinc is necessary for growth and sexual maturity, and retention of this nutrient increases significantly during the growth spurt. Studies show that many adolescents consume far less than needed. The richest sources of zinc are meat, seafood, eggs, and milk.

13.6 OVERWEIGHT IN INFANCY, CHILDHOOD, AND ADOLESCENCE

The standard clinical tool for identifying overweight and obesity is the body mass index (BMI), a height-to-weight scale, which is relatively easy to use. But, it takes no specific account of fat percentage, and it applies equally for both genders. In order to determine overweight in children or teenagers, a measurement called BMI age- and sex-specific percentile is used, because the amount of body fat changes with age and the amount of body fat differs between girls and boys. After BMI (weight in kilograms divided by height in meters squared) is calculated, the number is plotted in the BMI-for-age growth chart developed by the CDC (for either girls or boys) to obtain a percentile ranking. Percentile is the most commonly used indicator to assess the size and growth of children in the United States.[6] The percentile indicates the relative position of the child's BMI number among children of the same sex and age. Each of the BMI-for-age charts contains wavy lines indicating specific percentiles. If a child's weight falls between 50th and 60th percentiles, it means that his or her weight falls into the category occupied by 50%–60% of other children of the same age and gender. The CDC does not use the word "obesity" for children and teenagers. Instead, it uses two markers for overweight: (1) the 85th percentile, which they consider to be "at risk" level and which roughly corresponds to the overweight marker for adults (BMI of 25); and (2) the 95th percentile, which they consider to be the "overweight" level and which roughly corresponds to the obesity marker for adults (BMI of 30). For its own part, the American Obesity Association utilizes the 85th percentile as a reference point for "overweight" and the 95th percentile for "obesity." The weights that fall between the 5th and 85th percentiles are considered in the healthy weight range, and those that fall below the 5th percentile are considered underweight (Table 13.5). In many countries, a variety of reference data are used or recommended as part of the monitoring of children's growth. These are based on representative data from a given country.

In the United States, the prevalence of overweight (BMI-for-age values at or above 95th percentile) in children of age 6–11 increased from 4% in 1971–1974 to 17% in 2003–2006.[4,20] The prevalence of overweight in adolescents of age 12–19 increased from 6.1% to 17.5% during the same period. The percentage of infants considered significantly overweight increased 73.5% over the last two decades. In 1980, just 3.4% of infants <6 months of age were overweight. By 2001, 5.9% or about 242,000 of the 4.1 million born each year were overweight. Several trends may be behind the weight increase in infants. More newborns are large for their gestational age than a quarter century ago. The reason may be because more mothers are overweight and develop diabetes during pregnancy. In addition, more babies are rapidly putting on pounds in the first few months of life. One study has shown that babies who gain excessive weight during the first 6 months of life may be

---

TABLE 13.5
BMI-for-Age Weight Status Categories and Corresponding Percentiles

Weight Status	Percentile Range
Underweight	Less than 5th percentile
Healthy weight	5th percentile to less than 85th percentile
At risk of overweight	85th percentile to less than 95th percentile
Overweight	95th percentile or greater

---

more prone to obesity as toddlers. About 14% of U.S. toddlers are estimated to be overweight. Other studies have shown a connection between early weight gain and extra pounds in adolescence and later in life. It could be that overfeeding early in life may affect the brain's chemistry during the key developmental period and reprogram a person to eat excess.[15] Being overweight may have a genetic component that first expresses itself in infancy and remains a risk factor throughout life.

Childhood obesity is also a problem in many regions of the world including developing countries. An estimated 155 million school-aged children around the world are overweight or obese, according to the International Obesity Taskforce. The prevalence of childhood obesity is growing rapidly even in countries where hunger is also a problem. Numerous complications are associated with children being overweight or obese, even at a very young age. These include high blood pressure, high serum triglycerides, high fasting glucose, and central obesity. The risk factors for type 2 diabetes and heart disease—long considered to be diseases of adulthood—are now affecting children.[13] These obesity-related diseases are being seen at earlier ages among children making childhood obesity "the greatest single global public health problem of our time."

The reasons for the alarming increases in the prevalence of overweight children are not well understood, but changes in demographics, family structure, lifestyle, decrease in physical activity, greater accessibility to food as well as media influences are assumed to play a role. As in adults, there is no quick and easy way to lose weight in children. Instead, many overweight children end up becoming overweight and obese adults. While there are genetic factors related to childhood obesity, diet and physical activity-related causes are modifiable and have, therefore, been targets of obesity prevention efforts.

Formula-fed infants tend to be bigger than breast-fed infants in late infancy. There is strong evidence that breast-feeding has a protective effect against later childhood and adolescent obesity. Children aged 1–2 years require about 950 calories, but a study found the median intake for that age group is 1220 calories, an excess of nearly 30%. For those 7–11 months, the daily caloric surplus was about 20%. Even before their second birthday, many American children are developing the same bad eating habits. An 8-year study of 70 baby–mother pairs published in 2002 showed that food preferences are established early. Eight-year-olds usually like the same foods they did when they were 4 year olds, and preferences often form as early as age 2. If a mother does not like broccoli, chances are her child will not taste it.

Babies and toddlers are also learning early on to indulge their sweet tooth. Early exposure to intensely sweet foods can have long-term consequences. Intakes of sweetened beverages and high-fructose corn syrup may be contributors to the obesity epidemic as the increase in their consumption shows a pattern consistent with the rise in obesity.

Physical activity is on the decline among children and adolescents of all ages. Strong evidence links childhood obesity to television viewing through both observational studies and randomized controlled trials. Even among preschool children, television viewing is associated with risk of obesity.

The primary goal of treatment for children and adolescents who are overweight or at risk for overweight is to promote healthful lifestyle behaviors that will help the child or adolescent achieve and maintain desirable body weight. Unlike adults, children are still growing in height and require adequate calories for this growth. The main emphasis should be to prevent weight gain above what is appropriate for expected increases in height. A well-balanced healthy diet with low fat (<30% of calories) and regular exercise and physical activity each day is recommended. Avoiding frequent meals of fast prepackaged, processed foods, and limiting intake of sweetened drinks should be helpful.

Rickets in Breast-Fed Infant—A Case

A 9-month-old male infant whose parents were Saudi Arabian was brought to the emergency room because his father noticed that the baby cried whenever his right leg was touched or he had to support his body weight. There was no other history of illness or trauma. The patient was the second child of his parents. The father was on a student visa, and the mother had accompanied him as a housewife. The infant was breast-fed. By custom, she was always completely covered by clothing except for her eyes. She kept the baby similarly clothed, and because of her customs and fears, rarely left the apartment, essentially never exposing either herself or her baby to sunlight.

The infant had an uncomplicated full-term delivery and had normal weight. The parents visited the baby clinic regularly for 3 months and were told that he was growing normally. The parents were advised to visit the clinic in a month to start immunization, but the family did not return until the child was ill 6 months later, at which time he was admitted to the emergency room.

The patient weighed 17 pounds and was 28 inches long. The laboratory values revealed plasma calcium level of 9.2 mg/dL (normal 10 mg/dL), phosphate 2.9 mg/dL (normal 6 mg/dL), and alkaline phosphatase 1130 units/mL (normal 80–270 units/mL). The 25-hydroxy vitamin D level was depressed below the normal range. The right lower leg was slightly tender to palpation without redness or warmth. An X-ray film of the right leg showed mild bone demineralization, cortical thinning, flaring of the metaphyses, and slight widening of the epiphysial plate, consistent with moderately advanced rickets.

The patient was treated with calcium supplementation of 1 g/day and 10 μg of vitamin D per day. Breast-feeding was continued supplemented with progressively more solid foods. Two weeks after therapy was initiated, the plasma calcium level was 10.5 mg/dL, the phosphate was 3.5 mg/dL, and the alkaline phosphatase level was declining. There was no evidence of pain 4 months after treatment was initiated. A follow-up X-ray film of the right lower extremity showed healing of the bone defect.

The biochemical picture of rickets is[28,29] characterized by hypocalcemia, hypophosphatemia, elevated plasma alkaline phosphatase, elevated parathyroid hormone levels, and reduced concentrations of 25-hydroxy vitamin D. This case illustrates that rickets can develop in breast-fed babies without vitamin supplementation or exposure to sunlight. Breast milk is low in vitamin D (0.5–1 μg/dL) compared to the RDA of 10 μg/day. The risk factors for infantile rickets include malnutrition in the mother, prematurity, exclusive breast-feeding without nutritional supplements, dark skin, avoidance of sunlight, adherence to vegetarian diets, and avoidance of vitamin D supplemented cow's milk. Routine supplementation of breast-fed infants with 10 μg of vitamin D per day is necessary to reduce the risk of rickets.

REFERENCES

1. Chesney, R. W. 1988. Taurine: Is it required for infant nutrition? *J Nutr* 118:6.
2. Committee on Nutrition. 1983. Soy protein formulas: Recommendations for use in infant feeding. *Pediatrics* 72:359.
3. Crill, C. M., B. Wang, M. C. Storm, and R. A. Helms. 1999. Carnitine: A conditionally essential nutrient in the neonatal populations. *J Pediatr Pharm Pract* 4:127.
4. Dietz, W. H. 2004. Overweight in childhood and adolescence. *New Engl J Med* 350:855.
5. Ellis, L. A., and M. F. Picciano. 1992. Milk-borne hormones: Regulators of development in neonates. *Nutr Today* 27(5):6.
6. Flegal, K. M., C. J. Tabak, and C. L. Ogdea. 2006. Overweight in children: Definitions and interpretation. *Health Educ Res* 21:755.
7. Food and Nutrition Board, National Research Council. 1989. *Recommended Dietary Allowances*. 10th ed. Washington, DC: National Academy Press.
8. Grand, R. J., J. L. Sutphen, and W. H. Dietz. 1987. *Pediatric Nutrition*. Stoneham, MA: Butterworth Publishers.
9. Hamosh, M. 1989. Enzymes in human milk: Their role in nutrient digestion, gastrointestinal function, and nutrient delivery to the newborn infant. In *Textbook of Gastroenterology and Nutrition in Infancy*, ed. E. Lebenthal. New York: Raven Press, 121–134.

10. Heird, W. C. 1991. *Nutritional Needs of the Six to Twelve-Month Old Infant*. New York: Raven Press.
11. Jensen, R. G., A. M. Ferris, C. J. Lammikeefe, and R. A. Henderson. 1988. Human milk as a carrier of messages to the nursing infant. *Nutr Today* 23(6):20.
12. Kemsley, J. 2008. Unraveling breast milk. *Chem Eng News* 86(39):13.
13. Koopman, R. J., A. G. Mains, V. A. Dia, and M. E. Geese. 2005. Changes in age at diagnosis of type 2 diabetes mellitus in the United States 1988–2000. *Ann Fam Med* 3:60.
14. Kramer, M. S., F. Aboud, E. Miranova et al. 2008. Breast feeding and child cognitive development: New evidence from a large randomized trial. *Arch Gen Psychiatry* 65:578.
15. Lobstein, T., L. Baur, and R. Uauy for the International Obesity Taskforce. 2004. Childhood Obesity Working Group. *Obesity Res* 5(Suppl. 1):4.
16. Lucas, A., R. Morley, T. J. Cole et al. 1992. Breast milk and subsequent intelligence quotient in children born preterm. *Lancet* 339:261.
17. Mahan, L. K., and J. M. Ress. 1984. *Adolescent Nutrition*. St. Louis, MO: Mosby.
18. Newburg, D. S., and J. M. Street. 1997. Bioactive materials in human milk. Milk sugars sweeten the argument for breast-feeding. *Nutr Today* 32(5):191.
19. Newman, J. 1995. How breast milk protects newborns. *Sci Am* 273(6):76.
20. Ogden, C. L., M. D. Carroll, and K. M. Flegal. 2008. High body mass index for age among U.S. children and adolescents 2003–2006. *J Am Med Assoc* 299:2401.
21. Pipes, P. 1989. *Nutrition in Infancy and Childhood*. 4th ed. St. Louis, MO: C.V. Mosby.
22. Sanchez, C. L., J. Cubero, J. Sanchez et al. 2009. The possible role of human milk nucleotides as sleep inducers. *Nutr Neurosci* 12:2.
23. Sheard, N. F., and W. A. Walker. 1988. The role of breast milk in the development of gastrointestinal tract. *Nutr Rev* 46:1.
24. Sheng, H. P., and B. L. Nichols Jr. 1991. Body composition of the neonate. In *Principles of Perinatal–Neonatal Metabolism,* ed. R. M. Cowett, 650–70. New York: Springer-Verlag.
25. Sparks, J. W., and I. Cetin. 1991. Intrauterine growth. In *Neonatal Nutrition and Metabolism*, ed. W. M. Hay, 3–41. St. Louis, MO: Mosby Year Book Inc.
26. Sturman, J. A. 1988. Taurine in development. *J Nutr* 118:1169.
27. Zeiger, R. S. 1990. Prevention of food allergy in infancy. *Ann Allergy* 65:430.

CASE BIBLIOGRAPHY

28. Baron, K. A., and C. E. Phiripes. 1983. Rickets in a breast-fed infant. *J Fam Pract* 16:799.
29. Clinical Nutrition Cases. 1984. Rickets in a breast-fed infant. *Nutr Rev* 42:380.

14 Nutrition and Aging

Aging is a complex biological process in which there is reduced capacity for self-maintenance—a reduced ability to repair cells. More cells are being destroyed than are being produced and, in some instances cells are not replaced. It is a normal, progressive, and irreversible phenomenon throughout adult life and is associated with increased prevalence of chronic diseases[3] or degenerative conditions (e.g., cardiovascular disease [CVD], hypertension, diabetes, cancer, obesity, and osteoporosis). The process of aging begins with the cessation of growth and development and the changes that occur in body composition, organ function, and physical performance are seen in all humans; however, there is a general variability from person to person and even within individuals in whom various organs may age at different rates.

14.1 AGING

14.1.1 LIFE EXPECTANCY AND LIFESPAN

Life expectancy is a predictor of how long the average person would live if the death rates at the time of his or her birth lasted a lifetime. It is not a direct measure of how long people will live. The life expectancy for humans has increased over the centuries with improvements in sanitation, health care, and food quality and availability. In the United States, the average life in the population was 47.3 years in 1900, 72.5 years in 1975, 74.7 years in 1985, and 78.1 years in 2009. Despite the good news, the United States ranks 34th in life expectancy, according to the list by the CIA World Fact Book (2009 estimates). The life expectancy[21] for men and women is 75.15 and 80.69 years, respectively. The number 1 ranked country is Macau with a life expectancy of 84.56 (81.39 years for men and 87.47 for women). This is followed closely by Andorra, Japan, Singapore, San Marino, Hong Kong, Australia, and Canada. The life expectancy in the world is 66.67 years (64.52 years for men and 68.76 years for women). Swaziland has a life expectancy of 31.97 years. Many countries with the lowest life expectancies are suffering from high rates of HIV/AIDS infection with adult prevalence rates ranging from 10% to 38%.

Based on what history shows, worldwide women live longer than men. One of the reasons may be genetic inheritance, but there are also other factors involved.[18] In the United States, men outrank women in all of the 15 leading causes of death, except Alzheimer's. Men's death rates are at least twice as high as women's for suicide, homicide, and cirrhosis of the liver. American men have poorer health and a higher risk of mortality than women. More men smoke (26%) compared with 22% of women. They are twice as likely to be heavy drinkers and far more likely to engage in behaviors that put their health at risk. Men tend to work in more dangerous settings than women and they account for 90% of on-the-job fatalities, mostly in agriculture. In the United States, the gap between the life expectancy of men and women has narrowed since the peak gap of 7.8 years in 1979; it is now at 5.54. The trend appears to be driven by increases in death from diabetes, lung cancer, kidney failure, and heart disease. It may also represent the leading edge of the obesity epidemic.

There are racial differences in life expectancy in the United States. At the present time, white women have a life expectancy of 80.6 years followed by black women (77.4 years), white men (75.7 years), and black men (70.9 years). Location and income also affects lifespan in the United States. Millions of Americans who are worst off have life expectancies typical of developing countries.

According to the state data, Hawaii is the healthiest with an average lifespan of 80 years for men and women. The District of Columbia has the lowest life expectancy of 72 years.

One of the major contributing factors for this increased life expectancy has been the declining childhood mortality because of control and prevention of infectious diseases. Infant mortality rate in the United States hit a record low in 2009 at 6.42 infant deaths for every 1000 live births. This is a 2.6% decline from 6.59 deaths per 1000 births in 2008. Life expectancy at birth increased to 78.2 years in 2009, up from 78 years in 2008. What this means is that somebody born in 2009 can expect to live to an average of 78.2 years. This is a new record for life expectancy. In addition, the present era has seen a decreasing age-specific death rate in young adults and elderly persons because of lifestyle changes, increased standards of living, and improvements in medical technology and health care. As an example, between 1972 and 1992, the death rate in the United States from coronary heart disease decreased by 49% and from stroke by 58%. Age-adjusted death rates for the U.S. population fell for the tenth year in a row to an all time low of 741 deaths per 100,000 in 2009. This is down from 758.7 deaths in 2008. There were 2,436,682 deaths in the United States in 2009, down from 2,473,018 in 2008. Death rates for 10 of the 15 leading causes of death decreased significantly between 2008 and 2009. Death rates declined for heart disease (down 3.7%), cancer (1.1%), chronic lower respiratory diseases (4.1%), stroke (4.2%), accidents (4.1%), Alzheimer's disease (4.1%), diabetes (4.1%), influenza and pneumonia (4.7%), septicemia (1.6%), and homicide (6.8%). Thus, with each continuing year, the number of aged people increases. The proportion of people 65 years old and older (an arbitrary designation of old age) varies from less than 5% in some underdeveloped areas of the world to over 15% in many parts of Western Europe. In the United States, the proportion of elderly people has increased from 4% in 1900 to 11% in 1978, to 12% in 1985. The number of elderly has increased elevenfold from 3.1 million in 1900 to 34 million in 2000. It is projected that in 2020, one out of five people will be in this group (Table 14.1). There are currently 3.5 million in the United States who are 85 years of age or older. One estimate is that this number will increase to 8.8 million in 2020 and 24 million or more in 2040. There are more women than men among the older population. Among persons ≥65 years old in 1997, 59% were women. In the oldest group, 71% of persons ≥85 years old were women. The most rapidly growing segment of elderly in the United States is the age group over 85 years. According to a 2000 census report, the number of Americans 100 years old or older was 50,454—up about 13,000, or 25%, from a decade earlier; As of November 1, 2008, the number has gone up to 96,548, the greatest number of centenarians in the world. The world's oldest person, Edna Parker, who lives in a nursing home in Indiana, is 115 years of age. The second largest number, 36,276, of centenarians is in Japan. Okinawa has several times more centenarians than the rest of Japan. Elderly Okinawans have among the lowest mortality rates in the world from a multitude of diseases of aging and, as a result, enjoy not only what may be the longest life expectancy but also the longest health expectancy. Many experts attribute the high life expectancy in Okinawa to the Japanese diet, which

TABLE 14.1
Percent of U.S. Population 65 Years and Older

Year	%
1900	4
1978	11
1985	12
2000	14
2020	20 (expected)

is particularly low in fat, high in grains, fish, fruits, and vegetables and light on meat, eggs, and dairy products; a low-stress lifestyle; and a high level of activity. The oldest Japanese person is a 113-year-old woman who lives in Okinawa.

Lifespan is the greatest possible age that a person can attain within a specific hereditary potential—has remained unchanged over time at about 115 years. However, there were two individuals in Japan and one in South America who lived to 116–118 years. The record lifespan is held by a recently diseased French woman, Jeanne Calment, who reached 122 years and 4 months. Despite impairment of vision and hearing, she appeared cognitively intact. She smoked until the age of 117, only 5 years before her death. She ascribed her longevity and relatively youthful appearance for her age to olive oil, which she said she poured on all her food and rubbed into her skin, as well as a diet of port wine and nearly 2 pounds of chocolates eaten every week.

14.1.2 THEORIES OF AGING

Various factors may affect the aging process. These include genetic, physical, and/or biological factors within the environment such as exposure to sunlight, smoking, radiation, infectious organisms, nutrition, and physical activity. Nutrition may be among the more significant factors. It may influence aging in two ways: first, it may affect the course of age-related degenerative diseases such as CVD and cancer, and second, an adequate diet may help postpone chronic diseases and improve life expectancy and perhaps lifespan. Nutrition may influence aging and lifespan by interacting at the structural and functional level of the gene by influencing translational events and/or posttranslational processes. Most tissue functions decrease during adult life. The frequency of many chronic diseases increases with advancing age, and there is a large body of evidence relating to the role of nutrition in the etiology of these conditions.

14.2 EFFECTS OF NUTRITION, DRUGS, SUPPLEMENTS, AND GENES

14.2.1 NUTRITION

Several studies in rodents have shown that restricting calories will increase longevity.[13] The first such study was reported by McCay et al. in 1933, who restricted the caloric intake of weanling rats. They observed that animals that survived the first year on a restricted food intake had reduced skeletal growth, delayed sexual maturation, and increased lifespan. Other studies also showed that moderate as well as severe restriction of calories increased lifespan. One other study reported that severe restriction of tryptophan, an essential amino acid, in the diet also increased the lifespan in rats. In all these studies, there was a higher mortality rate during the initial period of the experiment, and the animals that survived this period lived longer. The relevance of these findings in animals to humans is questionable. Chronic dietary restriction during early phases of growth and development at the level used in animal studies is neither practical nor an ethical approach to increasing the lifespan in human subjects because of the increased mortality observed in early phases of the experiment in animals and the possible untoward consequences of undernutrition during infancy and childhood. In one experimental study, in rats given food ad libitum, it was observed that those animals that ate less lived longer. With reference to the restriction of other nutrients such as proteins, fats, or minerals, no significant effect on longevity was observed.

Lifespan has been extended by low-calorie diets in several species of animals. Whether caloric restriction will increase survival in humans remains to be seen. Still observations in some populations offer indirect evidence that caloric restriction could be of value. Many people on Okinawa island in Japan consume diets low in calories but adequate in other nutrients. The incidence of centenarians there is high—up to 40 times greater than that of any other Japanese island. Epidemiological surveys in the United States and elsewhere indicate that cancers occur less frequently in people consuming fewer calories. Also, researchers have observed that moderate calorie reduction lowers blood pressure and blood glucose levels. Ongoing studies at the University of Wisconsin in rhesus monkeys have shown that calorie-restricted diet lowers blood pressure, blood glucose, insulin, and triglyceride levels.[10] Also it blunts aging and significantly delays the onset of age-related disorders, such as cancer, diabetes, CVD, and brain atrophy. Brain health is better overall. In particular, the regions of the brain responsible for motor control and functions such as working memory seem to be preserved in animals that consume fewer calories. The Wisconsin study is likely to provide the most detailed insight into the phenomenon and its potential application to human health as it has traced in greatest detail the diets and histories of an animal that closely resembles humans.

There is no proof yet that "caloric restriction" will extend life for humans.[20] But the lack of certitude hasn't stopped people from experimenting on themselves. About 2000 such enthusiasts are members of the Calorie Restriction Society, a California-based group that promotes the Spartan diet as offering immediate health benefits and supports those who try it. About 200–300 members have cut their consumption by at least 30%, while others are restricting to a lesser degree. The first study of people who voluntarily imposed a low-calorie diet (10%–25% fewer calories than required) on themselves found that their cholesterol levels, blood pressure, and other major risk factors for heart disease—the biggest killer—plummeted, along with risk factors for diabetes and possibly other leading causes of death such as cancer and Alzheimer's disease. While the people in the study do have an extremely low risk of heart disease, no one knows yet if they might be unhealthy in other ways. For example, eating less might weaken their bones or throw off their hormones. Aside from a few corroborating clues from historical records of famine, the only evidence from humans came in 1991 when eight subjects in the sealed biosphere laboratory in the Arizona desert unintentionally tested the theory when their food ran short. Their health appeared to improve markedly, according to a number of measures.

Small-scale studies[11] on humans are going on. But because of the long lifespan of people and the rigors of the diet, the data are not available yet to show that people live longer with low-calorie diets.

Many of the hormonal changes of caloric restriction are similar to the changes seen with aging, raising the question of whether or not caloric restriction is a form of "premature" aging. An important negative effect of caloric restriction is a reduction in bone mineral density. While the enthusiasm for a modest level of caloric restriction in humans is reasonable, it is important to remember that anorexia of aging and its subsequent weight loss represents one of the major clinical problems of older persons.

How caloric restriction works to increase lifespan and retard chronic diseases remains a mystery. One school of thought relates to the possible link between oxidative damage by free radicals and aging. It has been hypothesized that caloric restriction reduces the generation of free radicals. Lowered intake of calories may somehow lead to less consumption of oxygen by mitochondria, and less free radical formation and slower aging process. A different view is that caloric restriction provokes a shift in the metabolic strategy in cells that somehow favor longevity. It has been reported that caloric restriction extends lifespan in yeast, a widely studied laboratory organism whose metabolism is similar to that of animals in many fundamental ways. Caloric restriction appears to work through the silent information regulator No. 2 (SIR2) gene pathway. The gene codes for SIR2 proteins that deacetylate the lysine group of histones as well as other proteins. Histones are components of chromatin, the tightly bundled complexes of DNA, RNA, and proteins that make up chromosomes. When SIR2 deacetylates histones, it compresses the structures of chromatin, silencing various stretches of DNA by making the regions less accessible for gene transcription. Yeast cells grown with very little of their food, glucose, lived longer than normal but not if their SIR2 gene was disrupted. The reason seems to be that the cell's glucose metabolism system and the protein made by the SIR2 gene compete for nicotinamide adenine dinucleotide (NAD). Thus, SIR2 protein cannot perform its silencing duty unless it has NAD to help it, but when the cell is busily converting glucose to energy, there is less NAD available for the SIR2 protein. These studies have led to the general conclusion that the silencing protein SIR2 is a limiting component of longevity. Deletions of SIR2 gene in yeast cells shorten their lifespan while those given an extra copy of SIR2 live longer.

Recent studies have spurred interest in SIR2 as a candidate longevity factor in a broad spectrum of eukaryotic organisms. SIR2 gene homologs have been found in a very wide variety of organisms ranging from bacteria to humans. The mammalian version of SIR2 is SIRT1, a member of the sirtuin family of enzymes. It is a key regulator of cell defenses and survival in response to stress. Cells attempt to repair and defend themselves in response to damage or stress, but if unsuccessful, they often undergo programmed cell death, or apoptosis. A calorie-restricted diet increases SIRT1 in rats, and they are less prone to stress-induced apoptosis. The effects of calorie restriction are observed in nearly all species in which it has been tested. Despite this impressive body of experimental results, it remains unknown whether it can impact positively in humans.

14.2.2 DRUGS AND SUPPLEMENTS

Calorie restriction involves eating about 30% fewer calories less than normal. But its hunger-inducing regimen is too demanding for most people. Researchers are trying to find out other interventions such as new drugs that can slow down the progression of some chronic diseases and retard aging. One leading candidate, resveratrol, present in red wine and peanuts, has been found to extend the lifespan of yeast, human cells, *Caenorhabditis elegans*, and fruit flies and mice that are nourished with normal amounts of food.[19] Thus, resveratrol might yield calorie restriction's gain without pain. The big question is, can it work the same magic in humans?

Animals were given a much higher dose of resveratrol than humans could get from drinking red wine. A person would need to drink 200 glasses of wine a day to get the amount of resveratrol the mice got. Dietary supplements containing concentrated resveratrol extracts, mostly obtained from the Japanese herb, knotweed, let people ingest higher doses. But it is not known how many pills are needed for health-promoting effects in humans, like those observed in mice. Some studies in animals have shown that high doses inhibit formation of new blood vessels, wound healing, and blood clotting. It may have other deleterious effects. The results from small studies boost hopes that resveratrol may eventually be able to ameliorate many diseases of aging and possibly extend human life, but that would be many years and many studies away.

Several drugs and supplements have been shown to reverse the biological effects of aging in animal models; none has yet been proved to lengthen life in humans. A group of drugs, trimethadione and ethosuximide, used to treat childhood "absence" epilepsy, also called petit mal seizures, extends the lifespan of worms by an average of 47% and 17%, respectively, when given during the worm's adulthood. The drugs affect the activity of neurons, suggesting that the nervous system may play a significant role in controlling aging. Trimethadione can cause birth defects, and both drugs are toxic at high doses.

The antibiotic rapamycin, already in use for suppressing the immune system in transplant patients and treating cancers, has recently been found to delay aging in mice.[13] But any drug that suppresses the immune system may have adverse effects. 4-Phenylbutyrate, currently used to treat several diseases such as sickle cell anemia and cystic fibrosis, has been shown to extend the life and maintain the vigor of fruit flies. The compound is an inhibitor of histone deacetylase that may work by affecting chromatin structure and thus gene transcription.

Dietary supplements acetyl carnitine and lipoic acid improve vigor, metabolic function, resistance to oxidative stress, and memory in old rats. It has been reported that worms live about 60% longer if they are given coenzyme Q. Nerve growth factor is a small, secreted protein that induces differentiation and survival of particular target neurons. It is critical for the survival and maintenance of sympathetic and sensory neurons. It has been suggested that nerve growth factor may contribute to increased longevity and mental capacity. Acetylcarnitine, lipoic acid, coenzyme Q, and nerve growth factor are being used by some people to keep them in better health.[12]

There has been much enthusiasm for hormones and other supplements. The levels of many hormones decline with aging, but at present it is uncertain whether replacement of these hormones will extend life and improve its quality. Long-term effects of various supplements are not known.

14.2.3 GENETIC FACTORS

A number of genetic components of aging have been identified using model organisms, ranging from yeast, worms, and fruit flies to mice.[26] Gene expression is imperfectly controlled, and it is possible that random fluctuation in the expression levels of many genes contribute to the aging process.[24] Gene therapy in which artificial genes are inserted into an organism to replace mutated or otherwise deficient genes has been proposed as a future strategy to prevent aging.

Genetically engineered mice with an overactive gene called Klotho lived 20%–30% longer than normal without any signs of ill effects. The gene codes for a small peptide that is shown to modulate biological pathways involved in basal metabolic functions. The lifespan of roundworm *C. elegans* has been increased by lowering the activity of a single gene known as daf-2 from 2 weeks to an average of 12 weeks. The gene codes for a receptor for insulin, and insulin growth factor 1 (IGF-1) also helps regulate the production of superoxide dismutase and catalase. These free-radical scavengers ward off oxidative damage that can contribute to aging. A study using nematode worms has revealed that a gene called *pha-4* is essential for the longevity response to a calorie-restriction diet. Should the longevity link also apply to humans, it could open the door to the development of drugs that mimic the effects of calorie restriction while allowing people to maintain their normal diet.

Researchers are trying to identify genes that help people reach very old age. Individuals with exceptional longevity have a lower incidence and/or significant delay in the onset of age-related disease, and their family members may inherit biological factors that modulate aging process and disease susceptibility.

A study involving about 300 Ashkenazi with an average age of a little over 98 years and more than 200 of their offspring has identified mutation in the gene for cholesteryl ester transport protein (CETP).[7] The enzyme transfers cholesterol among lipoproteins in the blood. The mutation appears to increase the size of high-density lipoprotein (HDL) and low-density lipoprotein (LDL) particles and increase plasma HDL—the good cholesterol. Researchers also found that possessing larger HDL and LDL particles was associated with a lower prevalence of age-related diseases including hypertension, CVD, and a constellation of risk factors for type 2 diabetes and CVD. A polymorphism, or mutation, in the gene that produces CETP was significantly more common in individuals who had exceptional longevity and offspring than in control subjects (offspring of parents who had lived a normal lifespan). As shown by a standardized test of cognitive status in adults, centenarians who had higher than normal HDL levels also showed little cognitive decline.[2]

Another gene[6,16] appears to figure in the area of aging involving telomeres, relatively short protective structures of DNA and protein that cap the ends of chromosomes. Telomeres have been compared to the plastic tips at the ends of shoe laces that prevent laces from unraveling. Along with the rest of the cell's DNA, telomeres are copied during cell division. However, the replication machinery is unable to copy the very tip of the DNA molecules. This means that the telomeres become shorter every time a cell divides. After several cycles of the cell division, the telomeres become too short to protect the remaining DNA. The cell then stops dividing (a stage referred to as senescence) and ages, and is more susceptible to dying. It has been suggested that shortened telomeres may be responsible for some of the changes associated with aging. The enzyme telomerase can repair the telomeres preventing them from shrinking.

Recently, it has been reported that the same group of very old individuals described above and their offspring had a mutation in the gene that codes for telomerase.[4,8] Because of the mutation, these individuals had higher levels of telomerase and significantly longer telomeres than those in the control group, and the trait was strongly heritable. These findings suggest that telomere length and variants of telomerase gene combine to help people live long lives perhaps by protecting them from the disease of the old. It may be possible to develop drugs that mimic the telomerase that the centenarians of the Ashkenazi family are blessed with. However, there may be a downside to the plan of boosting telomerase activity in other populations because giving the cells more chance to divide may increase the chances of developing and causing cancer. But the studies provide evidence that people with long telomeres have less age-related disease and this could be the reason for longevity.

Researchers have developed a genetic test[22] that they claim can identify those who can look forward to an exceptionally long life. They scanned the genomes of 1065 centenarians and compared them with scans from 1267 normal healthy people. They found 150 DNA variants that were more common in the old-aged group and seemed to make their bodies healthier and resilent. The scientists identified 19 patterns among 150 genes and said these patterns predicted with 77% accuracy who would be in the extreme old-age group. The study looked at only Caucasians, but scientists should now look for DNA markers in other populations such as Africans and Asians.*

In another recent study, Japanese scientists engineered female mice from 2 female genes (so they had no genetic father). These biomaternal mice lived an average of 186 days longer, a lifespan boost of 30% longer than the normal female mice (normal mix of maternal and paternal genes). The bimaternal mice were smaller in size and had more eosinophils, white blood cells that improve immune function, than the normal female mice. The female genes, body weight, and improved immune function may contribute to longevity.

14.3 ROLE OF ANTIOXIDANTS

Epidemiological and experimental studies have demonstrated a reduced risk of some chronic diseases including atherosclerosis and cancer in individuals with high-antioxidant status (e.g., β-carotene, vitamins C and E, and the trace element selenium). Experimental evidence suggests a role for oxygen free radicals in the development of chronic diseases and in the aging process. Free radicals are toxic compounds containing one or more unpaired electrons produced during cellular metabolism that can damage body cells resulting in death of vital cells if not stopped by an anti-oxidant. Oxidative damage from free radicals is increasingly implicated in degenerative diseases of aging. Antioxidant systems that would normally protect against oxidant mechanisms decline with aging. For example, blood levels of vitamin E, carotenoids, and selenium decline with aging. In addition, antioxidant enzymes such as glutathione peroxidase and superoxide dismutase decrease in activity. Such changes make tissues more vulnerable to various types of toxicity.

Excessive oxidative stress remains a major theory of aging. Experiments in the worm *C. elegans* have demonstrated that mutations that activate an antioxidant pathway prolong life. Similarly, Drosophila strains that have extended longevity have higher antioxidant activity.

According to the free-radical hypothesis, the degenerative changes associated with aging may be produced by the accumulation of deleterious side reactions of free radicals. Oxygen free radicals (e.g., superoxide, hydroxyl, and peroxyl radicals), which are produced during normal metabolism, can contribute to the aging process. Free radicals can induce DNA cross-links that, in turn, can lead to somatic mutations and loss of essential enzyme expression. In a study that bolsters the free radical theory of aging, scientists recently have genetically engineered mice with higher levels of

---

* Sebastiani et al. (2010) is an interesting study, but soon after the paper was published, some experts in this field criticized the study because the control samples and samples from centenarians were analyzed in slightly different ways. Earlier studies had suggested that tiny contributions from several genetic factors combine to account for about 25% of variation in human longevity and that the remaining 75% are attributable to diet and other environmental factors. The authors were working to address the issue, and on July 21, 2011, they officially retracted the paper. The authors acknowledged the problem with original analysis and stated that "the specific details of new analysis change substantially from those originally published online to the point of becoming a new report. Therefore, we retract the original manuscript and will persue alternative publication of the new findings." (Sebastiani et al. 2011. Retraction. *Science* 333:404.)

catalase in their mitochondria. These mice lived 5.5 months longer than the controls whose average lifespan is about 2 years.

Proponents of the free-radical hypothesis promote supplements of β-carotene, vitamins C and E, and the mineral selenium, but there is no evidence that these antioxidants prolong lifespan in humans. However, health is known to improve when people eat antioxidant-rich fruits and vegetables.

14.4 FACTORS AFFECTING NUTRITION STATUS

14.4.1 PHYSIOLOGIC CHANGES

Aging is associated with loss of physiological functions and with the declining of concentrations of several anabolic hormones such as growth hormone (GH) and insulin-like growth factors (IGF-1 and IGF-2). IGF-1 stimulates glucose metabolism, improves nitrogen balance, and is the mediator of most of the functions of GH. Human aging is associated with increased fasting and lipid-induced cholecystokinin concentration and decline in adrenal and gonadal sex steroids.

Alterations in body composition occur throughout adult life. There is a continuous decline in total body potassium and nitrogen as age advances, which is indicative of a decrease in total body cell mass. The loss of potassium exceeds the loss of nitrogen, and because potassium is more concentrated in muscle than in nonmuscle lean tissue, the reduction in skeletal muscle is thought to be greater than nonmuscle protein mass. At birth, the skeletal muscle has approximately 200 g protein per kilogram body weight. This rises to about 450 g between 21 and 30 years of age, and then diminishes slowly through advancing age until age 70 when it returns nearly to the level seen at birth. In general, after the third decade, there is a 6.3% decrement in lean body mass for each 10-year period.

There are two urinary metabolites of muscle origin that are used as measures of body muscle content (Figure 14.1): creatinine and 3-methyl histidine (3MH). The most commonly used is creatinine, which is formed by muscle cells from the breakdown of creatine and its high-energy form, creatine phosphate, which is produced in the largest amounts in muscle. Creatinine is formed from these precursors by a nonenzymatic chemical reaction that occurs at a constant rate of 1.5%/day. The term creatinine equivalence (kilograms muscle mass per gram of urinary creatinine excreted per day) ranges from 17 to 22 and is an approximate index of muscle mass. 3MH is an amino acid residue formed only in cells that contain actin and myosin. During the breakdown of these

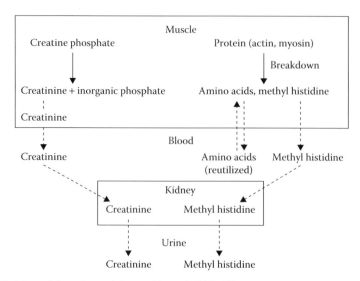

FIGURE 14.1   Origin and fate of creatinine and 3-methyl histidine.

myofibrillar proteins, 3MH is released; it is not recycled or degraded, but is excreted unchanged in the urine. Since muscle is by far the largest reservoir of actin and myosin, the amount of 3MH excreted in the urine is considered the measure of body muscle mass. The excretion of both creatinine and 3MH in the urine decreases progressively with age, and at 90 years of age is about 50% of that at 20 years of age. In a recent study, it has been shown in *C. elegans* that a specific enzyme called P13 kinase has to be present for sarcopenia to occur, suggesting that there may be a simple way to delay age-related muscle deterioration in humans.

There are age-related decreases in functional capacity and strength that are due chiefly to a reduction in the muscle component of lean body mass. This may be related in part to decreased physical activity. Exercise can cause a significant increase in functional capacity and reverse, to some extent, the body composition changes seen with aging. Increased physical activity has been shown to increase life expectancy even into advanced old age.

The decline in lean body mass that occurs during aging is accompanied by a concomitant increase in total body fat even though the body weight may remain the same. There is also a centralized shift of subcutaneous fat from the limbs to the trunk in elderly persons. Total body water is decreased in older persons. This change is significant for the disposition of water-soluble drugs, detoxified metabolites, and thermal regulation.

By age 70, there is a reduction in weight of some organs. For example, the kidneys undergo a 9% reduction in weight, the lungs 11%, the liver 18%, and bone decreases by about 12% in men and up to 25% in women.

There is a reduction in the function of many organs and tissues. The natural process of aging affects both structure and function of the kidneys. Older kidneys excrete sodium load much slower than do young kidneys. There is age-related decrease in glomerular filtration rate and the kidney's capacity to maximally concentrate urine. Although the aging kidney can maintain an adequate internal environment for daily function acute stresses from infections, toxic insults or other organ dysfunction may slow decrease in function. The prevalence of moderate to severe renal failure in population 65 years and older is estimated at 10.8% in nondiabetic and nonhypertensive individuals. Between 30 and 70 years of age, cellular enzymes fall by 15%, cardiac output by 30%, renal blood flow by 50%, and so on. Aging is associated with increased thresholds for taste and smell. There is decreased secretion of hydrochloric acid and pepsin in the gastric juice (about 20%) and a 30% decrease in trypsin in the pancreatic juice. Jejunal lactase activity decreases with advancing age, although the activities of other disaccharidases remain constant throughout adult life.

There is a well-characterized decline in immune function with advancing age. In addition, the immune system is compromised by nutritional deficiencies. Thus, the combination of old age and malnutrition makes older people vulnerable to infectious diseases.

14.4.2 Malabsorption and Gastrointestinal Disorders

The intestinal wall loses strength and elasticity with age, and secretions of gastrointestinal hormones are diminished. These age-related alterations slow motility. Constipation is much more common in the elderly than in the young.

Because of the reduced level of some enzymes in the gastrointestinal tract, the efficiency of digestion and absorption of nutrients may be affected. In addition, the prevalence of digestive disorders is increased in the elderly. In younger populations, about 4.6% of individuals have digestive disease, but after age 45 this increases to 25%.

The most important change with aging is the reduction in gastric acid output in a subgroup of older people who have atrophic gastritis. It affects about one-third of those over 60 years of age. It is characterized by an inflamed stomach, bacterial overgrowth, and a lack of hydrochloric acid and intrinsic factor—all of which can impair the digestion and absorption of nutrients, especially vitamin B_{12}, but also biotin, folic acid, calcium, iron, and zinc.

14.4.3 METABOLISM

There is a decrease in the basal metabolic rate (BMR) of about 20% between the ages of 30 and 90. There is age-related alteration in the metabolism of various nutrients. Epidermal 7-dehydrocholesterol, a precursor of vitamin D, decreases from 5 µg/6.25 cm² of skin at age 50 to 2.5 µg at age 90. The absorption of both calcium and vitamin D declines substantially with age. Also, the efficiency of conversion of vitamin D to its active form by the kidney is decreased. Normal aging is associated with a progressive impairment in carbohydrate tolerance with a modest increase in fasting glucose of about 1 mg/dL/decade and substantial elevations of blood glucose levels after oral or intravenous glucose challenge. This is attributed to diminished sensitivity of peripheral tissues to insulin. Therefore, the use of glucose tolerance curves developed for younger adults may not be appropriate for the diagnosis of diabetes in the elderly. Metabolism of some drugs may be reduced. The plasma half-life of the drug diazepam (Valium) increases substantially with aging, rising from 55 hours in 50-year-old persons to as long as 90 hours in 80-year-olds.

14.4.4 DRUGS

Although the elderly are 10%–12% of the population, they account for more than 25% of all prescribed and over-the-counter drugs. Use of medication can compromise the nutritional status of elderly individuals by altering their food intake, digestion, absorption, and utilization of nutrients. The drugs they take can cure some diseases, reduce symptoms of many others, and provide better health; however, excessive use of drugs can affect the manner in which the body handles nutrients.

Aspirin is the most common self-prescribed drug; it is used as an analgesic for all types of pain and is an anti-inflammatory agent used in certain kinds of arthritis. In some individuals, however, it can cause microscopic bleeding in the gastrointestinal tract that results in the loss of iron. The use of some laxatives, which is common in the elderly, can decrease the absorption of some nutrients such as vitamin D and phosphorus. Mineral oil, for example, is known to interfere with the absorption of fat-soluble vitamins. Antacids such as aluminum hydroxide can react with dietary phosphate and make it unavailable for absorption. Diuretics, which are prescribed for treating high blood pressure, induce sodium and water loss via the kidney. Along with the loss of sodium, a desirable effect, many diuretics also promote loss of potassium and calcium, an undesirable effect.

14.4.5 DISEASES

Diseases, especially chronic ones such as CVD, diabetes, hypertension, and cancer, are more prevalent in the elderly. Many of these diseases may modify nutrient requirements and may profoundly affect how the body can use nutrients.

14.4.6 OTHER FACTORS

Disability, inadequate or improperly fitted dentures, poverty, social and personal problems, and so on, may also affect nutritional status.

14.5 NUTRIENT REQUIREMENTS

Many of the above-mentioned physiological changes that occur during aging may affect the nutritional needs of the elderly population in general.

14.5.1 ENERGY

Because muscle is metabolically highly active, a change in muscle mass has important implications in terms of energy homeostasis. The BMR, which accounts for a major portion of total daily energy expenditure, is directly related to muscle mass. A progressive decline in lean body mass, along with the decreased physical activity, causes the reduction of energy needs in the aged compared to younger individuals. For people of 51–75 years of age, energy allowances decrease to about 90% of that required for young adults (i.e., a reduction of 300 Cal/day for men and 200 Cal/day for women). For persons over 75 years old, there is a further reduction to about 75%–80% of the energy consumed by young adults. In fact, a major characteristic of aging is a progressive decrease in voluntary intake of energy.

14.5.2 PROTEIN

There is controversy regarding the amount of protein necessary to maintain nitrogen balance in the elderly. On the one hand, because of the possible decrease in the efficiency of digestion, absorption, and utilization of dietary protein, some feel that the need for protein is more in the aged population; however, because of the decreased skeletal muscle mass, the loss of daily total body protein is also less. Therefore, the need for protein may be less for older individuals. The Food and Nutrition Board recommends that the elderly consume about 12%–14% of their energy intake as protein.

14.5.3 OTHER MACRONUTRIENTS

Dietary fat is a source of essential fatty acids and is a carrier of fat-soluble vitamins. These functions can be ensured by daily consumption of 15–25 g of fat. There are no recommended daily allowances (RDA) for carbohydrates, but because of the decreased glucose tolerance, the inclusion of more complex carbohydrates and less refined sugar is recommended, and a minimum intake of 50–100 g of total carbohydrate is suggested. Dietary fiber serves an important function in the intestinal tract by promoting the elimination of waste products. The elderly should not have to rely on products such as laxatives. Their need should be met by moderate intake of dietary fiber (20–35 g/day) from sources such as fruits, vegetables, and whole grains.

The elderly are more susceptible to water imbalance. The number of nephrons in the aging kidney is less and increases the solute load per nephron. Because of the lower body water, even mild stresses such as fever or hot weather can precipitate rapid dehydration in older adults. Use of diuretics and laxatives can cause water loss. Dehydrated adults seem to be more susceptible to urinary tract infection and pneumonia. To prevent dehydration, older adults need to drink six to eight glasses of water per day. Milk and juices may replace this water, but beverages containing caffeine or alcohol should be limited because of their diuretic effect.

14.5.4 MICRONUTRIENTS

For most of these nutrients, the needs for the elderly are essentially the same except for thiamin and riboflavin, which are expressed in terms of total caloric intake. The need for vitamin D may be higher because of the reduced capacity of their skin to produce 7-dehydrocholesterol (the precursor of vitamin D), decreased efficiency of conversion of the vitamin to its active form, and their limited exposure to sunlight. Vitamin D deficiency is associated with muscle weakness and is common in elderly individuals. Vitamin D metabolites directly influence muscle cell maturation and functioning through a vitamin D receptor. Supplementation in vitamin D–deficient elderly people has been shown to improve muscle strength, walking distance, and functional ability, resulting in reduction in falls and nonvertebrate fractures. Vitamin D receptors are present in a variety of cells including neurons and the glial cells associated with them. Vitamin D deficiencies are associated with higher risk of osteoporosis, dementia, immune-related disease, heart disease, diabetes, and cancer. Having low blood levels of vitamin D[5] is independently associated with an increase in all-cause mortality in the general population. Among many factors that may be responsible for vitamin D's apparent protection against all-cause mortality is its effect on telomeres and its potential effect on slowing aging.[15] Shortening leukocyte telomeres is a marker for aging. A recent study found that people with the highest blood levels of vitamin D had significantly longer telomeres—equivalent to 5 years of normal aging—than those with the lowest vitamin D levels. Healthy vitamin D blood levels may protect against many age-related diseases and slow the aging process. An intake of 10 µg daily is recommended to prevent bone loss and maintain vitamin D stores, especially for those who engage in minimal outdoor activity. Some studies have revealed an age-related decline in plasma pyridoxal phosphate and vitamin B_{12}. Vitamin B_6 nutriture in the elderly is important because it plays a role in homocysteine metabolism and because deficiencies of vitamin B_6 have been associated with impairments of immune function. This vitamin is also necessary for the maintenance of glucose tolerance and normal cognitive functions. The requirements for this vitamin appear to be higher for older adults than for young men and women and higher for men than women. Thus, the RDAs for vitamin B_6 in adults 51 years of age and older are 1.7 mg/day for men and 1.5 mg/day for women as compared to 1.3 and 1.2 mg/day for younger men and women, respectively.

Because between 10% and 30% of older Americans lose their ability to absorb adequate vitamin B_{12} from food, the RDAs include specific recommendations that elderly individuals consume foods fortified with this vitamin. Dietary calcium and the efficiency of calcium absorption decrease with age. Since calcium deficiency is a contributing factor to osteoporosis, it is advisable to take about 1200 mg calcium per day to maintain calcium equilibrium.

Data from several surveys reveal that the food intake of adults diminishes with age, and with it the consumption of essential nutrients is expected to decrease. The efficiency of nutrient absorption and utilization by the body may be lower in the aged and, as a consequence, the intake of some nutrients can fall below RDA. A multitude of sensory losses and other physical problems can also interfere with an older person's ability to obtain adequate nourishment.

Therefore, the elderly must select foods with a higher nutrient density (higher nutrient to energy ratio) than the diets of younger persons. To assure adequate intake of micronutrients, a daily, multi-vitamin–mineral supplement may be used. Use of supplements by the elderly is discussed in Section 30.8 of Chapter 30.

14.6 LIFESTYLE

A long, healthy life is no accident. Studies are already yielding important clues on what produces healthy aging. It begins with good genes. Some people, including a proportion of centenarians, live most of their lives free from frailty and disability. Genes play a healthy role in their long and healthy life. Identifying variations in genes in this subgroup of humans holds a great potential for improving public health. A long and healthy life also depends on good habits that include diet and exercise.

Seventh-day Adventists eat a vegetarian diet, don't smoke, and spend a lot of time with family and church groups, which help reduce stress. They routinely live to 88 or so, which suggests that these are ages most people could attain with a healthy lifestyle.

It is known that obese people live, on average, less time. Recently, a relationship has been reported between body weight and telomere length; the length decreases with increase in body weight. A similar relationship exists with smoking, with the length of telomeres shortening with the number of cigarettes smoked. According to a study on 20,000 healthy adults in the United Kingdom, people who followed four healthful habits lived an average of 14 years longer than those who did not. These habits are avoiding smoking, eating lots of fruits and vegetables, exercising regularly, and drinking alcohol in moderation. Those who eat more than 2 servings a day of vegetables have about 40% less mental health decline than those who eat few or no vegetables; leafy vegetables are the most effective. Adding six to eight walnuts in an otherwise healthy diet may help older people improve performance on tasks that require motor and behavioral skills. Walnuts are rich in essential fatty acids, polyphenols, and other antioxidants.

A balanced diet should consist of 55%–60% carbohydrate, less than 30% fat (25%–30%), and 15%–20% protein. The carbohydrates should be in the form of fruits and vegetables. Protein should be primarily from plant sources (e.g., whole grain, beans, etc.) with no more than one-third from animal sources. Fat should be mostly from vegetable oils such as olive oil. Refined sugar should be used as little as possible, if at all.

Being physically active reduces the risk of heart disease, cancer, and other diseases, potentially extending longevity.[25] It has recently been found that people who did a moderate amount of exercise—about 100 minutes a week of activities such as tennis, swimming, or running—had telomeres that on average looked like those of someone about 5 or 6 years younger than those who did the least—about 16 minutes a week. Those who did the most—doing about 3 hours a week of moderate to vigorous exercise—had telomeres that appeared to be about 9 years younger than those who did the least. Length of telomeres is considered a marker for biological age.

Seniors who walk regularly, or who otherwise have the highest levels of physical activity, have nearly one-half to one-fifth the risk of developing dementia and Alzheimer's disease than those who are sedentary.[1] Even in very elderly individuals, a little physical activity, such as walking 4 hours a week, goes a long way toward extending life.

Short mental exercises, to boost reasoning skills, memory, and mental processing skills, staves off mental decline in middle-aged and elderly people.

Good genes are known to provide a healthy and long life. Individuals with a gene that expresses more telomerase have longer telomeres. Mutation in the gene that expresses CETP is associated with large-sized HDL and LDL particles and high-HDL levels. These changes are associated with longevity. High-telomerase levels, the length of telomeres, and high HDL levels can be achieved by increased intake of vitamin D, maintaining ideal body weight, increasing activity, and not smoking. Thus, good habits that include diet and exercise can also provide some benefits for long life. One example is the lifestyle of Okinawan centenarians.

Okinawa, the southern group of islands located between Japan's main islands and Taiwan, has the highest proportion of centenarians in the world: 39.5 for every 100,000 people. Elderly Okinawans generally have clean arteries and low plasma cholesterol. Heart disease, breast cancer, and prostate cancer are rare. Good health is attributed to the consumption of locally grown fruits and vegetables, fish, pork, huge quantities of tofu and seaweed, rigorous activity, and low-stress lifestyle. When asked about the secret of longevity, one 102-year-old individual said that the key to his healthy long life is a special drink he takes before going to bed: a mixture of garlic, honey, turmeric, and aloe poured into *awamori*, the local distilled liquor. Okinawans do not have a genetic predisposition to longevity. When they grow up in other countries, they take on the same disease risks as those in their new home.

Defect of Myostatin Function in a Toddler—A Case

During 2004 in Berlin, a baby boy was born with bulging arm and leg muscles. The doctor became concerned that the infant's unusually well-defined muscles might be a sign of illness. A pediatric neurologist examined the boy and found him normal. At age 5 the boy could hold 7-pound weights with his arm extended, which is something many adults cannot do. He has muscles twice the size of other kids his age and half their body fat. Doctors read a paper on myostatin published a few years earlier. Researchers had created a strain of myostatin "knock-out" mice and named them "mighty mice." These mice had twice as much muscle as normal mice. The doctors wondered whether the boy had an abnormal myostatin gene. DNA testing confirmed the suspicion.

The protein myostatin is produced in skeletal muscle cells and acts on muscle tissue by binding to a cell-bound receptor. In humans, myostatin is encoded by the MSTN gene.[29] The protein normally restrains muscle growth ensuring that muscles do not grow too large. Animal studies have shown that mutations that reduce the production of functional myostatin lead to an overgrowth of muscle tissue. Animals treated with chemicals that block the binding of myostatin to its receptor have significantly larger muscle.[28]

The boy's mother is somewhat muscular. Her brother and three other close male relatives all are unusually strong, with one of them, a construction worker, able to unload heavy cornerstones by hand. In the mother, one copy of the gene is mutated and the other is normal. The boy has two mutated copies, one came from his father. The mutation is very rare in people.

An American boy born in 2005 was diagnosed with a clinically similar condition but with a slightly different cause. His body produces a functional myostatin but has a defect in its receptor; his muscles do not respond to the myostatin signal.

For now, the little boy is healthy and very strong. But doctors worry that he could eventually suffer heart and other health problems. Inhibitors of myostatin, a negative regulator of muscle mass, are being developed to mitigate aging-related muscle loss and as potential therapeutic targets for muscular dystrophy.

REFERENCES

1. Abbott, R. D., L. R. White, G. Webster Ross et al. 2004. Walking and dementia in physically able elderly men. *J Am Med Assoc* 292:1447.
2. Arai, Y., and N. Hirose. 2006. Aging and high-density lipoprotein metabolism. *Aging Health* 2:611.
3. Arking, R. 2003. Aging: A biological perspective. *Am Sci* 91(6):508.
4. Atzmon, G., M. Cho, R. M. Cawthon et al. 2009. Genetic variation in human telomerase is associated with telomere length in Ashkenazi centenarians. *Proc Natl Acad Sci* Epub, 2009 Nov 13.
5. Autier, P., and S. Gandini. 2007. Vitamin D supplementation and total mortality: A meta-analysis of randomized controlled trials. *Arch Int Med* 167:1730.
6. Baird, D. M. 2006. Telomeres. *Exp Gerontol* 41:1273.
7. Barzilai, N., G. Arzmon, C. Schechter et al. 2003. Unique lipoprotein phenotype and genotype associated with exceptional longeivity. *J Am Med Assoc* 290:2030.
8. Butler, R. N., M. Fossel, S. M. Harman, C. B. Heward, S. J. Olshansky, T. T. Perls, D. J. Rothman, S. M. Rothman, H. R. Warner, M. D. West et al. 2002. Is there an antiaging medicine? *J. Gerontol* 57A:B333.
9. Colman, R. J., R. M. Anderson, S. C. Johnson et al. 2009. Calorie restriction delays disease onset and mortality in rhesus monkeys. *Science* 325:201.
10. Frasseto, L. A., M. Schloeter, M. Mietus-Snyder et al. 2009. Metabolic and physiologic improvements from continuing a paleolithic, hunter-gatherer type diet. *Eur J Clin Nutr* 63:947.
11. Hagen, T. M., J. Liu, J. Lykkesfeldt et al. 2002. Feeding acetyl-L-carnitine and lipoic acid to old rats significantly improves metabolic function while decreasing oxidative stress. *Proc Nat Acad Sci* 99:1870.
12. Harrison, D. E., R. Strong, Z. D. Sharp et al. 2009. Rapamycin fed late in life extends lifespan in genetically heterogenous mice. *Nature* 460:392.
13. Heilbron, L. K., and E. Ravussin. 2003. Caloric restriction and aging: Review of the literature and implications for studies in humans. *Am J Clin Nutr* 78:361.
14. Janssen, H. J., M. M. Samson, and H. J. J. Verhaar. 2002. Vitamin D deficiency, muscle function and falls in elderly people. *Am J Clin Nutr* 75:611.
15. Joeng, K. S., E. G. Song, K. J. Lee, and J. Lee. 2004. Long lifespan in worms with long telomeric DNA. *Nat Genet* 36:607.
16. Kang, H., S. Benzer, and K. Min. 2002. Life extension in Drosophila by feeding a drug. *Proc Nat Acad Sci* 99:838.
17. Kawahara, M., and T. Kono. 2010. Longevity in mice without a father. *Hum Reprod* 25(2):457.
18. Khaw, K., N. Wareham, S. Bingham et al. 2008. Combined impact of health behaviours and mortality in men and women: The EPIC-Norfolk prospective population study. *PLOS Med* 5:e12.
19. Meyer, T. F., S. G. Kovacs, A. A. Ehsani et al. 2006. Long-term caloric restriction ameliorates decline in diastolic function in humans. *J Am Coll Cardiol* 47:398.
20. National Center for Health Statistics. 1999. Health, United States, 1999 with Health and Aging Chartbook. Hyattsville, MD.
21. Richards, J. B., A. M. Valdes, J. P. Gardner et al. 2007. Higher serum vitamin D concentrations are associated with longer leukocyte telomere length in women. *Am J Clin Nutr* 86:1420.

22. Sebastiani, P., N. Solovieff, A. Puca et al. 2010. Genetic signatures of exceptional longevity in humans. *Science* doi:10.1126/Science 1190532.
23. Schriner, S. E., N. J. Linford, G. M. Martin et al. 2005. Extension of murine lifespan by overexpression of catalase targeted to mitochondria. *Science* 308:1909.
24. Sinclair, D., and L. Guarante. 2006. Unlocking the secrets of longevity genes. *Sci Am* 294(3):48.
25. Stessman, J., R. Hammerman-Rozenberg, A. Cohen et al. 2009. Physical activity, function, and longevity among the very old. *Arch Int Med* 169:1476.
26. Tyner, S. D., S. Venkatachalam, J. Choi, S. Jones, N. Ghebranious, H. Igelmann et. al. 2002. p53 mutant mice that display early aging-associated phenotypes. *Nature* 415:45.
27. Willis, S., S. I. Tennestedt, M. Marsiske et al. 2006. Long-term effects of cognitive training on everyday functional outcomes in older adults. *J Am Med Assoc* 296:2805.

CASE BIBLIOGRAPHY

28. McPherson, A. C., A. M. Lawler, and S. J. Lee. 1997. Regulation of skeletal muscle mass in mice by a new TGF-β superfamily member. *Nature* 387:83.
29. Schuelke, M., K. Wagner, L. Stotz et al. 2004. Myostatin mutation associated with gross muscle hypertrophy in a child. *New Engl J Med* 350:2682.

Part III

Nutrition and Specific Disorders

15 Nutritional Assessment

The maintenance of optimal health requires adequate tissue levels of essential nutrients. Nutritional disorders result from an imbalance between the body's requirements for nutrients and energy, and the supply of these substrates of metabolism. This imbalance may take the form of either deficiency or excess of a particular nutrient(s) and may be attributable either to an inappropriate intake or to a defective utilization. The depletion of body nutrient stores and, ultimately, the loss of specific cellular functions are common to many acute and chronic diseases. With nutritional therapy, the loss of nutrients can be prevented or reversed, and the risk of clinical complications can be minimized or eliminated.

Nutritional assessment is the evaluation of nutritional status (i.e., the health condition of an individual as influenced by food consumption and assimilation and utilization of nutrients). Malnutrition, which affects morbidity, mortality, and the length of stay in hospitals, can respond quickly to appropriate therapy.[1,2] Therefore, it is essential to view the assessment of the patient's nutritional status to be as important as the many diagnostic tests currently available. The evaluation of nutritional status is the first step in the development of a satisfactory plan for the nutritional care of an individual. It can provide valuable clinical assistance in the treatment of acute diseases and can provide the basis for the prevention of chronic diseases later in life.

The assessment of nutritional status would be easier if one could always associate a specific symptom or characteristic with a given nutrient deficiency or excess. Unfortunately, with a few exceptions (e.g., enlargement of thyroid in iodine deficiency), the lack of specificity of clinical signs and the unlikelihood that an individual is deficient in only one nutrient make a direct association impractical; however, any sign or symptom can help direct further investigation toward the assessment of nutritional status.

The evaluation of nutritional status, in common with other aspects of clinical medicine, utilizes history, physical examination, and laboratory tests to provide the data on which an effective diagnosis can be made.[3,4,5] Complete nutritional assessment includes the following: anthropometric measurements, clinical evaluation, laboratory assessment, and dietary evaluation.[6] Each of these components has important strengths and limitations and no single technique will provide a thorough assessment of nutritional health. Not everyone agrees that all the components are always essential and on how much detail should be incorporated into any one of these components when used.

15.1 ANTHROPOMETRIC MEASUREMENTS

Anthropometry is a technique developed by anthropologists in the late 19th century. It uses measurements of body thickness to estimate fat and lean tissue mass.[8] It is the simplest and most quantitative measure of nutritional status. It is useful in monitoring normal growth and nutritional health in well-nourished individuals as well as in detecting nutritional inadequacies or excesses. The main advantages of anthropometry are that it is simple, safe, and inexpensive, and it can be applied at the bedside. The limitation of the technique is that it can detect only those nutrient abnormalities that result in measurable changes in body size or proportion. The measurements most commonly used are length (infants and young children) or height, weight, calculated body mass index (BMI), head circumference (infants and young children), triceps skinfold thickness (SFT), and mid upper arm circumference. Body size, as assessed by weight and SFT, is closely related to food intake and the utilization from the time of conception to the geriatric period.

15.1.1 BODY WEIGHT

Body weight is one of the most convenient and useful indicators of nutritional status. At birth, the low birth weight of an infant suggests that the child is at risk. Frequently, a low-birth-weight infant is the offspring of a poorly nourished mother. The weight should be measured using a beam or lever balance-type scale and the patient should be in a gown or in underwear. Reference tables provide standard weights based on height, age, and sex, and in some cases, there is an adjustment for frame. The patient's weight is compared using these tables. The most commonly used is the Metropolitan Insurance reference weights table (MET). It is derived from actuarial data and, therefore, represents the recommended or desirable weight for height that is associated with maximum lifespan. The MET does not tell what weight makes one the healthiest while alive. The Health and Nutrition Examination Survey (HANES) normative values are higher than the MET reference weights, indicating that the general population may be heavier than recommended in MET tables. If the patient has edema at the time of weighing, the weight may be falsely high.

15.1.2 LENGTH AND HEIGHT

In the case of infants and toddlers, length is measured with the subject in supine position, looking straight up, using an apparatus with a fixed headboard and a sliding footboard. For older children and adults, height is measured using a horizontal arm that moves vertically on a calibrated scale. The patient should be without shoes, heels together, against a straight surface, and with the head level and erect.

15.1.3 BODY MASS INDEX

BMI, the weight in kilograms divided by the height in meters squared, is being used recently as a nutritional measure because the same standards apply to male and female patients. The following BMI values are used: normal nutrition, 20 to less than 25; significant protein–energy malnutrition (PEM), less than 18.5; overweight, from 25 to less than 30; obesity, 30 or greater; and morbid obesity, 40 and above.

15.1.4 SKINFOLD THICKNESS

A skinfold consists of two layers of subcutaneous fat without any muscle or tendon. Approximately 50% of body fat is subcutaneous. As a correlation exists between subcutaneous fat and the fat within the body, SFT measurements are used to estimate total body fat. SFT can be measured at several sites (e.g., triceps, biceps, subscapular, and supraliac), but the triceps are usually employed in assessing the fat stores in adults for practical reasons (i.e., easy access) and because edema is not usually present at this site. Special calipers are available for SFT measurements and the most commonly used is the Lange skinfold caliper. A fold of skin in the posterior aspect of the non-dominant arm midway between shoulder and elbow is grasped gently and pulled away from the underlying muscle. The SFT reading is taken 2–3 seconds after applying the caliper. Normally, three readings are taken and the average is compared with reference standards to assess fat reserves. Standards for skinfold thickness measurements are available from the National Health and Nutrition Examination Surveys I and II and were derived from a probability sample of the U.S. population.

There are limitations in the use of SFT for predicting body fat content. The thickness may vary according to the subject's age, sex, and ethnic origin. Body fat tends to increase with age; therefore, it may not correlate as well with subcutaneous fat. In men, values of thickness less than 12.5 mm suggest undernutrition, and values over 20 mm suggest excess fat and overnutrition. In women, values less than 16.5 mm suggest undernutrition, while values greater than 25 mm indicate excessive body fat and overnutrition. When correlated with midarm circumference (MAC), SFT yields information regarding lean body mass.

15.1.5   HEAD CIRCUMFERENCE

Head circumference is a good index of brain growth. It is usually measured from infants and children as a screening test for microcephaly and macrocephaly. As a nutritional indicator, head circumference may not add significantly to the nutritional information gained from weight, height, SFT, and midarm muscle circumference (MAMC), but the measurement is a standard procedure in pediatric practice.

15.1.6   MIDARM MUSCLE CIRCUMFERENCE

MAMC can serve as a general index of nutritional status. It reflects both caloric adequacy and muscle mass. MAC is measured at the midpoint of the left upper arm by a fiberglass, flexible-type tape. True muscle mass circumference can be calculated from SFT and MAC because the total circumference includes two layers of skinfold. It is assumed that the upper arm is a perfect cylinder. The MAMC is calculated by the following formula:

$$MAMC = MAC - (3.14 \times SFT)$$

Protein–calorie malnutrition and negative nitrogen balance induce muscle wasting and decrease muscle circumference. The MAMC values can be compared to reference graphs available for both sexes and all ages. The MAMC is particularly valuable to patients in edematous states in whom weights are inaccurate or insensitive.

15.2   CLINICAL EVALUATION

General malnutrition may result from primary factors attributable to deficient dietary intake or from secondary factors due to defects in the utilization of nutrients (e.g., gastrointestinal disorders, metabolic disorders). Malnutrition from any cause, if prolonged, results in the following sequence of events: (1) a gradual decrease in tissue levels of the nutrients that are deficient; (2) a biochemical lesion such as an altered activity of the enzyme dependent on a specific nutrient and/or the accumulation of a metabolite; (3) an anatomical lesion; and (4) cellular diseases.

Many of the clinical signs and symptoms of malnutrition often appear late in the process of undernutrition. These are preceded for weeks—and sometimes months—by a gradual depletion of tissue reserves. Clinical examination may identify individuals with overt signs of malnutrition; however, persons with subclinical or marginal malnutrition would be overlooked. Even the presence of a clinical sign may not be a reliable indicator of a given nutrient deficiency because such a sign may not be specific to a particular nutrient. Angular legions, for example, may result from the deficiency of three or four vitamins and may even be due to a local infection. Despite these limitations, the clinical examination provides an overall impression of nutritional health and can reveal specific signs of malnutrition when these exist. Clinical evaluation includes medical history and physical examination.

15.2.1   MEDICAL HISTORY

Contributing factors to malnutrition may be uncovered from the history of chronic illness, weight loss, and weight gain. History is geared to identify underlying mechanisms that put patients at risk for nutritional depletion or excess. From the history, the physician may detect reasons for an existing nutritional problem or assess the likelihood of a nutritional problem developing in the future.

For example, a strong family history of heart disease will alert the physician to seek serum lipid levels and to encourage the patient to decrease excess body weight. Alternately, if the patient reports recent appetite changes, weight changes, digestive problems, and so on, these are symptoms of medical problems that can cause the patient's nutritional status to deteriorate. Nutrient utilization may be affected if an individual is on prescribed drugs with antinutrient or catabolic properties, or consumes alcohol regularly. A certain medical history is helpful (e.g., birth weight for infants and children, occurrence of serious illness, presence of chronic diseases or other disorders that may interfere with ingestion and/or utilization of nutrients).

The unintentional weight loss of more than 10 pounds indicates a need for thorough nutritional assessment. Weight loss of more than 10% of usual weight should be considered to represent PEM that may impair muscle strength and endurance. Weight loss in excess of 20% is considered severe protein–calorie malnutrition that will impair most organ systems. If major elective surgery is planned, the patients should be given adequate feeding preoperatively or at least postoperatively.

15.2.2 PHYSICAL EXAMINATION

The physical examination for determining nutritional status is the same as the usual clinical examination except that the physician looks for physical signs and symptoms from a nutritional point of view. Many deficiencies have more than one cause, and it should be recognized that there are very few key signs that signify a deficiency of a single, specific nutrient. Clinical symptoms are seldom diagnostic for specific nutritional deficiencies and require confirmation by means of biochemical testing and dietary data. Symptoms frequently reflect more than one nutritional deficiency. Taste abnormality may be due to zinc deficiency, but taste also declines with age and can be affected by drugs or smoking. Dermatitis can be due to a deficiency of zinc, essential fatty acids, or some vitamins. Edema, especially of the lower extremities, may be due to a deficiency of vitamin B_1 and/or proteins. Some of the signs may be quite clear. An observation of the patient can indicate obvious obesity, wasting, or apathy; this can provide essential information regarding general nutritional status.

During the physical examination, special attention is given to the areas where signs of nutritional deficiency appear. The hair, eyes, mouth, mucous membranes, tongue, teeth, thyroid, skin, skeleton, tendon reflexes, and neuromuscular excitability provide clues to the presence or absence of nutritional defects. The hair, skin, and mouth are susceptible because of the rapid turnover of epithelial tissues.

Mucosal changes of the gastrointestinal tract are reflected in problems such as diarrhea. The color of the mucous membranes (e.g., those on the undersides of the eyelids in which the blood supply is close to the surface) provides an opportunity to observe the pigmentation of the blood. A pale mucous membrane suggests anemia, whereas more a highly colored membrane is typical of persons with adequate hemoglobin levels. Deficiencies of some of the vitamins manifest themselves in varying forms and degrees of dermatitis. Lesions on areas of the skin exposed to sunlight occur in niacin deficiency. General dryness or roughness due to follicular hyperkeratosis may suggest vitamin A or essential fatty acid deficiency. Chronic wasting accompanied by loss of subcutaneous fat—the result of calorie or protein deficiency—results in fine wrinkling of the skin, especially in older patients in whom the skin has lost its elasticity. A tendency to excessive bruising may occur with a deficiency of vitamin K and the loss of protective fat. Hemorrhages are seen in vitamin C deficiency.

Cracks at the corner of the mouth referred to as angular stomatitis and vertical cracks followed by redness, swelling, and ulceration in areas other than the corner of the lips reflect riboflavin deficiency. A smooth pale tongue may be associated with severe iron deficiency, and in folate deficiency, the tongue is fiery red. Hair as an epidermal structure can sometimes reflect a state of nutritional deficiency. Thin, dyspigmented, easily pluckable hair without normal luster may reflect protein or protein–calorie deficiency. Some of the clinical signs used in the physical examination for

TABLE 15.1
Clinical Nutritional Assessments

Organ Systems	Physical Signs	Nutrient Consideration
General	Wasted, skinny	Energy
	Loss of appetite	Protein–energy
Hair	Thin, sparse, dry, dyspigmented	Protein–energy
	Easily pluckable	Protein–energy
Face	Pale	Iron, thiamin
	Swollen, edema	Protein
Mouth	Tongue—glossitis	Riboflavin, niacin
	Tongue—magenta	Riboflavin
	Lips—cheilosis, inflammation	Riboflavin
	Teeth—mottled enamel	Excess fluoride
Eyes	Xerophthalmia, keratomalacia	Vitamin A
	Bitot's spots	Vitamin A
	Pale	Iron
Neck	Goiter	Iodine
Skin	Xerosis (dryness)	Vitamin A
	Flaking dermatitis	Protein–energy, niacin
	Eczematous scaling	Zinc
	Bruising	Vitamin K, vitamin C
	Pigmentation changes	Niacin
	Thickening, dryness	Linoleic acid
Nails	Ridging, brittle	Iron
Central nervous system	Apathy—kwashiorkor	Protein
	Irritability—marasmus	Protein–energy
	Tetany	Calcium, magnesium
	Peripheral neuropathy	Thiamin, cobalamin
Bones	Bowlegs	Vitamin D

nutritional assessment are listed in Table 15.1. By noting physical changes in the patient, the physician may have a clinical impression of the nutritional status, which objective anthropometric and laboratory measurements can confirm.

15.3 LABORATORY ASSESSMENT

Laboratory evaluation can identify specific nutrition-related abnormalities such as anemia, iron deficiency, or protein deficiency.[10,13] Biochemical tests provide the first indication of nutritional abnormality before clinical or anthropometric changes occur. These tests are specific for the particular nutrient being investigated, and therefore, one must have a suspicion on clinical grounds that a particular deficiency may exist so that the appropriate test can be undertaken. For many micronutrients, techniques have been developed and employed in evaluating nutritional status. These include a measurement of blood levels of the nutrient, a measurement of the urinary excretion rate with or without a test dose of the nutrient administered, a measurement of diminished enzyme activity in the blood, and changes in the level of certain metabolites or increases in abnormal metabolites, which may result from a more advanced deficiency. Laboratory measurements for vitamin and mineral deficiencies are of limited use in the nutritional evaluation of patients except when the clinical presentation is highly suggestive of a specific nutrient deficiency (e.g., zinc in a patient with hypogeusia). For most sick patients, an assessment of protein and calorie status is, by far, the most important issue.

15.3.1 Assessment of Body Protein Status

For purposes of nutritional assessment, body protein can be considered as being divided equally between muscle (somatic) and nonmuscle (visceral) components.[14] In patients with protein malnutrition without calorie deprivation, the measurements of nonmuscle or visceral protein (e.g., serum albumin) may be severely substandard while the anthropometric measure or somatic protein (MAMC) may be normal. The reverse is true in patients with calorie deprivation (i.e., all anthropometric measurements may be severely substandard, while the visceral protein measurements may be normal). Thus, in classifying patients according to the type of malnutrition (e.g., marasmus or calorie-deprived vs. kwashiorkor or protein-deprived), it is useful to have measurements of both the somatic and visceral protein components.

15.3.1.1 Visceral Protein Component

This component is composed of proteins that act as carriers, binders, and immunologically active proteins. Circulating proteins that are commonly used to estimate the size of the visceral protein component include albumin, transferrin, thyroxine-binding prealbumin (PA), and retinol-binding protein (RBP), all of which are synthesized by the liver. Serum albumin is a convenient laboratory test and is the most commonly used. Albumin is the protein present in the highest concentration in the serum. It has two well-known functions. One is its property to bind various substances in the blood. For example, albumin binds bilirubin, fatty acids, metals, cortisol, aspirin, and some other drugs. The other function is the contribution albumin makes to the osmotic pressure of the intravascular fluid. Its concentration makes it a major contributor (approximately 80%) of this pressure, which maintains the appropriate fluid distribution in the tissues. Therefore, hypoalbuminemic states commonly are associated with edema and transudation of extracellular fluid. A lack of essential amino acids from either malnutrition or malabsorption, or impaired synthesis by the liver can result in a decreased serum albumin concentration. The normal range for albumin is 3.5–5.5 g/dL serum. In general, it is believed that an albumin concentration between 2.8 and 3.5 g/dL is suggestive of mild visceral protein depletion, between 2.1 and 2.7 g/dL suggests moderate depletion, and less than 2.1 g/dL suggests severe depletion. A low serum albumin level may be seen in conditions other than protein deficiency, including those due to loss of protein (e.g., as in renal and gastrointestinal disease) or reduced synthesis (e.g., as in liver disease); however, it is difficult to consider a patient with hypoalbuminemia as well nourished, whatever the cause.

As the half-life of albumin is approximately 18 days, its value does not reflect acute protein depletion. Serum transferrin, a β-globulin that transports iron in the plasma, has a half-life of 8–10 days and thus more accurately reflects acute changes in the status of visceral protein. It can be readily estimated in routine laboratory experiments by a measurement of the total iron-binding capacity (TIBC). It is calculated by using the following equation:

$$\text{Transferrin} = 0.8\ \text{TIBC} - 43$$

The normal values for transferrin are 250–300 mg/dL plasma. A value of 150–250 mg/dL is suggestive of mild depletion, 100–150 mg/dL suggests moderate depletion, and less than 100 mg/dL suggests severe depletion of visceral protein. Transferrin levels correlate with nitrogen balance and thus are useful in monitoring patients receiving nutritional support. Transferrin levels must be evaluated in the context of iron stores as iron deficiency leads to an increase in transferrin levels. In addition, transferrin levels may also be increased during pregnancy, hepatitis, and with the use of oral contraceptives. It has also been reported that transferrin levels decrease with high-dose antibiotic therapy.

PA is so named because it migrates ahead of albumin in the customary electrophoresis of serum or plasma proteins. It is also known as transthyretin. PA plays a major role in the transport of thyroxine and is a carrier protein for RBP. Its half-life is about 2 days, but any sudden demand for protein synthesis, such as trauma and acute infection, depresses serum PA. Therefore, a careful interpretation of the data obtained must be made before nutritional depletion can be inferred. The normal serum concentration of PA is 15.7–29.6 mg/dL; a level of 10–15 mg/dL suggests mild depletion, 5–10 mg/dL suggests moderate depletion, and less than 5 mg/dL suggests severe protein depletion.

RBP is the specific protein for retinol transport and is linked with PA in a constant molar ratio. Normal values for RBP are 2.6–7.6 mg/dL. The RBP is catabolized in the kidney, leading to elevated levels in patients with renal failure. Additionally, RBP levels have been reported to increase initially in a patient with hepatitis possibly because of release from the damaged liver. Conditions that lead to decreased RBP levels include vitamin A and zinc deficiency, stress or injury, and hyperthyroidism. The half-life of RBP is about 10 hours and thus can best reflect acute changes in protein malnutrition, but it is too sensitive and can change with even minor stress. Therefore, it has little clinical use as a determinant of visceral protein nutriture.

Other proteins such as fibronectin[11] and somatomedin C (insulin-like growth factor-1, IGF-1) have been used in nutrition assessment and as markers of nutrition support. Fibronectin is a glycoprotein found in the blood, lymph, and many cell surfaces, with structural functions as well as functions in host defense. Plasma fibronectin levels have been shown to drop rapidly in response to starvation in healthy volunteers and to return to normal soon after refeeding. Decreased levels have been found in patients with major burns. Fibronectin levels have been found to increase significantly after 1–4 days of adequate parenteral or enteral feeding. The normal range for fibronectin is 0.3–0.35 mg/mL serum. Plasma fibronectin has a half-life of approximately 15–22 hours.

IGF-1 has important functions in regulating growth and has been found to respond to both fasting and refeeding.[15] The normal range for IGF-1 is 200–350 ng/mL serum, and its half-life is 8–12 hours. IGF-1 concentrations are markedly lowered by energy and/or protein deprivation. Both energy and protein are critical in the regulation of serum IGF-1 concentration. After fasting, an optimal intake of both energy and protein is necessary for the rapid restoration of circulating IGF-1. In adult humans, energy may be somewhat more important than proteins in this regard.

Although fibronectin and IGF-1 appear to have potential uses in nutrition assessment, they are not currently readily available and it may be costly to justify routine usage at this time.

15.3.1.2 Somatic Protein Component

The most widely used biochemical marker for estimating body muscle mass is the 24-hour urinary creatinine excretion.[17] Creatinine is derived from active muscle at a constant rate in proportion to the amount of muscles a patient has. Thus, in a protein-malnourished individual, urinary creatinine will decrease in proportion to the decrease in muscle mass. Creatinine excreted is expressed in terms of height—the creatinine height index (CHI), which combines biochemical and anthropometric measurements—and is used to assess chronic protein–calorie malnutrition in adults. The rationale is that in long-term protein malnutrition, height will remain constant while muscle protein stores will be gradually depleted. As muscle mass diminishes, creatinine excretion will decrease proportionately, and the ratio of creatinine to height will drop. The index is calculated as a percentage of normal as follows:

$$\frac{\text{Milligram of creatinine excreted by the subject in 24 hours} \times 100}{\text{Milligram of creatinine excreted by a normal subject of the same height and sex}}$$

Tables are available for predicted urinary creatinine values for adult men and women of different heights. Values of 80%–90% of normal indicate a mild deficit, 60%–80% of normal indicate a moderate deficit, and values less than 60% indicate a severe deficit of muscle mass.

Dietary creatinine from meat consumption may affect the value of urinary creatinine. CHI is not useful in patients with renal disease.

Another measurement to assess total body somatic protein mass is that of 3-methyl histidine (3MH) excreted in the urine in 24 hours. 3MH is an amino acid that is present exclusively in myofibrillar protein. Upon breakdown of this protein, the 3MH released is not recycled but is entirely excreted in the urine. The amount excreted is proportional to the muscle mass, but it does not reflect all muscle protein breakdown. It does not change with the breakdown of sarcoplasmic protein. Its estimation requires an amino acid analyzer, which is not routinely available.

15.3.2 BODY FAT

Total body water and lean body mass determination from dilution techniques provide an indirect estimation of the fat component of the body:

$$\text{Body fat} = \text{body weight} - \text{lean body mass}$$
$$\text{Lean body mass} = \frac{\text{Body water}}{0.72}$$

Total body water is determined using antipyrene, deuterium oxide, or some other tracer, which dissolves in all the water of the body and is not rapidly metabolized. An intravenous injection of the exactly known amount of the tracer is given. After time is allowed for uniform distribution, a blood sample is drawn and the concentration of the tracer in the water of the blood is measured. Water represents a fixed fraction (approximately 0.72–0.73) of the lean body mass.

Body fat can also be determined by the measurement of impedance. Bioelectric impedance[9] (BEI) or total body electrical conductivity assessment is based on the conductivity properties of an electrolyte-based medium. It relies on differences in electrical properties of the fat-free mass and the fat mass. Lean body mass has more water and associated electrolytes and therefore demonstrates greater electrical conductivity; the leaner the person, the less the resistance to the electrical current. Impedance is the pure resistance of a biological conduction to the flow of an alternating current. The technique involves connecting electrodes to the hands and feet and passing a mild electric current through the body. The measurement of electrical resistance is then used in a mathematical equation to estimate the percentage of body fat. BEI measurements have been found to correlate well with deuterium isotopic dilution measurements in both obese and nonobese normal volunteers.

The BEI technique is safe, noninvasive, and requires little or no patient cooperation. The instrument is portable and fairly easy to operate. The impedance method seems to be valid for assessing current body composition in subjects without large disturbances in fluid and electrolytes distribution. Edema and dehydration lead to alterations in resistance measurements.

15.3.3 IMMUNE FUNCTION

Malnutrition affects the immune system. The best studied in humans is PEM, which often involves deficiencies of other nutrients. Almost all of the body's defense mechanisms are damaged by nutritional deficiencies. The systems affected include immunoglobulins and antibody production, phagocytosis, complement activity, and secretory and mucosal immunity. Of the several tests that can be done, only lymphocyte count and skin tests are routinely employed for an assessment of nutritional status.

The total lymphocyte count is derived from the complete blood count. The normal value is greater than $1500/\text{mm}^3$. The total lymphocyte count decreases progressively with various states of PEM. It can also be affected by an acute stress response or by the presence of a large wound. Delayed cutaneous hypersensitivity is evaluated by the response of the patient to recall antigen. The antigens commonly used are streptokinase/streptodornase (SK/SD), mumps, *Candida*, and purified protein derivative (PPD). A positive skin test is defined as an induration at the site of injection of 5 mm or more in 24–48 hours after the administration of any one of these antigens. A lack of response or redness and an induration of less than 5 mm suggest immune incompetence or anergy and are associated with PEM; however, a variety of drugs and diseases can interfere with the skin reaction.

15.3.4 NITROGEN BALANCE

Although this is not a test for nutritional assessment, it is useful to evaluate the progress of nutrition therapy. During the treatment of malnourished patients, the anthropometric and biochemical parameters are slow to improve, and the information usually is needed quickly for effective patient management. The determination of nitrogen balance is the most useful clinical study to assess whether the anabolic state has been achieved in response to therapy. In patients with no renal impairment or small bowel disease associated with protein-losing enteropathy, nitrogen balance is determined by calculating the difference between nitrogen intake and nitrogen excreted:

$$\text{Nitrogen balance} = \frac{N_i}{6.25} N_c + 4^a$$

4^a = consideration for other nonurea nitrogen loss, where N_i = dietary protein intake, grams per 24 hours; N_c = urinary urea nitrogen, grams per 24 hours.

An individual with a positive nitrogen balance is retaining more nitrogen than is being excreted (anabolic state). The negative nitrogen balance indicates the severity of the catabolic state. With an adequate intake of protein and calories, nitrogen losses can be matched with nitrogen intake and a nitrogen balance (or positive nitrogen balance) can be achieved.

15.3.5 LIPIDS

Cholesterol and triglyceride concentrations in blood samples obtained after a 12-hour fast are indices of fat nutrition. Cholesterol values in excess of 220–240 mg/dL are considered abnormally high and indicate metabolic problems in lipid metabolism. Triglycerides in excess of 150 mg/dL are indicative of an abnormality in lipid handling because of the individual's sensitivity to dietary fat and/or carbohydrate. Essential fatty acid deficiency can be diagnosed by a determination of the levels of trienes and tetraenes in plasma. The ratio of triene/tetraene is normally less than 0.4 but is much higher in essential fatty acid deficiency.

15.3.6 OTHER NUTRIENTS

A laboratory assessment of nutritional status with respect to individual nutrients is based on measurements of fluid or tissue content of nutrients, nutrient-containing compounds (e.g., hemoglobin for iron), or functional indices (e.g., the activity of transketolase, a thiamin-dependent enzyme for thiamin, or an accumulation of metabolites due to a deficient activity of some enzymes dependent on the nutrient). Assessments for individual vitamins are discussed in the Chapters 8–10.

15.3.7 NUTRIENTS INVOLVED IN HEMATOPOIESIS

15.3.7.1 Iron

The packed cell volume of whole blood (hematocrit) is often used to diagnose iron deficiency. Hematocrit is lowered in iron deficiency due to insufficient hemoglobin formation of microcytic hypochromic red blood cells. A measurement of hemoglobin itself is a more direct means of estimating iron deficiency; however, hemoglobin levels also fall in PEM due to decreased production of globin, deficiencies of vitamin B_6 and copper, and nutritional megaloblastic anemia. The direct determination of iron and the estimation of the degree of saturation of transferrin are extremely useful in detecting the iron-deficiency status. The normal hemoglobin and hematocrit values for men are greater than 14 g/dL and greater than 40%, respectively. For women, the corresponding values are 12.5 g and 36%. Values lower than these figures are seen in anemic conditions.

15.3.7.2 Folic Acid

Folic acid deficiency is characterized by macrocytic anemia, megaloblastosis of the bone marrow, diarrhea, and glossitis. A measurement of folic acid concentration in the serum is useful in the diagnosis of deficiency. Levels below 6 ng/ml indicate deficiency. Folic acid is required for one step in the conversion of histidine to glutamic acid. In the deficiency of folic acid, the intermediate, formimino glutamic acid (FIGLU), accumulates and is excreted in the urine. The normal excretion of FIGLU is only in trace amounts, but in folic acid deficiency, its excretion is increased considerably. Therefore, the measurement of FIGLU in the urine is used to assess folate nutrition.

15.3.7.3 Vitamin B$_{12}$

A deficiency of vitamin B$_{12}$ is associated with macrocytic anemia and megaloblastosis of the bone marrow. The serum cobalamin level is generally considered a sensitive index for the detection of clinical disorder caused by cobalamin deficiency. Low serum concentration of vitamin B$_{12}$ is also associated with an increased urinary excretion of methyl malonic acid (MMA).[12] The conversion of MMA to succinic acid is dependent on vitamin B$_{12}$. In vitamin B$_{12}$ deficiency, MMA accumulates and is excreted in the urine. In normal individuals, only a trace amount of MMA is found in the urine. Therefore, the measurement of urinary MMA is useful in the diagnosis of vitamin B$_{12}$ deficiency.

15.4 DIETARY ASSESSMENT

Dietary evaluation is an important adjunct to the other three assessments because it provides the description of dietary intake background, which may help to explain any observed clinical or biochemical abnormalities and may suggest proper remedial steps.[7,16] Twenty-four-hour recall is one of the most common methods of dietary assessment. As the name implies, the individual is asked to recall all food and beverages consumed over the preceding 24 hours and sometimes the physical activity level during this period. The advantage of the 24-hour recall is that it requires little effort on the part of the respondent, but the consumption in a single 24-hour period may not be representative of current weekly or monthly consumption; in addition, the data are subject to inaccuracies due to faulty memory and quantitative errors in assessing how much food has been eaten. Diet history by recall can be corroborated by asking specific questions about the patient's consumption and the family's purchases of individual food items such as bread, milk, vegetables, eggs, beverages, and so on.

A more accurate assessment is performed by the dietitian by having the patient maintain a 1-week diet diary. All foods and fluids ingested with approximate quantities are recorded at the time of actual consumption. The data obtained from these records are then evaluated. Understanding an individual's dietary practices and food consumption patterns allows the medical professional to identify nutrient deficiencies, imbalances, and excesses.

REFERENCES

1. Alberda, C., A. Graf, and G. A. McCarger. 2006. Malnutrition, consequences and assessment of a patient at risk. *Best Pract Res Clin Gastroenterol* 20:419.
2. Baker, J. P. 1982. Nutritional assessment: A comparison of clinical judgement and objective measurements. *N Engl J Med* 306:969.
3. Charney, P. 1995. Nutrition assessment in the 1990's: Where are we now? *Nutr Clin Pract* 10:131.
4. Forse, R. A., and H. M. Shizgal. 1980. The assessment of malnutrition. *Surg* 88:17.

5. Grant, A., and S. DeHoog. 1991. *Nutritional Assessment and Support*. 4th ed. Seattle, WA: Grant/DeHoog Publications.

6. Grant, J. P., P. B. Custer, and J. Thurlow. 1981. Current techniques of nutritional assessment. *Surg Clin North Am* 61:437.

7. Guthrie, H. A. 1989. Interpretation of data on dietary intake. *Nutr Rev* 47:33.

8. Himes, J. H., ed. 1991. *Anthropometric Assessment of Nutritional Status*. New York: Wiley-Liss Inc.

9. Holt, T., C. Cui, B. J. Thomas et al. 1994. Clinical applicability of bioelectric impedance to measure body composition in health and disease. *Nutr* 10:221.

10. Jensen, T. G., D. Englert, and S. J. Dudrick. 1983. *Nutritional Assessment: A Manual for Practitioners*. Norwalk, CT: Appleton-Century-Crofts.

11. Mckone, T. K., A. T. Davis, and R. E. Dean. 1985. Fibronectin: A new nutritional parameter. *Am Surg* 5:336.

12. Savage, D. G., J. Lindenbaum, S. P. Stabler, and R. H. Allen. 1994. Sensitivity of serum methylmalonic acid and total homocysteine determination for diagnosing cobalamin and folate deficiencies. *Am J Med* 96:239.

13. Shizgal, H.M. 1980. Nutritional assessment with body composition measurements. *JPEN, J Parenter Enteral Nutr* 88:17.

14. Solomons, N. W., and L. H. Allon. 1983. The functional assessment of nutritional status: principles, practice, and potential. *Nutr Rev* 41:33.

15. Thissen, J. P., J. M. Ketelslegers, and L. E. Underwood. 1994. Nutritional regulation of the insulin-like growth factors. *Endocr Rev* 15:80.

16. Wansink, B., and P. Chandon. 2006. Meal size, not body size, explains errors in estimating calorie content of meals. *Ann Intern Med* 145:326.

17. Weinsier, R. L., and S. L. Morgan. 1993. Nutritional assessment. In *Fundamentals of Clinical Nutrition*, 133. St. Louis, MO: Mosby-Year Book.

16 Obesity and Eating Disorders

Adipose tissue is a normal constituent of the human body that serves the important function of storing energy as fat for mobilization in response to metabolic demands. Also, subcutaneous fat constitutes the only means of the body's insulation. The tissues are susceptible to temperature fluctuation and the insulation provided by subcutaneous fat not only conserves energy but also facilitates thermal regulation. We do need some fat. Simply having body fat does not imply obesity. Obesity is the medical term for overfatness frequently resulting in a significant impairment of health.[36,43]

The terms *overweight* and *obesity* are often used interchangeably; however, they are not synonymous. Overweight is defined as the excess weight for height by standards such as actuarial tables. Obesity, on the other hand, refers to excess body fat. In most individuals, overweight and obesity are related, but there are exceptions. Some football players, for example, may be overweight because of their increased lean body mass, but not obese or overfat. And some inactive individuals with little muscle may be obese but not overweight.

Ideal body weight is the body weight for a given height that is statistically associated with the greatest longevity. The Metropolitan Life Insurance Company and a number of other groups publish tables of ideal body weight derived from longevity statistics. Since the Metropolitan Life Insurance Company statistics were published in 1959, the average body weight in the United States, and hence the prevalence of obesity, has increased. The mortality rate, however, has decreased, particularly in women over the age of 45 years (the group with the highest prevalence of obesity). Recent statistics on ideal body weight and longevity have reflected that trend, and the ideal body weight of the American population has been increased by 10%–15%.

The normal proportion of body weight as fat is 15%–20% for men and 20%–25% for women. The human body has two kinds of fat: essential fat and storage fat. Essential fat is vital to health in many ways; for example, it cushions and protects the body's organs. The average college-age man has 15% body fat: 3% essential fat and 12% storage fat. A woman of the same age has about 25% body fat: 13% essential fat and 12% storage fat. Adipose tissue is difficult to measure clinically, however, and the precise cut-off between normality and obesity has been a subject of debate for years. It is clear that many adverse consequences are associated with severe obesity, but because of difficulties inherent in quantifying adipose tissue, the precise amount needed to increase risks of health is not known. A 1985 National Institutes of Health Consensus Panel convened to discuss the health implications of obesity concluded that a body weight of 20% over the desirable weight clearly has adverse effects on health and longevity.

The pattern of fat distribution throughout the body also affects metabolic consequences and may be a more important factor than total adipose tissue mass. Thus, a person with fat located predominantly in the abdominal region may be at greater risk of some chronic diseases than another person with a greater total amount of adipose tissue that is located predominantly in the gluteal area.

16.1 CLASSIFICATION

Obesity has been classified in various ways.[48] One classification is based on the number and the size of adipose cells. At the cellular level, there are at least two distinct forms of obesity. Many individuals, often those with a mild or moderate obesity beginning in middle age, have an adipose tissue depot that is made up of a normal number of adipocytes but contains large quantities of fat in each cell (see Figure 16.1). This type is called *hypertrophic* obesity. Other individuals, often those with

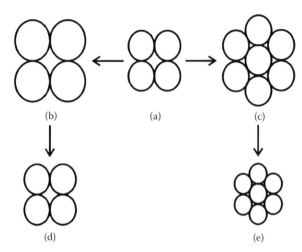

FIGURE 16.1   (a) Normal, nonobese. (b) Hypertrophic obesity—a normal number of adipocytes characterized by enlarged cells. (c) Hyperplastic obesity characterized by an excess number of adipocytes; the cell size may be normal. (d) After weight reduction in hypertrophic obesity, the fat cell size is normal. (e) After weight reduction in hyperplastic obesity, the fat cell size is too small (abnormal), and there is no reduction in fat cell number. (Modified from Winick, M., *Nutrition in Health and Disease*, John Wiley and Sons, New York, 1980.)

marked obesity and with a history dating to early childhood, have an adipose depot made up of too many adipocytes, each containing fat that is reasonably normal in quantity. This type is called *hyperplastic* obesity. During weight reduction, the number of fat cells is not affected, but the size of the fat cells is reduced. Thus, an obese individual whose fat cells are just too large (hypertrophic) can reduce the size of each fat cell to normal and will then have adipose tissue identical in every respect to that in average-weight individuals. By contrast, an obese individual who has too many fat cells that are normal in size will have to reduce the size of those fat cells to below normal in order to maintain a normal quantity of adipose tissue. These individuals will still have too many fat cells and will now be in the doubly abnormal state of having too many, too small fat cells. These individuals have a particularly difficult time maintaining the reduced body weight. It has been suggested that there are two critical periods of life when many fat cells are developed: infancy and adolescence. Overfeeding during these critical periods may lead to a permanent abnormality with which a person must struggle throughout life. Therefore, preventive measures must be taken early in life if hyperplastic obesity is to be avoided.

Obesity can also be classified by the regional fat distribution. Recent evidence suggests that where fat is distributed in the body is a strong determinant of health risk and perhaps also of the etiology of obesity and the ease of weight loss.[49] Excessive fat located in the central abdominal area of the body, so-called *android, apple-shaped*, or *upper body* obesity (Figure 16.2a), is statistically associated with increased risk of diabetes, hypertension, and cardiovascular disease (CVD). This type of obesity is most common in men. In contrast, fat distributed in the lower extremities around the hips or femoral region, characterized as *gynoid, pear-shaped*, or *lower body* obesity (Figure 16.2b), is relatively benign and is common in women. A simple determination of waist-to-hip circumference can identify the two types of obesity. A ratio of about 0.7 is considered normal. A ratio below 0.7 indicates lower body obesity, while a ratio above 0.7 indicates upper body obesity. Fat below the waist is more difficult to lose than fat above the waist so that those who are predominantly lower-body obese find it very difficult to lose weight even when they adhere to a diet faithfully. A woman who is obese over all her body might find that her upper body will be reduced dramatically by dieting while her lower body will not be much affected.

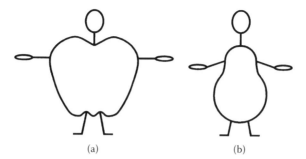

FIGURE 16.2   (a) Apple-shaped or upper-body obesity common in men. (b) Pear-shaped or lower-body obesity common in women.

16.2   PATTERN OF FAT DEPOSITION

The patterns of fat deposition throughout life are different in men and women,[46] with men being leaner than women from the first year of life through childhood and throughout the fifth decade of life. During the preschool years, the average male shows a loss of subcutaneous fat, while the average female maintains the same amount of subcutaneous fat. Girls continue to deposit fat subcutaneously throughout puberty. A minimum level of fat is considered to be necessary to initiate menarche and to maintain a normal menstrual cycle. This directly influences reproductive ability. In boys, the prepubertal increase in subcutaneous fat is less than in girls and is followed by a decrease until age 18 years. At the end of the second decade of life, adipose tissue expressed as a percentage of total body weight is approximately 1.5 times greater in women than in men. Lean body mass increases in both sexes during adolescence. The increase in males is greater because of the greater increase in skeletal muscle.

16.3   PREVALENCE

Obesity is the most common nutritional problem in the United States. The prevalence rates for overweight and obesity in the United States are obtained from the National Health and Nutrition Examination Surveys (NHANES), carried out by the National Center for Health Statistics. So far, there have been five data "cycles" covering the years 1960–1962, 1971–1974, 1976–1980, 1988–1994, and the latest, which was conducted from 1999 to 2000. In these surveys, overweight is defined as a body mass index (BMI) > 25.0 and obesity is defined as BMI > 30.0. The BMI is calculated by dividing individuals' weight in kilograms by the square of their height in meters. According to these surveys, in 1962, 12.8% of the population was obese. The prevalence of obesity increased only modestly in the next two decades, rising to 14.1% in 1971–1974 and to 14.5% in the NHANES of 1976–1980. Since then, the body weights in the United States have been inflating at an alarming rate (and the rest of the world seems to be following suit). As per the NHANES completed in 1994, the prevalence of obesity increased by more than 50% between 1980 and 1994. In 1980, 14.5% of the population was obese. By 1994, that number had increased to 22.5%. As per the latest NHANES conducted in 1999–2000, the age-adjusted prevalence of obesity among U.S. adults increased from 22.5% in 1988–1994 to 30.5% in 1999–2000. According to the recent survey (NHANES 2003–2004), the prevalence of obesity among adults in the United States was 32.9%, and the prevalence of obesity and overweight was 66.2%. The prevalence of morbid obesity (BMI > 40) increased from 0.8% in 1990 to 2.2% in 2000. About 55% of the population was officially considered overweight. Many public health experts call this the "obesity epidemic." If the current trend continues, 75% of adults in the United States are projected to be overweight and 41% obese by 2015. From 1971 to 2004, there was an increase in the amount of calories consumed. For women, the average increase was 335 Cal/day, and for men the increase was 168 Cal/day. Most of these calories were from sweetened beverages, which now account for almost 25% of daily calories in young adults in the United States. A 12-ounce can of soda provides the equivalent of 10 teaspoons of sugar. An extra intake of just one can a day can pile on 15 pounds of body weight in a single year. Consumption of sweetened drinks is believed to be contributing to the rising rates of obesity.

For children and adolescents, the BMI indicating overweight varies with age, so definitions of overweight and obesity for adults do not apply. Instead, those who are over the age-specific 85th percentile of weight from the earliest survey are considered overweight and those who are above the 95th percentile are considered obese. As per the most recent NHANES, more than 25% of children are overweight or obese. The prevalence of overweight children (>95th percentile of sex-specific BMI for age) increased in 1999–2000 compared with 1988–1994. The prevalence of over-weight children in 1999–2000 was 15.5% among ages 12–19, 15.3% among ages 6–11, and 10.4% among ages 2–5. Approximately 17.5% of children (ages 6–11 years) and 17% of adolescents (ages 12–19 years) were overweight in 2004. Childhood obesity is a critical public health problem in the United States. Over the past 3 decades, obesity has soared among all age groups, tripling among children ages 2–11 years. Today, more than 23 million children and teenagers are overweight or obese. Among certain racial and ethnic groups, the rates are still higher. One in seven low-income preschool children is obese, but the obesity epidemic may be stabilizing. Overweight children are more likely than their peers to be overweight adults and thus contribute to a further increase in the prevalence of obesity in the near future.

A recent study on the spread of the obesity epidemic in the United States between 1991 and 1998 showed a steady increase in all states. The magnitude of the increased prevalence varied by region (ranging from 31.9% for mid-Atlantic to 67.2% for south Atlantic—the area with the great-est increases) and by state (ranging from 11.3% for Delaware to 101.8% for Georgia—the state with the greatest increase). The most recent survey reported by the Centers for Disease Control and Prevention (CDC) found that 18% of adults aged 18 and over in Colorado were obese in 2009, making it the only state, along with Washington, DC, with an obesity rate below 20%. By contrast, 34.4% of adults in Mississippi were obese. Ten years ago, 28 states had obesity rates below 20% of their adult population, the CDC report said. Also, no state had an obesity rate above 30% in 2000, whereas more states are above that threshold today. These are Alabama, Arkansas, Kentucky, Louisiana, Mississippi, Missouri, Oklahoma, Tennessee, and West Virginia. Overall, the report found that 26.7% of adults nationwide are obese. This is up from 25.6% in a 2007 survey and sug-gests an additional 2.4 million Americans joined the ranks of the obese in the 2-year interim. In 2000, the comparable number was 19.8%.

The CDC said that the overall obesity probably is much higher; it relied on telephone surveys with about 400,000 adults who were asked to self-report their height and weight, the information that people often misrepresent. The CDC pointed to a report it issued in January 2010 that found the prevalence of obesity was 33.8% nationwide (32.2% for men and 35.5% for women). The earlier study was based on actual measurements of height and weight among 5555 adults in 2007 and 2008.

The high prevalence occurs in all ethnic and racial groups and at all ages and in both sexes. It is even higher among persons with lower levels of education and in certain ethnic or racial groups. For men and women, the prevalence of overweight increases with each 10-year increment of age until 50–59 years of age when it begins to fall progressively at older ages. The percent of adult men who are overweight or obese (59.4%) is somewhat greater than that of women (50.7%). There is a high prevalence (almost 60%) among middle-aged African American and Mexican American women. The value for white women is 33.5%. Blacks have a 51% higher prevalence of obesity, and Hispanics have a 21% higher prevalence of obesity compared with whites. A greater prevalence of obesity for blacks and whites is found in the South and Midwest than in the West and Northeast. During the past decade, the average American gained 3.6 kg, and the proportion of persons with healthier, lighter weight decreased significantly. Health care costs directly attributed to obesity are estimated to be $147 billion/year, and an additional $40 billion/year is spent on weight reduction programs and special foods.[4] The medical costs for an obese individual are estimated at $1429 higher per year than for an individual of normal weight. It has been estimated that more than 300,000 people die each year from obesity-related diseases.[1,31] Americans have increased their life expectancy by cutting back on cigarette smoking 20% in the last 15 years. This is expected to increase life expectancy by 0.31 years. However, growing BMI rates would also mean that there would be a reduced life expectancy by 1.02 years giving a net life expectancy reduction of 0.71 years, according to a recent study. Although life expectancy may still increase in the future—because of factors such as overall health care improvements, nutrition, and education—rising obesity rates will eventually slow that progress.

Over half of adults living in European Union (EU) countries are now overweight or obese according to the Health at a Glance Europe 2010 report just released by the European Commission and the Organization for Economic Co-operation and Development (OECD). The rate of obesity has more than doubled over the past 20 years in most EU Member States. The United Kingdom turns out to be the most obese (just over 25% of the population), closely followed by Ireland and Malta. Currently, one in seven children in the EU is overweight or obese—and the figures are set to rise even further. In the EU, only one in five children exercises regularly. Physical activity tends to fall between the ages of 11 and 15 in most EU Member States. More than one-third of African women and a quarter of African men are overweight.

Weight problems have long been recognized as a health hazard in the United States, Europe, and other industrialized places. But in recent years, the same worry has emerged in many less well-off places. According to the 2007 report of the World Health Organization (WHO), there are more than 1.6 billion overweight and obese people worldwide, a number that is twice the number of people who are suffering from starvation and undernutrition.

In some countries, there is a growing "weight gap." Well-off minorities in India, China, Brazil, and some other developing countries are gaining weight as the poor go hungry. America and other wealthier countries have the opposite problem. The richer and better-educated tend to eat right, while the poor often balloon from a diet of cheap and fatty fast foods. In 1989, less than 10% of Mexicans were overweight. But, in 2006 the National Surveys found that 71% of Mexican women and 66% of Mexican men were overweight or obese. Diabetes was almost nonexistent in Mexico 15 years back, but now about one-seventh of the country's people suffer from type 2 diabetes, and the disease is quickly growing in number. In China, the percentage of overweight and obese rose from 12.9 in 1991 to 27.3 in 2004, and in Brazil the percentage of obese and overweight rose from 20 in 1975 to 36.7 in 1997.

Concerning childhood obesity, it has been estimated that worldwide over 22 million children under the age of 5 are severely overweight, as are 155 million children of school age.[41] One in 10 children worldwide is overweight. Environmental factors, lifestyle preferences, increased sugar intake in the form of soft drinks, increased portion size, and steady decline in physiological activity have been playing major roles in the rising rates of obesity all around the world.[33,34]

The WHO predicts that overweight and obesity may soon replace more traditional public health concerns such as undernutrition and infectious diseases as the most significant cause of public health.

16.4 CAUSES OF OBESITY

Obesity results from an interaction between several environmental factors. Consumption of energy-dense foods and a sedentary lifestyle are thought to explain most cases of obesity. Causes such as inadequate sleep, decreased rate of smoking (known to reduce weight), use of some medicines such as antipsychotic medications, infectious agents, and eating more processed food have been suggested to contribute to obesity. Some factors are described in the following sections.

16.4.1 CALORIES

The first law of thermodynamics leads inevitably to the conclusion that for adipose stores to increase, more calories must be assimilated than are required to meet metabolic demands. This provides a common definition of obesity as a situation wherein the body contains an excess of calories as storage triglycerides in adipose tissue; however, the simplistic view that obesity is due solely to overeating and may be treated successfully through caloric restriction alone does not appear valid. Other causes, in addition to excess caloric intake, have been suggested. Using advanced brain imaging, researchers have found that extremely obese people in the study have fewer dopamine D_2 receptors, which can lead to an impaired ability to feel satisfied or to experience the sensation of having enough food. This can cause compulsive patterns of overeating—food addiction—in a lot of individuals.

16.4.2 GENETICS

Several recent studies provide strong support for a genetic influence on human fatness and obesity. Observations that obesity runs in families suggest that some individuals may be genetically predisposed to this disorder. It has been estimated that two obese parents have a 73% chance of having an obese offspring; one obese and one lean parent have a 41.2% chance; and two lean parents have only a 9% chance of having an obese offspring. Twin studies indicate a strong correlation of body weight and body fatness between identical twins, and it appears that heredity plays a substantial role in the development of obesity in this case. Family studies show that obesity runs in families, but they do not critically separate environmental from genetic factors.

Studies are underway to link the differences in obesity susceptibility among subgroups of people to differing versions of particular genes. Recently, scientists have discovered the first clear genetic link to obesity that is carried by significant numbers of people. Genome-wide scans performed on nearly 40,000 study subjects around the world identified a gene called FTO whose variation was associated with obesity. In every country studied, carriers of one copy of the gene were about 2.6 pounds heavier while those carrying 2 copies were about 6.6 pounds heavier. The finding is significant because the changed version of the gene is relatively common at least in the European populations studied so far. Researchers report that around half of the people have one copy of the offending version while 16% have 2 copies. Those with 2 copies are 67% more likely to be obese. More recently, scientists have discovered that genetic differences among people can stem from lost or duplicated sections of chromosomes, called copy number variants (CNVs). The CNVs have been implicated in disorders such as autism that slow mental development or cause learning disabilities. Autistic patients sometimes have an extra segment on chromosome 15 or are missing a section of chromosome 16. Such patients often are heavy as well, suggesting a connection between CNVs and weight. A study has found that a number of CNVs are more common in obese children than in a group of children with normal weight.[9] The most prevalent of these is the deletion from chromosome 16. The missing segment of chromosome 16 holds 9 genes, including one known as SH2B1, which has already been linked as a possible culprit in obesity. Mice lacking this gene become extremely fat and develop insulin resistance. This suggests that CNVs can cause a metabolic disease like obesity.

16.4.3 BROWN FAT

Some people seem to be able to eat much more than others without gaining weight, and they do not appear to be any more active. According to one hypothesis, this is because of brown fat. It is the cytochrome-pigmented brown adipose tissue (which gives brown fat its name) found in rodents, hibernating animals, and various other mammals, including the human embryo and newborns. Brown adipose tissue does not develop after birth and occurs only in certain areas of the body. A normal adult may have small areas of brown fat in and around the neck and chest (Figure 16.3). Brown fat is rich in mitochondria and produces heat. It is, in fact, a minifurnace that burns up calories either to provide the body with needed heat or to help keep the body's energy input and outflow in balance. In normal animals, brown adipose tissue appears to serve as a caloric buffer that disposes of excess energy when food intake is high and that conserves energy when food intake is low.

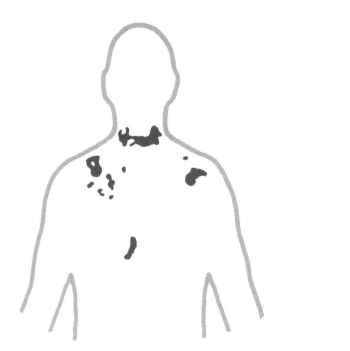

FIGURE 16.3   Brown adipose tissue lies in the neck and back in adults.

Consistent with the theory that obesity results from a problem with metabolism, it has been proposed that a defect in the function of brown adipose tissue may be responsible, in part, for obesity, at least in experimental animals. An obese mouse becomes obese when, because of a genetic defect, its brown adipose tissue does not function. On the other hand, the well-fed rat remains lean, despite excess food ingestion, because its brown adipose tissue grows and hyperfunctions, disposing fuel by burning it. The relevance of this theory to adult humans is uncertain, but it is possible that obese individuals are endowed with fewer brown fat cells than those of normal or slimmer weight, or that perhaps the brown fat of these obese people is not working as it should in its function to burn up extra calories.

Recently, nuclear medicine specialists used integrated positron emission tomography and computed tomography (PET-CT) scans to identify brown fat in humans and measure its activity. Because brown fat rapidly burns glucose to produce heat, it lights up the PET scans. Samples of brown fat from a few subjects showed that these cells express mitochondrial uncoupling protein 1 (UCP 1), which give the cell's mitochondria an ability to uncouple oxidative phosphorylation and utilize substrates to generate heat rather than ATP. Researchers found that thinner people have more brown fat than heavier people, young people more than older people, and people with lower blood glucose levels (reflecting higher metabolic rates) have more than those whose metabolism[30] is sluggish. Brown fat appears to be more active in women than men even though obesity is more prevalent in women. The new studies add to the emerging view that brown fat is involved in the complicated energy balance and may play a role in diseases such as type 2 diabetes that can arise when that balance is thrown off.[44]

16.4.4   LIPOPROTEIN LIPASE

It has been proposed that the activity of lipoprotein lipase (LPL) in adipose tissue can potentiate hunger by altering the availability of circulating metabolites. This hypothesis is based on the fact that the obese hypoglycemic mouse and the Zucker fatty rat both have early-developing hyperplastic–hypertrophic obesity. The earliest metabolic changes seen in the Zucker fatty rat, which may predispose to obesity, have increased LPL activity in adipose tissue and have increased fat cell size during the first week of life. LPL is the enzyme that hydrolyzes the triglyceride moieties of circulating chylomicrons and very low-density lipoproteins to free fatty acids, which are then transported across cell membranes, reesterified, and stored within the cell. Increased LPL activity precedes the development of hyperphagia. The activity of this enzyme controls the concentration of triglycerides that enter adipose cells and, by default, removes them from access to other cells. The reduction in availability then triggers further food consumption.

16.4.5 ATPᴀꜱᴇ

ATPase exists in all cells in the body and helps to burn off 15%–40% of all calories not used during physical activity. The obese individual has 20%–25% less ATPase than a person of normal weight. The more obese the person is, the lower is the ATPase level in red blood cells. The energy used by the red blood cells of severely obese patients is about 22% less than the energy used by the red blood cells of individuals with ideal body weight. Some obese people may burn up fewer calories than a thinner individual. Obese people may generally be more fuel efficient than thin ones and end up with more pounds stored as adipose tissue.

16.4.6 Sᴇᴛ Pᴏɪɴᴛ

According to one theory, each individual has a biologically predetermined "set point" for body weight, namely, that the body weight is programmed or receives information from fat cells (or hormones or enzymes) to maintain a given body weight, amount of fat, and lean body mass. Obesity results when the body's set point acts to defend body weight and fatness at a higher-than-normal level. Attempts to lose weight below the set point may be biologically resisted. The set point theory is yet to be proven.

16.4.7 Rᴏʟᴇ ᴏꜰ Hᴏʀᴍᴏɴᴇꜱ

Recent research reveals that adipose tissue that specializes in fat storage also functions as an endocrine organ releasing hormones that send signals to the brain and regulate food intake, energy expenditure, insulin sensitivity, and fat and carbohydrate metabolism.[6,27,35] Some hormones of the gastrointestinal tract also have important sensing and signaling roles in regulating body weight and energy expenditure. The balance between caloric intake and expenditure under most circumstances is accurate. Current evidence suggests that nutrient and hormonal signals from the gut and adipose tissue converge and directly act on brain centers leading to change in fuel metabolism and thus, stable body weight. Over time, the central nervous system responds to peripheral signals to orchestrate changes in both energy and glucose homeostasis. In this way, the central nervous system ensures that the nutrient demand of all tissues is being met. Dysfunction of the ability of the central nervous system to integrate fuel-sensing signals may underlie the etiology of metabolic diseases such as obesity.

16.4.7.1 Leptin

Leptin[10] is a protein hormone secreted primarily in adipose tissue that circulates in all parts of the body. The name leptin is derived from the Greek word *leptos*—meaning thin. Within the arcuate region of the hypothalamus, two regions are labeled as the "feeding" center and "satiety" center. In the feeding center, neurons produce neuropeptide Y (NPY) and agouti-related protein (AgRP); both stimulate feeding and promote obesity. Leptin acts on its receptors in the feeding center and decreases the secretion of NPY and AgRP. In the satiety center, one set of neurons produce a peptide called α-MSH. Neurons that produce α-MSH connect to neurons elsewhere in the hypothalamus that carries a surface protein known as the melanocortin 4 receptor (MC4R), whose activation reduces appetite and promotes weight loss. AgRP, which promotes feeding, is an antagonist of this receptor; it prevents receptor activation. Thus, leptin acts to trigger MC4R receptors both by stimulating them directly via α-MSH-producing neurons and by inhibiting their antagonist. A group of cells in the lateral hypothalamus produces a small protein called melanin-concentrating hormone (MCH). It promotes food intake and obesity. Another group of nerve cells in the same region secretes two neuropeptides when they sense a need to eat, such as after a drop in blood glucose level. They are named orexins. Both MCH and orexins are inhibited indirectly by leptin. The net action of leptin is to inhibit appetite, stimulate thermogenesis, enhance fatty acid oxidation, decrease glucose, and reduce body weight and fat.

Investigators have identified and cloned the gene for leptin dubbed Ob (for obesity), which when mutated causes a severe hereditary obesity in mice. Leptin is required to keep the animal's weight under control. Mice with an absence of Ob gene/or mutated Ob gene are characterized by an early onset of severe obesity. They eat excessively, show inappropriately low energy expenditure, and have an inherited form of diabetes.

Despite these pronounced effects in animals, the role of leptin in the regulation of energy balance in humans is less clear.[17] Leptin is thought to act as an afferent satiety signal in the brain to regulate body fat mass. Serum leptin levels are highly correlated with BMI and body fat. The average plasma leptin level in obese humans is 31 ng/mL compared with 7.5 ng/mL in normal-weight individuals. But it is not clear why, despite having high leptin levels, obese people do not eat less. The vast majority of obese people do have mutations related to either leptin or its receptor. They appear, therefore, to have a form of functional "leptin resistance," a defect in the blood–brain transport system for bringing leptin into the brain, or a postreceptor defect in the transmission of the signal to the hypothalamus. The mechanism for leptin resistance, and whether it can be overcome by raising leptin levels, is not established.

Leptin receptors are also expressed in many peripheral tissues, including liver, kidney, skeletal muscle, pancreas, and immune cells suggesting other actions of leptin outside the brain. The presence of receptors in the pancreas has led some researchers to hypothesize that serum leptin may regulate insulin metabolism. Women have higher circulating leptin levels than men even when adjustments are made for differences in body fat. Women with low body fat, including athletes and those with eating disorders, often stop menstruating, developing a condition called hypothalamic amenorrhea.[2] These women may not have enough leptin because of low body fat. Administration of leptin has restored menstrual period in these women.[45] This hormone may serve as a treatment for women who suffer from infertility. Higher leptin levels may speed sexual maturity and may make the body better at conserving energy.[14] Recent studies suggest that leptin also benefits brain function. People with low leptin levels have greater risk of developing Alzheimer's disease compared with those with the highest leptin levels. Leptin plays an important role in regulating bone growth.

16.4.7.2 Insulin

Insulin and its receptor have traditionally been studied for their role in glucose homeostasis. There is mounting evidence that the central actions of insulin parallel that of leptin. Central administration of insulin reduces food intake and body weight, whereas impairment of hypothalamic insulin receptors cause hyperphagia and insulin resistance. In healthy individuals, insulin levels rise after a meal. In a manner similar to leptin, insulin interacts with specific receptors in the arcuate nucleus of the hypothalamus and reduces food intake by decreasing the expression of NPY. Obesity in the vast majority of humans is associated with both hyperinsulinemia and hyperleptinemia, indicative of insulin and leptin resistance, respectively.

16.4.7.3 Visfatin

Visfatin is a newly discovered protein secreted by visceral fat. It has an insulin-like ability to lower blood glucose. At similar concentrations, visfatin and insulin have comparable ability to stimulate glucose uptake. Visfatin normally circulates at concentrations 3%–10% that of insulin. Intriguingly, visfatin mimics insulin by binding to the insulin receptor without interfering with the binding of insulin itself.

16.4.7.4   Adiponectin

Adiponectin is a 244–amino acid protein that is derived from adipose tissue. However, people who are obese have reduced concentrations of this protein. Decreased concentrations are also seen in patients with type 2 diabetes. Administration of adiponectin in animals increases insulin sensitivity and glucose tolerance and suppresses gluconeogenesis by the liver. It also causes weight loss in obese animals.[3] Adiponectin has thus been proposed as an important mediator of insulin resistance in people who are obese.

16.4.7.5   Resistin

Resistin is a 94–amino acid polypeptide secreted by adipocytes.[42] Its level is increased by diet-induced and genetic obesity and is causally connected to obesity-associated insulin resistance. Resistin regulates preadipocyte differentiation to adipocytes through a negative feedback mechanism to limit adipose tissue formation in response to increased energy intake. It also functions as a regulator of glucose homeostasis and a physiological antagonist to hepatic insulin action.

16.4.7.6   Ghrelin

Ghrelin is a 28–amino acid peptide secreted primarily by the stomach and duodenum and has been implicated in both mealtime hunger and the long-term regulation of body weight.[24,40] In humans, plasma ghrelin levels rise shortly before and fall shortly after every meal, a pattern that is consistent with a role in the urge to begin eating. Fasting ghrelin levels appear to be inversely proportional to BMI. Compared to normal-weight controls, ghrelin levels are lower in obese patients. The levels are higher in patients with anorexia nervosa but tend to normalize when these patients manage to put on weight. Drugs that suppress ghrelin might be developed, and these could provide valuable additional means to treat obesity.

Patients with Prader–Willi syndrome, a complex disease with many defects, develop extreme obesity associated with uncontrollable and voracious appetite. The plasma ghrelin levels are exceptionally high in comparison to patients similarly obese due to other causes. It may be that excessive ghrelin production contributes to the appetite and obesity components.

16.4.7.7   Obestatin

Obestatin is an appetite-suppressing hormone produced by the same gene that expresses ghrelin in the stomach. Obestatin is not a "statin" like the well-known class of cholesterol-lowering drugs. The name combines the Latin words for devour and suppression. The hormone has been tested in laboratory rats.[20]

16.4.7.8   Cholecystokinin

Cholecystokinin is a peptide hormone secreted in the duodenum, the first segment of the small intestine, in response to the presence of nutrients (specifically fat) within the gut lumen. It causes the release of digestive enzymes and bile from the pancreas and gall bladder, respectively. It also acts as a hunger suppressant. The satiating effect of cholecystokinin (CCK) is mediated by the vagus nerve. The activated vagus in turn stimulates cells in the brain stem leading to signals in other areas of the brain that cause the individual to stop eating.

16.4.7.9   Peptide yy3-36

Peptide yy3-36 is secreted by cells of the stomach, small intestine, and large intestine in response to a meal and in proportion to calories ingested.[7] The hormone acts on the arcuate nucleus of the hypothalamus, and stimulating neurons that create a sensation of satiety and inhibiting neurons that stimulate feeding behavior. In response to the ingestion of nutrients, plasma peptide yy3-36 (Pyy) levels increase within 15 minutes, peak around 60 minutes after a meal, and remain elevated for up to 6 hours.

Endogenous levels of Pyy are low in obese subjects, suggesting that peptide deficiency may contribute to the pathogenesis of obesity.

16.5 ASSESSMENT OF OBESITY

Obesity is defined as an excess accumulation of adipose tissue in the body; however, measuring body fat and deciding what is normal and what is excessive fat presents some problems. There are several methods used in the determination of obesity.

16.5.1 Body Weight

For lack of a better database, life insurance industry statistics have been used to develop so-called tables of normality. These tables give ideal or desirable weight ranges for height, frame size, and sex and are associated with greatest longevity. The definition of overweight is accepted as 10% above ideal body weight, and the definition of obesity is 20% above ideal body weight. The tables have been used on the assumption that whatever weight is desirable at age 21 years is also desirable at age 65. In Western society, there is generally an increase in body weight as well as a change in body composition with age. Therefore, it is not clear whether the desirable weight should be the same from 21–65 years.

16.5.2 Body Mass Index

To clarify the confusion about how to classify overweight, Garrow proposed the use of BMI (Figure 16.4). This expression of the ratio of weight in kilograms (with minimal clothing) to height (without shoes) in square meters has a better correlation with body fat than other weight–height relationships. BMI can be approximated by multiplying weight in pounds by 703, then dividing by height in inches squared. For both men and women, the degree of obesity is classified as follows: individuals whose BMI is between 20 and 24.9 are considered to be in the desirable weight

Weight (lb)

Height (ft/in)	100	105	110	115	120	125	130	135	140	145	150	155	160	165	170	175	180	185	190	195	200	205
5'0"	20	21	21	22	23	24	25	26	27	28	29	30	31	32	33	34	35	36	37	38	39	40
5'1"	19	20	21	22	23	24	25	26	26	27	28	29	30	31	32	33	34	35	36	37	38	39
5'2"	18	19	20	21	22	23	24	25	26	27	27	28	29	30	31	32	33	34	35	36	37	37
5'3"	18	19	19	20	21	22	23	24	25	26	27	27	28	29	30	31	32	33	34	35	35	36
5'4"	17	18	19	20	21	21	22	23	24	25	26	27	27	28	29	30	31	32	33	33	34	35
5'5"	17	17	18	19	20	21	22	22	23	24	25	26	27	27	28	29	30	31	32	32	33	34
5'6"	16	17	18	19	19	20	21	22	23	23	24	25	26	27	27	28	29	30	31	31	32	33
5'7"	16	16	17	18	19	20	20	21	22	23	23	24	25	26	27	27	28	29	30	31	31	32
5'8"	15	16	17	17	18	19	20	21	21	22	23	24	24	25	26	27	27	28	29	30	30	31
5'9"	15	16	16	17	18	18	19	20	21	21	22	23	24	24	25	26	27	27	28	29	30	30
5'10"	14	15	16	17	17	18	19	19	20	21	22	22	23	24	24	25	26	27	27	28	29	29
5'11"	14	15	15	16	17	17	18	19	20	20	21	22	22	23	24	24	25	26	26	27	28	29
6'0"	14	14	15	16	16	17	18	18	19	20	20	21	22	22	23	24	24	25	26	26	27	28
6'1"	13	14	15	15	16	16	17	18	18	19	20	20	21	22	22	23	24	24	25	26	26	27
6'2"	13	13	14	15	15	16	17	17	18	19	19	20	21	21	22	22	23	24	24	25	26	26
6'3"	12	13	14	14	15	16	16	17	17	18	19	19	20	21	21	22	22	23	24	24	25	26
6'4"	12	13	13	14	15	15	16	16	17	18	18	19	19	20	21	21	22	23	23	24	24	25

Less Risk — More Risk

FIGURE 16.4 BMI (number in squares) varies with weight and height. BMIs of 27–29 carry moderate health risks, with risk increasing as BMIs rise.

range; individuals with a BMI of 25–29.9 have a low relative risk; those with a BMI of 30–40 have a moderate risk; and those with values above 40 are described as morbidly obese and are clearly in the high-risk category. The major weakness of the use of body weight and BMI is that individuals such as some football players may be classified as obese when they may not be.

16.5.3 SKINFOLD THICKNESS

About half of body fat is deposited under the skin, and the rest is around organs and between muscle fibers. By measuring the subcutaneous fat, it is possible to evaluate one's fat level. Fat is not distributed evenly (under the skin) throughout the body. Therefore, the measurement should be made at some selected sites to reveal information about the individual's fat content. The skin is pinched together and pulled away from the muscles. The thickness of the skin and the underlying fat tissue is then measured with the caliper and expressed in millimeters. There are several sites that one can choose, but the tricep skinfold is the most commonly used. The measurement is taken midway between the shoulder and the elbow at the back of the dominant arm held in a relaxed position. Average readings for those between the ages of 25 and 45 years are about 18 mm for men and 23 mm for women. Fat arms appear to run in families even when the rest of the body may have a much lower level of fat. Therefore, it is advisable not to rely on tricep skinfold measurement alone; but if the thickness at other skinfold sites is also above average, the individual is considered to have a higher fat level.

The other sites commonly used are the suprailiac skinfold (the top of the hip bone just above the crest) and the abdominal skinfold. Skinfold thickness provides a more direct estimation of body fat than weight-for-height values alone, but skinfold thickness measurements vary significantly between observers and within a single observer at different sites in the body. Thus, accurate assessment requires measurements of multiple skin sites.

The distribution and the amount of subcutaneous fat change with age and are also quite different by sex. As people lose weight, skinfold thickness decreases, and as people put on weight, skinfold thickness increases. Crash and fad diets cause more water loss, and skinfold thickness is not affected much. Because the amount of fat distribution from place to place in the body varies, some investigators have suggested that using the sum of skinfolds from different sites would better reflect total body fat.

16.5.4 OTHER TECHNIQUES

There are other techniques for evaluating body fat, but these are more difficult, expensive, and time-consuming and have generally been used only for research purposes.[12] Total body water can be estimated from the dilution of antipyrine as well as from tritiated water or deuterium oxide. Water is assumed to be a fixed proportion of body fat-free mass (FFM), which is equal to (water mass)/0.73. The FFM is subtracted from total body weight to get total body fat.

Total body potassium can be measured by the use of ^{40}K, and it gives an index of lean body mass because potassium is present only in fat-free components of the body. Using the estimated value for potassium in lean body, one can calculate the lean body mass and then derive the total body fat. Body fat can also be directly measured from the dilution of xenon or cyclopropane. Underwater weighing is based on the principle that body fat weighs less (is less dense) than lean body mass. Bones and muscles will easily sink in water. Fat tissue is much less dense and floats in water. Therefore, the more body fat one has, the more buoyant one is in water. People can be weighed in special underwater tanks to determine the amount of fat on their bodies in relation to body mass. Although this procedure is considered to be accurate, it has practical limitations, which make it inappropriate for routine use.

During the last few years, a number of new techniques have been developed to quantitate body fat. These include the measurement of impedance or body conductivity and the use of ultrasound.

For bioelectrical impedance analysis (BIA), two conductors are attached to a person, and a small electric current is sent through the body. The resistance between the conductors provides a measure of body fat since the resistance varies between fat and muscle. FFM has electrolytes and about 73% water and is a good conductor while fat is a poor conductor. Based on BIA principles, several tools are now available, including bathroom scales that measure body weight as well as the percentage of muscle, body fat, and water.

16.6 MEDICAL COMPLICATIONS

Clinical observations suggest that obesity is associated with a number of chronic diseases including adult-onset diabetes, hypercholesterolemia, high plasma triglycerides, hypertension, heart disease, cancer, gallstones, arthritis, and gout. (It must be stressed, however, that not all obese individuals are unhealthy and the health problems are not evenly distributed among obese individuals.) In addition, there may be undesirable social, psychological, and economic consequences of obesity.

A strong association exists between overweight and adult-onset diabetes.[23] The prevalence of diabetes is about 2.9 times higher in overweight persons than in normal-weight individuals. Obesity is associated with increased insulin secretion apparently due to the presence of insulin resistance. Fasting blood glucose increases approximately by 2 mg/dL for every 10% excess above ideal body weight. It has recently been reported that adipocytes secrete a unique signaling molecule named resistin (for resistance to insulin). Circulating resistin levels are decreased by the antidiabetic drug rosiglitazone and are increased in diet-induced and genetic forms of obesity. The administration of antiresistin antibody improves blood sugar and insulin action in mice with diet-induced diabetes. Resistin is thus a hormone that potentially links obesity to diabetes.

Obese patients commonly have an increase in plasma triglycerides and/or cholesterol levels. It is estimated that there is an increase in blood cholesterol of about 2 mg/dL for each kilogram of excess body weight. These individuals also overproduce very low-density lipoprotein. The data from the Framingham study show a linear association between body weight and blood pressure. In many instances, body weight reduction lowers blood pressure and normalizes blood glucose in obese people.

C-reactive protein (CRP), a biomarker for inflammation, predicts the risk of CVD and future cardiovascular events. CRP is secreted primarily by the liver after its synthesis is triggered by pro-inflammatory cytokins such as interleukin 6 (IL-6) derived from monocytes, macrophages, or adipose tissue. Approximately one fourth of circulating IL-6 is estimated to be released by adipose tissue in individuals of normal weight. People who are obese or overweight tend to have elevated levels of CRP. Weight loss studies have shown that decreasing body weight significantly decreases CRP.[11] Reducing inflammation through weight loss could be associated with reduced risk of CVD and other obesity-associated diseases.

In test-tube studies, researchers recently found that CRP binds leptin. They also found that mice given leptin alone ate less and lost weight. Animals that received both leptin and CRP kept eating and gained weight. CRP may block the action of leptin in the body. How it does is not clear. One possibility is that CRP, by attaching to leptin, prevents the hormone from reaching the brain or binding to its receptors. The studies also found that liver cells, where CRP is made, produce increased levels of the protein when exposed to leptin. This suggests that CRP, leptin, the brain, and liver are part of a feedback loop that regulates appetite.

Research based on data from more than 320,000 Northern California Kaiser members, whose weight and height were tracked between 1964 and 1985, revealed a strong association between obesity and kidney disease. Even moderately overweight people had a higher risk of kidney failure than people whose weight was in the normal range. And for morbidly obese, the risk was more than 70% greater. Being overweight was seen as a risk factor after adjusting for high blood pressure, diabetes, and other known factors.

A government study has found that people who are overweight at age 50 face significantly increased risk of premature death.

Childhood obesity in the United States appears to be causing girls to reach puberty at an early age. A multiyear study that followed 354 girls found that those who were fatter at age 3 and who gained weight during the next 3 years reached puberty, as defined clinically, by age 9. Early onset of puberty in girls is associated with a number of adverse outcomes including psychiatric disorders and deficits in psychosocial functions, early indications of alcohol use, and teenage pregnancy.

In a disturbing twist on the obesity epidemic, some overweight teenagers were found to have severe liver damage caused by too much body fat, and a handful needed transplants. Many more may need a new liver by their 30s or 40s, some experts believe. The American Liver Foundation and others in the field estimate 2%–9% of American children over 5 who are obese or overweight have nonalcoholic liver disease.

16.6.1 WAIST CIRCUMFERENCE

Over the past 10 years, a raft of new studies has shown that predicting a person's long-term health may be as simple as taking a waist measurement.[22] Fat around the waist has been linked to a greater risk of heart disease, diabetes, stroke, hypertension, breathing problems, disability, some cancers, and higher mortality rates. Federal health surveys show that over the past four decades the mean waist size for men has grown from 35 to 39 inches and for women from 30 to 37 inches. Nearly 39% of men and 60% of women are carrying belly fat.

A study has shown that among about 27,000 people in 52 countries waist circumference more accurately predicted which men and women would have heart attacks than did any other body measure, including weight and BMI. Central fat cells are actually little endocrine factories, producing hormones that send messages to many organs. Central fat is metabolically most active. It produces insulin resistance; increases insulin levels, appetite, and triglycerides; and decreases high-density lipoprotein levels. This cascade of events leads to increased risk for coronary heart disease. People with a substantial waistline may run an elevated risk of cognitive decline as they age. A large waist raises the risk of early death in women. Hip fat appears to be protective in reducing CVD and death among women but not in men. But not all researchers agree that hip fat is beneficial and if it is no one yet knows why.

A bigger waist also means higher health care costs.[50] It is estimated that in the U.S. patients with 41-inch waists pay about $2600 more per year. Abdominal adiposity as assessed by waist circumference may be a better predictor of health care costs than the more widely used BMI.

According to the U.S. Department of Health and Human Services, women with a waist circumference of more than 35 inches and men with a waist circumference of more than 40 inches are at increased risk of developing chronic diseases. However, lower thresholds for waist circumference have been recommended for Asian populations by the WHO, due to recent findings. Those at increased risk of developing chronic diseases include Asian women with a waist circumference of more than 31 inches and Asian men with a waist circumference of more than 35 inches.

It will be decades before we know the metabolic puzzle of fat. In the meantime, the important action to take is to stop waist expansion. Regular moderate exercise—doing 30 minutes of walking 5 or 6 days a week—can prevent an increase in abdominal fat and waist size. People who engage in this level of moderate exercise live as much as a year and half longer than those who do not. More vigorous exercise can reduce waist size and add as much as four years of life.

Obesity may be associated with heavy menstrual blood flow and menstrual cycle irregularities. Gout and arthritis appear to be more common in obese individuals than in those with normal body weight. The risk of gallbladder disease is higher in obese patients and may be related to increased cholesterol synthesis and its biliary excretion associated with increased lithogenicity of bile. Numerous epidemiological studies on obesity and site-specific malignancies show higher mortality from cancer of the colon and cancer of the prostate in men and cancer of the breast in women.

Recent life insurance statistics reveal that when body weight is 10% above average, life expectancy decreases by 11% in men and by 7% in women. For individuals who are 20% above ideal weight, life expectancy decreases even further by 20% for men and by 10% for women.

16.7   DIET AND OTHER STRATEGIES FOR WEIGHT REDUCTION

Many strategies for losing weight are in use. These include diet, exercise, behavioral modification, appetite suppressants, and surgical treatment. Bariatric surgery is indicated for selected patients with severe obesity when other methods of weight control have failed.

Surgical techniques involve either creating a smaller bowel to produce a malabsorption of ingested calories, or creating a smaller stomach so that the reduced reservoir for food can prevent large calorie intake at any one time, or both. Gastric bypass triggers weight loss in part by reducing the blood levels of ghrelin. Dietary treatment is particularly effective for initial weight loss.

Body weight represents the balance between energy intake and energy expenditure, each of which is influenced by a variety of factors. The major components of caloric expenditure are the use of energy for maintaining body functions at rest or basal metabolic rate (BMR), which amounts normally to about 60%–70% of total energy expenditure; dietary thermogenesis (the energy required for the digestion and the absorption of food), which uses about 5%–10% of calories ingested; and physical activity, which accounts for 25%–35% of calories expended in an average individual. Obesity results from a prolonged period of positive energy balance during which energy intake exceeds expenditure. Reducing body weight requires that negative energy balance is produced.

The caloric requirement varies according to the individual's body weight and activity. A simple formula for estimating the homeostatic caloric requirement is to multiply a person's ideal weight in pounds by 12–14 for women and by 14–16 for men. This gives a rough estimate of the number of calories required to maintain the body weight at an average level of physical activity. To lose 1 pound, a person must take in 3500 fewer calories than expended. For example, to lose 1 pound each week, the individual has to maintain a negative energy balance of 500 cal a day. This can be done by decreasing caloric intake and/or by increasing physical activity. Any one of the following activities can result in the expenditure of about 500 cal: running for 45 minutes, playing tennis for 60 minutes, walking for 75 minutes, bicycling for 90 minutes, or playing golf for 120 minutes.

It is important to realize that body weight reduction means the reduction of body fat and not lean body mass. The normal diet provides a balanced energy source (e.g., calories comprise 50%–55% carbohydrates, 10%–15% proteins, and 30%–35% fats). Carbohydrates are not considered a dietary essential because glucose can be formed from amino acids and the glycerol moiety of fat; however, a minimum of 100 g/day carbohydrate is required in the diet to prevent ketosis and excessive loss of electrolytes and water in the urine. A minimum of 0.8 g/kg body weight or about 55 g of good-quality protein for a 70-kg individual is required to preserve lean body mass. The remaining calories in the diet can be adjusted accordingly. Because food intake is less in a weight-reducing diet, the intake of other essential nutrients may also be reduced, although the requirements for most nutrients are not altered. Therefore, it is advisable to take a multivitamin–mineral pill daily to prevent deficiencies of these nutrients.

Hypocaloric diets range from a moderate reduction in daily calories, 200–500 cal/day, to 1000–1200 cal/day. A realistic treatment goal is usually a loss of 5%–10% of initial body weight over a 6–12-month period followed by long-term maintenance of reduced weight. Most cardiovascular risk factors are improved even at this level of moderate weight reduction because of the predominant loss of visceral fat leading to disproportionate decrease in the risk of developing complications. The recent Diabetes Prevention Programs found that a mean weight loss of 5–6 kg achieved by diet and exercise reduced the risk of progression from impaired glucose tolerance to type 2 diabetes by 58% over a 4-year period.

Very low-calorie diets are diets that provide 500–800 cal/day, which require a follow-up by a nutritionist and a physician to avoid electrolyte disorders and symptomatic cholelithiasis.

During rapid weight loss, the risk for cholesterol gallstone formation increases. Patients with higher BMI and greater absolute rate of weight loss seem to have the highest rate of gallstone formation. Despite short-term success, these diets provide no greater weight loss at 1 year than do low-calorie diets. Analysis of published data on long-term weight loss maintenance showed that approximately 50% of the initial lost body weight is regained within the first 1–2 years and 95% or more by 5 years after completion of the calorie reduction phase.

The high frequency of relapse and limited weight loss with nonsurgical therapies are among the frustrations experienced by the obese patient. Investigations of the energetics of weight loss and weight gain demonstrate that maintenance of a reduced weight is associated with decreases in energy expenditure that are greater than can be accounted for by reductions in metabolic mass. Physical activity increases energy expenditure and is a key component of any weight maintenance program, countering the reduction in total energy expenditure that occurs with weight loss.

16.8 FAD DIETS

There are hundreds of diet programs currently available, and new ones continue to appear in the scientific literature and in the popular press, many with attractive titles including Prudent Diet, La Costa Spa Diet, Drinking Man's Diet, TOPS (Take Off Pounds Sensibly) Diet, Wine Diet, Do-It-Yourself Wise Woman's Diet, Dr. Atkins' Diet Revolution, Calories Don't Count Diet, Ed McMahon's Slimming Down Diet, I Love New York Diet, and Champagne Diet. These are categorized as balanced, low-carbohydrate, high-carbohydrate, high-protein, and high-fat diets. There are also "one emphasis diets" based on the premise that the one food they feature can lead to weight loss. One of the most popular of these is the grapefruit or Mayo diet. In addition, there are "miraculous pills and amazing devices" claiming to help individuals lose excess weight effortlessly.

Special diets with unusual food combinations such as low carbohydrates, high proteins, and other radical measures carry considerable risk and do not offer any advantage in a weight-reducing program. The best approach to lose weight is to follow a balanced mildly hypocaloric diet. Any diet with less than 1000 Cal/day should be used only under medical supervision. Once the excess weight is lost, it should be maintained. Data from experiments on animals suggest that repeated cycles of weight loss and regain—so-called yo-yo dieting—make it take a longer time to lose a certain amount of weight and a shorter time to regain it when the cycles are repeated. This is attributed, at least in part, to the adaptation of BMR as a result of dieting.[29] Frequent intentional weight loss or "weight cycling" (yo-yo dieting) may have long-term adverse effects on immune function and is known to weaken the immune system,[39] leaving the dieters more susceptible to illnesses such as cold and infections. Longer periods of weight stability are linked to better immune function. Exercise is one way dieters can keep weight off. It can also boost the immune system and blunt the negative effects weight loss could have on one's immune system.

16.9 ALTERNATIVE MEDICINE FOR WEIGHT REDUCTION

16.9.1 SEAWEEDS FOR DIETERS

Kanten, known as agar-agar in the West, is an ancient vegetable gelatin traditionally made by completely freezing and drying extracts of various red sea vegetables. It contains 81.2% fiber, which is the highest among all foods. It contains calcium, iron, and phosphorus and supplies no calories. Kanten has long been used as part of an Asian diet. It can be used as an ingredient in combination with other seasonings. Recently, it has been a favorite with health-conscious cooks around the world.

Kanten expands after it is ingested, tripling in mass as it absorbs fluids in the stomach. The bulk gives a feeling of fullness and in turn makes the individual eat less. Though research on the impact of Kanten on dieters is limited, recent results are promising.

A study was done in Japan on 76 overweight patients divided into two groups. Each group received a balanced diet designed to help them lose weight. But one group got a small serving of Kanten before their dinner. The Kanten group consumed on average 325 fewer calories at their evening meals. They lost 4.4% of their body weight over 12 weeks, while the other group lost 2%.

There is a debate on the amount of Kanten to be ingested, but some Japanese doctors recommend dieters consume 2 g of thoroughly dissolved Kanten in liquid three times a day, eat a balanced diet, and exercise.

16.10 PHARMACOTHERAPY

Weight-loss medications include appetite suppressants, inhibitors of fat absorption, enhancers of energy expenditure, and stimulators of fat mobilization, which act peripherally to reduce fat mass or to decrease triglyceride synthesis.[5] The hypothalamus is the major appetite and eating control center in the brain and is sensitive to a variety of facilitatory and inhibitory neurotransmitters and peptide neurohormones from the brain and the gastrointestinal tract.

Appetite suppressants reduce food intake by modulating the concentration of serotonin and/or norepinephrine in the brain. The modulation can occur at the level of neurotransmitter release or reuptake, or both. An appetite-suppressant medication generally produces an average weight loss of about 10% of the initial body weight and maintains its effectiveness for as long as it is used. As soon as it is discontinued, however, weight rapidly rebounds to pretreatment levels. The first appetite suppressants used were amphetamines, which increase norepinephrine release from nerve terminals. Amphetamines used over long periods can cause physical dependence. They are presently not recommended for use as appetite suppressants. Phentermine is another appetite suppressant that augments more norepinephrine but has a lower incidence and a lesser severity of side effects. It can help reduce food intake enough to lose, on average, about 10% of the initial body weight.

Serotonergic weight control drugs include fenfluramine (Pondimin), dexfenfluramine (Redux), and fluoxetine (Prozac). Fenfluramine and dexfenfluramine decrease food intake and also may increase energy expenditure. Fenfluramine often was combined with low doses of phentermine (fen-phen) after initial reports suggested that the combination might be useful in reducing the adverse effects associated with each individual drug while maintaining or enhancing therapeutic efficacy. Several placebo-controlled studies reported that the long-term use of this combination effectively maintained weight loss, and during the 1990s, many weight loss clinics were opened for the sole purpose of prescribing fen-phen. This resulted in widespread prescribing (up to 5.8 million dieters) and often in the indiscriminate, long-term use of these medications in mildly obese people. However, fenfluramine and dexfenfluramine were removed from the U.S. market in 1997 due to findings linking their usage to valvular heart disease and irreversible pulmonary hypertension.

After the recall of fenfluramine, some tried a combination of phentermine and Prozac (fen-pro). Many fen-phen fanatics are touting "herbal fen-phen," a combination of the herbal antidepressant St. John's wort and the herb ephedra, which contains ephedrine. The latter increases energy expenditure in humans. Ephedrine, in combination with caffeine and/or aspirin, has shown promise as a treatment for obesity. However, some of the ephedrine-containing supplements have been implicated in several cases of heart attacks, seizures, and some deaths.

A drug, sibutramine (Meridia), has been approved by the U.S. Food and Drug Administration (FDA). The drug inhibits the reuptake of serotonin and norepinephrine by nerve cells. It does not stimulate an additional release of serotonin as the banned products did. Meridia is proving to be a very popular drug. In clinical studies, sibutramine (5–30 mg/day) caused a significant dose-related weight loss in obese patients. In a 12-month study of obese subjects, those who were given a daily dose of 10 mg of the drug had an average weight loss of 4.8 kg, and with a dose of 15 mg/day, the weight loss was 6.1 kg compared with 1.8 kg for placebo treatment. Sibutramine may increase blood pressure and heart rate in some individuals. Frequent blood pressure and pulse rate monitoring is recommended because these are dose-related effects. The long-term safety of this drug has not been established. In April 1999, a new weight loss medication, orlistat (Xenical), was approved by the FDA. The drug is a lipase inhibitor that acts in the intestine to block the digestion and the absorption of about one-third of dietary fat. The drug works directly in the gastrointestinal tract and does not enter the bloodstream or the brain. Weight losses of 9%–11% of the initial body weight have been reported when orlistat was combined with a moderate calorie-restricted diet. These losses have been shown to be maintained up to 2 years and are associated with reductions of plasma low-density lipoprotein cholesterol and insulin levels compared with those of the placebo groups. The most common side effects associated with orlistat include gastro-intestinal problems, for example, more frequent stools and steatorrhea and reduced absorption of fat-soluble vitamins. Patients on orlistat should receive a daily supplement containing fat-soluble vitamins given at least 2 hours before or after each dose of the drug. Alli, the reduced strength version of orlistat, is approved for over-the-counter sale to overweight adults 18 years and older. Alli is meant to be used in conjunction with a low-calorie, low-fat diet, and regular exercise. Meridia and Xenical are likely to be only the front line in what may become an entire army of new drugs launched to fight obesity. Leptin may be the next new type of obesity drug to reach the market. In the hypothalamus, peptides that stimulate appetite (e.g., NPY, orexins, AgRP, melanin-concentrating hormone), as well as those that reduce appetite (melanocyte-stimulating hormone, cocaine- and amphetamine-related transcript, corticotropin-releasing hormone, oxytocin), are secreted.

Rimonabant is a cannabinoid receptor antagonist. Cannabinoid receptors are believed to play a role in appetite and body weight regulation. Rimonabant has been studied as a potential treatment for both obesity and smoking cessation. It produces modest but clinically significant weight loss in obese patients. In 2006, it was approved in Europe for treating obesity. In October 2008, the European Medicines Agency recommended a temporary suspension of Rimonabant sales in Europe, concluding that the drug's benefits no longer outweighed its risks. Its adverse effects include mood disorders, dizziness, and psychiatric effects. The drug has not been approved in the United States.

Some medications approved for other indications are known to affect appetite and body weight. A few antidepressants and antianxiety medications can cause weight gain. Antidiabetic agent metformin is associated with weight loss. The anticonvulsant drug topiramate (Topamax) is known to induce weight loss.[26]

Several approaches to the development of obesity drugs are being pursued based on the numerous pathways for regulating appetite and weight that have been discovered in recent years. Potential therapies include inhibitors of the appetite-stimulating peptides NPY, ghrelin, and MCH or molecules that stimulate the action of appetite-suppressing peptides.[25] And even agents that do the opposite—stimulating appetite or suppressing satiety—may have therapeutic potential to treat patients with eating disorders such as anorexia nervosa, for example, or to stimulate the appetite of people receiving certain kinds of cancer chemotherapy.

Recently, one study in rats and mice found that N-acylphosphatidylethanolamines (NAPEs) are secreted from the small intestine into circulation in response to eating a high-fat meal and travel to the hypothalamus and suppress the appetite. NAPE is also an intermediate in the biosynthesis of endocannabinoids by neurons in the brain. Mice and rats injected with NAPE eat less than normal and lose weight. Another study found that a high-fat meal causes mice to produce the protein adropin (derived from Latin roots *aduro*—to set fire to—and *pinquis*—fat and oils) in the liver and brain.[28] It is encoded by the Energy Homeostasis Associated gene Enho. Liver Enho expression is regulated by energy status and dietary nutrient content. Animals that become obese after eating a high-fat diet for 3 months do not produce adropin normally. However, injecting these obese mice with synthetic adropin causes them to consume less food and lose weight. If these compounds function in a similar manner in humans, they may form the basis for the development of new therapeutic targets to prevent or treat obesity.

16.11 EATING DISORDERS

Eating disorders refer to a heterogeneous group of conditions characterized by severe disturbances in eating behavior.[8,13] During the past few years, eating disturbances have captured the interest of both health professionals and the general public. The main characteristic of some of the common disorders is an overwhelming desire to become and to remain thin.[18] The marked increase in these disorders within recent years is due, in part, to our society's infatuation with slimness, encouraged largely by the advertising media. Beauty pageants are another tradition through which society defines its ideal of beauty, including body weight and shape. During the last few years, the BMI of an increasing number of winners of Miss America pageants has fallen in the range of undernutrition (<18.5), with some having a BMI as low as 16.9 (Figure 16.5).[37] Eating disorders can be found in both men and women, but the incidences are more than 10 times as common in women than men. Once considered to affect only those in their second and third decades, these conditions are increasingly being first diagnosed in their 30s and 40s. The current sociocultural emphasis on thinness and on physical fitness as a symbol of beauty and success has apparently contributed to this age distribution. The two common ones are anorexia nervosa and bulimia nervosa. The latter has gained attention recently because some well-known personalities have come forward to admit that they were suffering from this eating disorder. More recently, a fourth-year medical student wrote a letter (unsigned) to a medical journal, entitled *My Secret*, describing her personal experiences with this disease. According to her, about 18% of college women in this country suffer from bulimia and all keep it a secret. Soon after this letter was published, a physician who completed her residency 10 years previously wrote a letter (signed) entitled "Bulimia: My Secret No More." She described the problems she faced and how she was treated by the medical community. Another medical student chronicled her struggle with anorexia, physicians' attitudes toward eating disorders, and society's ideals for women in a book, *Stick Figure—A Diary of My Former Self.*

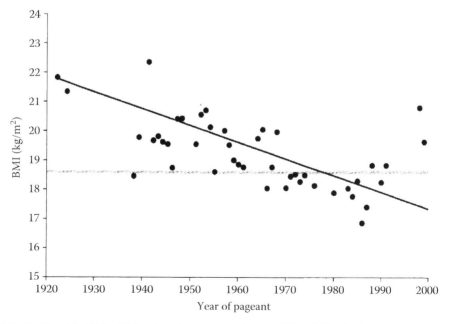

FIGURE 16.5 Trend in BMI of Miss America pageant winners, 1922–1999. The horizontal line represents the World Health Organization's BMI cutoff point (18.5) for undernutrition. (Courtesy of Benjamin Caballero, Center for Human Nutrition, Johns Hopkins University.)

16.11.1 ANOREXIA NERVOSA

Anorexia nervosa is a clinical syndrome of self-induced starvation characterized by a voluntary refusal to eat due to an intense fear of fatness and a disturbed perception of body size. The syndrome was first described in 1874 in England and was coined "anorexia nervosa," meaning lack of appetite. This is a misnomer because most patients with this disorder do not seem to have lost appetite at least in the early stages of the illness. These patients experience hunger, but they suppress the sensation because not eating is more pleasurable. It occurs 15–20 times more frequently in females than in males. This lower incidence in males may, in part, be due to less pressure on males in our society to be thin. Some young men in contact sports, especially wrestling, are likely to try extreme methods of reducing in order to squeeze into a lower weight class.

The preillness personality in anorexia nervosa varies considerably. A typical patient with this disorder is a white female from a middle- to upper–middle class family. The patient tends to be conscientious, a perfectionist, highly motivated, and very successful academically. Male anorectics tend to be underachievers, working hard but often in a misdirected fashion. Among women, in more than half of the cases, the syndrome begins before age 20 years; and in about three-fourths, it occurs before age 25 years. According to recent estimates, about 1% of Americans between the ages of 12 and 25 years will develop anorexia nervosa to some degree. The typical patient before the illness is quiet and cooperative, without weight or eating problems. Then, an emotional crisis of some sort leads the individual to go on a diet.

Anorexia nervosa may begin as a simple attempt to lose weight. A comment from a well-meaning friend or relative suggesting that the person seems to be gaining weight or is too fat may be all that is needed. The early phase of dieting may pass unnoticed. The diet soon becomes an irrational quest to lose all traces of body fat. It is a potentially life-threatening disorder characterized by the patient's refusal to maintain a body weight above 85% of what would be expected based on age and height.

The specific cause(s) of the disease is still not known, but both biological and psychological factors may be involved. There is an increased risk of anorexia nervosa among siblings (6%), with a four- to fivefold difference in concordance rates for monozygotic twins; this suggests a predisposing role for genetic factors. There are strong family influences. A child's risk is greater if another family member also had an eating disorder. Recent studies suggest that a hypothalamic abnormality may exist, which may lead to physiological and behavioral changes characteristic of the disorder. Slow gastric emptying may also be a factor, but this disturbance may be secondary to malnutrition. It remains unclear why an individual goes against a profound physiological drive to normal nutritional status and chooses instead self-induced starvation.

Anorexia nervosa is considered a diagnostic challenge as the patient may disguise the symptoms and/or have complaints suggestive of other medical conditions. A thorough history, along with physical and mental examinations, however, is usually sufficient to differentiate anorexia nervosa from other medical psychiatric conditions. In addition to the skeleton-like appearance, several complications (including any of the consequences of starvation) are possible in this disorder. These tend to reflect the duration and the severity of reduced food intake and degree of the body weight loss. One of the most consistent physiological changes is amenorrhea. This occurs in about 30% of anorectics prior to significant weight loss and may be related to stress. The loss of fat causes a reduction in estrogen level and can lead to osteoporosis, even in young individuals. Other metabolic changes include decreased BMR, lowered heart rate, hypotension, hypothermia, decreased white blood cell count, hypoproteinemia, and anemia.

Anorexia nervosa is a chronic illness that requires a multidisciplinary management approach using medical, psychiatric, nutritional, and other support staff. Severe malnutrition is not only life-threatening, but it also impairs thinking, so psychological treatment is not possible until nutritional status is improved. In most cases, nothing short of hospitalization and intravenous feeding will help. Modest, steady weight gain is an adequate goal in the early phase of treatment. Weight gain alone by no means corrects the underlying psychological problem of the anorectic; consequently, long-term psychotherapy is usually indicated. The goal of treatment is to resume the normal eating pattern and to achieve and maintain a desirable body weight status. The outcome of anorexia nervosa remains uncertain. With nutrition and psychotherapy, as many as two-thirds of anorectics may recover normal or near-normal weight, but many continue to struggle with the emotional problems that began their illness. Real progress may depend on working out these problems with competent professional help.

16.11.2 BULIMIA NERVOSA

Bulimia nervosa is defined as recurrent episodes of rapid, uncontrollable ingestion of large amounts of food in a short period of time usually followed by purging, either by forced vomiting and/or by abuse of laxatives or diuretics. The purging techniques are used to "undo" the threatened weight gain, relieve fullness, and restore the individual's self-control. Similar to anorectics, they have an exaggerated fear of fatness and intend to pursue slimness as a means of bringing control and a sense of effectiveness into their lives. Although bulimia was first described as a distinct psychiatric illness only in 1979, its prevalence is very high and it has probably existed for a long time. Literally, bulimia means "ox hunger" or voracious appetite, but this is a misnomer as most bulimics do not report such feelings of hunger. Riddled with shame for being unable to control their disorder, they hide binges and purges even from their closest friends. Less than a third discuss their behavior with their physicians, and only about 25% are under medical care.

Although the actual incidence of bulimia nervosa has not been clearly established, this eating disorder is recognized as a significant problem for about 8% of adolescents and young adult females. Unfortunately, no well-controlled studies have been conducted to determine the incidence in the general population. Bulimia, however, is suspected to be more prevalent than anorexia nervosa. Bulimics generally have problems with impulse control, are chronically depressed, are intolerant of frustration, and have an exaggerated sense of guilt and recurrent anxiety. They may think of food constantly and turn to food during a crisis or problem—not away from food as anorectics do. They generally look healthy, and their behavior is unnoticed by their friends and families. The patients who seek help do so because of feelings of guilt, anxiety, depression, or because they can no longer continue the habit and still function in daily activities.

The typical bulimic is a white, college-educated female of normal weight for height in her mid-20s who has been involved in bulimic behavior for 4–6 years before seeking treatment. Often, it is not the eating disorder per se that leads them to seek treatment but the development of secondary symptoms such as medical complications, depression, or poor job or school performance. Bulimics are more aware that their behavior, although secretive, is aberrant, and they may be more willing to accept treatment.

The cause of bulimia remains unknown. According to some investigators, individuals at risk appear to be biologically vulnerable to affective instability (fluctuating mood), live in a highly conflicted family environment, and possess personality traits that result in difficulty with self-esteem during childhood or adolescence. The onset of bulimia is associated with a conscious desire to diet. At some point, the patients lose control of their compulsion to eat large amounts of food and binge, and their purge is a convenient method of re-establishing weight control. Thus, a binge–purge cycle becomes established. A possible role for CCK[19] (a satiety-inducing nerve gut peptide) has been implicated in bulimia. When compared to healthy individuals, bulimics have a blunted meal-induced secretion of CCK. As in anorexia nervosa, societal influences seem to play a prominent role in the desire to be thin.

There are no clinical signs of bulimia except for the frequent fluctuation in body weight. The diagnosis, therefore, usually is based on self-reported symptoms with few supported physical findings or laboratory data. Medical complications are the consequences of vomiting and laxative abuse. Physical examination may reveal the following: salivary gland hypertrophy due to vomiting; bruising of the knuckles from their rubbing against the upper incisors during the induction of vomiting; and dental erosion due to prolonged and repeated exposure of the dental enamel to an acidic environment. Irregular menses is frequent. Metabolic alkalosis, hypochloremia, and hypokalemia due to loss of hydrochloric acid and potassium are the most common metabolic complications and may lead to cardiac arrhythmias. Secondary metabolic disturbances may produce weakness and tetany.

For treatment, the main goals are to interrupt the binge–purge cycle by normalizing the patient's eating patterns and to change the patient's attitude toward food, eating, and body size. Recent studies suggest that inositol may be possible nutritional therapy as both an alternative and an additive to conventional therapy. Published reports suggest that of the various psychotropic medications, antidepressant drugs show the most promise in decreasing the frequency of binge activity and in increasing the patient's sense of well-being. Bulimia patients recognize their behavior as maladaptive. Compared to anorectics, they are more aware of associated psychological difficulties and are more willing to work with physicians and counselors.

16.11.3   BINGE EATING

Binge eating is the most recently recognized eating problem and could well be the most common. In this case, the binges are not followed by purges as in bulimia nervosa; those affected usually become obese. Binging is nearly always done in private; in public, sufferers tend to eat normal or even less than normal amounts. The individual with this disease, if untreated, will fail at all attempts at permanent weight loss.

16.11.4   NIGHT EATING DISORDERS

Two night eating disorders[47] have recently been reported. Some individuals who had been sleep-walkers in childhood may develop another problem as adults. This time their nightly rambles take them to the kitchen for cookies, candy, and potato chips, which they bring to bed and devour while still sleeping (sleep eating). They wake up feeling exhausted and sick from all the junk food. This condition is called sleep-related eating disorder (SRED). The other is night eating syndrome (NES) in which patients wake up on average twice a night and are unable to fall asleep again unless they eat something. They eat about 35% of their calories after dinner and do not feel hungry in the morning. It is not clear what causes NES, but it affects more women than men and often begins during periods of stress.

Although the two disorders differ in some important ways—most notably, whether the person is conscious or not—they share many similarities. Both are hybrids of sleep and eating disorders. In addition to sabotaging good-quality sleep, both conditions seriously undermine attempts to maintain a well-balanced diet. This disorder often causes depression and weight gain. The two conditions may affect 1% of the U.S. population—nearly 3 million Americans. The antidepressant Zoloft appears to help some patients with SRED and NES.

16.11.5   BARYPHOBIA

Baryphobia—the fear of becoming obese—is a relatively new disorder. This occurs when children themselves and parents put their children on the same low-caloric diet that they follow. Parents do this in an attempt to prevent their children from developing obesity. Children do not get adequate calories for growth.

16.11.6   PICA

Pica denotes the compulsion for persistent ingestion of unsuitable substances having little or no nutritional value. Pica during pregnancy is most often reported as consumption of dirt, clay, or laundry starch. Recent studies suggest that some forms of pica may be related to iron deficiency because treatment with iron improves the condition.

16.11.7 Miscellaneous Eating Disorders

A most recent study has shown that many Americans suffer an eating disorder and struggle with related psychiatric disorders, including suicidal tendencies. Researchers analyzed data collected by the National Comorbidity Survey Replication Adolescent Supplement, which included the results of in-person interviews conducted with more than 10,000 adolescents between the ages of 13 and 18. The results indicated that the prevalence rates of eating disorders ranged from less than 0.5% of those interviewed to as much as 2.5%.

While boys and girls appeared to be equally susceptible to anorexia, girls were found to be more likely to develop bulimia and/or binge-eating disorders. The majority of those with any eating disorder had at least one other mental health issue. This was the case with about 9 of 10 bulimic adolescents and 8 of 10 of those with a binge-eating problem. Eating disorders were most commonly linked to social impairment, a problem that affected 9 in 10 anorectic adolescents. And all eating disorders were associated with a higher lifetime risk for suicidal tendencies. Researchers noted that only a minority of adolescent patients with an eating disorder received treatment to deal with their food issues.

Afflicted teens can go months to years undetected due to secrecy surrounding the illness. The disease can become chronic and can lead to death. Prior research has suggested that adults plagued with the problem are also susceptible to higher rates of associated medical complications. The prevalence of these disorders appears to be higher than previously expected, and they represent a major public health concern.

Orderly Dieting and Disorderly Eating—A Case

A 49-year-old black woman entered a nutrition and weight control clinic for an evaluation and the treatment of her obesity. She weighed 184 pounds (132% of her ideal body weight), and her BMI was 28.3 (desirable BMI is 20–25). Her waist/hip ratio of 0.8 indicated a lower-body obesity. Her stated goals were to lose 20 pounds, learn new eating habits, find any medical problem she might have and control her hypertension without medication, if possible. The patient claimed that she had maintained a normal weight throughout childhood and early adulthood, including three pregnancies through age 26 years. Then, she gradually began to gain weight, especially after she quit smoking at the age of 35 years. At age 37 years, she weighed 170 pounds, and by 41 years, she weighed 200 pounds. She then lost 31 pounds during the next 7 months using an appetite suppressant but regained the lost weight upon the discontinuation of the drug. Since then, she has tried weight loss programs unsuccessfully and has followed a variety of fad diets.

Her physical examination was unremarkable except for her obesity and mild hypertension. Her food records indicated that her average dietary intake was 1800 Cal (range 1000–2400 Cal). A restricted 1000-Cal balanced diet was prescribed, and she was seen weekly for several months in individual counseling sessions with a dietician or a behavior analyst. Throughout this period, she reported no physical, behavioral, or emotional difficulties, and she adhered closely to her dietary plan. She lost 22.5 pounds (3.7 lb/week) in the first 6 weeks and 10 pounds (1.6 lb/week) over the next 6 weeks. After this initial weight loss, which was due entirely to dietary restriction, she began a gradual and modest exercise program. Nine weeks later, she lost an additional 21.5 pounds (2.4 lb/week). She was advised to increase her caloric intake and to maintain her current weight of 130 pounds.

The patient returned to the clinic 5 1/2 months later after her family told her she had an eating disorder and insisted that she go back for follow-up; by this time, she had lost an additional 14 pounds (0.63 lb/week) in 22 weeks, weighing 108 pounds or 86% of her ideal body weight. She said that although her family and some friends were concerned that she had become too thin, she herself was happy and felt well at her current weight. She described her highly restricted eating habits, a vigorous exercise routine of brisk daily walks in place of lunch, and spending about 50 min/day on a stationary exercise bicycle. Her family constantly watched what she ate, discussed her eating habits, and pressured her to eat more. The body composition by bioelectric impedance analysis revealed a body fat content of 17%. She was advised to eat more and to return to the clinic after 4 weeks. However, she cancelled all subsequent visits and maintained a weight of 108 pounds for the next 4 months.

Discussions with the patient's family members indicated that the patient had characteristics of an unspecified eating disorder resembling anorexia. She was generally secretive about her weight and about how little she ate (sometimes <800 Cal/day). She often argued with her family about these matters, did not accept that there was any reason for concern, and resisted offers of help. Her family noted severe mood swings, and she sometimes became angry or depressed for no apparent reason. She was encouraged to seek counseling but continued to deny any problems.

This case emphasizes that some individuals may develop eating disorders after entering weight control programs for obesity.[51] It is also possible that this patient may have had an eating disorder, for example, bulimia or anorexia, in the past, which was not known. Physicians may encounter individuals, like this patient, who do not appear to be in the high-risk age or racial categories but may show several personality characteristics commonly associated with formal eating disorders.

REFERENCES

1. Adams, K. F., A. Schatzkin, T. B. Harris et al. 2006. Overweight, obesity, and mortality in a large prospective cohort of persons 50 to 71 years old. *N Engl J Med* 355:763.
2. Ahima, R. S. 2004. Body fat, leptin and hypothalamic amenorrhea. *N Engl J Med* 351:959.
3. Ahima, R. S. 2006. Metabolic actions of adipocyte hormones: Focus on adiponectin. *Obesity* 14:95.
4. Andreyeva, T., R. Sturm, and J. S. Ringel. 2004. Moderate and severe obesity have large differences in health care costs. *Obes Res* 12:1936.
5. Atkinson, R. L. 1997. Use of drugs in the treatment of obesity. *Annu Rev Nutr* 17:383.
6. Badman, M. K., and J. S. Flier. 2007. The adipocyte as an active participant in energy balance and metabolism. *Gastroenterology* 132:2103.
7. Batterham, R. L., M. A. Cowley, C. J. Small et al. 2002. Gut hormone PYY_{3-36} physiologically inhibits food intake. *Nature* 418:650.
8. Becker, A. E., S. K. Grinspoon, A. Klibanski, and D. B. Herzog. 1997. Eating disorders. *N Engl J Med* 340:1092.
9. Bochukova, E. G., N. Huang, J. Keogh et al. 2010. Large, rare chromosomal deletions associated with severe early onset obesity. *Nature* 463:666.
10. Considine, R. V., and J. F. Caro. 1996. Leptin in humans: Current progress and future directions. *Clin Chem* 42:482.
11. Dietrich, M., and I. Jialal. 2005. The effect of weight loss on a stable biomarker of inflammation, C-reactive protein. *Nutr Rev* 63:22.
12. Drahl, C. 2009. Weighing options. *Chem Eng News* 87(15):11.
13. Edwards, K. I. 1993. Obesity, anorexia and bulimia. *Med Clin North Am* 77:899.
14. Farooqi, I. S., S. A. Jebb, G. Langmack et al. 1999. Effects of recombinant leptin therapy in a child with congenital leptin deficiency. *N Engl J Med* 341:879.
15. Fiorito, L. M., M. Marini, L. A. Francis et al. 2008. Beverage intake of girls at age 5 years predicts adiposity and weight status in childhood and adolescence. *Am J Clin Nutr* 90:935.
16. Frayling, T. M., N. J. Timpson, M. N. Needon et al. 2007. A common variant in the FTO gene is associated with body mass index and predisposes to childhood and adult obesity. *Science* 316:889.
17. Friedman, J. M. 1998. Leptin, leptin receptors and the control of body weight. *Nutr Rev* 56:S38.

18. Gale, S. M., V. D. Castracane, and C. S. Mantzoros. 2004. Energy homeostasis, obesity and eating disorders: Recent advances in endocrinology. *J Nutr* 134:295.

19. Geracioti, T. D., and R. A. Liddle. 1988. Impaired cholecystokinin secretion in bulimia nervosa. *N Engl J Med* 319:683.

20. Gillum, M. P., D. Zhang, X. Zhang et al. 2008. A gut-derived circulating factor induced by fat ingestion inhibits food intake. *Cell* 135:813.

21. Hill, J. O., J. Hauptman, J. W. Anderson et al. 1999. Orslistat, a lipase inhibitor, for weight maintenance after conventional dieting: A 1-year study. *Am J Clin Nutr* 69:1108.

22. Hojgaard, B., D. Gyrd-Hansen, K. R. Olsen et al. 2008. Waist circumference and body mass index as predictors of health care costs. *PLOS One* 3(7):e2619.

23. Hossan, P., B. Kawar, and M. E. Nahas. 2007. Obesity and diabetes in the developing world—a growing challenge. *N Engl J Med* 356:213.

24. Inui, A. 2001. Ghrelin: An orexigenic and somatotrophic signal from the stomach. *Nat Rev Neurosci* 2:551.

25. Jeanrenaud, B., and F. Rohner-Jeanrenaud. 2001. Effects of neuropeptides and leptin on nutrient partitioning: Dysregulation in obesity. *Annu Rev Med* 52:339.

26. Kirov, G., and J. Tredget. 2005. Add-on topiramate reduces weight in overweight patients with affective disorders: A clinical case series. *BMC Psychiatry* 5:19.

27. Korner, J., and R. L. Leibel. 2003. To eat or not to eat—how the gut talks to the brain. *N Engl J Med* 349:926.

28. Kumar, K. G., J. L. Trevaskis, D. D. Lam et al. 2008. Identification of adropin as a secreted factor linking dietary macronutrient intake with energy homeostasis and lipid metabolism. *Cell Metab* 8:468.

29. Leibel, R. L., M. Rosenbaum, and J. Hirsch. 1995. Changes in energy expenditure from altered body weight. *N Engl J Med* 332:621.

30. Lowell, B. B., and J. S. Flier. 1997. Brown adipose tissue, β3-adrenergic receptors and obesity. *Annu Rev Med* 48:307.

31. McTigue, K., J. C. Larson, A. Vakoski et al. 2006. Mortality and cardiac and vascular outcomes in extremely obese women. *J Am Med Assoc* 296:79.

32. Meda, H., R. Yamamoto, K. Hirao, and O. Tochikubo. 2004. Effects of agar (Kanten) diet on obese patients with impaired glucose tolerance and Type 2 diabetes. *Diabetes Obes Metab* 7(1):40.

33. Moreno, M. A. 2009. Sugary drinks and childhood obesity. *Arch Pediatr Adolesc Med* 163:400.

34. Olsen, N. J., and B. L. Heitmann. 2009. Intake of calorically sweetened beverages and obesity. *Obes Res* 10(1):68.

35. Powel, K. 2007. The two faces of fat. *Nature* 447:525.

36. Rosenbaum, M., R. L. Leibel, and J. Hirsch. 1997. Obesity. *N Engl J Med* 337:396.

37. Rubenstein, S., and B. Caballero. 2000. Is Miss America an undernourished role model? *J Am Med Assoc* 283:1569.

38. Sakurai, T., A. Amemiya, M. Ishii et al. 1998. Orexin and orexin receptors: A family of hypothalamic neuropeptides and G-protein-coupled receptors that regulate feeding behavior. *Cell* 92:573.

39. Shade, E. D., C. M. Ulrich, M. H. Wener et al. 2004. Frequent intentional weight loss in associated with lower natural killer cell cytotoxicity in postmenopausal women: possible long term immune effects. *J Am Diet Assoc* 104:903.

40. Strader, A. D., and S. C. Wood. 2005. Gastrointestinal hormones and food intake. *Gastroenterology* 128:175.

41 Strauss, R. S., and H. A. Pollack. 2001. Epidemic increase in childhood overweight 1986–1998. *J Am Med Assoc* 286:2945.

42. Steppan, C. M., S. T. Bailey, S. Bhat et al. 2001. The hormone resistin links obesity to diabetes. *Nature* 409:307.

43. Van Itallie, T., and A. Simopoulos, eds. 1995. *Obesity: New Directions and Assessment in Management.* Philadelphia, PA: The Charles Press.

44. Virtanen, K. A., M. E. Lidell, J. Orava et al. 2009. Functional brown adipose tissue in healthy adults. *N Engl J Med* 360:1518.

45. Welt, C. K., J. L. Chan, J. Bullen et al. 2004. Recombinant human leptin in women with hypothalamic amerorrhea. *N Engl J Med* 351:987.

46. Winick, M. 1980. *Nutrition in Health and Disease.* New York: John Wiley and Sons.

47. Winkelman, J. W. 2006. Sleep related eating disorder and night eating syndrome. *Sleep* 29(7):876.

48. Wolf, C., and M. Tanner. 2002. Obesity. *West J Med* 176:23.
49. Young, T. K., and D. E. Gelskey. 1995. Is noncentral obesity metabolically benign? Implications for prevention from a population survey. *J Am Med Assoc* 274:1939.
50. Zhang, C., K. M. Rexrode, R. M. Van Dam et al. 2008. Abdominal obesity and the risk of all-cause, cardiovascular, and cancer mortality: Sixteen years of follow-up in U.S. women. *Circulation* 117:1658.

CASE BIBLIOGRAPHY

51. Andronis, P. G., and R. F. Kushner. 1991. Orderly dieting and disordered eating: A case report. *Nutr Rev* 49:16.

17 Cholesterol and Dyslipidemia

In the first two decades of the last century, the majority of deaths resulted from infectious diseases, but deaths from heart disease now exceed the combined total deaths from infection, cancer, and accidents. Epidemiologists have identified about 10 risk factors in the general population, which have been found to correlate significantly with death rates from coronary heart disease (CHD), and three of these occupy a position of preeminence: hypercholesterolemia, high blood pressure, and smoking. Diabetes, heredity, age, gender, and personality type are also important, but these are the ones on which we have no control.

A new factor has recently been identified. It is a mutation in the heart protein gene MYBPC3, which increases the risk for heart disease sevenfold. The mutation is carried by 1% of the world's population and by around 4% of people from the Indian subcontinent. The World Health Organization estimates that in 2010, India will have 60% of the world's heart disease cases—nearly 4 times its share of the world's population. The mutated protein causes severe hypertension, inflammation, and weakening of the heart muscle. In younger people, the body seems to have an effective mechanism to break down the protein. But with age, the mechanism stops working efficiently, which is why heart disease in people carrying the gene develops in middle age. Undoubtedly, hypercholesterolemia has received the greatest share of attention not only by epidemiologists but also by clinical investigators as well. The relationship of plasma cholesterol levels to CHD is ultimately related to the plasma lipoproteins, which are the vehicles for transporting lipids from the site of origin to their site of utilization. Before discussing the lipoproteins, a brief description of the biochemistry of cholesterol follows.

17.1 CHOLESTEROL

The compound now known as cholesterol was described for the first time in the latter half of the 18th century. De Fourcroy in 1789 mentioned that more than 20 years earlier, Poulletier de la Salle had obtained from the alcohol-soluble part of human gallstones "Un substance feuilletè, lamelleuse, brillante, assez semblable à l'acide boracique." Fourcroy prepared a larger quantity of the substance, which he believed was the same as "blanc de baleine," that is, spermaceti. During the time between Poulletier's observation and Fourcroy's publication, other researchers had extracted the substance from gallstones and made observations regarding its solubility. In 1816, Chevreul introduced the designation *cholesterine* from Greek: chole, bile; and steros, solid.[3] Cholesterol was found to be present in human and animal bile in 1824, human and animal brain in 1834, human blood in 1838, and hen's eggs in 1846. It was thereafter gradually recognized as a normal constituent of all animal cells and several secretions, as well as a component of certain pathological deposits. It was found in atheromatous arteries in 1843.

17.1.1 Food Sources

Cholesterol is found in all animal tissues so that some is present in all foods of animal origin, but eggs are the only common foods rich in cholesterol. Principal dietary sources include meat (liver, 370 mg; veal, lamb, and beef, 80–85 mg/3 oz serving), eggs (one large, 252 mg), shellfish (shrimp, 128 mg/3 oz serving), poultry (chicken, 74 mg/3 oz serving), fish (45–60 mg/3 oz serving), and dairy products (whole milk, 34 mg/8 oz; ice cream, 54–98 mg/cup; American cheese, 28 mg/oz). It is virtually absent in foods of plant origin, which do, however, contain other sterols.

17.1.2   Body Cholesterol

Cholesterol is present in every body cell in humans. A 150-pound male has about 140–145 g of cholesterol, most of which is in the brain, nervous system, connective tissue, and muscle. Blood contains about 8% of body cholesterol.

17.1.3   Functions

Cholesterol is a necessary metabolite, but not a dietary essential, because it is synthesized in the body normally at a rate sufficient to meet body needs. Its functions have still not been fully elucidated, but several important roles for this sterol have been described.

- It is a major constituent of all cell membranes throughout the body and is essential for their normal structure and function. The protein/phospholipid pattern of membranes may be modified by cholesterol with functional consequences such as membrane permeability.
- Cholesterol regulates the assembly of a cytosolic multiprotein complex (CMC) that controls an important cell-signaling pathway. This CMC contains a cholesterol-binding protein known as OSBP, as well as two different protein phosphatase enzymes. The intact complex is required to properly dephosphorylate a key signaling protein known as extracellular-regulated protein kinase (ERK), and cholesterol is necessary to keep this complex together.[28] When cellular cholesterol levels are lowered, the complex falls apart and phosphorylated ERK builds up.
- As much as 50% of myelin that surrounds the nerves is cholesterol, and it is suggested that cholesterol is necessary for proper nerve conduction and brain function.
- It is the precursor of bile acids, which are synthesized in the liver and which aid in the digestion and the absorption of fat. In the absence of bile acids, the absorption of fats and fat-soluble vitamins is negligible.
- It is the precursor of adrenal and reproductive steroid hormones.
- It is an essential component of plasma lipoproteins, which are vehicles by which fat-soluble material is transported from one part of the body to another.
- Cholesterol is the precursor of vitamin D.
- Neurons in the brain communicate with one another through specialized junctions called synapses. It has been known for several years that neurons in the brain need a factor that is produced in another type of brain cell (glial cell) in order to form their full complement of synapses. Researchers have recently identified this factor to be cholesterol. Neurons produce enough cholesterol to survive and grow, but without additional cholesterol provided by glial cells, their production of synapses is limited. The brain cannot pick up cholesterol supply from blood because lipoproteins carrying cholesterol do not cross the blood–brain barrier. The finding may have implications for understanding and treating Alzheimer's disease since a cholesterol-carrying brain lipoprotein is suspected of playing a role in the synaptic plasticity that occurs in Alzheimer's disease.

17.1.4   Synthesis

Virtually every mammalian cell with the exception of mature erythrocytes can produce its own cholesterol, but at different rates. In humans, more of the cholesterol is derived from de novo synthesis than from dietary cholesterol. For a 70-kg adult, the total cholesterol synthesis ranges from 500 mg to about 1 g daily. More than 90% of the cholesterol formed in the body probably is synthesized in the liver and the intestine, with the liver being the major site. The extrapolation of data from primates indicates that about 50% of the total body cholesterol synthesis (350–450 mg) takes place in the liver. Cholesterol synthesized by the liver is unique because only the hepatocyte secretes cholesterol into the systemic circulation for use by other cells. All of the carbon atoms of cholesterol

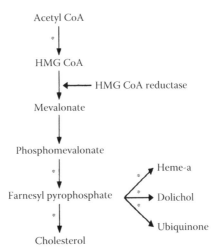

FIGURE 17.1 Pathway for the biosynthesis of cholesterol. * Indicates two or more steps.

are derived from acetyl coenzyme A (CoA), a common metabolite of carbohydrate, fat, and protein metabolism. More than 25 enzymes are involved in the formation of cholesterol from acetyl CoA. The principal steps include the conversion of acetyl CoA to β-hydroxy β-methyl glutaryl CoA (HMG-CoA), which is reduced to mevalonic acid by the enzyme HMG-CoA reductase. Mevalonic acid is converted by several steps to squalene and then to cholesterol (Figure 17.1).

The cholesterol pool of the body is derived from two sources: absorption of dietary cholesterol and de novo synthesis, primarily in the liver and the intestine. When the amount of dietary cholesterol is reduced, its synthesis is increased in the liver and the intestine to satisfy the needs of other tissues and organs. The primary site for control of cholesterol biosynthesis is the HMG-CoA reductase, which catalyzes the step that produces mevalonic acid. This is the committed step and the rate-limiting reaction in the pathway of cholesterol biosynthesis. In humans, dietary cholesterol absorbed from the intestine exerts feedback inhibition on its synthesis by inhibiting the activity of HMG-CoA reductase in the liver but not in the intestine. The dietary cholesterol that suppresses HMG-CoA reductase activity and cholesterol synthesis emerges from the intestine in the form of chylomicrons. The feedback potential for cholesterol from other sources such as newly synthesized cholesterol or that released from storage is not understood. Bile acids may also play a role in the formation of cholesterol in the liver and intestines because the intake of bile salts reduces the total body cholesterol synthesis, but the mechanism is not known. Total energy intake is another factor that may influence cholesterol synthesis in the liver, with higher intake of calories favoring and restricting calories, reducing cholesterol synthesis. In normal individuals, sensitive feedback mechanisms are in operation to regulate cholesterol synthesis and the body pool remains relatively constant.

Deficiency of mevalonate kinase, which converts mevalonate to phosphomevalonate, was the first enzyme defect in cholesterol biosynthesis to be recognized. See the case study at the end of Chapter 17. Nine other enzyme deficiencies have since been identified in this pathway. They are associated with skeletal and organ malformation, skin abnormalities, and some other effects.

17.1.5 Cholesterol Degradation

Cholesterol output from the body is accomplished mainly by its conversion to bile acids but also by formation of steroid hormones and by excretion in the feces. Quantitatively, the conversion of cholesterol to bile acids (which takes place solely in the liver) is the major pathway by which cholesterol is removed from the body. Humans convert about 0.5 g of cholesterol to bile acids per day, and the total bile acid pool in the enterohepatic circulation is estimated to be about 3.5 g (Figure 17.2).

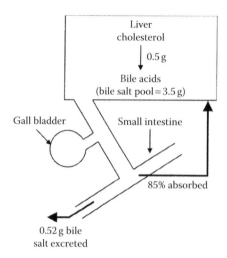

FIGURE 17.2 Enterohepatic circulation of bile acids.

Approximately 85% of the bile salts are reabsorbed. The formation of bile acids by the liver is under negative feedback control (i.e., the bile acids returning to the liver following absorption from the intestine inhibit the synthesis of the new bile acids). If the enterohepatic circulation is interrupted, the rate of bile acid synthesis increases.

17.2   LIPOPROTEINS AND LIPID TRANSPORT

The two main lipids in blood are cholesterol and triglycerides. As lipids, they are not soluble in aqueous solutions such as the blood and must, therefore, be transported by other macromolecular complexes known as lipoproteins. These dynamic particles are in a constant state of synthesis, degradation, and removal from the plasma. They are composed of an inner core of nonpolar lipids (triglycerides and/or cholesteryl esters) surrounded by a polar coat of phospholipids, free cholesterol (unesterified), and proteins known as apoproteins. The apoproteins serve as sites for cell-surface receptors and serve as activators or coenzymes for enzymes involved in lipoprotein metabolism. Lipoproteins are classified according to their physical–chemical properties (Table 17.1). Major classes of lipoproteins are separated by means of ultracentrifugation and electrophoresis. In order of increasing density, protein, and phospholipid concentration, and decreasing triglyceride concentration, these include chylomicrons, very low–density lipoproteins (VLDLs), intermediate-density lipoproteins (IDLs), low-density lipoproteins (LDLs), and high-density lipoproteins (HDLs). Normally, about 65% of the plasma cholesterol is carried by LDLs, 20% is carried by HDLs, 14% is carried by VLDLs, and about 1% is carried in chylomicrons.

Hyperlipidemias are disorders of the rate of synthesis or clearance of lipoproteins from the bloodstream. Usually, they are detected by measuring plasma triglycerides and cholesterol. The increases in these lipids can be dietary, genetic, or secondary to other conditions. Dietary hyperlipidemias tend to be mild while genetic disorders can be severe. Secondary lipidemias can result from various metabolic disorders and can be due to certain drugs. Lipidemias are classified on the basis of which lipoproteins are elevated: Type 1 hyperlipidemia is due to an accumulation of chylomicrons; Type 2a is characterized by increased LDL (familial hypercholesterolemia), while in Type 2b both VLDL and LDL are increased (familial combined hyperlipoproteinemia); Type 3 is a condition due to an elevation of IDL; Type 4 is the abnormality in which there is an elevation of VLDL; and Type 5 hyperlipidemia is due to an increase in both chylomicrons and VLDL particles. Dyslipidemia is probably a better term than hyperlipidemia because it includes abnormally high and low lipoprotein levels as well as abnormalities in the composition of these particles.

TABLE 17.1

Properties and Functions of Major Plasma Lipoproteins

Lipoprotein	Origin	Density Range	Major Lipid	Major Protein	Function
Chylomicrons	Small intestine	<0.94	Triglycerides	B-48, A-I, A-II	Absorption and transport of dietary fat
VLDL	Liver	0.94–1.006	Triglycerides	B-100, C-I, C-II, C-III, E	Transport of triglycerides from liver to other tissues
IDL	Plasma, VLDL	1.006–1.019	Triglycerides and cholesterol esters	B-100, E	Cholesterol transport, precursor of LDL
LDL	Plasma, IDL	1.019–1.063	Cholesterol esters	B-100	Cholesterol ester transport
HDL	Liver, small intestine	1.063–1.21	Phospholipid and cholesterol	A-I, A-II	Removal of cholesterol from extrahepatic tissues

17.2.1 CHYLOMICRONS

Chylomicrons are assembled in the small intestinal mucosal cells when fat is ingested and carry dietary triglycerides, cholesterol, and other lipids. The apoprotein that is essential for the assembly and the secretion of these particles is apo B-48, which is synthesized in the small intestine. It is so named because it constitutes 48% of the amino terminal end of apo B-100, which is the major apoprotein of VLDL, IDL, and LDL. The particle released by the intestinal mucosa is called a nascent chylomicron. When it reaches the plasma, it receives C apoproteins (C I, C II, and C III) from circulating HDLs. When the chylomicrons reach the capillaries of adipose tissue and muscle, they are acted on by lipoprotein lipase (LPL) that is bound to the surface of endothelial cells. Apo C II is an essential activator of LPL—the enzyme that degrades the triglycerides contained in chylomicrons. The liberated fatty acids cross the endothelium, enter the adipocytes and muscle cells, and are esterified again to form triglycerides for storage or are oxidized to provide energy. Apo C III is an inhibitor of LPL and may modulate the degradation of triglycerides.

After most of the triglycerides are removed, the chylomicron enters the circulation again with its size diminished. It then returns the C apoproteins to HDL and accepts apo E. This particle is called chylomicron remnant, which can be removed from the circulation by the liver. The liver cell membranes contain receptors that recognize the two protein components of chylomicron remnant, apo E, and apo B-48. The receptor-bound remnant is taken up into the hepatic cell by receptor-mediated endocytosis, is digested by lysosomes, and the cholesteryl esters are cleaved to generate free cholesterol. The free cholesterol has several fates including its conversion to bile acids and its utilization for membrane synthesis.

Chylomicrons are present normally only after a fatty meal. In the fasting serum, the presence of chylomicrons is always abnormal and may be due to genetic factors or to other disease states. Genetic defects (rare) in LPL or its cofactor apo C II affect the rate of triglyceride degradation and result in chylomicronemia, a form of hypertriglyceridemia (Type 1 hyperlipoproteinemia). Abdominal pain and pancreatitis are frequent presenting symptoms. This condition is treated by reducing dietary fat intake to less than 20 g/day.

17.2.2   VERY LOW–DENSITY LIPOPROTEIN

The VLDL lipoproteins are the main transporters of endogenous triglycerides. They are assembled and secreted by the liver as nascent particles containing apo B-100. In the circulation, they receive apo C II and apo E from HDL. Like chylomicrons, the triglycerides in VLDL are hydrolyzed by the same LPL and then transfer apo C II and apo E to HDL. In doing so, the particles become smaller and are called VLDL remnants or IDL.

About 50% of the IDL particles are cleared by the hepatic receptor-mediated endocytosis and require the apo E as ligand. The other 50% loses most of the remaining triglycerides, and their density increases further until they become LDLs that contain only one apo protein, apo B-100. Hepatic triglyceride lipase plays a role in removing triglycerides from IDL.

In general, VLDL triglyceride concentrations are highly correlated with plasma triglyceride level during the postabsorptive state except when the LPL system is deficient or overwhelmed. The presence of chylomicrons is simply evaluated by the appearance of a creamy layer on the surface of plasma or serum that has been stored overnight in the cold. The elevation of plasma VLDL (Type 4 hyperlipidemia) is a common abnormality, but the underlying disorder is unknown. It may be due to an overproduction of these particles.

A high-caloric diet (especially rich in carbohydrates), obesity, alcohol consumption, insulin resistance (as seen in obesity), and hyperinsulinemia are associated with VLDL overproduction. Elevated levels of these particles can saturate LPL and lead also to increased chylomicrons in the plasma, a phenotype called mixed lipemia (Type 5 hyperlipidemia). This is also a fairly common disorder.

17.2.3   INTERMEDIATE-DENSITY LIPOPROTEIN

The IDL particles are formed in the plasma during the conversion of VLDL to LDL. They contain amounts of triglycerides and cholesterol that are intermediate between those of VLDL and LDL. Normally, the conversion of VLDL to LDL proceeds so efficiently that appreciable quantities of IDL usually do not accumulate in the plasma after an overnight fast. The IDL may be increased in a rare inborn error of metabolism—dysbetalipoproteinemia (Type 3 hyperlipidemia). The defect is due to an abnormal form of apo E. This disorder is associated with an increased risk of peripheral vascular disease and coronary disease. Patients often have palmar xanthomas (yellow-orange discoloration in the creases of the palms and fingers) and tuberoeruptive xanthomas (small raised lesions in areas of pressure, particularly the elbows and knees).

17.2.4   LOW-DENSITY LIPOPROTEIN

The LDL particle contains only one apo protein, apo B-100; LDLs constitute the major carrier of cholesterol in the blood and account for 60%–70% of cholesterol. When the liver and other tissues require cholesterol for the synthesis of membranes, hormones, bile acids, and so on, they synthesize LDL receptors and obtain cholesterol by the receptor-mediated endocytosis of LDL. On the other hand, when tissues no longer require cholesterol, they decrease their synthesis of LDL receptors and LDLs remain in circulation. Serum LDL levels are closely allied to the etiology of coronary disease. This is why LDL cholesterol is the primary target of cholesterol-lowering therapy. Thyroid hormone appears to be necessary for the maintenance of the LDL receptor; in hypothyroidism, LDL levels are elevated because of defective catabolism. Genetic defects in the structure of the LDL receptor or its synthesis and processing cause abnormally high plasma levels of LDL. This disorder is termed *familial hypercholesterolemia* (Type 2a hyperlipidemia) and occurs in either a heterozygous form (1 in 500) or a homozygous form (extremely rare). Heterozygotes of this disorder inherit one defective LDL receptor gene. Consequently, they possess approximately half the number of functioning LDL receptors and double the LDL cholesterol level of unaffected patients. Total cholesterol usually exceeds 300 mg/dL, and LDL cholesterol is more than 200 mg/dL. Premature CHD and a strong family history of hypercholesterolemia are common. Clinically, heterozygous patients may deposit cholesterol in the iris, leading to *arcus senites*. Cholesterol deposits in the tendons, particularly the Achilles tendons and extensor tendons of the hands, lead to tendon xanthomas. Untreated heterozygous patients have approximately a 5% chance of myocardial infarction by age 30, 50% chance by age 50, and 85% chance by age 60. Homozygotes for this disorder inherit a defective LDL receptor gene from both parents and generally have LDL cholesterol >500 mg/dL. This rare disorder results in CHD by age 10–20 years.

Patients with homozygous disorder respond poorly to cholesterol-lowering drugs currently available in the market, such as statins. The standard care for these patients is LDL aphoresis. It is a process of physically removing cholesterol from the blood every 1–2 weeks in a clinic or hospital and is not widely available. The procedure can transiently reduce the total cholesterol levels by more than 80% and may delay the onset of atherosclerosis. The microsomal triglyceride transfer protein (MTP) is responsible for transferring triglycerides onto apolipoprotein (apo) B within the liver in the assembly of VLDL, the precursor of LDL.[4] In the absence of functional MTP, as in the rare recessive genetic disorder abetalipoproteinemia, the liver cannot secrete VLDL leading to the absence of all lipoproteins containing apo B in the plasma. A similar phenotype is observed in MTP knockout mice. Thus, the inhibition of MTP is the therapeutic strategy for reducing LDL production and plasma LDL cholesterol levels. Researchers have developed MTP inhibitor BMS 201038, which has been found in small clinical trials to reduce plasma LDL by 50%, triglycerides by 65%, and apo B levels by 56%. However, the therapy is associated with gastrointestinal and liver side effects. Studies are continuing to determine the long-term effects of small doses of several MTP inhibitors on LDL cholesterol levels.

Familial defective apo B-100 is a genetic disorder clinically indistinguishable from heterogenous familial hypercholesterolemia. These patients have normally functioning LDL receptors but a defective apo B receptor, which results in a reduced binding to LDL receptors. This disorder results in LDL cholesterol levels between 250 and 450 mg/dL. In familial combined hyperlipoproteinemia, both VLDL and LDL are elevated (Type 2b hyperlipidemia). The genetic defect underlying this phenotype is not known, but the secretion of VLDL in most cases is increased about twofold above normal. It occurs in about 15% of CHD patients before 60 years of age.

LDL particles vary in size and density. Small, dense LDL particles called pattern B are more atherogenic than larger and less dense particles (pattern A). This is because the small particles are more easily able to penetrate the endothelium. Most LDL particles have I (I for intermediate) size that is close to normal gaps in the endothelium. People with dense LDL particles frequently have high plasma triglyceride levels and diabetes, and people with lower triglyceride levels have more large, dense LDL particles. It is more expensive to measure the subtypes and facilities are not widely available. So, a common lipid profile is routinely done.

17.2.5 High-Density Lipoprotein

Newly synthesized HDLs are disc-shaped particles containing predominantly unesterified cholesterol, phospholipid, and the major proteins, apo A I and apo A II. Lesser amounts of other proteins (e.g., apo C_S and apo E_S) are also sequestered in HDLs for transfer later to chylomicrons and VLDL. HDLs perform several important functions:

- These particles are excellent acceptors of free cholesterol from extrahepatic tissues, including macrophages, and other circulating lipoproteins via ATP-binding cassette transporter Al. The free cholesterol is then immediately esterified by lecithin cholesterol acyl transferase, a plasma enzyme synthesized by the liver, which is activated by apo AI of HDL. As the cholesteryl esters are synthesized, they begin to form a core of the lipoprotein, forcing it to assume a spherical particle called HDL_3. As HDL_3 acquires new cholesterol, it

is reconstructed into a still larger particle, HDL$_2$. Conversely, HDL$_2$ particles are converted to HDL$_3$ particles by the hydrolysis of triglycerides, through the action of hepatic lipase. The HDL$_2$ levels provide the best estimate of the antiatherogenic effect of HDL.
- They transfer cholesteryl esters to VLDL and LDL in exchange for triglycerides. This transfer is mediated by cholesteryl ester transfer protein (CETP).
- They carry cholesteryl esters to the liver where HDL is degraded by receptor-mediated endocytosis and cholesterol is released.

The process by which HDL promotes the removal of cholesterol from peripheral cells and facilitates its delivery back to the liver for excretion is referred to as reverse cholesterol transport. Men tend to have lower serum HDL levels with and lower cholesterol content than women. Men also have increased incidence of CHD. Epidemiologic studies have shown that high concentrations of HDL cholesterol (over 60 mg/dL) have protective value against cardiovascular diseases such as myocardial infarction and stroke. This is the reason why HDL-bound cholesterol sometimes is called "good cholesterol." Low concentrations of HDL cholesterol (below 40 mg/dL in men, below 50 mg/dL in women) increase the risk for atherosclerotic disease.

Plasma levels of HDL above the average do not produce untoward clinical manifestations and are associated with below-average risk of atherosclerosis. Those with high HDL cholesterol levels are also less likely to have dementia. Low levels are associated with a sharply increased risk of atherosclerosis but do not appear to produce other clinical manifestations. In the genetic disorder termed *familial hypoalphalipoproteinemia*, there is a deficiency of HDL and its apoprotein apo AI and the disorder is associated with an increased risk of coronary disease. In a very rare disorder, Tangier disease, HDL levels are almost undetectable. These patients may have neuropathies and enlarged orange-pigmented tonsils.

17.2.6 LIPOPROTEIN (A)

Several other minor lipoproteins that are important in normal or disease states exist. Of these, lipoprotein (a) [Lp (a)] has received attention recently because of its positive relationship with CHD. Lp (a) is identical in structure to LDL but has an additional protein called apo (a) that is covalently linked to apo B-100. About 80% of the amino acids in apo (a) are the same as those of plasminogen, the precursor of plasmin, whose target is fibrin. It is capable of occupying the binding sites for plasminogen on the endothelium and on the fibrin, interfering with fibrinolysis. Elevated plasma levels of Lp (a) have been suggested to increase the risk of CHD by the deposition of lipids in the arterial wall and the inhibition of fibrinolysis.

17.3 PLASMA CHOLESTEROL AND RISK OF HEART DISEASE

There is a general agreement that a high plasma cholesterol level is one of the major risk factors for CHD. Evidence relating cholesterol to an increased risk of atherosclerosis and CHD is derived from many different types of study.[12,14,17,24] One important factor is that in arterial disease, there are blockages that form in the arteries known as plaques, which are growths or masses of chemical products deposited in the walls of the artery. Biochemical analysis of the plaque material shows that it contains large amounts of lipids, a big portion of which is cholesterol.

Hypercholesterolemia induced in a wide variety of experimental animals, including nonhuman primates, produces atherosclerosis and occasional cases of myocardial infarction. Individuals with a low blood cholesterol level have a low risk of CHD, while those with high blood cholesterol levels are at high risk. When populations that have a lower incidence of CHD than Americans migrate to the United States, their blood cholesterol level and risk of CHD approach that of the host country. Studies that involve the lowering of blood cholesterol by drugs or diet therapy have been shown to reduce the frequency of atherosclerotic lesions in men who have previously had heart disease. Clinical and epidemiological evidence links elevated blood cholesterol level to coronary artery disease (CAD). The relationship is sharpened when LDL and HDL cholesterol levels are also compared. The LDL cholesterol is directly related to the risk of CAD. An inverse relationship exists between HDL and vascular disease, with the HDL_2 subtraction being more highly correlated than the total HDL cholesterol. Species with most of their blood cholesterol carried as HDL (such as rats and dogs) do not normally develop coronary disease. Victims of heart attack have lower levels of HDL than healthy people. In the Framingham study, the risk for men in the lowest quintile (HDL cholesterol <35 mg/dL) is more than four times as great as for those in the highest quintile (>54 mg/dL). A steep inverse dependence of risk is also observed among women, with those in the uppermost quintile (HDL >69 mg/dL) having less than 33% of the risk of those in the lowest quintile (HDL <45 mg/dL).

These observations on cardiovascular disease incidence have now been demonstrated in postmortem studies by the use of coronary angiography, which shows that the degree of coronary atherosclerosis and the increased risk for cardiovascular events—both at younger and older ages—are linked to HDL and LDL concentrations. Thus, it is important to measure the total plasma cholesterol and the two major risk variables, LDL and HDL cholesterol, in order to define the risks of a specific individual or group.

The optimal level of cholesterol in the blood is a disputed subject, but most authorities consider that the lower the level, the less risk of premature CHD. Blood cholesterol level may be 3%–5% higher in winter than in summer, and there is a weak inverse relationship between birth weight and blood cholesterol level. According to the National Cholesterol Education Program Adult Treatment Guidelines, a total blood cholesterol level of less than 200 mg/dL is desirable, whereas a level of greater than 240 mg/dL is high. For a whole population, the risk of CHD at a blood cholesterol level of 240 mg/dL is almost twice that at 200 mg/dL. To prevent early CHD, all the other risk factors that can be controlled should also be considered. For example, a plasma cholesterol of 200 mg/dL in a smoker can be equivalent to 275 mg/dL in a nonsmoker as far as the risk of CHD is concerned. Thus, for the prevention of heart disease, elimination of smoking, treatment of hypertension, diabetes, and so on, as well as lowering of cholesterol levels should be done simultaneously. Normal levels of LDL cholesterol or "bad cholesterol" should be under 130 mg/dL; optimal is 100–129 mg/dL, borderline high is 130–159 mg/dL, and very high is 190 mg/dL and above.

The risk of CHD is further refined by a ratio developed from epidemiological data, which is determined by comparing the total plasma cholesterol value with the HDL cholesterol concentration. This ratio relates the atherogenic aspect of total cholesterol to the reportedly antiatherogenic aspect of HDL cholesterol. The ratio averages 5.8 in men with CAD and 5.1 or less in those without disease. This suggests that decreasing the total plasma cholesterol and increasing the HDL cholesterol may prevent or delay arterial disease. The average ratio would be about 4.5. Ideally, we want to be better than average if we can. Thus, it is better to keep the ratio below 3.5.

As HDL has become important as an index to risk, what can be done to change its level in blood? There are several factors that are found to affect plasma HDL levels. Male sex hormone, progesterone-containing oral contraceptives, obesity, diets very high in carbohydrates, uncontrolled diabetes, hypertriglyceridemia, and cigarette smoking are associated with reduced levels of plasma HDL cholesterol. Estrogen tends to increase the HDL level. Exercise is known to have a beneficial effect on HDL cholesterol. Alcohol consumption also causes an increase in HDL fraction. It has been suggested that by drinking three 12-ounce cans of beer a day, nonexercisers can maintain HDL levels similar to those of persons who jog regularly; however, alcohol may adversely affect blood pressure and has other adverse consequences.

17.4   THE NATIONAL CHOLESTEROL EDUCATION PROGRAM

The National Cholesterol Education Program (NCEP) was officially launched by the National Heart, Lung, and Blood Institute in 1985 after the lowering of high serum cholesterol levels was shown to reduce the risk of nonfatal myocardial infarctions and coronary heart disease (CHD) deaths in the Lipid Research Clinic's Coronary Primary Prevention Trial. In 1988, the Expert Panel on Detection, Evaluation and Treatment of High Blood Cholesterol in Adults (Adult Treatment Panel [ATP]) released guidelines for cholesterol evaluation and treatment in adults; in 1993, revised guidelines (ATP II) were released. In 1991, the Expert Panel on Blood Cholesterol Levels in Children and Adolescents released guidelines for primary prevention in this population group and for detecting and treating children and adolescents from high-risk families.

The Third Report of the Adult Treatment Panel (ATP III) published in 2001 gives evidence-based guidelines for cholesterol management. The NCEP has updated recommendations in 2004 and calls for extensive cholesterol treatment, especially in patients at high risk of CHD. The message from the updated report is that lower cholesterol levels are better for high risk patients. It is calling for LDL cholesterol treatment targets of <100 mg/dL and further lowering to <70 mg/dL in very high-risk patients as a therapeutic option for clinicians. ATP III recognizes the metabolic syndrome (MS) as a secondary target of therapy after LDL cholesterol, the primary target, has been addressed. MS is diagnosed when three or more of its five determinants are present; it is described in Chapter 19 on diabetes.

If these guidelines are fully adhered to, 11.1 million U.S. adults would either need to start or intensify their current statin treatment. It is predicted that this would prevent around 20,000 myocardial infarctions and 10,000 coronary disease–related deaths per year and at a cost of about $3.6 billion.

17.5   PLASMA TRIGLYCERIDES AND RISK OF HEART DISEASE

Triglycerides are derived from two sources: the diet and the liver, which incorporates these molecules in the core of VLDL for secretions into the bloodstream. Triglycerides have not been traditionally considered the cornerstone of lipid risk factors for CHD. Yet, emerging evidence from epidemiological, clinical, genetic, and molecular studies suggests otherwise, namely that triglycerides and triglyceride-rich lipoproteins such as VLDL are indeed independent risk factors of CHD.[1,27] The relationship is stronger and more consistent in women and in the elderly. When other lipid abnormalities such as increased LDL cholesterol or low HDL cholesterol are included in the multivariant analysis, triglycerides sometimes lose their independent predictive power. Patients with high serum triglyceride levels almost always have a low serum HDL cholesterol, which also predicts CHD risk.

A serum triglyceride concentration of more than 200 mg/dL is considered somewhat elevated and a concentration of more than 400 mg/dL is considered high according to the NCEP guidelines. A reasonable target is a triglyceride concentration of 200 mg/dL or less, preferably near 150 mg/dL, because higher values are associated with an increased risk for CHD when serum total cholesterol exceeds 240 mg/dL and the ratio of serum LDL cholesterol to HDL cholesterol exceeds 5.1. Reasonable targets for HDL cholesterol concentrations are 45 mg/dL in men and 55 mg/dL in women.

Overweight and obesity, physical inactivity, smoking, excessive alcohol intake, and a high-carbohydrate diet can elevate serum triglyceride levels in the range of 200–300 mg/dL. Triglycerides in this range may add to the CHD risk of individuals with elevated serum LDL cholesterol. Serum triglycerides in the high range, 400–500 mg/dL, may signal an increased CHD risk. The causes generally include genetic factors, as well as lifestyle habits. Quite often, individuals who have triglycerides in this range have other risk factors, including low HDL, elevated LDL, obesity, and diabetes. When triglycerides are higher than 500 mg/dL, there is usually a genetic defect in LPL. With triglyceride levels >1000 mg/dL, the patient is at risk of pancreatitis. Patients who develop CHD most often have atherogenic triglyceride-rich lipoproteins.

17.6   DIETARY MANAGEMENT

To treat hyperlipidemia, dietary measures are always initiated first and may obviate the need for drugs. The primary objective of dietary management is to reduce elevated levels of plasma cholesterol including LDL fraction. At least three factors appear to be responsible for altering plasma cholesterol level. These include dietary cholesterol, fat, and calories. Dietary cholesterol induces hypercholes-terolemia possibly by suppressing hepatic LDL receptors. Metabolic ward studies generally show a positive association between dietary cholesterol and blood cholesterol levels. The average intake of cholesterol in the U.S. diet is about 400 mg/day. It has been estimated that an increase in cholesterol intake from 250 to 500 mg/day can raise plasma cholesterol levels by an average of 10 mg/dL, although there may be variability between individuals. Some may show appreciable increases in plasma cholesterol while others may show little or no increase when dietary cholesterol is raised. Several health professional organizations recommend that cholesterol intake be reduced to less than 300 mg/day.

The quantity and the quality of dietary fats are also important. Various types of investigations have demonstrated that a low-fat diet reduces blood cholesterol levels and that the hypocholes-terolemic effect is related more to the amount of saturated fatty acids relative to polyunsaturated and monounsaturated fatty acids. Like cholesterol, saturated fatty acids increase LDL levels by suppressing the liver LDL receptors; however, all saturated fatty acids are not alike in their effect on plasma cholesterol. Stearic acid appears to be neutral or much less hypercholesterolemic than lauric, myristic, and palmitic acids. The estimated saturated fatty acid intake in the United States is 20–60 g/day. The ingestion of 10 g/day saturated fatty acid for several weeks raises total and LDL cholesterol levels by 8–10 mg/dL. Most of these increases occur entirely at the plasma LDL level. The plasma VLDL and HDL levels do not change. Polyunsaturated fatty acids (PUFAs) of either the ω_6 (linoleic acid) or ω_3 (α-linolenic acid) family tend to lower plasma cholesterol levels including the LDL fraction, possibly by increasing the activity of LDL receptors. Many epidemiologic and controlled interventional studies have shown the antiatherogenic effect of both α-linolenic acid and its long-chain fatty acids. ω_3 fatty acids have unique triglyceride lowering properties, not shared by ω_6 fatty acids. PUFAs, although effective in lowering both total and LDL cholesterol, have a tendency to lower HDL cholesterol, which is protective against CHD. These fatty acids are also very liable to peroxidation and thus increase the requirements for anti-oxidants. The intake of ω_6 PUFA in the United States is in the range of 10–30 g/day, and for ω_3 it is 0–5 g/day. Monounsaturated fatty acids were once thought to be neutral with regard to their effect on plasma cholesterol. More recent studies have shown that oleic acid, when substituted for saturated fatty acids, decreases plasma cholesterol level. Therefore, the present recommendation is to decrease saturated fatty acids and increase the intake of monounsaturated fatty acids. Such a diet has been consumed in the Mediterranean region where the concentration of plasma choles-terol and the rates of CHD are low. The estimated monounsaturated fatty acid intake in the United States is 20–50 g/day. *Trans* fatty acids are produced by bacterial action in ruminant animals (cattle, sheep) and when vegetable oils are hydrogenated. They make up about 6% of the total fatty acid intake in the U.S. diet, or in the range of 6–8 g/day. Ingestion of 8 g of *trans* fatty acid daily can raise total and LDL cholesterol levels by 5–7 mg/dL.

Excess energy intake accompanied by obesity causes an overproduction of VLDL, which can raise plasma LDL and total cholesterol. The Framingham study has estimated that for every 10 pounds of body weight gain, total cholesterol level increases by 7 mg/dL in men and 5 mg/dL in women. Obesity is also associated with lower HDL cholesterol. Whether these changes in plasma cholesterol and lipoprotein levels are due to an excess energy intake per se, or to an increase in total fat or saturated fat is unknown. Body weight loss is found to lower both LDL and total cholesterol and to increase HDL. The addition of exercise to the weight loss program enhances the increase in HDL cholesterol. Weight loss is considered to be an effective means of lowering plasma cholesterol in obese individuals. Therefore, the recommendation to decrease the intake of saturated fatty acids and cholesterol and to maintain ideal body weight seems to be justified.[7,8] Among other factors, dietary fiber, especially the water-soluble type (e.g., oat bran, pectin, guar gum), is found to have a hypocholesterolemic effect. Some fiber components bind bile salts, which are then excreted in the stool. The reduction in bile salts in the enterohepatic circulation causes the liver to increase the conversion of cholesterol to bile acids to maintain a normal bile acid pool (see Figure 17.2). This results in a reduction of plasma cholesterol. The total dietary fiber intake in the United States is in the range of 5–20 g/day. A daily intake of 2 ounces of oat bran (11 g total fiber; 6 g soluble fiber) can lower total and LDL cholesterol levels by about 5 mg/dL. Among other factors, dietary fiber, especially the water soluble and viscous type (e.g. oats, pectin, guar gum, barley, eggplant, okra), is found to have a hypocholesterolemic effect.

Recently, plant stanol and sterol esters have been made available in margarine. One of the products is Benecol spread. These products, when ingested two to three times a day, lower total and LDL cholesterol by 6%–15% by reducing the absorption of cholesterol in the intestine. The use of 25–40 g/day of soy protein can lower LDL cholesterol levels by an additional 5%. The oxidative modification of LDL is important and possibly obligatory in the formation of atherosclerotic plaques. Therefore, inhibiting the oxidation of LDL by the intake of antioxidant-rich foods may decrease or prevent atherosclerosis. An adequate amount of dietary fiber, as well as antioxidants, can be obtained by the consumption of fruits, vegetables, cereals, grain, and legumes.

Nuts (almonds, peanuts, pecans, walnuts) have hypolipidemic effects. Consumption of nuts (5 servings/week) is found to reduce the risk of CHD incidence by about 35%. Nuts are rich in fiber as well as plant sterols. Recent studies have found that individuals who follow a low-fat vegetarian diet, along with a moderate exercise plan and stress management, improve the functions of their endothelium, the key to preventing heart attacks.[16,25]

Although diet, smoking, and other factors contribute to the risk of CHD—the leading cause of death in the Western world—air pollution may play a role too. Recently, studies conducted on human cells as well as on mice have shown that microscopic particles in diesel exhaust combine with cholesterol to activate genes that trigger hardening of the arteries. People with high cholesterol may be especially vulnerable to heart disease when they are exposed to diesel exhaust and other ultrafine particles that are common pollutants in urban air. These studies emphasize the importance of controlling air pollution as another tool for preventing CHD.

17.7   DRUG THERAPY

Treatment with drugs is generally initiated when a diet that is low in cholesterol, fat, and saturated fat is not able to lower plasma cholesterol and triglycerides to satisfactory levels. The commonly used drugs include bile acid–sequestering agents, nicotinic acid, fibric acid derivatives, and HMG-CoA reductase inhibitors. Cholestyramine and colestipol are bile acid–binding resins. Taken orally, they are not absorbed from the gastrointestinal tract but bind bile acids in the intestinal lumen and increase their excretion along with sterols in the stools. The decrease in the level of bile acids in the enterohepatic circulation causes a compensatory increase in the conversion of cholesterol to bile acids by the liver. This in turn depletes the cellular pool of cholesterol and increases the hepatic LDL receptor activity and receptor-mediated catabolism. Low-density lipoprotein cholesterol is reduced approximately by 15% with 5 g/day of colestipol (equivalent to 4 g of cholestyramine), by 23% with 10 g/day, and by 27% with 15 g/day.

The vitamin nicotinic acid, when used in pharmacological doses, decreases the hepatic synthesis of VLDL and LDL and increases the level of plasma HDL. This action of nicotinic acid is not shared by nicotinamide. One predictable side effect of nicotinic acid that occurs consistently during the initiation of therapy is cutaneous flushing, but the duration and intensity diminish with prolonged therapy and can be minimized by starting with low doses and by taking the medicine with food. The primary action of niacin is to inhibit the mobilization of free fatty acids from peripheral tissues, thereby reducing the hepatic synthesis of triglycerides and the secretion of VLDL. It lowers serum triglycerides by 30%–60% and total and LDL cholesterol by 15%–20%. The ability of niacin to increase HDL cholesterol concentration by up to 30% at the maximum dose exceeds that of all other drugs.

Akira Endo and his group started research on inhibitors of HMG-CoA reductase. This team reasoned that certain microorganisms may produce an inhibitor of this enzyme to defend themselves against other organisms—as mevalonate is a precursor of many substances required by organisms for the maintenance of their cell walls or cytoskeleton. In 1973, they isolated the first agent mevastatin produced by the fungus (*Penicillium citrinum*). Endo's two interests—fungi and cholesterol—spurred the discovery and the development of cholesterol-lowering drugs called statins. Of the handful of drugs that have fought cardiovascular diseases, statins are right at the top of the list. Endo received the 2006 Japanese prize for his work on the development of statins and the Clinical Medical Research Award from the Lasker Foundation in 2008. More than 25 million people worldwide take statins to lower cholesterol, creating an over $20 billion market in the process.

The fungal-derived compounds lovastatin (mevinolin), mevastatin (compactin), and their chemically modified versions provastatin, simvastatin, and others are extremely effective in lowering the plasma concentration of LDL. These drugs reduce the conversion of HMG-CoA to mevalonic acid (see Figure 17.1) and the synthesis of cholesterol in the liver. This leads to a compensatory increase in the number of LDL receptors and in LDL catabolism.

These agents separately reduce total and LDL cholesterol concentrations by 20%–40%. For patients with a very high concentration of LDL, combined therapies with drugs exhibiting such mechanisms of action are the most effective. The potential benefits of statins may extend well beyond their ability to lower cholesterol. They reduce the level of C-reactive protein (CRP), a marker for inflammation of blood vessels. Elevated levels of CRP have been associated with increased risk of heart attack. They have antioxidant properties. They have shown promise in combating a number of other ailments. They may be effective against Alzheimer's disease by reducing amyloid plaques in the brain. They may limit the progression of multiple sclerosis by blocking the immune response that damages nerve tissue. Studies have shown that statins increase bone formation in rodents. If these benefits hold up in humans, statins may prove to be useful in the treatment of osteoporosis. Statins may reduce the risk of age-related macular degeneration and other eye conditions.[11] These diseases are thought to be associated with problems in circulation in the eye.

The statin drugs could also reduce the risk of type 2 diabetes, according to recently published data from the 5-year West of Scotland Coronary Prevention Study. In this study,[10] data from 5974 men, aged 45–64 years, were analyzed to assess the risk of diabetes. About 2.6% of these men developed the disease, and there was a 30% risk reduction for diabetes among provastatin users. If this effect is due to cholesterol and triglyceride reduction, then all statins may be expected to share this effect. If, however, it is more related to some specific property of provastatin, it may be a unique attribute of this drug. The anti-inflammatory properties of provastatin could play an important part.

Fibric acid derivatives and other related compounds lower triglyceride levels by 20%–50% and raise HDL cholesterol by 10%–15%. The mechanism by which fibric acid derivatives exert their effects is not completely understood. Fibrates increase the activity of LPL in capillaries, thus reducing the triglyceride levels by increasing VLDL and IDL catabolism. Patients with severe triglyceridemia are best treated with diet and/or fibrate, alone or in combination with niacin.

17.8   RECENT STUDIES ON HDL

The quest for new drugs to increase HDL levels efficiently has been a major driver of HDL research. A small group of people in an island in northern Japan have very high HDL, often exceeding 100 mg/dL. They are also deficient in CETP. This discovery in 1990 led investigators to develop inhibitors of CETP.[2] Studies found that blocking the action of CETP raises HDL levels as much as 66%. However, clinical trials of torcetrapib, a drug developed by Pfizer, failed to reduce deaths and had other adverse effects. Most CETP inhibitors increase HDL and some appear to show benefits. Researchers are pursuing other drugs in the same class as torcetrapib.

In a small northern village in Italy, there are people with dangerously low average HDL (7 mg/dL) and average triglycerides of 319 mg/dL. Despite these values, the arteries of people in the island are clear. Further work has revealed that the people have a mutation in HDL's protein apo A1. The mutant version is dubbed apo A1 Milano. The villagers are linked to common ancestors (a couple) who had lived there in the 1700s and passed the gene on to their offspring, and they live a longer, healthier life as a result.

Because the Milano variant may be especially good, a biotech firm developed a way to synthesize the protein and put it into artificial HDL. In a small study, researchers gave 57 heart patients infusions of synthetic HDL or saline. They then used an ultrasound probe to measure the effect on their arterial plaques. In about a month, the volume of plaque shrank an average of about 4% in those receiving apo A1 Milano, compared with only a slight increase in those who got the placebo. Unfortunately, there are practical obstacles. Making the Milano version is tedious, and the treatment is costly and inconvenient, requiring weekly intravenous infusion instead of a daily pill. Researchers are pursuing other strategies.

17.9   HYPOCHOLESTEROLEMIA

A low total cholesterol concentration of <100 mg/dL in an adult can be due to rare hereditary traits or secondary to a number of diseases. Mutations in the gene for apo B-100 that disrupt synthesis or produce truncated forms of apo B-100 are associated with hypocholesterolemia. These mutations are inherited as codominant traits. Heterozygotes have plasma levels in the range of 50–100 mg/dL with reduced LDL, but normal HDL, and are asymptomatic. Homozygotes have even lower total and LDL cholesterol concentration and may have a malabsorption of fat and fat-soluble vitamins.

Patients with hypobetalipoproteinemia have mutations in one or both apo B alleles that lead to truncated apo B proteins. Because of defective synthesis, there are markedly reduced levels of apo B–containing lipoproteins in plasma. Heterozygotes may have LDL cholesterol levels less than 50 mg/dL. Usually these patients are asymptomatic. Patients with the rare autosomal recessive disorder of abetalipoproteinemia have a total inability to release apo B-48 from intestinal cells or apo B-100 from the liver. They have a normal apo B but lack a microsomal triglyceride transfer protein gene, which is required for the assembly of lipoproteins. Because they cannot make chylomicrons, they may have a malabsorption of fat and fat-soluble vitamins. Vitamin E deficiency in infancy and early childhood can result in neurological problems. If vitamin replacement is adequate, individuals with abetalipoproteinemia can live a normal life.

A number of systemic diseases can lower serum cholesterol concentration. Malnutrition, often associated with alcoholism or gastrointestinal disease, can cause low levels of total and LDL cholesterol.

17.10   EFFECTS OF LOW BLOOD CHOLESTEROL

Low blood levels of cholesterol seem to correlate with a modest increase in cancer risk in some studies. Whether low blood cholesterol is an independent risk factor or a result of cancer is not known.[5] Lowering blood cholesterol concentration is also associated with increased deaths due to violence,[9] accidents, trauma, and suicide. Low brain serotonin is suggested as a possible factor in the association of blood cholesterol, with personality characteristics predisposing to aggression and suicidal behavior.

It is important to stress that the association between high blood cholesterol and heart disease appears to be far greater than the possible relation of low cholesterol levels to cancer and behavioral changes. Therefore, patients with blood cholesterol levels higher than 240 mg/dL should attempt to lower cholesterol, but if the blood levels are less than 200 mg/dL, it may be wise to avoid further reduction until the matter of unusually low cholesterol level and its relationship to cancer and behavioral changes is further clarified.

17.11   ALTERNATIVE MEDICINE TO LOWER CHOLESTEROL

A number of foods and food components have been found to reduce cholesterol. Foods containing viscous fiber, ω_3 fatty acids, and nuts are mentioned earlier. Policosanol, berberine, and plant sterols are described below.

17.11.1 POLICOSANOL

Policosanol is a mixture of alcohols made from plants, most often the sugarcane. It is sold in the United States as a dietary supplement under dozens of brand names. It is also an ingredient in Bayer AG's One-A-Day Cholesterol Plus Multivitamin, which claims to help "maintain healthy cholesterol." Several Cuban studies show policosanol 10 mg/day taken for 3 months lowers cholesterol by about 24%. However, two recent studies from South Africa and Germany raise doubt about the efficacy of policosanol.

17.11.2 BERBERINE

Berberine is a plant alkaloid with a long history of medicinal use in both Ayurvedic and Chinese medicines. It has a bright yellow color that is easily seen in most of the herb materials that contain significant amounts of this compound. Berberine structure is presented in Figure 17.3. It can be found in the roots, rhizomes, stem, and bark of the plants. Among Chinese herbs, the primary sources are *phellodendron* and *coptis* (goldthread). It has long been used as a dye. It is currently known as "natural yellow 18," being one of about 35 yellow dyes from natural sources.

Berberine extracts have demonstrated significant antimicrobial activity against a variety of organisms. The predominant clinical uses of berberine include bacterial diarrhea, intestinal parasite infections, and ocular trachoma. It is also known for its immune-enhancing properties and has been used as a treatment for diabetes. In recent years, it has become an ingredient in several Western herbal products for treatment of gastrointestinal disorders. It has been found to reduce high blood pressure at doses of 1 g/day.

It has recently been reported that berberine lowers cholesterol through a mechanism different than that of the statin drugs, suggesting potential use both as an alternative to the statins and as a complementary therapy that might be used with statins in an attempt to gain better control over cholesterol.[19]

In a controlled Chinese study, it was shown that berberine administered twice a day in 500 mg dose for 3 months reduced total blood cholesterol levels by 18%, LDL cholesterol by 20%, and triglycerides by 28%, while there was no change in people using placebo. The effect of berberine was even more pronounced in people who were not taking any other cholesterol-lowering treatment: a 29% drop in total cholesterol levels, a 25% drop in LDL-cholesterol levels, and a 35% drop in triglycerides.

Berberine increases the activity of ERK, with the end result that more receptors of LDL are formed on the surface of liver cells without adverse side effects typical of statins.

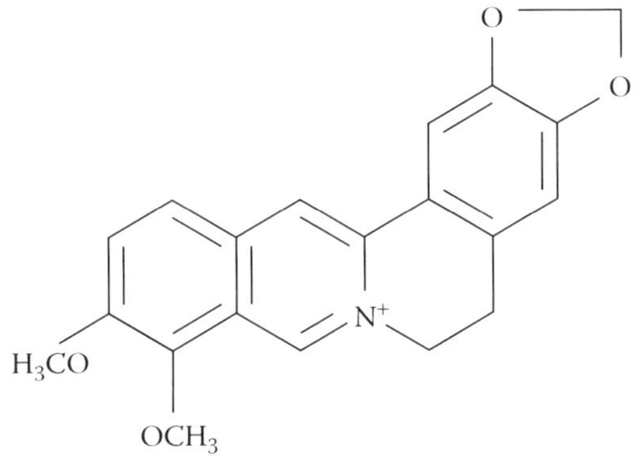

FIGURE 17.3 Chemical structure of berberine.

17.11.3 PHYTOSTEROLS

Phytosterols are plant sterols structurally similar to cholesterol. There are two types: sterols that have a double bond in the sterol ring and stanols that lack a double bond in the sterol ring. The most abundant sterols in plants and in the human diet are sitosterol and campesterol. Stanols comprise only about 10% of total dietary phytosterols.

Like cholesterol, phytosterols must be incorporated into mixed micelles before they are taken up by the enterocytes. Once inside the enterocytes, absorption of phytosterol is inhibited by the activity of efflux transporters consisting of a pair of ATP-binding cassette (ABC) proteins known as ABCG5 and ABCG8. Each of these form one half of the transporter that secretes phytosterol and unesterified cholesterol from the enterocyte into the intestinal lumen. Phytosterols are secreted back into the intestine by these transporters at a much greater rate than cholesterol, resulting in lower intestinal absorption of dietary phytosterols than cholesterol. Within the intestine, phytosterols are not as readily esterified as cholesterol, so they are incorporated into chylomicrons at a much lower concentration. Phytosterols incorporated into chylomicrons enter the circulation and are taken up by the liver where they are rapidly secreted into bile by hepatic ABCG5/G8 transporters. Phytosterol secretion into bile is much greater than cholesterol secretion. Thus, the lower blood concentration of phytosterol relative to cholesterol can be explained by decreased intestinal absorption and increased secretion into bile. In the intestinal lumen, phytosterol displaces cholesterol from mixed micelles and inhibits cholesterol absorption.

In humans, the consumption of 1.5–1.8 g/day of plant sterols or stanols reduces cholesterol absorption by 30%–40%. At higher doses (2.2 g/day) of phytosterol consumption, cholesterol absorption is reduced by 60%. In response to decreased cholesterol absorption, LDL receptor expression is increased resulting in increased clearance of circulating LDL cholesterol.[22]

Foods rich in phytosterols include wheat germ, rice bran, crude vegetable oils, and avocado. Two new margarines, Benecol spread (856 mg/tablespoon) and Take Control (1000 mg/tablespoon), and other products with added plant sterols and stanols are available in many countries around the world. Some countries allow health claims for such products. For information on the nutrient content of specific foods search the USDA Food Composition Database.

Numerous clinical trials have found that daily consumption of foods enriched with phytosterols or stanols lowers plasma cholesterol.[22] The NCEP Adult Treatment Panel III has included the use of 2 g/day of plant sterol or stanol esters as a component of maximal dietary therapy for elevated LDL cholesterol. Some studies have shown that dietary phytosterols can lower β carotene in blood but not fat-soluble vitamins. The effect of long-term use of foods enriched with plant sterols on CHD risk is not known. Children and pregnant and lactating women should not take supplements enriched with phytosterols.

Sitosterolemia is a rare hereditary disease that results from inheriting a mutation in both copies of the ABCG5 and ABCG8 genes.[20] Individuals who are homozygous for a mutation in either transporter proteins have dramatically elevated serum phytosterol concentration due to increased intestinal absorption and decreased biliary secretion of phytosterols. Although serum cholesterol concentration may be normal or only mildly elevated, individuals with sitosterolemia are at high risk for premature atherosclerosis. People with sitosterolemia should avoid foods or supplements with added plant sterols.

17.12 INBORN ERRORS OF CHOLESTEROL BIOSYNTHESIS

17.12.1 SMITH–LEMLI–OPITZ SYNDROME

Smith–Lemli–Opitz syndrome (SLOS) is an inherited disorder marked by the body's inability to make its own cholesterol. The abnormality is harmful even during the first few months after conception, for cholesterol is critical to the formation of basic biological structures, including the brain. As a consequence, SLOS babies may be born with a variety of serious birth defects, including cleft palate, heart defects, mental retardation, inhibited growth, and general malformations. SLOS, also known as RHS syndrome, affects an estimated 1 in 20,000 children and is believed to be the second most common autosomal recessive disorder, after cystic fibrosis. In SLOS, a defect in cholesterol synthesis is the culprit. The defect is in the enzyme delta-7-sterol reductase, which is needed to convert 7-dehydrocholesterol (7DHC) into cholesterol.[29] The 7DHC accumulates in certain sites of the body such as the eyes, where the buildup can lead to cataract formation. Cholesterol therapy appears to offer many benefits, including enhanced physical growth, to SLOS patients.

Mevalonic Aciduria—A Case

A 2-year-old boy was admitted to a hospital because of failure to thrive, mental retardation, and cataracts. He weighed 8.8 pounds. The child was delivered 4 weeks prematurely with a birth weight of 4.4 pounds. This was his mother's fourth pregnancy, and she had lost 20 pounds in the first trimester of this pregnancy. During the neonatal period, the infant had episodes of acidosis associated with diarrhea and fever. Laboratory investigation showed, among other parameters, iron deficiency anemia, hemoglobin of 8 g/dL (normal: 11–14 g/dL), hematocrit of 28 mL/dL (normal: 32–45 mL/dL), and cholesterol of 75 mg/dL. Mevalonic acid was identified in the blood and the patient excreted about 9 g of this metabolite in the urine per day. A deficiency of mevalonate kinase was demonstrated in the patient's fibroblasts. The patient died a few months later. In a subsequent pregnancy of his mother (her fifth pregnancy), the concentration of mevalonic acid in amniotic fluid was found to be elevated and a therapeutic abortion was performed at 19 weeks.

Mevalonic aciduria is an inherited disorder of cholesterol biosynthesis and the molecular defect in the above-described case is in the activity of the enzyme mevalonate kinase.[31] The overproduction of mevalonate in this patient is due to the removal of feedback inhibition by cholesterol of HMG-CoA reductase, which is the rate-limiting enzyme of cholesterol biosynthesis. The excretion of about 9 g of mevalonic acid each day represents a sizable loss of nutrients and is consistent with the observed failure to thrive. The pathway that leads to the formation of cholesterol from mevalonic acid is important not only to cholesterol biosynthesis but also for the formation of at least four additional isoprenoid compounds (Figure 17.1).[15] These are ubiquinone (present in the mitochondria as an electron transporter), heme A (present in cytochrome oxidase in the mitochondria), dolichol (a membrane lipid involved in glycoprotein synthesis), and isopentenyl adenine (found in transfer RNA). Cholesterol and isoprenoid compounds become essential nutrients for patients with a defect in mevalonate kinase.

REFERENCES

1. Anonymous. 2001. Cholesterol and triglycerides. Numbers to count on. *Mayo Clin Health Lett* 19(7):1–3.
2. Brousseau, M. E., E. J. Schaeffer, M. L. Wolfe et al. 2004. Effects of an inhibitor of cholesteryl ester transfer protein on HDL cholesterol. *New Engl J Med* 150:1505.
3. Cook, R. P., ed. 1958. *Cholesterol, Chemistry, Biochemistry, and Pathology*. New York: Academic Press.
4. Cuchel, M., L. T. Bloedon, P. O. Szapary et al. 2007. Inhibition of microsomal triglyceride transfer protein in familial hypercholesterolemia. *New Engl J Med* 356:148.
5. Dalen, J. E., and W. S. Dalton. 1996. Does lowering cholesterol cause cancer? *J Am Med Assoc* 275:67.
6. Dandapany, P. S., S. Sadayappan, Y. Xue et al. 2009. A common MYBPC3 (cardiac myosin-binding protein C) variant associated with cardiomyopathies in South Asia. *Nat Genet* 41:187.
7. Denke, M. A. 1994. Diet and lifestyle modification and its relationship to atherosclerosis. *Med Clin North Am* 78:197.
8. Dod, H. S., R. Bhardwaj, V. Sajja et al. 2010. Effect of intensive lifestyle changes on endothelia function on inflammatory markers of atherosclerosis. *Amer J Cardiol* 105:362.

9. Fowkes, F. G. R., G. C. Leng, P. T. Donnan et al. 1992. Serum cholesterol, triglycerides, and aggression in the general population. *Lancet* 340:995.

10. Freeman, D. J., J. Norrie, N. Sattar et al. 2001. Provastatin and the development of diabetes mellitus. Evidence for a protective treatment effect in the West of Scotland Coronary Prevention Study. *Circulation* 103:357.

11. Gehibach, P., T. Li, and E. Hataf. 2009. Statins for age-related macular degeneration. *Cochrane Database Syst Rev* (3):Art No. CD006927. Doi 1002/14651858.

12. Ginsberg, H. N. 1994. Lipoprotein metabolism and its relationship to atherosclerosis. *Med Clin North Am* 78:1.

13. Golomb, B. A., and M. A. Evans. 2008. Statin adverse effects: A review of the literature and evidence for a mitochondrial mechanism. *Amer J Cardiovas Drugs* 8:373.

14. Grundy, S. M. 1994. Disorders of lipids and lipoproteins. In *Internal Medicine*, ed. J. H. Stein, 1436–1456. St. Louis, MO: Mosby.

15. Haas, D., and G. F. Hoffmann. 2007. Mevalonate kinase deficiency and autoimmune disorders. *New Engl J Med* 356:2671.

16. Halliwell, B. 1995. Oxidation of low-density lipoproteins: Questions of initiation, propagation, and the effect of antioxidants. *Am J Clin Nutr Suppl* 61(suppl.):670s.

17. Kane, J. P., and R. J. Havel. 2001. Disorders of the biogenesis and secretion of lipoproteins containing B apoproteins. In *Metabolic and Molecular Basis of Inherited Disease*, Chap. 115, 8th ed., ed. C. R. Scriver, A. L. Beaudet, W. SI Sly, and D. Valle, 2717–2752. New York: McGraw-Hill.

18. Knoop, R. H. 1999. Drug treatment of lipid disorders. *N Engl J Med* 341:498.

19. Kong, W., J. Wei, P. Abidi et al. 2004. Berberine is a novel cholesterol-lowering drug working through a unique mechanism distinct from statins. *Nat Med* 10:1344.

20. Lee, M., K. Lu, and S. B. Patel. 2001. Genetic basis of sitosterolemia. *Curr Opin Lipidol* 12:141.

21. Mauch, D. H., K. Nagler, S. Schumacher et al. 2001. CNS synaptogenesis promoted by glia-derived cholesterol. *Science* 294:1354.

22. Mauch, W. H., K. Nagler, S. Schumacher et al. 2005. Plant stanol and sterol esters in the control of blood cholesterol levels: Mechanism and safety aspects: *Amer J Cardiol* 96(suppl 1):15.

23. Saji, J., A. V. Sorokin, and P. D. Thompson. 2007. Phytosterols and vascular disease. *Curr Opin Lipidol* 18:35.

24. Schaefer, E. J. 2002. Lipoproteins, nutrition and heart disease. *Am J Clin Nutr* 75:191.

25. Shireman, R. 1996. Overview—formation, metabolism and physiologic effects of oxidatively modified low density lipoprotein. *J Nutr* 126:1049S.

26. Soudijn, W., I Van Wijngaarden, and A. P. Ijzerman. 2007. Nicotinic acid receptor subtypes and their ligands. *Med Res Rev* 27:417.

27. Sprecher, D. L. 1998. Triglycerides as risk factor for coronary artery disease. *Am J Cardiol* 82:49U.

28. Wang, P. Y., J. Weng, and R. G. W. Anderson. 2005. OSBP is a cholesterol-regulated scaffolding protein in control of ERK ½ activation. *Science* 307:1472.

29. Wassif, C. A., C. Maslen, S. Kachilele-Linjewile et al. 1998. Mutations in the human sterol delta-7-reductase gene at 11q 12–13 cause Smith–Lemli–Opitz syndrome. *Am J Human Genet* 63:55.

30. Witztum, J. L. 1994. The oxidation hypothesis of atherosclerosis. *Lancet* 344:793.

CASE BIBLIOGRAPHY

31. Hoffman, G., K. M. Gibson, I. K. Brandt, P. I. Bader, R. S. Wappner, and L. Sweetman. 1986. Mevalonic aciduria—an inborn error of cholesterol and nonsterol isoprene biosynthesis. *N Engl J Med* 314:1610.

18 Osteoporosis

There are two skeletal disorders related to nutrition: (1) osteoporosis and (2) osteomalacia. Osteoporosis or "porous bones" is an age-related disorder characterized by a decrease in the amount of bone to such a critical level that bones become susceptible to fractures with minimal trauma. It can be divided into two epidemiological types: (1) Type I (postmenopausal) occurs in women between the ages of 48 and 55 years in whom bone loss is associated with estrogen deficiency. (2) Type II is seen in both men and women over the age of 70; bone loss is not accelerated at any specific age but occurs at a slow, steady rate over many years. The composition of the remaining bone in osteoporosis is chemically normal. Osteomalacia is characterized by inadequate bone mineralization as a result of vitamin D deficiency. In contrast to osteoporosis, individuals with osteomalacia have lower bone calcium to protein ratio.

18.1 OSTEOPENIA AND BONE MINERAL DENSITY

Osteopenia is the thinning of bone mass. It is considered a risk factor for the development of osteoporosis. It is commonly seen in people over the age of 50 who have lower than average bone density but do not have osteoporosis. Osteopenia is due to deficiencies of calcium, vitamin D, magnesium, and other vitamins and minerals. The difference between osteopenia and osteoporosis is the measure of bone density.

Bone mineral density (BMD), a measure of bone density, reflects the strength of bones as represented by their calcium content.[21] This measure can determine if a patient has osteopenia or osteoporosis and estimate the risk of bone fractures. BMD measurements are noninvasive and painless procedures usually done on the hips, spine, wrist, fingers, shin bone, or heel. Bone density is measured using any of several techniques. The most commonly recognized is called the "dual energy X-ray absorptiometry" or DEXA test. It can detect bone density before a fracture occurs, confirm the diagnosis of osteoporosis, predict the chance of fracture in the future, determine an individual's rate of bone loss, and monitor the effects of treatment. Bone density is interpreted by comparing the patient's results to those of control populations as T- and Z-scores. The T-score compares the patient's bone density to that of a mean value of young Caucasians of the same gender, while Z-score compares the patient's bone density to the mean value of a matched population in terms of age, sex, and ethnicity. The more negative the score, the greater the severity of the disease and the greater one's risk of fracture. Several organizations have developed mean values for bone density. The T-scores are used to assess men over the age of 50 and postmenopausal women. Children and young adults are assessed using Z-scores. The World Health Organization defines osteopenia as a condition in which bone density is between 1 standard deviation (SD) and 2.5 SD below the mean density of a normal young adult. Osteoporosis is defined as a condition in which bone density is more than 2.5 SD below the mean.

18.2 EPIDEMIOLOGY OF OSTEOPOROSIS

Osteoporosis is called a "silent disease" because it progresses gradually over many years, often without symptoms or detectable and measurable changes.[7] It is common in postmenopausal women and in elderly persons of both sexes and constitutes an important public health problem. Currently it is estimated that over 200 million people worldwide suffer from the disease. Approximately 30% of all postmenopausal women in the United States and Europe have osteoporosis. At least 40% of these women and 15%–30% of men over 50 years of age will sustain one or more fractures in their remaining lifetime. In the United States, 5.3% of all hospitalized patients over 65 have the diagnosis of bone fracture, and this figure increases to 10.2% in patients over 85 years of age. Osteoporosis affects an estimated 20–25 million people over the age of 45 in the United States. The incidence of the disease is greater (approximately twice as high) in women than in men and is more common in Caucasian women than in black people and other ethnic groups. The risk of developing osteoporosis increases with age; 30% of women between the ages of 70 and 79 and 70% of women 80 years of age and older will develop osteoporosis without medical intervention. It is a major cause of disability in the United States among middle-aged and advanced-aged individuals. More than 1.5 million Americans have fractures, including more than 700,000 vertebral fractures, 250,000 hip fractures, and 250,000 wrist fractures, related to the disease each year. Patients who suffer from hip fractures have a 12%–20% higher mortality rate than persons of the same sex and similar age without fractures. In 1995, the annual cost of treating osteoporosis and osteoporosis-related fractures in the United States was estimated to be US$13.8 billion. This figure may double in the next 20 years if prevention and early intervention measures do not reduce the incidence of these diseases. Thus, the impact of osteoporosis on the health-care system as the baby-boom generation ages and as lifespan increases is potentially staggering.

18.3 DISEASE PROCESS

The skeleton has been likened to a wall whose individual bricks are continually being removed and replaced (Figure 18.1). Discrete sections of bones are removed by bone-resorbing cells, the osteoclasts, and replaced with new bone laid down by bone-forming cells, the osteoblasts. A balance between osteoblast and osteoclast activity results in a continuous remodeling process. In the normal adult, resorption is accomplished over the course of several weeks and replacement is accomplished over several months. The entire remodeling sequence is completed in 4–5 months. Under normal conditions, a perfect balance exists between the activities of bone-resorbing osteoclasts and bone-forming osteoblasts. All the common diseases of bones, as well as the bone changes seen during aging, are superimposed on the normal remodeling sequence. Bone loss under any circumstance results from a disturbance in the activity of the osteoclasts or osteoblasts.

A variety of compounds expressed by bone cells or released during bone formation or resorption enter the circulation and provide information about bone health. Tartrate-resistant acid phosphatase (TRAP) is released during resorption, and its serum level provides information about the activity of osteoclasts. Osteocalcin originates from osteoblast activity. Circulating osteocalcin is considered a marker of bone formation. The levels of these markers are used to monitor patients after the initiation of treatment to assess if turnover is accelerated.

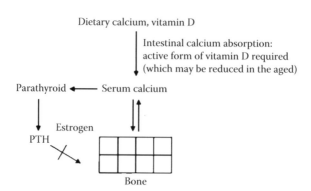

FIGURE 18.1 Factors affecting serum calcium levels and calcium exchange between bone and circulation.

The primary source of calcium is dietary and its absorption requires the active form of vitamin D (1,25-dihydroxycholecalciferol). The conversion of vitamin D to its active form is reduced in the elderly, and this in turn may affect calcium absorption. A low level of serum calcium increases the secretion of parathyroid hormone (PTH) that acts on the bone to release calcium into the circulation. Estrogen inhibits this PTH action. There is a reduction of estrogen in postmenopausal women.

Up to the age of 18 years or so there is linear growth of bones, and 10–15 years thereafter bone building continues. The peak bone mass is achieved by 25–30 years of age; up to this point, bone accretion exceeds bone resorption and the individual remains on a positive calcium balance. The peak bone mass is maintained without much change until about 35–40 years, and during this period the individual remains on calcium balance. Thereafter, bone resorption exceeds bone accretion and all persons (both men and women) progressively lose bones (0.3%–0.5% yearly) with advancing age, with the rate differing among individuals. The most important factor influencing fracture susceptibility in the elderly is the amount of bone mass present at maturity. Because everyone starts to lose bone after the age of 40, those with denser skeleton (peak bone mass) may be expected to take longer to reach the critically reduced level of bone mass at which bone can break easily than do individuals with a relatively small bone mass at skeletal maturity.

Because of the important influence of early lifestyle factors on maintaining healthy bones later in life, osteoporosis is often viewed as a pediatric disease with a geriatric outcome. However, recent research has demonstrated that in older persons, both dietary and lifestyle approaches not only retard age-related bone loss but also actually increase BMD.[3,9]

18.4 FACTORS CONTRIBUTING TO BONE MASS

18.4.1 GENETIC FACTORS, BODY, AND BUILD

White and Asian women in the United States are generally at greater risk for osteoporosis, especially those who are of small stature and those who are proportionally underweight for their height. Blacks have greater bone density and a lower risk of fracture compared to white Americans. People with lower body weight have lower BMD. Excess weight and obesity reduce the risk of developing osteoporosis.

There is evidence for a strong hereditary role in the development of bone mass by the age of 25 years or so that is independent of the consumption patterns of calcium and other nutrients, although dietary and some other factors can modulate or fine-tune the predetermined quantity, size, and shape of bones. Certain populations, such as Northern European and Asian women, are at high risk for the development of osteoporosis. The lower rate of osteoporosis in black people may be related to their greater bone and muscle mass.

The significance of heredity as a risk factor for osteoporosis is currently being studied. It has been proposed that approximately 75% of the genetic effect on a person's chance to develop osteoporosis is due to a particular allelic variant in the gene that is responsible for encoding the 1,25-dihydroxyvitamin D receptor. Osteoporosis is likely to be a polygenic disease involving a large variety of gene products implicated in bone modeling (growth) and remodeling (loss). Heredity may be important in the development of osteoporosis.

Recently, researchers in Omaha, Nebraska, came across an 18-year-old female patient with bones that had 50% greater BMD than average. The researchers began tracing 200 members of the patient's family up to 85 years old. They identified 17 people with exceptionally dense bones but who were otherwise phenotypically normal. None of them had suffered a broken bone. This high bone mass (HBM) trait is localized to chromosome 11q12–13. A systematic search for mutations uncovered an amino acid change in a β-protein module of the low-density lipoprotein (LDL) receptor–related protein. The gene and the mutation that were discovered were likened to "nature's cure for osteoporosis." This is an example of a mutation having apparently a beneficial effect.[13] The understanding of how HBM mutation confirms a unique estrogenic activity in bone remodeling may facilitate the development of therapies for the treatment of osteoporosis. Studies on the development of medication to duplicate the mutation are in progress.

18.4.2 Sex

Women are more prone to osteoporosis than men because of their lower peak bone mass in adulthood and the dramatic impact of menopause on bone mass. A deficiency of the female hormone estrogen caused by either menopause or removal of the ovaries results in accelerated bone loss. Estrogen deficiency at menopause also decreases calcium absorption. As a consequence, bone mass decreases. The critical role that estrogen plays in maintaining bone health is evidenced by several observations, perhaps the most important of which is the marked loss of bone mass during the years immediately prior to and following menopause. At menopause, women undergo an accelerated rate of bone loss (2%–3% yearly) that is most apparent over the subsequent decade and is superimposed on age-related bone loss; this loss then gradually decreases over 8–10 years until annual bone loss is similar to premenopausal rates. There is individual variation in the rate and duration of bone loss. Body fat, a nonovarian source of circulating estrogen, influences the rate of bone loss with higher amounts of body fat protecting against menopausal bone loss. Weight loss in women around menopausal age is associated with an increased loss of bone density. But it may be possible to reverse this to some extent using supplementary calcium.

Further support for the role of estrogen in maintaining bone health is the ability of estrogen, alone or in combination with progestin, to prevent bone loss at the hip and spine and to reduce hip fracture rates. Estradiol, originating in the ovary, is the primary circulating estrogen in premenopausal women, and estrone, synthesized mainly in adipose and muscle tissues, is the primary estrogen in postmenopausal women. Estrogen normally inhibits the action of PTH, which increases bone resorption (Figure 18.1). Recent work also suggests that estrogen interacts with bone cells and regulates cytokine production and thereby controls the rate or extent of osteoclast formation and activity. Of interest is the fact that both estrogen receptor α (ER α) and estrogen receptor β (ER β) are present in bone cells.[27] In men, low testosterone levels, alcoholism, and excessive use of steroids can cause low BMD but can often be treated.

18.4.3 Calcium Intake

Calcium metabolism plays a significant role in bone turnover, and deficiency of calcium and vitamin D leads to impaired bone deposition. In addition, parathyroid glands react to low serum calcium levels by secreting PTH, which increases bone resorption to ensure sufficient calcium in the blood. Epidemiological evidence supports the concept that increased calcium intake during growth and early adulthood results in higher peak bone density. A comparison was made between two groups of people living in two different geographical regions in Yugoslavia—one distinguished by traditionally high calcium intake (800–1100 mg/day) and the other known to consume lower amounts of calcium (350–500 mg/day). Those who consumed a high level of calcium had both a greater skeletal mass and relatively fewer hip fractures than did those who consumed low levels of calcium. The age-related bone loss for the two groups of individuals was similar, but the greater peak mass of the inhabitants consuming high levels of calcium was apparently responsible for their fewer fractures. Japanese women whose calcium intake averaged 400 mg/day had the highest frequency of fractures, whereas Finnish women with a calcium intake of about 1300 mg/day had the lowest frequency of fractures. Studies conducted in the United States also show that women who consumed more milk (e.g., main dietary source of calcium) and other dairy products during childhood and adolescence had significantly higher bone densities later in menopause than did women who consumed dairy products in lesser amounts.

Recent studies have shown that many American girls do not get enough calcium in their diet after the age of 11. Many women of all ages in the United States do not get enough calcium either.

Much of this is blamed on the substitution of sodas in their diet for milk. But there may be other reasons. Soda itself can negatively affect calcium utilization. Research on several thousand men and women found that those who regularly drank cola-based sodas—three or more times per day—had about 4% lower BMD on the hips even though their calcium and vitamin D intakes were controlled. Phosphoric acid, a major component of sodas, may interfere with calcium utilization, and caffeine inhibits calcium absorption. For people who have trouble digesting dairy products (due to lactase deficiency), lactose-free dairy products and lactase enzyme pills are available. Calcium-fortified foods, such as juices and cereals, and calcium supplements are helpful for people who are unable to get adequate calcium from their diets.

Calcium, in conjunction with vitamin D, is needed to strengthen bones, increase bone mass, and decrease fracture rates. The National Research Council's Institute of Medicine published recommendations for calcium intake based on age. For example, it has recommended 1000 mg/day of elemental calcium for young women. Individuals older than 51 years of age should consume at least 1200 mg/day of calcium. Calcium is best ingested from the diet, but if the diet is low in calcium, supplements can be used. Calcium supplements most commonly come in 2 forms: (1) calcium carbonate and (2) calcium citrate. Calcium carbonate is less expensive than the latter, but needs to be taken with food for better absorption. Calcium citrate is better absorbed than calcium carbonate and can be taken without food. Patients who take proton inhibitors do not absorb calcium well. Calcium citrate is the supplement of choice for this population.

18.4.4 PHOSPHORUS INTAKE

Phosphorus is present in most foods in the American diet and the usual intake is nearly 50% more than the recommended daily allowance (RDA) of 800 mg. Some studies have shown the adverse effects of excess dietary phosphorus or low calcium-to-phosphorus ratio on plasma PTH, calcium utilization, and bone health. It is generally recommended that the calcium-to-phosphorus ratio in the diet should be between 1:2 and 2:1, although the optimum ratio is not defined.

18.4.5 LACTOSE INTAKE

Studies in humans have demonstrated that the milk sugar lactose has a beneficial effect on calcium absorption, although not all investigators have confirmed these findings. Lactose intolerance appears to have little effect on calcium absorption from dairy products consumed in moderation and from nondairy products. Although there are reports of greater prevalence of osteoporosis in individuals with lactase deficiency, the cause-and-effect relationship between lactase deficiency, calcium absorption, and osteoporosis has not been established.

18.4.6 PROTEIN INTAKE

A high-protein intake at levels exceeding the RDA for this nutrient is known to increase urinary excretion of calcium. Several mechanisms have been proposed to explain the hypercalciuric effect of excess dietary protein. One may be the increased excretion of sulfate arising from the catabolism of sulfur-containing amino acids. Other suggested mechanisms include an increased glomerular filtration rate and reduced renal tubular reabsorption of calcium, both of which contribute to increased urinary calcium excretion. However, adequate protein intake is necessary to reduce BMD loss and the risk of fracture, especially in elderly women.[1]

Some studies have shown a positive relationship between protein intake from foods of animal origin and risk of hip fracture. In one study, women with higher meat intake (five or more servings a week) had a significantly increased risk for forearm fracture compared with women who ate meat less than once a week. In another study, elderly women whose diets contained a high ratio of animal protein to vegetable protein had more rapid bone loss and a greater risk for hip fracture than those with a low ratio. Other studies found that bone mass was inversely associated with animal-protein intake and positively related to the intake of vegetable protein.

18.4.7 VITAMIN D INTAKE

Adequate vitamin D levels are essential for the efficient utilization of dietary calcium. Both the liver and the kidney are involved in the hydroxylation of the vitamin and the conversion to its metabolically active form, which is needed to facilitate the intestinal absorption of calcium. The vitamin D status of an individual depends on the dietary intake of this vitamin and/or exposure to sunlight (ultraviolet rays), which transfers the precursor present on the skin to vitamin D. The elderly may not get adequate vitamin from the diet or may not get adequate exposure to sunlight. The hydroxylation of the vitamin by the aged kidney is less efficient. Low levels of circulating vitamin D are common among the elderly worldwide. Mild vitamin D deficiency is associated with increased PTH production. PTH increases bone resorption, leading to bone loss. A positive association exists between serum 1,25-dihydroxy cholecalciferol levels and BMD, while PTH is negatively associated with BMD. There is some evidence that administration of small amounts (6.5 μg/day) of synthetic calcitriol (the active form of vitamin D) to the elderly and to postmenopausal women increases the efficiency of intestinal calcium absorption and improves calcium balance.

For elderly persons who have limited exposure to sunlight because of minimal outdoor activities or because they live in areas where winters are long, supplementation may be needed. In addition, patients with renal or hepatic disease may need supplementation with an appropriate vitamin D metabolite.

18.4.8 VITAMIN C INTAKE

Impaired collagen synthesis may be a cause of osteoporosis because this process is integrated with the deposition of minerals during bone formation. In vitamin C deficiency, the ability to form mature collagen fibers is lacking due to defective hydroxylation of proline. One of the most clinically pertinent reports on the relationship between vitamin C and osteoporosis is that of Hyams and Ross (1963). They described a 54-year-old menopausal woman with severe osteoporosis and low back pain that remained undiagnosed for about a year. After admission to the hospital, she was found to have frank scurvy. X-rays confirmed osteoporosis, which was arrested, and her back pain responded to the provision of 500 mg/day of ascorbic acid.[10] Aging, as well as smoking, decreases vitamin C levels in the blood and may predispose the individual to osteoporosis for precisely the same reason.[11]

18.4.9 VITAMIN K INTAKE

Osteocalcin, a vitamin K–dependent protein, accounts for 15%–20% of noncollagenous protein in the bone. It is produced by osteoblasts during bone matrix formation and appears in bones with the onset of hydroxyapatite deposition. Osteocalcin synthesis is increased by vitamin D, and its concentration in the bone is directly proportional to the amount of calcium in bone. Some studies have found that serum concentrations of vitamin K are reduced in populations at risk for osteoporosis and in individuals with fracture.

Epidemiological studies have demonstrated a relationship between vitamin K and age-related bone loss. The Nurses' Health Study followed 72,000 women for 10 years. In an analysis of the cohort, women whose vitamin K intakes were in the lowest quintile had a 30% higher risk of hip fracture than women with vitamin K intakes in the highest four quintiles. The Framingham Health Study conducted over 7 years found that men and women with dietary vitamin K intakes in the highest quartile had a 65% lower risk of hip fracture than those with dietary vitamin intakes in the lowest quartile. Circulating levels of undercarboxylated osteocalcin were found to be higher in postmenopausal women than in premenopausal women and to be markedly higher in women over the age of 70. In a study of 7560 elderly women, circulating undercarboxylated osteocalcin appeared to be predictive of fracture risk.

Supplementation with 1 mg/day of phylloquinone in the 55- to 75-year-old population decreases bone loss and reduces urinary calcium excretion. Studies in women 40–78 years old found that supplementation with 45 mg of vitamin K per day resulted in 60%, 77%, and 81% lower risk for vertebral, hip, and nonvertebral fractures, respectively. Thus, vitamin K deficiency might be associated with increased skeletal fragility and vitamin supplementation may offer protection. However, the precise role of vitamin K in maintaining bone health remains to be determined.

18.4.10 MAGNESIUM INTAKE

About two-thirds of the body's magnesium is present in the skeleton. Magnesium in bone is not an integral part of the hydroxyapatite lattice structure, but rather appears to be located on the crystal surface. Normal serum magnesium levels are necessary for proper calcium metabolism because hypomagnesemia results in hypocalcemia, peripheral resistance to the effects of vitamin D, and resistance to the effects of PTH. Thus, adequate calcium intake alone may not ensure proper bone health if magnesium status is abnormal. Significant reductions in serum and bone magnesium content have been described in several studies of postmenopausal women with osteoporosis. Recently, in a community-based study in elderly men and women, dietary magnesium was found to be positively associated with BMD. Thus, magnesium therapy may prevent fractures. More studies are necessary to better understand the role of magnesium in ensuring bone health. Plasma homocysteine levels can be lowered by folic acid and vitamin B_{12}.

18.4.11 OTHER NUTRIENTS—FOLIC ACID, VITAMIN B_{12}, VITAMIN A, AND SODIUM

A role for hyperhomocysteinemia in the etiology of osteoporosis has been suggested by the findings of two separate studies.[4] One study found that men with the highest blood homocysteine levels were four times as likely to develop hip fractures as men with the lowest levels. The second study found that men and women with the highest levels of homocysteine had twice the risk of suffering a fracture compared with those with the lowest levels. It is still not clear whether homocysteine actually causes bone loss and whether lowering homocysteine levels can reduce the risk of osteoporosis. Homocysteine can be added to the growing list of risk factors for osteoporosis.

Results of several epidemiological studies suggest that long-term intakes of more than 5000 IU/day of vitamin A are associated with decreased BMD and an increased risk of osteoporotic fracture in older men and women. Some studies have found that regular high intake of sodium increases urinary calcium loss and markers of bone resorption.

18.4.12 FIBER AND RELATED SUBSTANCES

Several studies have demonstrated that dietary fiber has a chelating effect on calcium, thereby making it unavailable for intestinal absorption. As a result, there is negative calcium balance in individuals receiving high fiber such as cellulose, whole wheat, fruits, and vegetables from their normal diet, despite adequate calcium intake. It is estimated that a fiber intake of 26 g increases calcium requirements by about 150 mg/day. Oxalate in foods such as spinach and phytic acid (in wheat bran) may reduce the efficiency of calcium absorption; however, in the amounts present in the normal diet, these constituents (e.g., fiber, oxalate, phytate) appear to have little significance in calcium absorption.

18.4.13 VEGETARIAN DIET

Vegetarians lose less bone than omnivores. This is attributed to the lower percentage of sulfur-containing amino acids in proteins from foods of plant origin than in meat. The sulfur-containing amino acids, when present in amounts higher than that required for the body's needs, are metabolized to sulfate and excreted in the urine, making the urine more acidic. In general, vegetarians have less-acidic urine than those eating a nonvegetarian diet. Vegetarian diet also increases the recycling of steroids such as estrogens, which are secreted in the bile and are reabsorbed through the intestinal mucosa.

Several studies have found that higher intakes of fruits and vegetables, particularly those rich in potassium, are associated with higher BMD and lower risk for fracture in older adults.[26] Dietary approaches to stop hypertension (DASH) studies have also reported that high intakes of fruits and vegetables, in addition to having positive effects on blood pressure, reduce calcium loss and lower biochemical markers of bone turnover, particularly resorption (loss). Green leafy vegetables are rich in vitamin K, a low intake of which may contribute to osteoporosis by causing undercarboxylation of osteocalcin. Fruits and vegetables are good sources of folic acid, which is critical for reducing blood levels of homocysteine that is linked to osteoporotic fracture.

The inclusion of soybean products in the diet decreases urinary calcium excretion and favorably affects BMD. In a study published recently, intakes of fruits and vegetables showed a protective cross-sectional association in both men and women. Fruits and vegetables are important sources of potassium and magnesium. Potassium promotes renal calcium retention, and magnesium is essential for maintaining calcium balance.

18.4.14　Caffeine Intake

Caffeine and caffeine-containing beverages such as coffee increase urinary calcium excretion, although caffeine's effect on bone health is unknown. Excessive caffeine ingestion may increase the risk of osteoporosis via increased calcium excretion. A lifetime ingestion of caffeine has been shown to decrease BMD in postmenopausal women. In a study in which 980 postmenopausal women were enrolled, BMD was decreased in the hip and lumbar spine as demonstrated by dual-energy X-ray absorptiometry. Women who ingested the equivalent of two cups of coffee daily throughout their adult lives were found to be at an increased risk for decreased BMD, but the deleterious effect of caffeine on bones could be offset by the daily consumption of one or more glasses of milk.

18.4.15　Alcohol, Cigarette Smoking, and Drugs

Bone loss and osteoporosis have been observed in relatively young and middle-aged males with a history of chronic alcoholism.[15] Usually osteoporosis does not occur in males of these age groups. Chronic alcohol feeding in rats causes a decrease in trabecular bones despite normal levels of calcium, phosphorus, and testosterone. The cause of osteoporosis in chronic alcoholics may be due to a direct toxic effect of alcohol on the bone and/or poor dietary intake of some nutrients including calcium, phosphorus, vitamin D, and protein. Malabsorption of calcium due to pancreatic insufficiency, steatorrhea, increased urinary loss of calcium induced by alcohol, alcohol-induced hypercorticoidism, and parathyroid stimulation secondary to calcium-binding proteins in cirrhosis are other mechanisms by which altered bone metabolism may contribute to clinical musculoskeletal diseases in alcoholic populations, but the site or sites involved and their importance remain to be clarified. Alcoholics also may be at risk for increased falls.

Cigarette smoking has been reported to induce calcium loss.[11,28] Smoking inhibits the activity of osteoblasts and is an independent risk factor for osteoporosis. Women who smoke, especially those who are thin, are at increased risk for fractures compared with nonsmokers. In addition, premenopausal smokers have lower estrogen serum concentrations and undergo menopause earlier than nonsmokers, while postmenopausal smokers using exogenous estrogen have lower estrogen serum concentrations than expected.

Drugs such as corticosteroids, diuretics, and certain antitubercular drugs are known to induce calcium loss. Aluminum-containing antacids cause calcium loss and extensive demineralization.

The development of osteoporosis has been associated with the administration of >20,000 U/day of heparin for 6 months or longer. Various mechanisms have been suggested, but the pathophysiology of this rare adverse effect remains unclear. Affected patients may present with bone pain and/or radiographic findings suggestive of fractures. The possibility of the development of osteoporosis should be considered in patients undergoing long-term, high-dose heparin therapy.

Statins, a class of cholesterol-lowering drugs, have been shown to increase new bone formation in rodents and in human cells in vitro. A recent population-based study in women aged 60 years and older found statins to be protective against nonpathological fracture. If the use of statins in humans is associated with increased bone formation, these agents offer a promising treatment option for osteoporosis.[5]

Drugs called selective serotonin reuptake inhibitors (SSRIs) have been used for treating depression, and scientists have observed that people taking these medications have reduced BMD. Circulating levels of serotonin are inversely related to bone mass in women, according to a new study. Serotonin is yet another player in the complex physiology of bone.[14,23]

18.4.16 TRACE ELEMENTS

18.4.16.1 Manganese

Manganese deficiency has been suggested as a potential underlying factor in the development of osteoporosis, although the deficiency of this trace element has not been reported in free-living human populations. Manganese-dependent glycosyl tranferases are required for the synthesis of mucopolysaccharides of collagen. The deficiency of manganese in rats results in the inhibition of both osteoclast and osteoblast activity. The implication of this observation in regard to human bone disease needs to be ascertained.[17,18]

An individual who had followed a bizarre macrobiotic diet experienced repeated fractures and was found to have no manganese in the blood. More recently, young men between the ages of 19 and 22 were fed a semipurified manganese-deficient diet for 39 days. Among other findings, serum calcium and phosphorus levels in these young men were found to increase. Similar findings of elevated serum calcium and phosphorus were observed in rats maintained on a manganese-deficient diet for 1 year. The bones of these animals were found to be low in manganese and exhibited an osteoporotic condition. Interesting in this connection are the observations that serum manganese levels in osteoporotic women are only 25% of the level seen in normal women. The findings in both human and animal studies suggest that bone manganese stores are mobilized in the deficiency of this trace metal. The dissolution of bones to supply manganese also releases other bone constituents including calcium and phosphorus, increasing their levels in blood. Tea is the richest source of manganese.

18.4.16.2 Boron Intake

Boron is not yet classified as an essential nutrient for humans; however, it has been recently suggested that inadequate dietary boron may be one factor that enhances the susceptibility of bone loss and osteoporosis because of the mineral's possible effect on calcium metabolism.

A study was done in postmenopausal women (between the ages of 48 and 82 years) housed in a metabolic unit. The individuals were first fed a diet low in boron (0.25 mg/day) for 120 days, and they were then continued on the same diet supplemented with boron (3 mg/day) for the next 4 months. Boron deprivation caused an increase in urinary calcium, and a decrease in serum 17β-estradiol (the most biologically active form of native human estrogen) and testosterone, its precursor. Boron supplementation markedly elevated the serum concentrations of 17β-estradiol and testosterone, and decreased the urinary excretion of calcium.[16,19]

The administration of estrogen is the known effective means to slow down the loss of calcium from the bone, which occurs after menopause. How boron may reduce the loss of urinary calcium or increase serum estrogen and testosterone is not known. Boron may be involved in hydroxylation steps in the synthesis of specific steroid hormones. Therefore, this trace element may be an important nutritional factor that may prevent or reduce the incidence of osteoporosis. Foods rich in boron include fruits and leafy vegetables, nuts, legumes, wine, and beer.

18.4.16.3 Silicon Intake

Silicon has been claimed to participate in bone calcification. It is present in mucopolysaccharide-rich tissues, and a proportion of silicon is bound tightly and can be released only by strong acidic or alkaline treatment. In experimental silicon deficiency, there is a reduction of glycosaminoglycans in cartilage. Silicon is present in high concentrations in collagen (and part is firmly bound), and collagen concentration in bones is depressed in silicon deficiency. It is apparently required for the maximal activity of prolyl hydroxylase (one of the enzymes catalyzing posttranslational modification of collagen). This suggests that silicon has a role in bone collagen biosynthesis. Silicon is specifically concentrated in bone-forming cells, the osteoblasts, and its concentration within the mitochondria exceeds that of calcium. The concentration of silicon in the aorta and cartilage decreases with age. There are no studies reported on the effect of aging on the silicon content of bones and whether silicon is involved in several human disorders including osteoporosis. There is a need to study the nutritional significance of silicon as it relates to age-related diseases.

18.4.16.4 Fluoride Intake

Mineralized tissues contain approximately 99% of total body fluoride, with most of it found in bone. The fluoride ion is able to substitute for the hydroxyl ion in apatite and form fluorapatite, which is more resistant to dissolution by acid. Several years back, it was reported that the incidence of osteoporosis was much lower in areas where water supplies had a higher fluoride content than those areas where the fluoride content in water supplies was low. This suggested that fluoride had a positive influence on bone mass; however, the study made no adjustments for other possible factors such as genetics, exposure to sunlight, and dietary patterns in this population.

Fluoride is a powerful stimulator of osteoblasts and increases spinal bone mass in a dose-dependent manner; but the level of this component required to produce an increase in bone mass versus the level that can cause fluorosis is not well defined. Fluoride has been in use as a therapeutic agent for treating osteoporosis in the amount of 40–75 mg/day, administered orally in divided doses because of gastrointestinal side effects. More recent studies have shown that although bone density increases in individuals receiving fluoride, there is no reduction in spinal fractures and, in fact, a higher number of nonspinal fractures is observed. Bones with excess fluoride content have an abnormal structure and their fragility may be increased. Thus, increased bone mass is not necessarily equivalent to increased bone strength. Some have suggested that the dose of fluoride in this study was too high, resulting in fragile bones. At present, the use of fluoride should be considered an experimental treatment and should be administered only within a clinical trial.

18.4.17 Organ Transplant

Over the last few years, organ transplant has been established as a therapy for certain end-state diseases. Improved outcome of this therapy has meant that many patients are living several years after their transplants. Therefore, long-term complications not related to graft function are of increasing clinical importance. Osteoporosis is a common posttransplant disorder that is garnering much attention.[6] Various epidemiological and cross-sectional studies estimate that as many as 7%–11% of nondiabetic kidney transplant recipients, 45% of diabetic kidney transplant recipients, 18%–50% of heart transplant recipients,[12] and 24%–65% of liver transplant recipients develop osteoporosis in their posttransplant period.

Factors responsible for bone loss in organ transplant recipients depend on the underlying disease and the particular organ system transplanted. For example, potential kidney transplant recipients commonly have at least some evidence of renal osteodystrophy. Potential heart transplant recipients with congestive heart failure suffer from specific conditions that may contribute to low BMD. These include vitamin D deficiency, dietary calcium deficiency, therapy with diuretics, and hypogonadism. Several drugs used to prevent organ rejection predispose patients to osteoporosis. Corticosteroids and cyclosporine have been associated with promoting bone loss after transplantation. The high incidence of osteoporosis in posttransplant patients highlights the need for more effective therapies in high-risk patients.

18.4.18 PHYSICAL ACTIVITY

There is a general agreement that exercise results in increased bone mass, and physical inactivity associated with aging or immobilization appears to contribute to bone loss. The bone mass of athletes exceeds that of sedentary people, and exercise reduces age-related bone loss. The optimal type and the amount of physical activity that can prevent osteoporosis have not been established. Bone loss is dramatic and continues in the weightless environment of outer space and in individuals confined to a wheelchair or to continuous bed rest. Weight-bearing activities such as walking, jogging, and running are more beneficial than non-weight-bearing activities such as swimming and cycling. The evidence in favor of the beneficial effect of exercise is strong enough to recommend it in any program of prophylaxis or treatment of osteoporosis.

18.4.19 TOXIC EFFECTS OF SOME MINERALS

There are several minerals to which we are exposed, and some at higher levels may produce toxic effects. These include cadmium, lithium, and lead. Cadmium is present in tobacco smoke and also can enter the body as a result of industrial pollution. Certain kinds of intestinal parasites appear to increase cadmium absorption. The kidney is a target tissue for its accumulation, and it can produce adverse effects on the skeleton by causing renal damage and subsequent alterations in vitamin D metabolism. Cadmium inhibits 1-hydroxylase, which is required for the conversion of vitamin D to its active form. The treatment of patients with large doses of vitamin D (20,000–100,000 IU/day) relieves the symptoms of cadmium toxicity. Cadmium also inhibits the activity of lysyl oxidase, a copper-containing enzyme essential for collagen formation. Lead impairs the formation of the active form of vitamin D. Lithium has a variety of uses in medicine, including the treatment of some psychiatric disorders and as a substitute in low-sodium diets. Lithium is retained readily in the bones due to its physicochemical similarity to calcium and magnesium and can interfere with the action of PTH on the bone. Chronic lithium therapy can produce osteoporosis, especially in women.

Osteoporosis and Calcium Balance—A Case Study

A 75-year-old woman was admitted to a hospital for the evaluation of osteoporosis. The diagnosis of osteoporosis had been made in another clinic 2 years earlier after the onset of severe back pain and an evidence of demineralization of the spine. At that time, her physician treated her with 50,000 IU of vitamin D twice weekly, 1 g of calcium carbonate daily, and 50 mg of sodium fluoride daily. Three months later, vitamin D was discontinued because of hypercalcemia. All treatments were stopped 6 months before the present admission.

Physical examination revealed that she was well developed and moderately well nourished. Her height was reduced 3 inches below her normal of 5 feet 6 inches, and the skeletal X-ray showed diffuse osteoporosis. Besides showing kyphosis, the X-ray of her chest was otherwise within normal limits. Routine laboratory blood tests, urine analysis, and liver function tests were in the normal range. There was no renal disease.

Serum calcium was 9.5 mg/dl (normal: 8.9–10 mg/dl), phosphorus was 3.6 mg/dl (normal: 2.5–4.5 mg/dl), and PTH was 84 U/ml (normal: 0–45 U/ml). Serum 25-hydroxy vitamin D and 1,25-dihydroxyvitamin D were in the normal range.

Metabolic studies showed that on her usual calcium intake of 290 mg/day, she excreted 296 mg in the feces and 72 mg/day in the urine, which gave a balance of −78 mg/day and a net absorption of 0.8%. After treatment with 0.5 μg/day of 1,25-dihydroxyvitamin D for 5 days, her serum calcium increased to 10.1 mg/dl and her PTH level decreased only slightly to 77 U/ml. Her negative calcium balance improved to −27 mg/day and calcium absorption increased to 27%. Because of the persistently elevated levels of PTH, she underwent exploration of her parathyroid glands, which were found to be enlarged. A subtotal parathyroidectomy was performed. The pathological diagnosis was chief cell hyperplasia. Treatment with 1,25-dihydroxyvitamin D was continued. Two months later, the serum calcium level was 9.1 mg/dl and PTH was 42 U/ml. The patient did well and her back discomfort was progressively decreased.

Studies by some investigators have shown that most patients with postmenopausal osteoporosis show levels of PTH that are either normal or low.[29,30] However, about 11% of the patients show an increase in PTH. The patient described here belongs to this group. It has been hypothesized that in these patients, age-related decreases in the formation of 1,25-dihydroxyvitamin D in the kidney, deficiencies of gonadal steroids, and other factors are responsible for the exaggerated disorder. Malabsorption of calcium follows and a reduced flow of calcium into the blood stimulates an increase in PTH, which in turn increases the renal formation of 1,25-dihydroxyvitamin D. The fact that the level of 1,25-dihydroxyvitamin D is normal in the presence of elevated PTH suggests a failure of hydroxylation in the kidney. In a different case reported by other authors, it was shown that following subtotal parathyroidectomy, the patient did well with no new fractures and back discomfort. It is, therefore, important to determine serum PTH levels in postmenopausal women with osteoporosis.

The treatment of osteoporosis is difficult, but hyperparathyroidism, if present, can be corrected. None of the agents recommended for treatment of osteoporosis is fully effective. At the present time, the only rational approach is prevention. Current data indicate that patients with osteoporosis consume less calcium, require more calcium to achieve balance, and have lower plasma 1,25-dihydroxy vitamin D than controls. Some investigators found that postmenopausal women require 1.5 g/day of calcium to attain balance compared with 1 g in premenopausal controls. It is recommended that 1200 mg of calcium be consumed daily.

REFERENCES

1. Bell, J., and S. J. Whiting. 2002. Elderly women need dietary protein to maintain bone mass. *Nutr Rev* 60:337.
2. Berg, K. M., H. V. Kunins, J. L. Jackson et al. 2008. Association between alcohol consumption and both osteoporotic fracture and bone density. *Amer J Med* 121:406.
3. Binkley, N. C., and J. W. Suttie. 1995. Vitamin K nutrition and osteoporosis. *J Nutr* 125:1812.
4. Cashman, K. D. 2005. Homocysteine and osteoporosic fracture risk: A potential role for B vitamins. *Nutrition Rev* 63:29.
5. Chan, K. A., S. E. Andrade, M. Boles, D. S. M. Buist, G. A. Chase, J. G. Donahue, M. J. Goodman, J. H. Gurwitz, A. Z. Lacroix, and R. Platt. 2000. Inhibitors of hydroxymethylglutaryl-coenzyme A reductase and risk of fracture among older women. *Lancet* 355:2185.
6. Delmas, P. D. 2001. Osteoporosis in patients with organ transplants: A neglected problem. *Lancet* 357:325.
7. Ebeling, P. K. 2008. Clinical practice: Osteoporosis in men. *New Engl J Med* 358:1474.
8. Fleel, J. C. 2000. Leptin and bone: Does the brain control bone biology? *Nutr Rev* 58:209.
9. Harris, S. T. 1993. Osteoporosis: Pharmacologic treatment strategies. *Adv Intern Med* 38:303.
10. Hyams, D. E., and E. J. Ross. 1963. Scurvy, megaloblastic anemia, and osteoporosis. *Br J Clin Pract* 17:332.

11. Kiel, D. P., J. A. Baron, J. J. Anderson, M. T. Hannan, and D. T. Felson. 1992. Smoking eliminates the protective effect of oral estrogens on the risk for hip fracture among women. *Ann Intern Med* 116:716.

12. Leidig-Bruckner, G., S. Hosch, P. Dodidou et al. 2001. Frequency and predictors of osteoporotic fractures after cardiac or liver transplantation: A follow-up study. *Lancet* 357:342.

13. Little, R. D., J. P. Carulli, R. G. D. Mastro et al. 2002. A mutation in the LDL receptor–related protein 5 gene results in the autosomal dominant high-bone-mass trait. *Am J Hum Genet* 70:11.

14. Modder, U. I., S. J. Achenbach, S. Amin et al. 2010. Relation of serum serotonin levels to bone density and structural parameters in women. *J Bone Mineral Res* 25:415.

15. Moniz, C. 1994. Alcohol and bone. *Br Med Bull* 50:67.

16. Nielsen, F. H. 1992. Facts and fallacies about boron. *Nutr Today* 27(3):6.

17. Nieves, J. W. 2005. Osteoporosis: The role of micronutrients. *Amer J Clin Nutr* 51:1232.

18. Poole, K. E., and J. E. Compston. 2006. Osteoporosis and its management. *Brit Med J* 333:1251.

19. Prestwood, K. M., and M. E. Werksler. 1997. Osteoporosis: Up-to-date strategies for prevention and treatment. *Geriatrics* 52:92.

20. Recker, R. R. 2008. Autosomal dominant high bone mass: The phenotype. A brief description. *J Musculoskelet Neuronal Interact* 8:294.

21. Richards, J. B., F. Rivadeneira, M. Inouye et al. 2008. Bone mineral density, osteoporosis, and osteoporotic fractures: A genome-wide association study. *Lancet* 37:1505.

22. Riggs, B. L., and L. J. Milton III. 1992. The prevention and treatment of osteoporosis. *N Engl J Med* 327:620.

23. Rosen, C. J. 2009. Serotonin rising—the bone, brain, bowel connection. *New Engl J Med* 360:957.

24. Sojka, J. E. 1995. Magnesium supplementation and osteoporosis. *Nutr Rev* 53:71.

25. Tolstoi, L. G., and R. M. Levin. 1992. Osteoporosis—the treatment controversy. *Nutr Today* 27(4):6.

26. Tucker, K. L., M. T. Hanna, H. Chen et al. 1999. Potassium, magnesium, and fruit and vegetable intakes are associated with greater bone mineral density in elderly men and women. *Am J Clin Nutr* 69:727.

27. Vidal, O., L. G. Kindblom, and C. Ohlsson. 1999. Expression and localization of estrogen receptor-β in murine and human bone. *J Bone Miner Res* 14:923.

28. Wong, P. K., J. J. Christie, and J. D. Wark. 2007. The effect of smoking on bone health. *Clin Sci* 113:233.

CASE BIBLIOGRAPHY

29. 1983. Clinical Nutrition Cases: Osteoporosis and calcium balance. *Nutr Rev* 41:83.

30. Riggs, B. L., J. C. Gallager, H. R. DeLuca, A. J. Edis, P. W. Lambert, and C. D. Amaud. 1976. A syndrome of osteoporosis, increased serum immunoreactive parathyroid hormone, and inappropriately low serum 1, 25-dihydroxyvitamin D. *Mayo Clin Proc* 53:701.

19 Nutritional Aspects of Diabetes

Diabetes mellitus is a spectrum of inherited and acquired disorders that is characterized by elevated circulating blood glucose levels. This condition results from an absolute or a relative deficiency of insulin (the hormone secreted by pancreatic β cells) and/or insulin action with a consequent deranged metabolism of carbohydrate, fat, and protein. Diabetes is a major health problem affecting 5%–6% of the U.S. population. It is a leading cause of blindness, amputation, and renal failure (16 million in 1995) and a major cause of heart attack and stroke. Diabetes can be controlled and the patients with this disease can lead a productive life. Nutrition plays a key role in the management of this disease.

19.1 CLASSIFICATION

Two common types of diabetes that differ in both clinical manifestations and etiology are well recognized: (1) type 1 or insulin-dependent diabetes (IDD), formerly called juvenile-onset diabetes; and (2) type 2 or non-insulin-dependent diabetes (NIDD), formerly called maturity-onset diabetes (Table 19.1).

Type 1 diabetes usually, but not always, begins before 20 years of age. It constitutes about 5% of all cases of diabetes. The peak age of onset is 11–13 years, which usually coincides with puberty. The next peak age of onset occurs at 6–8 years of age, around the start of grade school. The frequency is similar in boys and in girls. Approximately 7.4% of adults who are diagnosed with diabetes between 30 and 74 years of age have type 1 diabetes. Patients with this type of diabetes have virtually no capacity to secrete insulin after the disease is established. Type 1 diabetes is characterized by a tendency toward ketosis and an absolute dependence on insulin for the maintenance of health and survival. The presentation of diabetes is often acute because of a sudden reduction in insulin secretion that is usually related to autoimmune damage to pancreatic β cells in a genetically susceptible individual. Some patients with type 1 diabetes have a strong family history of autoimmune conditions such as autoimmune thyroid or adrenal disease.

The genetics of type 1 diabetes are incompletely understood. There is concordance in about 50% of identical twins; however, the pattern of inheritance is not complete, implying that several genes as well as unknown environmental factors may be involved.

The environmental trigger may cause an uncontrollable autoimmune response that attacks insulin-producing β cells.[11] Some epidemiological studies suggest that breast-feeding reduces the risk for developing the disease later in life, presumably by protecting against infections, enhancing the infant's immune system and delaying exposure to foreign food antigens. Cow's milk protein has been suggested as a trigger for the disease, but it has not been proven conclusively. Epidemiological studies have shown that supplementing infant diets with gluten-containing foods before 3 months of age is associated with an increased risk of developing the disease. Giving children 2000 IU of vitamin D per day during their first year of life is associated with a reduced risk for type 1 diabetes. Populations living at or near the equator, where there is abundant sunshine, have low incidence rates of type 1 diabetes. Conversely, populations at higher latitudes, where available sunshine is more scarce, have higher incidence rates. Thus breast-feeding, avoiding cow's milk and gluten-containing foods, and daily supplementation of vitamin D may protect against the disease.

TABLE 19.1
Comparison of the Two Types of Diabetes

	Insulin-Dependent Type (Type 1)	Non-Insulin-Dependent Type (Type 2)
Age of onset	Usually before the age of 20 years	Usually after the age of 40 years
Nutritional status (prior to diagnosis)	Generally malnourished	Mostly obese
Genetic predisposition	Moderate	Strong
Prevalence	Less than 6% of all diabetics	About 95% of all diabetics
Plasma insulin	Very low or absent	Low, normal, or high
Ketosis	Common in untreated patients	Rare
Acute complications	Ketosis	—
Insulin treatment	Always necessary	Usually not required

There are some forms of type 1 diabetes that have no known etiology. Some of these patients have permanent insulin deficiency and are prone to ketoacidosis, but have no evidence of autoimmunity. This form is more common among individuals of African and Asian origin. In another form found in Africa, the absolute requirement for insulin replacement therapy in affected individuals may come and go and patients periodically develop ketoacidosis.

Type 2 diabetes is usually associated with an older age of onset, around 40 years of age or more.[10] In the United States, approximately 95% of all individuals with diabetes have type 2 diabetes, and of these about 80% are obese. Both the incidence and the prevalence of diabetes increase dramatically with age. For example, the prevalence of self-reported diabetes is 1.1% among individuals 20–39 years of age, and is almost 25% among individuals 60 years of age or older. It is the most common of all metabolic disorders. It has a slow, insidious course and may be present several years before diagnosis.

There is a consistent genetic predisposition for type 2 diabetes; there is nearly 90% concordance among identical twins in which one member has the condition. Individuals who have both parents with type 2 diabetes have a 50% chance of having the disease. Recently, researchers identified a gene that affects susceptibility to type 2 diabetes in some diabetes-prone populations. The gene encodes calpain-10, a member of the protein family called calpains (calcium-activated neutral proteases), which are regulatory proteins found in all human cells.[13] Variations in the gene are associated with up to a threefold increase in the risk of developing type 2 diabetes. In humans, at least eight versions of calpain-10 are expressed in different tissues. One form is found in pancreatic islets. Variations in calpain-10 affect the rate of insulin-stimulated glucose oxidation.

Type 2 diabetes appears to start with the resistance of insulin to stimulate glucose uptake in insulin-sensitive tissues (e.g., muscle, adipose tissue). Insulin resistance is a decreased ability to respond to the effects of normal amounts of circulating insulin. As a result, higher levels of insulin are needed to produce its effects.

The pancreas tries to compensate by producing and secreting more than the normal amounts of insulin to maintain normal blood sugar levels. During this process, the β cells eventually will require higher levels of blood sugar to signal the secretion of insulin, resulting in impaired glucose tolerance (IGT). At some future time, the pancreas may not be able to maintain these compensatory high levels of insulin secretion.

Conditions associated with the development of insulin resistance, especially central obesity (as estimated clinically by a high waist-to-hip ratio), greatly increase the risk of type 2 diabetes, although some lean individuals are insulin resistant. Even in insulin-resistant individuals, impaired insulin secretory capacity appears to be responsible for the diabetic state. Both genetic and environmental factors contribute to the etiology of type 2 diabetes. Vitamin D deficiency has been shown to alter insulin synthesis and secretion in both humans and animal models.[1,6] It has been reported that vitamin D replenishment improves glycemia and secretion in patients with type 2 diabetes with established vitamin D deficiency, thereby suggesting a role for vitamin D in the pathogenesis of type 2 diabetes.[24] The presence of vitamin D receptors (VDRs) and vitamin D–binding proteins (VDBPs) in pancreatic tissue and the relationship between certain allelic variations in the VDR and VDBP genes with glucose tolerance and insulin secretion have further supported this hypothesis.

Recent studies have linked consumption of meat, fish, and fish oils to insulin resistance and diabetes. A low-fat vegetarian diet has been shown to improve diabetes. Although there can be limitations on secretory capacity in type 2 diabetes, together with the presence of insulin insensitivity, these patients do not have an absolute dependence on injectable insulin for their survival in the early stages of the disease. The hyperglycemia can often be controlled by dietary means only and physical activity, or with an oral hypoglycemic drug. Some insulin is detectable in the plasma of nearly all patients in this category and they are, therefore, less prone to ketosis. In this sense, the disease is less severe than type 1 diabetes, but long-term complications occur in both types. Most persons with type 2 diabetes may become insulinopenic later on and may have to inject insulin.

In addition to the aforementioned two types of diabetes, there is a category that constitutes heterogeneous groupings of patients for whom a designation of either of the two traditional forms of diabetes appears inappropriate. These are all categorized as secondary diabetes. These include carbohydrate intolerance as a result of pancreatic insufficiency following chronic recurrent pancreatitis and secondary to the administration of certain drugs. Pregnant women with no previous history of abnormal carbohydrate metabolism may develop IGT or overt diabetes mellitus (gestational diabetes). Most patients will return to normal glucose tolerance in the postpartum state.

About 2%–4% of pregnant women in the United States or 135,000 women annually develop gestational diabetes, according to the American Diabetes Association. High blood sugar during pregnancy results in the baby being overfed in the womb. The result of this overfeeding may be that children become metabolically imprinted or programmed to become obese.

A recent study included 9439 women who gave birth in Oregon, Washington, and Hawaii between 1995 and 2000. All the women were screened for gestational diabetes during pregnancy, and their children's weights were recorded between the ages of 5 and 7 years. A child's weight during this period is strongly predictive of his or her weight later in life. Compared with children born to mothers with normal blood sugar during pregnancy, children born to mothers with poorly controlled high blood sugar were 89% more likely to be overweight and 82% more likely to be obese between the ages of 5 and 7 years. Conversely, children born to mothers with gestational diabetes that was adequately treated were no more likely to be overweight or obese than children born to mothers with no evidence of gestational diabetes. Individuals at high risk for gestational diabetes include older women, those with previous history of glucose intolerance, and those with a history of babies who are large for their gestational age.

19.2 EPIDEMIOLOGY

The prevalence of type 1 diabetes in the United States is 1.7 per 1000 in individuals younger than 19 years of age and 2.1 per 1000 in adults. The disease affects an estimated 1.4 million people in the United States and 10–20 million people globally. One of the most striking characteristics of type 1 diabetes is the large geographic variability in its incidence.[9] It varies from 0.1/100,000 people/year in China and Venezuela to 39.5/100,000/year in Finland. A child in Finland is 400 times more likely to develop diabetes than a child in China. A clear difference appears between the northern and southern hemispheres, with no countries below the equator having an incidence greater than 15/100,000. In contrast, above the equator the disease is common in Europe. It is highest in Finland and lowest in Greece. In the United States, non-Hispanic whites are about 1.5 times as likely to develop type 1 diabetes as African Americans and Hispanics.

A report by the Centers for Disease Control and Prevention (CDC) based on data from 2007 show that the number of Americans with diabetes has grown to 24 million people, or roughly 8% of the U.S. population. The CDC estimates that another 57 million people have blood sugar abnormalities called "prediabetes," which put people at increased risk for the disease. Over 600,000 people are newly diagnosed with diabetes each year in the United States. There are major ethnic differences in susceptibility to type 2 diabetes, which are probably largely genetically determined. The prevalence of the disease is highest among Native Americans; adult Pima Indians have a prevalence of about 50%. Relative to white people, the prevalence of type 2 diabetes is higher in African Americans (1.6 times) and Mexican Americans (1.9 times). The overall prevalence of diabetes among women aged 20 years and older is estimated to be 10.2% and for men 11.2%. According to the report by the CDC, the prevalence of diagnosed cases of diabetes increased by a third (from 4.9% to 6.5%) between 1990 and 1998. As the American population becomes increasingly nonwhite and obese, the number of diabetics is likely to rise. From 2005 to 2007, the number of diabetics increased by 3 million. The CDC predicts that the national incidence of diabetes will rise by 37.5% by the year 2025.

Diabetes is a serious condition that places people at risk for greater morbidity and mortality relative to the nondiabetic population. For example, compared with the general population the mortality rate for people with type 1 diabetes is 5–12 times higher, and for adults with type 2 diabetes, it is two times higher. In 1993, approximately 400,000 deaths from all causes were reported in individuals with diabetes. This figure represents 18% of all deaths of individuals aged 25 years and older in the United States. According to the National Center for Health Statistics, diabetes was the seventh leading cause of death by disease type. Diabetes is the fourth leading cause of death in African American women and the third leading cause of death in Hispanic women aged 45–74 years and in Native American women aged 65–74 years. Morbidity also is greater for people with diabetes and is primarily related to acute and chronic complications associated with the condition.

In 1997, the annual per capita health-care expenditure for people with diabetes was approximately three times that for individuals without diabetes (US$10,071 versus US$2,699). An estimated US$77.7 billion, or approximately 8% of all U.S. health-care dollars, was spent on people with diabetes, and hospitalization accounted for 62% of the direct health-care costs.[2] The total cost for diagnosed diabetes in 2007 was US$115 billion for direct medical costs and US$58 billion for indirect costs (disability, work loss, premature mortality).

The number of people around the world suffering from diabetes has skyrocketed in the last two decades from 30 million to 230 million, claiming millions of lives and severely taxing the health-care systems that are dealing with the epidemic, according to data released recently by the International Diabetes Federation (IDF). The number of diabetics is expected to rise to 360 million by 2030.[30] While the growing problem of diabetes in the United States and other developed countries has been well documented, the IDF's data show that 7 of the 10 countries with the highest number of diabetics are in the developing world. China has the largest number of diabetics over the age of 20, around 39 million people or about 2.7% of the adult population. India has the second largest number of cases with an estimated 20 million people, or about 6% of the adult population. In some countries in the Caribbean and the Middle East, the percentage of diabetic people ranged from 12% to 20%; the highest ratio was posted in Nauru, an island in the South Pacific.

While type 2 diabetes was traditionally thought of as affecting only older people, in recent years it has been showing up in individuals of younger and younger ages. Diabetes in children is routinely assumed to be type 1. However, recent studies have reported marked increases in the prevalence of type 2 diabetes in children and adolescents, lowering considerably the age at which people are affected by diabetes today with the largest number now being found to be between the ages of 40 and 59, as opposed to the previous age of 60 and older.

There are many factors driving the growth of diabetes worldwide, but most experts agree that changes in lifestyle and diet are the chief culprits, in addition to genetic predisposition. As developing countries rapidly industrialize, people tend to do work involving less physical activity. At the same time, the availability of food that is cheap but high in calories becomes more common. This combination causes weight gain, which leads to a greater risk of developing type 2 diabetes. The increase in prevalence of the disease in developing countries parallels the increase in obesity.

19.3 DIAGNOSIS OF DIABETES

Patients with type 1 diabetes can be usually recognized by the abrupt appearance of polyuria (frequent urination), polydipsia (excessive thirst), and polyphagia (excessive hunger), which is often triggered by stress or illness. These symptoms are usually accompanied by rapid weight loss and weakness, and an unequivocal elevation of blood glucose (200 mg/dl). Fasting plasma glucose levels above 140 mg/dl on two occasions are diagnostic for both types of diabetes.

An oral glucose tolerance test (OGTT) is indicated for those with fasting plasma glucose close to 140 mg/dl. The patient is given 75 g of glucose orally following an overnight fast. Plasma glucose levels are determined at 30 minutes and at 2 hours after glucose ingestion. Fasting plasma glucose level is initially higher (greater than 125 mg/dl) in the diabetic person and rises to concentrations greater than 200 mg/dl 2 hours following the oral administration of glucose. The rate of glomerular filtration of glucose exceeds that of tubular reabsorption in the kidney (approximately 180 mg/dl) and glucose appears in the urine. In contrast, normal individuals show a fasting plasma glucose level of 70–90 mg/dl and a rise to only about 140 mg/dl following glucose load. The diagnosis of diabetes is made when two fasting plasma glucose levels are 126 mg/ml or higher. Other options are a value of 200 mg/dl or higher 2 hours after oral glucose administration. Persons with fasting plasma glucose levels ranging from 110 to 125 mg/dl are said to have impaired fasting glucose (IFG), while those with levels of 200 mg/dl or higher 2 hours after oral glucose administration are said to have IGT. Both IFG and IGT are considered prediabetes and are associated with increased risk for diabetes.

The ability of glucose to react nonenzymatically with free amino groups in proteins has led to the development of several tests that can be used to assess the level of blood glucose over a period of days or months. Glucose condenses with the amino terminal valine residue of the β chain of hemoglobin to form glycohemoglobin (GH), also called HbA1c. The amount of nonenzymatic glycated protein formed is proportional to the glucose concentration and the time of exposure. Diabetics have a higher percentage of GH than do normal individuals (6%–15% compared to 3%–5%). A 1% change in GH can represent a 25–35 mg/dl change in mean plasma glucose. The half-life of modified hemoglobin is equal to that of erythrocytes. Thus the measurement of GH provides an index of the average plasma glucose level over about 2 months. Tests are also available for the assessment of glycosylated albumin (GA), and since albumin's half-life is shorter than that of hemoglobin, the GA value reflects plasma glucose levels over only a few weeks. Both of these tests are extremely useful measurements of glucose control in diabetics, but neither is as sensitive as OGTT in the diagnosis of diabetes.

19.4 ROLE OF ADIPONECTIN, OSTEOCALCIN, FETUIN-A, AND MELATONIN

19.4.1 ADIPONECTIN

Adiponectin is a protein hormone secreted from adipose tissue into the bloodstream. However, paradoxically, people who are obese have reduced concentrations of the hormone. Weight reduction increases circulating adiponectin levels.

Mounting physiological and genetic evidence strongly implicates adiponectin in the development of type 2 diabetes.[18] Reduced levels are documented in obese, insulin-resistant, and type 2 diabetes–affected patients. But adiponectin levels are higher in patients with type 1 diabetes. Insulin-sensitizing antidiabetic drugs given to insulin-resistant individuals cause an increase in adiponectin levels. Administration of adiponectin increases insulin sensitivity in animals. Adiponectin has thus been proposed as an important mediator of insulin resistance in people who are obese.

Preclinical and metabolic studies in humans have suggested that adiponectin might decrease the risk of type 2 diabetes. Proposed mechanisms include suppression of gluconeogenesis and stimulation of fatty acid oxidation, glucose uptake, and insulin secretion. Studies done on the Pima Indian population suggest that those who have high levels of blood adiponectin are less likely to develop type 2 diabetes than those with low levels of this protein hormone.

19.4.2 Osteocalcin

Osteocalcin, the second most abundant protein in bone after collagen, is involved in the mineralization of bone and calcium homeostasis. A recent study has revealed a novel metabolic role for this protein in the regulation of blood glucose and fat deposition.[14] Osteocalcin is shown to influence pancreatic β cell function and insulin sensitivity, adiponectin production, energy expenditure, and adiposity.[17,31]

Mice lacking the gene that encodes osteocalcin, an osteoblast-specific secreting protein, exhibited glucose intolerance, insulin resistance, and impaired insulin secretion compared with wild-type mice. Osteocalcin-deficient mice also had high serum triglycerides and adiposity. Administration of purified osteocalcin to osteocalcin-deficient animals corrected their glucose tolerance and enhanced their insulin secretion. In addition, osteocalcin caused an increase in the secretion of adiponectin from adipose tissue. When mice receiving osteocalcin were fed a high-fat diet, they gained significantly less weight and had normal serum triglyceride levels compared with mice not given osteocalcin.

Studies in postmenopausal women demonstrated that subjects in the highest quartile for serum osteocalcin had reduced fasting glucose and HbA1c levels compared with subjects in the lowest quartile. Serum osteocalcin levels were lower in type 2 diabetes patients and patients treated with oral antidiabetic drugs or insulin. Serum osteocalcin levels were negatively correlated with body mass index. Several other studies in humans have shown that people with type 2 diabetes have low serum osteocalcin levels.

It is known that exercise plays an important role in lowering blood glucose levels. It is also true that a sedentary lifestyle is partly responsible for the rise in the incidence of diabetes. It may be possible that building bone mass by exercise, especially working with weights, increases osteocalcin levels and in turn boosts insulin production and insulin sensitivity. So, this is another good reason to exercise regularly. The understanding of the role of osteocalcin as a hormone may help find newer approaches for the treatment of diabetes and obesity.

19.4.3 Fetuin-A

Fetuin-A is a protein produced in the liver and secreted into the bloodstream. For a long time it has been known to have an important function in protecting against vascular calcification by keeping calcium and phosphorus solubilized in serum. Animal and human studies suggest that the protein may play a role in the pathogenesis of type 2 diabetes.

Fetuin-A[15] was found to be an endogenous inhibitor of the insulin-stimulated insulin receptor tyrosine kinase. Administration of fetuin-A to rodents inhibited insulin-stimulated tyrosine phosphorylation of insulin receptor. In addition, fetuin-A knockout mice exhibited increased insulin sensitivity and were resistant to the adipogenic effect of high-fat diet, supporting the hypothesis that fetuin-A is involved in the pathogenesis of insulin resistance in rodents.

In a recent study,[28] researchers measured the levels of fetuin-A in 519 diabetes-free individuals aged 70–79 years and followed them for 6 years for the development of diabetes. Participants with the highest levels of plasma fetuin-A showed a high risk of developing diabetes when compared to those with low levels of this protein. The association between fetuin-A and diabetes was independent of individuals' levels of physical activity and other risk factors for diabetes. In another study of 27,548 subjects (16,644 women and 10,904 men) between the ages of 35 and 65 years, investigators followed them from 1998 to 2005 for the development of diabetes. They found that high plasma fetuin-A levels at baseline predicted the incidence of diabetes independently of other established risk factors for the disease, thus supporting the hypothesis that fetuin-A may play a role in the development of type 2 diabetes. Several groups are currently studying fetuin-A's actions in the body, and there is interest in developing a drug to neutralize fetuin-A. Ideally, the drug needs to disable fetuin-A's action on the insulin receptor while not disturbing its blood calcium duties.

19.4.4 MELATONIN

Scientists have recently found a surprising connection between sleep and the regulation of glucose levels in blood. A common variant of MTNR1B, a gene that codes for the human melatonin receptor, was found to be associated with higher fasting glucose levels and risk of diabetes.[5] Melatonin receptor was thought to be primarily expressed in the brain. But recently it has been shown to be also present in pancreatic β cells in humans, mice, and rats. Secretion of melatonin, a neurohormone that regulates circadian rhythm, is lowest during the day and peaks at night, which is opposite to the pattern of insulin secretion.

The presence of melatonin receptor on the insulin-secreting cells makes it likely that the receptor is directly controlling the output of insulin. When researchers added melatonin to human β cells in vitro, insulin production went down. That melatonin and insulin are connected makes sense, because in the middle of the night when melatonin levels are high the need for insulin should be low.

Population studies have shown that diabetes rates rise as sleep declines. A study has found that people who get less than 5 hours of sleep a night were significantly more likely to have type 2 diabetes. Experiments on sleep performed in the laboratory confirm this trend. Healthy young adults who were prevented from entering deep sleep for just three nights could not properly regulate blood sugar levels. And the subjects became more resistant to insulin during the study, eventually reaching the level of insulin sensitivity that resembled the insulin resistance of diabetic people.

Several studies have identified melatonin receptor mutations that are associated with increased average blood glucose level and about 20% increased risk of developing type 2 diabetes. The observations on melatonin's impact on insulin-producing cells are interesting. More studies are needed to fully understand how melatonin affects blood sugar levels and the development of diabetes. It would also be important to study the glucose levels in people who take melatonin supplements to aid sleep and to track the incidence of diabetes in this group of people.

19.5 MECHANISM OF INSULIN ACTION

Insulin activates the transport system and the enzymes involved in intracellular utilization and storage of glucose, amino acids, and fatty acids; it increases the permeability of many cells to potassium. It also inhibits catabolic processes such as the breakdown of glycogen, fat, and protein. The actions of insulin are initiated by binding to cell surface receptors, which are ligand-activated tyrosine protein kinases.

The receptor is a plasma membrane glycoprotein. It consists of two α subunits and two β subunits linked by disulfide bonds to form a β-α-α-β heterotetramer. The α subunits are entirely extracellular and contain the insulin-binding domain, while the β subunits are transmembrane proteins that possess tyrosine-specific protein kinase activity. Insulin binding to the α subunits stimulates the tyrosine kinase activity of the β subunits, which in turn results in receptor autophosphorylation, conformational changes in the β subunits, and activation of the receptor kinase toward other substrates. These and other adaptor proteins initiate a complex cascade of phosphorylation reactions, ultimately resulting in the widespread metabolic effects of insulin.

The function of insulin is to control carbohydrate metabolism. Homeostatic mechanisms maintain plasma glucose concentrations between 55 and 110 mg/dl. A minimum concentration of 40–60 mg/dl is required to provide adequate fuel for the central nervous system, which uses glucose as the primary energy source and is independent of insulin for glucose utilization. Muscles and adipose tissues also use glucose as a major source of energy, but these tissues require insulin for glucose uptake. If glucose is unavailable, these tissues are able to use other substrates such as amino acids and fatty acids for fuel.

Normally we experience an increased blood glucose level shortly after food is ingested, a postprandial hyperglycemia. The β cells of the islets of Langerhans sense the increased levels of circulating glucose and secrete insulin. This hormone lowers the concentration of glucose in the blood by inhibiting glucose production (glycogenolysis and gluconeogenesis) and by stimulating the uptake of glucose by muscles and adipose tissues. The liver does not require insulin for glucose transport, but insulin inhibits gluconeogenesis and facilitates the conversion of glucose to glycogen and free fatty acids. The latter are esterified to triglycerides, which are transported as very low-density lipoproteins (VLDLs) to adipose tissue. In muscle, insulin promotes the uptake of glucose and its conversion to glycogen. It also stimulates the uptake of amino acids and their conversion to protein and inhibits protein degradation in muscle and other tissues. It thus causes a decrease in the circulating concentration of most amino acids, except alanine. Insulin does not lower alanine concentration because it enhances the rate of transamination of pyruvate to alanine.

In adipose tissue, glucose is converted to free fatty acids and stored as triglycerides. Insulin inhibits hormone-sensitive lipase in adipose tissue and prevents the breakdown of triglycerides stored in adipose tissue to free fatty acids that may be transported to other tissues for utilization. This counteracts the lipolytic action of glucagon, epinephrine, and other hormones, and also reduces the concentration of glycerol (a substrate for gluconeogenesis) and free fatty acids (substrates for the production of ketone bodies).

As blood glucose concentration drops to normal during fasting, insulin release is inhibited and simultaneously a number of counterregulatory hormones that oppose the effect of insulin are released (e.g., glucagon, epinephrine). As a result, several processes maintain normal blood glucose for the central nervous system.

19.6   COMPLICATIONS OF DIABETES

In diabetes mellitus, either insufficient insulin levels or insufficient insulin action reduces the transport of glucose into muscle and adipose tissue. As the glucose is not rapidly taken up by these tissues in the absence of insulin, the inability to clear the blood of glucose is a typical characteristic of diabetes. In an untreated type 1 diabetic patient, the level of insulin is too low and that of glucagon is too high relative to the needs of the patient. Under these conditions, glycolysis is inhibited and gluconeogenesis is stimulated. The high glucagon to insulin ratio also promotes glycogen breakdown; therefore, the hyperglycemic state is exaggerated. Blood glucose is often elevated to such a point that the renal threshold (about 180 mg/dl) is exceeded and the glucose spills in the urine (glucosuria). Thus, the potential energy of the excreted glucose is lost to the body, resulting in hunger, weight loss, and fatigue. Excessive thirst and urination result from body water being utilized for the excretion of glucose.

Amylin is a peptide hormone also secreted by pancreatic β cells in parallel with insulin secretion during meals. Amylin has been found to complement the effects of insulin in postprandial glucose control.[26] Amylin acts to delay gastric emptying and inhibit glucagon secretion. It decreases food intake by causing the central nervous system to signal satiety. Amylin knockout mice fail to achieve the normal anorexia following food consumption.

In diabetes, adipose tissue is deficient in glucose (no transport) and therefore has a reduced supply of the glycerol-3-phosphate required for the synthesis of triglycerides. In the absence of insulin, there is no (negative) control of the hormone-sensitive lipase and there is increased breakdown of fat and oxidation of fatty acids to acetyl coenzyme A (CoA); however, much of the acetyl CoA cannot enter the citric acid cycle because of the inadequate supply of oxaloacetate required for the condensation steps. Consequently, acetyl CoA is converted to acetoacetic and h-hydroxybutyric acids (i.e., ketone bodies). Muscle tissues may use some ketone bodies for energy metabolism. Usually, there is excessive production and loss of these substances from the blood by way of the lungs and the kidneys. Acetoacetate readily breaks down into acetone, which is exhaled in the breath. Hence, a characteristic acute phase of the diabetic patient is the so-called acetone breath. Urinary excretion of ketone bodies results in the loss of sodium, and a state of acidosis occurs. Some of the metabolic complications of diabetes are listed in Table 19.2.

Ordinarily, a normal person on a mixed diet excretes less than 0–1 g of ketone bodies in 24 hours. In ketosis (excessive ketone bodies in blood), values as high as 100 g/day or even higher have been

TABLE 19.2
Metabolic Complications of Diabetes

Protein	Carbohydrate	Fat
Decreased synthesis	Glucose availability in muscles and fat cells is decreased	Decreased synthesis
Increased catabolism	—	Increased lipolysis
Urinary increase in nitrogen and potassium	Decreased glycogenesis, increased glycogenolysis, increased gluconeogenesis	Increased blood lipids
Increased gluconeogenesis	Hyperglycemia, glucosuria; increased volume of urine, dehydration	Ketonemia, ketonuria; loss of urinary sodium, acidosis

reported. This is an acute consequence of diabetes and is treated by the administration of insulin and the management of fluid, acid–base, and electrolyte balances.

The chronic consequences of diabetes involve tissues that do not require insulin (e.g., ocular lens, peripheral nerves, renal glomeruli). In these tissues, the intracellular level of glucose parallels that in plasma. Among the many complications of diabetes are kidney disease, gangrene, cardiovascular disease, retinopathy, and damage to the blood vessels and the nervous system. Kidney disease is 17 times more common among diabetics than among nondiabetics, and 75% of chronic kidney disease cases are due to diabetes and/or hypertension. Scientists have long attributed diabetic kidney disease (DKD)—the leading cause of renal failure—to high glucose levels in the blood and defects in the kidney microvasculature. A recent study[29] suggests that there is a "direct effect of insulin" on epithelial cells (known as podocytes) in the kidney. And DKD likely results from defective insulin signaling in the kidneys. Heart disease and stroke are twice as common, and blindness is 25 times as common among diabetics as among nondiabetics. The life expectancy of a diabetic patient is about a third less than that of the general population.

The risk of cardiovascular disease is significantly higher in patients with diabetes mellitus. The most common lipid abnormality in type 2 diabetes is hypertriglyceridemia with lower levels of high-density lipoprotein (HDL) cholesterol. Poor control of type 1 diabetes also is associated with elevated LDL cholesterol levels as well as hypertriglyceridemia. Lipoproteins may be glycosylated (because of high plasma glucose), resulting in their abnormal function. All of these lipid abnormalities contribute to the risk of cardiovascular disease. Coronary heart disease (CHD) is the leading cause of premature death in individuals with type 2 diabetes. Compared with nondiabetic individuals, those with diabetes are 2–3 times more likely to develop CHD, and their risk of death following a myocardial infarction also is 2–3 times higher than their non-diabetic counterparts. These sobering figures point to the importance of minimizing or eliminating all other preventable risk factors for cardiovascular disease in patients with diabetes (e.g. smoking, hypertension, obesity) through the prescription of exercise, diet, and appropriate medication.

Hypertension occurs more frequently in patients with diabetes compared with the nondiabetic population, but the cause is unknown. Patients with type 1 diabetes are usually normotensive in the absence of nephropathy, but the blood pressure rises within 1–2 years following the onset of nephropathy. Thus, hypertension in a type 1 diabetic patient is usually of renal origin. The relationship between hypertension and type 2 diabetes is more complex and is not as closely correlated with the presence of nephropathy. Hyperinsulinemia may contribute to the pathogenesis by decreasing the renal excretion of sodium or through some other mechanism.

Metabolic syndrome (MS; insulin resistance syndrome), also known as syndrome X, is a term used to describe a constellation of derangements that includes insulin resistance,[16,19] hypertension, dyslipidemia, central obesity, endothelial dysfunction, and accelerated cardiovascular disease.

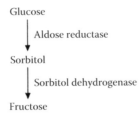

FIGURE 19.1   The synthesis of fructose from glucose via sorbitol.

Epidemiological evidence supports hyperinsulinemia as a marker of coronary artery disease, although an etiological role has not been demonstrated.

Although the mechanisms accounting for the development of diabetic complications are probably multifactorial, most authorities accept a correlation between the degree and duration of hyperglycemia and the frequency of complications; but the precise pathogenic mechanisms for the development of diabetic complications are poorly understood. The toxic effects of hyperglycemia may be the result of nonenzymatic protein glycation, increased formation of sorbitol, and decreased level of myoinositol.

Hyperglycemia may promote the condensation of glucose with cellular proteins in a reaction analogous to the formation of GH. These glycated proteins may mediate some of the early microvascular changes of diabetes and nerve disorders. GH may not release its oxygen normally and this may lead to blood vessel diseases, which in turn may damage the eyes, kidneys, and other organs.

Individuals with diabetes are at increased risk for cataracts. Control of blood glucose, blood pressure, and blood cholesterol reduces the onset and progression of retinopathy. Elevated intracellular glucose concentrations and an adequate supply of reduced nicotinamide adenine dinucleotide phosphate (NADPH) cause the formation of sorbitol; this is catalyzed by aldose reductase. Sorbitol may also be converted to fructose by NAD-dependent sorbitol dehydrogenase (Figure 19.1). Sorbitol (and also fructose) diffuses poorly across cell membranes and thus accumulates inside the cell, causing osmosis-induced disturbances. An increased concentration of sorbitol is seen in the human lens and other tissues in diabetics. Some of the pathological alterations associated with diabetes may be attributed to this phenomenon, including cataract formation, peripheral neuropathy, and vascular problems. There are inhibitors of aldose reductase that prevent the accumulation of sorbitol in these tissues. These may prove useful in the treatment of the symptoms of nerve injury in humans.

Another metabolic disturbance in nerves is a reduction in myoinositol content. Inositol is a component of the membrane phospholipid phosphatidyl inositol and of the second messenger inositol triphosphate. The mechanism for decreased tissue myoinositol levels in diabetics is not known; however, aldose reductase inhibitors, which decrease the formation of sorbitol, also increase the level of inositol in nerves. The myoinositol depletion in diabetics may be, in part, due to the competition between glucose (and sorbitol) and myoinositol for intracellular transport because of their structural similarity.

Several other medical conditions are associated with diabetes. The Nurses' Health Study has found that postmenopausal women with diabetes had a slightly greater risk for breast cancer. People with diabetes face a risk of old-age dementia that is roughly 50% greater than those without diabetes. One study showed that for every percentage point increase in HbA1c—on average glucose control over a few months—there was a small drop in tests for memory, the ability to multitask, and other cognitive tests. Diabetes increases the risk for Alzheimer's disease. Diabetes is associated with depression. In addition, persons who are depressed are at increased risk for diabetes.

19.7   DIETARY MANAGEMENT

Diet is the cornerstone of treatment for both forms of diabetes.[12,21] In general, diabetics have the same nutritional requirements as do nondiabetic individuals of the same age, sex, height, and activity; however, the patient's nutritional intake must be carefully monitored in order to minimize the load placed on the blood sugar–regulating mechanism. For this reason, the treatment of all diabetics involves some form of dietary modification, and any of the following three programs may be selected depending on the severity of the disorder: (1) diet alone, (2) diet and oral hypoglycemic agents, and (3) diet and insulin. Patients with type 1 diabetes are treated with insulin and diet modification, whereas those with type 2 diabetes are treated with diet alone, oral hypoglycemic drugs, or insulin, depending on the severity of the disease. Persons with mild type 2 diabetes can frequently be controlled by diet therapy.

There are several classes of oral medications available for type 2 diabetes: Sulfonylureas stimulate the pancreas to secrete more insulin. The most widely used are glibenclamide and gliclazide. Biguanidines work by reducing the release of glucose from glycogen stores and by provoking an increase in the cellular uptake of glucose in body tissues. One of the most widely used is metformin. Triazolidines increase insulin sensitivity, and an example is rosiglitazone. The α-glucosidase inhibitors such as acarbose inhibit the digestion of dietary starch, reducing the amount of absorbed glucose.

The diet should meet all the nutritional needs compatible with good health practices in the general population. The use of special "diabetic foods" appears to offer no advantage because the dietary prescription can be met with commonly used foods. The ultimate goal of nutrition intervention is a healthy individual with normal longevity. Nutritional therapy attempts to diminish the effects of the disease by maintaining a normal metabolic state. This is done by normalizing blood glucose levels through the enhancement of insulin sensitivity and optimization of glucose use and glucose production. This helps maintain normal blood levels of other fuel sources such as fatty acids, ketone bodies, and amino acids. For patients receiving insulin, special attention needs to be given to the timing of meals and the distribution of foods to avoid a large variation in blood glucose levels. Hypoglycemic episodes are harmful to the brain and should be avoided at all costs in patients receiving insulin or oral hypoglycemic agents. For all diabetic individuals, meals and snacks should be well integrated with activity and exercise, because exercise increases insulin availability and insulin sensitivity. A readily absorbable form of carbohydrates, such as fruit juice, candy, sugar, or glucose solution, should be readily available.

19.8 DIETARY FACTORS

19.8.1 Energy

Probably the most effective dietary management for NIDD is caloric restriction for weight reduction, because most individuals with this type of diabetes are obese. It has been shown that the higher the average bodyweight in the population, the greater the prevalence of diabetes. In many patients, the disease disappears after as little as a 10% weight loss even in those who were as much as 30% overweight at the time of diagnosis; however, a program for energy restriction must be tailored to individual needs. A diabetic person who is at, or near, the ideal weight must still control his or her energy intake. In this case, the goals are adequate nutrient intake, maintenance of weight, and prevention of obesity. Children with type 1 diabetes do not require caloric limitation. The nutrients must provide sufficient energy for normal growth and development, otherwise growth retardation occurs. Patients with type 2 diabetes who are young should be treated as adults except that their energy intake must be adequate for normal growth and development without gaining excess weight. Children with good control of sugar will gain weight rapidly if they overeat beyond their energy needs. Regular exercise is a valuable adjunct to therapy. Exercise increases caloric expenditure and is of value in achieving weight loss in overweight patients. Both diet and exercise have a major effect on increasing insulin sensitivity in individuals with type 1 or type 2 diabetes. Exercise also tends to lower plasma triglyceride levels with concomitant increases in HDL cholesterol, both of which may be beneficial in preventing atherosclerosis.

19.8.2 Carbohydrate

Historically, the primary goal of diet therapy for diabetics has been the reduction of carbohydrate intake. A high-carbohydrate diet is known to cause higher postprandial blood glucose levels, temporary worsening of glycemic control, and an increase in fasting serum triglycerides. The recent trend, however, has been to liberalize dietary carbohydrate intake in patients with diabetes mellitus, and it appears that the plasma glucose response to a standard oral glucose challenge is improved if patients with diabetes ingest a high-carbohydrate diet for several days. Individuals are more sensitive to insulin when consuming high-carbohydrate diets as opposed to high-fat diets, because they have an increased number of insulin receptors. Of greater importance is the enhanced intracellular glucose metabolism associated with high-carbohydrate diets. As loss of normal insulin sensitivity seems to characterize patients with type 2 diabetes, a high-carbohydrate diet would seem to be the treatment of choice for these patients.

It is generally recommended that 55%–60% of calories be supplied by carbohydrates. This level of carbohydrate intake facilitates diabetes management in children as well as adults with IDD and NIDD. Complex carbohydrates (found in grain products and root vegetables) should account for a major portion of total carbohydrate calories. Sucrose and other caloric sweeteners with a high glycemic index should be limited to 10% of the calories at each meal. The glycemic response (the ability to contribute to the concentration of blood glucose) to 50 g of glucose, maltose, or sucrose is much higher than the response to 50 g of starch. Fructose offers an advantage over sucrose for diabetic individuals because it is about 1.7 times sweeter, is metabolized without insulin, and produces less hyperglycemia. It produces only 20% of the glycemic response of glucose and 33% of the response of sucrose. Fructose is present in fruits, honey, and corn syrup.

Inositol is a six-carbon sugar that is related to glucose in terms of configuration. It is widely distributed in foods of both plant and animal origin as part of the phosphatidyl inositol of the cell membrane and as free inositol. It can be endogenously synthesized from glucose. Diabetics have an intracellular deficiency of inositol, especially in the nerves. The deficiency is attributed to increased urinary excretion; decreased formation of inositol, because less glucose is available inside the cell and one of the enzymes involved in the synthesis, glucokinase, is insulin dependent; and competition between glucose and sorbitol for the intracellular transport of inositol.

There are reports suggesting that the secondary complications of diabetes (i.e., renal disease) can be ameliorated by dietary inositol supplementation. Some investigators have shown a reversal of the diabetes-induced increased glomerular filtration rate with a sevenfold to tenfold increase in dietary levels of inositol. Thus, diabetics may have a significantly greater need for inositol than nondiabetics. There may be a broad range of inositol requirements as there is a range of severity of diabetes. There is an increased interest to learn more about the role of inositol in cell function and dietary requirements of this sugar in diabetics.

Alternative sweeteners such as sorbitol, aspartame, saccharin, and acesulfame K have been advocated as substitutes for sucrose to provide sweetness without hyperglycemia or increased calories for individuals with diabetes. Sorbitol, a sugar alcohol, is used as a sweetener because it is poorly absorbed from the gastrointestinal tract and thus reduces the prompt increase in plasma glucose characteristic of dietary carbohydrate. Sorbitol is half as sweet as sucrose but provides calories equal to those of sucrose.

The artificial sweeteners presently available for use in the United States include aspartame (Nutrasweet), saccharin, sucralose, and acesulfame K. Aspartame is a dipeptide made up of aspartyl-phenylalanyl methyl ester. It is about 200 times sweeter than sugar. Technically, it is a nutritive sweetener that provides 4 Cal/g, but compared to the sweetness of sucrose the amount required would only supply about 0.5% of the calories provided by sugar. Saccharin is 300 times sweeter, sucralose is 500 times sweeter, and acesulfame K is 200 times sweeter than sugar. The risks, benefits, and effects of these sweeteners in individuals with diabetes have not been fully tested. Because diabetics are likely to ingest greater quantities of these sweeteners than the general population, there is a need for extensive research to determine the long-term effect of these sweeteners on appetite, weight gain, blood glucose, and insulin levels in diabetic individuals.

19.8.3 FAT

High-fat diets have metabolic disadvantages. They cause insulin resistance and impair intracellular glucose metabolism in several tissues, thus decreasing glucose transport into muscle and adipose tissues and decreasing the activity of insulin-stimulated processes. A high-fat diet increases the risk of atherosclerosis. Because diabetics are much more likely to develop atherosclerosis at an early age and be more severely affected by the condition than nondiabetic individuals, the restriction of dietary fat and cholesterol by substituting carbohydrate seems to be wise. The fat intake, therefore, should represent no more than 30% of calories and should contain a good ratio (1:1:1) of polyunsaturated to monounsaturated to saturated fatty acids, in order to delay the development of atherosclerosis. Cholesterol intake must be restricted to less than 300 mg/day. Vegetable fats are preferred over fats of animal origin. The recommended cholesterol intake is <300 mg/day for diabetic patients with normal plasma cholesterol concentrations. For patients with elevated LDL, <7% of total calories should be from saturated fat and cholesterol intake should be restricted to <200 mg/day.

19.8.4 PROTEIN

The amount of protein required by the average diabetic is similar to that for a normal person. Proteins should be of reasonably high quality and should provide all the amino acids necessary for adequate nutrition. Proteins should provide about 15% of the total calories, or 0.8 g/kg desirable body weight for adults. Protein consumption should be about 20% of the total calories, or 1.5 g/kg body weight daily in children and in pregnant and lactating women. With the onset of nephropathy, a lower protein intake of 0.6 g/kg/day is considered sufficiently restrictive.

19.8.5 ALCOHOL

The metabolism of alcohol does not require insulin, and it would appear to offer some theoretical advantages; however, alcohol is high in calories (7 Cal/g) and is of no other nutritive value. It tends to promote hypertriglyceridemia. In a small minority of patients who have high blood sulfonylurea (hypoglycemic drug) levels, alcohol produces distressing symptoms. Even so, in most patients an occasional drink can be permitted. A convenient way is to trade fat calories for alcohol calories. Excess alcohol should be avoided because it inhibits gluconeogenesis.

19.8.6 DIETARY FIBER

Dietary fiber influences glucose assimilation and reduces serum cholesterol. Research has shown that certain plant fibers delay the absorption of carbohydrate and result in less postprandial hyperglycemia. Increased fiber in the diet is associated with reduced insulin resistance. An increase in fiber from whole grains, legumes, and vegetables may appear to be beneficial for diabetics. It is recommended that adult diabetics consume about 40 g/day of dietary fiber.

19.8.7 VITAMINS AND MINERALS

Special vitamin and mineral supplementation is ordinarily not required by diabetics. These nutrients should be provided at the recommended dietary allowance (RDA) levels. Recent studies have shown that people with diabetes mellitus have at least 30% lower vitamin C concentration in the blood than persons without diabetes. Vitamin C supplementation (1 g/day) for 3 months has little effect on blood glucose concentration, but does lower glycosylated hemoglobin by 18%. Vitamin C may inhibit the glycosylation of proteins in vivo by a competitive mechanism. Vitamin C supplementation (2 g/day) for 3 weeks lowers erythrocyte sorbitol levels by 44.5% and reduces capillary fragility. Fruits and vegetables are the main sources of vitamin C. Eating even a small quantity of fruits and vegetables may be beneficial. Also, recent studies have shown that the protection against diabetes increases progressively with the quantity of fruits and vegetables consumed.

Vitamin C supplementation may provide a simple means of preventing and ameliorating the complications of diabetes without the use of drugs. Vitamin D deficiency appears to be common among people with type 2 diabetes. Studies have shown a significant positive correlation between serum 25-hydroxy-vitamin D (a measure of vitamin D nutritional status), insulin sensitivity, and pancreatic β cell function.[1] Vitamin D supplementation should be of benefit to patients with diabetes.

Chromium reportedly affects insulin secretion and glucose metabolism. Chromium or brewer's yeast (which contains a high concentration of chromium complex) has been given to adults having NIDD with variable results. Some investigators found an improvement in glucose tolerance, but in others no change in glucose metabolism was noted. These data suggest that in some patients chromium deficiency may be a factor in impaired glucose metabolism but there is as yet no clinical indication for the use of chromium in the treatment of diabetes.

19.9   PHYSICAL ACTIVITY

Exercise is an integral component of comprehensive diabetes care that can have positive benefits, particularly in type 2 diabetes because obesity and inactivity contribute to the development of glucose intolerance in genetically predisposed individuals. A regular program of physical activity contributes to body fat reduction, improves blood lipids, and lowers blood pressure. For individuals with type 1 and type 2 diabetes, exercise is also useful for lowering plasma glucose (during and following exercise) and for increasing insulin sensitivity.

Despite these benefits, exercise presents severe challenges for individuals with diabetes because they lack glucose regulatory mechanisms. The skeletal muscle is a major site for metabolic fuel consumption during resting states, and increased muscle activity during moderate to heavy exercise greatly increases glucose requirements. Muscle glycogen stores are depleted quite rapidly, after which glucose is derived from the peripheral circulation. To meet the increased glucose demands, hepatic glycogenolysis and gluconeogenesis increase. This is mediated primarily through the suppression of insulin secretion and the increased secretion of counterregulatory hormones such as glucagon. Low permissive levels of insulin are required for glucose uptake by the muscle. Peripheral glucose utilization remains high after exercise has been discontinued; this is thought to be related to the replenishment of glycogen stores in the liver and muscle. In nondiabetic individuals, hepatic glucose output and peripheral utilization are balanced such that normal plasma glucose level is maintained during and after exercise.

In type 1 diabetic individuals, exercise may cause hyperglycemia or hypoglycemia, depending on preexercise plasma glucose concentration, the circulating insulin level, and the levels of exercise-induced counterregulatory hormones. If the insulin level is low when the individual starts exercising, hepatic glucose output will increase and peripheral glucose utilization will decrease, and hyperglycemia will ensue. This can promote ketone body formation and possibly lead to ketoacidosis. Patients whose plasma glucose concentrations are more than 250 mg/dl should delay exercise because these levels indicate insulin deficiency. Conversely, if the circulating insulin level is excessive, this relative hyperinsulinemia may reduce hepatic glucose production (decreased glycogenolysis and gluconeogenesis) and increase glucose entry into muscles, leading to hypoglycemia. Hypoglycemia is more likely to occur if the blood glucose level is 100 mg/dl or lower just before exercise. Thus, the individual should eat a carbohydrate snack or decrease the dose of insulin.

To avoid exercise-related hyperglycemia or hypoglycemia, individuals with type 1 diabetes should monitor plasma glucose before, during, and after exercise and adjust insulin dose and food intake accordingly. In general, exercise should be avoided at times corresponding to peak insulin action because high insulin levels can suppress the action of counterregulatory hormones.

For patients with type 2 diabetes who are treated with diet alone, exercise is unlikely to cause hypoglycemia. Individuals who take oral hypoglycemic agents or insulin may become hypoglycemic if plasma insulin levels are high enough to increase peripheral utilization of glucose and to suppress hepatic glucose output. Individuals whose plasma glucose is less than 100 mg/dl before exercise should consider increasing their carbohydrate intake. Because patients with type 2 diabetes do not absolutely lack insulin, they are less likely to become hyperglycemic in response to exercise. A light regular exercise routine such as walking or stationary cycling is safe and effective.

19.10   METABOLIC SYNDROME

Metabolic syndrome involves the dysregulation of several measures of health. According to the definition released by the World Health Organization in 1998, it consists of glucose intolerance and/or insulin resistance, plus two or more of the following criteria: hypertension, dyslipidemia, central obesity, and microalbuminuria. The definition developed by the National Cholesterol Education Panel is slightly different, but shares the same general features. It requires three of the following criteria: abdominal obesity as measured by waist circumference, hypertriglyceridemia, low HDL cholesterol, high blood pressure, and elevated fasting glucose (see the definition given in Section 19.10.1). In both definitions, individuals with diabetes are included.

Using either of these definitions, MS is quite prevalent in the United States, but the clinical adoption of MS as a diagnosis seems to be occurring slowly. It is unclear how well the clinical community has adopted MS at this point in time. Partly this may be because physicians do not routinely measure waist circumference, and that value seems to be a better measure of obesity for diagnosing MS than the more commonly used body mass index calculation. Larger waist circumference is an important factor driving the increasing prevalence of MS in the United States.

In healthy individuals, insulin sensitivity varies from sixfold to eightfold along a continuously distributed range. There is no other physiological variable that has that degree of variation in a healthy population. The main causes of this variation include obesity, physical fitness, and genetic factors, with ethnicity playing a particularly important role in modulating risk. Whatever the cause of their insulin resistance, these individuals have hyperinsulinemia, some level of glucose intolerance, and dyslipidemia, which in turn put them at risk for type 2 diabetes, cardiovascular disease, and a number of other health problems, including polycystic ovary syndrome, prostate and breast cancers, and sleep-disordered breathing. Metabolic syndrome in itself is not a disease, but the metabolic abnormalities it encompasses undoubtedly put affected individuals at increased risk for cardiovascular disease.

Metabolic syndrome affects approximately one quarter of the U.S. population, and its prevalence is increasing. Comparing data from 1999–2000 with data from 1988–1994, the overall age-adjusted prevalence of MS increased from 24% to 27% with an even more significant increase among women—from 23.5% to 29%. With the rapidly rising incidence of obesity among children and teenagers, the number of adults with MS is likely to swell. According to the CDC, about 16% of 6–19 year olds in 1999–2002 (more than 9 million youngsters total) were overweight. Studies show that MS is highly prevalent in this group.

19.10.1   DEFINITION OF METABOLIC SYNDROME

According to the National Cholesterol Education Program's ATP III definition, MS involves three or more of the following five criteria:

1. Central/abdominal obesity as measured by waist circumference (men—greater than 40 inches [102 cm]; women—greater than 35 inches [88 cm])
2. Fasting triglycerides greater than or equal to 150 mg/dl (1.69 mmol/L)

3. HDL cholesterol (men—less than 40 mg/dl [1.04 mmol/L]; women—less than 50 mg/dl [1.29 mmol/L])
4. Blood pressure greater than or equal to 130/85 mm Hg
5. Fasting glucose greater than or equal to 110 mg/dl (61 mmol/L)

One study gathered dietary information on more than 9500 men and women ages 45–64 years and tracked their health for 9 years.[19] Overall, a Western dietary pattern—high intakes of refined grains, fried foods, and red meat—was associated with an 18% increased risk for MS, while a "prudent" diet dominated by fruits, vegetables, fish, and poultry correlated with neither an increased nor a decreased risk. Those who ate the most fried foods increased their risk for MS by 25% compared with those who ate the least. And surprisingly the risk of developing MS was 34% higher among those who drank more than one can of soda a day compared with those who drank none.[23]

Another study in more than 6000 middle-aged white residents of Framingham, Massachusetts, found that those who consumed more than one soda per day either regular or diet had a 48% higher risk of having MS.[8] A third study found that diet soda consumption was associated with a 36% greater relative risk of incident MS and a 67% greater relative risk of incident type 2 diabetes compared with nonconsumption of soda. Researchers were uncertain why regular or diet soda seemed to have such a large effect. According to them, it was unlikely that an ingredient in soda caused the effect. It is more likely that consuming sweet sodas can increase the craving for more sweets and that people who indulge in sodas probably have less healthy diets.

Several strategies have been proposed to prevent the development of MS. These include increased physical activity (such as walking 30 minutes a day) and a healthy, reduced-calorie diet.

19.11   LIFESTYLE MODIFICATION TO REDUCE THE RISK OF TYPE 2 DIABETES

Nutrition can also reduce the incidence of diabetes. Two randomized, controlled trials—one conducted in the United States and the other in Finland—have recently been completed. Individuals with IGT were randomly allocated to an intensive lifestyle intervention program or a standard control group. The intervention programs were aimed at achieving a weight reduction of 5% or more; an intake of total and saturated fat of less than 30% and 10% of total energy intakes, respectively; an increase in fiber intake of at least 15 g/1000 Cal; and moderate exercise for at least 30 min/day. Frequent ingestion of whole grain products, fruits, vegetables, low-fat milk, and vegetable oils rich in monounsaturated fatty acids were recommended. Moderate intakes of fish (some oily) and lean meats (and for vegetarians vegetable sources of proteins) were also encouraged. In Finland, these lifestyle programs were associated with a 58% reduction in the risk of developing diabetes, and the 4-year cumulative incidence of diabetes was 11% in the intervention group and 23% in the control group. The results in the United States were similar, with 29% of the control group developing diabetes during the 3-year average follow-up period compared with 14% in the intervention group. To reduce the risk of diabetes, people of all ages should avoid excess weight gain, and those who are overweight should lose weight. This lifestyle management also applies to treatment for people who already have coronary heart disease and diabetes.

19.12   ALTERNATIVE MEDICINE FOR DIABETES

Several herbs may help in managing the symptoms associated with diabetes. These include gardenia fruit extract, bitter melon, cinnamon, aloe, ginseng, and several others. Gardenia fruit extract has been traditionally used in Chinese medicine for centuries to treat the symptoms of diabetes. Recent studies have identified a chemical, genipin, in the extract. Genipin is known for its ability to cross-link proteins.[32] Researchers have found that the chemical also blocks the function of the enzyme called uncoupling protein (UCP2). In both animals and humans, high concentrations of UCP2 appear to inhibit insulin secretion from the pancreas and increase the risk of type 2 diabetes.

Pancreas cells taken from normal mice secrete insulin when treated with genipin or gardenia fruit extract, whereas the cells of mice that lack UCP2 do not. These results suggest that the extract works through its effect on UCP2 enzyme. These findings could lead to the development of genipin-related drugs for diabetes.

Bitter melon is a common vegetable consumed by many people in the Far East and Central and South American countries. It has also been used in India for the treatment of diabetes for a long time. Eating bitter melon as fried slices, water extract, or juice may improve blood sugar control in people with type 2 diabetes according to some clinical trials. Researchers have identified at least four components in bitter melon that stimulate the enzyme called AMP-activated protein kinase (AMPK). The enzyme plays a role in energy metabolism and glucose uptake, processes that are impaired in diabetes. Exercise also activates AMPK in the muscle that in turn mediates the movement of glucose transporters to the cell surface, which is an important step in the uptake of glucose from circulation. Thus, bitter melon has an effect similar to that of exercise on AMPK. A recent scientific study has proved that bitter melon increases insulin sensitivity. In 2007, the Philippine Department of Health issued a circular stating that bitter melon, as a scientifically validated herbal medicinal plant, can lower elevated blood sugar levels.

Cinnamon is commonly used as a spice. It is also known for its potential diabetes benefits. Studies have shown that this spice may lower blood sugar by decreasing insulin resistance in people with type 2 diabetes. In one study, volunteers ate from 1 to 6 g of cinnamon for 40 days. Cinnamon was found to reduce blood sugar levels by 24% and cholesterol levels by 18%. The active compounds are found in the water-soluble portion of cinnamon. The herb can be taken in the form of tea or can be added in juice. Other studies have reported no significant effects after taking 1.5 g of cinnamon for 6 weeks.

Studies done on these and other herbs are only on small groups of people, and they have not explored the long-term benefits of such herbs. There is a need for more research in this field to determine the benefits and safety of these herbs.

Vinegar has been used for its healing properties for thousands of years. It is also used in the kitchen to enhance flavor. It has several health benefits. One of its many uses in the health industry is for dieting purposes. It is said to be a very good appetite suppressant, which increases the feeling of a full stomach, thus causing one to eat less and lose weight. It is also helpful for diabetics. Studies have shown that vinegar can improve insulin sensitivity in healthy or insulin-resistant subjects.

More recently, scientists examined 10 subjects with type 1 diabetes who had an average age of 32 years. Subjects were randomly assigned to consume vinegar (30 ml vinegar and 20 ml water) or placebo (50 ml water) 5 minutes before a meal of bread, cheese, turkey, ham, orange juice, butter, and a cereal bar. At 30 minutes after eating, compared to placebo, vinegar consumption reduced blood glucose by about 20%. Researchers say that patients with type 1 diabetes may supplement their diets with two tablespoons of vinegar, such as in a salad dressing, to lower blood sugar levels.

Diabetes Mellitus in an Obese Woman—A Case

A 38-year-old woman with a history of gradual weight gain over a period of 15 years to her present weight of 468 pounds was hospitalized. Physical examination revealed a well-developed, very obese, middle-aged woman with a height of 5 feet 8 inches. She had no distress except for a pendulous abdomen and massive skin folds. Her blood pressure was 150/100 mm Hg (normal: <125/85 mm Hg).

Routine laboratory tests showed that her blood hemoglobin, hematocrit, electrolytes, total protein, and albumin levels were in the normal range. Blood glucose was 180 mg/dl (normal: 60–100 mg/dl), cholesterol was 265 mg/dl (normal: 150–240 mg/dl), and triglyceride was 267 mg/dl (normal: 25–150 mg/dl). Urinalysis revealed 1+ glycosuria.

After the baseline studies, the patient was fed a 3500-Cal diet daily containing 15% protein, 40% fat, and 45% carbohydrate. On the fourth day, blood was drawn for glucose, insulin, and insulin binding (using radioactive iodine-labeled insulin) studies. On the fifth day, OGTT (100 g of glucose) was performed. The high-calorie diet was succeeded by four 4-day periods of starvation (less than 50 Cal/day), alternating with four 7-day periods of severe caloric restriction (600 Cal/day). After 60 days, a 3500-Cal diet was restored and the OGTT was repeated. The patient lost 29 pounds during the 2-month trial.

Insulin binding studies were carried out using lymphocytes at insulin concentrations between 0.1 and 1 ng/ml. Over this range, the patient's lymphocytes bound between 1.1% and 1.4% of labeled insulin per 56×10^6 cells before weight reduction. Insulin receptors of lymphocytes respond in vivo to the same metabolic influence as do receptors in the liver and fat cells, and are, therefore, suited for the study of the physiology of insulin receptors.

Before weight reduction, the fasting blood glucose level was 155 mg/dl, which increased after ingesting 100 g of glucose to a peak of 250 mg/dl at 90 minutes and remained at this level for 180 minutes. The fasting blood insulin level was 28 μU/ml, which went up to 100 μU and remained elevated during the OGTT. After the period of caloric restriction, the insulin binding of lymphocytes per 56×10^6 cells increased from 1.3% to 3.2%, indicating that the deficit in insulin binding was restored to essentially normal by the caloric restriction. Fasting plasma glucose declined from 155 to 82 mg/dl, and when the OGTT was repeated the peak glucose level was 140 mg/dl. In 180 minutes, it was down to 110 mg/dl. Fasting plasma insulin decreased from 28 to 10 AU/ml.

This very obese patient with mild type 2 diabetes mellitus demonstrated classic insulin resistance, which resolved after a weight loss of 29 pounds.[33,34] Despite being still very obese, the negative caloric balance was a more significant factor in restoring the number of insulin receptors. It is important for physicians to identify obese individuals and to plan for them weight reduction programs with caloric restriction and exercise. This simple remedy may forestall the appearance of more serious disorders of type 2 diabetes mellitus.

REFERENCES

1. Alvarez, J. A., and A. Ashraf. 2010. Role of vitamin D in insulin secretion and insulin sensitivity for glucose homeostasis. *Int J Endocrinol* 2010:351385.
2. American Diabetes Association. 1998. Economic consequences of diabetes mellitus in the U.S. in 1997. *Diabetes Care* 21:296.
3. Aune, D., G. Ursin, and M. B. Valerod. 2009. Meat consumption and the risk of type II diabetes: A systematic review and meta-analysis of cohort studies. *Diabetologia* 52:2277.
4. Berdanier, C. D. 1992. Is inositol an essential nutrient? *Nutr Today* 27 (2):22.
5. Chambers, J. C., W. Zhang, D. Zabaneh et al. 2009. Common genetic variation near melatonin receptor MTNRIB contributes to raised plasma glucose and increased risk of type II diabetes among Indian Asians and Europeans Caucasians. *Diabetes* 58:2703.
6. Danescu, L. G., S. Levy, and J. Levy. 2009. Vitamin D and diabetes mellitus. *Endocrine* 35:11.
7. Davie, S. J., B. J. Gould, and J. S. Yudkin. 1992. Effect of vitamin C on glycosylation of proteins. *Diabetes* 41:167.
8. Dhingra, R., L. Sullivan, P. F. Jacques et al. 2007. Soft drink consumption and risk of developing cardiometabolic risk factors and the metabolic syndrome in middle-aged adults. *Circulation* 116:480.
9. Dyck, R., N. Osgood, T. H. Lin et al. 2010. Epidemiology of diabetes among first nations and non-first nations adults. *J Can Med Assoc* 10:1503.
10. Edelman, S. V. 1998. Type II diabetes mellitus. *Adv Int Med* 43:449.
11. Eisenbarth, G. S., J. Connelly, and J. S. Soeldner. 1987. The "natural history" of Type I diabetes. *Diabetes Metab Rev* 3:873.

12. Franz, M. J., J. P. Bantle, C. A. Beebe et al. 2002. Evidence-based nutrition principles and recommendations for the treatment and prevention of diabetes and related complications. *Diabetes Care* 25:148.

13. Horikawa, Y., N. Oda, N. J. Cox, X. Li et al. 2000. Genetic variation in the gene encoding calpain-10 is associated with type 2 diabetes mellitus. *Nat Genet* 26:163.

14. Im, J. A., B. P. Yu, J. Y. Jeon, and S. H. Kim. 2008. Relationship between osteocalcin and glucose metabolism in postmenopausal women. *Clin Chim Acta* 396:68.

15. Ix, J. H., C. L. Wassel, A. M. Kanaya et al. 2008. Fetuin-A and incident diabetes mellitus in older persons. *J Amer Med Assoc* 300:182.

16. Kelley, D. E. 2000. Overview. What is insulin resistance? *Nutr Rev* 58:S2.

17. Lee, N. K., H. Sowa, E. Hinoi et al. 2007. Endocrine regulation of energy metabolism by the skeleton. *Cell* 130:456.

18. Li, S., H. J. Shin, E. L. Long, and R. M. Van Dam. 2009. Adiponectin levels and risk of type II diabetes. *J Amer Med Assoc* 302:179.

19. Lutsey, P. L., L. M. Stiffen, and J. Stevens. 2008. Dietary intake and the development of the metabolic syndrome: The Atherosclerosis Risk in Communities study. *Circulation* 117:754.

20. Lissenco, V., C. L. Nagomy, M. R. Erdos et al. 2009. Common variant in MTNR1B associated with increased risk of type II diabetes and impaired early insulin secretion. *Nat Genet* 41:82.

21. Narayan, K. M. V., B. A. Bowman, and M. E. Engelgau. 2002. Prevention of type 2 diabetes. *BMJ* 323:63.

22. Nathan, D. M. 1993. Long-term complications of diabetes mellitus. *N Engl J Med* 328:1676.

23. Nettleton, J. A., P. L. Lutsey, Y. Wang et al. 2009. Diet soda intake and risk of incident metabolic syndrome and type II diabetes in the Multi-Ethnic Study of Atherosclerosis (MESA). *Diabetes Care* 2:688.

24. Ozfirat, Z., and T. A. Chowdhury. 2010. Vitamin D deficiency and type II diabetes. *Postgrad Med J* 86:18.

25. Porte Jr., D., and M. W. Schwartz. 1996. Diabetes complications: why is glucose potentially toxic? *Science* 272:699.

26. Roth, J. D., H. Hughes, E. Kendall et al. 2006. Antiobesity effects of the β-cell hormone amylin in diet-induced obese rats: Effects on food intake, body weight, composition, energy expenditure and gene expression. *Endocrinology* 147:5855.

27. Sardesai, V. M., and T. H. Waldshan. 1991. Natural and synthetic sweeteners. *J Nutr Biochem* 2:236.

28. Stefan, N., A. Fritsche, C. Weikert et al. 2008. Plasma fetuin-A levels and the risk of type II diabetes. *Diabetes* 57:2762.

29. Welsh, G. I., L. J. Hale, V. Eremina, et al. 2010. Insulin signaling in the glomerular podocyte is critical for normal kidney function. *Cell Metabolism* 12:329.

30. Wild, S., G. Roglic, A. Green et al. 2004. Global prevalence of diabetes estimates for 2000 and projections for 2030. *Diabetes Care* 27:1047.

31. Winhofer, Y., A. Handi Surya, A. Tura et al. 2010. Osteocalcin is related to enhanced insulin secretion in gestational diabetes mellitus. *Diabetes Care* 25:139.

32. Zhang, C. Y., L. E. Parton, C. P. Ye et al. 2006. Genipin inhibits UCP2-mediated proton leak and acutely reverses obesity- and high glucose-induced b-cell dysfunction in isolated pancreatic islets. *Cell Metab* 3:417.

CASE BIBLIOGRAPHY

33. Archer, J. A., P. Gorden, and J. Roth. 1975. Defect in insulin binding to receptors in obese man; amelioration with calorie restriction. *J Clin Invest* 55:166.

34. Clinical Nutrition Cases. 1987. Diabetes mellitus in an obese woman. *Nutr Rev* 45:51.

20 Nutritional Aspects of Kidney Disease

Renal disease is one of the major sequelae of common disorders such as diabetes and hypertension. Diabetes is the most common cause of chronic kidney disease (CKD) and accounts for nearly 44% of the new cases. About 54% of patients on kidney dialysis have diabetes.

Since the kidney is the major excretory organ for the end products of metabolic processes involved in the utilization of many exogenous nutrients, the nutritional management of a patient with kidney disease is a critical factor in reducing mortality and morbidity. The most common renal problems necessitating careful dietary management are chronic renal failure, acute renal failure, and nephrotic syndrome. The management of kidney stones also requires dietary modifications even though strictly speaking this condition is not due to kidney disease. Each of these conditions requires dietary management whose strategy is quite different and is based on pathophysiological changes present in a particular disease.

20.1 KIDNEY FUNCTIONS

The kidneys are involved in many critical bodily functions. They regulate fluid, electrolytes, and acid–base status by filtration of blood, followed by selective reabsorption from or secretion to the tubular fluid. The kidneys are critical in elimination of waste products, and alteration in renal function is one of the major causes of drug toxicity because of inadequate excretion of drugs or their metabolites. Kidneys also have endocrine functions. They release three important hormones: (1) erythropoietin, which stimulates the bone marrow to make red blood cells; (2) renin, which regulates blood pressure; and (3) the kidney converts vitamin D to 1,25 dihydroxy D, or calcitriol—the hormonally active form of vitamin D—which has a role in the regulation of bone and mineral metabolism. These various functions can best be thought of as related to specific functional subunits of the kidney.

The functional unit of the kidney is the nephron. Each kidney is composed of approximately 1 million nephrons. Its chief function is to regulate the concentration of water and soluble substances like sodium and to filter the blood by absorbing what is needed and excreting the rest as urine. The initial portion of the nephron, the glomerulus, functions to selectively filter blood. It allows water and low molecular weight substances to pass through but retains large compounds such as plasma proteins. With normal glomerular function, approximately 180 L of plasma ultrafiltrate reach the proximal tubule each day. This filtrate contains both waste products and essential plasma constituents such as glucose, electrolytes, amino acids, and minerals. The function of the tubules is to selectively retain essential components filtered by the glomerulus and reabsorb water and electrolytes to maintain normal fluid and electrolyte status. Of the 180 L of water filtered, the kidneys reabsorb all but 1 to 2 L

Currently, determination of serum creatinine and blood urea nitrogen (BUN) and the estimation of glomerular filtration rate (GFR) remain the most important tests to assess kidney function. The values of creatinine and BUN may vary with muscle mass and protein intake as well as the functional status of the liver. Therefore, kidney function is calculated using serum sample and a formula to get the estimated GFR (eGFR). The eGFR corresponds to the percentage of kidney function available. People with healthy kidneys have 100% of their kidney function.

When GFR is decreased due to functional or structural damage to the kidney, a variety of functions and also the structure of the kidney are altered. When GFR is below normal but not low enough, the kidneys try to maintain normal fluid, electrolyte, and acid–base balance. But when GFR is severely decreased, the kidneys retain sodium, water, potassium, magnesium, phosphorus, and hydrogen ions resulting in edema, either hyponatremia or hypernatremia, hyperkalemia, hyperphosphatemia, and severe metabolic acidosis. Hypocalcemia results from decreased formation of calcitriol. The patients also develop hypertension due to retention of sodium and water. Anemia and bone disease are commonly seen in patients with low GFR.

Many organic compounds accumulate when renal failure occurs. Most are the products of amino acid and protein metabolism. Quantitatively, the most prominent are urea, creatinine, and uric acid. Some of these compounds are considered toxic in high concentrations. Accumulation of these compounds and the clinical signs and symptoms that result from renal failure are referred to as uremia. The many symptoms of uremia include weakness, loss of appetite, nausea, vomiting, and diarrhea. If these conditions are not treated by hemodialysis, peritoneal dialysis, or renal transplantation, death will supervene.

People have two kidneys. Humans can live a normal, healthy life with just one kidney as one kidney has more functioning ability than is needed to survive. Every year, thousands of people donate one of their kidneys for transplantation to a family member or a friend. The two forms of renal failure are CKD and acute renal failure.

20.2 CHRONIC KIDNEY DISEASE

Most kidney diseases attack nephrons, causing them to lose filtering capacity. Damage to the nephron can happen quickly, often as a result of injury or poisoning. But most kidney problems happen slowly. A person may have "silent kidney disease" for years. Gradual loss of kidney function is called CKD or chronic renal insufficiency. It is an irreversible, usually progressive diminution in renal function to a degree that has damaging consequences for the patient. People go on to develop permanent kidney failure. They also have a high risk of death from a stroke or heart attack.

About 70% of CKD cases are due to diabetes mellitus and/or hypertension. Other risk factors include family history of kidney disease, glomerulonephritis, use of some drugs, and chronic urologic disorders.

There are 5 stages of CKD. Knowing the different stages helps physicians to determine the type of treatment necessary for patients. The National Kidney Foundation has classified CKD in 5 stages based on glomerular filtration rate, which are shown in Table 20.1.

The U.S. Renal Data Service states in a 2008 report that 31 million Americans have some degree of CKD. Of these, about 300,000 have stage 5 or end-stage kidney failure. They are on dialysis or have a GFR of <15 ml/min. Another 400,000 people have stage 4 (severe disease), and about 7.5 million are at stage 3 (moderate disease). The rest have some kidney damage but have normal or

TABLE 20.1
Stages of Chronic Kidney Failure

Stage	Description	GFR (mL/min)
Normal	Healthy kidneys	≥90
1	Slight kidney damage with normal GFR	≥90
2	Mild kidney failure	60–89
3	Moderate kidney failure	30–59
4	Severe kidney failure	15–29
5	End-stage renal failure	<15

only mildly reduced kidney function. Many people with CKD do not know they have the disease because symptoms are normally subtle until late in the course. With early detection the course of CKD can usually be slowed. In the United States, African Americans have significantly higher rates of CKD than other racial groups. This may be partly due to higher rates of hypertension in this group.

In 2005, care of patients with kidney failure in the United States cost over $32 billion. The number of cases is expected to rise as obesity and diabetes mellitus continue to increase worldwide.

20.2.1 NUTRITIONAL MANAGEMENT

The wide spectrum of clinical disturbances that characterize CKD results primarily from an imbalance between excretory capacity and the intake of food and water. For most ingested substances, intake becomes excessive in patients with renal failure, leading to accumulation and resulting clinical disturbances. For other ingested substances, intake may become inadequate because of renal wastage, increased requirements, or dietary restrictions. The goal of nutritional management is to adjust the intake of nutrients to meet the profoundly altered needs and capacities of the patient.

Nonexcretory functions of the kidney are also impaired in CKD. Most important among these are the hormonal functions of the kidney, such as its role in blood pressure regulation, erythropoiesis, and vitamin D activation.

20.2.1.1 Protein

The kidneys are the principal organs responsible for the elimination of the nitrogenous products of protein catabolism with urinary loss of nitrogen accounting for approximately 70% of dietary nitrogen intake, fecal loss accounting for about 10%–20%, and skin loss for the remainder. The common denominator in all patients with CKD is the inability to excrete nitrogen properly. As a result, the levels of nonprotein nitrogen products increase in the blood. As the levels of these products increase, particularly urea, the patient begins to develop certain symptoms. Under these conditions, the major aim of therapy is to prevent further strain on the system by limiting the amount of exogenous nitrogen ingested. In addition, it is important to create conditions that minimize the breakdown of endogenous proteins (from muscle and other sources). The first aim is accomplished by limiting the amount of protein in the diet.[8,9,12] It should be adequate to maintain nitrogen balance. Some studies suggest that restricting protein intake to 0.6–0.75 g/kg of body weight per day may delay the need for renal replacement therapy. Reduced protein intake also reduces mortality from CKD by 31% compared with higher intake or unrestricted protein intake. Protein should be of high biological value to satisfy requirements for all essential amino acids. An additional requirement for nitrogen balance is adequate caloric intake. Otherwise, the efficiency of nitrogen utilization is significantly diminished.

20.2.1.2 Electrolytes and Acid–Base Balance

It is important for a CKD patient to be normovolemic. Dehydration may increase the degree of insufficiency, producing uremic symptoms. Overhydration may contribute to hypertension and congestive heart failure. A patient's volume status is primarily determined by the kidney's ability to handle sodium appropriately. The ability must be determined on an individual basis. Some patients may be salt wasters and require large amounts of sodium in order to prevent depletion. Other patients may handle sodium loads poorly and rapidly develop edema. In order to prevent or ameliorate these problems, the daily urinary sodium excretion should be measured. When the patient is normovolemic or minimally edematous, this amount of sodium (equal to the excreted amount) should be given in the diet.

Although hyperkalemia is a common cause of death in patients with chronic renal insufficiency, potassium retention is usually not seen until the GFR is severely compromised, that is, GFR < 5 ml/min, or when sodium intake is severely restricted. Large intakes of potassium should be avoided.

Acid–base disturbances may be seen in CKD patients. These patients may develop metabolic acidosis due to either the presence of renal tubular acidosis or the inability of the kidneys to excrete fixed acids. Correction of acidosis requires administration of sodium bicarbonate.

20.2.1.3 Phosphate, Calcium, and Vitamin D

Control of serum phosphate concentration is an important part of the management of patients with CKD. High levels of dietary phosphate may accelerate the progression of renal insufficiency. Hyperphosphatemia does not manifest until GFR falls below 20 ml/min. Then it leads to the retention of phosphate. This causes hypocalcemia, which in turn stimulates increased parathyroid activity. Elevated levels of parathyroid hormone (PTH) increase the clearance of phosphate and result in normal phosphorus and calcium levels in the blood along with elevated PTH levels. Later, PTH secretion is no longer sufficient to lower serum phosphate and increase calcium to a normal level. Persistent hypocalcemia then results in a sustained elevation of PTH concentration.[10] This induces bone resorption. The chronically diseased kidney cannot convert vitamin D to calcitriol. Daily doses of calcitriol over many weeks slowly correct the serum calcium level.[14] Bone pain disappears. Control of dietary phosphate is achieved by restricting the intake of dairy foods and decreasing protein intake. The usual intake of phosphorus in the United States varies from 1.3–2 g/day. With the restriction of dairy foods and proteins, the intake of phosphorus can be reduced to 600–900 mg/day.

20.2.1.4 Magnesium

The kidney is the major organ responsible for the maintenance of serum magnesium within normal levels. Hypermagnesemia is often present in patients with advanced CKD. Patients with uremia should limit excessive dietary intake of magnesium to avoid dangerous hypermagnesemia that may develop.

20.2.1.5 Vitamins

Patients with moderate renal failure may have normal or reduced levels of calcitriol, but they manifest abnormalities in the functional integrity of target organs for vitamin D. These patients need supplements of 0.5–1.0 µg/day of calcitriol. Low-protein diets may increase the risk for deficiency of certain vitamins. Low levels of vitamin B_1, B_2, B_6, and vitamin C have been reported in some patients with CKD. Therefore, multivitamin supplements have been suggested.

20.2.2 Nutritional Management for Patients Treated with Dialysis

End-stage kidney disease (stage 5) is the end result of CKD and is characterized by severely limited kidney function that is not adequate to maintain life. Patients need renal replacement therapy via dialysis or kidney transplantation. Dialysis patients have substantially different dietary requirements than those of undialized uremic patients.[17] Once maintenance dialysis begins, the intake of protein is liberalized so that patients can be kept as nutritionally healthy as possible.

Amino acid losses have been estimated to be approximately 1–2 g/h of dialysis, and about 25% of these losses are essential amino acids. If a glucose-free bath is used, amino acid losses are about 50% higher. The recommended dietary protein intake is 1–1.25 g/kg of body weight per day (70–90 g). At least 70% of the protein should be of high biological value. Intake of calories should be those prescribed prior to the initiation of dialysis (30–35 Cal/kg of body weight per day).[6] High sodium intake should be avoided. Hypertension in dialysis patients is attributed to positive sodium balance and volume expansion. An appropriate amount of fluid is allowed so that patients do not gain more than 0.5 kg/day between dialysis treatments. The typical fluid allowance is 500–800 ml/day plus urine output. Strict control of sodium and fluid is essential in patients with marked hypertension.

Individuals undergoing dialysis cannot excrete potassium. Therefore, they should avoid potassium-rich foods. Hypophosphatemia is treated with phosphate binders and hypocalcemia with calcium supplements and calcitriol. Water-soluble vitamins are dialyzable and patients may have a decrease in blood levels of these vitamins. They should be supplemented.

Most people with chronic uremia and those treated with dialysis frequently have high serum triglycerides and very-low-density lipoprotein (VLDL) cholesterol and low levels of high-density lipoprotein (HDL) cholesterol; they are also at increased risk for cardiovascular disease. Diets with lower carbohydrate content (about 35% of the total daily calories) are effective in lowering fasting triglycerides. Several studies have found toxic effects of star fruit, *Averrhoa carambola*, in patients with both CKD and end-stage renal failure on dialysis.[3] The symptoms are neurological and include vomiting, asthenia, muscle twitching, insomnia, mental confusion, and coma. The exact cause is cannot be determined, but some of the symptoms may be due to oxalate, which is more concentrated in carambola than in other foods.

20.3   ACUTE KIDNEY INJURY

Acute kidney injury (AKI), previously called acute renal failure, is a complex and increasingly common syndrome. The condition is generally recognized as the abrupt loss of kidney function that leads to fluid retention, accumulation of metabolic waste products, and dysregulation of extracelluar volume and electrolytes.

AKI can result from a variety of causes. Common causes of AKI range from decreased renal perfusion and contrast-induced nephropathy to sepsis and nephrotoxicity from medications such as aminoglycoside antibiotics and nonsteroidal anti-inflammatory drugs. Problems happen quickly such as when an accident injures the kidney. Losing a lot of blood can cause sudden kidney failure. Some drugs or poisons can make the kidneys stop working. It affects about 5% of people who are hospitalized for any reason. It most often occurs as a complication of surgery or trauma and can result in the patient's demise. AKI is even more common in those receiving intensive care (25%–30% of patients in an intensive care unit). Depending on its severity, AKI may lead to a number of complications, including metabolic acidosis, high serum potassium, changes in body fluid balances, and effects on other organ systems. Nationally, AKI-related medical costs are estimated at about $10 billion annually.

In hospitalized patients the mortality rate ranges from 10%–80%, depending on patient population studies. Patients with uncomplicated AKI have a mortality rate of about 10%. In contrast, patients with AKI and multiorgan failure have rates of over 50%. If dialysis is required, the mortality rate rises further to as high as 80%.

AKI is diagnosed on the basis of clinical history such as elevated BUN and creatinine levels. Usually there is oliguria. On occasion there is no decrease found in urinary volume, but there is failure to excrete the waste products of catabolism. AKI may be brief with spontaneous recovery or prolonged (two to three weeks or more).

Treatment for AKI primarily relies first on treating the underlying cause and maintaining the patient until kidney function has recovered.[16] Clinical presentation may range from an uncomplicated monoorgan failure to a critically ill patient with multiorgan dysfunction syndrome. Thus, the treatment will be determined not only by AKI but also the underlying disease process. Initially, the patient is often unable to tolerate oral feedings. Because of fluid restriction (conditioned by oliguria), the intake of calories and nutrients is not sufficient. During this period (usually 2 to 3 days), 100 g of glucose in 500 ml of solution is given. If the patient can eat, the intake for energy is set at 30–35 Cal/kg body weight/day and 0.25 g/kg body weight of protein of high biological value. If oral feeding cannot be given and if BUN rises rapidly, dialysis may be required. As soon as oral feedings are feasible, the patient can be started on a diet similar to the kind recommended for CKD and uremia. Fluid intake should equal urinary output and other extrarenal losses of water (diarrhea or vomiting), plus 400 ml/day. Salt intake may range from 3 to 5 g/day unless hypertension or congestive heart failure is present. In that case, salt intake should not exceed 1 g. Potassium intake should be restricted.

If the patient is hypercatabolic, dialysis is needed to prevent hyperkalemia and other uremic manifestations. With dialysis, daily intake of protein (1–1.25 g/kg body weight) is possible together with energy (40–45 Cal or more/kg of body weight). For most individuals, there is eventually adequate recovery. Dietary adjustments of protein, water, and electrolytes are made as the patient recovers.

20.4   NEPHROTIC SYNDROME

Nephrotic syndrome is typically due to damage to epithelial cells or basement membranes or both, causing massive proteinuria (protein loss of more than 3.5 g/day). The amount of protein lost exceeds the liver's synthetic ability and leads to lower plasma protein levels. Clinically, low serum albumin, generalized edema, and increase in serum lipids (cholesterol and triglycerides) accompany this disorder. Decreased vascular oncotic pressure, due to proteinuria, leads to increased lipoprotein production by the liver. Lipid catabolism is decreased due to low levels of lipoprotein lipase. VLDLs and low-density lipoproteins (LDLs) are increased in serum, and HDLs are decreased. These abnormalities are associated with increased risk of coronary heart disease. γ-globulin is also lost in the urine, and this may contribute to a susceptibility to bacterial infections commonly found in patients with nephrotic syndrome.

The main dietary strategy is to compensate for protein loss by taking adequate amounts of protein. In the past, high-protein diets (more than 100 g/day) were often prescribed for nephrotic syndrome patients to restore serum albumin levels. But this high level of protein intake is found to increase urinary protein loss and decrease serum albumin concentration. Studies suggest that excessive protein intake makes kidneys function vigorously to filter the surplus protein. This can cause tubular damage in the kidneys. The current approach is to offer a diet with moderate amounts of protein (not less than 0.6 g/kg of body weight per day) of high biological value supplemented with the amount of protein equal to urinary loss. This strategy preserves renal function. Chicken and fish sources of protein may be of more benefit than beef or pork. Vegetarian sources of protein such as soy and flaxseed are found to reduce proteinuria and hyperlipidemia more than animal proteins.

To lower serum lipid levels, one must avoid saturated fat such as butter, cheese, fried foods, and egg yolks and increase the intake of fruits and vegetables. People suffering from nephrotic syndrome may not be able to regulate their water balance. Hence, these people are often advised to restrict their fluid intake.

20.5   KIDNEY STONE DISEASE

Kidney stone disease is a common disorder characterized by the formation of crystalline aggregates (kidney stones) that can develop anywhere along the urinary tract. Urolithiasis is a medical term used to describe stones occurring in the urinary tract.[4] Another frequently used term is nephrolithiasis.

The less-soluble constituents of urine sometimes precipitate in the urinary tract. They may form minute particles or masses and be passed readily, or they may become larger aggregates, varying in size from "sand" or "gravel" to good-sized stones. Patients with kidney stones typically present with an episode of severe pain. A stone may stay in the kidney or break loose and travel down the urinary tract. A small stone may pass all the way out of the body without causing too much pain. If the stone becomes large enough to block the flow of urine out of the kidney, it can cause pressure, pain, and infection. If the stone moves out of the kidney with the flow of urine, it can cause severe pain as it moves through the ureters—the tubes that carry urine from the kidney to the bladder. If the stone gets stuck, infection can occur.

20.5.1 EPIDEMIOLOGY

Upper (renal) stones are common in Western industrialized countries. An estimated 1 million cases of symptomatic kidney stones occur per year in the United States and comprise 1% of all hospitalizations. More than $2 billion is spent each year in treating this painful condition. For some unknown reason, the number of people in the United States with kidney stones has been increasing over the past several years. In the late 1970s, less than 4% of the population had stone-forming disease. By the late 1990s, more than 5% of the population suffered from kidney stone disease. Caucasians are more likely to develop the disease than African Americans. Stones occur much more frequently in men. The prevalence of kidney stones rises as men reach the age of 40 and continues to rise into their 70s. For women the prevalence peaks in their 50s. About 5% of American women and 12% of American men will develop a kidney stone at some time in their life and the prevalence has been increasing in both sexes. In the United States, there is an increased prevalence in the southeastern region of the country. This variation might be related to differences in temperature and sunlight exposure. Renal stone disease is one of the common problems in countries in tropical Asia. It accounts for 40% of renal problems in Pakistan, which is a country in the "stone belt." The hot climate and dietary factors play important roles. The prevalence is also high in India, Israel, and the Middle East.

20.5.2 CAUSES

Stone formations do not have a single, well defined cause but are the result of a combination of factors. For the formation of kidney stones the concentration of a dissolved salt has to exceed its solubility in urine, a condition referred to as supersaturation. The development of supersaturation depends on the solubility of the dissolved substance, its amount excreted in urine, the volume of the urine, and its pH. Changes in any one of these factors affect stone formation. Normally, urine contains components that prevent or inhibit the crystals from forming. When these substances fall below their normal proportion, stones can form out of an accumulation of crystals. These inhibitors also do not seem to work for everyone, so some people form stones. Being obese or overweight may increase the risk of developing painful stones, and women may be especially vulnerable to these added risks, according to recent studies.[5] Researchers found that women who weighed more than 220 pounds were 90% more likely to develop kidney stones than those who weighed less than 150 pounds.[22,23] Men and women who gained more than 35 pounds since they were 21 years old also had a 39%–82% higher risk of kidney stones.

Investigations have suggested that an organic matrix is the one essential component of all urinary stones (calculi). This matrix is a mucoid, containing about 65% protein, 14% carbohydrate, 11% inorganic elements, and 10% "bound" water. Certain nutritional factors and a number of pathological states appear to trigger the matrix-forming mechanism and thus the formation of urinary calculi. Clinical and dietary studies have shown a positive association between the excessive consumption of animal protein and renal stone disease. Presumably an accompanying increase in the acidity of urine would be involved.

Certain other factors have been suggested as contributing to the formation of urinary calculi. Among them are hyperparathyroidism, hypervitaminosis D, hypovitaminosis A, and hypvitaminosis B_6.

Hyperparathyroidism results in a removal of calcium salts from bone with a rise in blood calcium and urinary calcium. Kidney stones are quite prevalent in tropical countries, hence the suggestion that the overproduction of vitamin D by sunlight is a causative factor. The effect of high vitamin D in producing a calcium imbalance, coupled with a possible low vitamin A intake, might induce the formation of calcium stones. Vitamin A deficiency regularly produces bladder stones in rats. Vitamin B_6 deficiency causes increased urinary oxalate excretion in some animals and in humans. Feeding large amounts of glycine or tryptophan causes increased oxalate excretion that can be corrected by taking vitamin B_6. However, there are many types of stones without calcium.

20.5.3 CLASSIFICATION

Stones can be formed from a variety of substances excreted in the urine. Stones can be classified according to their chemical compositions. The most common types are calcium stones, magnesium ammonium phosphate stones, uric acid stones, and cystine stones. Physical characteristics may help in identifying the type of stone. Calcium oxalate stones are very hard, often of a dark brown to black color, and typically have a rough surface. Phosphate stones are usually pale and friable. Uric acid stones are typically yellow to reddish brown and are moderately hard. Cystine stones are yellow or greenish yellow and rather soft. Specific dietary and drug therapy will vary depending on the composition of the urinary stone.

Modification of urine pH also prevents the formation of kidney stones. Acidic urine helps prevent stones of calcium and magnesium phosphate and carbonate, while an alkaline urine helps prevent oxalate and uric acid stones. The diet should support therapy with alkalinizing or acidifying agents by supplying acid-producing or alkaline-producing foods. Fruits and vegetables contribute to the formation of alkaline urine, while meat, fish, and poultry contribute to the formation of acidic urine. Most importantly, to prevent all types of urinary stones a liberal intake of fluid is necessary.

20.5.3.1 Calcium Stones

Calcium-based stones are the most common, causing more than 75% of cases, and calcium oxalate is the most common type of stone overall (36%), followed by calcium phosphate (6%–20%), and mixed stones (11%–31%). Metabolic defects leading to their formation include hypercalciuria in over 65% of cases and less frequently hyperoxaluria, hypocitraturia, or a combination thereof.

Calcium homeostasis is maintained by PTH and vitamin D. Both affect bone resorption by osteoclasts. PTH causes a diminution of phosphorus reabsorption and an increase in calcium reabsorption by renal tubular cells. It also causes increased synthesis of an active form of vitamin D that acts upon the small intestinal mucosa, causing increased absorption of calcium and phosphorus. About 40% of patients with calcium stones will have hypercalciuria. Increased calcium in urine may result from an increase in intestinal calcium absorption, a lack of appropriate renal tubular reabsorption of calcium, loss of calcium from bone, or a combination of these factors. In a few instances of hypercalciuria, the underlying disease process can be identified. About 5%–10% of calcium stones are associated with primary hyperparathyroidism. In most cases, however, it is primary or idiopathic hypercalciuria (IH). The exact mechanism of hypercalciuria is unknown.

Normally, men excrete less than 300–400 mg of calcium/day in their urine and women excrete even less. In IH, there is increased increased urinary excretion of calcium. It is accompanied by normal serum calcium, a tendency toward reduced serum phosphate, and renal stone formation. The majority of calcium stones contain oxalate. Some of the oxalate in urine is dietary in origin from vegetables (rhubarb, spinach) beverages (tea, cocoa, coffee, cola), nuts, berries, and other fruits. Oxalate is also formed from an excess intake of vitamin C. The gastrointestinal tract plays an important role in oxalate homeostasis. Oxalate absorption increases when calcium and magnesium intake decreases.[15] Disorders of the small bowel such as Crohn's disease and ileal resection may result in excessive oxalate absorption, with its subsequent excretion in urine. Other causes of hyperoxaluria include pyridoxine deficiency and primary hyperoxaluria. The latter is a rare inherited autosomal recessive disease with oxoglutarate carboligase deficiency. Individuals who tend to form oxalate stones experience an increase in urinary oxalate excretion. Foods and beverages rich in oxalate should be restricted in any patient who has elevated levels of urinary oxalate excretion and has passed a calcium oxalate stone.

Urinary citrate binds calcium by chelating, inhibits calcium oxalate formation, and interferes with calcium oxalate crystallization. However, hypocitraturia is common among many stone formers. Hypocitraturia can be caused by chronic metabolic acidosis due to bicarbonate loss from chronic diarrhea or laxative abuse, small bowel pathology, and metabolic acid loads from high animal protein intake. Some drugs such as angiotensin-converting enzyme inhibitors decrease urinary citrate excretion. Citrate supplements (e.g., potassium citrate) are commonly prescribed for patients with low citrate levels in urine. Fruits, vegetables, and especially lemon juice are found to increase urinary citrate and reduce stone recurrence.[11]

A low fluid intake results in low urine volume and an increased concentration of urinary solutes. Central to all the treatments regardless of the stone type or the metabolic abnormality that has led to stone formation is the ingestion of large amounts of fluid.[20] This is necessary because all the types of stones result from an increased concentration of a particular substance in the urine. Simply diluting the urine then will reduce the concentration of the offending substance. Most individuals can be trained to drink 2.5–3 L of fluid per day. They should drink fluid before going to bed and again when they get up. This is important because overnight urine normally tends to be concentrated.

High sodium intake increases urinary calcium excretion and facilitates calcium stone formation. High meat intake causes significant increase in the urinary excretion of calcium, oxalate, and uric acid, three of the urinary risk factors for calcium stone formation. Compared with individuals eating 50 g or less of animal protein per day, those eating 77 g or more have a 33% higher risk for kidney stones.[1] A diet restricted in animal protein and sodium reduces the risk by about 50% for stone recurrence.[2] A vegetarian diet increases urinary pH and decreases urinary calcium excretion. Studies have shown that the risk for stone formation is 40%–60% lower in individuals following a vegetarian diet compared with those eating the standard Western diet.

20.5.3.2 Magnesium Ammonium Phosphate (Struvite) Stones

These stones constitute about 10% of all stones and occur in patients with recurrent urinary infection involving urea-splitting organisms. The ammonia thereby generated produces highly alkaline urine in which magnesium ammonium phosphate precipitates in the form of crystals. The mainstay of therapy is permanent eradication of the infection. Intake of 8–12 g/day of methionine or 500 mg of ascorbic acid 2–3 times a day can acidify the urine. However, these agents should be used only for short periods of time and have only limited usefulness.

20.5.3.3 Uric Acid Stones

Excessive excretion of uric acid in urine may be due to the increased intake of foods rich in purines (organ meats, dried beans, some types of fish) or due to various disease processes. Endogenous uric acid production is increased in gout and some other conditions. The average uric acid excretion by adults is 500 mg/day. Solute concentration as well as pH appears to be important in the solubility of uric acid and urate. Uric acid is insoluble at a lower pH. The amount of free uric acid decreases as the pH rises, and at pH 7 uric acid is more soluble as urate (combination with sodium and potassium). In patients with uric acid stones, the mainstays of therapy are adequate fluid intake, a low-purine diet, and the use of alkalinizing salt solutions to maintain urinary pH between 6 and 6.5. The most widely used is oral sodium citrate and citric acid in the form of solution.

20.5.3.4 Cystine Stones

This rare type of renal stone occurs in patients with cystinuria who have a genetic defect in cystine, lysine, arginine, and ornithine transport in the renal tubules, which causes large amounts of these products to be excreted in urine. Of these only cystine forms crystals and stones. Cystine does not become soluble until the urine pH is 7.4, and stones form over a range of normal urinary pH. There is no effective dietary therapy. Fluid intake must be increased and urinary alkalinization is useful.

20.5.3.5 Other Rare Stones

Stones containing sulfanilamides have been described in humans and silica calculi have been reported in patients ingesting silica gel over a long period of time. Rare adenine stones have been described in children with an inherited enzyme deficiency disorder and hyperuricemia.

REFERENCES

1. Borghi, L., T. Schianchi, T. Meschi et al. 2002. Comparison of two diets for the prevention of recurrent stones in idiopathic hypercalciuria. *New Engl J Med* 346:77.
2. Chai, W., and M. Liebman. 2005. Effect of different cooking methods on vegetable oxalate content. *J Agric Food Chem* 53:3027.
3. Chen, L. L., J. T. Fang, and J. L. Lin. 2005. Chronic renal disease patients with severe star fruit poisoning: Hemoperfusion may be an effective alternative therapy. *Clin Toxicol* 43:197.
4. Coe, F. L., A. Evan, and E. Worcester. 2006. Kidney stone disease. *J Clin Invest* 115:2598.
5. Corhan, G. C., W. C. Willett, E. L. Kight et al. 2004. Dietary factors and the risk of incident kidney stones in younger women. Nurses' Health Study II. *Arch Intern Med* 164:885.
6. Cuppart, L., and C. M. Avesani. 2004. Energy requirements in patients with chronic kidney disease. *J Ren Nutr* 14:121.
7. Ekerno, W. O., Y. H. Tan, M. D. Young et al. 2004. Metabolic risk factors and the impact of medical therapy on the management of nephrolithiasis in obese patients. *J Urol* 172:159.
8. Fouque, D., M. Leville, and J. P. Boisselle. 2006. Low protein diets for chronic kidney disease in non-diabetic adults. *Cochrane Database Syst Rev* 19(2):CD001892.
9. Ideura, T., M. Shimazui, H. Morita, and A. Yoshimura. 2007. Protein intake of more than 0.5g/kg BW/day is not effective in suppressing the progression of chronic renal failure. *Contrib Nephrol* 155:40.
10. Joy, M. S., P. C. Karagiannis, and F. W. Peyerl. 2007. Outcomes of secondary hyperparathyroidism in chronic kidney disease and the direct costs of treatment. *J Manag Care Pharm* 13:397.
11. Kang, D. E., R. L. Sur, G. E. Haleblian et al. 2007. Long-term lemonade based dietary manipulation in patients with hypocitraturic nephrolithiasis. *J Urol* 177:1358.
12. Knight, E. L., M. J. Stampfer, S. E. Hankinson et al. 2003. The impact of protein intake on renal function decline in women with normal renal function or mild renal insufficiency. *Ann Intern Med* 138:460.
13. Lentine, K., and E. M. Wrone. 2004. New insights into protein intake and progression of renal disease. *Curr Opin Nephrol Hypertens* 13:333.
14. Levin, A., and Y. C. Li. 2005. Vitamin D and its analogues: Do they protect against cardiovascular disease in patients with kidney disease? *Kidney Int* 68:1973.
15. Lewandowski, S., and A. L. Rodgers. 2004. Idiopathic calcium oxalate urolithiasis: Risk factors and conservative treatment. *Clin Chim Acta* 346:17.
16. Molitoris, B. A., A. Levin, D. Warnock et al. 2007. Improving outcomes of acute kidney injury: Report of an initiative. *Nat Clin Pract Nephrol* 3:439.
17. Mehrotra, R., and J. D. Kopple. 2001. Nutritional management of maintenance dialysis patients. Why aren't we doing better? *Annu Rev Nutr* 21:343.
18. Pak, C. Y., K. Sakhaee, O. Moe et al. 2003. Biochemical profile of stone-forming patients with diabetes mellitus. *Urol* 61:523.
19. Pedraza-Chaverri, J., D. Barrera, R. Hernandez-Pando et al. 2004. Soy protein diet ameliorates renal nitrotyrosine formation and chronic nephropathy induced by puromycin aminonucleoside. *Life Sci* 74:987.
20. Qiang, W., and Z. Ke. 2004. Water for preventing urinary calculi (Cochrane Review). *Chochrane Database Syst Rev* 3:CD004292.
21. Reynolds, T. M. 2005. ACP Best Practice No. 181: Chemical pathology clinical investigation and management of nephrolithiases. *J Clin Pathol* 58:134.
22. Semins, M. J., A. D. Shore, M. A. Makary et al. 2010. The association of increasing body mass index and kidney stone disease. *J Urol* 183:571.
23. Taylor, E. N., M. J. Stampfer, and G. C. Curhan. 2005. Obesity, weight gain and the risk of kidney stones. *J Amer Med Assoc* 293:455.
24. Valasquez, M. T., S. J. Bathena, T. Ranich et al. 2003. Dietary flaxseed meal reduces proteinuria and ameliorates nephropathy in an animal model of type II diabetes mellitus. *Kidney Int* 64:2100.
25. Weir, M. R., and J. C. Fink. 2005. Salt intake and progression of chronic kidney disease: An overlooked modifiable exposure? A commentary. *Amer J. Kidney Dis* 45:176.
26. Wolf, M., A. Shah, O. Gutierrez et al. 2007. Vitamin D levels and early mortality among incident hemo-dialysis patients. *Kidney Int* 72:1004.

21 Nutritional Aspects of Genetic Diseases

The uniqueness of each person's genetic makeup suggests that each of us may have differences in metabolism and nutritional needs and responses. These are often obvious where enzyme deficiency occurs but more subtle where the properties of an enzyme are only slightly altered. Because proteins are complex structures subject to a variety of alterations ranging from absence to alleles, which cause no phenotypic change, there is often a wide range of severities for a particular genetic disease. Many genetic diseases are silent until elicited by an environmental factor. This chapter focuses on those situations where diet influences genetic disease or where nutritional therapy is useful.

Foods undergo a series of reactions in the body. They traverse a metabolic path that often has minor branches. Blocking a pathway leads to an accumulation of precursor and to a deficiency of products (Figure 21.1). The precursors frequently flood minor pathways, inhibit other reactions, act as unusual substrates for normal reactions, or compete with other substances for transport proteins. These effects lead to obvious nutritional therapies including supplying metabolites missing beyond the block, supplying substances that will aid in the removal by the minor pathways, and increasing the substances affected by competitive actions so that the reaction proceeds in a more normal fashion. Sometimes the excess metabolite is stored rather than secreted, and in those cases it is this accumulation that causes the symptoms of the disease. Where the offending substance is not essential, the disease can be ameliorated by avoiding this substance and its precursors.[3,5,7,15]

21.1 CARBOHYDRATE METABOLISM

Dietary carbohydrates include simple sugars such as glucose and fructose; the disaccharides sucrose, lactose, and maltose; and polymeric carbohydrates, primarily starch. Some components of fiber are polymeric carbohydrates, but they are indigestible. A variety of other carbohydrates is found in the diet, but usually makes up only a minor portion. The larger carbohydrates are broken into simple sugars before being absorbed in the intestine. A number of enzymes are involved. Fructose and galactose are converted to intermediates of the glucose pathways and undergo anaerobic glycolysis, form other sugars, or undergo storage as glycogen. Genetic disorders of carbohydrate metabolism often disrupt the metabolism of specific sugars and are treated by eliminating those sugars from the diet.

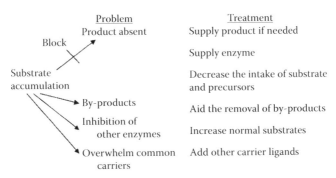

FIGURE 21.1 Consequences and treatment of a metabolic block.

21.1.1 Sucrose and Fructose Metabolism

Sucrase deficiency is a rare disease. Intestinal sucrase and isomaltase activities come from a single precursor and in many cases both are absent. Deficiency of sucrase–isomaltase results in the inability to digest dietary sucrose. Both conditions (sucrase and isomaltase deficiencies) manifests during infancy on the introduction of sucrose-containing formulas. A later onset deficiency has also been described in adults. The inability to digest sucrose produces signs and symptoms of malabsorption, including diarrhea, increased gas production, and abdominal distention. Avoiding sucrose permits normal development. Sucrase preparations from yeast taken by mouth can be used for enzyme replacement.

Fructose is transported across the apical intestinal brush-border membrane by a sodium-independent facilitated-diffusion mechanism involving GLUT 5 transporter. GLUT 2 may assist in the absorption of excess luminal fructose. The inherited form of fructose malabsorption is rare. But recently, malabsorption of fructose and sorbitol has been found in a number of patients. This may be related to the deficiency of GLUT 5, but no assessments of intestinal GLUT 5 or its controlling gene have been made in any patients. Symptoms of fructose malabsorption include diarrhea, flatulence, and abdominal pain. Patients experiencing significant symptoms should reduce or eliminate their dietary fructose.

Fructose is metabolized by conversion to fructose 1-phosphate by fructokinase followed by aldolase cleavage to dihydroxyacetone phosphate and glyceraldehyde (Figure 21.2). The glyceraldehyde is phosphorylated by glyceraldehyde kinase. It can then combine with dihydroxyacetone phosphate to form fructose 1,6-bisphosphate by the action of aldolase. Three aldolases exist. Although each can react with both fructose 1-phosphate and fructose 1,6-bisphosphate, aldolase B, the one found in liver, has by far the most activity toward fructose 1-phosphate. In its metabolism, fructose is also phosphorylated to fructose 6-phosphate, especially in adipose tissue and skeletal muscle.

Defects in fructokinase cause essential fructosuria, a benign condition. It is a rare, autosomal recessive disorder. It is not associated with any long-term or short-term complications. Essential fructosuria is detected by routine screening of urine for reducing sugars. Fructose gives a positive test for reducing sugars and a negative reaction with glucose oxidase. Ingested fructose is partly (10%–20%) excreted as such in urine, and the rest is slowly metabolized by an alternative pathway—conversion to fructose 6-phosphate by hexokinase in adipose tissue and muscle. Dietary treatment is not indicated, and the prognosis is good. Defects in aldolase B give rise to hereditary fructose intolerance (HFI). It is the most frequent inborn error of fructose metabolism.

Patients with aldolase deficiency may have vomiting, hypoglycemia, cataracts, and liver and kidney failure.[8,22] Consumption of fructose by patients with fructose intolerance results in the accumulation of fructose 1-phosphate and depletion of inorganic phosphate in the liver. Tying up inorganic phosphate in the form of fructose 1-phosphate makes it impossible for liver mitochondria

Sucrose (glucosyl fructose) + water $\xrightarrow{\text{sucrase}}$ glucose + fructose

Fructose + ATP $\xrightarrow{\text{fructokinase}}$ fructose 1-phosphate + ADP

Fructose 1-phosphate $\xrightarrow{\text{aldolase B}}$ dihydroxyacetone phosphate + glyceraldehyde

Glyceraldehyde + ATP $\xrightarrow{\text{glyceraldehyde kinase}}$ glyceraldehyde 3-phosphate + ADP

Glyceraldehyde 3-phosphate + dihydroxyacetone phosphate $\xrightarrow{\text{aldolase}}$ fructose 1,6-bisphosphate

FIGURE 21.2 Digestion of sucrose and principal steps in the metabolism of fructose.

to generate adenosine triphosphate (ATP) by oxidative phosphorylation. Hence, the ATP levels fall. Fructose 1-phosphate inhibits glycogenolysis and some steps in gluconeogenesis, leading to hypoglycemia. The hypoglycemic effects and vomiting cause these patients to avoid sweet-tasting substances. Treatment involves the elimination of fructose, sucrose (which contains fructose along with glucose), and sorbitol (which is converted to fructose) from the diet. Care must be taken to avoid substances sweetened with sucrose such as certain medications. Patients live a normal life if fructose and substances that form fructose are avoided.

Defects in fructose 1,6-biphosphatase, the key enzyme in gluconeogenesis, impair the formation of glucose from all gluconeogenic precursors, including dietary fructose. Thus, hypoglycemia is likely to occur when glycogen reserves are limited (as in newborns) or exhausted (as in fasting). The defect also causes accumulation of the gluconeogenic substrates pyrurate, lactate, glycerol, and alanine. Avoiding fasting (i.e., avoiding gluconeogenesis) is the major issue, but limitation of sucrose and fructose intake is also recommended.

21.1.2 Lactose and Galactose Metabolism

The most common difficulty with carbohydrate digestion is the deficient breakdown of lactose[16] (milk sugar). Lactase, the enzyme responsible, is one of seven carbohydrases found in the brush-border of the small intestine, and while present in infants of all races and adults of Northern European descent, it is often absent in adult blacks and Asians. In patients with lactase deficiency, lactose remains in the gut where it is attacked by bacteria to form lactic acid, carbon dioxide, and hydrogen. The acid causes cramping and contributes to diarrhea brought on by the osmotic movement of water into the intestine. Most people with this problem avoid milk and foods that contain large amounts of milk. Small amounts are tolerated.

Transient lactase deficiency often follows intestinal infections and is an important problem in infants. Soybean milk is usually used, but milk treated with lactase is reported to be better tolerated. Even a 50% depletion of lactose in milk products abolished the symptoms in five of six subjects examined. Yogurt contains lactase and the bacteria that produce it and is a good food to supply milk products to those with lactase deficiency. Pasteurization after fermentation of milk products makes them less useful.

Galactose is phosphorylated by galactokinase to galactose 1-phosphate; a transferase moves the uridine diphosphate moiety of uridine diphosphoglucose (UDPG) to form uridine diphosphogalactose and glucose 1-phosphate (Figure 21.3). An epimerase interconverts the two uridine diphosphosugars. Deficiencies of any of the enzymes can occur. Transferase deficiency is the most common. Kinase deficiency is fairly rare and epimerase deficiency is represented by a single case. Galactosemia occurs in kinase and transferase deficiencies, and the elimination of galactose and its sources, primarily milk, is required. Other foods containing galactose should also be avoided. For infants, nonmilk protein sources are needed and soybean milk or casein hydrolysates are often used. Symptoms include failure to thrive, vomiting, and diarrhea in infants followed by evidence of liver

$$\text{Lactose (galactosyl glucose)} + \text{water} \xrightarrow{\text{lactase}} \text{glucose} + \text{galactose}$$

$$\text{Galactose} + \text{ATP} \xrightarrow{\text{galactokinase}} \text{galactose 1-phosphate} + \text{ADP}$$

$$\text{Galactose 1-phosphate} + \text{UDP glucose} \xrightarrow{\text{transferase}}$$

$$\text{UDP galactose} + \text{glucose 1-phosphate}$$

$$\text{UDP galactose} \xrightarrow{\text{epimerase}} \text{UDP glucose}$$

FIGURE 21.3 Digestion of lactose and principal steps in galactose metabolism.

damage, cataracts, and mental retardation. Liver damage is associated with transferase deficiency but not with kinase deficiency. Cataracts occur in both deficiencies and are caused by the conversion of galactose to its alcohol galactitol, which brings water into the lens of the eye by osmosis. The symptoms, except for mental retardation, are reversed by the elimination of galactose-containing foods. Because some galactosemics have cataracts at birth, pregnant mothers who have had a galactosemic child are advised to restrict their galactose intake.

21.1.3 GLUCOSE METABOLISM

Deficiency of the transporter that carries glucose and galactose from the small intestine is very rare. The system functions by cotransport of Na^+ ions. The elimination of these sugars and their precursors from the diet, the use of specially prepared formulas during the first few months of life, and the gradual introduction of foods free of these sugars are used in treatment.

Glucose 6-phosphate dehydrogenase (GPDH) deficiency is the most common disease-producing enzyme defect in humans (estimated to affect about 400 million people worldwide), often giving rise to hemolytic anemia. The anemia results from red blood cell destruction because of oxidative damage. Normally, this is minimized by reduced levels of glutathione. Glutathione reduction requires the presence of reduced nicotinamide adenine dinucleotide phosphate (NADPH), the product of the GPDH reaction. Patients with GPDH deficiency are generally quite healthy, provided their red blood cells are not subjected to oxidative stresses. Consumption of fava beans by these patients can precipitate a dramatic acute hemolytic anemia (most likely because these beans contain oxidants). In addition, the intake of oxidant drugs such as primaquine (used to treat malaria) and sulfa drugs can also cause hemolytic anemia. GPDH mutants provide an example where the elimination of a specific food (i.e., fava beans) avoids a disease. Not all patients with the mutant enzyme are at risk because a variety of mutant forms occur, but all persons with favism have an altered GPDH.

21.1.4 GLYCOGEN METABOLISM

Glycogen is the principal storage form of carbohydrates in animals. It is synthesized from uridine diphosphoglucose by glycogen synthase, and the long chains formed are cut and the ends moved to form a treelike structure. During breakdown, a phosphorylase breaks an end bond and adds phosphate to form glucose 1-phosphate, which is changed to glucose 6-phosphate (Figure 21.4). The glucose 6-phosphate then moves to the endoplasmic reticulum where in the liver it is converted to glucose by glucose 6-phosphatase.

A deficiency of this enzyme causes the most common form of glycogen storage disease and is referred to as type I or von Gierke's disease. Glucose 6-phosphate accumulates and floods its breakdown path anaerobic glycolysis. An overproduction of lactate causes lactate acidosis. Gout also occurs. The inability of liver glycogen to maintain the blood glucose level causes severe hypoglycemia. The disease is treated by frequent feedings of small meals during the day and by the administration of an uncooked starch suspension at bedtime, which by its slow digestion keeps the glucose level high during the night. Uncooked cornstarch can be given in milk every 3–4 hours

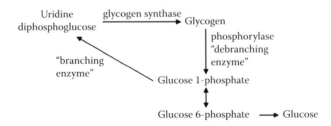

FIGURE 21.4   Principal steps in the biosynthesis and metabolism of glycogen.

during the day to children 9 months to 2 years old; this gives good control of blood glucose, uric acid, cholesterol levels, and normal growth rates.[14] Long-term (i.e., 5–9 years) studies show that uncooked cornstarch gives as good a result as nasogastric feedings. An optimal schedule is three meals a day with cornstarch administered 3 hours after each meal. The recommended daytime distribution of nutrients is 65% carbohydrate, 10%–15% protein, and 25% fat.

The group of disorders occurring when liver phosphorylase is deficient or poorly activated causes milder but similar symptoms. It is treated in the same manner, but less stringent regulation is required. Debranching is also required in glycogen breakdown. This involves moving three glucose residues adjacent to a 1,6-link to the end of a 1,4-linked chain and scission of the remaining 1,6-linked glucose to form free glucose. Most cases of liver debrancher deficiency have hypoglycemic episodes, but the disease is usually milder than glucose 6-phosphatase deficiency. A high-protein diet promotes gluconeogenesis and frequent feedings help maintain normal blood glucose levels. In some, a high carbohydrate intake exacerbates the disease. Muscle phosphorylase deficiency is a separate entity where severe exercise causes cramping and loss of muscle protein in the urine. Dietary carbohydrate improves the status of these patients, but avoiding strenuous exercise is the major recommendation.

21.2 AMINO ACID METABOLISM

21.2.1 PHENYLALANINE

Phenylalanine is used in protein synthesis and as a precursor of tyrosine. When its conversion to tyrosine is blocked, an increase in blood phenylalanine occurs.[17,20] The excess phenylalanine transaminates to form phenylpyruvate, the phenyl ketone found in urine in phenylketonuria (PKU). PKU is the most common disorder of amino acid metabolism and is most frequently caused by a deficiency in phenylalanine hydroxylase[12] (Figure 21.5). But defects in the reductase that converts dihydrobiopterin to the tetrahydro form also occur; defects in the three enzymes involved in the formation of biopterin are rare.[10]

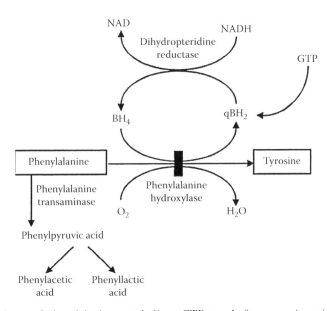

FIGURE 21.5 Pathway of phenylalanine metabolism: GTP stands for guanosine triphosphate, qBH_2 for quinoid dihydrobiopterin, BH_4 for tetrahydrobiopterin, and the dark bar indicates a deficiency of the enzyme in classic phenylketonuria. (Reproduced with the permission of Dr. David Valle.)

Treatment involves limiting phenylalanine intake to levels that are required to maintain protein synthesis and growth. Breast milk supplemented by phenylalanine-free formula can be used, although the precise amount of breast milk obtained from weighing before and after feeding is required. The artificial sweetener aspartame (Nutrasweet), aspartyl phenylalanine methyl ester, is another phenylalanine source that must be avoided. But studies with patients 11–23 years old indicate that a single 12-oz. serving of an aspartame-sweetened drink had a rather small effect on the blood phenylalanine level.

It is important that dietary restriction be started as soon as possible. One study found that the intelligence quotient (IQ) of patients decreased by four points for each 4-week delay. Maintaining careful control is difficult but important. Blood phenylalanine concentrations below 120 μmol/l or above 300 μmol/l correlated with lowered IQ levels. Although low-phenylalanine diets initially were discontinued after 5–8 years, a number of studies suggest that control should be extended into adolescence or be lifelong. Patients who have had their phenylalanine levels carefully controlled have normal IQs, but some cognitive defects (e.g., in arithmetic skills) may still occur. Most patients show changes in the white matter of the brain by nuclear magnetic resonance even if carefully treated. Older phenylketonurics who have been off their diet may benefit from dietary restriction with improvement in behavioral problems or psychiatric disturbances.

As larger numbers of patients with PKU have reached childbearing age, maternal PKU has become important. Most of these mothers have abandoned dietary treatment. Untreated hyperphenylalaninemics have children with microencephaly, mental retardation, low birth weight, and often congenital heart defects. To eliminate these hazards, the mother should be on a low-phenylalanine diet at the time of conception. There is an inverse linear relationship between increased blood phenylalanine levels and head size and birth weight.

Several studies have examined the trace elements in the diets prescribed for PKU. In one, balance studies were repeated at 3–4-week intervals for infants between the ages of 2 and 16 weeks. The diets exceeded breast milk in copper, iron, and manganese, and further supplementation was not recommended. A different study found some children with decreased iron parameters, while one-third of children were found to have intakes higher in copper and iron but lower in selenium in patients than their siblings. Low carnitine levels have also been reported.

Patients with defects in biopterin synthesis require additional treatment. Because biopterin is also a cofactor of tyrosine and tryptophan hydroxylases, it must be supplied or the products of the reactions given. In some patients, the essential amino acids that share the transporter with phenylalanine are used, and an enzyme, phenylalanine ammonia lyase, which breaks down phenylalanine inside the intestine, is also given.

21.2.2 Tyrosine

Two well-recognized forms of hereditary tyrosinemias have been reported. Type I tyrosinemia is due to fumarylacetoacetate hydrolase deficiency (Figure 21.6). It varies in severity and frequently causes liver disease and death. The anemia associated with the disease is due to the accumulation of succinylacetone, which inhibits porphobilinogen synthase, an enzyme involved in the formation of heme. A high plasma methionine level is frequently found. Type I disease is treated by restricting phenylalanine and tyrosine intake. They are not eliminated from the diet because both are required for protein synthesis and tyrosine is also used to make melanin and hormones such as epinephrine and thyroxin.

A deficiency of tyrosine transaminase causes type II tyrosinemia, which is characterized by ocular and skin lesions. Reducing protein intake to 2–3 g/kg/day is recommended. A pregnancy treated with a protein-restricted diet and a tyrosine/phenylalanine-free supplement had a good outcome.

Alkaptonuria is caused by the absence of homogentisate oxidase. Homogentisate accumulates and is excreted in the urine, which turns dark on standing as homogentisate is oxidized and

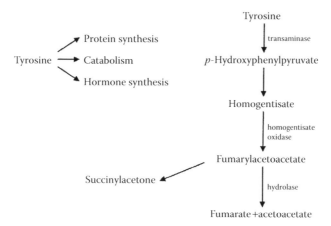

FIGURE 21.6 Tyrosine catabolism.

polymerized to a melanin-like substance. Alkaptonuria is a relatively harmless condition. Late into the disease, there is generalized pigmentation of connective tissues and a form of mild arthritis. In 1902, Archibald Garrod showed that this disease is transmitted as a single recessive Mendelian trait. He perceived the direct relationship between genes and enzymes, and it formed the basis for his classic ideas concerning heritable metabolic disorders.

21.2.3 HISTIDINE

Although some patients have severe mental deficiency, a vast majority of histidinemia patients do not require treatment. Histidase, the enzyme that forms urocanic acid from histidine, is most frequently at fault. In its absence, histidine and the imidazole derivatives of pyruvate, lactate, and acetate are found in urine. Diets low in histidine decrease the blood levels of histidine and imidazole derivatives, but most patients show little clinical change.

21.2.4 ARGININE AND ORNITHINE

Gyrate atrophy of the choroid and retina is caused by deficient ornithine δ-aminotransferase (ornithine transaminase). A surprisingly large number of different defects at the gene level have been found. The eye is the major organ affected, with a gradual onset of blindness by mid-adulthood. The aminotransferase uses pyridoxal phosphate as a cofactor. Pharmacological doses of pyridoxine and the restriction of arginine intake have been tried, each with mixed results. Vomiting and lethargy after eating occur in the hyperornithinemia, hyperammonemia, and homocitrullinuria syndromes. The clinical symptoms are related to hyperammonemia and resemble those of urea cycle disorders. The cause of the disease is probably a defect in ornithine transport into the mitochondria, with ornithine accumulation in the cytoplasm and reduced intramitochondrial ornithine causing impaired ureagenesis and orotic aciduria. Adding ornithine or its precursor, arginine, often improves the hyperammonemia.

21.2.5 UREA CYCLE

On a high-protein diet, the carbon skeletons of amino acids are oxidized for energy or stored as fat and glycogen, but the amino nitrogen must be excreted. The synthesis of urea in the liver is the major route for the removal of ammonia, a highly toxic metabolite derived from ingested protein or from normal or augmented protein turnover. To facilitate the process, enzymes of the urea cycle are controlled at the gene level. The urea cycle, which consists of a series of five biochemical reactions, has two roles. In order to prevent the accumulation of toxic nitrogenous compounds, the urea cycle incorporates nitrogen that is not used for net biosynthetic purposes into urea, which serves as a waste nitrogen product in humans. The urea cycle also contains several biochemical reactions for the de novo synthesis of arginine. Amino acid degradation releases ammonia that is utilized to form carbamyl phosphate (CP), which is catalyzed by CP synthase (CS). N-acetylglutamate, an essential cofactor for CS, is formed from acetyl coenzyme A (CoA) plus glutamate catalyzed by N-acetylglutamate synthetase (NAGS). The formation of CP is not part of the urea cycle proper, but rather an entry reaction. The formation of urea requires the following successive steps:

1. ornithine + CP → citrulline (catalyzed by ornithine carbamylase)
2. citrulline + aspartate → arginosuccinate (AS; catalyzed by AS synthase)
3. AS → arginine + fumarate (catalyzed by lyase)
4. Arginine → urea + ornithine (catalyzed by arginase)

Ornithine released in the last reaction is used in the first reaction to complete the cycle. The enzymes NAGS, CP synthetase, and ornithine carboxylase are found in the mitochondrion and AS synthetase, lyase, and arginase are found in the cytoplasm.

The overall incidence of urea cycle disorders is considered to be around 1:36,000 live births. Defects in any of the enzymes in the cycle usually lead to severe hyperammonemia and ammonia intoxication. The chief symptoms include lethargy, behavioral changes, and vomiting. Most people with mild urea cycle disorders have learning disabilities and reading and writing difficulties.

A complete lack of any of the enzymes involved in the urea cycle will result in infant death. However, deficiencies of each of the enzymes have been identified. While many cases occur in neonates and infants, some forms are not seen until adulthood. Infants with severe urea cycle disorders typically show symptoms after the first 24 hours of life. Those with mild to moderate enzyme deficiencies may not show symptoms until childhood. Some who have less severe deficiencies show symptoms in adulthood.

Although specific additional treatments (e.g., activation of other pathways of waste nitrogen synthesis and excretion) are useful for each deficiency, regulating protein intake and providing proteins of good quality are the cornerstones of treatment. Alternate pathways of nitrogen excretion include conjugation with glycine to form hippurate that is rapidly excreted in the urine. Glycine is synthesized rapidly and derives its nitrogen from the same pool as ammonia.

21.2.6 METHIONINE

Methionine is adenosylated on its sulfur to form S-adenosylmethionine, which serves as a major methylating agent and as a precursor of spermine and spermidine. S-adenosylhomocysteine, the demethylated product, forms homocysteine, which combines with serine to form cystathionine, a precursor of cysteine (Figure 21.7).

Thus, while methionine is an essential amino acid, cysteine is not. Patients may have a deficiency of any one of the three enzymes involved: (1) methionine adenosyltransferase, (2) cystathionine β-synthase, and (3) γ-cystathionase; the latter two enzymes are dependent on pyridoxal phosphate. Synthase deficiency, the most common of the three disorders, causes homocystinuria, which is accompanied by eye, bone, and brain derangements. Diets low in methionine and supplemented with cysteine are used in treatment. Some patients with residual activity are treated with pyridoxine, but many of these still require some restriction of methionine intake. Methionine adenosyltransferase deficiency is rare and benign. γ-cystathionase deficiency also causes few problems and requires no treatment, although pyridoxine is given to some patients.

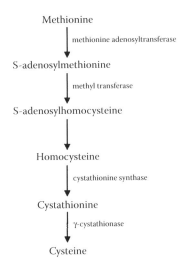

FIGURE 21.7 Formation of cysteine from methionine.

21.2.7 VALINE, LEUCINE, AND ISOLEUCINE

The most common disorder of branched-chain amino acid metabolism is the failure to convert the products of transamination, α-keto acids, to CoA derivatives by oxidative decarboxylation (Figure 21.8). The keto acid decarboxylase, a thiamin pyrophosphate–dependent enzyme, catalyzes the decarboxylation reaction common to the catabolic pathway for the keto acids of all three branched-chain amino acids. Maple syrup urine disease, or branched-chain ketoaciduria, results and causes mental and physical retardation. Specially prepared diets that are free of valine, leucine, and isoleucine are commercially available. These must be started in the first few days after birth to avoid the disease. Because the branched-chain amino acids are essential, adequate amounts must be provided. Some patients with partial activity benefit from thiamin, which appears to stabilize the decarboxylase. In pregnancy, protein-restricted diets and carnitine have been useful. Some diets for the treatment of maple syrup urine disease have been deficient in isoleucine.

Each of the three branched-chain amino acids traverses a separate path during its catabolism. The paths share similar steps such as transamination, oxidative decarboxylation, dehydrogenation, dehydration, reduction, and thiolysis. Many patients present with episodes of acidosis. Most of these diseases are treated by moderate restriction of protein intake while others are refractory to intervention. In the leucine path, deficiencies of isovaleryl CoA dehydrogenase, 3-methylcrotonyl CoA carboxylase, and mild deficiencies of 3-methylglutaconyl CoA hydratase are successfully treated by decreasing protein intake, but the severe form of the third disease is not responsive to treatments used so far. Mitochondrial 3-hydroxy 3-methyl glutaryl CoA is a ketone body precursor. Deficiency of 3-hydroxy 3-methyl glutaryl CoA lyase is treated by restricting dietary protein and fat and by avoiding fasting conditions, which would elicit ketosis in normal individuals. Some patients self-impose these restrictions. Isoleucine catabolism can be defective at the 2-methylacetoacetyl CoA thiolase step, but again these patients are responsive to the restriction of protein intake.

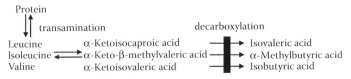

FIGURE 21.8 The metabolic block in maple syrup urine disease. (Reproduced with the permission of Dr. David Valle.)

Disturbances of valine catabolism are extremely rare. A patient with 3-hydroxyisobutyryl CoA deacylase deficiency had multiple developmental abnormalities and died when 3 months old.

21.2.8 GLUTARYL COENZYME A ACCUMULATION

Lysine, hydroxylysine, and tryptophan give rise to glutaryl CoA in the course of their metabolism. A block in its further metabolism leads to its accumulation and the excretion of glutaric acid. Muscle and nervous system abnormalities occur. Restriction of dietary lysine brings down the glutaryl CoA level, but little clinical improvement occurs, usually because the damage is done (which is irreversible by the time the diagnosis is made). Early supplementation with carnitine; vigorous treatment of the incurred infection with fluids, glucose, and insulin; and (perhaps) dietary restriction of glutarigenic amino acids (lysine and tryptophan) can prevent neurologic symptoms in patients without striated damage at diagnosis.

21.2.9 CYSTINURIA

Cystinuria is due to a defect in the transporter for basic amino acids and characterized by the occurrence of cysteine stones in the urinary tract. Dibasic amino acids also share this transporter. Although restriction of sulfur amino acids would seem a reasonable approach, results have been found to vary.

21.2.10 LYSINE

Lysinuric protein intolerance is caused by a transport protein defect. Lysine and other basic amino acids are lost, leading to defective function of the urea cycle and hyperammonemia. Patients avoid protein but become malnourished. Treatment involves adjusting protein intake to minimum requirements. Supplementation with citrulline, a component of the urea cycle, is beneficial.

21.3 DISORDERS OF LIPID METABOLISM

Most of the energy of the body is stored as triglycerides (i.e., three fatty acids linked to glycerol). These fatty acids may be obtained from the diet or synthesized in the body. Genetic difficulties occur in the transport or in the catabolism of fatty acids. Two major treatments are helpful: (1) In some patients where there is an inability to catabolize, prevention of fatty acid mobilization by frequent feeding of carbohydrates is helpful. (2) In others where the difficulty is specifically in the transport or catabolism of long-chain fatty acids, feeding triglycerides of medium- or short-chain fatty acids is recommended.

Triglycerides are hydrolyzed into fatty acids and glycerides, mostly monoglycerides, in the small intestine. Emulsifying agents such as bile salts and lipase and its adjunct colipase are used. Small and medium-length fatty acids can enter the circulation directly, but longer-chain fatty acids are reesterified to triacylglycerides and transported as chylomicrons through the lymphatics into the systemic circulation. In abetalipoproteinemia, lipids accumulate within the intestinal cells. Mental retardation, retinal and spino-cerebellar degeneration, and steatorrhea also occur along with spiny red blood cells, acanthocytes, and abnormal blood clotting. The defect is not in the gene or processing of either of the two forms of apolipoprotein B, a protein component of chylomicrons, very-low-density lipoproteins, or low-density lipoproteins, but in a triglyceride transfer protein found in the endoplasmic reticulum. The elimination of long-chain fatty acids from the diet is essential. Large doses of vitamin E are used probably because vitamin E is normally carried by the very-low-density lipoproteins. This indicates the importance of preventing oxidative damage to the nervous system, as does the finding of defective superoxide dismutase in amyotrophic lateral sclerosis. Sometimes it is helpful to give short- and medium-chain fatty acids containing 8 to 14 carbons that can enter the circulation directly.

These fatty acids are transported bound to serum albumin; however, there are reports of liver cirrhosis following the administration of medium- and short-chain fatty acids, so they should be given with caution.

Fatty acids are hydrolyzed from chylomicrons by the lipoprotein lipase. Deficiency of this enzyme, its cofactor, apoprotein C II, or occurrence of an inhibitor are rare but cause a marked increase of chylomicrons and very-low-density lipoproteins in homozygotes. Many different alterations of the lipoprotein lipase gene have been found. Bouts of pancreatitis are frequent. Restriction of dietary fat intake to 20 g/day usually prevents symptoms.

Smith–Lemli–Opitz syndrome (SLOS) is a recessively inherited disorder of cholesterol biosynthesis that results in decreased levels of plasma cholesterol and accumulation of the cholesterol precursor, 7-dehydro cholesterol (7DHC). The disease is the result of mutations in the human sterol 7-delta reductase gene. Cholesterol is critical in the formation of basic biological structures, including the brain. The estimated daily synthetic need for cholesterol during infancy is 20–40 mg/kg of body weight per day based on the isotopic analysis of newly synthesized cholesterol following the infusion of deuterium water.[1] In adults, the daily synthetic requirements decrease to approximately 10 mg/kg of body weight per day or between 500 and 900 mg/day in the average adult. Treatment with cholesterol supplementation of 50 mg/kg of body weight per day either in the natural form (eggs, cream, meat, and meat-based formulas) or as purified food-grade cholesterol has been shown to improve plasma sterol levels and result in improved growth and development in many patients.[9] Photosensitivity, apparently caused by the increased level of 7DHC in the skin, is a common problem in children with SLOS exposed to the sun or even just bright light. It is easily remedied by standard sun-blocking creams.

Antenatal treatment of SLOS by cholesterol supplementation is feasible and results in the improvement of fetal plasma cholesterol levels and red blood cell volume. SLOS may be one of the growing numbers of genetic disorders for which prenatal diagnosis is available and therapeutic intervention may be possible.

21.3.1 PROPIONATE AND METHYLMALONATE

Propionyl CoA is formed from the catabolism of valine, isoleucine, methionine, threonine, odd-chain fatty acids, propionate, and cholesterol. A carboxyl group is added by the biotin-dependent enzyme propionyl CoA carboxylase (Figure 21.9). The D-methylmalonyl-CoA formed is converted to the L-form by a racemase. The L-methylmalonyl CoA is converted into succinyl CoA, a component of the citric acid cycle, by methylmalonyl CoA mutase, an enzyme that requires vitamin B_{12} as a cofactor. Propionyl CoA carboxylase deficiency can occur as a specific isolated defect or as a defect involving all biotin-dependent carboxylases. Combined carboxylase deficiency may be due to defective coupling of biotin to the carboxylases (holocarboxylase synthetase deficiency) or to incomplete release of biotin from degraded carboxylases (biotinidase deficiency). Severe neonatal metabolic acidosis occurs in many of these patients. Biochemically, the situation is complex because the enzyme has two nonidentical subunits, either of which may be affected.

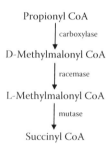

FIGURE 21.9 Metabolism of propionyl CoA to succinyl CoA.

There are often marked differences in the severity of symptoms within a family for reasons that are not known. While treatment for the specific enzyme disorders is difficult, for biotinidase deficiency the intake of supplemental amounts of biotin on a daily basis can prevent all symptoms of this potentially devastating disorder. Low-protein diets with special attention to lowering the precursors of propionyl CoA are used. Some patients lose large amounts of propionylcarnitine in their urine and are helped by carnitine supplementation. Isoleucine deficiency in some of the diets used for this treatment has been reported.

Methylmalonyl CoA mutase deficiency is one of a number of causes of methylmalonyl acidemia. Other causes are due to defects in the enzymes involved in the metabolic alterations needed for vitamin B_{12} to function in this pathway. As with most genetic diseases, the defect can be due to point mutations and to the inability to make the enzyme. Some have defects in cobalamin metabolism prior to the point where the derivatives for methylmalonyl CoA metabolism occur. Cobalamin supplementation and avoiding methylmalonyl CoA precursors are used in the treatment as appropriate.

21.3.2 CARNITINE

Carnitine can be made in the liver and muscle, but a dietary source is also needed. Carnitine deficiency occurs if the transport protein in the intestine is deficient. Long-chain fatty acids are carried into cells and their organelles especially in the heart, skeletal muscle, and adipose tissue by carnitine, while those with medium length and short chains do not need carnitine for transport. Fatty acids form their CoA derivatives before oxidation, which occurs in the mitochondria. Fatty acid CoA derivatives (in cytosol) are converted to carnitine derivatives by carnitine palmitoyl transferase I (in the outer mitochondrial membrane), moved across the inner mitochondrial membrane by a translocase, and made back into CoA derivatives by a second transferase (within the mitochondrial matrix; Figure 21.10). Deficiencies in each of these steps can occur with that of the last step, carnitine palmitoyl transferase II, being the most common.[23] It causes myoglobinuria after stress or exercise and is seen especially in older children and young adults.

Normal muscle can use either glucose or fatty acid as fuel, with fatty acid predominating at rest and the amounts of glucose employed increasing with increasing exercise severity. In carnitine palmitoyl transferase deficiency,[11] glucose is the fuel under all circumstances and, accordingly, performance is enhanced by high glucose intake. Those with translocase deficiency cannot recover carnitine filtered in the kidney and have the symptoms of carnitine deficiency. Carnitine deficiency symptoms can also occur in type II deficiency because acylcarnitines accumulate and deplete the pool of free carnitine. Treatment involves limiting prolonged exercise, avoiding fasting situations, and bringing in dietary modifications including the replacement of long-chain with medium-chain triglycerides supplemented with carnitine.[18]

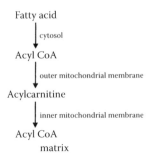

FIGURE 21.10 Movement of fatty acid coenzyme A across the cell membrane.

21.3.3 OTHER ABNORMALITIES

After fatty acids have been carried into the mitochondria, they are broken down two carbons at a time by β-oxidation in a repetitive sequence of steps: (1) Removal of hydrogens by dehydrogenase hydration, and (2) a second dehydrogenation yielding β-ketoacyl CoA (Figure 21.11). The β-ketoacyl CoA reacts with CoA to form acetyl CoA and an acyl CoA with two fewer carbons. The new acyl CoA undergoes additional rounds of acetyl CoA formation until it is entirely converted to acetyl CoA. Acyl CoA dehydrogenases are a set of enzymes rather than a single entity, and deficiencies of specific members can exist. While deficiencies of each have been described, those of the medium-chain acyl CoA dehydrogenases are very common and in some cases lead to sudden death in a previously asymptomatic child. Lethargy induced by fasting, vomiting, and coma are often presenting symptoms. Hypoglycemia, a low level of ketone bodies for the blood sugar level, and organic dibasic aciduria are among the results. Treatment involves avoiding fasting and taking in adequate calories. Long-chain acyl CoA dehydrogenase deficiency is less common and is treated with frequent carbohydrate-rich feedings that are supplemented by medium-chain triglycerides. Some deficiencies of fatty acid metabolism respond to pharmacological doses of riboflavin. Multiple acyl CoA deficiency and 3-methyl 3-hydroxy glutaryl CoA lyase deficiency are both treated with frequent meals, and additional carnitine and riboflavin are given for the former. In contrast to many other genetic diseases, 85%–90% of patients with this disease have the same mutation.

In addition to transporting fatty acids, lipoproteins also carry cholesterol in the plasma and genetic defects of lipoprotein receptors are associated with hypercholesterolemia and atherosclerotic heart diseases in both homozygotes and heterozygotes. Restriction of dietary cholesterol intake is recommended, but treatment with drugs that lower cholesterol levels is also required. In heterozygotes, medications that stimulate the activity of the normal receptor gene are also used.

In the course of transporting lipids in the plasma the larger lipoproteins lose fatty acids to tissues, and rearrangement of lipoprotein to decrease the amount of amphipathic lipid on the surface must occur. Lecithin-cholesterol acyltransferase (LCAT) allows this rearrangement by moving a fatty acid residue from lecithin to cholesterol. Deficiency of LCAT is rare. Dietary fat restriction is recommended.

Fatty acid catabolism causes the formation of enzyme-linked reduced flavins. These send their electron to the electron-transport system through an electron-transport protein that couples flavin enzymes to ubiquinone reductase. When this protein is deficient, glutaric acidemia type II occurs. Severe forms are fatal, but milder cases can be helped by diets low in fat and proteins, which are substances that can reduce flavoproteins.

Branched-chain fatty acids are not converted to carnitine derivatives in the outer face of mitochondria, and their initial breakdown occurs in peroxisomes. Refsum's disease is a deficiency of phytanic acid α-hydroxylase activity that causes phytanic acid to accumulate; neurological disease

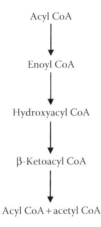

FIGURE 21.11 Generation of β-ketoacyl coenzyme A.

results. Phytanic acid has a methyl group on its third carbon and cannot be oxidized in the normal manner by β-oxidation. Phytanic acid is a metabolite formed in ruminants from chlorophyll. When dairy products and meat from ruminants are eliminated from the diet, considerable improvement in neurological dysfunction occurs.

21.4 MISCELLANEOUS GENETIC DISEASES

Phytosterolemia is characterized by the accumulation of plant sterols and coronary heart disease. It is rare and treated by avoiding plant and shellfish sterols.

Wilson's disease is associated with the accumulation of copper. Liver cirrhosis and behavioral disorders are common. The disease is due to insufficient excretion of copper in bile. While removing copper with a chelating agent is the mainstay of treatment, keeping copper intake low is also important. Zinc supplements can be used for maintenance. A vegetarian diet has been suggested as one way of maintaining a low copper intake. Organ meats, shellfish, chocolate, nuts, beans, and cereals are among the foods prohibited.

Adenine phosphoribosyl transferase (an enzyme in the purine salvage pathway) deficiency is characterized by the formation of stones from adenine metabolites in the urinary tract. Restriction of dietary intake of purines is suggested.

A heterozygote having a 50% reduction in porphobilinogen deaminase is at risk for developing acute intermittent porphyria, although only about 10% of such people will have an attack. Environmental factors play an important role in precipitating an attack. Abdominal pain with vomiting is a common finding. Often, the attack can be aborted by a high carbohydrate intake.

Peroxisomes are organelles in which a variety of reactions occur. Very-long-chain fatty acids are broken down, bile acids are formed, and many other biosynthetic and oxidative reactions occur. Deficient peroxisomal function can result from a variety of events and is called Zellweger's syndrome. It is usually a fatal disease in infants. Milder forms can be treated by decreasing the levels of very-long-chain fatty acids by giving oleate as their triglyceride; preventing phytanic acid accumulation through dietary restrictions; and providing either phospholipids or plasmalogens, which are normally made in the peroxisomes.

X-linked adrenoleukodystrophy is a peroxisomal disease resulting from the mutation of a transporter and associated with a synthetase for very-long-chain CoA fatty acids. The transporter is adjacent to the genes for red–green color vision, and deletions and rearrangements frequently affect the function of the genes. Adrenal hormone replacement and administration of trioleyl glyceride or erucic acid (a 22-carbon monounsaturated fatty acid) to decrease very-long-chain fatty acids are dietary aspects of treatment.

21.5 SUMMARY

This chapter has attempted to survey genetic diseases where single defined deficiencies occur. Only those where diet plays an important role in inducing the disease or treating the disease have been considered. It may be helpful to reiterate the general principles along with some applications of each.

If a metabolic pathway is blocked, intermediates prior to the block accumulate. These may cause no symptoms as in essential fructosuria, mild symptoms as in alcaptonuria, or severe disease as in PKU. The precursor or its by-products may interfere with other enzymes and transport proteins, as occurs in PKU and glucose 6-phosphatase deficiency, or accumulate, as in Refsum's disease. Accumulation of excess precursor in the intestinal tract in lactase and other disaccharidase deficiencies allows bacterial fermentation, lactate formation, and osmotically induced diarrhea. The excretion of excessive amounts of precursor may aid in initial diagnosis, but sometimes causes dysfunction, as occurs with deposits in the urinary tract in adenosine phosphoribosyltransferase deficiency and cystinuria. Precursor accumulation may deplete other metabolites as in fructose aldolase deficiency where the inorganic phosphate level of the liver is drastically lowered.

Where the precursor has essential functions in the body it must be given in regulated amounts. Examples are phenylalanine in PKU and leucine, valine, and isoleucine in maple syrup urine disease. These amino acids are needed for protein synthesis.

Deficiency of a product occurs if the product cannot be made in the body and must be supplied. Thus, in PKU tyrosine becomes essential, and in cystathionine β-synthase deficiency cysteine is required in the diet. Most genetic difficulties of carbohydrate metabolism can be treated by omitting the offending sugar because the needed sugars can be synthesized from glucose. Although sugar inter-conversions supply specific sugars for syntheses, they are inadequate to meet energy requirements so that in these situations a source of useable calories must be supplied. In glucose 6-phosphatase deficiency, uncooked starch and frequent feedings prevent ketosis and hypoglycemia. In muscle phosphorylase deficiency carbohydrate feeding extends endurance, and in fructose 1,6-bisphospha-tase deficiency frequent carbohydrate feedings prevent abortive attempts at gluconeogenesis. The presence of defects in medium-chain acyl CoA dehydrogenase is another situation where adequate caloric intake is an important aspect of treatment.

Diet can bring on or exacerbate genetic diseases. Fava beans precipitate episodes of hemolytic anemia in GPDH deficiency. Protein in excess of minimal requirements worsens diseases of the urea cycle, and propionate precursors increase the severity of propionyl CoA carboxylase and meth-ylmalonyl CoA mutase deficiencies. Pregnancy in patients with metabolite elevation often leads to difficulties for the fetus. Galactosemic mothers may bear infants with cataracts, while hyperphenyl-alaninemics have children with decreased head size and birth weight.

Fava Beans and Acute Hemolysis—A Case Study

A 34-year-old Iraqi male was admitted to the hospital because of severe anemia, renal failure, and jaundice. Four days before admission he had fever, anorexia, and vomiting. At the time he was admitted to the hospital, he could not walk without assistance. He reported having maroon-colored urine, dryness in his mouth, and yellowness in his eyes. He did not have any pain other than discomfort in his eyes. The patient had no history of kidney disease or hepatitis.

At admission his temperature was 99.3°F, pulse rate 117, blood pressure 141/67 mm Hg, and weight 140 pounds. Hematology analysis revealed he had a hemolytic disease with result-ing jaundice and acute renal failure. He had elevated white blood cell count. Initial possible diagnosis included an inherited membrane abnormality (e.g., spherocytosis), deficiency of glu-cose 6-phosphate dehydrogenase (GPDH), hemoglobinopathy, or an infectious disease such as malaria. Additional laboratory studies showed no sign of spherocytosis, hemoglobinopathy, or malaria.

During the initial and follow-up assessments on medical and dietary history, his female friend reported that the patient had eaten "really big beans" the day before he began to have the aforementioned symptoms. She did not know what kind they were, but said that she had never seen him eat that type of bean before. When fava beans were shown to the patient, he confirmed that they were the type of beans he had eaten. This suggested that his hemolysis crisis might have been due to consuming fava beans. This was confirmed when the patient's red blood cell GPDH activity was found to be 2–6 U/g of hemoglobin (normal is 4.6–13.6 U/g hemoglobin). The patient was diagnosed with favism, an acute hemolytic episode caused by sensitivity to fava beans. His treatment included blood transfusion, hemodialysis, multivitamin injection, and so forth for 2 weeks and he was discharged after receiving dietary instructions.

Clinical favism presents characteristically with the sudden onset of acute hemolytic ane-mia within 24–48 hours of ingesting the beans.[24,25] GPDH deficiency is by far the most com-mon congenital defect affecting more than 400 million people throughout the world. The highest prevalence rates (with gene frequencies in the range of 5%–25%) are found in tropi-cal Africa, the Middle East, tropical and subtropical Asia, some areas of the Mediterranean, and Papua New Guinea. The remarkable correlation between the prevalence of GPDH and the past and present endemicity of malaria strongly suggests that the former confers resistance against the latter. The high prevalence in malaria-endemic areas of GPDH mutants that have arisen independently corroborates this notion; indeed, it constitutes an example of convergent evolution through balanced polymorphism.

Hereditary Fructose Intolerance—A Case Study

A healthy 2-month-old female infant, who had previously been exclusively breast-fed, vomited when given supplementary feeds of sweetened cow's milk. She reacted similarly when given fruit juice and sometimes became quiet and sleepy after such a feed. Her mother experimented with various feeds and learned to avoid those that made her child ill. The child grew up with an aversion to sweet foodstuffs and fruit. Her brother, born 2 years later, had a similar history.

Later, when both became medical students they wondered if their aversion was due to HFI. They volunteered to take the test. They were given fructose orally 0.5 g/kg of body weight. Blood samples were taken at 0 and 90 minutes after the administration of fructose. Blood analysis revealed hypoglycemia, dramatic fall in serum phosphate to 60% of normal value, and increase in serum lactate and uric acid in both of them, characteristic of HFI.

In HFI, deficiency of aldolase B causes the accumulation of fructose 1-phosphate (FIP). FIP inhibits phosphorylase, which causes a decrease in the formation of glucose[8] from glycogen.

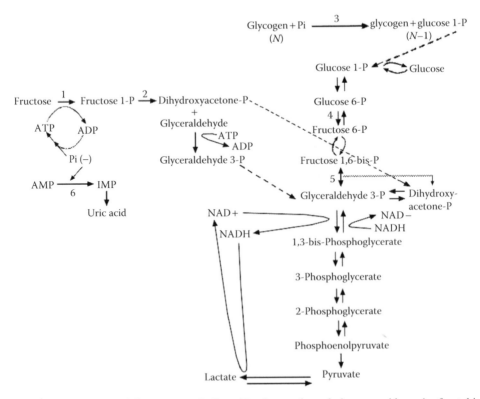

FIGURE 21.12 Summary of fructose metabolism: N—the number of glucose residues, 1—fructokinase, 2—aldolase B, 3—phosphorylase, 4—phosphoglucoisomerase, 5—aldolase A, and 6—AMP deaminase. Curved reaction arrows ($\circlearrowright$) indicate that forward and reverse reactions are catalyzed by different enzymes.

FIP also inhibits two gluconeogenic enzymes, glucose-6-phosphate isomerase and aldolase (Figure 21.12). Thus, the overall effect is a decrease in blood glucose concentration after the ingestion of fructose.

Unregulated activity of fructokinase in the absence of sufficiently active aldolase B leads to the depletion of ATP. Much of the inorganic phosphate (Pi) then remains bound to FIP. This explains the decrease in Pi after fructose intake.

Decrease in Pi inhibits phosphorylase and also triggers the increased rate of degradation of adenosine monophosphate (AMP) by releasing inhibitory effect of Pi on AMP deaminase, ultimately leading to an increase in serum uric acid. The true incidence rate of HFI is not known but may be as high as 1 in 23,000. The gene for aldolase B is on chromosome 9—several mutations causing HFI have been identified. A single mutation, which results in substitution of proline for alanine in position 149 of the polypeptide, is the most common one identified in Northern Europe. This mutation plus two other point mutations account for 80%–85% of HFI in Europe and in the United States.

Symptoms become manifest only when patients ingest fructose or sorbitol. The primary symptom is vomiting, and other features of hypoglycemia present within 20–30 minutes after the ingestion of fructose. Other symptoms include poor feeding, failure to thrive, and liver dysfunction. Continued fructose use can lead to liver and kidney failure and death.

Treatment consists of the complete elimination of all sources of sucrose, fructose, and sorbitol from the diet. With this treatment, liver and kidney dysfunctions improve and catch-up growth is common.

REFERENCES

1. Bradley, L. A. 1999. Antenatal therapy of Smith–Lemli–Opitz syndrome. *J Fetal Diagn Ther* 14:133.
2. Cockburn, F., and R. Gitzelmann, eds. 1982. *Inborn Errors of Metabolism in Humans*. New York: Alan R. Liss.
3. Crenn, P., and F. Maillot. 2007. Dietary advice for treatment of inborn errors of metabolism in adult neurology: Principles and limitations. *Rev Neurol* 163:936.
4. Desnick, R. J., ed. 1991. *Treatment of Genetic Disease*. New York: Churchill Livingstone.
5. Fernandes, R. J., J. M. Saudubray, and G. Van Den Bergue, eds. 1995. *Inborn Metabolic Diseases*. 2nd ed. Berlin: Springer-Verlag.
6. Hoffman, G. F., S. Athanassopoulos, A. B. Berlins et al. 1996. Clinical course, early diagnosis, treatment and prevention of disease in glutaryl-CoA dehydrogenase deficiency. *Neuropediatrics* 27:115.
7. Holton, J. B., ed. 1987. *The Inherited Metabolic Disease*. New York: Churchill Livingstone.
8. Hommes, F. A. 1993. Inborn errors of fructose metabolism. *Am J Clin Nutr* 58(suppl.):788S.
9. Irons, M., E. R. Elias, D. Abuelo et al. 1997. Treatment of Smith–Lemli–Opitz syndrome: Results of a multicenter trial. *Am J Med Genet* 68:311.
10. Irons, M. B., J. Nores, T. L. Stewart et al. 1983. Phenylketonuria and its variants. *Adv Hum Genet* 13:217.
11. Isackson, P. J., M. J. Bennett, and G. D. Vladutiu. 2006. Identification of 16 new disease-causing mutations in the CPT2 gene resulting in carnitine palmitoyltransferase deficiency. *Mol Genet Metab* 89:323.
12. Koch, R., and E. Wenz. 1987. Phenylketonuria. *Annu Ret Nutr* 7:117.
13. Merrill Jr., A. H., and J. Michael Henderson. 1987. Diseases associated with defects in vitamin B_6 metabolism or utilization. *Annu Rev Nutr* 7:137.
14. Parker, P. H., M. Ballew, and N. L. Greene. 1993. Nutritional management of glycogen storage diseases. *Annu Rev Nutr* 13:83.
15. Raghuveer, T., U. Garg, and W. Graf. 2006. Inborn errors of metabolism in infancy and early childhood: An update. *Am Fam Physician* 73:1981.
16. Saavedra, J. M., and J. A. Perman. 1989. Current concepts in lactose malabsorption. *Annu Rev Nutr* 9:475.
17. Scriver, C. R., A. L. Beaudet, W. S. Sly, and D. Valle, eds. 2001. *Metabolic and Molecular Basis of Inherited Disease*. New York: McGraw Hill.

18. Stanley, C. A., D. E. Hale, G. T. Berry et al. 1992. A deficiency of carnitine-acyl carnitine translocase in the inner mitochondrial membrane. *N Engl J Med* 327:19.
19. Tada, K., J. P. Combo, and R. J. Desnick, eds. 1987. *Recent Advances in Inborn Errors of Metabolism.* New York: Karger.
20. Valle, D. L. 1983. Inborn errors of metabolism. In *Manual of Clinical Nutrition*, ed. D. M. Paige, 36.1. Pleasantville, NJ: Nutrition Publications.
21. Winick, M., ed. 1979. *Nutritional Management of Genetic Disorders.* New York: John Wiley & Sons.
22. Wong, D. 2005. Hereditary fructose intolerance. *Med Genet Metab* 15:165.
23. Yasuno, T., H. Kaneoka, T. Tokuyaso et al. 2008. Mutations of carnitine palmitoyltransferase II (CPT II) in Japanese patients with CPT II deficiency. *Clin Genet* 73:496.

CASE BIBLIOGRAPHY

24. Arese, P., and A. De Flora. 1990. Pathophysiology of hemolysis in glucose 6-phosphate dehydrogenase deficiency. *Semin Hematol* 27:1.
25. Hampl, J. S., K. A. Holland, J. T. Marple, M. R. Hutchins, and K. K. Brockman. 1997. Acute hemolysis related to consumption of fava beans: A case study and medical nutrition therapy approach. *J Am Diet Assoc* 97:182.

22 Nutritional and Metabolic Effects of Alcohol

Hundreds of thousands of years ago, humans presumably realized that when fruits and other plant materials were well mixed with water and left in the warmth of the sun a strange product was formed. This substance became known as alcohol or, more properly, ethyl alcohol. There is no historical record of either who discovered alcohol or the substance from which the first alcohol originated. However, there is evidence to indicate that alcohol has played a role in the social development of human beings for many thousands of years.

The oldest alcoholic drinks were fermented beverages of relatively low alcohol content such as beers and wines. In about 800 AD, an Arabian known as Jabir Iban Hayyan succeeded in developing the technique of distillation. The word alcohol is derived from the Arabic term *al-kohl*, meaning "finely divided spirit," because vapors of fermented products were removed in an invisible form.

Alcohol (or alcoholic beverages) has been used in social, religious, and symbolic events for many years.[21] In its various forms, alcohol has been a part of the medical profession's armamentarium since the Middle Ages. It was considered a remedy for practically all diseases, as evidenced by the word whiskey, which in Gaelic "usquebaugh" means "water of life."

By ancient tradition, wine and beer were considered as food, which were acceptable by the sick when solid food could not be tolerated. When spirits became available, they too were accepted by the medical profession and the laity as appropriate nourishment both for debilitated persons and for those who refused to eat in times of sickness.

22.1 EPIDEMIOLOGY

Until the beginning of the nineteenth century, the use of alcohol remained under reasonable control. Since then, its use has come to increasing prominence. Alcoholism—the compulsive uncontrollable drinking of alcoholic beverages—is a disease that ranks third in the world behind heart disease and cancer in incidence. The medical and social effects of excess alcohol consumption comprise one of the largest groups of problems encountered by physicians. The yearly cost of alcohol-related problems in the United States is as much as $300 billion, including health problems, lost productivity, accidents, crime, and treatment. In 1997, a national household survey reported that two of three adult Americans (19 years of age and over) drink at least occasionally, 1 in 8 drinks to excess, and 1 in 16 drinks enough to be classified as a problem drinker.

Excessive alcohol consumption ranks as the third leading preventable cause of death in the United States after cigarette smoking and obesity.[23] More than 100,000 deaths per year in the United States are attributed to alcohol use disorders. According to a 2003 survey, 13.6% of the population drove vehicles under the influence of alcohol at least once in the 12 months prior to the survey. Binge drinking (consuming 5 or more drinks on one occasion) has steadily increased in the United States with an estimated 1.5 billion episodes in 2001. Rates of binge drinking are higher for young adults (aged 18–25 years) with resultant higher rates of motor vehicle accidents in this population. Although sociodemographic features, such as young age, low income, and low education levels, have been associated with an increased risk for problem drinking, alcohol use disorders are prevalent throughout all sociodemographic groups.

22.2   ABSORPTION

Alcohol can enter the body in several ways, but its common entry is through the mouth. Unlike carbohydrates, fats, and proteins, alcohol does not require prior digestion. No active processes are involved in its absorption, which begins almost immediately after ingestion. About 30% of the alcohol taken orally is absorbed from the stomach and the rest from the small intestine.

The rate of absorption from the stomach and the rate of passage into the small intestine are influenced by several factors. If the stomach contents do not pass into the small intestine, for example, because of delayed emptying, the rate of absorption will slow and may even cease. Alcohol is absorbed fastest if the stomach is empty. The presence of food in the stomach, especially food rich in fat, slows the absorption of alcohol and delays its passage in the small intestine. Hence, drinking alcoholic beverages during or after a meal reduces the likelihood of intoxication. The higher the concentration of alcohol (up to 30%) in a beverage, the faster the absorption. In general, alcohol is absorbed rapidly from distilled spirits such as whiskey, slowly from wines, and more slowly from beers. Carbonated alcoholic beverages are usually absorbed more rapidly than those not containing carbon dioxide, which hastens the emptying time of the stomach into the intestine. After the alcohol reaches the small intestine it is quickly absorbed. It does not accumulate in the small intestine as may happen in the stomach.

23.3   DISTRIBUTION

Alcohol enters the bloodstream from the stomach and the small intestine. It then distributes throughout the body including the brain and cerebrospinal fluid in proportion to the water content of individual tissues. Thus, the amount of alcohol per unit of water in these various tissues and body fluids will essentially be the same. The average water content of the body is 65% and that of blood is about 83%, and so after equilibrium, the alcohol content of a unit of blood will be approximately 1.27 times that of the unit of the whole body. It is, therefore, possible to calculate the amount of alcohol in the body by determining the alcohol levels in the blood or other biological fluids. The commonly accepted figures for the urine-to-blood alcohol ratio is 1.25, for saliva to blood alcohol the ratio is 1.20, and for spinal fluid to blood alcohol the ratio is 1.14. Alcohol levels in the brain are difficult to measure. Blood alcohol content is commonly used as a metric of intoxication for legal and medical purposes.

Because of its ready volatility, alcohol can also be determined from the breath. There is a constant relationship between the amount of alcohol in the blood and that in the alveolar air. The latter contains close to 5.5% carbon dioxide by volume (or 190 mg in 2100 mL of alveolar air). The alveolar air–to-blood alcohol ratio is close to 1/2100. The weight of alcohol in 1 mL of blood should therefore be equal to the quantity of alcohol in the breath that accompanies 190 mg of carbon dioxide. There are instruments available that can quickly determine alcohol and carbon dioxide in the breath air and relate them to blood alcohol.

22.4   NUTRITIONAL SIGNIFICANCE OF ALCOHOL

Alcohol possesses several properties that make it an excellent energy food. No other food item taken orally acts as swiftly as alcohol. It does not change chemically in the gastrointestinal tract and is ready for absorption the moment it is ingested. It follows relatively short and simple metabolic routes and is broken down completely, with only a small percentage being eliminated in the urine and expired air. Acetate as acetyl–coenzyme A (CoA), an intermediate in the oxidation of alcohol (described in Section 22.5), is also an active participant in the process, which allows the tissues to utilize proteins, fats, and carbohydrates and is not toxic.

Approximately 7 Cal (30 kJ) are liberated in the complete oxidation of 1 g of alcohol and, therefore, it is a more concentrated energy food than either proteins or carbohydrates. Only fat, liberating

TABLE 22.1
Sources and Approximate Amounts of Energy in Alcoholic Beverages

Beverages	Serving Size (oz.)	Alcohol (g)	Alcohol Energy Cal (in kJ)	Total Energy Cal (in kJ)
Light beer (alcohol 3.25%)	12.0	11.3	79 (330)	99 (414)
Beer (alcohol 3.7%)	12.0	12.8	89 (372)	146 (611)
Table wine (alcohol 9.4%)	4.5	12.3	86 (360)	90 (377)
Desert wine (alcohol 15.4%)	4.5	20.2	141 (590)	203 (849)
Whiskey (80 proof)	1.5	14.0	98 (410)	98 (410)
Vodka (90 proof)	1.5	15.0	105 (439)	105 (439)

9 Cal/g (38 kJ), exceeds it in this respect. During its stay in the stomach, alcohol appears to stimulate appetite and digestion in unhabituated subjects, a process that must be considered a part of its nutritive value. There is no physiological need for alcohol, which by strict definition is not a nutrient.

Some of the major beverages are beers, table wines, port and sherry, cocktail and dessert wines, liqueurs, and distilled spirits. The concentration of alcohol varies from one kind of drink to another. For example, most regular American beers contain about 4% alcohol; for table wines, the range is from 8% to 10% alcohol. Port and sherry are strengthened by the addition of extra alcohol to bring the alcohol concentration to 15%. Dessert wines have 20% alcohol, and liqueurs contain 22%–50% alcohol. The alcohol content of American distilled spirits varies from 40% to 50%. Beer and wine are labeled with the percentage of alcohol, but distilled spirits are labeled by proof. Standards for proof vary from country to country. In the United States, proof is twice the alcohol concentration expressed as percentage. Therefore, 80 proof whiskey contains 40% alcohol.

Distilled spirits contain little nutritional value besides calories. Beer and wine contain unfermented carbohydrates and trace protein, but like distilled spirits, they have negligible minerals. Other than beer, which contains small amounts of riboflavin and niacin, alcoholic beverages have negligible amounts of vitamins.

One serving of an alcoholic beverage is roughly equivalent to 12 ounces (350 mL) of beer, 4 ounces (115 mL) of unfortified wine, and 1.5 ounces (43 mL) or a jug of 80 proof distilled spirit. The amount of alcohol and energy of some common beverages are shown in Table 22.1. Note that a typical serving of beer has less alcohol but more calories than a typical serving of whiskey.

Of the total alcohol consumed in the United States, about 50% is in the form of beer, 40% as distilled spirits, and the remainder as wine.

22.5   ALCOHOL METABOLISM

The major amount of ingested alcohol is completely metabolized in the liver, but a certain quantity of the total, between 2% and 4% after moderate drinking and as high as 10% after excessive drinking, is eliminated as such primarily by way of the kidneys and lungs and to some extent by perspiration. Sections 22.5.1 through 22.5.3 describe three possible pathways for alcohol metabolism.

22.5.1   CYTOSOLIC ALCOHOL DEHYDROGENASE PATHWAY

This important pathway is responsible for 80%–90% of alcohol metabolism in the body. The initial oxidation of alcohol to acetaldehyde is catalyzed by alcohol dehydrogenase (ADH), a zinc-containing enzyme present primarily in the cytoplasm of the hepatic cell. This reaction requires nicotinamide adenine dinucleotide (NAD) as a cofactor (22.1). Acetaldehyde is a very toxic substance that, fortunately, is quickly metabolized to acetate by mitochondrial aldehyde dehydrogenase (ALDH), known as ALDH2. This reaction also requires NAD as a cofactor (22.2). ALDH is present in most cells of the body, but its highest activity is in the liver. Most of the acetate is released into the blood and is oxidized by extrahepatic tissues to carbon dioxide and water.

$$CH_3CH_2OH + NAD \quad \rightarrow \quad CH_3CHO + NADH + H^+$$

Ethanol   ADH   Acetaldehyde   (22.1)

$$CH_3CHO + NAD + H_2O \quad \rightarrow \quad CH_3COOH + NADH + H^+$$

Acetaldehyde   ALDH Acetic Acid   (22.2)

The rate of alcohol metabolism by ADH is relatively constant as the enzyme is saturated at low blood alcohol levels (BALs) and thus exhibits zero-order kinetics (constant amount oxidized per unit time). The metabolism is proportional to body weight (and probably liver weight) and averages approximately 7 g of alcohol per hour.

ADH is also found in gastric mucosa. In some situations, a portion of the absorbed dose of alcohol does not appear to enter the systematic circulation, suggesting first-pass metabolism. The relative contribution of hepatic versus gastric ADH to this response continues to be debated. The ADH may be capable of exerting modest metabolic effects at alcohol concentrations found in the stomach after a drink. Gastric ADH also may play a role in the effect of food in reducing alcohol bioavailability. Food, by delaying gastric emptying, allows for more extensive gastric metabolism.

22.5.2 MICROSOMAL ETHANOL-OXIDIZING SYSTEM

This pathway occurs in the hepatocyte smooth endoplasmic reticulum. It is responsible for the metabolism of about 10% or more of alcohol at high BALs. The cytochrome P-450 enzymes in the presence of oxygen and the reduced form of nicotinamide adenine dinucleotide phosphate (NADPH) oxidize alcohol to acetaldehyde (22.3). The latter is then metabolized by ALDH as described in Section 22.5.1 under the ADH pathway. One cytochrome P-450 isoform designated P-4502E1 (CYP2E1) appears to be the most important, accounting for 30% of microsomal ethanol-oxidizing system (MEOS) activity. At high BALs, ADH is saturated and CYPE2E1 (which produces metabolic tolerance to alcohol) is stimulated.

$$CH_3CH_2OH \xrightarrow[\text{NADPH}+H^+ \quad \text{NADP}^-]{\quad \frac{1}{2}O_2 \quad\quad H_2O \quad} CH_3CHO$$

Ethanol   Acetaldehyde   (22.3)

An important feature of CYP2E1 is that it is inducible by chronic alcohol use and it may contribute to the increased rate (more than 50%) of alcohol elimination in heavy drinkers. This may account, in part, for the greater tolerance of alcohol by regular drinkers. CYP2E1 and other cytochrome P-450 isoenzymes that can oxidize alcohol also metabolize certain drugs. Alcoholics, when sober, exhibit increased metabolism of these drugs; however, because alcohol competes with these drugs for metabolism, there is decreased rate of drug elimination when the patient drinks.

22.5.3 PEROXISOMAL CATALASE

Most of the catalase in the liver is localized in the peroxisomes. It can mediate the oxidation of alcohol by hydrogen peroxide (22.4) to acetaldehyde, which is further eliminated by ALDH as described in Section 22.5.1. This pathway does not seem to be important in terms of bulk elimination of alcohol. Whether it is clinically important in other ways in humans is unknown.

$$CH_3CH_2OH \quad + \quad H_2O_2 \quad \rightarrow \quad CH_3COOH + 2H_2O \qquad (22.4)$$

| Ethanol | Hydrogen Peroxide | Acetic acid | Water |

Ethanol ... Hydrogen Peroxide ... Acetic acid ... Water

22.6 RATE OF ALCOHOL METABOLISM

The level of alcohol in blood is expressed in milligrams per deciliter. In general, blood alcohol peaks 30–45 minutes after ingestion. In a person weighing 150 pounds (70 kg), the rate of alcohol metabolism is approximately 7 g/h and the BAL decreases by nearly 15 mg/100 mL/h. Table 22.2 presents the relationship between the number of drinks taken in 1 hour and the peak BAL. The values given are approximate and may vary with age, body weight, height, and gender, as well as the rate of consumption, prior drinking habits, and intake of various foods. Heavy drinkers, for example, can have elevated rates of alcohol metabolism due to higher than normal activities of alcohol-metabolizing enzymes in such individuals. If the rate of alcohol consumption exceeds the rate at which alcohol can be metabolized, then the BAL rises and the individual may become intoxicated. A person consuming two drinks in an hour would have blood alcohol concentrations of 20–35 mg/dL, and with five drinks the BAL will be about 100 mg/dL. This figure is legally defined as intoxication in most states.[15] There is, however, enormous variation in the published data on the rate of disappearance of alcohol from blood among individuals. The range is 10–20 mg/dL/h in nonalcoholics and possibly greater than 20 mg and as high as 36 mg in chronic drinkers. Older people may have higher BALs than young adults after consuming the same amount of alcohol because of age-related changes. These include a marked decrease in muscle mass and body water and decreased metabolism. Older people may also be taking certain medications that may affect metabolic rate. Thus, blood alcohol concentration may vary considerably among persons who consume these amounts.

There are important differences among gender and ethnic groups in the amounts and types of the metabolizing enzymes ADH and ALDH, and this may be important in determining an individual's alcohol use patterns.

22.6.1 GENDER DIFFERENCE

Young females develop higher BALs than their male counterparts after equal alcohol consumption.[7] This can be explained by the smaller size of women and the distribution of alcohol in a smaller water space, which varies inversely with their larger proportion of body fat. It has also been suggested that some alcohol is metabolized in the stomach.[27] The ADH activity of gastric mucosa is about 40% less in women (at least under the age of 50) than in men. As a result, less alcohol is

---

TABLE 22.2
Relationship between the Number of Drinks and Blood Alcohol Concentration

Number of Drinks Consumed in 1 Hour	Peak BAL (mg/100 mL)
1	10
2	25
3	45
4	70
5	100

Note: Values are approximate and may vary with alcohol content of the drink and several factors such as body weight, gender, prior alcohol consumption, and food intake.

metabolized in the stomach and high BAL occurs for any amount imbibed, possibly chronically exposing the liver to higher levels of alcohol. This subject is still in dispute and some recent studies did not show a gender-related gastric first-pass difference.

In comparing the weight of the human stomach (50 g), weight of the human liver (1500 g), and level of enzyme activity in these two organs, it appears that the liver has 300 times the capacity for alcohol oxidation than does the stomach. This suggests that a high BAL in females may be because of slightly slower hepatic alcohol metabolism in females. This could be related to hormonal status.

The amount of alcohol considered as moderate drinking for men is not necessarily moderate for women. Moderate drinking presently defined is not more than two drinks per day for men. Moderate drinking for women should be no more than one drink per day.

22.6.2 ETHNIC DIFFERENCE

After alcohol ingestion, in most people there is no buildup of acetaldehyde to any great extent. However, some 30%–50% of Chinese, Japanese, Koreans, Vietnamese, and Indonesians and about 40% of South American Indians have an atypical ALDH, with a single amino acid substitution of glutamine for a lysine residue in position 487 of the polypeptide chain of mitochondrial enzyme with near-zero activity. In these individuals, acetaldehyde is oxidized by a cytosolic enzyme, which has much lower activity than the mitochondrial enzyme. Levels of acetaldehyde in these persons after ingestion of alcohol may be 10 times higher than in individuals with normal mitochondrial variants of ALDH. In such persons, even a small amount of alcohol can produce the so-called Asian flush response with vasodilation, facial flushing, tachycardia, headaches, nausea, and vomiting (Figure 22.1a and b). These symptoms resemble those seen following the ingestion of alcohol in patients taking Antabuse (disulfiram), which inhibits ALDH. Interestingly, the presence of the less efficient ALDH isoenzyme is associated with lower drinking frequencies and amount of alcohol consumed, suggesting that the ALDH variant protects against heavy drinking and alcoholism. The presence of the less efficient ALDH appears to be very uncommon in Caucasians, African Americans, and North American Indians.

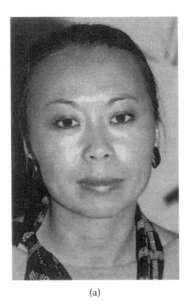 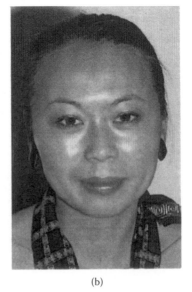

(a)   (b)

FIGURE 22.1 Flushing response after alcohol intake in aldehyde dehydrogenase–deficient individuals: A Japanese female before (a) and after (b) drinking a mild dose of ethanol. The facial flush was visible about 15 minutes after alcohol consumption. (Courtesy of Dr. D. P. Agarwal, Institute of Human Genetics, Hamburg, Germany.)

Some people with the deficiency of ALDH2 view it as a lifetime inconvenience and try to be more tolerant of alcohol with repeated moderate drinking, thereby perhaps increasing the enzyme activity. Acetaldehyde is a known carcinogen. Recent studies suggest that alcohol-flux-afflicted individuals consuming alcohol regularly may be at a higher risk for alcohol-related diseases such as esophageal cancer.

A chemical called Alda-1 has recently been indentified and found to bind defective ALDH2 and restore its structure allowing it to convert acetaldehyde to nontoxic acetate.[1,22] In addition to its role in acetaldehyde oxidation, ALDH2 is involved in the detoxification of other toxic aldehydes that accumulate in the body and bioactivation of nitroglycerine, which is used to treat angina. The effectiveness of nitroglycerine is reduced in patients with ALDH2 deficiency. The work on the action of Alda-1 on ALDH2 opens up the possibility of designing analogs that can selectively affect the metabolism of other molecules that are detoxified by ALDH2.

22.7 METABOLIC EFFECTS OF ALCOHOL

Because there is no way to store alcohol and no feedback control for the rate of alcohol oxidation, its metabolism dominates other oxidative pathways, producing dramatic metabolic changes.[5,14,16,25] There are several effects of the products of alcohol metabolism. These products include elevated NADH:NAD ratio, generation of acetaldehyde, and induction of CYP2E1.

The large load of NADH generated in the cytoplasm and mitochondria during alcohol oxidation shifts the equilibrium of several enzyme reactions toward the formation of reduced metabolites (Figure 22.2). Pyruvate is reduced to lactate. Increased lactate formation results in mild hyperlactic

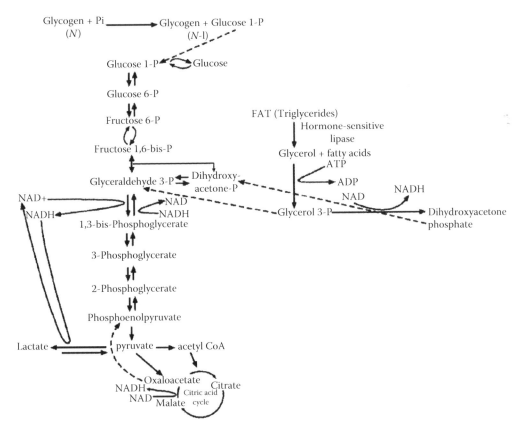

FIGURE 22.2 The effect of alcohol metabolism on blood glucose: N is the number of glucose residues. Curved reaction arrows ⮂ indicate forward and reverse reactions catalyzed by different enzymes.

acidemia and contributes to hyperuricemia owing to impaired renal excretion of uric acid. This explains, at least in part, the common clinical observation that excessive consumption of alcoholic beverages aggravates or precipitates gouty attacks in susceptible individuals.

The enzymes of β-oxidation are inhibited, blocking the oxidation of fatty acids. This is the major cause of fatty liver, increased export of very-low-density lipoproteins (VLDLs), and hypertriglyceridemia associated with alcohol use. Dehydrogenase reactions dependent on NAD in the citric acid cycle are impaired, thereby slowing the overall activity of the cycle. This results in the accumulation of citrate, which positively regulates the level of acetyl-CoA carboxylase and fatty acid synthesis. Increased NADH also favors the conversion of dihydroxyacetone phosphate to glycerol-3 phosphate, which provides the glycerol component in the synthesis of triglycerides. Thus, a high NADH:NAD ratio stimulates the syntheses of both fatty acid and the glycerol component of triglycerides and promotes the secretion of VLDLs. This raises the level of serum triglycerides, especially in obese people or in those having a lipolytic defect. In the latter group, ingestion of alcohol even in moderate quantities can cause significant hypertriglyceridemia. This condition together with the slowing of fatty acid oxidation contributes to fat accumulation in the liver that develops in alcoholism. When alcohol consumption ceases after a long binge, free fatty acids are high and the rate of ketogenesis increases as fatty acid oxidation resumes, resulting in ketosis.

The availability of pyruvate and dihydroxyacetone phosphate is decreased. Glutamate dehydrogenase activity is diminished by elevated NADH levels, decreasing the availability of α-keto glutarate, which is necessary for the transamination of amino acids before their conversion to glucose. This condition together with low levels of pyruvate and dihydroxyacetone phosphate impairs gluconeogenesis and may result in hypoglycemia.

Acetaldehyde generated from alcohol metabolism is chemically reactive and has been implicated as a key factor in hepatic injury. Acetaldehyde reacts readily with nucleophiles to form adducts. These adducts may directly damage a key function of the cell or may act as a neoantigen stimulating the immune system and leading to immune-mediated cell injury. Acetaldehyde can also deplete cellular glutathione by reacting with it or by oxidizing other molecules that in turn oxidize glutathione. This can cause cellular injury through oxidative stress. One of the metabolic complications in alcoholic patients is alcoholic ketoacidosis. Alcoholics who fast while drinking heavily exhibit metabolic alterations similar to an insulin-deficient state, with high levels of serum free fatty acids, low insulin levels, and high glucagon and catecholamine levels. Alcohol-induced impairment of fatty acid oxidation coupled with vomiting and dehydration at the end of a binge can lead to the accumulation of β-hydroxybutyric acid and lactic acid. Glucose levels may be low, normal, or elevated.

Alcohol oxidation by way of CYP2E1 produces an array of metabolic effects. The enzyme generates reactive oxygen species (ROS), including hydroxyl radical, superoxide anion, and hydrogen peroxide. Thus, CYP2E1 is a major source of oxidative stress. The enzyme also has an unusual capacity to activate many xenobiotics to toxic metabolites, thereby contributing to a wide spectrum of alcohol-related pathology.

22.8 EFFECT OF ALCOHOL ON THE BODY

Heavy alcohol consumption exerts deleterious effects on almost every organ of the human body.[19,28] Excessive drinking (three or more drinks a day) is associated with the increased incidence and severity of hypertension, which is reversible if alcohol consumption decreases. The risk of osteoporotic fractures in both sexes is about 40% higher among those having more than two drinks a day compared with those having less than that amount. Chronic alcohol consumption can suppress osteoblast function and enhance bone resorption. Alcohol consumption is associated with decreased fertility in both men and women.[6] In males, alcohol contributes to a reduction in blood testosterone concentration. Congeners found in alcoholic beverages may contribute to body damage with heavy drinking. These include low-molecular-weight alcohols (e.g., methyl alcohol and butanol), aldehydes, esters, histamine, phenols, tannins, lead, and cobalt. Persistent heavy drinking may damage the central nervous system (CNS), liver, cardiovascular system, and the digestive tract. It has been estimated that one in five hospital beds is occupied as a result of diseases or disorders in which alcohol plays a major contributing role. There is a linear dose–response relationship between alcohol consumption and the risk of death from homicide, suicide, and traffic and other accidents. A substantial proportion of violent crimes, including rape and murder, are committed under the influence of alcohol. Additionally, a substantial proportion of accidents in the home, at work, and on roads alcohol related. The 1990 World Health Organization report, "Diet, Nutrition, and Prevention of Chronic Diseases," proposed that the greatest public health challenge posed by alcohol was to bring down average consumption in industrialized societies to 4% of total energy and to eliminate alcohol abuse. A few examples of the major disorders associated with alcohol consumption are discussed in Sections 22.8.1 through 22.8.7.

22.8.1 NEUROLOGICAL DISORDERS

The brain is very sensitive to alcohol. Its normal functions of judgment, reasoning, and muscle control are affected by the amount of alcohol in the brain. Neurological effects of alcohol can be observed in the brain, the peripheral nerves, or both and can be acute or chronic in nature. Some key adverse medical aspects of alcohol's effect on the CNS are loss of proper coordination and impairment of emotional control. These are the common causes of motor vehicle accidents and violent behavior, respectively. At low concentrations in the blood alcohol may act as a stimulant to the CNS, but as the concentration increases there is a depressant effect. The intoxicating effect of alcohol depends mainly on BAL. Tolerance to higher doses of alcohol occurs in regular drinkers and is primarily due to an increase in metabolic rate and the direct adaptation of CNS tissues to alcohol. Persons who have achieved tolerance through habitual drinking may tolerate a very high level of alcohol, one that may be fatal in a novice drinker.

On average, at a BAL of 25–40 mg/dL there are generally no effects or only mild alterations of feelings. At 50 mg/dL, impairment of reaction time and coordination may be observed. At a BAL of 80–100 mg/dL, there is usually an increase in feelings of relaxation, sedation, and/or euphoria. This is because of alcohol's effect on the brain cortex, depressing the inhibitory center and lessening inhibitions. This effect manifests as a feeling of confidence and power. Because of these effects, many people consider alcohol to be a stimulant. At levels between 100 and 200 mg/dL, most drinkers show visible signs of intoxication and physical and mental impairment affecting perception and performance. Motor coordination deteriorates, judgment is impaired, and reaction time increases; visual and auditory discrimination also is affected. The walk may be unsteady. Slurred speech may show at around 150 mg/dL. Unless a person has developed a high tolerance for alcohol, a BAL of 200 mg/dL represents very serious intoxication. At a BAL over 200 mg/dL, most people are quite sedated. They have trouble standing up and staying awake. At concentrations of 400 mg/dL, the person is in coma.

Although legal intoxication limits for alcohol vary from 80 to 100 mg/dL among states, lower alcohol concentrations are known to impair driving skills. The risk for a single-vehicle fatal crash for drivers with an alcohol level of 20–40 mg/dL is estimated to be 1.4-fold that of an abstainer, and for levels of 50–100 mg/dL it is 11.1 times higher. At concentrations of 150 mg/dL, the risk rises to 380 times greater. Two to four drinks over an hour may raise the BAL to about 40–50 mg/dL. Thus, the likelihood of accidents is significantly increased after consuming even moderate doses of alcohol.

Long-term excessive use of alcohol can result in premature aging of the brain.[20] Whereas some difficulties with cognitive function clear up after a period of abstinence, residual problems can remain, usually due to a combination of nutritional deficiencies and the degeneration of nerve and tissue cells. A recent study has shown that drinking alcohol has both pluses and minuses when it comes to three types of brain abnormalities: (1) silent strokes, (2) brain atrophy, and (3) white matter lesions. Those who drank at least 15 drinks a week had a 41% lower risk for silent stroke than abstainers, but those who drank one to six drinks weekly had fewer white matter lesions than either abstainers or people who drank more than 15 times a week. White matter lesions are linked to mental weakness and motor difficulties. One surprising result in this study was that the brain seems to shrink for all drinkers, and the more a person drank the more the brain shrank. The study highlights again that consumption of alcohol has a bewildering array of associations.

In the brain, alcohol seems to affect a variety of receptors including γ-aminobutyric acid (GABA), N-methyl-D-aspartate, and opioid receptors. After chronic exposure to alcohol, some brain neurons seem to adapt to this exposure by adjusting their response to normal stimuli. The adaptation is thought to be responsible for the phenomenon of tolerance, whereby increased intakes of alcohol are needed over time to achieve desired effects. The risk of greatly increased tolerance and development of addiction seems greater in those who consume an average of about four or more drinks per day. The increase in tolerance and the development of addiction are gradual processes that usually progress over a period of a few months or years.

Alcohol withdrawal syndrome can occur when individuals decrease their alcohol use or stop using alcohol altogether. The severity of symptoms can vary greatly. The clinical manifestations include hyperactivity resulting in tachycardia, anxiety, insomnia, and in the most severe cases delirium tremens.

22.8.2 Liver

The liver is the most significant target organ in alcoholism with the clinical spectrum of diseases ranging from fatty liver to alcoholic hepatitis to cirrhosis and death. Alcohol-induced liver disease is the single most common form of hepatic damage in the United States and probably accounts for some 50% of clinical liver diseases.[3] Alcoholic liver disease results in 12,000 deaths per year in the United States. Unfortunately, many patients become symptomatic only after severe liver disease is present. The fatty liver condition is usually reversible with abstinence from alcohol and a nutritionally adequate diet. Alcohol-induced hepatitis and cirrhosis are more serious disease processes. Each of these ailments is thought by some to be because of the direct effects of alcohol on the liver tissue and may occur even in the presence of an adequate diet. Cirrhosis is the most common cause of alcohol-related death, after traffic accidents. About one quarter of heavy drinkers develop cirrhosis over many years, and the process of liver disease is accelerated in female alcoholics. Why severe liver disease is observed only in about 25% of those with long-term alcohol abuse is unknown. There does seem to be some relationship to total alcohol consumption. For men, those who develop advanced liver injury have typically ingested the equivalent of 80 g/day or more of alcohol for 10 years or more. This is approximately equivalent to 8 bottles of beer or 6 ounces of distilled spirits daily. For women, the threshold seems to be lower, or approximately 40 g of alcohol per day or more. Women may also present clinically with alcoholic liver disease at an earlier age compared with men. What makes women more susceptible is unclear. Combination of alcohol and acetaminophen (Tylenol) should be avoided as acetaminophen toxicity is greatly increased with the concomitant ingestion of alcohol.

22.8.3 Cardiovascular System

It has been estimated that about one quarter of people with alcoholism develop disease of the heart or the cardiovascular system. This occurs because alcohol is a striated muscle toxin that produces heart inflammation or cardiomyopathy. With abstinence and bed rest, the tissues return to normal and the individual recovers. Heart problems also develop as a consequence of alcohol-induced hypertension and elevation of blood lipids including cholesterol. Thus, coronary diseases occur at as high as a sixfold increased rate in individuals who are alcohol dependent. Those who drink alcohol to excess have at least an additional 20% risk of dying from cardiovascular disease.

Light-to-moderate alcohol consumption appears to protect against coronary heart disease (CHD). The protective effect may be because of increased high-density lipoprotein (HDL), which is a well-established protective factor for CHD. Alcohol also reduces the tendency for thrombosis. Antioxidants in some alcoholic beverages such as wine may protect against the oxidation of low-density lipoprotein (LDL) cholesterol. The reduced risk for CHD has been found at the level of one drink every second day, and there is little additional reduction of risk beyond consumption levels of about one drink per day.[24]

22.8.4 GASTROINTESTINAL DISORDERS

Alcohol is an irritating substance, and in strong solutions can damage the mucosa and result in esophagitis and gastritis. Erosion and ulceration of the mucosa can occur, and gastritis and duodenal ulcers are a frequent result. The stomach problems reflect high levels of gastric acid output especially prominent with beer and wine intake. Alcohol can also cause hemorrhagic lesions of the duodenal villi and diarrhea, secondary to increased small bowel motility and decreased water and electrolyte absorption. About 10% of chronic alcoholics commonly develop acute and chronic pancreatitis. The severity of these problems is related to the extent and duration of alcohol misuse.

22.8.5 IMMUNE SYSTEM

Alcohol-dependent individuals frequently have a lowered resistance to infections of all types because of the depressing effect of alcohol and acetaldehyde on the immune system.[32] Alcoholics are particularly prone to pneumonia. Immune responses are relatively well preserved in well-nourished alcoholics, but tend to be impaired in those alcoholics without nutritional supplementation.

22.8.6 CANCER

Alcohol intake is associated with a linear increase in the incidence of breast cancer up to five drinks a day. Even one drink daily increases the risk by about 10%. Hormonal mechanisms and direct carcinogenic effects of alcohol have been postulated. The rate of cancer in alcoholics is 10 times higher than in the general population.[29] Alcohol abuse is associated with a high risk of cancer of the upper digestive and respiratory tracts. It also appears that this risk increases with greater alcohol consumption. The mechanism behind the higher risk for cancer with alcohol abuse is possibly multifactorial and not fully understood.

22.8.7 FETUS

Alcohol abuse during pregnancy has detrimental effects on the fetus. The infant may be born addicted and may experience withdrawal symptoms within the first week of life. The more dramatic consequence, fetal alcohol syndrome (FAS), is clearly associated with heavy and chronic alcoholism in the mother. Most common in FAS are prenatal and postnatal growth deficiencies persisting through early childhood. Often the infant has an abnormally small head. Mental deficiency and developmental delay are almost always present. A high BAL during a critical period of embryonic development probably is necessary to produce FAS. There is probably no safe level of alcohol ingestion in pregnancy, although lower levels have not been shown to be harmful.

Alcohol and acetaldehyde readily cross the fetus, which does not have an efficient metabolizing system for alcohol and its metabolite, and these substances are likely to stay in the fetus over an extended period of time. It has been suggested that alcohol and/or acetaldehyde may have a direct teratogenic action. However, several environmental factors such as improper prenatal care, multiple-drug abuse, and inadequate nutrition, including alcohol-induced maternal and fetal nutritional deficiencies, are also possible potential causes for the anomalies observed in children of alcoholic mothers.

22.9   NUTRITIONAL IMPLICATIONS

The effect of alcohol on the nutritional status of an individual may range from insignificant to catastrophic depending on the amounts, regularity, and direction of its use as well as the foods that may be consumed in conjunction.[31] There seems to be little significant impact on nutrition as a result of light-to-moderate alcohol consumption. Clinical studies have shown that low (<1 ounce of alcohol), short-term alcohol consumption increases appetite and food consumption; however, at high doses (2 ounce or more) alcohol decreases appetite. In particular, heavy drinkers who are in energy balance will have markedly lower intakes of macronutrients and may consume a diet that is poor in other respects; they may, for example, eat only small amounts of fruits and vegetables. Poor dietary intake is responsible for the general malnutrition frequently seen in those taking alcohol in excess. Alcohol-related pathology further contributes to malabsorption and the metabolism of some nutrients.

Gastrointestinal mucosal cells have a rapid turnover. There is increased regeneration of these cells and increased secretion of gastric juice and some enzymes at low alcohol consumption. At high doses, mucosal cell turnover is impaired, thus affecting normal absorption. These alterations generally revert to normal with abstinence. Alcoholics have a high incidence of liver injury, which contributes to abnormalities in intestinal absorption. Absorptive defects are accentuated further by altered bile and pancreatic secretions in patients with liver disease and pancreatic disorders.

The dietary intake of alcoholic patients consists mostly of carbohydrates with inadequate amounts of protein and vitamins. During a drinking spree, food intake is negligible. Alcohol may so displace protein-rich foods that a state of protein-calorie malnutrition may occur. Even in a state of early alcoholism, the mean albumin level is lower, usually between 3.5 and 4 g/dL, in contrast to the normal range between 3.8 and 5.2 g/dL. As tissue injury and subsequent protein malnutrition progresses, the albumin level may fall further.

Alcoholics are frequently deficient in both water-soluble and fat-soluble vitamins. Certainly, poor intake of vitamins is a primary cause of deficiency, but alcohol can affect their absorption, storage, metabolism, and excretion as well. In addition to lowering intake by decreasing appetite, alcohol-induced gastrointestinal injury leads to impaired active transport across the intestinal mucosa. Any vitamin absorbed through the small intestine by active transport may be deficient in even apparently well-nourished alcoholics.

Folic acid deficiency is most common, occurring in 50%–60% of those with chronic alcohol consumption. Inadequate dietary intake, intestinal malabsorption, and impaired storage in the liver all contribute to deficiency of this vitamin.[2] Thiamin deficiency can occur in long-term alcohol users as a consequence of both inadequate ingestion and malabsorption. Pyridoxine absorption is primarily passive and affected only by very high concentrations of alcohol. Once absorbed, it is taken up by the liver where it is converted to pyridoxal phosphate (PLP) and stored. Hepatic accumulation of PLP is markedly decreased by alcohol and is due to accelerated degradation of PLP caused by acetaldehyde. Urinary loss of pyridoxine is also increased by alcohol consumption and results in very low levels of both pyridoxine and PLP in the plasma of alcoholics, particularly with liver disease. Vitamin A storage in the liver is reduced by alcohol. One possible mechanism for this effect is increased conversion of retinol to retinoic acid because of the induction of the vitamin A–metabolizing microsomal enzyme system by alcohol. Through additional alcohol-related pathology, it is possible to find deficient levels of other vitamins in people with alcoholism. On the other hand, most people who are alcohol dependent do not show significantly altered blood levels of these vitamins. Thus, potential deficiencies are likely to be mild and easily corrected through abstinence, appropriate nutrition, and oral intake of multivitamins.

A number of alcohol-related neurological disorders are due to nutritional deficiencies, primarily the B vitamins including thiamin. Brain function can be affected by acute thiamin deficiency. Alcohol uses up the vitamin for its conversion to carbon dioxide and water, yet alcoholic beverages provide no thiamin. These deficiencies result from a decreased taste for food, decreased appetite, and malabsorption of nutrients, due to irritated lining of the stomach and small intestine. Peripheral polyneuropathy, a common nutritional deficiency disorder, is characterized by weakness, numbness, and partial paralysis of extremities; pain in the legs; and impaired sensory reaction and motor reflexes. This condition is reversible with an adequate diet and supplemental thiamin and other B vitamins. If the polyneuropathy is left untreated, it may progress to Wernicke's encephalopathy. This more serious disorder is also reversible. It is characterized by ophthalmoplegia, ataxia, apathy, drowsiness, confusion, and inability to concentrate. Without treatment, it can be fatal.

Low levels of potassium, calcium, phosphorus, magnesium, and zinc occur as a consequence of dietary deficiency and acid–base imbalances during excessive alcohol ingestion and withdrawal. These deficiencies play a significant role in the clinical syndromes seen in alcoholic patients. For example, hypokalemia can lead to muscle paralysis and areflexia. Decrease in serum phosphorous contributes to mental confusion and muscle weakness. Magnesium deficiency may be responsible for irritability and other neurological symptoms. Zinc deficiency results in delayed wound healing but is unassociated with other clinical symptoms.

Some mineral levels are found to be higher in alcoholics. Alcohol tends to increase iron absorption. Also, beverages such as certain wines may contain significant amounts of iron. Therefore, there is a potential for excessive iron deposition in the liver, producing tissue injury. High hepatic copper and nickel levels have been reported in patients with alcoholic cirrhosis, but the significance of these changes is unknown.

22.10 HEALTH BENEFITS OF ALCOHOL

Although alcohol is a risk factor for several diseases, it may also provide health benefits. Moderate drinkers tend to have better health and live longer than those who are heavy drinkers and abstainers. Alcoholic beverages, particularly red wine, are linked to healthier hearts.[8] Those who consume alcohol in moderation are less likely to have hypertension. Studies have shown that people who consume one to three drinks per day have a low risk for Alzheimer's disease[17] compared with those who do not drink. A study of more than 12,000 women found that those who consumed light (one-half drink)-to-moderate (one drink) amounts of alcohol daily had about a 20% lower risk of experiencing problems with their mental abilities later.[30] Low levels of alcohol appear to have cognitive benefits. While the study involved only women, the findings probably hold for men also. Another study in mice showed that sake,[13] a traditional Japanese beverage also known as rice wine, could have beneficial effects on the skin. Sake and one of its components, ethyl-D-glucoside, reduced epidermal permeability barrier disruption during ultraviolet irradiation. Sake has been used in skin care lotions historically, and anecdotal evidence suggests that skin complexions are smoother in areas with high sake consumption.

A most recent study found that women who drink moderate amounts of alcohol do not gain as much weight in midlife as those who do not drink. Typically alcohol consumption is not advised for people trying to lose or avoid gaining weight. A glass of wine contains about 125 Cal and a regular 12-ounce beer has about 150 Cal. Researchers examined data from 19,220 women enrolled in the Women's Health Study. The women, originally of healthy weight, provided health and lifestyle information over an average of 13 years. After adjusting for other factors that influence weight, the researchers found that compared with women who did not drink, women who drank 15–30 g of alcohol a day—the equivalent of a drink or two—were 30% less likely to be overweight or obese at the end of the study period. The effects were found for beer, red wine, and spirits, although the strongest association was found with red wine.[33]

It is unclear what accounts for women's moderate alcohol consumption and not gaining weight despite extra intake of calories from alcohol. It is speculated that women burn more alcohol after drinking than men do. It is also possible that women who drank alcohol in the study consumed fewer calories from foods. They were more likely to smoke and were more physically active. The findings are interesting. But alcohol should not be used as the primary way toward weight loss or weight maintenance.

Researchers in France have found bioactive compounds in oak-aged wine that are derivatives of ellagitannins, which are known natural products in oak.[4] Ellagitannins are extracted into wine during the aging process and are converted to a number of topoisomerase II inhibitors including vescalene. These compounds have the same type of activity as, but higher potency than, a commercial anticancer drug. The finding is significant for wine drinkers because a substantial amount of wine is aged in oak. A survey in 2005 found that 50%–80% of U.S. wineries age their wine in oak barrels. But it is not yet scientifically sound to drink wine for protection against cancer.

In 2004, the German brewer Nautilus GMGH Laboratoriumsbedarf introduced a beer containing nicotine that is advertised as the first smoking-cessation beer.[11] Called NicoShot, this beer contains 6.3% alcohol by volume and 3 mg of nicotine per each 250-mL "shot" can. The company claims that drinking three cans of NicoShot is comparable in nicotine intake to a pack of cigarettes. Similar to nicotine gum, NicoShot is considered a nicotine replacement therapy that provides a steady, controlled release of nicotine. It can be used to relieve withdrawal symptoms at the beginning of quitting or to avoid a relapse months after quitting when a new stress or situation may trigger a strong urge to smoke. With some European nations such as Sweden banning smoking in restaurants, bars, and cafés, the company hopes NicoShot can help improve one's social life by allowing one to relieve those nicotine cravings without having to walk out of the bar for a quick smoke. As more and more U.S. states and localities move to ban smoking in public places, it is likely that nicotine-containing beers will become available in the United States soon. It will be interesting to see how we deal with the double whammy of alcohol and nicotine in the same brew.

Health benefits attributable to alcohol consumption are interesting. However, the findings are based on observational studies and (because of other variables that may exist and that may affect individual health differently) the health effects may or may not be due to alcohol per se. One does not need to take a drink daily to avoid weight gain or reduce the risk of Alzheimer's disease, hypertension, or other diseases. The adverse effects of alcohol are well known. And because it is also well known that even a small amount of alcohol affects the brain adversely, taking a light drink daily of this addictive substance may very likely invite trouble for those who partake (especially in those predisposed genetically to becoming alcoholic) as it might then lead to moderate consumption and eventual dependence on alcohol. Consumption of alcohol daily for health maintenance is not recommended.

22.11   ALCOHOL DEPENDENCY

Alcohol dependency is a condition characterized by a pattern of compulsive alcohol use and physiological dependence on alcohol (i.e., tolerance and/or symptoms of withdrawal). Unlike alcoholics, alcohol abusers have at least some ability to set limits on their drinking.[10] However, their alcohol use is still destructive.[26] Abstainers are individuals who consume no alcohol.

For the vast majority of people, drinking alcohol is a pleasant experience. This is especially the case when people are engaged in recreational and social activities and when their drinking behavior can be considered moderate (up to two drinks for men and one drink for women). Drinking in moderation is not harmful for most adults. Nevertheless, the consumption of alcohol carries a risk of adverse health and social consequences related to its intoxicating and dependence-related properties. Millions of people may be able to handle the effects of alcohol without becoming abusers. But the number of American adults 18 years and older who are dependent on or abuse alcohol rose from 13.8 million in 1991–1992 to 17.6 million in 2001–2002, according to an epidemiological survey directed by the National Institute on Alcohol Abuse and Alcoholism (NIAAA). The largest percentage of drinking problems in the United States is found among young adults (18–29 years of age). Overall, more than 10% of these young adults surveyed in 2001–2002 were either alcoholics or alcohol abusers.

A recent study has shown that people who begin to drink alcohol before the age of 14 years are more likely to become alcoholics than those who stay away from alcohol until the age of 21; they also develop dependence on alcohol faster and face a longer struggle with alcohol throughout their lives.[12] The researchers analyzed the results of the 2001–2002 survey of 43,093 adults. They found that 47% of people who had started drinking before age 14 met the criteria for alcoholism, compared with 4% of those who started drinking at the age of 21. Twenty-seven percent of the men and women who started drinking before age 14 were alcohol dependent before the age of 25, compared with 4% of those who began drinking at 21. People who started drinking at an early age were 2.6 times more likely to have episodes of alcohol dependence lasting longer than a year, and nearly 3 times as likely to have 6–7 symptoms of alcohol dependence versus 3–5 symptoms. These findings underscore the dangers of early alcohol use, so that the efforts made over the years to help prevent drinking among teens—such as having raised the drinking age to 21 in some areas—are recommended in order to avoid or reduce the rates of alcohol dependence.

Over the past several years, studies of college students have shown that those who get tipsy after a drink or two are one-third to one-half as likely to develop alcoholism as those who drink a lot before they feel drunk. Scientists have recently identified a variation in a gene that may have an effect on how people respond to alcohol. About 10%–20% of the population carries a version of the gene that makes their brains especially sensitive to alcohol. The gene produces the enzyme CyP2 E-1[34] involved in alcohol metabolism (as described earlier) as well as Tylenol and nicotine. The people who carry the version of the gene linked to increased sensitivity to alcohol produce more of the enzyme and have lower risk for alcoholism. A low sensitivity to alcohol is associated with increased risk for alcoholism. CyP2E-1 could therefore be useful as a predictor of those who are at risk for alcoholism.

Alcohol abuse and dependence have a variable course characterized by periods of remission and relapse. There are anticraving medications that help some alcoholics. Disulfiram (Antabuse) inhibits ALDH, and the accumulation of acetaldehyde causes an unpleasant flushing reaction if taken with alcohol. Outcomes of patients taking disulfiram are improved when the drug is taken under supervision. Naltrexone (Revia), an opioid antagonist, and an acamprosate and glutamate antagonist, reduces alcohol consumption in alcoholics and is effective in reducing relapse rates when combined with psychosocial treatment. A new synthetic compound known as MTIP has shown promise in animal testing.[9] In rats genetically predisposed to develop alcoholism and in rats trained to be alcohol dependent, the compound curbed alcohol use, suggesting that it may be effective in treating a broad range of alcoholics. It inhibits the binding of corticotrophin-releasing factor (CRF) to CRF receptors. The levels of CRF rise in the brain after drinking alcohol and also during alcohol withdrawal. CRF has been linked to various psychiatric conditions, including alcoholism.

Alcoholism is a chronic relapsing condition with up to 90% of the patients returning to drinking after treatment. MTIP and any other intervention that can reduce the percentage of alcoholics going back to drinking would be welcomed.

22.12 ALTERNATIVE MEDICINE FOR ALCOHOLISM AND ALCOHOL HANGOVER

22.12.1 Alcoholism

Despite decades of research and dozens of treatments, alcoholism, America's most common addiction, remains notoriously difficult to overcome. More than 30% of American adults have abused alcohol or suffered from alcoholism at some point in their lives, according to a study in 2007 by the NIAAA. Yet, only a quarter of those afflicted received any treatment. And only a small fraction of those who seek treatment manages to abstain from alcohol for a year. There are traditional treatments for alcoholics such as the program pioneered by Alcoholics Anonymous that rely largely on peer support to encourage abstinence. There are a variety of behavioral and cognitive therapies employed by psychologists and psychiatrists to help patients avoid the triggers and thought patterns that urge them to drink. And there are posh inpatient rehabilitation centers. But despite all this variety of treatments there is no full-proof treatment that ensures success. This is because alcoholism, like addiction to narcotics, causes permanent changes in the brain that can at best be ameliorated but not permanently undone.

Several herbs can ease some alcohol withdrawal symptoms such as anxiety and insomnia. Kudzu, a plant with out-of-control growth and considered a pest in much of the South, is being studied as a treatment for alcoholism.[18] Kudzu extract has been used in traditional Chinese medicine as a treatment for alcoholism and hangover. Researchers at a hospital in Boston, Massachusetts, studied the effect of this herb on alcohol drinking in humans. They had no problem finding volunteers (men and women in their twenties) for the study, which required the volunteers to hang out in an "apartment" complete with television, recliners, and a refrigerator loaded with beer. The volunteers were told to spend a 90-minute session drinking beer and watching television. The individuals selected had said that they regularly consume three to four beers or drinks per day.

Some subjects received capsules of kudzu and others a placebo. Those who took kudzu pills drank an average of 1.8 beers per session compared with 3.8 beers by those who took the placebo. None of the subjects had any side effects from mixing kudzu with beer. Researchers speculated that drinkers (in the presence of kudzu) needed fewer beers to satisfy them and to take away their desire for more drinks.

Kudzu contains a substance called daidzin, which could make drinking alcohol an unpleasant experience. Daidzin has been synthesized and it shows promise in laboratory tests. It inhibits ALDH2-causing accumulation of acetaldehyde. Experiments have shown that kudzu extracts or synthetic daidzin decrease alcohol intake in alcohol-preferring golden hamsters and alcohol-dependent rats. Daidzin prevents alcohol-induced increase in dopamine in the brain's pleasure center. This additional finding about daidzin may help prevent relapse in recovering alcoholics by diminishing cravings—something Antabuse does not do.

Kudzu has a weak extrogenic-like activity and also interacts with methotrexate. The findings from animal and human studies suggest that kudzu and daidzin may have potential in the management of some aspects of alcohol abuse and alcoholism. More research is needed before they can be safely used for alcohol treatment.

22.12.2 Alcohol Hangover

Coconut water is the liquid inside young green coconuts (fruits of the coconut palm). As the fruit matures, most of the water is gradually replaced by coconut meat. A young coconut has very little meat, which is tender.

The hangover that follows a night of drinking is essentially the result of being dehydrated. Alcohol is a diuretic. Too much alcohol drinking causes dehydration, electrolyte imbalance, and hypoglycemia. People have tried several methods such as hot tea, fatty foods, and several herbs to combat hangover. But none of these methods work particularly well. Coconut water is a natural fat-free drink with the ability to rehydrate the body, and it contains all the electrolytes that are present in blood. In some developing countries, coconut water has been used as an intravenous drink but has proven to be the best natural hangover cure.

Long a dietary staple in the tropics, coconut water has become popular among younger people and athletes in several countries. Advocates of coconut water claim that it can do everything from boosting immune function to reducing menstrual cramps, but there are no significant studies to bolster many of these claims. Coca-Cola, Pepsi, and some other beverage companies have entered this market, and in 2008 its sales in the United States topped $50 million.

Alcoholic Hypoglycemia

A Case in an Adult

A 54 year-old male was known to be a chronic alcoholic. He spent the day normally and retired to bed at about 10 p.m. apparently sober. There was no admission of any immediate alcohol excess. The next morning at about 8 a.m. his daughter noticed that he was mentally very confused, and an hour later he was found completely unconscious. She called their family physician who came immediately to see him. When he was examined, there was a smell of ketones in his small, airless room. He was deeply comatose and lay flat on his back with open eyes and giving an occasional twist of his head. The skin was distinctly moist. The pupils reacted to light, all tendon reflexes were present and equal, abdominal reflexes were present, and no plantar reflexes were obtained. He was immediately taken to a nearby hospital. By this time, he had been in a coma for about 3 hours.

A catheter specimen of the patient's urine showed a strong positive test for ketones and a negative test for glucose. Treatment was based on a provisional diagnosis of diabetic—that is, hyperglycemic—coma without glycosuria. In view of some uncertainty, however, it was decided to administer dextrose intravenously before giving him insulin. At the conclusion of an injection of 25 mL of 25% dextrose, the patient at once regained consciousness in a dramatic manner. He was then kept in the hospital for further investigation. He was given regular food. The ketosis resolved after 36 hours without specific treatment, although he was encouraged to eat. Tests showed that he had no diabetes but had mild hepatitis.

Five months later, a similar incident of hypoglycemia occurred in which the brother of the previously described patient became mentally confused and disoriented. He did not go into coma, and his blood sugar was 53 mg/dL. Frank ketosis was again present. Treatment was with dextrose administration and subsequent progress was similar as seen earlier.

Hypoglycemic coma after alcohol intoxication in association with poor diet has been reported by several investigators.[36] Blood glucose levels in their patients were in the range of 20–40 mg/dL. Usually, this type of hypoglycemia occurs 12–14 hours following alcohol ingestion. The frequent history of inadequate diet with resulting hepatic glycogen depletion undoubtedly is an important factor. In most patients, the hypoglycemia can be completely reversed by a single intravenous administration of 20–50 mL of 50% dextrose solution.

A Case in a Child

A 3-year-old girl had been entirely well when put to bed in the evening. The next morning her parents found her to be comatose. They assumed that she had ingested cologne because of the odor in her breath and the presence of the cologne bottle nearby. This was probably ingested in the early morning hours by the girl who usually wandered around at night. Lavage was performed at an army dispensary and then the patient was sent to the hospital.

Physical examination revealed a semicomatose child who weighed 32 pounds. Her blood glucose level was 22 mg/dL. Urinalysis showed no sugar, but the presence of acetone was indicated. The child began to have convulsions, which were mainly tonic, with intermittent chronic movement. She was then administered 10 mL of 50% dextrose intravenously. Immediately following the administration of dextrose, there were no further convulsions. Thirty minutes later the child opened her eyes and became much more alert. The patient was discharged in 2 days.

The patient in this case had ingested methyl alcohol. However, in the same report the author described the case of a 6-year-old boy who drank an unknown quantity of gin. He was hypoglycemic and had convulsions and died.[35,37] There are several reports involving children intoxicated with alcohol causing hypoglycemia and convulsions. Sensitivity of children to alcohol is well known. The death of an infant has been reported after the infant had been dressed with a diaper dipped in alcohol. Another child became intoxicated after breast-feeding; his mother had previously ingested a large amount of an alcoholic drink.

Blood glucose examination is required in any child suffering from coma and convulsions, especially when the history is not clear. In the case of hypoglycemia, immediate administration of glucose is more urgent than any other schedule of treatment. Intravenous administration of hypertonic glucose solution must be added to the conventional treatment in any case of alcohol intoxication, with the probability that the procedure will be lifesaving.

Biochemical Basis

Hypoglycemia usually results in an inadequate supply of glucose to the brain, which can then cause the derangement of cerebral function and death. Alcohol does not affect glycogenolysis. Alcoholic hypoglycemia classically occurs in persons whose important daily source of calories over a period of days is alcohol, which cannot be metabolically converted to glucose and may inhibit gluconeogenesis. The increase in the NADH:NAD ratio in the liver as a result of alcohol metabolism is probably the major factor in the suppression of gluconeogenesis. The pathway from fructose 1,6-bisphosphate is not blocked by alcohol, and fructose rapidly overcomes the hypoglycemia induced by alcohol. The increase in NADH:NAD ratio, characteristic of the oxidation of alcohol, may affect the gluconeogenic sequences in several different ways (see Figure 22.2):

- The availability of oxaloacetate for conversion to phosphoenol pyruvate is reduced following the slowdown of the citric acid cycle that occurs during alcohol oxidation. This is because an increase in the NADH:NAD ratio tends to suppress several oxidative reactions of the cycle, such as oxidation of isocitrate to α-ketoglutarate and of malate to oxaloacetate.
- The availability of pyruvate for conversion to oxaloacetate and then to phosphoenol pyruvate is decreased by the rapid reduction of pyruvate to lactate under the impact of high concentrations of NADH.
- Glycerol produced by adipose tissue during lipolysis is a known source of glucose, especially during fasting. The conversion requires the formation of dihydroxyacetone phosphate from glycerol-3-phosphate (requires NAD) and is depressed by high levels of NADH.
- The glucose-lowering effect of alcohol can augment that of other hypoglycemic agents such as insulin and sulfonylureas, and when these compounds are administered in the presence of alcohol severe hypoglycemia with irreversible neurological changes may result.

Alcohol is a potent hypoglycemic agent. Under certain circumstances, it exerts a more profound sugar-lowering effect than insulin or other well-recognized hypoglycemic agents. Diabetic patients may be even more vulnerable to this effect of alcohol. Thus, diabetics should not consume alcohol on an empty stomach. Abnormal behavior in a diabetic should not automatically be equated with drunkenness; hypoglycemia also should be considered. Despite these potential problems, moderate alcohol intake in the setting of a mixed meal is not contraindicated in diabetes.

REFERENCES

1. Arolfo, M. P., D. H. Overstreet, L. Yao et al. 2009. Suppression of heavy drinking and alcohol-seeking by a selective ALDH-2 inhibitor. *Alcohol Clin Exp Res* 33:1935.
2. Ballard, H. S. 1998. The hematological complications of alcoholism. *Alcohol Health Res World* 56:52.
3. Bloor, J. H., J. E. Mapoles, and F. R. Simon. 1994. Alcoholic liver disease: New concepts of pathogenesis and treatment. *Adv Int Med* 39:49.
4. Borman, S. 2005. Anticancer agents found in aged wine. *Chem Eng News* 83 (44):36.
5. Crabb, D. W. 1995. Ethanol oxidizing enzymes: Roles in alcohol metabolism and alcoholic liver disease. *Prog Liver Dis* 13:151.
6. Eggert, J., H. Theobald, and P. Engfeldt. 2004. Effect of alcohol consumption on female fertility during an 18-year period. *Fertil Steril* 81:379.

7. Frezza, M., C. Di Padova, G. Pozzato, M. Terpin, E. Baraona, and C. S. Lieber. 1990. High blood alcohol levels in women. The role of decreased gastric alcohol dehydrogenase activity and first-pass metabolism. *N Engl J Med* 322:95.

8. German, J. B., and R. L. Walzem. 2000. The health benefits of wine. *Annu Rev Nutr* 20:561.

9. Gehlert, D. R., A. Cippitelli, A. Thorsell et al. 2007. 3-(4-Chloro-2-morpholin-4-yl-thiazol-5-yl)-8-(1-ethylpropyl)-2,6-dimethyl-imidazo[1,2-b]pyridazine: A novel brain-penetrant, orally available corticoptropin-releasing factor receptor 1 antagonist with efficacy in animal models of alcoholism. *J Neurosci* 27:2718.

10. Grant, B. F. 1997. Prevalence and correlates of alcohol use and DSM-IV alcohol dependence in the United States: Results of the National Longitudinal Alcohol Epidemiologic Survey. *J Stud Alcohol* 58:464.

11. Hanson, D. 2005. Nicotine fix from beer. *Chem Eng News* 83(44):53.

12. Hingson, R., T. Heeren, and M. Winter. 2006. Age at drinking onset and alcohol dependence: Age at onset, duration, and severity. *Arch Pediatr Adolesc Med* 160:739.

13. Hirotsune, M., A. Haratake, A. Komiya et al. 2005. Effect of ingested concentrate and components of sake on epidermal permeability barrier disruption by UVB irradiation. *J Agric Food Chem* 53:940.

14. Hoffman, R. S., and L. R. Goldfrank. 1989. Ethanol-associated metabolic disorders. *Emerg Clin North Am* 7:943.

15. Jones, A. W. 1993. Disappearance rate of ethanol from the blood of human subjects: Implications in forensic toxicology. *J Forensic Sci* 38(1):104.

16. Lieber, C. S. 1995. Hepatic and other medical disorders of alcoholism and alcoholic liver disease. *Prog Liver Dis* 13:151.

17. Luchsinger, J. A., and R. Mayeux. 2004. Dietary factors and Alzheimer's disease. *Lancet Neurol* 3:579.

18. Lukas, S. E., D. Penetr, J. Berko et al. 2005. An extract of the Chinese herbal root Kudzu reduces alcohol drinking by heavy drinkers in a naturalistic setting. *Alcohol Clin Exp Res* 29:756.

19. McGrandy, B. S., and J. W. Langenbucher. 1996. Alcohol treatment and health care system reform. *Arch Gen Psychiatry* 53:737.

20. Mukamal, K. J., W. T. Longstreth, M. A. Mittleman, R. M. Crum, and D. S. Siscovick. 2001. Alcohol consumption and sub-clinical findings on magnetic resonance imaging of the brain in older adults. *Stroke* 32:1939.

21. Orten, J. M., and V. M. Sardesai. 1971. Protein, nucleotide and porphyrin metabolism in the biology of alcoholism. In *The Biology of Alcoholism*, ed. B. Kissin and H. Begleiter, 229–261. New York: Plenum.

22. Perez-Miller, S., H. Younus, R. Vanum et al. 2010. Alda-1 is an agonist and chemical chaperone for the common human aldehyde dehydrogenase 2 variant. *Nat Struct Mol Biol* 17:159.

23. Rouse, B. A. 1997. *Substance Abuse and Health Statistics Sourcebook*. Washington, DC: U.S. Department of Health and Human Services.

24. Sacco, R. L., M. Elkind, B. Boden-Albala et al. 1999. The protective effect of moderate alcohol consumption on ischaemic stroke. *J Am Med Assoc* 281:53.

25. Sardesai, V. M., ed. 1969. *Biochemical and Clinical Aspects of Alcohol Metabolism*. Springfield, IL: Charles C. Thomas.

26. Schuckit, M. A. 2000. *Drug and Alcohol Abuse: A Clinical Guide to Diagnosis and Treatment*. New York: Academic/Phenum.

27. Seitz, H. M., and C. M. Oneta. 1998. Gastrointestinal alcohol dehydrogenase. *Nutr Rev* 56:52.

28. Schenker, S., and M. K. Bay. 1998. Medical problems associated with alcoholism. *Adv Int Med* 43:27.

29. Singletary, K. W., and S. M. Gapstur. 2001. Alcohol and breast cancer: Review epidemiologic and experimental evidence and potential mechanisms. *J Amer Med Assoc* 286:2143.

30. Stampfer, M. J., J. H. Kang, J. Chen et al. 2005. Effects of moderate alcohol consumption on cognitive function in women. *New Engl J Med* 352:245.

31. Suter, P. M. 2001. Alcohol and mortality: If you drink, do not forget fruits and vegetables. *Nutr Rev* 59:293.

32. Szabo, G. 1997. Alcohol's contribution to compromised immunity. *Alcohol Health Res World* 21:30.

33. Wang, L., I. Lee, J. E. Manson et al. 2010. Alcohol consumption, weight gain and risk of becoming overweight in middle aged and older women. *Arch Int Med* 170:453.

34. Webb, A., P. A. Lind, J. Kalmijn et al. 2011. The investigation into CyP2E-1 in relation to the level of response to alcohol through a combination of linkage and association analysis. *Alcoholism Clin & Expt Res* 35:10.

CASE BIBLIOGRAPHY

35. Cummins, L. H. 1961. Hypoglycemia and convulsions in children following alcohol ingestion. *J Pediatr* 58:23.
36. Taylor, J. S. 1955. Hypoglycemia in chronic alcoholism. *Br Med J* 1:648.
37. Tolis, A. D. 1965. Hypoglycemic convulsions in children after alcohol ingestion. *Pediatr Clin North Am* 12:425.

23 Nutritional Epidemiology

The word epidemiology is derived from the Greek words *epi* (upon), *demios* (people, as in democracy and demography), and *logia* (from *legein*, meaning to speak). Epidemiology is a fundamental medical science that focuses on the incidence and the distribution of disease frequency in human populations. It is a process to identify and control health problems. It uses biostatistics, statistical processes, and methods applied to the analysis of biological phenomena to describe and quantitate health events and the factors that place individuals at risk for health events. Basically, epidemiologists are interested in how and why diseases are distributed or vary in frequency in populations according to time (clustering in time; short-term variations), places (geographical distribution between regions and nations; rural versus urban), and people (specific characteristics of people such as ethnic origin, occupation, and dietary intake). Specifically, epidemiologists examine patterns of illness in a population and then try to determine why certain groups or individuals develop a particular disease whereas others do not. As a comparative quantitative science, epidemiology is interwoven with many diverse disciplines such as demography, sociology, economics, biology, and nutrition. Medical and public health disciplines use epidemiological study results to solve and control human health problems.[4,6]

Nutritional epidemiology is the study of different dietary patterns and disease patterns among various populations in the world. It uses epidemiological approaches to determine relations between dietary factors and the occurrence of specific diseases.[14] It depends on a valid assessment of exposures of individuals to foodborne factors. If one group tends to develop certain diseases while another group does not, speculation can occur about the role the diet plays in this difference. Of relevance in nutritional epidemiology is the association between a specific dietary constituent and the distribution of a disease.

23.1 HISTORICAL PERSPECTIVE

Historically, epidemiology was generally restricted to and evolved from the study of infectious diseases. The tallying of population-based vital statistics dates back to the bubonic plague, which killed approximately one-fourth of Europe's population between 1346 and 1352. During this period, officials began keeping records of the number of persons dying each week. In the 17th century, John Graunt used life tables to summarize the mortality experience in terms of numbers, percentages, and probabilities, and noted urban–rural differences in mortality, high mortality rates in children (one-third died before the age of 5 years), and discrepancies in morbidity and mortality rates in men and women. Men experienced higher mortality rates but lower morbidity rates than women. In 1775, Percival Pott reported high rates of scrotal cancer among chimney sweeps. He attributed this increase in cancer rates to the lodging of soot in the rugae of the scrotum. This work was the first example in the field of occupational epidemiology.

In 1798, Edward Jenner found that smallpox could be prevented by an inoculation with the substance from cowpox lesions. This was the first documented case of actively preventing a disease through vaccination. During the London cholera epidemic of 1854, John Snow, a physician, used relatively simple population-based methods to show that cholera was transmitted by impure water.

Although nutritional epidemiology is relatively new as a formal area of research, investigators have used basic epidemiological methods for more than 200 years to identify numerous essential nutrients.[12] In the mid-eighteenth century, observations that fresh fruits and vegetables could cure scurvy led English physician James Lund in 1753 to conduct one of the earliest controlled clinical trials of a nutrition-based disease, scurvy, which was common on all long trips by sea. Lund devised a modern intervention trial with five strategies. Sailors with the disease received daily one of the following: a quart of apple cider; two spoons of vinegar; a half pint of seawater; two oranges and one lime; or a mixture consisting of nutmeg, garlic, mustard, and other herbs. The men who consumed oranges and lemon had the most "sudden and good effects" on the cause of this disease. The sailors recovered rapidly and reported to duty after 6 days. This experiment resulted in a health policy in 1795 that required that limes or lime juice be included in the diet of all sailors.[13] These sailors were nicknamed "limeys." Scurvy was ultimately found to be the result of vitamin C deficiency.

In an example from the late nineteenth century (1878–1883), the unusual occurrence of beriberi among sailors subsisting largely on polished rice led Takaki in Japan to hypothesize that some factor was lacking in their diet; the addition of canned milk and vegetables to their ration effectively eliminated this disease.

In 1923, Joseph Goldberger conducted what is considered a classical epidemiological investigation that altered the belief that pellagra was an infectious disease primarily associated with the cornmeal subsistence diet in the southern United States.[7] Goldberger observed that healthcare personnel attending to patients with pellagra did not develop the disease. By studying individuals with and without this disease, he hypothesized and proved that diet initiated the disease.

These classical studies and events led to the groundwork for nutritional epidemiology.[2] On the basis of epidemiological observations, the prevention of scurvy, beriberi, and pellagra (each of which is caused by a deficiency of a single dietary factor—vitamin C, vitamin B1, and niacin, respectively) was accomplished prior to the identification of the actual biochemical and nutritional entities. During the past few years, a vast number of epidemiological studies in human populations have revealed an association between several variables, including certain diets, and the occurrence of chronic degenerative diseases such as coronary heart disease (CHD) and certain types of cancer.

23.2 TECHNIQUES/APPROACHES

Epidemiological research describes and seeks to explain the distribution of health and illness within human populations. The techniques used are based mainly on comparative observations made at the level of whole populations, special groups (such as migrants or vegetarians), or individuals within the population, who are investigated by methods using varying degrees of control. By relating the differences in the incidence of disease, associations that may be causal are identified. Various approaches are available to study the relationship between diet and disease. Each method makes a distinctive contribution in elucidating the etiological factors in a disease. Every type of study has particular strengths and weaknesses. Confident judgments are normally possible when the lines of different types of evidence converge.

23.2.1 DESCRIPTIVE STUDIES

These studies describe the patterns of disease occurrence in one or more populations, in the components of some population, or in a single population over time. The observed patterns may be related to certain environmental variables or characteristics of the population, such as demographical factors, industrial pollution, or diet. Data from descriptive studies are suggestive rather than definitive, and serve primarily to identify population groups at risk and to generate hypotheses for further investigation.

23.2.2 CORRELATION STUDIES

These studies, based on aggregate exposure data and observed outcomes, provide the next step in establishing meaningful associations. In these studies, broad, between-population differences in patterns of exposure to a particular agent or consumption of a particular nutrient or food are compared with the population incidence rates (IRs) of the disease of interest. This approach seeks to determine the extent to which two characteristics (risk factor and disease occurrence) are related. This type of comparison is also referred to as an ecological study because the analysis is at the level of an entire population rather than at the level of individuals. The study investigates diet and disease at the population level and entails comparisons of disease rates with the consumption of nutrients, foods, or other aspects of diet. The per capita consumption of specific dietary factors in such studies is based on disappearance data, meaning the national figures for food produced and imported minus the food exported, fed to animals, or otherwise not available to humans. This type of analysis is frequently able to utilize existing data and is a valuable tool for generating new hypotheses.

Migration studies enable an assessment of whether the correlations observed are due to genetic inheritance or environmental factors. For example, migration studies that attempted to separate genetic from environmental or lifestyle factors have revealed that heart disease and many types of cancer are more likely to involve environmental than genetic factors.

In free-living populations, ecological studies are usually simple, relatively inexpensive, and easy to perform. For some research questions, ecological studies may be the only way to test a hypothesis. These studies have special strengths, especially when conducted between populations either internationally or cross-culturally among contrasting populations within a country. Interpopulation ranges in intakes of foods and dietary constituents are sometimes wider than, or different from, intrapopulation ranges. For example, in industrialized countries virtually all individuals consume between 23% and 50% of their calories in the form of fat, whereas the mean fat intake for the whole population throughout the world varies from less than 15% to 42% of calories.

Because these studies focus on populations or large groups, findings may not be applicable to individuals. An obvious limitation of most correlation studies is the inability to control for potential confounding factors (discussed in Section 23.3). Many variables can influence the development of diseases, and populations differ in a variety of aspects, any of which could explain the differences observed in the occurrence of a disease. For instance, diets high in meat (of the type eaten in industrialized societies) are associated with an increased risk of some cancers common in such societies. But diets high in meat are also likely to be high in fat, and they may also be high in sugar and alcohol.

23.2.3 OBSERVATIONAL STUDIES—CASE–CONTROL

Unlike correlational studies, case–control studies enable investigators to collect data for individuals rather than for groups and they are designed to control for confounding variables. These studies are backward directional (Figure 23.1), which compare a group with disease (cases) with a group of noncases (controls). The investigator attempts to identify factors from each group's past that differentiate the case participants from the control ones. Controls are selected from persons who do not have the disease of interest but who are as much like the cases in other respects as possible. The past histories of cases and controls are examined and the frequency of various items in the two groups is compared to elucidate antecedent exposures to agents that may have caused the disease. A group of, say, cancer patients (cases) is compared with a similar cancer-free population (controls) to help establish whether the past or recent history of a specific exposure, such as smoking, alcohol consumption, and dietary intake, is causally related to the risk of disease. Because case–control studies look to the past to identify a contributing factor that may affect an individual's health, they are often referred to as retrospective studies.

Case–control studies are relatively inexpensive to conduct. They generally provide information more efficiently and rapidly than cohort studies (described in Section 23.2.4) because the

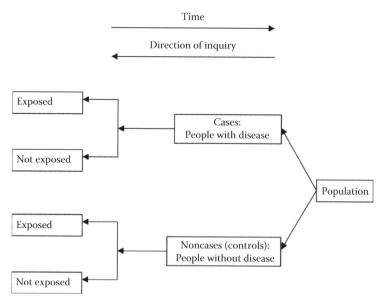

FIGURE 23.1 Design of a case–control study.

number of subjects can typically be smaller because the study is initiated by the identification of cases. This type of approach can investigate a wide variety of potential risk factors simultaneously. If a disease is rare, the relative risk, called an odds ratio (Table 23.1), can be estimated by this method.

Among the disadvantages are that the information about past events (e.g., diet) may be unavailable, incomplete, or inaccurately recalled, and the information supplied by cases and/or controls may be biased (discussed in Section 23.3). Selection bias can also be a shortcoming of these studies. Another important point is that one may not know whether the disease preceded or followed changes in exposure to a suspected agent, and thus incorrect associations may occur. In retrospective studies, the relative risk can be estimated only indirectly and approximately as it is not possible with this method to calculate incidence rates in persons exposed and not exposed to a given factor. Once an etiological factor has been uncovered in retrospective studies, prospective investigations are desirable to confirm or deny the findings.

TABLE 23.1
Summary of Data in a Case–Control Study[a]

Exposure to Dietary Factors of Interest	Presence of Disease		
	Yes	No	Total
Yes	a	b	a + b
No	c	d	c + d
Total	a + c	b + d	n

Notes: Odds ratio = (a/c)/(b/d); relative risk = [a/(a + b)]/[c/(c + d)].

[a] Entries denote the number of subjects in the study who fall into the specific category of disease status and dietary patterns.

23.2.4 OBSERVATIONAL STUDIES—COHORT

A comparison of historical exposures reported by cases and controls (case–control studies) can provide suggestive evidence for a cause-and-effect relationship. This type of information, however, may be distorted or biased by the fact that the ability of cases and controls to recall earlier exposures differs. Such bias could be avoided by using a cohort study design in which exposure is assessed among unaffected persons, and subjects are then observed for a subsequent development of illness.

A cohort study is also called a follow-up study of a (usually large) group of people who are initially disease free. It is usually prospective, that is, exposure to the risk factor and the subsequent outcomes are observed after the beginning of the study (Figure 23.2). An alternative name for such a cohort study is longitudinal study.

The research involves a group of individuals called a cohort, who do not yet have the disease under investigation. Researchers follow the cohort over a period of time while collecting specific information regarding habits or factors such as diet suspected to be related to the development of the disease. The frequency of disease among subjects exposed to a suspected cause of disease is then compared with the frequency among those who were not exposed. A higher rate of disease in the group exposed to a suspected cause suggests an association between the exposure and the disease.

Cohort studies avoid most of the methodological problems of other studies and can produce more definitive results. Among the advantages of prospective studies is that the relative risk of developing a disease in individuals exposed to a specific factor can be determined directly as incidence rates of the disease are known. As the cohort is classified according to a specific factor (e.g., high fat intake) prior to the development of the disease, bias is reduced as this classification (high-fat versus low-fat intake) cannot be influenced by the knowledge that disease exists. In prospective studies, more than one disease may be followed. For example, a study may be initiated to determine the factors influencing CHD, and in the course of the disease an association for cancer may be noted.

The main limitations of prospective studies are practical. Even for common diseases in industrialized societies, it is necessary to enroll tens of thousands of subjects to have reasonable statistical power to determine relative risk. They take a long time to study diseases that take many years to develop. Such studies are long, expensive, large-scale undertakings. If the disease has a low incidence and a long induction period (time between exposure and outcome), a large cohort must be followed over a prolonged period of time to obtain meaningful results. Some individuals may drop out

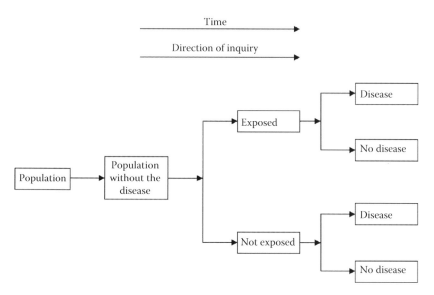

FIGURE 23.2 Design of a cohort study.

of studies. Because such studies are expensive, they are of value mainly as a means of investigating diseases common in economically developed countries.

23.2.5 Experimental Epidemiology

Two types of experiments are possible: (1) clinical trials and (2) community trials. These are controlled studies where some type of intervention (dietary constituents, nutritional supplement, or exercise) is used to determine its impact on certain health parameters. Studies include an experimental group (subjects who are given intervention) and a control group (subjects who are not given intervention). The control group receives a placebo (inactive substance) that looks the same as the experimental treatment but has no effect, such as a sugar pill.

The preferred experimental method is the randomized controlled trial in which people are assigned to an intervention or control group at random. In clinical trials, the study factor is randomly assigned at the individual level. In community trials, the unit of random assignment is the group. Random assignment reduces the risk of introducing bias into either group. The strength of evidence from experimental studies is increased if they are conducted blind, meaning that the subjects do not know whether they belong to the intervention or to the control group. Thus, they would be less inclined to alter their responses or report symptoms based on what they think should happen. If the trial is designed so that neither the subjects nor the investigators collecting the data are aware of the subjects' group assignments (treatment or placebo), the study is called double blind. In this case, another member of the research team holds the code for subject assignments and does not participate in the data collection. This reduces the possibility that the researchers will see the results they want to see even if the actual data may be different.

Other than their ability to randomize the study factor, experimental designs are similar to cohort studies in directionality and analysis. Therefore, they are also called experimental cohort studies. In a randomized trial, the potential confounding variables should be distributed at random between the treatment and control groups, thus minimizing the possibility of spurious differences in outcome because of extraneous factors. Experimental studies provide more definitive proof of the causation of disease than observational studies. However, due to ethical constraints, the study of factors believed to increase the risk of disease in humans cannot usually be assessed experimentally by deliberately exposing groups of people to a risk factor. More often, experimental studies are used to test preventive or therapeutic measures of diseases.

23.3 EPIDEMIOLOGICAL MEASURES

Measures of association in epidemiological studies discussed here are used to investigate the etiology, treatment, and prevention of diseases:

- Incidence rate (IR) is the number of new cases of a certain disease appearing during a certain period of time in a specified population. It measures the rapidity with which newly diagnosed cases of a disease develop. It is estimated by observing a population, counting the number of new cases of the disease in that population (A), and measuring the net time (PT) that individuals in the population at risk for developing the disease are observed. A subject at risk for a disease followed for 1 year contributes 1 person-year of observation. The incidence rate is given by $IR = A/PT$. Using a hypothetical example, if 1000 cigarette smokers are followed for 10 years (for an aggregate duration of 10,000 years) for the occurrence of the first myocardial infarction and 20 show signs of that condition, the incidence rate is 20 myocardial infarctions per 10,000 person-years. If 1000 nonsmokers are followed for the same duration and 10 have myocardial infarctions, the incidence rate is 10 myocardial infarctions per 10,000 person-years.

- Prevalence is the number of existing cases of a condition among a given population at a particular point in time (e.g., on a given day). Prevalence rate (P) is a proportion estimated by dividing the number of existing affected individuals (C) by the number of persons in the population (N), given by $P = C/N$. It ranges between 0 and 1 and has no units. If there are 100 individuals with a disease in a population of 100,000, the prevalence rate is 0.001.
- Risk is the likelihood that an individual will contract a disease within a specified period of time. More precisely, risk is the proportion of unaffected individuals who, on average, will contract the disease of interest over a specified period of time. It is estimated by observing a particular population for a defined period of time—the risk period. The estimated risk (R) is a proportion. The numerator is the number of newly affected persons (A) with the disease, and the denominator is the size (N) of the population under observation:

$$R = \text{number of new cases/persons at risk} = A/N$$

- All members of the population are free of the disease at the start of observation. Risk, which has no units, lies between 0 (when no new occurrence arises) and 1 (when the entire population is affected) during the risk period. Alternately, risk can be expressed as a percentage by multiplying the proportion by 100. If 100 cigarette smokers (all free of disease) are followed for a 10-year period for the occurrence of the first myocardial infarction and 4 show signs of that condition, the 10-year risk for the disease is 0.04 or 4%. If 2 of 100 nonsmokers have a first myocardial infarction over 10 years of follow-up, the risk is 0.02% or 2%. Risk factor is an attribute or an agent suspected to be related to the occurrence of a particular disease. Risk ratio is the likelihood of the occurrence of a particular disease among persons exposed to a given risk factor divided by the corresponding likelihood among unexposed persons.
- Relative risk is a measure that shows the extent of association between a disease and an exposure. It is the ratio of the risk for those exposed to the risk for those not exposed. The relative risk for the aforementioned risk data is 2.0. This means that cigarette smokers had twice the risk of myocardial infarctions of nonsmokers. If there had been no difference in the risk between cigarette smokers and nonsmokers, the relative risk would have been 1.0. If those exposed had a lower risk than those not exposed, the relative risk would have been less than 1.0.
- Odds ratio. The relative risk cannot be directly obtained from a case–control study. In this study design, participants are not followed over time, which is necessary to measure risk. As the purpose of doing a case–control study is to examine the association between a disease and an exposure, a measure of association other than the relative risk must be used. This measure is the odds ratio. It is the odds of a particular exposure among persons with a specific disease divided by the corresponding odds of exposure among persons without the disease of interest. The odds ratios obtained from case–control studies can closely approximate the relative risk, particularly if the condition is rare (Table 23.1).
- Bias is a systematic error in the design or conduct of a study that leads to a distortion of the results. Observational studies are generally more subject to bias than are clinical trials, because the latter are undertaken under more controlled conditions. Case–control studies may be dependent on the recall of study participants. The faulty recall of participants can lead to recall bias. The study can be biased if the control group is not selected with care, leading to selection bias. These and a number of other kinds of bias can affect studies.
- A confounding variable is a variable that, within a specific epidemiological study, is associated with both the disease of interest and the exposure of interest, thus distorting the relationship. An example is that age is related to both smoking history and the risk of lung cancer, and thus it must be accounted for (controlled) in studies of smoking as a cause of

lung cancer. Another example is that obesity is related to both high serum cholesterol levels and the risk of myocardial infarction, and thus obesity is a potential confounder and must be accounted for. Confounding does not always lead to an overestimation of an association between a condition and an exposure, in that it can also have the opposite effect and obscure an association that is actually present.[9]

23.4 SIGNIFICANCE OF EPIDEMIOLOGICAL STUDIES

The major objective of epidemiology in nutrition is to identify factors (e.g., dietary components) contributing to disease occurrence, leading eventually to intervention measures for disease control or prevention.[15] Through epidemiology, diet–disease relationships can be examined at the level of free-living populations and clinically defined subgroups. Each of the techniques on its own provides only circumstantial evidence of how a disease is caused. Most conclusions regarding causality based on the demonstration of an epidemiological association include a substantial element of judgment. Although the evidence is circumstantial, it may be possible to substantiate it or discard it by relevant data from other types of studies. When findings from several methods (other epidemiological studies, human clinical trials, and animal experiments) confirm an association derived from epidemiological data, the conclusion made regarding causality is on much firmer ground and the hypothesis becomes more probable. If an association is found to be causal (i.e., the factor causes the disease), comprehensive or multidisciplinary studies in which epidemiological studies are combined with information from other scientific disciplines is the preferred approach for determining (or confirming) causality.

Epidemiology can provide the basis for developing and evaluating preventive measures such as nutrition education, food supplementation, food fortification, and financial assistance for needy people to purchase healthy food. The effectiveness of nutrition programs can be monitored and evaluated by epidemiological studies, which involve a surveillance of the nutritional status of participants.

23.5 A FEW EXAMPLES OF NUTRITIONAL STUDIES

Although excellent epidemiological studies were conducted before the twentieth century, a systematic body of principles by which to design and judge such studies began to form only in the last century and more so after the Second World War. Several of these studies have had far-reaching influence on health. In 1915, endemic goiter was named as the easiest known disease to prevent, and the use of iodized salt for goiter control was proposed in the same year in Switzerland. The first large-scale clinical trials with iodized salt were carried out shortly afterward in Akron, Ohio, on 5000 girls aged between 11 and 18 years. The prophylactic and therapeutic effects were impressive and iodized salt was introduced on a community scale in many countries in 1924. The community intervention trials of fluoride supplementation in water that were started during the 1940s have led to a widespread primary prevention of dental caries.[7]

The Framingham study, perhaps the most frequently cited diet–heart study in the United States, represents an extensive prospective population study of CHD and its associated risk factors.[8] The study showed that hypercholesterolemia, hypertension, and cigarette smoking are three major risk factors in CHD. The study has included a biannual follow-up since its start in 1948. A total of 2283 men and 2844 women aged 30–62 years were included in the initial sample. The study found a correlation between serum total cholesterol levels and the development of CHD in a diet study group as well as the entire population sample. Individuals with serum cholesterol levels greater than 260 mg/dL were three times more likely to develop a heart disease than were individuals whose cholesterol levels were less than 200 mg/dL. When compared by an elevated total cholesterol level, the data confirmed the notion that high-density-lipoprotein cholesterol concentration is a potent lipid predictor of CHD. This remarkable study is continuing to produce other valuable findings more than 50 years after it began.

The most influential study on diet and CHD was the work of Keys (1970) relating the intakes of dietary factors of 16 defined populations in seven countries to the incidence of heart disease in those same groups.[11] For populations demonstrating high mean serum cholesterol levels and a high prevalence of CHD, the proportion of dietary calories from saturated fat was 15% or more. For those populations demonstrating a low prevalence of CHD, the saturated fat content of the diet averaged 10% of the total calories. Also, populations with low serum cholesterol levels were associated with intakes of protective, nonincriminated foods such as whole grain bread and cereals, vegetables, fruits, and fish. These populations exhibited lower coronary death rates. Recent research has substantially expanded the classic cholesterol–heart disease relationships by indicating a significant protective impact and a potential therapeutic role for vitamin C, vitamin E, β-carotene, other antioxidant phytochemicals, vitamin B_6, vitamin B_{12}, and folate.

Another example of an observational cohort study is the one conducted by Folson and his group[5] published in 1993. A cohort of 41,837 Iowan women from 55–69 years old was followed for 5 years. During this time, 1504 deaths occurred. Body mass index (BMI) was associated with mortality following a J-shaped curve. This means that death was highest among two groups—the women with the lowest BMI and the most obese women. The waist-to-hip circumference ratio had a significant positive correlation with mortality, which increased in increments. This ratio emerged as a better marker of the risk of death among older women than the body mass index.

Epidemiological studies have yielded data to answer many questions about cancer incidence and the role of eating patterns. It has been estimated that at least a third of cancer mortality is related to dietary factors.[10] Various studies indicate that a high intake of total fat and meat increase the risk of some types of cancer. Other dietary factors, including smoked salt–cured and nitrate-cured foods, alcohol, and naturally occurring contaminants such as aflatoxins also pose a potential cancer risk. Dietary patterns emphasizing foods high in fiber are associated with low rates of certain types of cancer, especially breast and colon cancers. Fruits and green leafy vegetables, which are important sources of antioxidants, vitamins, protective and chemoprotective phytochemicals like phenols and indoles, as well as fiber, are also associated with a reduced risk of several forms of cancer.

A number of epidemiological studies have suggested that the consumption of soybeans and soy foods is associated with a lowered risk of several cancers, including breast, prostate, and colon cancers. One prospective study has shown that the consumption of tomatoes one to four times a week is associated with a lower risk of developing prostate cancer. It is evident that diet has a role in the prevention of cancer, but there is limited information available for intervention studies. As a result, some of the evidence is weak.

Nutritional epidemiology has contributed significantly to understanding the etiology of many other diseases. As our attention is increasingly focused on the role of diet in chronic, degenerative diseases, epidemiology is becoming central to the field of nutritional sciences. A number of diseases such as cataracts, osteoporosis, stroke, diabetes, and congenital malformations such as neural tube defects are now considered to have important dietary determinants. Epidemiological evidence to support the benefits of a variety of vegetables and fruits is strong, and there is abundant biological protective plausibility for a preventive/protective role played by numerous constituents of these foods. When interpreted appropriately, findings from epidemiological research can play a major role in efforts to improve public health.

REFERENCES

1. Ast, D. B. 1965. Dental public health. In *Preventative Medicine and Public Health*, ed. P. E. Startwell. New York: Meredith.
2. Bendich, A., and R. J. Deckelbaum, eds. 1997. *Preventive Nutrition: The Comprehensive Guide for Health Professionals*. Totowa, NJ: Humana Press.
3. Doll, R., and R. Peto. 1981. The cases of cancer. *J Natl Cancer Inst* 66:1191.
4. Eley, J. W., and J. R. Boring. 2001. Medical Epidemiology. New York: McGraw-Hill.

5. Folsom, A. R., S. A. Kaye, T. A. Seller, C. P. Hong, J. R. Cerhan, J. D. Potter, and R. J. Prineas. 1993. Body fat distribution and 5-year risk of deaths in older women. *J Am Med Assoc* 269:483.

6. Gerstman, B. B. 1998. *Epidemiology Kept Simple*. New York: Wiley-Liss.

7. Goldberger, J. E. 1964. Goldberger on Pellagra. Baton Rouge, LA: Louisiana State University Press.

8. Gordon, T., and W. B. Kennel. 1971. Premature mortality from coronary heart disease. The Framingham Study. *J Am Med Assoc* 215:1617.

9. Greenland, S., and H. Morgenstern. 2001. Confounding in health research. *Annu. Rev. Public Health* 22:189–212.

10. Greenwald, P. 1996. The potential dietary modification to prevent cancer. *Prev Med* 25:41.

11. Keys, A. 1970. Coronary heart disease in seven countries. *Circulation* 41(Suppl. 1):1.

12. Lilienfeld, A. M., and D. E. Lilienfeld, eds. 1980. *Foundation of Epidemiology*. 2nd ed. New York: Oxford University Press.

13. Lind, J. 1953. *A Treatise on the Scurvy* (Reprinted). Edinburgh: Edinburgh University Press.

14. MacMahan, B., and T. F. Pugh. 1970. *Epidemiology: Principles and Methods*. Boston: Little Brown.

15. Tarasuck, V. S., and A. S. Brooker. 1997. Interpreting epidemiologic studies of diet–disease relationships. *J Nutr* 127:1847–1852.

16. Willett, W., ed. 1998. *Nutritional Epidemiology*. Oxford: Oxford University Press.

Part IV

Special Topics

24 Dietary Fiber

The role played by fiber in health and disease has become the subject of increased public attention in recent years. This food component was considered an inert and insignificant part of human diet because it was not digested, absorbed, or metabolized by the body and is passed directly through as human waste. Interest was stirred, however, when it was reported that rural Africans whose diets were high in fiber seemed to have a lower incidence of certain diseases than people living in developed countries consuming low-fiber diets. Recent epidemiological and experimental observations have suggested the important roles of fiber in maintaining human health.

24.1 FIBER

24.1.1 DEFINITION

Until the mid 1970s, all data concerning the fiber content of food were expressed in terms of crude fiber. Crude fiber is a chemist's concept and refers to what is left after a treatment with boiling sulfuric acid, strong alkali, water, and alcohol. This obviously has little to do with human nutrition. In this procedure, some of the fiber components are dissolved and are not included in the final measurements. Hence, fiber levels based on crude fiber determinations are misleadingly low. Fiber is often referred to as unavailable carbohydrate, but it is neither strictly unavailable nor entirely carbohydrate. Currently, the term dietary fiber is used as a generic term that includes those plant constituents that are resistant to digestion by secretions of the human gastrointestinal tract.[7,12] Therefore, dietary fiber does not have a defined composition but varies with the type of foodstuff and the makeup of the diet. In 1984, the new official fiber determination method was accepted by the Association of Analytical Chemists and recognized by the United States Food and Drug Administration (FDA).[8]

24.1.2 FOOD SOURCES

All foods of vegetable origin contain fiber, but in variable quantities.[21,22] Whole grain cereals are a major source. The average fiber contents of some cereal products are as follows: whole wheat—12.8%, white flour—3.3%, wheat bran—42.4%, corn bran—88.8%, and white rice—4.1%. Dry beans, lentils, and soybeans have over 4%; roasted nuts have 2.3%–6.2%; and most fruits and vegetables have 0.5%–1.0%.

24.1.3 COMPONENTS OF DIETARY FIBER

The major components of dietary fiber are nonstarch polysaccharides,[9] which include celluloses, hemicelluloses, pectins, gums, and mucilages (Table 24.1). The noncarbohydrate constituent that is included in most definitions of fiber is lignin. Cellulose is known to be the most abundant organic molecule on Earth and is the best known component of fiber. It is found in all plant cells. It consists of unbranched polymers of 1-4 β-glucose, containing approximately 2000 carbohydrate units with an average molecular weight of about 6×10^5. The α-amylase (i.e., salivary and pancreatic amylases) cannot break the β 1-4 bond in cellulose, and because humans do not have cellulase, we cannot digest it. Some ruminants harbor cellulase-producing bacteria in their digestive tract and thus can digest cellulose. It has hydrophilic or water-retaining property. Oats and barley are particularly rich sources of cellulose.

TABLE 24.1
Physicochemical and Biological Actions of Fiber

Type of Fiber	Chemistry	Physical Property	Biological Action
Celluloses	Linear glucose polymers (β 1–4 linkage)	Hydrophilic, water-insoluble	↓ Transit time, stool bulk
Hemicelluloses	Branched polymers of pentoses and hexoses	Hydrophilic, water-insoluble	↓ Transit time, stool bulk
Pectins	Mixture of colloidal polysaccharides	Can form viscous solutions	↓ Rate of small intestinal absorption (glucose, bile acids)
	Galacturonic acid linked to sugars	Water-soluble, gel-forming, binds bile salts	↓ Plasma cholesterol
Gums	Polymers of hexoses, deoxysugars, and uronic acids that may be methoxicated and acetylated	Can form viscous solutions, water-soluble	↓ Rate of small intestinal absorption (glucose, bile acids), ↓ plasma cholesterol
Mucilages	Branched carbohydrate polymers obtained from seeds and seaweed	Can form viscous solutions, water-soluble	↓ Rate of small intestinal absorption (glucose, bile acids), ↓ plasma cholesterol
Lignins	Polymers of aromatic alcohols (phenyl propane), noncarbohydrate	Water-insoluble, binds bile salts	↓ Plasma cholesterol

↓ Indicates a decrease in stated function.

Hemicelluloses are much more complex polysaccharides. They contain mixtures of pentoses and hexoses, many of which are branched, and uronic acids, which are sugars that contain a terminal –COOH group. Each hemicellulose molecule contains an average of 150–200 carbohydrate units and has a molecular weight of 3×10^4. It has hydrophilic and ion-binding properties.

Pectins are polymers of 1-4 β-D-galacturonic acid with several other sugars and with a molecular weight of about $6–9 \times 10^4$. In the presence of suitable concentrations of acids, sugar and pectin produce jelly. This is responsible for the gelling properties of fruits. Pectin has ion-binding properties.

Gums are water-soluble viscous polysaccharides of 10,000–30,000 units that are mainly glucose, galactose, mannose, arabinose, ramnose, and uronic acid. Gums are commonly used in the food industry and are obtained as exudates from stems or seeds of tropical and semitropical trees and shrubs. Mucilages are polysaccharides from flaxseeds, psyllium seeds, and seaweeds and are used as thickeners and stabilizers because they have water-holding and viscous properties. Lignins are aromatic and are made up of polymers of substituted phenyl propane units. The molecular weights and polymer sizes of lignins vary a great deal depending on the source. Estimates of molecular weight range between 1000 and 8000. It has bile salt–binding ability.

Resistant starch (the sum of starch that escapes digestion and starch degradation products not absorbed in the small intestine) contributes to the pool of dietary fiber. Resistant starches are found in legumes, as well as starches like potatoes, pasta, and rice that have been cooked and cooled (as in pasta or potato salad, or sushi), and barely ripe bananas. And they are also being added to pasta and energy bars. Resistant starch is a "prebiotic" that, when fermented in the large intestine, increases beneficial bacteria. The amount of resistant starch in a typical Western diet is not known. Legumes appear to be the single most important source of resistant starch, with as much as 35% of the legume starch escaping digestion.

Dietary fibers may be classified as water-soluble and water-insoluble.[15] Some plants contain significant amounts of both soluble and insoluble fibers. Celluloses, hemicelluloses, and lignins are insoluble in water. Wheat products are good sources of insoluble fiber, but fruits and vegetables also contain significant amounts. Other sources include legumes such as lentils (15–19 g/cup serving), bran (17 g/cup), prunes (12 g), peas (10 g), nuts, seeds, green beans, cauliflower, zucchini, celery, avocado, and bananas. The soluble fiber components include pectins, gums, and storage polysaccharides. The primary sources of soluble fiber include oat products, barley, legumes, some vegetables (broccoli, carrots, potatoes, sweet potatoes, onions), and fruits. An average serving of oat bran (0.33 cup) provides 2 g of soluble fiber. One cup of cooked oatmeal contains about 1.5 g of soluble fiber, and legumes and beans provide 3 g of soluble fiber per 0.5 cup of cooked serving.

There are several fiber-associated substances that are found in high-fiber foods that may have some nutritional importance. Chief among these are phytates, saponins, tannins, lectins, and enzyme inhibitors. In plants, these substances may protect against attacks by predators, parasites, and molds, and may inhibit autodigestion by the plants' own digestive enzymes. Phytate has the ability to bind certain metals and can, therefore, interfere with the absorption of minerals and trace elements. Saponins are triterpenoid molecules with sugar residues, and they have the ability to alter the surface characteristics of cell membranes. They may enhance the binding of bile acids to fiber and may reduce cholesterol absorption. Tannins are polyphenolic compounds that can bind proteins and reduce their digestibility. Lectins are glycoproteins that can bind specific sugars on the surfaces of cells, induce cell lysis, and adversely affect the intestinal absorption of nutrients. Enzyme inhibitors are ubiquitous in foods of plant origin, but beans and cereals are rich sources. Inhibitors of lipase, amylase, and trypsin have been identified.

24.1.4 METABOLISM OF FIBER

The human digestive tract does not have the enzymes necessary for the breakdown of dietary fiber. The plant material in food (fruits, vegetables) has two fractions: nutrients, which can be digested and absorbed, and fibers. From the mouth, the food contents enter the stomach relatively unchanged; the hydrochloric acid in the stomach helps to break the cellular structures of plant material and releases the protoplasmic matter containing digestible nutrients. In the small intestine, these digestible components are broken down by hydrolysis and the nutrients are absorbed through the mucosal cells. In vitro studies indicate that the various fiber sources can inhibit the activity of pancreatic enzymes involved in the digestion of carbohydrates, fats, and proteins. The mechanism for this inhibitory action is not understood, but it may be attributed to the presence of specific fiber components or associated substances (e.g., enzyme inhibitors) in food sources. Whether this effect causes an actual reduction in digestive enzyme activity in vivo is not clear because the enzyme secretions are generally in excess after a meal.

The various fiber components and associated substances pass from the stomach through the small intestine into large intestine virtually unaltered. In the colon, different fiber components are subject to varying levels of bacterial degradation.[2] Pectin, gums, and mucilages are almost completely fermented, while cellulose and hemicellulose are only partly degraded. Because of its noncarbohydrate nature, most of the lignin passes through unchanged. Bacteria initiate the digestion and the metabolism of certain fractions, mainly hemicelluloses, pectins, and gums. There is a subsequent production of various by-products such as short-chain fatty acids (SCFAs) including acetate, propionate and butyrate, water, carbon dioxide, hydrogen, and methane. The combination of these products of microbial metabolism together with the physical presence of fiber in the colon may affect intestinal functions such as transit time, fecal weight, bowel habits, composition of bacterial flora, and the output of organic anions such as bile salts. Transit time—the time necessary for a substance to move through the entire gastrointestinal tract and be excreted in the feces—is known to be shortened by the ingestion of increased dietary fiber. A portion of SCFAs is used to support the colonic microbial population; some are absorbed and the remaining are excreted in the stools. As absorbed SCFAs can provide energy, it is possible that high dietary fiber intake may contribute significantly to the energy intake.

The amount of energy contributed by dietary fiber is the subject of considerable debate. Some researchers say that the contribution is negligible because dietary fiber interferes to some extent in the absorption of energy, yielding macronutrients coupled with a small amount of SCFAs derived from dietary fiber. Others believe that approximately 2 Cal/g (8.4 kJ/g) should be considered for soluble fiber. This can create inconsistencies when listing actual product nutrition labels. But as of 2009, there is no consensus on how much energy is actually absorbed. In some countries, fiber is not listed in nutrition labels and is considered to provide 0 Cal when the food's total calories are computed. In the United States, soluble fiber must be counted as 4 Cal/g, but insoluble fiber may be treated as 0 Cal and may not be mentioned in the label.

24.1.5 PHYSIOLOGICAL EFFECTS

The primary function of dietary fiber in the body is in the gastrointestinal tract,[3] but not all fiber components have the same physiological effects.[26] In the mouth, fiber stimulates the flow of saliva and increases the volume of food in the mouth. When the fiber reaches the stomach, it dilutes the contents. Water-soluble and viscous fiber components delay gastric emptying, while other fibers have no effect. In the small intestine, viscous fiber components may slow the digestion and the absorption of carbohydrates and fats. They tend to slow down intestinal glucose absorption and lower plasma cholesterol. In the large intestine, water-soluble fiber components are rapidly broken down (fermented) by bacteria. They do not appreciably increase stool weight and do not promote laxation. Fibers that are predominantly water insoluble are either not fermented or slowly fermented. They increase stool weight and promote laxation. There are at least two notable exceptions to these guidelines: Rice bran, which is virtually devoid of soluble fiber, also has been shown to lower plasma cholesterol. Psyllium is thought to be highly soluble and is effective in lowering plasma cholesterol. Many of the commercial laxatives are made from psyllium because it is extremely effective in laxation, a property usually associated with insoluble fiber.

24.2 FIBER AND DISEASE

Based mainly on epidemiological data, a low intake of dietary fiber has been associated with a broad spectrum of unrelated noninfectious diseases. A number of physiological claims have been made for the beneficial effects of fiber in the diet; some of the pieces of evidence for these claims appear to be justified, but some are simply anecdotal. The role of fiber in human disease can be grouped into diseases of the gastrointestinal tract, circulation-related diseases, metabolic diseases, and other diseases.

24.2.1 DISEASES OF THE GASTROINTESTINAL TRACT

24.2.1.1 Constipation

Constipation is common in our society especially among the elderly. It can be caused by several factors, one of which is thought to be the low dietary intake of fiber. Certain types of fiber have a marked effect on the output of fecal water and electrolytes and in the regulation of bowel functions. Various preparations of fiber form the basis of a large number of laxatives. Fiber behaves like a sponge as it passes along the gastrointestinal tract. Cellulose and hemicellulose have hydrophilic properties and are, therefore, effective in increasing stool bulk and weight. The main products of bacterial action on dietary fiber (especially hemicellulose and pectin) in the colon are volatile fatty acids, some of which have cathartic effects. These SCFAs also provide energy for bacterial growth. This increases fecal bulk. Indeed, feeding experiments have shown that for every gram of extra cereal fiber, the stool weight increases by 3–9 g. The increase in stool weight and bulk, together with the cathartic action, promotes colonic peristalsis and shortens transit time. The daily fecal weight for individuals in North America and Europe (low fiber intake) varies between 80 and 200 g, and for Africans living in their villages (high fiber intake) it is between 400 and 500 g. Fiber sources that contain insoluble fiber components such as wheat bran tend to have the greatest effect on stool weight, whereas the fibers in fruits and vegetables can be extensively fermented and are more likely to increase the microbial cell mass. Thus, dietary fiber clearly has an important physiological role in the normal functioning of the large bowel by providing bulk and substrates for fermentation. Several fiber components have been shown to be effective for the relief of constipation, including psyllium (Metamucil) and methylcellulose (Citrucil). The current treatment for constipation includes recommendations to increase the intake of dietary fiber, especially whole meal or whole wheat products that are high in cereal fiber.[19]

24.2.1.2 Diverticular Disease

Diverticular disease is characterized by small, "blow out"–type protrusions (diverticula) on the large intestine that can become inflamed, and the resulting condition is diverticulitis. It is caused as a result of an increased pressure inside the colon. It has been postulated that a fiber-deficient diet renders the colonic contents more viscous and hard to propel. The colonic lumen is narrower because of the lower bulk of the diet and builds up a higher intraluminal pressure. This increased pressure produces diverticula. There appears to be a strong negative correlation between the epidemiology of diverticular disease and fiber intake. In developed countries, the disease appears with increasing frequency in people who eat a diet from which the natural fiber has been removed by the milling of flour and the refining of sugar. Rural Africans who eat products that contain fiber do not develop diverticular disease. The low incidence of this disease among vegetarians in developed countries has been attributed to their higher intake of fiber, particularly of cereal origin. The traditional dietary management for patients suffering from this disease has been a low-fiber diet; however, recent clinical studies have shown that the symptoms of the disease are effectively alleviated by a high-fiber diet. It may exert its protective effect against diverticular disease by absorbing water. This permits the formation of larger and softer stools, which move quickly and do not cause an increased intraluminal pressure.

Studies in Greece do not give support to the association of dietary fiber deficiency to the etiology of diverticular disease; rather, the factors connected with city life and prosperity play important roles in causing the disease. Recent clinical trials also do not support the use of fiber in the treatment of the disease; however, in the last few years there has been a change from low-fiber diets that were once advocated in the management of the disease to high-fiber diets.[13]

The raised intraluminal pressure may be important in the causation of varicose veins, hemorrhoids, and hiatal hernia. Appendicitis has also been alleged to be the result of a low-fiber diet; however, in the United States and England, there has been a very definite decrease in the incidence of acute appendicitis over the past four decades, the same period in which the incidence of diverticular disease has been increasing.

24.2.1.3 Colon Cancer

Colon cancer is the second most frequent cause of cancer mortality in the United States, following lung cancer in males and breast cancer in females. It is thought to be related to diet because of the colon's direct contact with food residues. On the basis mainly of epidemiological evidence, some investigators have proposed a rationale for a protective role of fiber in relation to colonic cancer. In essence, it is theorized that fiber-depleted diets prolong the contact between concentrated stool content and the mucosa, and the same diet may favor the growth of bacterial flora capable of forming carcinogens or procarcinogens from the degradation of bile salts. It has been suggested that dihydroxy bile acids are converted to carcinogenic polynuclear hydrocarbons by bacterial action.

Fiber may protect against cancer in several ways: The ability of fiber to increase water content and fecal bulk can result in the dilution of potential carcinogens or cocarcinogens in the colon; fiber decreases the length of the time the mucosa is exposed to toxic materials by decreasing the transit time; it reduces the production of carcinogens by altering the bacterial flora or their functional activities; fiber can absorb the toxic materials, thus reducing their availability to the lining of the colon; and the production of SCFAs reduces colonic pH, which in turn may limit the uptake of ammonia by epithelial cells. A low pH may also reduce the conversion of bile acids by α-hydroxylation to potential carcinogens. The SCFAs provide energy for bacterial growth, which may help inactivate toxic substances. The SCFAs may also be antineoplastic. The most likely explanation for the protective effect of fiber may be some combination of these effects.

Correlation studies that compare colorectal cancer incidence or mortality rates among countries with estimates of national dietary fiber consumption suggest that fiber intake may be protective against colon cancer. Case–control studies of colorectal cancer rates and dietary practices also have shown that the intake of fiber-rich foods is inversely related to the risk of colon cancer.[24] Based on these studies, it is estimated that the risk of colorectal cancer in the U.S. population could be reduced by about 31% if fiber intake from food sources were increased by an average of about 13 g/day. The epidemiological studies can, however, be misleading. For example, the incidence of colon cancer in different countries and cultures correlates much better with the consumption of fat than with the consumption of fiber. Furthermore, there is no proven relationship between transit time and the incidence of colon cancer, and there is no proof that dietary fiber per se has a definable effect on the intestinal flora of humans. The SCFAs, which some consider as antineoplastic, can also stimulate large intestinal cell growth, which in turn can promote tumor formation when an initiator is administered in an animal model. The epidemiological associations are not as strong for fiber as they are for fats and proteins. Clinical trials using the incidence of adenomatous polyps as a marker for colon cancer risk have not supported these epidemiological associations. The Polyp Prevention Trial, a randomized multicenter trial of a low-fat, high-fiber, high-fruit, and high-vegetable diet, found no effect of diet on the recurrence of adenomas of the large bowel, even 8 years after randomization.[14] The possible relationship between dietary fiber and colon cancer remains a hypothesis that must be put to a rigorous test.

24.2.2 Circulation-Related Diseases

Increased serum lipids, especially triglycerides and cholesterol, are considered the primary risk factors in atherosclerosis and coronary heart disease (CHD). Some scientists put forth the hypothesis that a high consumption of starchy carbohydrates with fiber is protective against hyperlipidemia and CHD.[4] Vegetarians and Seventh-day Adventists generally consume high-fiber diets, have low levels of serum cholesterol, and have a low incidence of CHD; however, the diet of these groups is not only high in fiber but also low in animal fat. A diet high in soluble fiber may lower serum cholesterol levels by reducing the transit time, leading to decreased absorption of dietary cholesterol. The American Heart Association lists whole-wheat breads, wheat cereals, wheat bran, cabbage, beets, carrots, Brussels sprouts, turnips, cauliflower, and apple skin as foods high in insoluble fiber. Soluble fiber has been linked to lower levels of "bad" cholesterol. Viscous fibers like oat bran and beans seem to work particularly well because they form gel in the gut that slows down the absorption of fat and cholesterol. Fiber may also reduce serum cholesterol by another mechanism. Bile acids, which are synthesized by the liver, are required for emulsifying fats and oils during digestion and thus permit their absorption from the intestine. Some fiber components (e.g., pectin and lignin) bind bile salts and prevent their absorption, as well as the absorption of dietary cholesterol and fat from the intestine. This causes more of the bile salts, cholesterol, and fat to be excreted.[23] As bile acid excretion is the main elimination pathway of endogenously synthesized cholesterol, the increase in excretion may reduce the cholesterol pool and thus lower blood cholesterol levels. Another theory is that SCFAs (a product of fiber fermentation in the colon), after absorption, may inhibit the synthesis of cholesterol by the liver. Numerous studies in humans and in experimental animals have demonstrated that increased dietary fiber lowers plasma cholesterol. Fiber has been referred to as a hypocholesterolemic agent. Guar, pectin, lignin, oat bran, and locus bean gums have been tried in the treatment of types II and IV hyperlipidemic patients. Soluble fiber (guar and pectin) has been reported to lower low-density lipoprotein (LDL) cholesterol levels by 10%–15% with no reduction in high-density lipoprotein (HDL) cholesterol. Dried beans have been found to cause a 10% drop in cholesterol and a 20% drop in triglycerides in hyperlipidemic patients.

Dietary fiber, especially the soluble type, is thought to exert a preventive role against heart disease as it appears to have the ability to lower serum total and LDL cholesterol levels.[25] Many large epidemiological studies have demonstrated a reduced risk for CHD in both men and women who consume higher amounts of dietary fiber. In the National Heart, Lung, and Blood Institute family heart study, men and women who ate an average of 5.5 fruit and vegetable servings per day had LDL concentrations that were 6% and 7% lower, respectively, than those of individuals who ate on average only 1.5 servings each day.[11] It is now recognized that soluble fiber is a valuable intervention to decrease serum cholesterol levels by significant amounts, thereby reducing a known risk factor for CHD. Oats and psyllium have received a great deal of attention as sources with appreciable amounts of soluble fibers that have been shown to reduce serum cholesterol levels under controlled conditions. Supplementation with psyllium seed was found to lower total and LDL cholesterol levels by roughly 5% in men and 7% in women and enabled patients taking bile acid–binding resins or statins to reduce these medications by 50% to attain the same degree of lipid lowering.[16,17] The ingestion of fruits and vegetables that have a mixture of both soluble and insoluble fibers has also been shown to decrease serum cholesterol concentrations.

Recognizing the growing scientific evidence for the physiological benefits of increased fiber intake, the U.S. FDA has given approval to food products making health claims for fiber. The FDA allows producers of foods containing 1.7 g/per serving of psyllium husk soluble fiber or 0.75 g of oats or barley soluble fiber to claim that reduced risk of heart disease can result from regular consumption of these foods.

24.2.3 METABOLIC DISEASES

24.2.3.1 Diabetes

The increased consumption of fiber-deficient foods may have played an etiologic role in the increased incidence of diabetes. The incidence of diabetes in England and Wales has been correlated with the fiber content of the flour available for baking breads. A low-fiber diet may increase the risk of diabetes because such diets are usually more energy dense and promote obesity. Fiber has a role in the treatment of diabetes because it slows down the absorption of glucose in the small intestine. If postprandial blood glucose levels are elevated, incorporating soluble viscous fibers into the diet will minimize the abnormal glucose spike. The addition of fiber to the diet of diabetics results in a decrease in their postprandial glucose levels. The lowering of glucose appears to depend not only on the nature and the amount of fiber but also on its physical structure. For instance, when apples were given either whole, pureed, or as juice, an increased removal or disruption of fiber resulted in higher blood glucose levels. A high-fiber diet increases peripheral sensitivity to insulin,[20] the number of insulin receptors on circulating monocytes, and the apparent sensitivity of skeletal muscle to insulin. It appears that soluble fiber sources are more effective for patients with diabetes. They cause a reduction in glucose absorption rates and result in reduced levels of blood glucose and insulin.

24.2.3.2 Obesity

The lack of fiber digestibility gives people a feeling of satiety while adding minimal calories in the diet. Some studies suggest that high-fiber foods may help promote weight loss.[6] Breads containing high amounts of fiber frequently contain fewer calories per pound than standard bread. Fiber provides three major physiological obstacles to energy intake. First, it displaces available nutrients from the diet. Consuming food of the same weight of a less energy-dense food has been reported to increase satiety and to decrease energy intake in several short-term studies. Thus, by virtue of its ability to reduce energy density, fiber may reduce voluntary energy intake. Second, foods that are rich in fiber require chewing, which slows down food intake and also promotes a feeling of satiety, and therefore reduces food consumption. Third, soluble fiber delays gastric emptying by forming a viscous gel matrix that traps nutrients, retards their exit from the stomach, and slows digestion. The presence of fiber in the intestinal tract restricts the physical contact between nutrients and intestinal villi necessary for absorption. Thus, nutrient absorption occurs over an extended period during the consumption of diets high in soluble fiber. The delayed absorption of glucose results in lower post-prandial glucose and insulinemic responses, which are known to be linked to reductions in the rate of return of hunger and subsequent energy intake.

Under conditions of fixed energy intake, several studies in healthy adult subjects have demonstrated increased satiety, reduced hunger, reduced energy intake, and reduced body weight during the consumption of high-fiber diets. The beneficial effects of fiber on energy regulation were seen with both soluble and insoluble fibers when using foods high in fiber and fiber supplements.[10] Thus, increasing dietary fiber intake may help decrease the currently high national prevalence of obesity.

24.2.4 OTHER DISEASES

There is limited evidence that fiber intake may play a role in other diseases. A recent study has shown that eating fiber-rich fruits and vegetables and whole grain may reduce the risk of breast cancer. Fiber may bind unconjugated estrogens in the enterohepatic circulation (gastrointestinal tract) and reduce plasma estradiol. Also, a high-fiber diet helps keep blood glucose in the normal range and may reduce the risk of type 2 diabetes. High plasma glucose, estradiol, and diabetes have been linked to the increased risk of breast cancer.

In patients with chronic kidney disease, high fiber intake has been shown to reduce blood urea concentration. High fiber intake may have a beneficial effect on blood pressure.

24.3 RECOMMENDATIONS FOR FIBER INTAKE

The amount of fiber present in the human diet can vary geographically. In developed countries, fiber consumption is relatively lower than in other societies. For example, the average fiber intake in the United States is about 12–15 g daily. On the other hand, people in some African countries are known to consume as much as 50 g of fiber daily. The importance of an adequate dietary intake of fiber for health benefits is demonstrated by several studies on the effects exerted by the various components of fiber.

Currently, there is no established recommended daily allowance (RDA) for fiber. Recommendations for increasing the amount of dietary fiber in the United States have come from several health and professional organizations. A minimum fiber intake of 20 g/day with an upper limit of 35 g/day is recommended by the American Dietetic Association,[1] the National Cancer Institute, the U.S. National Academy of Sciences, Institute of Medicine, and the Federation of American Societies for Experimental Biology. Alternatively, 10–13 g of dietary fiber intake per 1000 Cal (4184 kJ) has also been suggested for American adults. The recommendation for children over 2 years of age is to include an amount equal to or greater than their age plus 5 g/day to achieve intakes of 25–30 g/day after the age of 20 years. No studies have defined desirable fiber intakes for infants and children younger than 2 years. A rational approach would be to introduce a variety of fruits, vegetables, and easily digested cereals as solid foods into the diet. A safe recommendation for the elderly is to encourage intakes of 10–13 g of dietary fiber per 1000 Cal (4184 kJ). However, the amount of fiber intake can be increased with age because energy requirements decline in older people. Intakes of up to 50 g/day are suggested for people with hypercholesterolemia and diabetes. To assure the intakes of all components, a variety of fiber-rich foods should be included in the diet. Thus, foods such as legumes, potatoes, turnips, green leafy vegetables, whole grain cereals, and fruits with edible skin should be part of the daily diet.

The British Nutrition Foundation has recommended a minimum fiber intake of 18 g/day for healthy individuals.

New research[18] suggests more fiber intake could equal more years of life. Analyzing data from nearly 400,000 men and women ages 50–71, researchers found that those who consumed the most fiber were 22% less likely to die from any cause during the 9 years they were studied. Men were 24%–56% and women 34%–59% less likely to die of heart and infectious or respiratory diseases, according to findings from the National Institutes of Health's AARP Diet and Health Study. How fiber reduces the risk of death is unclear. It may be because fiber lowers levels of "bad" cholesterol, improves blood glucose levels, reduces inflammation, and binds to potential cancer causing agents, helping to flux them out of the body.

Participants were found to get benefit only when fiber came from grains like oatmeal, cornmeal, and brown rice. Fibers from fruits, vegetables, and beans had no impact on risk of death. Whole grains are rich sources of fiber as well as vitamins, minerals, and antioxidants that may provide health benefits. Grains also have powerful anti-inflammatory properties.

24.4 OVERCONSUMPTION OF FIBER

Over the last few years, there have been several studies on the relationship between increased fiber intake and the prevention and treatment of certain diseases. Diabetes seems to be responsive to dietary fiber, especially the soluble variety. The blood cholesterol–lowering effect holds much promise for the prevention and/or treatment of CHD. However, consumption of fiber beyond the upper range of 40–50 g/day may cause problems for some individuals. Intestinal obstruction in susceptible individuals as well as fluid imbalance have occurred with high intakes of fiber, especially those with high water-holding capacity. A reduction in the efficiency of dgestion of energy-rich nutrients may also be experienced, although this is considered a positive from certain health perspectives such as therapeutic weight loss. A major concern with an overconsumption of fiber is the possible adverse impact on vitamin and mineral absorption. Phytate, which is generally present in foods rich in fiber, binds divalent cations and renders them unavailable. Therefore, there is the possibility of deficiencies in zinc, iron, calcium, and magnesium. Excessive intakes of insoluble fiber intake may pose the hazard of negative mineral balance, particularly among infants, children, adolescents, and pregnant women whose mineral requirements are greater than those for adult men and nonpregnant women. An increased fiber intake can also cause intestinal gas. Protease inhibitors that are frequently present in fiber-rich foods may be detrimental to the health of populations subsisting on a marginal diet.

Sucrase Deficiency and Protection against Colonic Disease—A Report

Epidemiological studies have shown that inflammatory bowel disease, colon cancer, and other noninfectious gastrointestinal diseases are rare in black Africans. This protection has been suggested to be due to their increased fiber intake. Epidemiological studies alone do not often establish the cause and effect of diseases, but they do result in further investigations to determine whether the epidemiological evidence represents the cause and effect or simply coincidence. Several studies have been published to determine the mechanisms behind the beneficial effects of fiber. The following report is an example.

The SCFAs are the principal end products of some of the fiber components in the large intestine. Low levels of SCFAs have been found in the presence of adenomatous polyps and colon cancer, diseases that are common among the Western population but rare in Africans. Fecal SCFAs are much higher and fecal pH values are relatively lower in black Africans than in Caucasians. These differences are assumed to be due to the differences in the levels of fiber intake in the two groups of population. However, in a section of Johannesburg, South Africa, where blacks and Caucasians both follow a Western lifestyle with a relatively low-fiber diet, differences in noninfectious gastrointestinal diseases between the two races have persisted.

In a recent study[27] of 23 black patients and 23 white patients in Johannesburg who had come to the hospital for routine upper gastrointestinal endoscopy for dyspepsia, duodenal biopsy specimens were collected and several parameters were determined. These included villus height, crypt depth, and activities of disaccharidases. There were no significant differences in villus height and crypt depth. Lactase activity (nanomole glucose per minute per milligram protein) was low in black patients (mean of 0.2 U) versus white patients (25.5 U) as was sucrase, with a mean of 22.8 U in black patients versus 43.5 U in white patients. No significant difference was observed for maltase in the two groups.

Primary lactase deficiency is a relatively common syndrome in Africans and they generally consume limited amounts of dairy products. The authors of this study suggest that undigested sucrose, like fiber, gives rise to increased colonic SCFAs in the black South African population. This may be one of a number of protective factors against noninfectious colonic diseases in this population.

REFERENCES

1. American Dietetic Association. 1997. Position of the American Dietetic Association: Health implications of dietary fiber. *J Am Diet Assoc* 97:1157.
2. Anderson, J. W. 1985. Physiological and metabolic effects of dietary fiber. *Fed Proc* 44:2902.
3. Anderson, J. W., P. Baird, R. H. Davis et al. 2009. Health benefits of dietary fiber. *Nutr Rev* 67:188.
4. Anderson, J. W., and T. J. Hanna. 1999. Impact of non-digestible carbohydrates on serum lipoproteins and risk for cardiovascular disease. *J Nutr* 129:1457S.
5. Anderson, J. W., B. M. Smith, and N. J. Gustafson. 1994. Health benefits and practical aspects of high-fiber diets. *Am J Clin Nutr Suppl* 59:1242S.
6. Berkow, S., and N. D. Bernard. 2006. Vegetarian diets and weight status. *Nutr Rev* 64:175.
7. Bingham, S. 1987. Definitions and intakes of dietary fiber. *Am J Clin Nutr* 45:1226.
8. Eastwood, M. A., and R. Passmore. 1984. A new look at dietary fiber. *Nutr Today* 19(2):6.
9. Heaton, K. W., 1983. Dietary fiber in perspective. *Hum Nutr Clin Nutr* 37C:151.
10. Howarth, N. C., E. Saltzman, and S. B. Roberts. 2001. Dietary fiber and weight regulation. *Nutr Rev* 59:129.
11. Jousse, L. D., D. K. Arnett, H. Coon et al. 2004. Fruit and vegetable consumption and LDL cholesterol: The National Heart, Lung, and Blood Institute Family Heart Study. *Amer J Clin Nutr* 79:213.
12. Kritchevsky, D. 1988. Dietary fiber. *Annu Rev Nutr* 8:301.
13. Lairon, D., N. Arnault, S. Bertrais et al. 2005. Dietary fiber intake and risk factors for cardiovascular disease in French adults. *Amer J Clin Nutr* 82:1185.
14. Lanza, E., B. Yu, G. Murphy et al. 2007. The Polyp Prevention Trial continued follow-up study. *Cancer Epidemiol Biomarkers Prev* 16:1745.
15. Lee, S. C., L. Prosky, and J. W. DeVries. 1992. Determination of total, soluble and insoluble dietary fiber in foods—enzymatic–gravimetric method, MES-TRIS buffer: Collaborative study. *J AOAC Int* 75:395.
16. Moreyra, A. E., A. C. Wilson, and A. Koraym. 2005. Effect of combining psyllium fiber with simvastatin in lowering cholesterol. *Arch Int Med* 165:161.
17. Neal, G. W., and T. K. Balm. 1990. Synergistic effects of psyllium in the dietary treatment of hypercholesterolemia. *South Med J* 83:1131.
18. Park, Y., A. F. Subar, A. Hollenbeck, A. Shcatzkin. 2011. Dietary fiber intake and mortality in the NIH-AARP Diet and Health Study. *Arch Intern Med* 171(12):1061.
19. Ramkumar, D., and S. S. Rao. 2004. Efficacy and safety of traditional medical therapies for chronic constipation. *Amer J Gastroenterol* 100:936.
20. Savaiano, D. A., and J. A. Story. 2000. Cardiovascular disease and fiber: Is insulin resistance the missing link? *Nutr Rev* 58:356.
21. Slavin, J. L. 1987. Dietary fiber: Classification, chemical analysis, and food sources. *J Am Diet Assoc* 87:1164.

22. Spiller, G. A. 1993. *Handbook of Dietary Fiber in Human Nutrition*. Boca Raton, FL: CRC Press.
23. Spiller, R. C. 1996. Cholesterol, fiber and bile acids. *Lancet* 347:415.
24. Story, J. A., and D. A. Savaiano. 2001. Dietary fiber and colorectal cancer: What is appropriate advice? *Nutr Rev* 59:84.
25. Theuwissen, E., and R. P. Mensink. 2008. Water-soluble dietary fibers and cardiovascular disease. *Physiol Behav* 94:285.
26. Trowell, H., and D. Burkitt. 1986. Physiological role of dietary fiber: A ten year review. *J Dent Child* 33:444.
27. Veitch, A. M., P. Kelly, I. Segal, S. K. Spies, and M. J. G. Farthing. 1998. Does sucrase deficiency in black Africans protect against colonic disease? *Lancet* 351:183.

25 Antioxidants and Health

During the past decade there has been an increased interest in the possible involvement of free radicals in many major disease processes as documented by a large number of publications related to this field. It has been suggested that the aging process, the effects of some environmental toxins, and various pathological events are mediated via free radical reactions. Epidemiological and experimental data have suggested that antioxidants present in food can effectively neutralize free radicals generated in the body and thus offer protection from many types of diseases. In addition to their presence in food sources, antioxidant supplements are easily available in the open market, and people are consuming them in mega quantities as a preventive measure.

25.1 FREE RADICALS

A free radical is defined as an atom or molecule that has one or more unpaired electron(s) in its outer orbit. It is this electron imbalance that gives rise in most cases to the high reactivity of the free radical because the radical tends to react with other molecules to pair the electron(s) and generate a more stable species. The common inorganic compounds nitric oxide (NO) and nitrogen dioxide (NO_2) are, by definition, free radicals. The presence of an unpaired electron in the outer orbit is represented by a superscript dot, $R^\bullet$. The most important free radicals in biological systems are derivatives of oxygen.

25.2 FORMATION OF FREE RADICALS

Free radicals are generated from sources inside the body as by-products of aerobic cellular metabolism. They are also produced on exposure to sunlight, ozone, radiation, smoking, alcohol, strenuous exercise, and environmental pollutants. One of the most commonly formed free radicals in the body is the superoxide anion ($O_2^{\bullet-}$). It is produced by the addition of an electron to molecular oxygen (Figure 25.1). This radical species is postulated to be formed in vivo through the activity of mitochondrial and microsomal electron transport chains and in the reactions involving certain flavoproteins such as xanthine oxidase and aldehyde oxidase. Activated phagocytes (e.g., neutrophils, eosinophils, monocytes, macrophages) generate superoxide anions as part of the process involved in killing foreign organisms. Also, heavy metals can accept an electron from free radicals and transfer it to molecular oxygen to form the superoxide anion radical. The superoxide anion radical itself can undergo a dismutation reaction in which one superoxide anion radical acts on another to produce hydrogen peroxide, which, by definition, is not a free radical. The addition of an electron to hydrogen peroxide forms hydroxyl radical ($OH^\bullet$), which is highly reactive and potentially more damaging on living systems. Hydroxyl radical can also be formed when hydrogen peroxide comes in contact with ferrous iron (Fenton reaction, (f) of Figure 25.1), or by an interaction between hydrogen peroxide and the superoxide anion radical catalyzed by ferrous salt (Haber–Weiss type reaction, (g) of Figure 25.1).

We eat on average about a pound (dry weight) of food per day and consume 1 pound of oxygen to provide the daily energy we need. It has been estimated that 1%–3% of oxygen consumed, or about 2 kg/year, is converted to superoxide.

An additional reactive metabolite of oxygen is singlet oxygen, which can be formed as an excited state of oxygen by energy capture. It is not a free radical. This form of oxygen can be generated in

(a) $O_2 + (e^-) \longrightarrow O_2^{\bullet-}$ (superoxide radical)

(b) $Fe^{+2} + O_2 \longrightarrow Fe^{+3} + O_2^{\bullet-}$ (superoxide radical)

(c) $O_2 + (e^-) + 2H^+ \longrightarrow H_2O_2$

(d) $O_2^{\bullet-} + O_2^{\bullet-} + 2H^+ \longrightarrow H_2O_2 + O_2$

(e) $H_2O_2 + (e^-) + 2H^+ \longrightarrow H_2O + OH^{\bullet}$ (hydroxyl radical)

(f) $Fe^{+2} + H_2O_2 \longrightarrow Fe^{+3} + OH^- + OH^{\bullet}$

(g) $O_2^{\bullet-} + H_2O_2 \xrightarrow[\text{Catalyst}]{\text{Fe salt}} O_2 + OH^{\bullet-} + OH^{\bullet}$

FIGURE 25.1 Generation of free radicals. (a) Addition of an electron to oxygen forms the superoxide anion radical. (b) In the presence of oxygen, ferrous iron is oxidized to ferric iron and oxygen is converted to superoxide. (c) Superoxide, in the presence of an electron and hydrogen ions, can form hydrogen peroxide nonenzymatically. (d) Superoxide can react with hydrogen ions (catalyzed by SOD) and form hydrogen peroxide. (e) Hydrogen peroxide, in the presence of an electron and hydrogen ions, can form water and hydroxyl radicals. (f) Hydrogen peroxide, in the presence of ferrous ions, can give rise to hydroxyl radicals. (g) Superoxide and hydrogen peroxide, in the presence of ferrous salt, can generate hydroxyl radicals.

tissues from lipid peroxidation of membranes and some enzymatic reactions. Oxygen free radicals, hydrogen peroxide, singlet oxygen, and hypochlorous acid (described in Figure 25.2) are considered reactive oxygen species (ROS) because they are much more reactive and capable of oxidizing many molecules, including polyunsaturated fatty acids.

Nitric oxide is another free radical that acts as an important biological signal in a large variety of physiological processes including smooth muscle relaxation, neurotransmission, and immune regulation.[5] Nitric oxide and other nitrogen-containing reacting compounds are nitrogen-reacting substances (NRS). Nitric oxide is formed in a variety of cell types by the action of nitric oxide synthase (NOS) on arginine. There are three main isoenzymes: (1) constitutive NOS, found primarily in endothelial cells and mediating vasodilation, (2) inducible NOS found in macrophages and neutrophils, and (3) brain NOS, which is involved in neurotransmission. At high concentrations, nitric oxide is cytotoxic and can cause tissue damage. If nitric oxide and superoxide are overproduced, they can react together to form a highly active cytotoxic species called peroxynitrite. Both peroxynitrite and its decomposition products cause tissue injury.

25.3 FREE RADICALS IN BIOLOGICAL SYSTEMS

Free radicals are unstable and react easily with essential molecules in the body. They try to reach a state of stability by giving away or receiving electrons from other molecules. When a free radical ($A^{\bullet}$) reacts with a nonradical compound (B), the free radical becomes a nonradical (A) and compound B becomes a free radical ($B^{\bullet}$). This in turn can react with another nonradical (C) and induce a chain reaction as follows:

$$A^* + B \rightarrow A + B^*$$
$$B^* + C \rightarrow B + C^*$$

The new free radical generated may be more reactive than the one responsible for initiating the reaction. The superoxide anion radical is not as reactive as the hydroxyl radical, which can abstract an electron from any biological molecule in its vicinity. The hydroxyl radical can damage protein, cause the breakage of DNA strands, and initiate lipid peroxidation. A single hydroxyl radical and molecular oxygen can react with a polyunsaturated fatty acid and alter its structure or functional integrity. This fatty acid free radical in turn can attack another fatty acid and, in the process, be transformed into a lipid hydroperoxide. This propagation reaction initiated by a single free radical results in damage to thousands of fatty acid molecules and the production of multiple fatty acid peroxyl radicals. These peroxyl radicals can react with other lipids, proteins, and nucleic acids and thereby propagate a chain reaction involving electron transfer. Fatty acid peroxide molecules break up and form dialdehydes (e.g., malonaldehyde), which can cause cross-linking between various types of molecules that lead to cytotoxicity, mutagenicity, membrane breakdown, and enzyme modification. Malonaldehyde also polymerizes with itself and other tissue breakdown products to form an insoluble pigment (lipofuscin), which accumulates in aging tissues. When two free radicals react with each other, a stable molecule is formed and this terminates the chain reaction.

25.4 PROTECTION FROM FREE RADICALS

Free radicals are produced in almost every cell of the human body at an astounding rate, but they do not normally cause damage to cells and tissues; generation of ROS is a carefully controlled process, and the reactions are compartmentalized. Our bodies have evolved various antioxidant defense mechanisms that combat their constant barrage. Antioxidants have the property to neutralize free radicals without becoming unstable free radicals themselves. The procedure leads to oxidation of antioxidants. This makes it necessary to replenish antioxidants on a constant basis.

There are two types of antioxidants in the body: (1) the antioxidant enzymes that prevent the accumulation of toxic substances, and (2) antioxidant small molecules that intercept any free radicals and singlet oxygen that are generated. These antioxidants exist in both the membranes and the aqueous compartments of cells.

25.4.1 ANTIOXIDANT ENZYMES

Antioxidant enzymes hunt for and neutralize the chain-initiating free radicals. The enzyme superoxide dismutase (SOD) is the first line of defense against oxygen toxicity.[8] It catalyzes the conversion of superoxide to less toxic hydrogen peroxide. Since superoxide is not membrane permeable, it can accumulate in the cellular fraction where it is produced. SODs exist in three forms to prevent this accumulation: a cytosolic copper/zinc SOD-1, a mitochondrial manganese-containing SOD-2, and an extracellular copper/zinc SOD-3.

There are two enzymes that catalyze the breakdown of hydrogen peroxide. Glutathione peroxidase (GP), a selenium-containing enzyme that is present in the cytosol and mitochondria, removes hydrogen peroxide by using it to convert reduced glutathione (GSH) to oxidized glutathione (GSSG).

$$2\,GSH + H_2O_2 \xrightarrow{\quad GP \quad} GSSG + 2H_2O$$

GP also catalyzes the reduction of lipid peroxides by glutathione and thus prevents the propagation of lipid peroxidation. The glutathione reductase (GR) regenerates GSH from GSSG in the presence of NADPH.

$$2\,GSH + Fatty\ acid - OOH \xrightarrow{\quad GR \quad} GSSG + Fatty\ acid - OH + H_2O$$

Catalase, a heme-containing enzyme located in the peroxisome organelles, also breaks down hydrogen peroxide to water.

$$2H_2O_2 \xrightarrow{\quad Catalase \quad} O_2 + 2H_2O$$

Manganese, copper, zinc, and selenium are commonly referred to as antioxidant nutrients, but these have no antioxidant action themselves and are instead required for the activity of antioxidant enzymes.

25.4.2 Antioxidant Small Molecules

The highly efficient antioxidant enzymes function to keep the free radicals in the cell at a minimum; however, enzymatic defenses against certain types of ROS (e.g., singlet oxygen and hydroxyl radical) are either ineffective or totally lacking. The body must rely on food-derived substances with antioxidant properties to effectively neutralize such species. These antioxidants scavenge various ROS directly; they include vitamins E and C, carotenes, and flavonoids from the diet and glutathione, uric acid, and taurine that are made endogenously.

Vitamin E refers to a group of related compounds (tocopherols). The molecule is highly lipophilic and resides almost exclusively in cell membranes and lipoproteins. It is thought to be one of the most important antioxidants found in lipid membranes in the body. It can react directly with a variety of radicals including peroxyl, hydroxyl, and superoxide radicals. It protects the polyunsaturated fatty acids in the membranes against peroxidation by scavenging peroxyl radicals. It is a chain-reaction-breaking antioxidant because it quenches the intermediate in the chain reaction. Tocopherols are widely distributed in nature, and the richest sources are vegetable oils.

Vitamin C (ascorbic acid) is a highly versatile antioxidant. It is capable of scavenging singlet oxygen and superoxide and hydroxyl radicals with the concurrent formation of dehydroascorbic acid. It can also regenerate vitamin E by reducing the tocopherol radical that is produced when vitamin E scavenges a peroxyl radical. Because it is highly water soluble, ascorbic acid functions in an aqueous environment, in contrast to vitamin E, which is lipid soluble. Fruits, especially citrus varieties and berries, tomatoes, lettuce, and green peppers are excellent sources.

Carotenes are a set of several hundred fat-soluble pigments present in yellow and green fruits and vegetables. In addition to being precursors of vitamin A, these pigments are also excellent antioxidants and radical trapping agents (especially for peroxyl and hydroxyl radicals). These pigments are also able to modulate endogenous levels of other antioxidants. Carotenes serve as another dietary source of lipid-soluble antioxidants.

Flavonoids are a large group of polyphenolic compounds that occur naturally in fruits and vegetables and in beverages such as tea and wine. The most important flavonoids are the anthocyanins, flavonols, and flavones. They are water-soluble scavengers of singlet oxygen and superoxide, peroxyl, and lipid peroxyl radicals.[24] There are several other phytochemicals (nonnutritive plant chemicals) that have antioxidant activity and protect cells against oxidative damage. Examples include allyl sulfides (onions, garlic), lycopene (tomatoes), and isoflavones (soy).

In addition to the dietary antioxidants, there are several endogenous substances that serve as important radical scavengers. Glutathione (GSH), a tripeptide, is synthesized intracellularly by all mammalian cells. The tissue concentration (at least in the liver) varies as a function of dietary sulfur-containing amino acids. Ascorbic acid can protect tissue GSH levels, and GSH in turn has sparing action on ascorbate. In addition to its role as a substrate for GP (which is involved in the destruction of hydrogen peroxide and lipid hydroperoxides), GSH can nonenzymatically scavenge singlet oxygen and superoxide and hydroxyl radicals.[19] It can act as a reductant, reducing species such as hydrogen peroxide directly to water.

Uric acid is a product of purine metabolism. It is present in blood, and its levels can be elevated by increased dietary purines; however, excessive levels of plasma uric acid can cause gout. Uric acid is a strong, circulating free radical scavenger and can directly interact with radicals such as the hydroxyl radical. It also protects vitamin C levels in blood. Humans have higher uric acid in blood than other mammals do, and this may account for the prolonged life span of humans. The amino acid taurine is an effective free radical scavenger and is normally concentrated in cells and tissues that possess considerable potential for producing oxidants. For example, there is a high concentration of taurine in the retina, a tissue in which various oxidants are generated photolytically and enzymatically, and in neutrophils, which enzymatically produce oxidants during the phagocytic process. There is no evidence that taurine levels can be increased by dietary means.

Bilirubin, the product of heme catabolism, is generally regarded as a potentially cytotoxic (causes jaundice) waste product that needs to be excreted. But recent studies show that it efficiently scavenges peroxyl radicals. It is considered to be the major protector of cell membranes.[23] Melatonin is produced in the pineal glands. Besides its function as a synchronizer of the biological clock, melatonin is now known to exert a powerful antioxidant activity. It is a direct scavenger of superoxide, hydroxyl, singlet oxygen, and nitric oxide. Coenzyme Q, a component of the electron transport chain, and lipoic acid, a coenzyme in energy metabolism, are also powerful antioxidants.[25]

25.5 BENEFITS OF FREE RADICALS

Free radicals cause many adverse reactions in vivo, which result in cell injury and dysfunction and subsequent degenerative disease states; yet free radical generation is critical for the normal operation of a wide spectrum of biological processes.[27] The catalytic action of many cellular enzymes involves the transfer of one electron; this yields free radical intermediates. Metabolism of arachidonic acid by cyclooxygenase to form prostaglandins is regulated by free radical reactions at certain sequential steps. One good example of favorable effect is that of activated phagocytes, which generate superoxide as part of their bactericidal role.

The process of phagocytosis involves engulfment of microorganisms, foreign particles, and cellular debris by cells such as neutrophils and macrophages (monocytes). The resting neutrophils mostly use glycolysis for their energy production and use very little oxygen, but during phagocytosis there is rapid consumption of oxygen by these cells and more glucose is metabolized via hexose monophosphate shunt (HMS). The severalfold increase in oxygen consumption is referred to as respiratory burst (Figure 25.2). The enzyme NADPH oxidase, located in the leukocyte cell membrane, catalyzes the reduction of molecular oxygen to superoxide, and the NADPH required in this reaction is provided by increased HMS activity.

The oxidase is normally dormant, but after phagocytosis occurs it becomes very active; this results in the production of superoxide and accounts for more than 90% of oxygen consumption by stimulated cells.

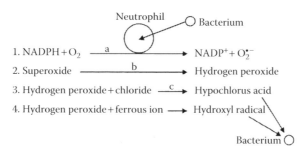

FIGURE 25.2 Bactericidal effect of neutrophil phagocytosis. (a) NADPH oxidase, present on leukocyte cell membranes, is activated by phagocytosis; it catalyzes the conversion of oxygen to superoxide. (The oxygen consumption increases several fold, which is known as the respiratory burst.) The NADPH required for this reaction is supplied by a simultaneous increase in the metabolism of glucose via the hexose monophosphate shunt and an increase in the level of glucose-6-phosphate dehydrogenase. (b) Superoxide dismutase catalyzes the conversion of superoxide to hydrogen peroxide. (c) Myeloperoxidase, in the presence of chloride ions, catalyzes the conversion of hydrogen peroxide to hypochlorous acid, which kills bacteria. Hydrogen peroxide, in the presence of ferrous ions, can form hydroxyl radicals, which has bactericidal actions.

The superoxide is converted to hydrogen peroxide by SOD. In the presence of chloride ions and myeloperoxidase, a lysosomal enzyme present within the phagolysosome, hydrogen peroxide plus chloride ions are converted to hypochlorous acid (HOCl). Hypochlorous acid (common in household bleach) is highly toxic to bacterial cells.

The importance of superoxide formation is appreciated by the fact that genetic deficiencies of NADPH oxidase in neutrophils cause chronic granulomatosis, a disease characterized by severe, persistent, chronic pyrogenic infections. Neutrophils from such individuals have a seriously impaired ability to kill microorganisms that have been ingested and often lead to septicemia and death at an early age.[2,13] Chronic granulomatous disease occurs in about 1 in 200,000 live births.

Another beneficial role of free radicals has been suggested by a recent study.[14] Superoxide is found to be important in the formation of calcium carbonate particles called otoliths that form above inner-ear sensory hair cells during embryonic development. The otolith-cell arrangements function as motion sensors that help animals sense the direction of gravity. A mutant mouse is known as "head-start" because of the awkward way it holds its head and body. Head-start mice hobble, fall over, and sometimes move about on their backs, as though they do not know which way is up. These animals have defective NADPH oxidase that reduces the ability to generate superoxide radicals during embryonic development when otoliths form. In normal animals, free radicals may help the vesicles in which otoliths form become permeable to calcium and other components involved in otolith formation.

Nitric oxide is a radical that acts as an important oxidative biological signal in a large variety of diverse physiological processes.[5] It activates the enzyme guanylate cyclase and produces the second messenger cyclic guanosine monophosphate (cGMP), which in turn mediates vascular smooth muscle relaxation.

A similar mode of action has been proposed for cell-to-cell signaling in the brain. Although there is no uniform agreement on the function of NO in the brain, evidence supports a role in long-term potentiation and memory formation. In addition, most nonadrenergic, noncholinergic (NANC) neurons are NO-activated via the same cGMP-dependent mechanism. NANC nerves subserving important roles in gastrointestinal motility and penile erection are among those functioning through NO signals.

The immune system seems to have harnessed the toxic properties of NO to kill invading organisms, pathogens, and tumor cells.

25.6   FREE RADICALS AND DISEASES

Under physiological conditions, the generation of free radicals is part of normal regulatory circuits and the cellular redox state is tightly controlled by antioxidants; however, increased production of these radicals can overwhelm the antioxidant defenses and may contribute to the development of many diseases. Circumstances that enhance oxidant exposure such as radiation, metabolism of environmental pollutants and some drugs that can compromise antioxidant capability are referred to as oxidative stress. The term *nitrosative* stress has been suggested to describe cellular consequences of excess NO. Actual determination of free radicals in vivo is difficult because they are highly reactive, short-lived, and normally present in low concentrations. Free radical reactions have been inferred by identifying the products of lipid peroxidation, particularly malonaldehyde, which reacts with thiobarbituric acid to give a colored compound; however, this test is not specific because malonaldehyde can be further metabolized by tissues.

Free radicals react with almost any compound of the cell, and if their target is DNA, the likelihood of cancer increases; if their target is low-density lipoprotein (LDL) in blood, arteriosclerosis may result. There are suggestions in the literature that oxygen free radical generation leads to a wide variety of conditions such as aging, cancer, arteriosclerosis, neurological disorders, cataracts, chronic inflammatory diseases, such as rheumatoid arthritis, and so on.[10] Additionally, many viral infections have been shown to generate ROS, which has been proposed to be involved in viral pathogenesis.[18]

25.6.1 AGING

Free radicals produced during normal metabolism of the cell over time can cause random damage to structural proteins, informational molecules, and DNA. The free radical theory of aging holds that advancing age is associated with an accumulation of low-level, free radical damage, which leads to physiological and clinical consequences associated with aging. The pigment lipofuscin associated with lipid peroxidation is known to accumulate with aging in all mammalian species, and the protective enzyme SOD declines with age. Also, age-related decreases in glutathione have been observed in the liver, kidney, heart, and blood in experimental animals and may be responsible for some aspects of the aging process.

A low-Cal diet is known to extend lifespan in some animals and may involve reduction in oxidative stress. There is some evidence to support the role of oxidative stress on aging in model organisms such as *Caenorhabditis Elegans*. But the evidence in mammals is less clear.[17] Diets high in fruits and vegetables that are rich in antioxidants promote health and reduce the effect of aging. But the beneficial effects of antioxidant supplementation for healthy individuals remain controversial and need to be evaluated.

25.6.2 CANCER

Free radicals are capable of oxidatively modifying DNA and may be the central cause of some cancers; however, a direct connection between oxidatively modified DNA and cancer is not available because of the limited understanding of the carcinogenic mechanism and because no single factor can explain the entire process. There is, however, extensive indirect evidence that supports a role of free radicals in carcinogenesis. The carcinogenic activity of polycyclic hydrocarbons has been correlated with their ability to form free radicals. The intake of metals such as iron, which facilitates the production of free radicals, is correlated with cancer development in humans and animals. Hepatocellular carcinoma may be related to severe iron overload in patients with homozygous hereditary hemochromatosis. Also, epidemiological studies point to the possibility of an association between moderately increased body iron and an increased risk of cancer in the general population. Epidemiological studies generally show an inverse relationship between cancer incidence and intake of foods high in antioxidants such as β-carotene and vitamins C and E. Low intakes of vegetables and fruits are consistently associated with increased risk of lung cancer. Dietary β-carotene is associated with decreased risk of several types of cancer.

Laboratory evidence from chemical, cell culture, and animal studies indicate that antioxidants may slow or possibly protect against cancer. The apparent benefit of antioxidants has prompted many people, including cancer patients, to turn to supplements with the hope that large amounts of these compounds will have even more protective effect. However, information from recent clinical trials is less clear. Some studies have found no effect on overall cancer risk in people who used antioxidants. And other studies have shown that antioxidants may actually increase lung cancer risk in smokers. It is not clear whether some antioxidants are more effective against disease than others. Different foods contain different types and amounts of antioxidants as well as other substances that could influence risk. At this time, there is not enough evidence to either recommend for or against taking supplements for cancer prevention.

25.6.3 CATARACTS

A cataract is a condition in which opaque regions develop within the normally transparent lens of the eye resulting in significant loss of visual acuity. Although the exact cause of this disease is unknown, intraocular generation of oxygen free radicals may constitute one of the significant risk factors in cataractogenesis. The lens is a highly susceptible target because it is continually exposed to the effect of light and a number of oxidizing metabolic products. Hydrogen peroxide is present in the aqueous humor and can give rise to hydroxyl radicals. Eye tissues, including the lens, have a high content of glutathione and vitamin C (30- to 35-fold over plasma level), presumably to prevent injury by free radicals. Epidemiological and experimental studies suggest that the risk of senile cataracts decreases with increased intake of vitamin C as well as other antioxidants such as β-carotene and vitamin E.

25.6.4 CARDIOVASCULAR DISEASE

Elevated levels of plasma LDL increase the risk for atherosclerosis; however, the precise mechanism(s) by which LDL promotes the development of this disease is still not clearly understood. It is currently believed that lipid peroxidation is involved in the oxidative modification of LDL, and this ultimately results in the initiation and progression of the atherosclerotic process. This hypothesis is supported by data from animal and human studies and from epidemiological investigations. The postulated mechanism for the development and progression of this disease is the production of oxidized LDL because of impaired antioxidant status. The oxidized LDL is taken up by monocytes that infiltrate the artery wall and differentiate into macrophages, which vigorously scavenge oxidized LDL to produce foam cells. The foam cells cause the initial fatty streak in the arterial wall, which builds up to form the plaque characteristic of vascular disease. The circulating antioxidants and antioxidants within LDL are believed to help prevent the LDL from being oxidized by fatty acid hydroperoxides.

The presence of oxidized lipids in atherosclerotic lesions is frequently observed, and a recent study has detected higher serum levels of lipid peroxides in patients with cardiovascular disease.[12] High iron stores are associated with excess risk of myocardial infarction apparently because of the possible role of iron in increasing the generation of free radicals. Indian immigrants in the United Kingdom consuming high amounts of clarified butter have higher-than-expected mortality from cardiovascular disease despite the absence of obvious risk factors.[11] Clarified butter contains large amounts of cholesterol oxides, whereas natural butter contains only trace amounts. The cholesterol oxides are assumed to be incorporated into LDL and may be responsible for high mortality rates among Indian immigrants. Epidemiological studies have shown a strong inverse correlation between plasma antioxidant status and risk of cardiovascular disease. The number of deaths attributed to coronary disease are reduced by 40% in subjects consuming 100 IU of vitamin E daily as compared to individuals whose dietary intake of this vitamin is much lower. Dietary carotenes and vitamin C are also inversely related to heart disease.

The support for antioxidants in slowing the progression of atherosclerosis also comes from other interesting observations. Mortality from coronary heart disease is lower in certain regions of France than in the United States and the United Kingdom despite the fact that individuals in all three countries have similar ranges of serum cholesterol levels. This "French paradox" cannot be explained by differences in other risk factors for heart disease. In France, there is regular consumption of moderate amounts of wine and other alcoholic beverages. Alcohol causes an increase in high-density lipoprotein cholesterol, which is considered to be antiatherogenic. Red wine is rich in flavonoids (which are more potent as antioxidants than vitamin E), and it is suggested that these compounds contribute substantially to the reduction of mortality from coronary heart disease in France.[7,20]

25.6.5 BRAIN

Polyunsaturated fatty acids, substrates for lipid peroxides, are major constituents in brain tissue, and in addition, some brain cells contain higher concentrations of iron, which facilitates free radical formation. Thus, the brain and the central nervous system seem to be particularly susceptible to free-radical-mediated damage. There is substantial evidence that oxidative stress is a causative factor in the pathogenesis of major neurodegenerative diseases.[6,15] A number of in vitro studies have shown that antioxidants can protect nervous tissue from damage by oxidative stress. Amyotrophic lateral sclerosis is a late-onset, progressive, degenerative disorder of motor neurons. It is characterized by varying degrees of weakness, atrophy, fasciculation, and spasticity. It is also called Lou Gehrig disease after the baseball hero who was afflicted by it. The disease is linked (in about 20% of cases) to defects in the SOD gene that encodes the cytosolic SOD.[21] Individuals with this disease apparently are unable to get rid of superoxide efficiently.

Reactive free radicals have been proposed to cause neuronal injury in several other neurological disorders. Necropsy studies have provided evidence of increased lipid peroxidation and reduced level of glutathione in substantia nigra in Parkinson's disease. In Alzheimer's disease, iron and ferritin content increase in cortical regions. Oxidative tissue degeneration also seems to be a key feature in Down syndrome and some other neurological disorders.

25.6.6 REPERFUSION INJURY

Reperfusion injury can be defined as the damage that occurs to a tissue during the resumption of blood flow following the episode of ischemia. This is distinct from an injury caused by the "ischemia" per se. Although other factors may be involved, most researchers agree that the deleterious effects actually occur during reperfusion and that free radicals play a major role in the pathogenesis of reperfusion injury. During the first 30–60 seconds of postischemic reperfusion there is generation of superoxide, which can combine with iron released by hypoxic cells to form hydroxyl radicals, the initiator of lipid peroxidation. Tissue function is better preserved if antioxidants such as vitamin E are incorporated in the reoxygenation medium at the end of ischemia.

25.6.7 NITRIC OXIDE AND DISEASE

Workers with heart disease in Alfred Nobel's dynamite factory in the 1860s found that their chest pains were relieved when they came to work. The reason, contemporary physicians quickly discovered, was that they were breathing in nitroglycerin, an ingredient in dynamite.

For a century or more, how nitroglycerin relieved the pain of angina was largely a mystery. About 25 years ago, the basic explanation began to take shape. The compound provides an external source for nitric oxide (NO), a signaling molecule that dilates blood vessels, providing relief from the effect of clogged arteries, a respite that lasts only a few minutes.

The enzyme, mitochondrial aldehyde dehydrogenase, converts nitroglycerin to 1,2-glyceryl dinitrate and nitrite (NO_2) predominately in mitochondria. Enzymes found within these specialized organelles can reduce nitrite to NO.

An excess of NO has been implicated in the pathophysiology of many inflammatory diseases including arthritis, myocarditis, colitis, nephritis, and a large number of pathological conditions such as amyotrophic lateral sclerosis, cancer, diabetes, and neurodegenerative diseases. The level of NO in endotoxin shock rises considerably. The clinically observed extreme hypotension in shock has been linked to elevated levels of NO and has been reversed by NOS inhibition in both animal models of shock and in humans. Postischemic damage to CNS neurons may also be due to elevated NO, perhaps resulting from the activation of neuronal NOS. Inhibitors selective for the neuronal NOS may find a role in the treatment of stroke.

Peroxynitrite is a potent oxidant with the potential to disrupt protein structures through the nitration of protein tyrosine residues. Nitration may in turn affect protein function. Nitrated mitochondrial SOD has been identified in rejected kidney transplant tissue. The degree of nitration in the tissue has been shown to parallel enzyme inactivity. Nitration has been shown in chronic inflammatory diseases, adult respiratory distress syndrome (ARDS), and atherosclerotic lesions.

A new study offers the first evidence that explains the link between cellular stress caused by free radicals and the protein misfolding that is associated with several neurodegenerative diseases.[26] Patients with these diseases, which include Parkinson's and Alzheimer's diseases, produce excess amounts of nitric oxide free radicals. Stuart A. Lipton of the Burnham Institute for Medical Research in LaJolla, California, and colleagues have reported that the NO group s-nitrosylates critical cysteine residues in protein-disulfide isomerase (PDI). The reaction alters PDI's structure and interferes with its role in fixing misfolded proteins in nerve cells. The misfolded proteins then accumulate and damage or kill off the affected neurons. The researchers suggest that the elevated levels of s-nitrosylated PDI in patients with Alzheimer's and Parkinson's diseases could serve as a biomarker for development of these diseases. Reducing levels of this damaged protein could have therapeutic benefit.

Interestingly, a relative deficit of NO also seems evident in a number of clinical conditions. A reduction in the bioavailability of NO is a very early and pervasive characteristic of the dysfunctional endothelium. The reduction in NO activity has been demonstrated in an experimental model of atherosclerosis, as well as in human subjects with coronary atherosclerosis. Loss of NO activity results in increased platelet adhesion and aggregation, increased monocyte adhesion and migration into the subendothelial space, formation of lipid-laden foam cells, and propagation of atherogenesis. Although the explicit lack of NOS or NO is not easy to demonstrate, clear clinical improvement occurs upon treatment with NO or NO-releasing drugs. While strategies to increase NOS activity in vivo are possible, the use of NO-releasing drugs represents a more expedient approach toward resolving clinical problems related to low NO levels. By far the most common example is oral nitroglycerin, which acts to augment NO in the coronary arteries and increases blood flow to ischemic myocardium. A more recent development is the addition of NO at very low levels (0.2–20 ppm) to the inspired air of acutely ill patients with ARDS, pulmonary hypertension, and neonatal respiratory prematurity. Because NO is a gas, it enters only those parts of the lung that are ventilated, dilating selectively the vessels of those areas and improving ventilation/perfusion ratios.

25.7   LARGE DOSES OF ANTIOXIDANTS

The human body is under constant assault by oxygen free radicals produced as a consequence of normal biochemical activity. Because the damage caused by free radicals can be life threatening, the body has many overlapping defense mechanisms to protect against oxidants.[22] These include antioxidant enzymes and scavengers of free radicals. A delicate balance is maintained between oxidants and antioxidants in healthy individuals. In some pathological conditions, the balance may be tilted toward the oxidant state. There is, therefore, a dietary need for antioxidants to neutralize excessive oxidants that may be formed endogenously, but the optimum amounts needed are yet to be determined.

There is considerable amount of epidemiological evidence revealing an association between those consuming diets rich in fresh fruits and vegetables and their lower risk of coronary heart disease and certain forms of cancer. It is generally assumed that the active dietary constituents contributing to these protective effects are the antioxidants. The fact that we need antioxidants for better health does not necessarily mean that their long-term (lifetime) intake in large doses is safe. The ingestion of excessive amounts of antioxidants is presumed to shift the oxidant–antioxidant balance toward the antioxidant side and prevent potential damage by free radicals; however, this may affect the key physiological processes that are dependent on free radicals. Data published recently on clinical trials indicate that antioxidant supplements do not reduce the incidence of tumors. In fact, the rates of lung cancer and number of deaths from heart disease increase with antioxidant supplements compared with rates and number of deaths in the groups receiving placebo.[3] Treatment for 4 years with either β-carotene or vitamin C does not seem to affect the rate of occurrence of adenomas in patients who had adenomas removed before entering the study. The lack of benefits with antioxidant supplements and the possible deleterious effects reported in these studies seem to conflict with reduced risk suggested by epidemiological investigations and short-term studies. A more recent review of several studies found no significant effect on mortality—good or bad—linked to taking antioxidants. Researchers found a higher risk of death for people taking vitamins: 4% for those taking vitamin E, 7% for β-carotene, and 16% for vitamin A.[1] These findings were based on an analysis of 47 studies involving 180,938 people who were randomly assigned to get real vitamins or dummy pills.

An estimated 80–160 million people take antioxidants in North America and Europe, about 10%–20% of adults. In 2006, Americans spent $2.3 billion on nutritional supplements and vitamins at grocery stores, drugstores, and retail outlets, according to Information Resources Inc., which tracks sales. Although there is little doubt that antioxidants are a necessary component for good health, it is not clear if supplements should be taken, and if so how much. Once thought harmless we now know that consuming megadoses of antioxidants can be harmful perhaps due to their toxicity and interactions with medicines. Therefore, the best approach for healthy individuals[4] is to avoid huge doses of a single antioxidant but rather to regularly consume antioxidant-rich foods, fruits, and vegetables.

REFERENCES

1. The Alpha Tocopheral, Beta Carotene Cancer Prevention Study Group. 1994. The effect of vitamin E and β-carotene on the incidence of lung cancer and other cancers in male smokers. *N Engl J Med* 330:1029.
2. Babior, B. M. 1991. The respiratory burst oxidase and the molecular basis of chronic granulomatous disease. *Am J Hematol* 37:263.
3. Bjelakovic, G., D. Nikolova, L. L. Gluud et al. 2007. Mortality in randomized trials of antioxidant supplements for primary and secondary prevention: Systematic review and meta-analysis. *J Amer Med Assoc* 297:842.
4. Block, G. 1992. Fruits, vegetables and cancer prevention: A review of the epidemiologic evidence. *Nutr Cancer* 18:1.
5. Davis, K. L., E. Martin, J. V. Turko, and F. Murad. 2001. Novel effects of nitric oxide. *Annu Rev Pharmacol Toxicol* 41:203.
6. Evans, P. H. 1993. Free radicals in brain metabolism and pathology. *Br Med Bull* 49:577.
7. Frankel, E. N., J. Kanner, J. B. German, and J. E. Kinsella. 1993. Inhibition of oxidation of human low density lipoprotein by phenolic substances in red wine. *Lancet* 341:454.
8. Fridovich, I. 1986. Superoxide dismutases. *Adv Enzymol* 58:61.
9. Greenberg, E. R., J. A. Baron, T. D. Tosteson et al. 1994. A clinical trial of antioxidant vitamins to prevent colorectal adenoma. *N Engl J Med* 331:141.
10. Halliwell, B. 1997. Antioxidants and human disease: A general introduction. *Nutr Rev* 55:S 44.
11. Jacobson, M. S. 1987. Cholesterol oxides in Indian ghee: Possible cause of unexplained high risk of atherosclerosis in Indian immigrant populations. *Lancet* 2:656.
12. Jialal, I., and S. Devaraj. 1996. Low-density lipoprotein oxidation, antioxidants, and atherosclerosis: A clinical biochemistry perspective. *Clin Chem* 42:498.
13. Jones, L. B., P. McGrogan, T. J. Flood et al. 2008. Special article: Chronic granulomatous disease in the United Kingdom and Ireland: A comprehensive national patient-based registry. *Clin Exp Immunol* 152:211.
14. Kiss, P. J., J. Knisz, Y. Zhang et al. 2006. Inactivation of NADPH oxidase organizer I results in severe imbalance. *Curr Biol* 16:208.
15. Knight, J. A. 1997. Reactive oxygen species and the neurodegenerative disorders. *Ann Clin Lab Sci* 27:11.
16. Palmer, H. J., and K. E. Paulson. 1997. Reactive oxygen species and antioxidants in signal transduction and gene expression. *Nutr Rev* 55:353.
17. Perez, V. I., A. Bokov, H. Van Remmen et al. 2009. Is the oxidative stress theory of aging dead? *Biochem Biophys Acta* 1790:1005.
18. Peterhans, E. 1997. Oxidants and antioxidants in viral diseases: Disease mechanisms and metabolic regulation. *J Nutr* 127:962S.
19. Reed, D. J. 1991. Glutathione: Toxicological implications. *Annu Rev Pharmacol* 30:603.
20. Renaud, S., and M. DeLorgeril. 1992. Wine, alcohol, platelets, and the French paradox for coronary heart disease. *Lancet* 339:1523.
21. Rosen, D. L., T. Siddique, D. Patterson, D. A. Figlewicz, P. Sapp et al. 1993. Mutations in Cu/Zn superoxide dismutase gene are associated with familial amyotrophic lateral sclerosis. *Nature* 362:59.
22. Sardesai, V. M. 1995. Role of antioxidants in health maintenance. *Nutr Clin Pract* 10:19.

23. Sedlak, T. W., and S. H. Snyder. 2004. Bilirubin benefits: Cellular protection by a biliverdin reductase antioxidant cycle. *Pediatrics* 113:1776.
24. Spencer, J. P., D. Vauzour, and C. Reindeira. 2009. Flavonoids and cognition: The molecular mechanisms underlying their behavioural effects. *Arch Biochem Biophys* 492:1.
25. Turunen, M., J. Olsson, and G. Dalloner. 2004. Metabolism and function of coenzyme Q. *Biochem Biophys Acta* 1660:171.
26. Uehara, T., T. Nakamura, D. Yao et al. 2006. S-Nitrosylated protein-disulphide isomerase links protein misfolding to neurodegeneration. *Nature* 441:513.
27. Valko, M., D. Leibfritz, J. Monkol et al. 2007. Free radicals and antioxidants in normal physiological functions and human disease. *Int J Biochem Cell Biol* 39:44.
28. Wieinacker, A. B., and L. T. Vaszar. 2001. Acute respiratory distress syndrome: Physiology and new management strategies. *Annu Rev Med* 52:221.
29. Westhuyzen, J. 1997. The oxidation hypothesis of atherosclerosis: An update. *Ann Clin Lab Sci* 27:10.
30. Witztum, J. L., and D. Steinberg. 1991. Role of oxidized low density lipoprotein in atherogenesis. *J Clin Invest* 88:1785.
31. Wu, G., and C. J. Meininger. 2002. Regulation of nitric oxide synthesis by dietary factors. *Annu Rev Nutr* 22:61.

26 Toxicants Occurring Naturally in Foods and Additives

Foods contain not only the nutrients we need (e.g., carbohydrates, proteins, fats, vitamins, inorganic elements) but also a large number of chemicals, some of which are toxic. Plants synthesize toxic chemicals apparently as a primary defense against bacterial, fungal, insect, and other animal predators. These are the normal components that constitute the genetically determined chemical profile of the plant that serves as food. Some toxic chemicals may enter the food supply by fortuitous natural mechanisms. These may be of microbial origin and may be environmental pollutants, including heavy metals. Chemicals sprayed into plants in the form of pesticides may be present in foods of plant origin and may be transmitted through feed grains to animals. There are also substances added to foods for functional purposes such as preservatives, antioxidants, and calorie reduction agents.

26.1 TOXICANTS IN FOOD

26.1.1 NATURALLY OCCURRING TOXICANTS

Foods of plant origin have a large number of microconstituents. For example, there are more than 392 chemicals identified in coffee, 314 in cocoa, 188 in tea, and 150 in potato. It is anticipated that more chemicals will be identified as the sensitivity of the analytical methods continues to improve.[19,25] A few of the toxicants found in some common foods are discussed in this section.

Table 26.1 lists toxicants present in some common foods. Potatoes contain solanine, which is an alkaloid with anticholinesterase activity. It interferes with the transmission of nerve impulses. It is estimated that 120 pounds of potatoes, an amount consumed by an average American per year, have about 10 g of solanine, which, if administered in a single dose, can be fatal. Lima beans, tapioca, cassava, and almonds contain cyanide (as cyanogenic glycosides). Cyanide inhibits cytochrome oxidase and causes fatal human poisoning after an ingestion of 0.5–3.5 mg/kg body weight, or approximately 50–350 mg of cyanide for an adult. Lima bean seeds of different varieties can produce 10–80 mg cyanide/100 g seeds. Oxalate is present in spinach and rhubarb to the extent of 10% of dry weight. It combines with dietary calcium and interferes with its absorption. Cabbage, cauliflower, Brussels sprouts, broccoli, kale, and turnips contain goitrogens. These substances interfere with iodine utilization and thus have antithyroid properties. Carrots, nutmeg, parsley, and pepper contain myristicene, a narcotic and psychomimetic. Phytates are present in many high-fiber foods such as cereals, legumes, and vegetables. They have the ability to bind calcium, zinc, and iron and cause the deficiencies of these nutrients.

Orange peel, which is used in the preparation of orange marmalade, is a rich source of citral, which is an antagonist of vitamin A. Linseed meal contains linetin, which interferes with pyridoxine utilization. Thiaminase, a vitamin B_1-destroying factor, is found in black berries, red cabbage, and some raw fish. Sweet clover and other related plants contain dicumarol, a vitamin K antagonist, and raw egg whites have avidin, which binds biotin. Protease inhibitors are found throughout the plant kingdom, mainly in legumes. Trypsin inhibitor is present in soybeans. Most of the harmful biological effects observed in raw soybeans disappear when the beans are cooked.

Lathyrus sativus is used as a cattle feed in some countries and also is used in making bread when wheat is in short supply. Eaten in small quantity, the seeds are a useful and valuable food. But if *L. sativus* is the main source of food, it can cause lathyrism—a neurological disease. This condition

TABLE 26.1
Natural Toxicants in Some Common Foods

Food	Toxicant	Biological Action
Potato	Solanine	Interferes with transmission of nerve impulses
Lima beans, cassava, almonds	Cyanide	Inhibit cytochrome oxidase
Spinach, rhubarb	Oxalate	Interfere with calcium absorption
Cabbage, cauliflower	Goitrogens	Interfere with iodine utilization
Cereal, legumes, vegetables	Phytate	Bind calcium, iron, and zinc and prevent their absorption
Orange peel	Citral	Vitamin A antagonist
Linseed meal	Linetin	Vitamin B_6 antagonist
Sweet clover	Dicumarol	Vitamin K antagonist
Egg white	Avidin	Biotin antagonist

usually develops in individuals between the ages of 15 and 30 years and more often in men. The first symptom is a feeling of heaviness of the legs with weakness setting in thereafter. The disease is caused by the toxic agent, β-aminopropionitrile, and related compounds present in the seeds of *L. sativus*. Cycads are palm-like trees growing mainly in the tropics. The seeds of these plants are used as a supplement in some parts of the world when food supplies become low. The seeds contain a toxin, methyl azoxymethanol, which is carcinogenic. Several herbs are commercially available for smoking and for preparing tea. They contain psychoactive agents, and thus the excessive use of these herbs can cause intoxication.

26.1.2   Food Contaminants

26.1.2.1   Heavy Metals

Some heavy metals such as lead, mercury, and cadmium are toxic when ingested in significant quantities. Small amounts of these metals regularly get into food.

26.1.2.1.1   Lead

Lead exposure occurs when lead dust or fumes are inhaled, or when lead is ingested via contaminated hands, food, water, cigarettes, or clothing. Before being banned in the mid-1990s, leaded gasoline was a major source of U.S. environmental exposure. Lead enters drinking water primarily as a result of corrosion of materials containing lead in the water distribution system and household plumbing. These materials include lead-based solder used to join copper pipe and brass faucets. In 1986, Congress banned the use of lead solder containing greater than 0.2% lead and restricted the lead content of faucets, pipes, and other plumbing materials to 8%. Older homes may still have plumbing that has the potential to contribute lead to drinking water. Lead may enter from the solder often to seam cans. Acidic foods such as fruits, fruit juices, and pickled products, which can leach out the solder, are more prone to contamination. After opening the can, if the contents are left in it, the lead concentration begins to increase. For example, an ounce of orange juice in a freshly opened can may contain about 80 mg of lead, and in 2 weeks, the lead concentration may be as high as 400 mg. Therefore, it is advisable to transfer the contents from the can into a glass container. More than 90% of the total body burden of lead is stored in the bones. Lead may be released in the blood, re-exposing organ systems long after the original exposure.

Symptoms of lead poisoning usually develop over weeks or months as lead builds up in the body during a chronic exposure, but acute symptoms from intake exposure can occur. Lead affects all organs and functions in the body to varying degrees. It interferes with several enzymes including two involved in heme synthesis. The common finding in severe poisoning includes hypochromic, microcytic anemia.

Typically, lead exposure is measured through blood samples. Because blood lead has a half-life of about 30 days, it reveals recent exposure. Bone lead has a half-life ranging from years to decades. The limit considered safe for lead, which can directly reduce IQ, has been lowered. The current reference range for acceptable blood lead concentration in healthy persons without excessive exposure to environmental sources of lead is less than 10 µg/dL for children and less than 25 µg/dL for adults. Blood concentrations in poisoning victims have ranged from 30 to >80 µg/dL in children exposed to lead paint in older homes and 90 to 137 µg/ dL in adults consuming contaminated herbal medicines. Approximately 250,000 U.S. children aged 1–5 years have blood levels greater than 10 µg/dL. Recent studies have shown that exposure to lead over a lifetime may increase the risk of dying prematurely. Older women with blood lead concentrations of 8 µg/dL or above had about 60% increased risk of dying prematurely.[13] Men who had the highest concentration of lead in their bones had a six times greater risk of dying from cardiovascular disease and 2.5 times greater risk of dying from all causes than men with the lowest lead levels.[31]

The first study to follow lead exposed children from before birth to adulthood has shown that even relatively low levels of lead permanently damage the brain and are linked to a higher number of arrests, particularly for violent crime.[32] Women should substantially increase their daily intake of calcium during pregnancy and even more during breast-feeding to offset dissolution of lead-affected bone into the bloodstream to provide calcium and other sustenance to developing children.

26.1.2.1.2 Mercury

Natural sources of atmospheric mercury include volcanoes, geologic deposits, and volatilization from the ocean. Alkali and metal processing, incineration of coal, medical and other waste, and mining of gold and mercury also contribute to mercury concentration in some areas.

The common way people in the United States are exposed to mercury is by eating fish containing methyl mercury. A recent study has provided new evidence linking high fish consumption to potentially unsafe levels of mercury. Scientists tested hair samples from 1449 people nationwide who volunteered to participate in the study. About 1 in 5 had mercury levels exceeding Environmental Protection Agency (EPA) safety guidelines. Almost half of the volunteers who had consumed large amounts of fish exceeded the EPA guidelines.

Most people have blood mercury levels below 5.8 µg/L, a value associated with possible adverse health effects. Mercury interferes with the brain and nervous system. Exposure of childbearing-aged women is of concern because of potential adverse neurological effects of mercury in fetuses. Consumption of fish with high mercury can lead to elevated mercury levels in the blood of unborn babies and young children and may harm their developing nervous system. The adverse effects have been documented by children's abilities to use language, to process information, and in visual/motor integration. According to National Health and Nutrition Examination Survey (NHNES) results for 1999–2002, approximately 6% of childbearing-aged women had blood levels of mercury at or above a reference value (5.8 µg/L), an estimated level assumed to be without appreciable harm. Based on this prevalence for the overall U.S. population of women of childbearing age and the number of births each year, it is estimated that about 300,000 newborns each year may have increased risk of learning disabilities associated with mercury exposure during pregnancy. The short-term strategy to reduce mercury exposure is to eat fish with low mercury levels and avoid or reduce consumption of fish with high mercury levels. The FDA advises that women who are or might become pregnant not eat shark, swordfish, king mackerel, and tile fish. State-based fish advisories and bans identify fish species contaminated by mercury and their locations and provide safety advice.

26.1.2.1.3 Arsenic

Arsenic enters drinking water supplies from natural deposits in the earth or from agricultural and industrial practices. Small amounts are present in plants and foods such as fish. At very low levels, there is relatively little concern. At high levels, arsenic attacks proteins that have a sulfur–sulfur bond, such as keratin found in hair and skin. The result is skin lesions and hair loss. Arsenic also interferes with some enzymes including those involved in energy production. Thus, persons suffering from chronic arsenic poisoning will slowly weaken. Other symptoms include cough and numbness in arms and legs. More serious is the connection between arsenic and cancer. The EPA has set the arsenic standard for drinking water at 10 parts per billion (ppb).

About 125 million people, mainly in developing countries, are being poisoned by arsenic in their drinking water. As many as half of the 4 million tube wells in Bangladesh are pumping groundwater contaminated with naturally occurring arsenic. In many contaminated wells, arsenic levels exceed 500 ppb, a level 50 times higher than the safety recommendation (10 ppb) from the World Health Organization (WHO). Large-scale contamination has also been found in some parts of West Bengal in India, China, Cambodia, Vietnam, Africa, and South America. Rice is usually grown in paddy fields flooded with water. Arsenic present in water accumulates in rice grain. Therefore, eating large amounts of rice grown in affected areas could be a health risk. This is a problem in countries such as Bangladesh where rice is a staple food. It is less of a problem in North America and Europe where water is provided by utilities.

Roxarsone is the most common arsenic-based additive used in chicken feed.[12] It is mixed in the diet of about 70% of the 9 billion broiler chickens produced annually in the United States. The purpose of this additive is to promote growth, kill parasites that cause diarrhea, and improve pigmentation of chicken meat. In its original organic form, arsenic in roxarsone is relatively benign. Some 2.2 million pounds of this arsenic compound is used in the nation's chicken feed each year. Part of the compound is converted by the bird to inorganic arsenic, and the rest is transformed into inorganic form after the bird excretes it. Chicken manure is spread in agricultural fields. Higher levels of arsenic are found in tap water in areas where chicken litter is spread in fields and lower levels in areas where chicken manure is not spread. It is estimated that people ingest 1.3–5.2 µg per day of inorganic arsenic from chicken alone. Those who eat much more chicken than average may ingest 21–31 µg of arsenic per day, which for some is greater than the tolerable daily intake recommended by the WHO. Tyson and Foster Farms have stopped using roxarsone in their chicken feeds, and McDonalds has asked its suppliers not to use arsenic additives. Many high-end and organic growers raise chickens quite successfully without this harmful compound additive. Banning the additive in feed would eliminate a substantial portion of arsenic from the human food chain and some of the arsenic in drinking water.

26.1.2.1.4 Cadmium
Cadmium is found in a number of industrial chemicals. Buildup of cadmium levels in water, air, and soil has been occurring especially in industrial areas. Fertilizers commonly contain cadmium, and grain and vegetable crops absorb the metal through polluted irrigation waters. The large source of most human exposure is dietary with an average daily intake of 10–30 µg/day. Smokers absorb an additional 1–3 µg/day.

Excess cadmium exposure adversely affects kidney, lungs, and bone. The WHO has established a provisional tolerable weekly intake for cadmium at 7 µg/kg body weight. This corresponds to a daily tolerable level of 70 µg for the average 70-kg man and 60 µg for the average 60-kg woman.

26.1.2.2 Nanoparticles
Nanotechnology is a new field of science in which particles with dimensions of 100 nanometers or less are manufactured by controlling matter on the molecular scale. Made from carbon, silver, zinc, gold, and other elements, these nanoparticles are used in electronics, medical equipment, and consumer products. Now, nanoparticles are increasingly being used by the food and agricultural industries and are finding their way into processed foods, food packaging materials, fertilizers, and storage containers. More than 150 foods and more than 400 food packaging materials containing nanoparticles are presently in the market internationally. Bottles are made with nanoparticles that

minimize the leakage of carbon dioxide out of the bottle; this increases the shelf life of carbonated beverages without having to use glass bottles or more expensive cans.

Nanoparticles are being developed to improve the taste, color, and texture of foods. They are used to deliver vitamins and other nutrients in food and beverages. Nanoparticles are also being developed to detect bacteria and pesticides in fruits and vegetables.

Studies have shown that these particles, because of their tiny size, can penetrate barriers and get into the system and enter liver, kidney, and even brain. Zinc oxide nanoparticles have been shown to be toxic to human lung cells in laboratory tests even at low concentrations. Silver particles have been shown to kill liver and brain cells from rats. The particles are chemically more reactive and bioactive.

There are very few published studies on the health and environmental impacts of nanoparticles. It is not known whether nanoparticles used in food packaging might leach into food or beverages, and it is also unclear what impact these particles might have on human health.[29] Consumers have virtually no way of knowing whether the food products they purchase contain nanoparticles. Under the present U.S. laws, it is up to manufacturers as to what they choose to put on their labels. The technology has the potential to deliver some significant benefits to the consumer, but there is a need for extensive research to determine potential health and safety implications.

26.1.2.3 Other Contaminants

26.1.2.3.1 Bisphenol A

Bisphenol A (BPA) is the highest-volume chemical in the world and is an industrial chemical that is used to harden plastic. Most of the 2–3 billion pounds produced in the United States per year is used in the manufacture of polycarbonate plastics and epoxide resins. It is found in numerous consumer products from compact discs to bicycle helmets to automotive parts. But it is the food, beverage, and dental applications of BPA that have some researchers and activist groups concerned. This is because it is found in baby bottles, refillable water containers, linings of most food and beverage cans, teethers, pacifiers, and dental sealants. It leaches out from all these products. It leaches into the contents of food containers, leaching more when the container is heated (such as in a microwave). Many people receive exposure of about 2.5 μg/kg body weight per day. The Centers for Disease Control and Prevention (CDC) has found measurable levels, 0.4–8 ppb, of BPA in urine samples from 93% of human subjects tested.

BPA is a weak estrogenic compound and is an endocrine disrupter—"an exogenous chemical that alters the structure or function of the endocrine system and causes adverse effects in individuals, offspring or population." Over the past decade, several studies have linked BPA to breast cancer, obesity, diabetes, neurological problems, and other disorders.[20] Much of the research on animals suggests that BPA has an effect at very low doses lower than the current safety standard set by the FDA, 50 μg/kg body weight/day. The standard was set 22 years ago and in the time since, scientists have learned more about the effects of even small amounts of BPA. Female mice dosed with BPA had serious reproductive problems, including defective eggs. Studies have linked fetal BPA exposure in rodents to mammary cancer, male genital defects, and neurobehavioral problems.

As a synthetic estrogen, BPA can mimic hormones and produce immense biological changes especially if a human being is exposed to it during critical periods of development, like the first trimester of pregnancy. Children are particularly vulnerable to such chemicals because their small bodies are developing rapidly and they eat and drink more relative to their body weights than adults. Recent studies have found that higher urinary concentrations of BPA are associated with an increased prevalence of cardiovascular disease, diabetes, and liver enzyme abnormalities. Male workers in China exposed to extreme levels of BPA consistently had a higher risk of sexual dysfunction.

The Canadian government has banned polycarbonated infant bottles. Some bottle makers have decided to drop the use of polycarbonate.

26.1.2.3.2   Phthalates

Phthalates are esters of phthalic acid used to soften polyvinyl chloride plastics. They are found in a large variety of products ranging from shower curtains to cosmetics to intravenous fluid bags, in addition to the enteric coating of pharmaceutical pills, nutritional supplements, and toys. They have been shown to disrupt hormones in animals and have been linked to reduced sperm count and other marks of feminization in male rodents. Higher levels of phthalates have been linked to earlier breast development in girls—a possible risk factor for breast cancer. High phthalate exposure during pregnancy results in decreased anogenital distance among baby boys. It is also linked to abdominal obesity and insulin resistance in men.

Phthalates are easily released into the environment because there is no covalent bond between the phthalates and plastics in which they are mixed. In some countries, there are restrictions for toys containing more than 0.1% of certain phthalates, especially those toys that can be placed in a child's mouth.

26.1.2.3.3   Melamine

Melamine is used to make plastics, laminates, fertilizers, and other products but is not approved as an ingredient in food. Milk dealers in China added the nitrogen-rich compound to boost the apparent protein content of diluted or substandard milk. The adulterated milk was then used to make powdered milk and infant formulas, as well as candies, cookies, flavored milk drinks, and other foods. The contaminated milk products killed at least six Chinese infants and sickened more than 300,000 other children[9,15] in 2008. In 2007, melamine was found in wheat gluten and rice protein concentrate exported from China and was used in the manufacture of pet foods in the United States. This caused the deaths of innumerable number of dogs and cats due to kidney failure. In 2008, eggs imported to Hong Kong from China were found to be contaminated with nearly twice the legal limit of melamine. China has adopted a regulation that requires producers to list additives on food labels. Chinese legislators also passed a food safety law that will enhance monitoring and supervision and toughen safety standards.

Trace levels of melamine were found in one or two infant formula samples (0.14–0.25 ppm). The FDA has declared that levels below 1 ppm do not pose a risk. The source of the chemical in U.S. infant formula is not known, but food packaging or sanitizers are possibilities.

26.1.2.3.4   Atrazine

The popular herbicide atrazine has been widely used to control broadleaf and grassy weeds in corn, grain, sorghum, and other agricultural crops for about 50 years. The widespread presence of atrazine in the environment poses a risk in humans, wildlife, and ecosystems. The chemical is known to be a potent endocrine disrupter, interfering with hormonal activity of animals and humans at extremely low doses. Research has shown that exposing frogs to as little as 0.1 ppm can cause severe health effects, including a kind of chemical castration. Studies have shown that atrazine can also impact the human reproductive system, decreasing sperm count and increasing infertility.

Atrazine use is controversial due to its widespread contamination of waterways and drinking water supplies. Atrazine has been banned in the European Union because of its persistent groundwater contamination. In the United States, approximately 76 million pounds are used each year. It is also used in about 80 countries worldwide. Its alleged endocrine disrupter effects, possible carcinogenic effects, and epidemiological connection to low sperm level in men and menstrual problems have led several scientists to call for banning it in the United States. The EPA is reevaluating the human health effects of the herbicide because of the recent studies that suggest a potential link between atrazine in drinking water, birth defects, and low birth weight in humans.

26.1.2.3.5   Perchlorate

Perchlorate is a highly soluble component of solid rocket fuel. It is also used in fireworks and explosives. Low levels of perchlorate have been detected in drinking water in 35 states in the United States. The chemical has been found in produce, including lettuce and melons. The substance has also been found in cow's milk, presumably because these animals drink water or eat feed contaminated with perchlorate.

Recent studies show that exposure to low levels of perchlorate is widespread throughout the United States, potentially affecting the health of tens of millions of women of childbearing age. Researchers at the CDC detected perchlorate in urine for each of the 2520 participants who were at least 6 years old. They also found that the concentration of perchlorate in children was generally higher than levels found in adolescents and adults. They also discovered that perchlorate exposure was associated with a decreased level of thyroid hormone among women with lower-than-normal concentrations of iodine in their urine. Perchlorate interferes with the thyroid uptake of iodine.

An estimated 43 million women in the United States have iodine levels low enough to put them at increased risk of developing goiter due to an insufficient amount of thyroid hormone. If these women become pregnant, they could have babies at risk of abnormal brain development. An embryo is completely dependent on maternal thyroid hormone during the first trimester of pregnancy. After that, the fetus begins to produce its own thyroid hormone but still receives about 30% of its total from the mother for the remainder of the pregnancy. Thyroid deficiency in the mother has repercussions for her fetus. Nursing infants have a special vulnerability to neurological problems from exposure. An infant can get substantial doses of perchlorate from breast milk. Also, perchlorate in a mother's body inhibits the movement of iodine into her breast milk. This creates double jeopardy for the nursing infant: low iodine intake at the same time that it is getting a risky level of perchlorate. Massachusetts became the first state in the nation to set a standard for perchlorate in drinking water at 2 ppb. California is the second state that set a standard at maximum contaminant level of 6 ppb. The states' standards will help guide clean up of perchlorate-tainted aquifers.

26.1.2.3.6 Benzene in Soft Drinks

Benzene is a cancer-causing chemical. Its levels are regulated in drinking water nationally and internationally and in bottled water in the United States, but only informally in soft drinks. In 2006, the FDA reported that many soft drinks had low levels of benzene (less than 5 ppb, the EPA's drinking water limit) while five contained levels greater than the EPA's limit. Two of these soft drinks contained amounts 15–18 times above the drinking water standard. The manufacturers of all five beverages agreed to reformulate their products. The same year Health Canada reported four soft drink products had levels above the Canadian guidelines of 5 µg/L in drinking water. The United Kingdom Food Standards Agency reported that 4 soft drinks had benzene levels above the drinking water standard (10 ppb) specified by the WHO. These four soft drinks were withdrawn. Some other countries also found higher levels of benzene in drinks.

Benzene is formed in soft drinks from benzoic acid, which is often added as a preservative in the form of its salt such as sodium benzoate. Benzoic acid is decarboxylated to form benzene in the presence of ascorbic acid (vitamin C) especially under heat and light.

Further, when considering the plethora of plastic bottles containing these benzene-laden soft drinks on the market and plastic that often contains other known chemical toxins like BPA that have been shown to adversely impact hormones, the two combined could likely result in exposure to both chemicals in a potentially more complex and harmful way, and therefore leave room for greater unknown potential risks to health and safety.

26.1.2.3.7 Toxins of Microbial Origin

Several compounds are produced by molds growing on food, but only a few of them appear to be of real or potential danger to human health. The best known are aflatoxins, which are produced by *Aspergillus flavus*. Aflatoxins are known to contaminate many foods, especially peanuts and other grains particularly in climates of high temperature and humidity. The toxins can cause liver damage and other symptoms such as enteritis. Food poisoning can also result from toxins produced by bacteria that get into the food supply because of poor sanitation, such as toxins derived from *Clostridium botulinum* and *Salmonella*. Canned foods that contain little or no acid are very good media for the growth of *C. botulinum*. The toxin has also developed in baked potatoes lightly wrapped in foil and allowed to stand for an extended period of time. The symptoms of botulism occur 8–12 hours after the ingestion of contaminated food and include headache, nausea, paralysis, and even death. Milk, eggs, fish, meat, and poultry that are eaten raw or that have been inadequately heated are most frequently implicated in salmonellosis. The toxin causes nausea, vomiting, abdominal pain, and diarrhea.

Among several seafood intoxications is that due to paralytic shellfish poisons produced by the plankton *Gonyaulax catenella* and other marine microorganisms.[8]

G. catenella is ingested by muscles, clams, and other shellfish. The toxic metabolite, saxitoxin, concentrates in the gills and the hepatopancreas of the shellfish. The shellfish show no disturbance as a result of the toxin. It survives ordinary cooking procedures. When contaminated seafood is eaten by humans, symptoms of toxicity usually develop in 1–3 hours. These include numbness of the lips and fingertips, an ascending paralysis, and, in severe poisoning, death from respiratory paralysis in 3–20 hours after eating the fish.

26.1.3 Substances That Are Toxic under Special Conditions

Some substances are toxic only under special circumstances. Tyramine is present in some foods such as cheese, wine, sherry, and beer. It is formed endogenously by the decarboxylation of tyrosine and is a potent vasopressor substance. Normally, it is metabolized by the action of the monoamine oxidase (MAO) system. Individuals who are on MAO inhibitor drugs, such as phenelzine (an antidepressant) and isoniazid, cannot metabolize tyramine, and it thus can act on blood vessels, producing severe hypertension.

Sensitivity to fava or broad beans (favism) is an example of an inherited metabolic disturbance. In sensitive individuals, inhalation of pollen from these plants or consumption of fava beans in either the cooked or raw state produces hemolytic anemia. Such individuals have a deficiency of glucose-6-phosphate dehydrogenase, which is inherited as a sex-linked trait. The cells are unable to maintain concentrations of reduced glutathione (GSH) sufficient to protect against oxidative damage. The GSH level in red blood cells of sensitive individuals is further reduced following the consumption of fava beans. Favism afflicts many young children and is endemic in the Middle East and in North Africa. The toxic substances in fava beans responsible for hemolytic anemia appear to be vicine and convicine, which are present to the extent of 0.5% of their dry weight.

Most people can consume wheat without any problem. However, individuals with celiac disease cannot tolerate certain fractions of wheat grain. When gluten is removed from the diet, improvement occurs in all aspects of the disease.

The ingestion of unripe ackee, a local Jamaican fruit, causes a highly lethal disease known as Jamaican vomiting sickness. Cooked ripe ackee fruits are nontoxic and have been a main staple in the diet of Jamaicans for centuries. The typical clinical course of the disease begins with vomiting and a sense of weakness, which abruptly occur in an individual who has been healthy. This episode lasts for several hours and is followed by a period of apparent improvement, which is usually followed by another attack of vomiting, convulsion, and coma, often leading to death. The unripe ackee contains the toxin hypoglycin, a seven-carbon amino acid with an unusual cyclopropyl propionic acid. It is metabolized to methylene cyclopropyl acetic acid, which exerts its toxic effect by inhibiting isovaleryl coenzyme A (CoA) dehydrogenase required for the metabolism of isovaleryl CoA. The latter compound, a metabolite of leucine, accumulates and causes vomiting.

There are several kinds of mushrooms. One variety—inky cap mushroom—is well tolerated by most people. However, if an alcoholic beverage is consumed during or shortly after a meal containing this variety of mushroom, the face of the individual becomes purplish red apparently because of the presence of a substance in this type of mushroom that inhibits the oxidation of acetaldehyde, a metabolite derived from alcohol.

For people allergic to some food components, the inadvertent addition of an allergenic substance can constitute a major hazard. The most common allergens are milk, eggs, peanuts, fish, shellfish, and soy. These can cause a variety of reactions including gastrointestinal problems, irritation, and breathing difficulties.

In some individuals, fish and shellfish are known to serve as possible allergens that may produce severe reactions. These include urticaria, angioneurotic edema, gastrointestinal disturbances, and migraine.

26.1.4 TOXICANTS PRODUCED DURING COOKING

26.1.4.1 Polyaromatic Hydrocarbons and Heterocyclic Amines

A series of toxic substances have been found in cooked meat and fish. Many cooking methods involve intense heat that can cause pyrolytic decomposition of some food components.[30] Major types of pyrolytic products are the polyaromatic hydrocarbons (PAHs) and the heterocyclic amines (HCAs). Both are known carcinogens. The PAHs are produced during cooking mainly by pyrolysis of fat, and HCAs are the products of amino acids, especially tryptophan. Beef grilled over a gas or charcoal fire has been found to contain a variety of PAHs. Up to 8 mg/kg benzopyrene has been found in charcoal-broiled steak. The source of PAHs is the smoke generated from pyrolyzed fat dripped from the meat onto the hot coals. The highest levels of PAHs are found in the meats with the highest fat content. When the meat is cooked in a way that prevents exposure to the smoke generated by dripped fat, the PAH level is either reduced or eliminated.

HCAs are primarily produced by high-temperature cooking of meats and fish. With uniform cooking methods, red meat such as beef and pork contain the highest concentrations of HCAs followed by chicken and fish. Nonmeat sources of protein such as eggs, cheese, and vegetables contain very low or undetectable concentrations of HCAs. High-temperature methods of cooking such as frying and broiling produce a much greater concentration of HCA than lower-temperature methods like boiling and microwaving. A well-done piece of meat contains more than 10 times the concentration of HCA than rare meat prepared by the same cooking method. These HCAs occur in very small quantities, but their mutagenic potencies raise concerns about possible carcinogenicity. Exposure to these toxic substances can be reduced by avoiding the charring of food during cooking, avoiding the direct contact of meat and fish with a naked gas flame or charcoal, and cooking meat and fish in aluminum foil. Mechanical separation of charred parts of meat and fish from the edible portion can also reduce the exposure level.

26.1.4.2 Formation of Toxic Aldehyde in Cooking Oil

When highly unsaturated vegetable oils such as soybean, sunflower, and corn oils are heated at frying temperatures (1850°C) for 30 minutes or longer healthy linoleic acid oxidizes to the highly toxic compound 4-hydroxy-2 trans-nonenal (HNE). This toxic aldehyde has been linked to a number of diseases, including Parkinson's and Alzheimer's diseases. The concentration of HNE in fried foods is directly proportional to its concentration in the cooking oil. The toxin accumulates with each heating cycle, underscoring the importance of not reusing these oils for frying.

26.1.4.3 Acrylamide

It has been discovered recently that acrylamide can be formed when starchy foods are cooked at high heat, particularly when they are fried. Acrylamide is also found in some raw, dried, and pickled foods such as olives, prunes, and dried pears. Studies show that heat and light can decompose polyacrylamide, the thickening agent used in commercial herbicides, into acrylamide. Acrylamide is a neurotoxin, a known carcinogen in rats, and a probable carcinogen in humans.

Scientists at Sweden's National Food Administration and the University of Stockholm were the first to discover acrylamide in cooked starchy foods. They found that acrylamide levels in potato chips, French fries, cookies, processed cereals, and bread are often hundreds of times higher than the maximum level (0.5 μg/L) considered safe for drinking water by the WHO and the EPA. The highest levels were found in potato chips (1200 ppb) and French fries (450 ppb). Subsequent studies on a few hundred samples in Norway, Switzerland, the United Kingdom, and the United States confirmed the results. On June 25–27, 2002, the WHO and the United Nations Food and Agriculture Organization held a meeting of 23 experts in Geneva to discuss scientific findings and to plan additional research. The WHO estimates that the total intake of acrylamide from the average Western diet and other sources such as cosmetics and cigarette smoke is about 70 μg/day for an adult, "a range significantly below that which is known to cause nerve damage in laboratory animals." The WHO estimates that the intake of acrylamide from the average Western diet is likely higher than that of PAHs from cooked meat and fish.

The FDA is currently analyzing several different foods for acrylamide. At present, the data are not sufficient to make a final determination regarding the public health impact of these preliminary findings. The agency has not altered its current dietary recommendations, but as further data are received, FDA's recommendations could change.

A Norwegian group has estimated that the acrylamide in all Norwegian foods could be responsible for 30 cancer deaths a year. Norway's National Food Authority has been working with food processors to find ways to reduce the production of acrylamide in food.[11] The agency also has recommended that people who eat a significant amount of potato chips—the food with the highest levels of the substance—should reduce their consumption to avoid possible harm.

How acrylamide gets in fried and baked food has been a puzzle for food chemists. However, most recently scientists have solved the mystery. At temperatures above 100°C, the amino acid asparagine—abundant in potatoes and cereal grains—bonds with reducing sugars like glucose according to the Maillard reaction.[18] In the acrylamide pathway, a Maillard product called N-glycoside cleaves at a carbon–nitrogen bond, yielding the carbon skeleton and terminal amide group at asparagine, which transitions to acrylamide. It is hoped that the food industry will be able to take immediate advantage of this information to find ways to remediate the problem.

Asparagine can also react with 2-deoxyglucose, which does not undergo the Maillard reaction, producing acrylamide. So, it is not necessarily the Maillard reaction that is producing acrylamide.

Amid concerns surrounding the identification of acrylamide in cooked starchy foods, a team of German food chemists is giving bread lovers something to smile about. They have shown that a novel protein modification displaying protective properties is generated when bread is baked. The bread crust, whose golden brown color results from the Maillard reaction between sugars and amino acids or proteins during baking, contains the highest levels of another Maillard reaction product: protein-bound pronyl lysine (PBPL). This product stimulates the activity of detoxication enzymes that can get rid of mutagens and endogenous toxins.[16] Rats fed PBPL experience the same protective effect.

26.1.5 SAFETY OF FOODS

Most foods do have various nonnutrient substances, including toxicants in microamounts, but many of these substances do not necessarily create a hazard because individual toxicants are not consumed alone and their concentrations are very low. Some are destroyed during cooking. In the amount present, almost all naturally occurring toxicants are detoxified in the body, and the toxicities of thousands of chemicals in our daily diet are not cumulative. There may be many antagonistic interactions between different toxicants in the diet so that the toxicity of one chemical may be offset by the presence of another chemical. Thus, consuming a variety of food ensures that there is little chance of any one chemical reaching the toxic level. Such antagonistic interactions support the concept of "safety in numbers."

But illness can result from the ingestion of food contaminated with certain toxins, even in small amounts (such as certain seafood microorganisms), and from eating abnormally high amounts of one food containing a naturally occurring toxin, and it also can occur in individuals who are susceptible to certain foods because of their physiological state.

The past few years have seen a host of food recalls in the U.S. due to food-borne pathogens: illness-causing strains of *Escherichia coli* in beef, spinach, and some other foods, and *Salmonella* contamination of peanuts, lettuce, and jalapeño peppers. Food-borne infections cause about 76 million cases of illness, 325,000 hospitalizations, and as many as 5000 deaths in the United States annually. U.S. consumers eat about 600 billion pounds of food annually, and an increasing amount of food is being imported from places where food standards may not be as strict as those in the United States. There is no single way to prevent all food-borne illness, but many food safety experts believe irradiation should be used much more widely as part of an overall program to enhance safety.[27] It is estimated that irradiating half of all ground beef, pork, poultry, and processed meat would prevent 900,000 cases of food-borne illness and 350 deaths in the United States each year. About 50% of Americans hold negative opinions about food irradiation. There is also evidence that treatment may degrade the flavor.

Several countries are also concerned about food safety. Toxic dyes in spices and pesticide-contaminated fruits have been found in Europe. In 2008, Japan recalled insecticide-tainted Chinese dumplings. Melamine in milk products created a firestorm in China in 2007 after tainted formula sickened thousands of infants.

The European Union and Japan have set standards for hundreds of trace-chemical contaminants. In China, a food safety law went into effect in June 2009. It raises safety standards, tightens regulations, and improves oversight of food production. In the United States, the FDA Food Safety Modernization Act is expected to be approved. The bill puts more focus on prevention of food-borne illnesses by requiring food facilities to develop risk-based preventative control plans that address identified hazards. The legislation also requires the FDA to inspect food facilities more frequently. It also requires importers to verify the safety of imported food. These measures should result in safer food supply and reduce the number of hospitalizations and recalls.

To protect the public from food-borne illness outbreaks, the FDA is responsible for approximately 80% of the nation's food, while other government bodies such as the Department of Agriculture oversee the remainder. The Center for the Public Interest released a list (Table 26.2) of what the organization called the top 10 riskiest foods based on reported cases of illness.

TABLE 26.2
Foods Likely to Cause Food-Borne Illness

Food Item	Number of Outbreaks	Number of Cases
Leafy greens	363	13,568
Eggs	352	11,163
Tuna	268	2341
Oysters	132	3409
Potatoes	108	3659
Cheese	83	2761
Ice cream	74	2594
Tomatoes	31	3292
Sprouts	31	2022
Berries	25	3397

26.2   ADDITIVES

Food additives play a necessary and beneficial role in the food supply.[21,28] A large variety of chemicals are added to food for many worthwhile or indispensable functions. Without food additives, it would be impossible for food to be safely produced in massive quantities and transported nationwide or worldwide. As preservatives, they can be categorized into three general types: (1) antibacterials that inhibit growth of bacteria, yeasts, or molds; (2) antioxidants that slow air oxidation of fats and lipids, which leads to rancidity; and (3) inhibitors that blocks the natural ripening and enzymatic processes that continue to occur in foodstuffs after harvest.

A food additive is defined as any substance that is not an inherent part of prepared foods. Additives are used intentionally (direct additives) to serve some functional purposes such as to maintain or increase the food's nutritional value, preserve freshness (e.g., antioxidants, antimicrobial agents), make food taste (e.g., sugar, salt) or look (e.g., colors) better, and aid in its processing and/or preparation (Table 26.3). Also included in this category are calorie reduction agents (e.g., fat replacers and high-intensity sweeteners). Food additives compose less than 1% of the weight of humans' dietary intake, and most of these additives occur naturally in foods or in the body. There are many additives made synthetically, but in terms of weight, they amount to a very small fraction in our diet.

Some additives used are nutrients (e.g., sucrose, starch, corn syrup, dextrose, vegetable gums, glutamic acid). Some are essential nutrients (e.g., sodium chloride and cobalt), but this does not exclude their possible toxicity at higher levels. Excessive salt content in the diet causes an increase in blood pressure among genetically susceptible individuals. To treat anemia, patients are administered 15–20 mg/day cobalt for a prolonged period with little or no toxicity. However, the presence of cobalt in beer (1.1–1.2 mg/L) has caused cardiomyopathy in some heavy beer drinkers. The disease was linked to cobalt in beer. Currently, some 2500—perhaps 3000—chemicals are used as direct additives.

Indirect additives (or unavoidable contaminants) are those chemicals that become part of the food in trace amounts as an unintentional result of some phase of production, processing, storage, or packaging.

Despite consumers' concerns about the safety of additives, additives are extensively studied and regulated. Moreover, most food additives have a large margin of safety. The FDA regulates food additives (direct and indirect) through the Federal Food, Drug, and Cosmetic Act passed in 1938. The passage of the Food Additive Amendment in 1958 and the Color Additives Amendment in 1960

TABLE 26.3
Common Food Additives

Categories	Examples
Preservatives	
Antioxidants	BHA, BHT, tocopherol
Antimicrobial agents	Sodium benzoate, sodium nitrite
Emulsifiers	Lecithin, egg yolk
Stabilizers and thickeners	Carrageenan, pectins
Colors	Carotene, caramel
Flavor enhancers	Vanillin, monosodium glutamate
Nutrient supplements	Vitamins, iron, iodine
Leavening agents	Yeast, baking powder
Anticaking agents	Ammonium citrate, baking powder
Nonnutritive sweeteners	Aspartame (NutraSweet)
Fat replacers	Olestra, Simplesse

makes it necessary for the food industry to demonstrate a proof of safety by the manufacturer based on extensive animal tests to get an approval by the FDA. Before 1958, it was the FDA's responsibility to prove that an additive was either safe or unsafe.

As part of the 1958 Food Additives Amendment,[3] the Delaney Clause prohibits the use of any additive that causes cancer in man and animals, regardless of the amount required to cause the disease. Some feel that the Delaney Law is not restrictive enough because it does not deal with other health risks that may be equally as dangerous as cancer. Some others believe that the law is too rigid in that some agents would have to be consumed in enormous amounts to reproduce the conditions that result in tumors under experimental conditions. Questions are also being raised as to whether a particular substance should be banned if proven harmful for only a few individuals.

The hundreds of additives used in foods before the 1958 Amendment were placed on FDA's generally recognized as safe (GRAS) list.[4] These substances were those regarded by expert scientists as safe, based on their extensive history of use in foods before 1958 or based on published scientific evidence. Some of these substances have been subsequently reviewed by the FDA and have been either approved for continued use, recommended for further study, or banned.

For reasons of potential toxicity, additives are also assessed by international bodies such as the Food and Agriculture Organization and the WHO Joint Expert Committee on food additives and other international and national bodies such as the Scientific Committee for Food of the European Union and the FDA. In Europe, each approved additive is assigned a number, termed "E number." This numbering system has been adopted by the *Codex Alimentarius Commission* to identify all additives regardless of whether they are approved for use. Countries outside Europe use only the number. For example, acetic acid is written as E260 on products sold in Europe, but is simply known as additive 260 in some countries.

As a general rule, additives found to be harmful in experimental animals, if permitted for use in food, are only allowed at levels far below those at which any experimental toxic effect is detectable. Thus, allowable daily intakes (ADIs) are determined by regulatory agencies typically at 1/100 of the no-effect level in animals.

Over the years, a substantial number of additives have been withdrawn from use on the basis of experimental studies showing unusual toxicity, including mutagenicity and carcinogenicity. Examples include a number of azo dyes now no longer used in countries that have their own regulatory bodies or that accept the findings of international bodies. One example is a dye known as Red 2G found in sausages and ground beef. Raw meat oxidizes to a brownish color, and the dye was used to make meat look fresher. The body converts the dye into aniline, which is found to be carcinogenic in mice. It is banned in the United States, Canada, Australia, and some other countries. The European Safety Authority has recommended food producers stop using the dye.

The use of other additives has been increasingly restricted (i.e., nitrates and nitrites as used in meat). Additionally, many additives are not permitted for use in foods and drinks manufactured for babies and small children.

Some additives commonly found in children's foods may increase the level of hyperactivity (inattention, impulsivity, and overactivity) at least into middle childhood, according to recent reports.[17] Researchers examined the effects of a variety of common food dyes and the preservative sodium benzoate—an ingredient in many soft drinks, fruit juices, and salad dressings. They found that these additives do cause some kids to become measurably more hyperactive and distractible. Studies have shown significant behavioral improvement on low-additive or additive-free diets compared with regular diets or behavioral deterioration on a placebo-controlled challenge with foods suspected of aggravating symptoms. The findings prompted Britain's Food Safety Agency to issue an immediate advisory to parents to limit their children's intake of additives if they notice an effect on behavior of their children. The American Academy of Pediatrics has concluded that a low-additive diet is a valid intervention for all children with attention-deficit hyperactive disorder.

A few of the more common but significant food additives that have become of public concern in recent years are considered below.

26.2.1 Nitrites

Nitrates and nitrites have long been used in the curing of meat and other food products. They provide foods such as ham, salami, and bacon their familiar cured flavor and pink color and have been found to protect them from the possible threat of botulin contamination. Botulin grows in an environment that contains little or no oxygen and has been found in improperly vacuum-packed foods (e.g., canned ham). As the presence of the bacterium and the toxin it produces cause no detectable change in the appearance, taste, or odor of food, there is no way for the consumer to know that the food is contaminated. The toxin can be deadly. The use of nitrites has been, nevertheless, of concern as it reacts with secondary amines (such as proline or polyamine derivatives found in foodstuffs) under stomach pH conditions to produce nitrosamines. They are potent carcinogens capable of producing a variety of different kinds of tumors in the animal system, and although there is no direct evidence, they are suspected of causing human cancers of the stomach and esophagus.

On the average, an American eats about 300 g/day vegetables containing about 85 mg of nitrate. More than half of this amount is supplied by 30 g of leafy vegetables. Celery, radishes, beets, and leafy vegetables are rich sources of nitrate, with some samples containing up to 15,000 ppm. Part of the ingested nitrate is converted to nitrite by bacteria in the oral cavity and the gastrointestinal tract. Nitrite from ingested foods amounts to 9–10 mg. This is about four times as much as that obtained from an average intake of cured meats in 1 day (1–2 mg). Nitrites also occur in cigarette smoke, polluted air, and drinking water. Nitrosamines occur in cigarette smoke, and a heavy smoker can get as much as 17 mg/day. The daily intake of nitrosamines, depending on certain exposures, can vary considerably (e.g., interiors of a new car, 0.2–0.5 mg; cosmetics, 0.4 mg; beer, 0.3–1 mg; scotch, 0.03 mg; and cured meats, 0.2 mg).

A high dietary intake of nitrate (e.g., in vegetables, drinking water) has been associated with a high rate of cancer in certain parts of the world. It has been found that vitamin C and vitamin E prevent nitrites from reacting with amines to form nitrosamines in rats. Vitamin C also has been shown to inhibit the induction of tumors by nitrosamines in rats.

Although nitrite may have deleterious effects, it prevents the growth of botulinum. It may be very difficult without nitrite to have normal storage, transport, and distribution of processed meat products. We may get more nitrite from ingested vegetables than in the form used as additive. One has to consider the risk/benefit ratio. Until another substance is proven equally effective, risks associated with the use of nitrites in cured meat products will remain acceptable because it prevents the growth of botulinum, a producer of a very lethal toxin. In 1978, the U.S. Department of Agriculture published a regulation specifying the amount of nitrite that can be added to cured meats as 120 mg/kg. Sodium ascorbate or erythorbate (a stereoisomer of L-ascorbic acid) must also be added in the amount of 550 mg/kg to prevent the formation of nitrosamines.[26]

A less benign aspect of nitrite ingestion, when high doses are involved, is the oxidation of circulating hemoglobin to methemoglobin in red cells. The oxidized Fe^{3+} in the heme group can no longer bind oxygen. A few cases of methemoglobinemia have been reported in infants consuming baby foods made with vegetables (e.g., like spinach and beets) that tend to accumulate nitrate during their growth (when fertilized with nitrates).

26.2.2 Butylated Hydroxyanisole and Butylated Hydroxytoluene

Butylated hydroxyanisole (BHA) and butylated hydroxytoluene (BHT) are two common synthetic preservatives added to food as antioxidants. They inhibit the degradative oxidation of polyunsaturated fats and prevent rancidity that can lead to undesirable flavor. Some investigators have reported an increased incidence of tumors in mice receiving a high quantity of BHT in their diet. Concerns have also developed regarding BHA; at high dietary levels, it has caused tumors in rats. On the other hand, there are several reports showing that both BHA and BHT inhibit carcinogenesis. These antioxidants have been tested and found to be acceptable at the level presently in use, but additional research is needed to evaluate the safety and efficacy of these compounds.

26.2.3 SULFITES

Like nitrates, sulfites have been used in foods for centuries. Six sulfiting agents—sulfur dioxide, sodium metabisulfite, potassium metabisulfite, sodium bisulfite, potassium bisulfite, and sodium sulfite—are considered GRAS for all uses in foods except fresh fruits and vegetables (other than potatoes). These agents are used in dry fruits (>1000 ppm), wines (100–150 ppm), and dehydrated vegetables (<100 ppm). Sulfites inhibit oxidative discoloration and flavor changes, and they also have antimicrobial effects. They serve all three functions as preservatives (antibacterials, antioxidants, and inhibitors of the natural ripening and enzymatic processes), which is one reason why they are found in so many household products.

There are several recent reports of adverse reactions and deaths associated with the consumption of sulfite-treated foods. About 8% of the asthmatic population was found to be sensitive to the ingestion of sulfites, but sulfites at levels currently used in foods would present no hazard to the majority of consumers. Sulfites were widely used in salad bars to keep fruits and vegetables looking fresh. Because of the unpredictable severity in sulfite-sensitive individuals, the labeling of foods containing sulfites appears to be necessary to protect those individuals. The FDA now requires that packaged foods that contain 10 ppm or more of sulfite must declare the presence of sulfite on the label. Because most of the reported sulfite reactions have occurred in restaurants, the FDA enacted a second regulation that prohibits the addition of sulfite on fruits and vegetables that are intended to be served or sold raw to consumers.

26.2.4 MONOSODIUM GLUTAMATE

Monosodium glutamate (MSG) has been used to enhance flavor and as a preservative since it was discovered in 1908 by Kikunae Ikeda, a chemistry professor in Tokyo. He isolated the substance from seaweed that for centuries Japanese cooks had been using to make food taste better and found that it was L-glutamate. It is produced by fermentation. Certain bacteria convert molasses or starch hydrolysate to L-glutamate, which is neutralized with sodium hydroxide to form MSG. Before fermentation was adopted, the main source of L-glutamic acid was extraction from wheat gluten, which contains as much as 25% of the amino acid by weight. It may be the most widely used flavor enhancer after salt and pepper. Annual worldwide demand is about 1.1 million tons. About 70% of the demand comes from Pacific Basin countries. The rest comes from South America (about 15%) and Europe and North America (about 15%).

MSG is commonly included in commercially processed foods in the United States in the amounts of 0.1%–0.6% by weight. In 1968, a syndrome (Chinese restaurant syndrome) associated with eating Chinese foods was reported. It was described as having a feeling of numbness over the back and neck, weakness, and palpitations lasting up to 2 hours but leaving no aftereffects. A few individuals are sensitive to this additive and encounter this syndrome when they eat some Chinese foods that are heavily seasoned with MSG. Pyridoxine pretreatment eliminates the symptoms caused by MSG with a concurrent increase in erythrocyte glutamate-oxaloacetate transaminase activity. Consumption of MSG could make a person more prone to being overweight or obese compared to people who do not use the flavor enhancer, according to a recent study.[10] The higher risk for becoming overweight was found even when researchers controlled for physical activity and total caloric intake.

26.2.5 Diacetyl

Diacetyl is a natural by-product of fermentation. Diacetyl and acetoin are two compounds that give butter its characteristic taste. At low levels, it gives beer and wine a slippery feel. As levels increase, it imparts a buttery or butterscotch flavor. Artificially produced diacetyl is added to a variety of food products, including microwave popcorn to give it a butter-like flavor.

Animal studies of exposure to butter-like flavoring including diacetyl have shown airway injury in rats after acute inhalation of these flavors. Since 2000, diacetyl exposure has been a concern in microwave popcorn facilities, when the Missouri's health department investigated a cluster of bronchiolitis obliterans (BO) cases in one factory producing this product. The National Institute of Occupational Safety & Health also investigated and found other clusters of disease that appeared to be associated with diacetyl. Since then, workers at several factories that manufacture artificial butter flavoring have been diagnosed with BO, a rare and serious disease of the lungs that causes shortness of breath, coughing, fatigue, and ultimately death.

Consumers may also be in danger of contracting the disease from fumes produced by microwaving popcorn containing (this man-made version of) diacetyl. The first case was reported in 2008. The individual ate at least 2 bags of buttery microwave popcorn daily for 10 years and was diagnosed with lung problems that were linked to breathing diacetyl vapors. Although rare, the individual's kitchen also had diacetyl levels comparable to those in popcorn. Since 2007, almost all major manufacturers no longer add diacetyl to their microwave popcorn. They have started replacing diacetyl with substitute ingredients of unknown toxicity. Despite the concern of adverse effects, government agencies consider diacetyl a safe substance because it occurs naturally in food such as butter and milk.

26.2.6 Carmine and Cochineal

Cochineal is a particular South and Central American insect from which the crimson-colored dye is derived. This insect produces carminic acid, which occurs as 17%–24% of the weight in the female of this insect. Carminic acid is mixed with calcium salts to make carmine dye. It is used as a fabric and cosmetic dye and a food coloring. The ingredient that gives Dannon Boysenberry Yogurt and Tropicana Ruby Red Grapefruit Juice their distinctive colors come from crushed female cochineal beetles: vivid red "carmine" and bright orange "cochineal." The pigment is also used in fruit drinks, some other yogurts, ice cream, gelatins, alcoholic drinks and other foods, shampoos, and cosmetics.

Under current FDA regulations, food labels must identify certain synthetic colorings by name such as FD&C Red No. 40. But for carmine, cochineal, and other naturally occurring ingredients, companies can use terms such as "color added" or oddly "artificial color." There are many other natural color additives in this group including beet powder and grape skin extract.

The Center for Science in the Public Interest (CSPI), a Washington public-health advocacy group, and a small group of consumers who are allergic to the insect ingredients, have pushed the FDA for stiffer rules. Joining the chorus were vegetarians who do not want to eat insects and consumers observing kosher dietary practices. There are a lot of people who will not be happy to know that they are eating products that contain dried beetles. The petition by the CSPI to the FDA suggested that the language on the label read "artificial color: carmine/cochineal extract (insect-based)." The food industry objected to both the word "insect" and the use of "artificial color" together with "carmine" and "cochineal."

According to the food industry, the lengthy description is unnecessary since it is not part of the requirement for other animal-derived ingredients. Lard is "lard" and it does not say "pork" after it. Milk and butter do not say "from cow." In January 2009, the FDA passed a regulation requiring carmine and cochineal extract to be listed by name on the label. This regulation is effective January 5, 2011. According to the FDA, the label will allow consumers who are allergic to these additives to identify and thus avoid products that contain these color additives.

Currently many food scientists are searching for preservatives in natural products. Some of the newest antimicrobials have been found in microorganisms themselves as they form their own chemical defenses when competing with each other for space and nutrients. For example, niacin and natamycin—cheese preservatives called bacteriocins—are harvested from microorganisms. Other potential sources include honey, milk, and even dried plums as scientists seek new sources and combinations of safe, effective preservatives.

26.2.7 Intense Sweeteners

26.2.7.1 Saccharin

Saccharin was the first synthetic sweetener available commercially and has been used since 1901. It is about 300 times sweeter than sucrose but has a slight bitter aftertaste. It provides no calories and thus appears to be ideally suited for diabetics and weight-conscious individuals. Based on a study from the Canadian Health Protection Branch, which showed evidence of bladder tumors in male rats fed high doses of saccharin, the FDA proposed to prohibit its use in 1977. As a result of public outcry and the need for a sugar substitute, Congress declared a moratorium on the ban, allowing continued use until additional research on saccharin's safety could be conducted. Several studies in humans showed no association between saccharin intake and cancer. In addition, leading health groups have reviewed the scientific research on saccharin and supported its safety. At the current intake levels, this sweetener is assumed safe for the general public and is approved for use in more than 90 countries. Saccharin continues to be in use in the United States, but is banned in Canada.

26.2.7.2 Cyclamate

Cyclamate was the second synthetic sweetener and became commercially available in 1951. It is 30 times sweeter than sucrose. In 1969, evidence from the study of saccharin/cyclamate mixture implicated cyclamate as a possible cancer-causing agent in rats, and in 1970, the FDA banned its use in the United States. In 1984, the FDA's Cancer Assessment Committee reviewed the scientific evidence and concluded that cyclamate is not carcinogenic; however, this sweetener is banned in the United States but is in use in Canada.

26.2.7.3 Aspartame

Aspartame (NutraSweet) is about 200 times sweeter than sucrose. It is a dipeptide that provides 4 cal/g (17 kJ), but the amount required for sweetness supplies only 0.5% of the calories provided by sugar. It became commercially available in 1981, and as of October 1, 1989, the FDA has received more than 4600 complaints about the side effects of aspartame including headaches, menstrual disorders, upper respiratory tract symptoms, and seizures. Some individuals may be sensitive to one or more metabolites of aspartame (e.g., aspartic acid, phenylalanine, and methanol).

26.2.7.4 Acesulfame-K

Acesulfame-K is a recent synthetic intense sweetener approved by the FDA for table use and use in dry mixes and chewing gums; it is awaiting clearance for other uses. It is marketed in the United States under the trade names Sunette and Sweet One. In the European Union, it is known under the E number (additive code) E950. It is not metabolized in the body, noncaloric, and 200 times as sweet as sucrose. Because of its structural similarity to saccharin, a suspected carcinogen, several individuals have registered concern against this sweetener's initial approval in the United States.

26.2.7.5 Sucralose

Sucralose is a chlorinated form of sucrose with a glycosidic linkage resistant to enzymatic hydrolysis. It is not metabolized and provides no calories. It is 400–800 times sweeter than sucrose. It has been approved in the United States and Canada for use in some foods. It is stable under heat and over a broad range of pH conditions. Therefore, it can be used in baking or in products that require a longer shelf life. It is also known as Splenda. In the European Union it is known under the E number (additive code) E955.

26.2.7.6   Alitame

Alitame, like aspartame, is a dipeptide containing aspartic acid. It is 2000 times as sweet as sucrose. In some countries, it is marketed under the name Aclame.

26.2.7.7   Neotame

Neotame is a relatively new nonnutritive sweetener that is 10,000 times sweeter than sugar. It is derived from aspartame and has a structure that prevents the peptide bond between phenylalanine and aspartic acid from breaking, making it safer for PKU patients. It is heat stable and can be used as a tabletop sweetener, in soft drinks, or in cooking. In addition to its role as a sweetener, neotame is a flavor enhancer.

26.2.7.8   Other Sweeteners and Enhancers

Several other intense sweeteners are in the early stages of development. These include dihydrochalcones derived from citrus fruits, sterioside from a South American plant, glycyrrhizin from licorice root (used as a flavor enhancer in the United States), and thaumatin, a mixture of proteins isolated from a West African fruit.

Sugar substitutes are great for reducing calories. However, they do not provide the exact sugar flavor and leave a bitter aftertaste when used in high concentrations.[23] More recently, chemicals have been developed that enhance the sweetness of sugar and sugar substitutes while keeping calories to a minimum. The chemicals[22] trick the taste buds into sensing sugar or salt even when it is not there. By adding one of these flavoring chemicals to their products, manufacturers can, for instance, reduce the sugar in a cookie, or salt in a can of soup, by one-third to one-half while retaining the same sweetness or saltiness. Kraft foods, Nestle, Coca-Cola, and Campbell Soup Company are in the process of using this technology in their products. A chemical that mimics MSG has received approval from the Flavor and Extract Manufacturers Association. Food items with this chemical are expected to appear in supermarkets in 2011.

Unlike artificial sweeteners, the chemical enhancers will not be listed on ingredient labels. Instead, they will be lumped into a broad category—"artificial flavors"—already found on most packaged food labels.

A 12-ounce can of chicken soup (2½ servings) has more than 2300 mg of sodium. That would probably be cut to about 1500 mg when the chemical is added. Food safety experts like the idea of sugar and salt reduction, but they are concerned about the new chemicals and would like more testing to be done before the chemicals are added in food products.

26.2.8   Fat Replacers

Preparations derived from carbohydrates such as starch, which provides 4 Cal/g, and cellulose (no calories) are used in place of fat, which supplies 9 Cal/g. Avicel, for example, is a cellulose gel introduced in the mid-1960s as a food stabilizer. Carrageenan, a seaweed derivative, was approved for use as an emulsifier, stabilizer, and thickener in foods in 1961. Its use as a fat replacer became popular in the early 1990s. A protein-based fat replacer called Simplesse, consisting of microparticulated egg whites and milk proteins, is classified by the FDA as GRAS for frozen desserts, cheeses, salad dressing, and mayonnaise. Other protein-based fat replacers are being tested. These include Trailblazer, which is made from natural ingredients, and Lita, which is based on microparticulate proteins from corn. But the use of these substitutes has been limited by heat stability, texture, and taste; none of these can be used for frying.

Olestra is a sucrose polyester containing six to eight fatty acids esterified to sucrose, instead of glycerol.[2] As it is larger than a typical molecule, it is not hydrolyzed by digestive enzymes and not absorbed, and therefore, it has no caloric value.[14] It has properties similar to those of naturally occurring fat, but it provides zero calories and no fat. Olestra reduces the absorption of fat-soluble nutrients, such as vitamins A, D, E, and K, and carotenoids, from foods eaten at the same time as olestra-containing products. To address these concerns, the FDA approved olestra on the condition that vitamins A, D, E, and K be added to olestra-containing foods.[1] The FDA approval limits olestra's use to savory snacks such as potato chips, tortilla chips, and cheese curls. The agency requires that package labels warn of potential digestive effects such as abdominal cramping and loose stools.

Some other fat-based replacers are being developed.[7] Salatrim (which stands for short-chain and long-chain triglyceride molecules) is the generic name for a family of reduced calorie fats that are only partially absorbed in the body. Salatrim provides 4 Cal/g. Several other synthetic fat replacers are in the early stages of development.

A Juicy Problem—A Case

A 68-year-old male presented at the hospital emergency department with acute urinary retention. His blood count and usual laboratory tests, including serum creatinine and prostate-specific antigen, were normal. Transurethral resection of the prostate was done, a long-term urinary catheter was left in place, and the patient was discharged. After 6 weeks, the patient presented to the emergency department with a 24-hour history of hematuria, oral petechiae, bleeding gums, and bruises on the shins. He was taking amlodipine for hypertension and low-dose aspirin. For the last 10 days, he had been drinking cranberry juice for symptomatic relief of discomfort associated with his indwelling urinary catheter. On physical examination, he appeared normal, normotensive, and with normal body temperature but had multiple oral petechiae and hemorrhages, extensive purpura on the shins, and bloodstained urine in the catheter bag. His blood hemoglobin and white cell counts were normal, but he had profound thrombocytopenia with a platelet count of 1×10^9/L (normal: $150–400 \times 10^9$/L). Examination of the blood film was unremarkable. There was no serological evidence of viral infection.

A diagnosis of immune thrombocytopenic purpura was made. The patient was treated with intravenous human immunoglobulin (400 mg/kg/day for 2 days) along with prednisolone, 1 mg/kg, daily. On the third day of treatment, the oral petechiae had resolved and the platelet count had risen to 12×10^9/L. On the eighth day, his platelet count was 200×10^9/L. The patient was discharged home on a reducing dose of steroids. The steroids were decreased and stopped over 6 weeks. Follow-up in the clinic during the next 18 months showed that his platelet count remained normal.

Because the patient was taking cranberry juice at the time of admission, further studies were done to determine any relationship between cranberry juice and the patient's thrombocytopenia. The regional poison center was contacted for advice. They said some brands might contain traces of quinine and its derivatives. Quinine is a known cause of immune-mediated thrombocytopenia. Cranberry juice of the same supermarket brand and batch as the patient had drunk was used in the study. No quinine was found in the juice. However, when dialyzed juice was added to the test system, both immunoglobulin M and immunoglobulin G antiplatelet antibodies were detected in the patient's serum. The detection of antiplatelet antibodies in the patient's serum only in the presence of dialyzed cranberry juice is evidence for an immune mechanism for the thrombocytopenia with a constituent of cranberry juice acting as the hapten.

There have been reports of thrombocytopenia as a result of milk and sesame seed consumption. This is the first case of thrombocytopenia related to cranberry juice. This case makes the point that common foods such as cranberry juice contain substances, some of which may cause deleterious effects in susceptible individuals.[33] It is well known by the general lay public that cranberry juice is helpful in treating and preventing urinary tract infections. In cases of thrombocytopenia, constituents of the patient's diet as a cause of platelet destruction should be borne in mind.

REFERENCES

1. Bergholz, C. M. 1992. Safety evaluation of Olestra, a non-absorbed, fat like fat replacement. *Crit Rev Food Sci Nutr* 32:141.
2. Cotton, J., J. Weststrate, and J. Blundell. 1996. Replacement of dietary fat with sucrose polyester: Effects on energy intake and appetite control in non-obese males. *Am J Clin Nutr* 63:891.
3. 1984. Food Additives Amendment of 1958, P.L. 85–292, 72 stat., 1984.
4. Food and Drug Administration. 1990. Direct food substance affirmed as generally recognized as safe: Microparticulated protein. *Fed Regist* 37:8384–8391.
5. Food and Drug Administration. 1996. Food additives permitted for direct addition to food for human consumption. *Olestra Fed Regist* 61:3118–3173.
6. Foster, E. M. 1982. How safe are our foods. *Nutr Rev Suppl* 40:28.
7. Gershoff, S. N. 1995. Nutrition evaluation of dietary fat substitutes. *Nutr Rev* 53:305.
8. Gessner, B. D., and J. P. Middaugh. 1995. Paralytic shellfish poisoning in Alaska: A 20-year retrospective analysis. *Am J Epidemiol* 141:766.
9. Guan, N., Q. Fan, J. Ding et al. 2009. Melamine-contaminated powdered formula and urolithiasis in young children. *New Engl J Med* 360:1067.
10. He, K., L. Zhao, M. L. Daviglus et al. 2008. Association of monosodium glutamate intake with overweight in Chinese adults. The intermap study. *Obesity* 16:1875.
11. Hileman, B. 2002. Acrylamide worries experts. *Chem Eng News* 80(27):9.
12. Hileman, G. 2007. Arsenic in chicken production. *Chem Eng News* 85(15):34.
13. Khalil, N., J. W. Wilson, E. O. Talbott et al. 2009. Association of blood lead concentrations with mortality in older women: A perspective cohort study. *Environ Health* 8:15.
14. Kirschner, E. M. 1997. Fake fat in real food. *Chem Eng News* 75(16):19–25.
15. Langman, G. 2009. Melamine, powdered milk, and nephrolithiasis in Chinese infants. *New Engl J Med* 360:1139.
16. Lindenmeir, M., V. Faist, and T. Hofmann. 2002. Structural and functional characterization of pronyl–lysine, a novel protein modification in bread crust melanoids showing in vitro antioxidative and phase I/II enzymes modulating activity. *J Agric Food Chem* 50:6997.
17. McCann, D., A. Barrett, A. Cooper et al. 2007. Food additives and hyperactive behavior in 3-year-old and 8/9-year-old children in the community: A randomized double-blinded placebo-controlled trial. *Lancet* 370:1560.
18. Mottram, D. S., B. L. Wedzicha, and A. T. Dodson. 2002. Acrylamide is formed in the Maillard reaction. *Nature* 419:448.
19. Newborne, P. M. 1988. Naturally occurring food-born toxicants. In *Modern Nutrition in Health and Disease*. 7th ed., ed. M. Shils and V. R. Young, 685–697. Philadelphia, PA: Lea & Febiger.
20. Patisaul, H. 2010. Assessing risks from bisphenol A. *Am Sci* 98(1):30.
21. Roberts, H. R. 1981. Food additives. In *Food Safety*, ed. H. R. Robert. New York: John Wiley and Sons, Inc.
22. Rovner, S. L. 2010. Sugary boost without calories. *Chem Eng News* 88(8):34.
23. Sardesai, V. M., and T. H. Waldshan. 1991. Natural and synthetic intense sweeteners. *J Nutr Biochem* 2:236.
24. Shiffman, M. H. 1990. Refried foods and the risk of colon cancer. *Am J Epidemiol* 131:376.
25. Strong, F. M. 1974. Toxicants occurring naturally in foods. *Nutr Rev* 32:225.
26. Tannenbaum, S. R., J. S. Wishmok, and C. D. Leaf. 1991. Inhibition of nitrosamine formation by ascorbic acid. *Am J Clin Nutr* 53:247s.
27. Tauxe, R. V. 2001. Food safety and irradiation: Protecting the public from food-borne infections. *Emerg Infect Dis* 7:516.
28. Thayer, A. M. 1991. Use of specialty food-additives to continue to grow. *Chem Eng News* 69(22):19–12.

29. Tiede, K., A. B. A. Boxall, S. P. Tear et al. 2008. Detection and characterization of engineered nanoparticles in food and the environment. *Food Addit Contam Part A* 25:795.

30. Wakabayashi, K., M. Nagao, H. Esumi, and T. Sugimura. 1992. Food-derived mutagens and carcinogens. *Cancer Res* 52:2092 S.

31. Weisskoff, M. G., N. Jain, H. Nie et al. 2009. A perspective study of bone lead concentration and death from all causes, cardiovascular diseases, and cancer in the Department of Veterans Affairs Normative Aging Study. *Circulation* 120:1050.

32. Wright, J. P., K. M. Dietrich, M. Douglas Ris et al. 2008. Association of prenatal and childhood blood lead concentrations with criminal arrests in early adulthood. *PLOS Med* 5(5):e101.

CASE BIBLIOGRAPHY

33. Davies, J. K., N. Ahktar, and E. Ranasinge. 2001. A juicy problem. *Lancet* 358:2126.

27 Vegetarianism and Other Popular Nutritional Practices

People have become increasingly conscious of health benefits related to nutrition. The heightened receptiveness of the "nutrition-conscious" population has created a fertile ground for food faddism to flourish. Food faddism is based on an exaggerated belief that certain diets and food supplements convey unique health benefits while certain foods should be eliminated from the diet because they are harmful. These fads are not always harmless. The consumer's misconception about health and nutrition and the vulnerability to misinformation are major contributors to an expanding market for quackery. Vegetarianism is becoming increasingly popular among health-conscious and environmentally conscious Americans. There is nothing wrong in following any diet as long as it provides adequate nutrition.

27.1 VEGETARIANISM

Vegetarianism is the consumption of a diet composed predominantly of plant foods.[8] It is widely practiced in many parts of the world and, therefore, is not considered as a special diet. Many vegetarians follow such a diet because of religious, cultural, economic, ethical, or other reasons. Traditional vegetarian diets and moderate avoidance of foods from animal sources pose fewer risks than do some of the newer regimes that involve extensive food avoidance and self-treatment for health problems. Recent epidemiological studies show that diet-related risk factors for several chronic diseases are lower among vegetarians than in those who include in their diet foods from animal sources.[7] Many people see it as a healthy way to eat, and the number of those who subscribe to vegetarianism is increasing considerably. These so-called new vegetarians comprise several diverse groups, differing from one another in their extremes of food avoidance and their affiliations with vegetarian-oriented groups. This has generated attention and concerns from the medical community.[6]

Dietary practices that fall under the heading of vegetarian are so varied that no broad generalization can be made about their safety and desirability. From the nutrition point of view, vegetarians can be classified as follows: vegans or strict vegetarians, who abstain from all forms of food from animal sources (e.g., red meat, poultry, fish, eggs, and dairy products); lacto-vegetarians (e.g., Trappist monks and vegetarians in India), who consume dairy products but not any of the other foods from animal sources; lacto-ovo vegetarians (e.g., Seventh-Day Adventists), who consume both dairy products and eggs; and pesco-vegetarians, who consume fish but abstain from other foods of animal origin. Individuals in each group can be well nourished, especially if reasonable precautions are taken to ensure an adequate intake of certain nutrients that may be limited in their diets, particularly in vegans; there are, however, some potential risks as well as benefits in vegetarian diets.[19]

27.1.1 POTENTIAL RISKS

27.1.1.1 Energy

Most vegetarian diets tend to be high in bulk and low in calories (Table 27.1). Therefore, meeting energy needs, particularly for growing children, may be difficult. As a group, vegetarians are leaner than nonvegetarians (those who do not restrict foods of animal origin).

TABLE 27.1
Potential Risks of a Vegetarian Diet

Nutrient Factor	Content in Plant Food Relative to Foods of Animal Origin
Calories	Generally low in plant foods
Protein	Low in one or more essential amino acids
Calcium	Generally low; milk and dairy products are major sources
Iron	Generally low; foods of animal origin are the best sources
Zinc	Bioavailability is low; foods of animal origin are good sources
Vitamin D	Absent
Vitamin B_2	Generally low; dairy products are good sources
Vitamin B_{12}	Absent in plant foods; foods of animal origin are the only sources for this vitamin

27.1.1.2 Protein

The protein quality in any single food from animal sources contains a favorable balance of essential amino acids required for growth and maintenance, and the proteins are considered complete. In contrast, proteins in any single plant food are partially or totally lacking in one or more of the essential amino acids and are considered as incomplete proteins. The biological value of such proteins is thereby reduced in proportion to their content of the limiting amino acids unless another protein is ingested to "complement" the amino acid imbalance. One exception is the protein found in soybeans, which is nearly as good as the protein found in foods of animal origin. The adequate intake of protein can be achieved by the inclusion of dairy products, eggs, or fish in a vegetarian diet. The vegan, however, deserves special attention, especially if protein needs are high, as they are in children and pregnant or lactating women. For their efficient use, all essential amino acids must be adequate at each meal. By simply combining different plant foods at the same meal, an adequate supply of complete proteins compatible to those present in foods of animal origin can be ensured. Examples are the consumption of nuts and seeds with legumes, legumes with cereal grains, and cereal grains with leafy vegetables.

27.1.1.3 Calcium

Milk and milk products are the major sources of calcium in American diets. Vegans and other vegetarians who avoid dairy products have low calcium intakes. Plant foods high in calcium include green leafy vegetables, legumes, almonds, and sesame seeds.

27.1.1.4 Iron

The best sources of iron are foods of animal origin. The heme form of iron present in meat is better absorbed by the body, while the iron from plant foods is not as well absorbed. The bioavailability may be further reduced by phytates in plant foods, but the relatively higher ascorbic acid content of most vegetarian diets promotes iron absorption by keeping the iron in reduced form. The prevalence of iron deficiency anemia is much higher among vegans than among nonvegetarians.

27.1.1.5 Zinc

A substantial amount of zinc is present in many plant foods, but the risk of deficiency is increased in vegans because phytates present in plant foods bind zinc and lower its bioavailability.

27.1.1.6 Vitamin D

Vitamin D is absent in plant foods but can be synthesized by an adequate exposure to sunlight and/or can be provided by fortified milk.

27.1.1.7 Vitamin B$_2$

Vegetarian diets are low in vitamin B$_2$, although usually not so inadequate as to produce clinical deficiency. Green leafy vegetables, legumes, and whole grains are relatively good sources of the nutrient.

27.1.1.8 Vitamin B$_{12}$

This vitamin is found almost exclusively in foods of animal origin.[9] Therefore, a vegan diet would lead to inadequate vitamin B$_{12}$ intake unless a vitamin supplement is taken.

27.1.1.9 Ensuring the Adequate Intake of Nutrients

The most important recommendation for all vegetarians is to maintain a wide variety in their diet. The greatest risk comes from relying on a single plant food source. Legumes are rich in protein, B vitamins, and iron; unrefined grains are good sources of carbohydrates, protein, vitamin B$_1$, iron, and trace minerals; nuts and other seeds provide protein, fat, B vitamins, and iron; and dark green vegetables are sources of calcium, riboflavin, and carotenes (the precursors of vitamin A).

27.1.2 POTENTIAL BENEFITS

A vegetarian diet is generally low in energy, saturated fat, and cholesterol, and high in fiber (Table 27.2). Therefore, it is thought that vegetarian populations tend to have ideal body weights, fewer diseases of the large bowel, and lower circulating cholesterol. Plant foods are also higher in magnesium, folic acid, and antioxidant nutrients such as vitamins E and C, carotenoids, and possibly other physiologically active substances that may have beneficial health effects. With reasonable caution, the vegetarian approach to eating can be well balanced nutritionally and can provide advantages that result in better health.

A vegetarian diet provides a wide range of health benefits.[14,17] A large body of scientific literature suggests that vegetarians have lower incidence of several chronic diseases such as hypertension, coronary heart disease, type 2 diabetes, obesity, osteoporosis, and diet-related cancers. According to studies in Dr. Dean Ornish's Multisite Cardiac Lifestyle Intervention Program, a low-fat vegetarian diet along with moderate exercise and stress management improves the function of the endothelium—the inner lining of arteries that is key to preventing heart attacks.[5,23] In African Americans, the consumption of nuts, fruits, and green salads is associated with a 40% lower risk of mortality. Large studies in England and Germany have shown that vegetarians are about 40% less likely to develop cancer compared to meat eaters. In the United States, studies of Seventh-day Adventists have shown that their lifestyle factors including a vegetarian diet increase longevity and quality of life.[26]

TABLE 27.2
Potential Benefits of a Vegetarian Diet

Nutrient Factor[a]	Benefit
Low in calories	May help maintain ideal body weight
Low in saturated fat	May reduce the risk of heart disease and cholesterol
High in folic acid	May reduce the risk of heart disease
High in potassium	May reduce the risk of hypertension
High in fiber	May reduce the risk of heart disease
High in antioxidants	May reduce the risk of several chronic diseases

[a] Nutrient content relative to foods of animal origin.

27.2 .MEDITERRANEAN DIET

Since the 1950s, health professionals have been collecting data on the diets of the people of the Mediterranean. The people of Greece, particularly Crete, had the longest life expectancy in the world until the 1960s, followed by Southern Italy, Spain, and France. Recent studies have confirmed that people who closely follow the Mediterranean diet live longer than other Europeans. There are at least six countries bordering the Mediterranean Sea and food habits vary between these countries according to culture, ethnic background, and region. But there are some characteristics common to all of them. These are listed as follows:

- Olive oil is used almost exclusively in Mediterranean cooking instead of butter, margarine, and other fats. More than any other food, olive oil represents the central position of the diet. It is rich in monounsaturated fats and antioxidants including vitamin E. Total fat in the Mediterranean diet is 25%–35% of calories with saturated fat at 8% or less of calories.
- High consumption of vegetables is a feature of this diet. Tomatoes have come under partic- ular scrutiny because they feature so heavily in Mediterranean food. Tomatoes are a major source of antioxidants, and heat processing such as cooking, as in the preparation of tomato sauces, increases the absorption of lycopene, one of the main antioxidants in tomatoes.
- High consumption of fruits is another major feature. Fresh fruit is the typical daily dessert.
- There is a high consumption of legumes, beans, nuts, and seeds in the diet.
- There is high consumption of unrefined cereal grains (including grain bread).
- Dairy products (principally cheese and yogurt) and poultry are consumed in low to moderate amounts.
- The consumption of eggs is zero to four weekly, and meat is consumed in lower amounts.
- Fish is consumed at least twice weekly. It is a source of ω-3 fatty acids.
- Wine is consumed in low to moderate amounts and usually taken with meals. Wine, especially red wine, contains a vast array of plant compounds with health-promoting properties.
- Lifestyle factors such as a relaxed attitude to eating, plenty of sunshine, and more physical activity are likely to be contributing factors to the overall healthy lifestyle of this region.

The benefits of the Mediterranean diet are as follows: Several studies have shown that the closer people followed the Mediterranean diet the less likely they were to die from either heart disease or cancer. Olive oil[4] with high levels of monounsaturated fatty acids and fruits and vegetables contain- ing beneficial fiber and antioxidants are protective against heart disease and cancer. Studies have also shown that five servings of fruits and vegetables daily reduce the risk of stroke by about 25%. People who mostly adhere to the Mediterranean diet are less likely to develop depression and age- related cognitive decline.[24] They have about a 40% lower risk of developing Alzheimer's disease. A recent study has shown that a calorie-restricted Mediterranean diet (as well as a low-carbohydrate diet) could be more effective for weight loss than a low-fat diet while also offering other benefits. Another study has shown that healthy people who follow the Mediterranean diet have a lower risk of developing type 2 diabetes.

Being physically active and eating a nutritious Mediterranean diet can help people control weight, lower blood pressure and cholesterol levels, reduce the risk of diabetes and heart disease, and basi- cally protect against chronic diseases.

27.3 KOSHER DIET

Kosher refers to a set of dietary laws that originated from the Old Testament and governs the selection and preparation of food.[18] Some foods, principally pork in the meat category and shellfish, are forbidden. Meat must come from animals that have been slaughtered in a ritually prescribed way. Blood must be extracted from the meat through salting or broiling. Fish do not have to be made kosher, but—probably out of superstition—even some fish are salted. Another dietary law prohibits cooking or eating meat and milk together. Two separate sets of utensils must be provided for the preparation, serving, and storing of milk and meat dishes. Kosher goods, whether sold by large companies or by corner butchers, must carry the certification of a rabbinical organization that has overseen the production and can vouch for its purity.

During the last 10 years, kosher foods have become popular among health-obsessed consumers of all faiths because they believe that kosher invariably means better. From the nutritional point of view, kosher meals, as long as they are well balanced, provide all the necessary nutrients in adequate quantities.

27.4 ZEN MACROBIOTIC DIET

The Zen macrobiotic diet was initiated by a native of Japan named Georges Ohsawa. This diet represents an example of a general trend toward natural and organic foods.[20,22] One of the reasons given for the popularity of these unusual diets is that they are considered to be a means of creating a spiritual awakening or rebirth. The dietary regimen proposed basically comprises 10 diets, ranging from the lowest level (diet −3), which includes 10% cereals, 30% vegetables, 10% soup, 30% foods of animal origin, 15% salads and fruits, and 5% desserts, to the highest level (diet 7), which is made up of 100% cereals. Followers of such diets believe that sequentially eliminating more and more specified foods from the diet as one progresses through the 10 stages will result in a happy, harmonious life.

The beginning level (diet −3) is a very well-balanced diet; but as it continues to the highest level (diet 7), animal products, fruits, vegetables, and so on are eliminated and so are essential nutrients. The Zen macrobiotic diet and philosophy are supposed to cure all diseases, but the individuals who persist in following the more rigid diet stand in great danger of incurring serious nutritional deficiencies, particularly as they progress to the highest level of dieting. The individual on such a diet is led to believe that any adverse condition that appears while following the diet is only temporary and disappears with continued adherence. Cases of scurvy, anemia, hypocalcemia, emaciation due to starvation, and other forms of malnutrition have been reported, including some deaths. The diet was quite popular in the 1970s, especially among young people, but has since faded.

27.5 ONE-EMPHASIS DIETS

There are many diets that are advertised on the premise that a particular food supposedly has magical powers and can lead to weight loss.[10] The one that became popular in the 1970s, and is still in use, is the grapefruit diet or the Mayo diet (no association to Mayo Clinic). While the diet consists of other foods, it calls for eating a grapefruit before each meal. It is claimed that grapefruits contain enzymes that are absorbed into the body and help to dissolve fat cells. There is no scientific basis for this theory because any enzyme would be digested in the intestinal tract like any other protein. Any weight loss can be explained by the boredom-related decrease in food intake. When an individual eats the same foods all the time, the quantity consumed is less. While these diets are convenient, relatively easy to follow, and may result in weight loss at least initially, little attention is given to weight maintenance. As such, any weight loss that occurs tends to be short-lived.

27.6 ORGANICALLY GROWN FOODS

The term organic traditionally refers to compounds of carbon. The use of the term organic in relation to food was originated by the late Jerome Rodale, an electrical contractor who decided to become an expert on farming and health. Organically grown foods are defined as foods grown without the use of any agricultural chemicals and processed without the use of food chemicals or additives.[16] The farming system excludes the use of synthetically compounded fertilizers, pesticides, growth regulators, and livestock feed additives. These foods are grown in soil supplemented only with natural matter (manure or compost) and mineral-bearing rocks, and depend on biological methods of pest control for protection. This is the way food was produced until the twentieth century when synthetic chemicals were introduced for the first time in food production. The recent style of food production using synthetic chemicals is referred to as "conventional."

The organic concept of farming has steadily gained popularity. It has been helped by an unfounded fear of pesticide residue in food and by misleading nutrition information. A few years back, organic farms were small family-run operations and organic food was available only in small retail stores or farmers' markets. Since the early 1990s, organic food production has grown at about 20% a year in the United States and many other countries. The public opinion that organic food is healthier than conventionally grown food is quite strong and is the main reason for the rapid growth in the organic food industry. In the United States in 2003, organic products were available in nearly 20,000 natural food stores and 73% of conventional grocery stores. In U.S. dollars worldwide, organic food sales jumped from $23 billion in 2002 to $52 billion in 2008. Many large food industries have entered the organic food business. Organic food accounts for about 2% of the food sales worldwide. The question is, however, do organically grown foods offer some kind of benefit?

27.6.1 NUTRITIONAL SUPERIORITY

It is often assumed that organic foods have special health-promoting properties. Claims are made that organically grown foods are nutritionally superior to foods grown under conventional agricultural methods. There is no consistent scientific evidence to support such an assumption; however, there is increasing evidence to support questions and concerns arising over the safety of foods grown by conventional farming methods.[27] The nutrient content of plant food (i.e., proteins, carbohydrates, fats, vitamins, and most minerals) is assumed to depend on the plant's genetic (hereditary) makeup and not on the environment in which it grows. Some foods labeled organic are not known to differ appreciably in nutrient composition from similar varieties grown in season using conventional methods. Regional soil patterns do reflect deficiencies of some trace minerals (i.e., these minerals are not required by plants, but they are essential for humans and animals) such as iodine, zinc, and selenium. Depending on geographic location, some of these specific mineral deficiencies may not change by following either method of farming. These deficiencies can be corrected by adding the lacking minerals to fertilizers or to food (i.e., iodide to salt).

The promoters of organic food suggest that all "natural" fertilizers (i.e., fertilizers without pesticides, herbicides, or any other added chemicals) are better able to nourish plants and therefore result in more nutritious, abundant, and quality-dense food. But, according to the opponents of the "organic debate," chemical fertilizers and genetic modifications are the most important contributors to the increase in world agricultural productivity over the past several years, and they are partly responsible for the abundance of food currently available to the growing population. Important questions remain, however; while conventional methods produce an abundance of food for a growing population, is that food measuring up to the same level of standards of quality and nutrition as 100% organically grown food?

Many factors impact the nutrient density of crops, whether they are grown organically or conventionally. Climate has an enormous impact on nutrient levels from one year to the next or from one region to the other. Patterns of rainfall and temperature, in particular, have a large impact on plant growth and development.

There are no well-controlled studies large enough to support any general conclusion regarding differences in nutrient levels of organic and conventionally grown foods.[21] But four analyses of U.S. and British nutrient content data have shown a decline in the content of some vitamins and minerals in fresh fruits and vegetables over the last 60 years during which the use of synthetic fertilizers and pesticides became common.[3] Other studies have shown lesser amounts but higher quality of proteins and higher amounts of carbohydrates in organic cereal grains. In addition, the vitamin C content was higher in the organic crop.

A study in Europe also found that organic food production methods result in high levels of nutritionally desirable compounds, such as vitamin C, iron, and magnesium. Organic animal products contain more polyunsaturated fatty acids. Some other studies report that there is no evidence that organic and conventional foods differ in concentrations of various nutrients. More well-controlled studies are needed to determine if there is any nutritional difference between the two types of foods.

When a plant is presented with a lot of nitrogen, it increases protein production and reduces carbohydrate formation. Because vitamin C is made from carbohydrates, the synthesis of vitamin C is also reduced. If there is more nitrogen than the plant can handle through increased protein production, the excess is accumulated as nitrate and stored in the green leafy part of the plant. This is the reason for higher content of nitrates in conventionally grown vegetables.

The use of chemical fertilizers has been shown to cause significant increase in protein content and decrease in amylose (carbohydrate) content in rice. This in turn may influence the texture, aroma, and flavor of cooked rice. Low-protein rice samples of the same culture are reported to be more flavorful than those with high protein. Basmati rice originated in India. It has a moderately firm cooked texture, is dry and not sticky after cooking, and has a unique aroma. It used to be grown only in certain regions of India and Pakistan. For the last 30 years, demand for Basmati rice has increased considerably worldwide. To meet this demand, rice is grown in different areas of India and some other countries with the use of fertilizers. The aroma has almost disappeared during recent years and the texture is not the same. These changes may be attributed to conventional methods of farming resulting in alterations in protein and amylose content, as well as the quality and taste of rice.

Thus, there is some evidence that major changes in agricultural methods may have an effect on the nutrient content of food. In view of the increasing demand for organic food, there is a need to collect and consider data in order to determine the differences between foods grown organically and conventionally.[15]

27.6.2 Safety of the Food Supply

The concern over the dangers of using pesticides,[2] inorganic fertilizers, and antibiotics in food production has encouraged people to turn to organically grown foods, which are produced without their use, although, of course, they are exposed to the same environmental pollutants as any other food. Even if a farmer grows his or her produce without pesticides or artificial fertilizers, there is no guarantee that it will be free of chemical residues, because pesticides can remain in the soil for years or can drift with rain from nearby farms. The nitrate levels in organic food are about 50% lower than those in conventional foods.

Organic foods may contain pesticide residues, perhaps as often as conventionally grown foods in some cases, although it is important to note that they may be present in much smaller amounts in organic foods (if at all, especially if grown on a 7-year-certified organic farm). However, all residues are within federal tolerance levels, which are set low to protect the consumers. More recent studies suggest that even small amounts of pesticides may have adverse health effects. Organic phosphate pesticides, while restricted or banned for home use, are widely used on a variety of crops. Residues of these pesticides are still routinely detected in food items consumed by young children. They can cause problems in neurological development during early childhood. A recent study has found the presence of pesticide metabolites in the urine samples of children consuming conventionally grown foods, and these metabolites were undetectable when children ate organic products. Higher levels of urinary pesticide metabolites have been linked to the incidence of attention deficit/hyperactivity disorder in children. Organic food seems to be a viable intervention to control pesticide exposure, at least in young children.

As far as poisons in the food supply go, many common "safe" foods contain naturally occurring toxicants, but these are usually present in minute amounts and pose no health hazard. Whether a food is poisonous is a matter of dosage. Thus, in this respect, those who consume organically grown foods may have no health advantage.

27.6.3 TASTE

It is also assumed that organically grown foods taste much better than conventionally grown foods. One study concluded by blind taste test that organic apples were sweeter. Firmness of organically grown apples was also rated higher than those grown conventionally. There are no objective tests to support or to disclaim the superior taste of organically grown foods.

27.6.4 COST

Organic farming techniques are relatively expensive. One major difference between organically grown and conventionally grown foods is that the former is often sold at relatively high prices to individuals who believe that this food is superior. People pay 50%–100% more for this type of foods than for their regular counterparts, and because these foods do not differ in looks, taste, or chemical analysis, the only assurance is the label stating that it is "organically grown." At the present time, there is more food being sold as organically grown than is actually grown organically, at least according to the 7 years it takes before a soil qualifies officially to be certified organic.

27.6.5 STANDARDS FOR ORGANICALLY GROWN PRODUCTS

Currently, the United States, Canada, European Union, Japan, and many other countries require producers to obtain special certifications to market food labeled as organic within their borders. In most countries, organic produce may not be genetically modified. Nanotechnology also may be excluded from certified organic food. In December 2000, the U.S. Department of Agriculture (USDA) released standards for organically grown agricultural products effective October 21, 2002.[11] The standards list the methods, practices, and substances that can be used in producing and handling crops, livestock, and processed products so that they can be labeled organic. It bans nearly all synthetic pesticides and fertilizers in the growing of organic foods, and bans the use of antibiotics and synthetic growth hormones in organic meat production. Foods cannot be called organic if ionizing radiation, sewage sludge fertilizer, or genetic engineering is used in its production. All agricultural products labeled organic must originate from farms or processors certified by a state or private agency accredited by the USDA, unless the farm or processor has annual sales less than US$5000.

Under the new regulations, the USDA has established four types of organic labels for foods: (1) "100% organic"—must contain only organic ingredients, and the USDA organic seal may be used on such products; (2) "organic"—must contain at least 95% organic ingredients by weight, and the USDA organic seal may be used on such products; (3) "products made with organic ingredients"—must contain at least 70% organic ingredients and up to three of them may be listed on the front of the package; and (4) "processed products with less than 70% organic ingredients"—this is listed on the information panel, but the word organic is not permitted on the front of the package.

Organic labeling is a marketing tool. It is not a statement about food safety. Nor is the term organic a value judgment about nutrition or quality. Currently, there are 12,200 organic farmers nationwide, and their numbers are increasing by 12% every year. Recent figures for the sales of various organic products and other relevant information are presented in Table 27.3.

Organic product sales in 2009 reached $26.6 billion. Of that figure, $24.8 billion represented organic food and $1.8 billion were for organic nonfoods. Organic fruits and vegetables,

TABLE 27.3
Organic Products for Consumer Use

Fruits	One of America's biggest organic products with >49,000 acres planted. Of the total organic fruits sold, grapes lead the pack with 39%, followed by apples (18%), citrus fruits (12%), and nuts (10%). From 1998 to 2000, fruit sales increased by 23%.
Vegetables	Second only to fruits as a mainstay of organic agriculture, with 48,000 acres in cultivation. The most popular is lettuce (12%), and tomatoes and carrots constitute 7% each of the acreage devoted to vegetables. From 1998 to 2000, sales increased by 23%.
Dairy	Milk and eggs are among the fastest-growing organic categories. Sales increased by 50% between 1994 and 1999, and by 96% between 1998 and 2000.
Grains	The market for organic wheat, rice, corn, barley, and oats has increased by 99% from 1998 to 2000 and now exceeds US$400 million/year. The demand for organic soybeans is increasing rapidly.
Meats	Organic livestock, except poultry, must be born on an organic farm. Two days after birth, the poultry must be moved to an organic farm. Livestock must consume 100% organic foods. Farmers may vaccinate livestock, but they may not use hormones or antibiotics. A sick animal treated with medicines is no longer organic. Access to outdoors is mandatory. From 1998 to 2000, the sales increased by 71%.
Snacks	Nutrition bars, chips, and salsa sales from 1998 to 2000 increased by 86%.
Wines and beers	Organic wine does not contain sulfites, and its grapes are grown without methyl bromide, an all-purpose pesticide. Wine and beer sales increased by 30% from 1998 to 2000.
Nonfood items	Sales of organic diapers, baby clothes and bedding, and organic personal care (aromatherapy) increased by 29% from 1998 to 2000.

which represent 38% of total organic food sales, reached nearly $9.5 billion in sales in 2009, up 11.4% from 2008 sales. Most notably, organic fruits and vegetables now represent 11.4% of all U.S. fruits and vegetables.

It is important to note that the soil currently used for conventional farming may take 5–7 years or longer to reform for pesticides to disappear. So if the same land is then used for organic farming immediately, even if the product is produced strictly with the use of organic practices it may still contain detectable levels of pesticides. Hence, because of the explosion in recent years of organic products in the market and with the variety of vendors jumping on the organic bandwagon for commercial purposes, there may be differences in quality, taste, color, and texture (tough or tender?) in some of these so-called organics, depending on whether the company producing the product took a full 7 years before rightfully labeling its product organic.

In any case, from a purely lay perspective, many people feel that any food grown in healthy soil over any time period without the use of chemicals, pesticides, herbicides, or GM seeds (which have not been fully researched) is food that is much safer to eat over strictly conventionally grown food using these man-made unnatural and toxic substances. Indeed, for many who have switched to buying organic produce, for example, a sweet and juicy pear or a head of purple cabbage, the "proof" is found in the richer taste, color, and added tenderness generally found in fully organically grown produce.

27.7 NATURAL FOODS

Natural foods are considered to be those foods that are grown naturally and are in their original state or have minimal refinement and processing. Canning, freezing, dehydrating, and using preservatives, emulsifiers, and artificial ingredients are regarded as processing of food. Traditional methods of smoking, roasting, drying, and curing meats, as well as salting and fermenting, are considered acceptable. Some examples of natural foods include whole grain breads and cereals, fresh fruits and vegetables, raw milk, unrefined sugar, honey, and molasses. Examples of foods that should not be labeled natural include salmon that contains the dyes cantaxanthin and astaxanthin and milk that contains added synthetic vitamins. Any coloring, even if it is from a natural source, precludes the natural label.

The Food and Drug Administration (FDA) does not have an official definition for the term "natural." It does not encourage the use of the term on food labels because the word is potentially ambiguous and may unjustifiably imply superior quality or safety. The claims made for organically grown foods, and arguments against such claims, apply equally well to natural foods. Because there is no legal meaning for natural foods, manufacturers can include ingredients that may not be considered natural by some consumers.

The word natural has become a sales gimmick. Sometimes the labels of natural or organic products can be misleading. For instance, rose hips vitamin C tablets may contain natural rose hips combined with synthetic ascorbic acid because natural extracts are too bulky for a pill or capsule. Rose hips contain only about 2% vitamin C. Without the addition of synthetic ascorbic acid, the tablet's size would be as big as a golf ball. Also, natural vitamins of the B group often consist of synthetic chemicals added to natural bases. The advocates of natural foods claim that they are healthier than ordinary foods.

From the standpoint of nutrition, vitamins from natural sources have no nutritional superiority over synthetic vitamins, nor do other natural foods, organic foods, or health foods possess unique nutritional attributes above and beyond those in conventional foods. Nutrients from both types of food react similarly in the body. Furthermore, all minerals are natural because the same elements are present in foods and in the earth.

Natural foods are heavily advertised and promoted. Consumers are misinformed that these foods are more nutritious and somehow better.[12] Like organic foods, natural foods are more expensive.

27.8 HEALTH FOODS

Health foods are self-prescribed food items that users believe have special properties to promote health, or to prevent or cure diseases. The connotation is that health foods are invested with special health-promoting properties. Emphasis is generally placed on particular foods rather than on nutrients. The term health food encompasses both organic and natural foods, along with certain other foods. The specific foods vary, but representative items include kelp (seaweed), ginseng, mineral water, royal jelly from beehives, buckwheat, yogurt, raw milk, honey, bran, raw sugar, sunflower seed, and wheat germ.

There is nothing wrong with the use of most items in the health food group; however, there are some that may have adverse effects if consumed in large quantities. The concern is regarding the unfounded and exaggerated claims that a certain food has attributes for maintaining health and for the prevention and cure of diseases. Their efficacy is usually attributed to the presence of some protective or accessory food factor that is necessary for health but is absent from other foods. There is neither any evidence that people who eat health foods enjoy better health nor that special deficiency diseases exist in the general population.

27.9 MEGADOSES OF VITAMINS AND NONVITAMINS

27.9.1 Megadoses of Vitamins

Megavitamin is a term used originally by nonmedical people to refer to large doses of vitamins. The megavitamin concept is based on the false assumptions that "If a little is good, more is better"; vitamins in large doses will prevent or cure diseases and will produce "optimal" health beyond that resulting from a nutritionally adequate diet; and individual or biochemical variability justifies the intake of high doses of vitamins. The dangers associated with high doses of fat-soluble vitamins are well documented. Most water-soluble vitamins are tolerated well in doses that exceed the amounts needed. This is because they are either degraded rapidly or are eliminated efficiently in the urine. Nevertheless, if a large dose is administered so as to increase the vitamin concentration in tissues, any vitamin may be toxic. Excess pyridoxine interferes with the utilization of riboflavin, and vitamin B_{12} may be inactivated by high doses of ascorbic acid. In doses higher than those recommended for nutritional needs but below the levels that result in toxicity, vitamins, like many other chemicals, may exert pharmacological actions. Examples include the ability of niacin to lower blood cholesterol and that of ascorbic acid to inhibit the growth of microorganisms in the urinary tract through the acidification of urine with ascorbic acid.

There are mechanisms available to protect against large doses of vitamins, but when the amount exceeds a certain limit the possibility for adverse effects exists. The protective mechanisms and adverse effects are described in Sections 27.9.1.1 and 27.9.1.2 with vitamin C as an example.

27.9.1.1   Protective Mechanisms

When large doses of vitamin C are consumed, there are usually no serious consequences because the body has mechanisms to prevent marked elevations of the levels of vitamins in the blood:

Nature's protection: Few natural foods contain vitamin C in high enough concentrations to cause toxicity. Foods such as lettuce and orange juice are rich in this vitamin, but there is a limit on the amount of these foods one can consume.

Absorption control: The absorption of the vitamin is very efficient in small doses, but the efficiency declines with higher doses.

Renal threshold: When the plasma level of ascorbic acid is low, very little of it is excreted in the urine because of the very effective tubular reabsorption. When plasma levels rise above the renal threshold for this vitamin (1.7 mg/dL), the rate of the vitamin excreted rises abruptly. This has the effect of limiting the level of ascorbic acid in the blood.

Induction of catabolic mechanism: The activity of the enzyme that inactivates the vitamin increases with higher blood levels of the vitamin. This explains the findings of near-normal blood levels of the vitamin in individuals who take large amounts. It also explains the occurrence of scurvy in individuals who reduce their intake of larger doses of the vitamin abruptly even though their intake level is adequate for a normal person.

27.9.1.2   Undesirable Effects

The undesirable effects of consuming vitamins in high doses are as follows:

Reproduction: There are reports that high doses of vitamins may be harmful in pregnancy. Also the newborn may develop scurvy due to the conditioning of its body to a high intake.

Diabetes: Large doses can lower the urinary pH and cause false-negative or false-positive tests for glucose in urine.

Anticoagulants: Ascorbic acid can reverse the anticoagulant effect of heparin.

Urinary stones: Ascorbic acid is metabolized to oxalate. Calcium oxalate is a common constituent of kidney stones. People predisposed to kidney stones should avoid high doses (>500 mg) of ascorbic acid.

High-altitude hypoxia: There is impaired high-altitude performance with high doses of the vitamin.

Iron: High doses of ascorbic acid enhance the intestinal absorption of iron.

The intake of very large doses of vitamins provides no unique nutritional benefit and can lead to numerous undesirable effects ranging from minor to serious.[13] Large doses are justified in certain conditions such as vitamin-dependent genetic diseases and in diseases associated with the defective transport of vitamins across cell membranes.

27.9.2   NONVITAMINS

27.9.2.1   Laetrile

Laetrile is a name applied to a substance found in the seeds of stone fruits such as apricots, peaches, plums, and to a lesser extent, almonds. This substance is amygdalin and is a cyanogenic glycoside. It contains 6% cyanide by weight. It has been incorrectly called vitamin B_{17}, although it bears no resemblance to a vitamin. Laetrile was originally espoused as a cancer cure and later was assumed to control rather than cure cancer. Several current studies on laetrile show that it does not benefit patients with cancer.

27.9.2.2   Pangamic Acid

Pangamic acid is an unidentified and variable product allegedly isolated from apricot kernels; it is erroneously referred to as vitamin B_{15}. There is no such vitamin. It is frequently recommended in lay press as an aid to athletic performance, as well as for the treatment of various diseases. The product is marketed as a dietary supplement as well as a drug for the treatment of cancer, hepatitis, heart disease, alcoholism, allergies, and some other conditions. Pangamic acid, however, has no known value for humans.

27.10   HAIR ANALYSIS

Hair analysis is based on the hypothesis that nutritional status (e.g., whether any deficiencies exist) can be determined by assaying the concentrations of vitamins and minerals in a hair sample. An increasing number of commercial laboratories have been set up to assess an individual's nutritional status by multielement hair analysis. In many cases, the finding of low levels of vitamins and metals in hair is exaggerated, and megadoses of these nutrients are prescribed to correct the so-called metabolic imbalances or alleged deficiencies uncovered by the analysis. Hair analysis has been used to detect certain types of heavy metal poisoning (i.e., lead, arsenic, mercury) in the population. However, very little is known about the extent to which hair concentrations of various elements correlate with their concentrations in the blood and the tissues. Furthermore, the relevance of hair vitamin and mineral concentrations to health and disease is unclear. For most minerals, even the normal range of concentration in the hair is unknown. One factor that interferes with the reproducibility and the validity of hair analysis is that hair is continuously exposed to the external environment. As shampoo contains zinc or selenium, this may significantly alter the hair content of these minerals. Dyeing, bleaching, and permanent waving procedures may also alter hair mineral concentrations.

To determine the value of hair analysis, an investigator sent identical hair samples from two healthy teenagers to several commercial hair analysis laboratories. The laboratories disagreed on the mineral content of the identical samples, as well as on what the "normal" values should be. The laboratories sent computerized interpretation of the presumed mineral deficiencies that these teenagers supposedly had. They recommended various quantities of different supplements to correct the deficiencies. Hair analysis is worthless for assessing vitamin status and is of limited value for assessing mineral content.[1]

L-Tryptophan Use and the Eosinophilia–Myalgia Syndrome—A Case

A 65-year-old man was admitted to a hospital in February 1990; he complained of skin rash, pruritus, and weakness. He was well until early October 1989, when he developed swelling of his hands and feet; diuretics provided no relief. Shortly thereafter, he noted pruritus and erythema, initially involving only the lower extremities, but gradually spreading to the trunk and the upper extremities, sparing the hands. He further reported a burning sensation and "shooting pains" in the legs and progressive muscular weakness, which was described as decreased strength in both hands, decreased stride length, and difficulty rising from chairs and climbing stairs. He reported taking tryptophan (3000 mg every night) for insomnia from May 1989. There was no other known toxic exposure or history of recent travel.

Physical examination showed an elderly man with prominent oral-buccal dyskinesia. The extremities were edematous, and the buttocks and the lower back were erythematous. Neurological examination showed a peripheral sensory neuropathy and weakness in the proximal muscle groups. Laboratory tests showed a hematocrit of 35% vol/vol (normal: 42%–50%), white blood cell count of 36,450/mm^3 (normal: 5,000–10,000 mm^3), and a normal platelet count. The eosinophil count was 13,851/mm^3. Other routine tests were normal.

The dyskinesia was attributed to the patient's medications, which were adjusted in dosage. The eosinophilia and neuromuscular abnormalities were recognized as a manifestation of eosinophilia–myalgia syndrome (EMS), and the patient was told to stop taking L-tryptophan supplements.[29,30] In the ensuing months, the patient's white blood cell count fell to 9100/mm^3, and the eosinophilia disappeared.

Background of Eosinophilia–Myalgia Syndrome

Tryptophan has been used for insomnia and depression, and to improve athletic performance. L-tryptophan was sold as a food supplement during the 1980s to induce sleep naturally, because this amino acid produced serotonin in the brain, similar to the role of milk as a sleep inducer. The compound 5-hydroxytryptophan has been available as an aid for insomnia, depression, obesity, and for children with attention deficit disorder.

Food supplements such as amino acids are often manufactured by the fermentative process, in which large quantities of bacteria are grown in vats and the food supplement is extracted from the bacteria and purified. Tryptophan has been produced in this way for many years. In the late 1980s, the company Showa Denko KK of Japan genetically engineered bacteria to greatly increase the production of tryptophan. These bacteria were used in the commercial production of tryptophan, and the product was introduced in the U.S. market in 1988.

In October 1989, the health department in New Mexico was notified of three female patients who sought medical treatment for sets of similar symptoms. These women had all taken L-tryptophan produced by the aforementioned Japanese company. Within weeks, a nationwide outbreak of this disease occurred. The disease was termed EMS because the initial symptoms were elevated eosinophils and myalgia (muscle pain). Over time, many other symptoms developed in patients that led, in some cases, to death; in many other cases, these led to serious paralysis and neurological problems, painful swelling, cracking of the skin, memory and cognitive defects, etc. The sale of all brands of L-tryptophan was banned in the United States in November 1989, and with that a precipitous fall was observed in the incidence of EMS. In 1989, for the purpose of nationwide surveillance, the U.S. Centers for Disease Control (CDC) defined this syndrome according to three criteria: (1) a blood eosinophil count of greater than 1000 cells/mm^3, (2) incapacitating myalgia, and (3) no evidence of infection (e.g., trichinosis) or neoplastic conditions that would account for these findings.

By July 1991, 1543 cases of EMS were reported to the CDC. However, estimates indicated that 5,000–10,000 people actually had EMS. At least 38 deaths were attributed to EMS. Of the patients reported to have EMS, 97% were white and 84% were females. The disease occurred most commonly in people aged 35–60 years. Patients with EMS were exposed to L-tryptophan from 2 weeks to 9 years, with a median dose exposure of 6 months. The daily dose varied from 500 to 11,500 mg, with a median dose of 1250 mg. No correlation was observed between the development of the disease and the duration or dose of L-tryptophan.

Several cases of EMS were reported in other parts of the world including the United Kingdom, France, Israel, Japan, Germany, and Canada. Cohort studies performed during the epidemic estimated the incidence rates for EMS among users of L-tryptophan to be 0.5%–0.9%, depending on the product lot of the L-tryptophan ingested. Since the epidemic of 1989–1991, only a few cases have been reported.

In epidemiological studies, more than 95% of the cases of EMS were traced to L-tryptophan supplied by Showa Denko KK. However, many people who consumed L-tryptophan from the implicated lot (44% in one study) did not develop the disease. Also, several cases of EMS and the related disease eosinophilic ascites have occurred prior to and after the 1989 epidemic. Clinical syndromes indistinguishable from EMS have been identified in persons consuming 5-hydroxytryptophan, which is not made in the same way as L-tryptophan (e.g., via fermentation). The EMS also has many similarities to the toxic oil syndrome, an epidemic disorder associated with the ingestion of adulterated rapeseed oil that swept Spain during the summer of 1981 and affected over 20,000 persons.[28] The responsible toxic compound and its mechanism of action are not known, but aniline and anilide–oil complex are suspected.

Numerous trace-level impurities have been identified in the L-tryptophan implicated in many of the EMS cases. The most prominent of these is 1,1-ethylidenebis (L-tryptophan; EBT). Studies in rats showed that EBT caused some, but not all, of the pathological effects associated with EMS. These data, as well as data from a number of experiments employing different strains or species of animals, suggest that EMS may be caused by L-tryptophan in high doses, impurities in L-tryptophan, or a combination of the two in association with other, as yet unknown external factors. Furthermore, results from published studies suggest that the risk of developing EMS may be linked in part to different patterns of xenobiotic metabolism and immune response genes in patients with EMS.

Tryptophan is an essential amino acid and its minimal daily requirement for adults is 3.5 mg/kg body weight. The average Western diet provides 1–3 g/day of tryptophan and there is no need to supplement this nutrient. Single amino acids do not occur naturally and offer no benefits; they can be harmful. The serious nature of the disease described in this case necessitates that caution be exercised in the use of tryptophan- and 5-hydroxytryptophan-containing nutritional supplements.

REFERENCES

1. Barrett, S. 1985. Commercial hair analysis. Science or scam? *J Amer Med Ass* 254:1041.
2. Bouchard, M. F., D. C. Bellinger, R. O. Wright, and M. G. Weisskopf. 2010. Attention-deficit/hyperactivity disorder and urinary metabolites of organophoshate pesticides. *Pediatrics* 125:1270.
3. Bourn, D., and J. Prescott. 2002. A comparison of the nutritional value, sensory qualities, and food safety of organically and conventionally produced foods. *Crit Rev Food Sci Nutr* 42(1):1.
4. Covas, M. I. 2007. Olive oil and the cardiovascular system. *Pharmacol Res* 55:175.
5. Dodd, H. S., R. Bharadwaj, V. Sajja et al. 2010. Effect of intensive lifestyle changes on endothelial function and on inflammatory markers of atherosclerosis. *Amer J Cardiol* 105:362.
6. Dwyer, J. T. 1994. Vegetarian eating patterns: Science, values and food choices—where do we go from here? *Am J Clin Nutr* 59:1255S.
7. Gu, Y., J. Nieves, Y. Stern et al. 2010. Food combination and Alzheimer's disease risk: A protective diet. *Arch. Neurol* 67:699.
8. Gustafson, N. 1997. *Vegetarian Nutrition.* 2nd ed. Eureka, CA: Nutrition Dimension.
9. Herbert, V. 1988. Vitamin B12: Plant sources, requirements, and assay. *Am J Clin Nutr* 46:852.
10. Herbert, V., and T. S. Kasdan. 1994. Misleading nutrition claims and their gurus. *Nutr Today* 29(3):28.

11. Hileman, B. 2001. After long struggle, standards for organic food are finalized. *Chem Eng News* (79)1:24.

12. Hiscow, H. B. 1983. Does being natural make it good? *N Engl J Med* 308:1474.

13. Jukes, T. H. 1975. Megavitamin therapy. *J Amer Med Ass* 233:550.

14. Key, T. M., P. N. Appleby, and M. A. Rosell. 2006. Health effects of vegetarian and vegan diets. *Proc Nutr Soc* 65:35.

15. Lairon, D. 2010. Nutritional quality and safety of organic food. A review. *Agron Sustain Dev* 30:33.

16. Leverton, R. M. 1974. Organic, inorganic: What they mean. In *Yearbook of Agriculture*, 70–73. U. S. Department of Agriculture, Washington, DC: Government Printing Office.

17. Mangels, M. R. 2009. Position of the American Dietetic Association: Vegetarian diets. *J Amer Diet Assoc* 109:1266.

18. Nathan, J. 1979. *The Jewish Holiday Kitchen*. New York: Schocken Books Inc.

19. National Institute of Nutrition (Canada). 1990. Risks and benefits of vegetarian diets. *Nutr Today* 25(3):27.

20. Ohsawa, G. 1991. *Macrobiotics: An Invitation to Health and Happiness*. San Francisco: Macrobiotic Foundation.

21. Paull, J., and K. Lyons. 2008. Nanotechnology: The next challenge for organics. *J Org Syst* 3(1):3.

22. Robson, J. R. K. 1982. Zen macrobiotic diets. In *Adverse Effects of Foods*, ed. E. F. P. Jellife and D. B. Jellife, New York: Plenum.

23. Shai, I., D. Schwartzfuchs, Y. Henkin et al. 2008. Weight loss with a low-fat diet. *New Engl J Med* 359:229.

24. Sanchez-Villegas, A., M. Delgado-Rodriguez, A. Alonso et al. 2009. Association of the Mediterranean dietary pattern with the incidence of depression. The Seguimiento Universidad de Navarra/University of Navarra Follow-up (SUN) Cohort. *Arch Gen Psychiatry* 66:2090.

25. Southgate, D. A. T. 1984. Natural or unnatural foods? *Br Med J* 288:881.

26. Walter, P. 1997. Effects of vegetarian diets on aging and longevity. *Nutr Rev* 55(11):561.

27. Williams, C. M. 2002. Nutritional quality of organic foods: Shades of grey or shades of green? *Proc Nutr Society* 61(1):19.

CASE BIBLIOGRAPHY

28. Kilbourne, E. M., J. G. Rigau-Perez, C. W. Heath, M. M. Zack, H. Falk, M. Martin-Marcos, and A. De Carlos. 1983. Clinical epidemiology of toxic-oil syndrome. *N Engl J Med* 309:1408.

29. Sairam, S., and J. R. Lisse. 2002. Eosinophilia–myalgia syndrome. *eMedicine* 1:1–10.

30. Shocker, I. D., and K. Golar. 1990. L-tryptophan use and the eosinophilia–myalgia syndrome. *Nutr Rev* 48:313.

28 Nutritional Aspects of Biotransformation

Our diet contains not only nutrients such as carbohydrates, fats, proteins, vitamins, and minerals, but also several nonnutrient substances, some of which have never been identified. The number and variety of chemicals occurring naturally in foods are enormous. We are also exposed to a variety of chemicals, including food additives, drugs, insecticides, industrial chemicals, and pollutants collectively called xenobiotics (from Greek: *xenos*, foreign; *bios*, life). In addition, we produce our own toxins as normal breakdown products of tissue components; bilirubin, a product of heme, is an example. Despite the continual barrage of toxic materials that enter our body, we manage to remain viable because of a number of enzymes that oxidize, rearrange, and conjugate these toxins and thereby prepare them for rapid elimination.

Substances that are lipid soluble tend to accumulate in mammalian organisms and can remain in the body for many months or even years. After filtration at the renal glomerulus, most lipid-soluble substances largely escape excretion from the body because they are readily reabsorbed from the filtrate by diffusion through the renal tubules. The primary purpose of detoxication is to convert toxic substances into more polar compounds, which are thus less lipid soluble. The object is to decrease the permeability of the compound through the lipid membranes, thus protecting the cell interior, and also to increase the water solubility and hence the excretion of the compound from the body via the urine or bile depending on molecular size. In general, the detoxication process decreases or abolishes the toxicity of the compound. In a number of examples, however, the detoxified products are more toxic than the parent compounds. This is particularly true of some chemical carcinogens, organophosphate insecticides, and a number of compounds that cause cell death in the lung, liver, and kidney. Therefore, biotransformation is the term commonly used for the process that involves not only a reduction in toxicity but also an increase in toxicity.

Nutrients in the diet are metabolized, used for energy or for the synthesis of some compounds of importance, and then are excreted. In patients with some genetically determined defects of intermediary metabolism, certain nutrients ingested in normal amounts may cause toxicity and/or deficiency of another nutrient. For example, in patients with phenylketonuria, the failure to metabolize phenylalanine by normal pathway results in mental retardation unless the intake of phenylalanine is restricted promptly when the disease is diagnosed after neonatal screening and maintained at least until 10 years of age. Tyrosine becomes an essential nutrient for these patients. In the case of nonnutrient substances, such as drugs that are taken for specific purposes, they have to be metabolized and excreted. If not, they can continue to act indefinitely. Likewise, other foreign compounds that may enter the body, such as food contaminants and industrial chemicals, are potentially toxic if they accumulate in the body and have to be metabolized. If there is a deficiency or an absence of a particular enzyme required for metabolism, the compound or its metabolite may remain in the body and may be toxic.

Refsum's disease is a rare, inherited neurodegenerative disorder in the catabolism of phytanic acid, a lipid of exogenous origin. Phytanic acid is a 20-carbon fatty acid, 16 of which are present in straight chain (Figure 28.1). It has four methyl bases occurring at carbon 3, 7, 11, and 15 (counting

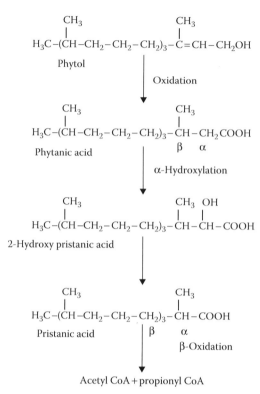

FIGURE 28.1 Metabolism of phytol and phytanic acid. Patients with Refsum's disease are deficient in a hydroxylase enzyme and accumulate phytanic acid in their tissues.

from the COOH group). It is formed from phytol, a component of many foods that are derived from plants. The structure of phytol corresponds to that of phytanic acid except that at carbon 1 there is an alcohol rather than the COOH group. When phytol is ingested, it is oxidized in the body to phytanic acid. This is part of a normal catabolic pathway for phytol, and further degradation of phytanic acid ensures that neither phytol nor any of its derivatives accumulate in the body. Normal human plasma contains traces of phytanic acid (less than 0.3 mg/100 mL) that are generally not detected.

Phytanic acid metabolism involves an initial α-hydroxylation followed by dehydrogenation and decarboxylation in which the COOH group is removed as carbon dioxide to yield α-hydroxy phytanic acid (pristanic acid), which undergoes a series of β-oxidation steps for the further degradation of this compound. β-oxidation of phytanic acid cannot occur prior to its conversion to pristanic acid because of the presence of a methyl group on the β-carbon. After α-hydroxylation, the newly formed pristanic acid does not have a methyl group on the β-carbon and, therefore, β-oxidation can proceed. Patients with Refsum's disease lack the α-hydroxylating enzyme and accumulate large quantities of phytanic[20] acid in their tissues and plasma (5%–30% of the total fatty acids in plasma). The accumulation of this acid has been suggested to cause slow but progressive neurological deterioration. It is not known at this time how this metabolic abnormality produces neurological damage, cerebellar degeneration, or peripheral neuropathy. The simplest hypothesis remains that the incorporation of the multiple-branched "thorny" phytanic acid molecule into tissue lipids in place of the normal straight-chain fatty acid interferes with the function of myelin or at least increases its susceptibility to damage. Serum phytanic acid levels may be controlled and symptoms alleviated by restricting its intake and that of phytol. The lipid is found primarily in dairy and ruminant fats and is derived from phytol of chlorophyll.

28.1 DETOXICATION PROCESS

Foreign compounds as well as toxins of endogenous origin are metabolized by a rather small number of reactions.[5] After absorption, the portal system delivers the xenobiotics to the liver, which primarily removes and metabolizes these compounds; however, metabolism in other tissues such as the intestine, kidney, lung, brain, and skin is also known to occur. The chemical reactions of enzymatic biotransformation are classified as either Phase I or Phase II reactions (Figure 28.2). Phase I reactions convert the parent compound to a polar metabolite by oxidation, reduction, or hydrolysis. The resulting metabolite may be nontoxic, less toxic, or occasionally more toxic than the parent compound. The substance acquires groups such as OH, COOH, NH_2, and SH, which enables it to undergo Phase II consisting of synthetic reactions. Phase II reactions involve the coupling of the parent substance or its metabolite with an endogenous substrate such as glucuronate, glycine, or glutathione. Nearly always, the conjugated compound is devoid of pharmacological (or biological) activity, but there are exceptions. Occasionally, a conjugated compound may be more toxic than the original substrate.

The net result of Phase I and Phase II reactions is to greatly decrease the toxicity and increase the excretability of toxic substances.

28.1.1 PHASE I REACTIONS

28.1.1.1 Oxidation

The oxidation of xenobiotics is achieved either by the removal of hydrogen (dehydrogenation) or the addition of oxygen. There are enzymes that catalyze the oxidation of a variety of aliphatic alcohols. Alcohol dehydrogenase, which is present in liver cytosol, in the presence of nicotinamide adenine dinucleotide (NAD) catalyzes the following reaction:

$$\text{Ethyl alcohol} + \text{NAD} \rightarrow \text{Acetaldehyde} + \text{NADH}$$

However, aldehydes are also toxic because of their chemical reactivity under physiological conditions. Acetaldehyde dehydrogenase converts acetaldehyde in the presence of NAD to acetic acid, which can be further oxidized to carbon dioxide and water or can be used for the synthesis of physiological compounds. Ethyl alcohol is an example of a compound that appears to be metabolized mainly by Phase I reaction. The fact that methyl alcohol yields intermediate toxic products (formaldehyde and formic acid) in the same kind of oxidation emphasizes that these reactions are general metabolic mechanisms that may fall short of total detoxication.

Monoamine oxidase (MAO), a mitochondrial enzyme found in all tissues except erythrocytes, oxidatively deaminates both endogenous amines (e.g., epinephrine, norepinephrine, and serotonin) and exogenous amines to their corresponding aldehydes. MAO has an important protective function in coping with our chemical environment such as the metabolism of tyramine that is present in cheese and some other foods.

The most important enzyme systems involved in Phase I reactions are the cytochrome P450-containing monooxygenases, also called mixed function oxidases (MFOs), which are localized in the hepatic endoplasmic reticulum. This system is composed of two enzymes: a heme protein called cytochrome P450 and a flavin enzyme called cytochrome P450 reductase. The enzyme

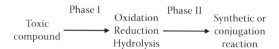

FIGURE 28.2 Phase I and Phase II of enzymatic biotransformation.

system requires NADPH and molecular oxygen. Cytochrome P450 gets its name from the fact that in its reduced form it binds carbon monoxide and then absorbs light most intensely at a wavelength of 450 nm.

Cytochrome P450 represents a family of heme-protein isoenzymes that have catalytic activity toward thousands of substrates. These include several drugs, small chemicals (e.g., benzopyrene present in city smog, cigarette smoke, and charcoal-broiled foods), biphenyl-halogenated hydrocarbons (e.g., polychlorinated and polybrominated biphenyls), insecticides, chemicals found in cosmetics, perfumes and hair dyes, and mutagens (e.g., nitrosamines). These enzymes also act on endogenously synthesized compounds such as steroids and fatty acids. The enzymes are present in all mammalian cell types except mature red blood cells and skeletal muscle cells. The liver has the highest concentration of total cytochrome P450 concentration of any organ and is thus the main site of xenobiotic metabolism. The reactions catalyzed by the monooxygenases include N- and O-dealkylation, aromatic ring and side-chain hydroxylation, sulfoxide formation, N-oxidation, N-hydroxylation, deamination of primary and secondary amines, and the replacement of a sulfur atom by an oxygen atom. In a single species of animals, there is only one cytochrome P450 reductase, but there are many different isoforms of cytochrome P450, which presumably are responsible for the variety of substrate specificity. Substrates of cytochrome P450 vary widely in structure, but all are highly lipid soluble. The enzyme is thus valuable in the initial conversion of xenobiotics to more polar compounds, which can be eliminated either directly or after conjugation.

Briefly, oxidized (Fe^{3+}) cytochrome P450 combines with a substrate to form a complex. NADPH donates an electron to the flavoprotein cytochrome P450 reductase, which, in turn, reduces iron to ferrous (Fe^{2+}) state in the cytochrome P450–substrate complex. The ferrous form of the iron then binds to a molecule of oxygen. A second electron is introduced from NADPH via the same flavoprotein reductase; this serves to reduce molecular oxygen and form an activated oxygen–cytochrome P450–substrate complex. This complex, in turn, transfers one atom of oxygen to the substrate to form the oxidized product, which is released, freeing the cytochrome P450 enzyme to repeat the cycle.

28.1.1.2 Reduction

Enzymes in the endoplasmic reticulum and cytosol of the liver and other tissues can catalyze the reduction of the nitro group (e.g., chloramphenicol → arylamine) and cleavage and reduction of an azo linkage (e.g., prontosil to sulfanilamide). The latter is an example of the transformation of an inactive form of the drug (prontosil) to the active form (sulfanilamide); however, most of the reactions lead to inactivation. The azo group is also present in food dyes, many of which are metabolized by this route.

28.1.1.3 Hydrolysis

Liver and other tissues contain a number of nonspecific esterases and amidases that can hydrolyze ester and amide linkages in foreign compounds. Procaine is acted upon by choline esterase to give p-aminobenzoic acid and diethylaminoethanol. Aspirin (acetylsalicylic acid) undergoes hydrolysis, forming acetate and salicylic acid. Acetate is either oxidized or used for the synthesis of physiological compounds, and salicylic acid is excreted as such or in conjugated form by the kidney.

28.1.1.4 Role of Epoxide Hydrolase

Cytochrome P450-containing monooxygenases can metabolize aromatic compounds to their corresponding epoxides. These are highly reactive chemical species able to form covalent bonds with nucleophilic functional groups of nucleic acids, proteins, or other biological macromolecules producing mutagens. An enzyme, epoxide hydratase (hydrolase), which is present in the endoplasmic reticulum, catalyzes the conversion of these epoxides to their corresponding dihydrodiols, which are less reactive and can be readily eliminated from the cells by undergoing conjugation with endogenous compounds. The close association of epoxide hydratase with cytochrome P450 in the endoplasmic reticulum may play an important role in the detoxication of these reactive epoxides.

28.1.2 Phase II Reactions

After xenobiotics are enzymatically oxidized, reduced, or hydrolyzed, the metabolites formed often contain one or more reactive chemical groups, which are amenable to conjugation reactions. The resulting newly formed compound is, in general, biologically inactive and more water soluble than the parent compound. Thus, conjugation reactions not only decrease the biological activity of xenobiotics but also increase their rate of excretion. The most common endogenous compounds used for conjugation are glucuronic acid, glycine, cysteine, and acetic acid, with sulfate as the best example of inorganic agent.

28.1.2.1 Glucuronyl Transferases

The most common and one of the most important reactions in Phase II is the formation of glucuronic acid derivatives of various substrates (foreign or endogenous such as steroids or bilirubin). Phenols, alcohols, carboxylic acids, and compounds containing amino or sulfhydryl groups may undergo glucuronide conjugation.[3,21] The reaction is catalyzed by a family of enzymes known as uridine diphosphate (UDP) glucuronyl transferases (GLTs). A required cofactor for these reactions is UDP glucuronic acid, which is formed from glucose. The enzymes are localized in the endoplasmic reticulum mainly in the liver, but are also present in the kidney, skin, brain, and spleen. Bilirubin is detoxified by forming glucuronide. The products of sex hormones are in a number of instances known to be excreted as glucuronides. About 150–200 mg of glucuronic acid is excreted as glucuronide per day in the urine of normal humans, and this amount increases considerably after administration of drugs that are excreted as glucuronides.

Patients with a disease known as the Crigler–Najjar syndrome are almost totally deficient in liver UDP GLT. These patients excrete no bilirubin glucuronide and are jaundiced. They frequently develop kernicterus, a syndrome characterized by irreversible damage to the central nervous system and usually die early in childhood. A lower-grade mild hyperbilirubinemia, known as Gilbert's syndrome, occurs in adults. Although this disease has not been as well characterized as the Crigler–Najjar syndrome, one of the findings is a moderate reduction in GLT activity.

28.1.2.2 Sulfotransferases

Sulfate conjugation is probably second only to glucuronic acid conjugation as an important Phase II reaction. The conjugation of foreign compounds with sulfate is catalyzed by a family of enzymes known as sulfotransferases (STs) found in the cytosol fraction of various tissues including the liver, kidney, and intestine. Phenols and alcohols are substrates for these enzymes. The cofactor required in these reactions is 3'-phosphoadenosine-5-phosphosulfate (PAPS) that is synthesized in the cytoplasm of all mammalian cells by a two-step reaction utilizing ATP and inorganic sulfate. The products formed in the conjugation reaction are the corresponding sulfate esters also known as ethereal sulfates.

28.1.2.3 Glutathione S-Transferases

These enzymes are present in the cytosol of the liver, and they catalyze the conjugation of glutathione with compounds containing electrophilic carbon and the sulfhydryl group of glutathione. The resulting conjugate successively loses glutamate and glycine from the glutathione and is then acetylated to form the mercapturic acid derivative of the parent substrate. The cofactor for the acetylation reaction is acetyl coenzyme A (CoA). Glutathione S-transferases (GSTs) contribute to inactivation of unstable and potentially toxic intermediates produced during some biotransformation reactions.

28.1.2.4 Amino Acid Conjugases

Glycine conjugation is characteristic of certain aromatic acids. The reaction depends on the availability of glycine and CoA. The enzyme that catalyzes the reaction of benzoic acid and other aromatic acids with CoA is located in liver mitochondria. In the case of benzoic acid, it is first converted to benzoyl CoA. The enzyme glycine N-acyltransferase present in both mitochondria and the cytosol catalyzes the transfer of benzoyl CoA to glycine to form hippuric acid, which is excreted in the urine. Benzoic acid enters the diet as a natural constituent in plants, with high amounts found in fruits and berries, and as a result of the widespread use of sodium benzoate as a food preservative. Another example of amino acid conjugase is the conjugation of glutamine with phenyl acetic acid to form phenyl acetyl glutamine.

28.1.2.5 Methyltransferases

Norepinephrine and epinephrine are metabolized in part to normetanephrine and metanephrine by o-methylation. Methylation does not generally increase the water solubility of the product in relation to the parent compound. The enzymes catalyzing these reactions are called methyltransferases and are found in either the cytoplasm or endoplasmic reticulum of the liver, lung, and kidney, and the cofactor required is S-adenosyl methionine. Methylation reaction is not important for foreign compounds.

28.1.2.6 N-Acetyltransferases

Acetylation is a common reaction of primary aromatic amines or hydrazines and some primary aliphatic amines. The enzymes carrying out acetyl transfer reactions are known as acetyl CoA:amine N-acetyltransferases, and they are present in the soluble fraction of organs such as the liver, intestine, kidney, and lung. The cofactor required for these reactions is acetyl CoA. The enzyme catalyzes the transfer of the acetyl group from acetyl CoA to the amine function of the foreign compound. Examples involving conjugation with the acetyl group include many sulfonamides and drugs such as isoniazid and procainamide. Acetylation sometimes results in the decrease in water solubility of the conjugated product.

The aforementioned individual reactions are generally more common for compounds with specific reactive groups; however, it is often possible for a compound to be detoxified by the action of more than one enzyme system that acts consecutively or concurrently on the compound or its metabolite. For example, benzene is oxidized to benzene oxide, a highly unstable compound, by the action of the cytochrome P450 system. Benzene oxide can be converted by the action of epoxide hydratase to its dihydrodiol, which can then be excreted as such. Benzene oxide can also spontaneously rearrange to phenol, which can be conjugated with glucuronic acid—the reaction is catalyzed by UDP GLT—or be conjugated with sulfate by the action of sulfotransferase. Benzene oxide can also be conjugated with glutathione by the action of GST and then be converted to its mercapturic acid derivative (Figure 28.3).

Aspirin (acetylsalicylic acid) is conjugated in part with sulfate. If the dose of the analgesic is increased progressively, the amount of sulfate-conjugated product excreted eventually reaches maximum, after which the aspirin is eliminated as the glucuronide or as other conjugate.

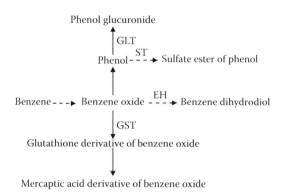

FIGURE 28.3 Detoxification of benzene. EH = epoxide hydratase; GLT = glucuronyl transferase; GST = glutathione S-transferase; ST = sulfotransferase.

28.1.3 MISCELLANEOUS REACTIONS

28.1.3.1 Free Radical Inactivation

Free radicals can be generated by normal aerobic cellular metabolism as well as by the metabolism of some xenobiotics. Oxygen is reduced by enzymatic and nonenzymatic processes to the superoxide radical (O_2). This species is postulated to be formed in vivo through the activity of some iron–sulfur oxidation–reduction enzymes and certain flavoproteins such as xanthine oxidase. The superoxide radical is highly reactive and can cause damage to cells in which it is produced. Divalent cations such as iron or possibly copper may cause catalyzed interaction between superoxide and hydrogen peroxide with the formation of the hydroxyl (*OH) radical. The hydroxyl radical is very highly reactive and potentially damaging in living systems because it can pluck an electron from any organic molecule in its vicinity and cause biochemical alterations that can lead to disease.

It is postulated that free radicals are involved in a variety of pathological events, and they appear to have a role in the general process of aging and tissue damage that results from radiation, reactive oxygen metabolites, and carcinogen metabolism. These radical species have also been proposed to cause atherosclerosis and neuronal injury in disorders such as Parkinson's disease and ischemic brain injury. Protection from free radical damage is provided by enzymatic and/or nonenzymatic components. The components of the enzyme system include superoxide dismutase (SOD), catalase (CAT), and glutathione peroxidase (GP). The nonenzymatic components include several antioxidants.

Enzymatic components: Humans contain three distinct SODs, each of which occurs in a different place: a SOD that contains copper and zinc is found primarily in the cytosol; a manganese-containing SOD is present in mitochondrial matrix; and a glycosylated SOD containing copper and zinc is present in the extracellular spaces. The superoxide radical is unable to cross the lipid bilayer except through anion channels, but the presence of SODs in different compartments prevents the accumulation of this free radical. SOD catalyzes the conversion of toxic superoxide to hydrogen peroxide, which is less reactive.

$$O_2^- + O_2^- + 2H^+ \xrightarrow{\text{SOD}} H_2O_2 + O_2$$

Hydrogen peroxide can be detoxified by the CAT or GP. CAT is present in all major body organs and is especially concentrated in the liver and erythrocytes. It catalyzes the following reaction:

$$2H_2O_2 \xrightarrow{\text{CAT}} 2H_2O + O_2$$

GP catalyses the oxidation of glutathione (GSH) to GSSG at the expense of hydrogen peroxide.

$$H_2O_2 + 2GSH \xrightarrow{\text{GP}} GSSG + 2H_2O$$

It also catalyzes the detoxication of lipid peroxyl radicals. High activity of GP is found in the liver and erythrocytes, moderate activity in the heart and lung, and relatively low activity in muscle. SOD along with CAT and GP constitutes the primary catalytic defense against metabolically generated free radicals.

Nonenzymatic components: The enzymatic reactions involving SOD, CAT, and GP are significant, but they are not 100% effective in eliminating the formation of all free radicals. For example, the very reactive hydroxyl free radical *OH is not eliminated by these enzymes. There are several compounds formed endogenously or present in the normal diet that serve as free radical scavengers. These include vitamin E, vitamin C, β-carotene, glutathione, uric acid, taurine, and flavonoids. These are described in Chapter 25.

28.1.3.2 Rhodanese

During the course of the normal metabolism of foods containing cyanogenic glycosides, the cyanide released is conjugated directly by a reaction catalyzed by the mitochondrial enzyme, rhodanese, found mainly in the liver. It is specific for cyanide ion and does not act on unhydrolyzed organic cyanides.

$$HCN + thiosulfate \rightarrow thiocyanate + sulfite$$

Thiocyanate is much less toxic than cyanide. Thus, the reaction catalyzed by rhodanese is a true detoxication reaction. Hydroxyocobalamin can also detoxify cyanide to form cyanocobalamin, which can be excreted in the urine.

28.1.3.3 Carnitine

Carnitine has an important role in the oxidation of long-chain fatty acids, but it can also promote the excretion of certain organic acids. Under some conditions (e.g., diabetes and anoxia), large amounts of organic acids can accumulate and form CoA esters. This can lead to reduction in the availability of CoA for natural metabolic processes. Carnitine can release CoA from acyl CoA forming acyl carnitine, which can be excreted in the urine. Of course, such removal of acyl carnitine from cells and blood carries the risk of producing a state of carnitine deficiency.

28.2 FACTORS AFFECTING DETOXICATION

Various factors affect the activities of the enzymes involved in detoxication. These include genetically determined polymorphism, age and sex, dietary and other environmental influences such as the entry of substances in the body that can cause induction or inhibition of enzyme(s), and diseases.

28.2.1 GENETICS

There is considerable interindividual variation in expression for the majority of xenobiotic metabolizing enzymes, and for a limited group of enzymes there is evidence for genetic polymorphism—genetic variation in a population when both gene variants exist with a frequency of at least 1%. Genetic polymorphism gives rise to distinct subgroups in populations that differ in their ability to perform a certain drug biotransformation reaction. Such differences in activity may have profound clinical consequences, especially when multiple drugs are given to a patient.

Individuals with deficient metabolism of a certain drug are called poor metabolizers (PM phenotypes) compared to normal or extensive metabolizers (EM phenotypes). The cytochrome P450 system plays a central role in the metabolism and disposition of an extremely wide range of compounds.[7,8] At least 18 human hepatic cytochrome P450 isoenzymes have been identified. Each is capable of catalyzing the oxidation of its own spectrum of substrates, and any single xenobiotic may be metabolized by more than one enzyme. Cytochrome P450 isoenzyme nomenclature uses the root symbol CYP, followed in order by an Arabic number to denote the gene family, an uppercase letter to designate a subfamily of highly related genes, and another Arabic number to identify the individual isoenzyme within the subfamily. These numbers usually reflect the order in which the isoenzymes were discovered. The cytochrome P450s involved in drug metabolism fall predominantly into three gene families termed CYP1, CYP2, and CYP3. The most abundant single cytochrome P450 in human liver is CYP3A4. It exhibits a broad substrate specificity and is responsible for the oxidation of many therapeutic drugs and a variety of structurally unrelated compounds including testosterone, estrogens, fatty acids, and xenobiotics. And it has been estimated that this specific cytochrome P450 may be involved in the metabolism of over 50% of the drugs used clinically.

The best characterized genetic difference is the one involving the isoenzyme called cytochrome P450 2D6, which is responsible for the oxidation of the hypertensive drug, debrisoquine. Extensive metabolizers excrete 10–200 times more of the urinary metabolite of this drug than poor metabolizers. Between 5% and 10% of Caucasians and about 1% of Chinese and Japanese have a deficiency of cytochrome P450 2D6, making them poor metabolizers of debrisoquine and more than 20 other prescribed drugs. On the average, debrisoquine metabolism is slower in Asians compared to Europeans. There is high expression of CYP2D6 in many persons of Ethiopian and Saudi Arabian origin. CYP2D6 is not inducible, so these people have developed a different strategy to cope with the (presumed) high load of alkaloids in their diet—multiple copies of the gene. These CYPs therefore rapidly break down a variety of drugs, making them ineffective—many antidepressants and neuroleptics are examples. Conversely, prodrugs, such as codeine, will be extensively activated and form large amounts of morphine. About 7% of the North American population lacks CYP2D6 needed to convert codeine to morphine.

African Americans who smoke consume fewer cigarettes than their white counterparts. A new study suggests a biological basis for this difference: reduced activity of cytochrome P450 2A6 (CYP2A6) that metabolizes nicotine.[16] As a result, active nicotine metabolite, cotinine, continues to circulate in the blood longer, delaying the smoker's feeling that he or she needs another "hit" on the cigarette.

This genetic difference may have several consequences. Adverse drug reaction may occur in individuals who lack a particular enzyme. Some xenobiotics may be activated by the enzyme to form metabolites with the potential of causing disease. A deficiency of a particular polymorphic enzyme involved in detoxification may be either a benefit or a risk in determining susceptibility to disease. For example, it has been shown that impaired debrisoquine metabolism is twice as common among patients with Parkinson's disease as in normal population. In contrast, there is evidence that the risk of lung cancer in cigarette smokers is considerably less in poor metabolizers. Polymorphism[2] of some other enzymes involved in detoxification has also been recognized. One enzyme involves N-acetyltransferase, responsible for the fast and slow acetylation phenotypes. Isoniazid (INH) is the drug widely used for the specific treatment of tuberculosis in children and adults, and acetylation is the most important pathway in INH elimination. After administration of a therapeutic dose, the slow acetylators have a higher concentration of INH in plasma for any specified period than the fast acetylators. Slow acetylators have increased risk of side effects of some drugs and of bladder cancer.

Approximately 5% of Canadian Eskimos, 50% of Europeans, and as high as 90% of Moroccans are slow acetylators. A combination of fast acetylator phenotype and high meat consumption increases the risk of colorectal cancer.[19] This may be because N-acetyltransferase catalyzes the formation of mutagenic products from heterocyclic amines derived from cooked meat. Conjugation reactions are believed to represent terminal inactivation events, and such have been viewed as true detoxication reactions. This concept must be modified since N-acetyltransferase is also involved in the conversion of precursor to reactive species.

The production of GSTs is controlled by a superfamily of genes that belong to at least six major gene classes. There is some evidence of polymorphism in each of the subclasses, but the best studied are the GSTM1 and GSTT1 genes. Lack of the GSTM1 gene is associated with increased susceptibility to lung and bladder cancers. The enzyme apparently participates in the metabolism of some components of cigarette smoke. Lack of the GSTT1 gene is associated with increased susceptibility to brain tumors.

There are racial differences in the distribution of these genes.[22] About 50% of Caucasians and Chinese people lack GSTM1. About 10% of South Indians lack GSTM1. The distribution of GSTT1 shows even greater differences between races.

28.2.2 AGE AND GENDER

The influence of age is most important in very young and very old patients. Early in fetal life, the activities of enzymes involved in biotransformation are absent or quite low. The enzymes begin to appear in the late fetal and early postnatal stages of life and later increase rapidly to reach adult levels. Neonatal hyperbilirubinemia results from the inability of newborns, particularly premature infants, to convert bilirubin to the more water-soluble and readily excretable bilirubin glucuronide. Normally, bilirubin in the plasma is either rapidly conjugated as the glucuronide and excreted in the bile or tightly bound to plasma protein. When conjugation is extremely limited, the ability of plasma protein to bind bilirubin is exceeded. Free bilirubin diffuses across the blood–brain barrier and can develop into a serious condition called kernicterus if the plasma bilirubin levels become sufficiently high. Brain damage, neurological disorder, and often death may ensue. The accumulation of bilirubin is caused by a relative deficiency of UDP GLT, which is not formed in sufficient amounts until the normal time of birth. Hence, the problem is particularly acute in premature infants. The level of plasma bilirubin decreases to normal level soon after birth as the synthesis of the enzyme increases in the liver. Hyperbilirubinemia can be reduced by exposing infants to fluorescent light—a so-called bilirubin reduction lamp. Apparently the lamp rays degrade bilirubin to products, possibly di- and monopyrrole derivatives, that are less toxic and can be metabolized or excreted by the infants.

Benzyl alcohol is commonly used as an antibacterial agent in a variety of formulations including solutions intended for intravenous administration. Benzyl alcohol is converted to benzoate and is then detoxified through conjugation with glycine to form hippuric acid. Neonates have very low activity of amino acid conjugase. Benzoic acidemia can result if newborns are given excess benzyl alcohol or benzoate.[4] The accumulation of benzoic acid causes the gasping syndrome, which consists of multiple-organ system failure, severe metabolic acidosis, and gasping respiration.[6] This potentially fatal syndrome is associated with cumulative benzyl alcohol doses >99 mg/kg body weight. Therefore, intravenous solutions and medications containing benzyl alcohol or benzoate should not be used in neonates. In general, Phase I detoxication pathways in newborns have one-third to one-half the adult activities but increase with both gestational age and postnatal age and reach adult levels in few months; the enzymes of Phase II reaction develop more slowly.

The elderly are a more heterogeneous group, and therefore, it is difficult to generalize about the effect of aging on the rate of detoxication; however, in the aged, the activity and capability of a multitude of physiological and biochemical processes abate, including metabolic rates. Among the most relevant to the handling of foreign compounds is a decline in liver mass and a reduction in liver enzyme affinity for some substrates.[13] In addition, elderly individuals may have reduction in renal function. Foreign compounds may persist in the body longer, in part because they may be detoxified somewhat slowly and excreted less efficiently. Lipid-soluble substances also tend to accumulate in the elderly to a greater degree because their body tissues contain a higher percentage of fat. The rate at which a drug or toxin disappears from the body is a function of both its rate of biotransformation and rate of excretion (i.e., renal, biliary, pulmonary). The decline in the concentration of the drug in the body can be mathematically described as the biological half-life, and it provides an estimate of the time required to reduce by one-half the quantity of drug present in a particular body compartment (plasma). The plasma half-life of diazepam (Valium), widely used in the management of anxiety, is found to exhibit a striking age dependency. At the age of 20 years, the average half-life is 20 hours, and it increases linearly with age to about 90 hours at 80 years. Several other drugs have been found to follow similar patterns.

There is little effect of age on most of the Phase II reactions in elderly humans except acetylation, which appears to decline slightly in the elderly. The antioxidant enzymes SOD, CAT, and GP, which protect against oxidant stress, decrease with age and may, in part, contribute to the process of aging.

Gender-dependent variation in detoxication may also be important in toxic response to various xenobiotics. There are clinical reports of decreased oxidation of estrogens, salicylates, and benzodiazepines in females relative to males. The rate of alcohol metabolism is lower in women than in men. But at this time generalizations about gender-specific differences in detoxication are premature.

28.2.3 DIETARY FACTORS

The availability of nutrients is important in the regulation of xenobiotic metabolism.[15] Phase I and Phase II reactions are catalyzed by enzymes that are proteins. Therefore, any nutritional state that reduces the availability of amino acids can be expected to reduce the formation of enzymes involved in detoxication. This can also occur when caloric intake is low because under this condition protein is catabolized and used as a source of energy, reducing the availability of amino acids for enzyme formation.

Phospholipids are needed for the synthesis of biological membranes including those of the endoplasmic reticulum where detoxication of most environmental chemicals takes place. Because polyunsaturated fatty acids derived from essential fatty acids (EFAs) are present in phospholipids, a deficiency of EFAs is expected to affect the rate of detoxication.

The cofactor NADPH is formed from niacin. Flavin mononucleotide (FMN) and flavin adenine dinucleotide (FAD), derived from riboflavin, are parts of cytochrome P450 reductase. Glycine (the precursor of heme of cytochrome P450), pantothenic acid (part of CoA), and pyridoxine (as pyridoxal phosphate) are required in the conversion of glycine to heme. Similarly, iron is a crucial component of cytochrome P450, and copper is required for iron metabolism. Therefore, deficiencies of these nutrients can affect Phase I metabolism and thereby cause an increase in the toxicity of some foreign chemicals.

In contrast to Phase I reactions where the role of nutrients is mostly catalytic, in Phase II reactions several nutrients are involved as substrates as well as in the production and composition of the enzyme systems that catalyze these reactions. GLT is the most versatile among the enzymes of conjugation reactions. UDP glucuronic acid availability is regulated by the presence of glucose, energy (UTP), and NAD. PAPS is primarily regulated by the availability of inorganic sulfate and ATP. Glutathione is the tripeptide derived from glutamate, cysteine, and glycine, and its formation requires vitamin B_6. It is a powerful nucleophile as well as an antioxidant.

During starvation, cellular metabolism shifts toward catabolism and the availability of important cofactors become limited. Studies with children in developing countries suggest that starvation may decrease the rates of detoxication. Children with protein deficiency metabolize a number of drugs less rapidly than normal children. Adequate protein given to these children brings the rate of metabolism to near-normal levels. A high-protein diet enhances the rate of oxidative metabolism in humans as judged by the clearance of antipyrine and theophylline from plasma.[11] On the other hand, high-carbohydrate and high-lipid diets cause reduction in the rate of detoxication. Vitamins C and E and carotenes serve as antioxidants. Selenium is part of GP, which detoxifies hydrogen peroxide and lipid peroxides produced in the body.

In addition to these nutrients, there are substances used as additives in food, and some of them may affect the rate of detoxication. Also, there are nonnutrient substances present in natural foods that are known to affect the activities of enzymes.[9] The way the food is cooked can also have an effect on the rate of detoxication.

The synthetic antioxidants butylated hydroxytoluene (BHT) and butylated hydroxyanisole (BHA) are used to inhibit lipid peroxidation of some processed foods. When consumed, these antioxidants also increase the activity of some enzymes responsible for the metabolism of xenobiotics and inhibit tumorigenesis. Thus, a minor component in the diet that is not a nutrient can have an influence on chemical carcinogenesis.

Some vegetables contain substances that are known to affect the enzymes of detoxication reactions. Substances such as caffeine, theophylline, and theobromine (found in beverages) inhibit oxidative metabolism by binding to cytochrome P450. Some foods contain phenols, which act as antioxidants and inhibit chemical carcinogenesis. Cruciferous vegetables (e.g., cabbage, cauliflower, and Brussels sprouts) contain indole derivatives, which are known to inhibit tumor formation by inducing activity of the cytochrome P450 system. These vegetables also contain aryl isothiocyanates, which induce glutathione S-transferase.

The ingestion of charred meat such as charcoal-broiled meat is shown to enhance oxidative metabolism of several drugs in humans. This effect is abolished by wrapping meat in aluminum foil during cooking. The induction effect is attributed to polycyclic hydrocarbons and other mutagenic pyrolysis products formed from amino acids as a result of incomplete combustion.

Chronic alcohol use results in the induction of one of the forms of cytochrome P450 known as II E_1, which can activate some xenobiotics to toxic reactive intermediates. Polycyclic aromatic hydrocarbons present in cigarette smoke as well as exposure to a variety of chemicals (i.e., insecticides, polycyclic hydrocarbons, and barbiturates) can induce the activity of some detoxifying enzymes. High concentrations of cobalt, cadmium, and other heavy metals can depress the activity of cytochrome P450 because they inhibit heme synthesis.

28.2.3.1 Role of Grapefruit Juice

After a drug is taken by mouth, it is absorbed in the small intestine and is partially metabolized by the intestinal and hepatic enzymes resulting in a significant reduction in the amount of drug reaching the systemic circulation. This is known as first-pass metabolism. The major enzyme in the small bowel enterocytes involved in metabolism is CYP3A4. Grapefruit and its juice contain phytochemicals identified as furanocoumarin derivatives, which have been found to exert inhibitory action on CYP3A4. This can lead to a higher level of drug entering systemic circulation. It can improve the bioavailability of a drug, thus increasing its efficacy or enhancing its adverse effects, particularly if the therapeutic window is narrow.

Grapefruit juice inhibits the enzyme in the small intestine and not in the liver, at least when consumed in normal quantities. This presumably reflects the very small concentration of furanocoumarins reaching the liver after absorption. So it does not impact injected drugs. The degree of the effect varies widely between individuals. The onset of the interaction can occur within 30 minutes following intake of a single glass of grapefruit juice, and the inhibitory effect can last up to 3 days following the administration of grapefruit juice.

Drugs used to lower blood cholesterol like Lipitor, Mevacor, and Zocor have increased potency when taken with grapefruit juice.[1] Excessive levels of these drugs in circulation can lead to a serious muscle disorder called rhabdomyolysis. Grapefruit juice can also interfere with the metabolism of drugs such as selective serotonin reuptake inhibitors like Prozac, which are used to treat depression, calcium channel antagonists, cyclosporine, and some other drugs. Grapefruit juice consumption is a clinically relevant issue, especially for the elderly, who are most likely to be taking the drugs affected by it. The drug may be taken when the grapefruit juice contents have been mostly metabolized.

In addition to the liver and the small intestine CYP3A4 is expressed in the breast, prostate, and colon. Inhibition of this enzyme can lead to increased levels of estrogen and testosterone in circulation and may have health consequences. According to one study, women who ate as little as a quarter of a grapefruit each day had a breast cancer risk that was 30% percent higher than average. Furanocoumarins reduce the breakdown of estrogen—thereby increasing blood estrogen levels.[17,18] High estrogen levels are associated with a higher risk of some types of breast cancer. However, the study has recently been called into question based on newer data.

Despite its effect on CYP3A4, grapefruit provides several nutrients including vitamin C, potassium, phosphorus, fiber, and the antioxidant lycopene. It also contains bioflavonoids that protect against cancer and heart disease.

In general, inhibition of enzymes involved in detoxication can have adverse effects when exposed to xenobiotics, while mild induction can help detoxify harmful substances at a faster rate and offer a positive protective effect when there is simultaneous exposure to toxicants.

28.2.4 Disease

A number of disease states may potentially alter the rate of detoxication. Acute or chronic liver disease affects the capacity of the liver to synthesize the enzymes responsible for detoxication and can have profound effects on the metabolism of toxic substances.[10] Such conditions include fatty liver, alcoholic hepatitis, alcoholic cirrhosis, hemochromatosis, chronic active hepatitis, biliary cirrhosis, and acute viral or drug-induced hepatitis. Cardiac disease, by limiting blood flow to the liver, may impair disposition of toxic substances whose metabolism is flow limited. Thyroid dysfunction has been associated with altered metabolism of some drugs and some endogenous compounds. Impairment of detoxication rate is also observed in patients with malaria and schistosomiasis.

REFERENCES

1. Bailey, D. G., and G. K. Dresser. 2004. Interactions between grapefruit juice and cardiovascular drugs. *Amer J Cardiovascular Drugs* 4:281.
2. Daly, A. K., S. Cholerton, U. Gregory, and J. R. Idle. 1993. Metabolic polymorphism. *Pharmacol Ther* 57:129.
3. de-Wildt, S. N., G. L. Kearns, J. S. Leder, and J. N. van den Anker. 1999. Glucuronidation in humans: Pharmacogenetic and development aspects. *Clin Pharmacokinet* 36:439.
4. Food and Drug Administration. 1982. Benzyl alcohol may be toxic to newborns. *FDA Drug Bull* 12:10.
5. Garrod, J. W., H. Oelschlager, and J. Caldwell, eds. 1988. *Metabolism of Xenobiotics*. Philadelphia, PA: Taylor and Francis.
6. Gershanik, J., B. Boecler, H. Ensley, S. McClosky, and W. George. 1982. The gasping syndrome and benzyl alcohol poisoning. *N Engl J Med* 307:1384.
7. Gonzalez, F. J. 1992. Human cytochromes P-450: Problems and prospects. *Trends Pharmacol Sci* 13:346.
8. Guengerich, F. P. 1993. Cytochrome P-450 enzymes. *Am Sci* 81:440.
9. Hidaka, M., M. Okumura, K. Fujita et al. 2005. Effects of pomegranate juice on human cytochrome P450 3A (CYP3A) and carbamazepine pharmacokinetics in rats. *Drug Metals Dispos* 33:644.
10. Howden, C. W., G. G. Birnie, and M. J. Brodie. 1989. Drug metabolism in liver disease. *Pharmacol Ther* 40:439.
11. Kappas, A., K. E. Anderson, A. H. Conney, and A. P. Alvares. 1976. Influence of dietary protein and carbohydrate on antipyrene and theophylline metabolism in man. *Clin Pharmacol Ther* 20:643.
12. Kim, H., Y. Yoon, J. Shon et al. 2006. Inhibitory effects of fruit juices on CYP3A activity. *Drug Metab Dispos* 34:521.
13. Kinirons, M. T., and M. S. O'Mahony. 2004. Drug metabolism and aging. *Brit J Pharmacol* 57:540.
14. Maskalyk, J. 2002. Grapefruit juice: Potential drug interactions. *J Can Med Assoc* 167:279.
15. Meydani, M. 1987. Dietary effects on detoxication processes. In *Nutritional Toxicology*, ed. J. N. Hathcock, Orlando, FL: Academie.
16. Molchan, E. T., F. H. Franken, and M. Jaszyna-Gasior. 2006. Adolescent nicotine metabolism: Ethnoracial differences among dependent smokers. *Ethnicity Dis* 16:239.
17. Monroe, K. R., S. P. Murphy, and L. N. Kolonel. 2007. Prospective study of grapefruit intake and risk of breast cancer in postmenopausal women: The multiethnic cohort study. *Brit J Cancer* 97:440.
18. Paine, M. F., W. W. Widmer, H. L. Hart et al. 2006. A furanocoumarin-free grapefruit juice establishes furanocoumarins as the mediators of the grapefruit juice-feladipine interaction. *Amer J Clin Nutr* 83:1097.
19. Roberts-Thomson, I. C., P. Ryan, K. K. Khoo, W. J. Hart, A. J. McMichael, and R. N. Butler. 1996. Diet, acetylator phenotype, and risk of colorectal neoplasia. *Lancet* 347:1372.
20. Steinberg, D., C. E. Maize, J. H. Herndon, H. M. Fales, W. K. Engel, and F. Q. Vroom. 1970. Phytanic acid in patients with Refsum's disease syndrome and response to dietary treatment. *Arch Intern Med* 125:75.
21. Turkey, R. H., and C. P. Strassburg. 2000. Human UDP-glucuronosyltransferases: Metabolism, expression, and disease. *Annu Rev Pharmacol Toxicol* 40:581.
22. Zhao, B., A. Seow, E. J. D. Lee, W. Poh, M. Teh, P. Eng, Y. Wang, W. Tan, M. C. Yu, and H. Lee. 2001. Dietary isothiocyanates, glutathione S-transferease-M1, T1 polymorphisms and lung cancer risk among Chinese women in Singapore. *Cancer Epidemiol Biomarkers Prev* 10:1063.

29 Nutraceuticals

29.1 INTRODUCTION

For thousands of years, it has been known that some foods contain something special that helps sick people get well and even keeps healthy people from getting certain diseases. For example, while vitamin A was not identified until the twentieth century, even in ancient times, foods rich in this nutrient have been used for treating night blindness—the most commonly recognized symptom of vitamin A deficiency. As far back as 1500 BC, it was recognized in the Egyptian medical literature that people unable to see properly at night should eat roast ox liver or the liver of a black cock. In India, it was known that night blindness was caused by bad and insufficient food. For several centuries, men have been aware that the disease scurvy could be prevented by including fruits and green vegetables in the diet. The recognition that there is a vital association between diet and human diseases has helped a great deal in identifying most of the nutrients.

Between 1910 and 1950, nutrition research focused solely on preventing nutrient deficiency diseases. The vitamins were discovered one by one and their biochemical roles were identified. The dietary need for essential fatty acids, amino acids, and some inorganic elements was also established during this period, which is often referred to as the golden age of nutrition. Recommended dietary allowances (RDAs) served as nutritional guidelines for the intake of nutrients important in a healthful diet. It is now assumed that all the nutrients required for the maintenance of optimal health have been discovered. The concept of food having medicinal functions other than those established for the presence of known nutrients fell out of favor among researchers in the field of nutrition. Food, of course, contains not only nutrients but thousands of substances which, for the most part, are considered inert or antinutrients.

Beginning in 1950, the need to consume adequate amounts of appropriate food groups to supply all the necessary nutrients was established. It has also been accepted that consuming more than the recommended quantities offers no benefit and can even be dangerous. The advice has been to limit certain nutrients to prevent the incidence of chronic diseases, for instance, reducing the consumption of fat and cholesterol for cardiovascular disease, salt for hypertension, and fat and calories for obesity.

The pendulum has started swinging back to the time before many of the nutrients were discovered. Recent attention has focused on the health effects of the diet devoid of overt clinical deficiencies. Specifically, inert, non-nutritive dietary compounds have been found to be associated with the cause or prevention of conditions as diverse as cancer, coronary heart disease (CHD), cataracts, etc. Diet-based disease prevention is increasingly seen as the wave of the future and there is currently a surge of interest and effort in the formulation of diets and foods tailored to meet specific health needs.[20,21]

Several sources have attempted to define and to distinguish the terms that are being used to describe foods and ingredients in foods that have health-promoting properties.[17,42] Some of the terms are described below

Functional foods. These were first introduced in Japan in 1989 to describe a class of food products containing ingredients that aid specific bodily functions in addition to being nutrients.

Designer foods. This term was coined by the National Cancer Institute to describe foods that naturally contain, or are enriched with, non-nutritive, biologically active chemical components of plants (phytochemicals; "phyto" connotes plants) that are effective in reducing cancer risk.

Nutraceuticals. This term is defined by the Foundation for Innovation in Medicine as any substance considered a food or part of a food that provides medical or health benefits, including the prevention or treatment of disease.

Pharmafoods. This term is used to describe any edible product for human consumption that is designed, produced, packaged, and sold to consumers, with claims that it achieves a well-documented health benefit that is therapeutic, prophylactic, or reduces the risk of disease.

Other terms for specially formulated foods include phytofoods, performance foods, smart foods, and phytochemical foods.

29.2   INTEREST IN NUTRACEUTICALS

People today are very much interested in foods that not only have good nutritional value but also may offer potential health benefits.[19] Generally these are becoming known as functional foods and by definition should demonstrate a beneficial effect on one or more target functions in the body (beyond adequate nutritional effects) in a way that is relevant to either improved state of health and well-being or a reduction in the risk of disease. Nutraceuticals, largely unregulated health-enhancing or disease-preventing products, until recently were mostly the province of small entrepreneurial companies. Several of the chemical industry's biggest companies have entered the nutraceutical market. The sales of these products increased from an estimated $11.3 billion in 1995 to $16.2 billion in 1999 and are projected to reach $49 billion by 2010.

Diet has been implicated in 6 of 10 leading causes of death in our society. These include heart disease, cancer, stroke, diabetes, atherosclerosis, and liver disease; heart disease and cancer account for about 70% of all deaths. It is commonly accepted that about one-third of the cancer cases and one-half of the heart disease, artery disease, and hypertension cases are related to diet.

The aging population has been steadily growing, but the lifespan has remained about the same. With this rapid growth, the incidence of chronic diseases is increasing—and with it the cost of health care is skyrocketing. There is epidemiological, experimental, and some clinical evidence that individuals with low fruit and vegetable intakes have an increased risk of some chronic diseases such as cancer and heart disease, so an increased intake of plant-based foods may contribute to the reduction in the risk of these diseases. This may increase the lifespan or at least increase the quality of life for older Americans.

While some foods have been linked to a reduction in the risk of certain diseases, it was only during the last 8–10 years that scientists have begun to identify specific food components whose beneficial effects may expand the role of diet in the prevention and treatment of diseases.[4,10] Most of the research work on dietary constituents is concentrated in the fields of cancer and heart disease. Food components may trigger enzyme systems that block or suppress DNA damage, reduce tumor size, and decrease the effect of estrogen-like hormones. Components have been identified in some foods that modulate the enzymes in the phase I and II reactions of detoxication, and help to inactivate and eliminate carcinogens and other toxicants, thus potentially offering protection against cancer. Some components with antioxidant properties may offer protection against cancer, heart disease, and some other chronic diseases. Some may offer protection against the oxidation of low-density lipoprotein (LDL) cholesterol, some may inhibit platelet aggregation, or some may be effective in reducing blood cholesterol and thus may have beneficial effects against heart diseases. Other food components may offer protection against various other diseases.

An enormous wealth of information is available from experimental studies, which show that specific dietary factors can significantly alter the likelihood of induction of cancer by known carcinogens in a variety of tissues and organs. Many of these modulatory effects observed in animals have also been reported in human epidemiological studies.[7,38]

The growth of malignant tumor is a long, slow process that involves three key steps:

1. The initiation of potentially cancerous changes in a cell's DNA;
2. The promotion of uncontrolled growth in a damaged cell; and
3. The progression of a cancerous lesion into a mass that can invade other tissues.

Initiation occurs when viruses, radiation, free radicals, and chemical carcinogens damage the DNA. Antioxidants in fruits and vegetables, tea, etc., help neutralize free radicals. Chemicals generally enter the body as procarcinogens and are converted to carcinogens by the action of phase I enzymes of detoxication. Compounds present in garlic and some other foods inhibit these enzymes. Phytochemicals present in broccoli and several other foods are potent inducers of phase II enzymes of detoxication, which convert carcinogens to inactive compounds (Figure 29.1). Substantial evidence supports the view that phase II enzyme induction is a highly effective strategy for reducing susceptibility to carcinogens.

In animal studies, linoleic acid (ω6 fatty acid family) appears to promote tumor growth while fish oil (ω3 fatty acid family) intake appears to reduce tumor growth. Phytoestrogens (in soybeans) may affect this step in some hormone-dependent tumors (Figure 29.2). Epidemiological and animal model studies have shown the effectiveness of nonsteroidal anti-inflammatory drugs (NSAIDs) in reducing cancer risk. The anticancer effect of NSAIDs is thought to be due to the inhibition of cyclooxygenase (COX), particularly COX2. COX2 has been found to be dramatically upregulated in various types of cancer cells. The premise that COX2 is involved in the pathological process of cancer growth and progression is supported by animal studies indicating that tumorigenesis is inhibited in COX2 knockout mice. Selective inhibitors of COX2 have been demonstrated to induce apoptosis (programmed cell death) in a variety of cancer cells, including those in the colon, breast, stomach, and prostate. The promotion step is dependent on the development of the tumor's own blood circulation. ω3 fatty acids as well as substances with COX2 inhibitor activity have been implicated in depressing the growth of this microcirculation (angiogenesis) in developing tumors. Resveratrol in grapes, curcumin in turmeric, and some compounds in blueberry, ginger, green tea, etc., exhibit COX2 inhibitor activity[42] (Figure 29.3) and thus have potential as cancer-preventive agents.

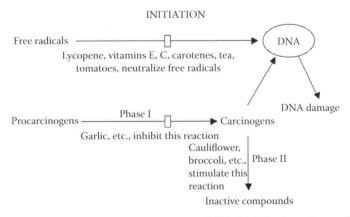

FIGURE 29.1   The role of diet in cancer process: INITIATION. Initiation is made up of a series of events whereby an exogenous or endogenous carcinogen induces alterations in the genetic make-up of the cell.

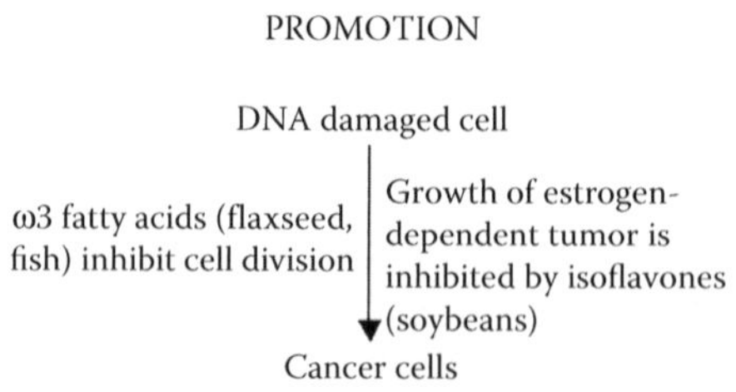

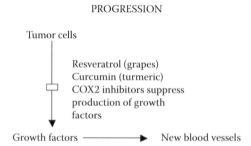

PROMOTION

DNA damaged cell

ω3 fatty acids (flaxseed, fish) inhibit cell division | Growth of estrogen-dependent tumor is inhibited by isoflavones (soybeans)

Cancer cells

FIGURE 29.2 The role of diet in cancer process: PROMOTION. Promotion involves alterations in gene expression and cell proliferation, which transform the initiated cell into a discernible population of cancer cells.

PROGRESSION

Tumor cells

Resveratrol (grapes)
Curcumin (turmeric)
COX2 inhibitors suppress production of growth factors

Growth factors ⟶ New blood vessels

FIGURE 29.3 The role of diet in cancer process: PROGRESSION. Progression involves increased growth and an expansion of a population of initiated and promoted cancer cells from a focal lesion to an invasive tumor mass.

29.3   FRUITS AND VEGETABLES WITH HEALTH-PROMOTING PROPERTIES

Plant foods such as fruits, vegetables, whole grain, spices, herbs, and beverages such as tea and wine contain many components (phytochemicals) that are beneficial to human health. Evidence supporting consumption of these foods on lowering the rates of many cancers and age-related diseases is extensive and consistent. For example, high consumption of fruits and vegetables is related to the prevention of osteoporosis by maintaining the body's bone density and reducing the risk of cardiovascular disease, prostate cancer, and lung cancer.

For the past decade and especially since 1994, attention has been focused on antioxidants present in foods of plant origin. Several chronic diseases, as well as the aging process, are attributed to the generation of free radicals in the body. Taking foods rich in antioxidants is expected to neutralize free radical damage and offer protection.[18]

Considerable evidence indicates that the liberation of, or generation of, free radicals within the cell is highly damaging and may directly or indirectly contribute to some chronic diseases. Several nutritive and non-nutritive antioxidants have been reported to be of benefit in protecting against free radical damage. In addition to vitamins C and E and β-carotene, some fruits and vegetables are rich in other antioxidants such as flavonoids. Dietary flavonoids are highly concentrated in some common foods such as cereals, tea, coffee, onion, apples, wine, beer, and nuts.

Several other compounds in fruits and vegetables have been identified and shown or postulated to offer protection against various chronic diseases (Table 29.1). Some of these compounds are widespread, whereas others are characteristic of particular classes of fruits and vegetables. A few of the fruits and vegetables classes and their components with beneficial health effects are described in Table 29.1.

Table 29.1   Foods with Disease-Fighting Properties

Food	Active Component	Disease-Preventive Role
Soy beans	Phytoestrogens, antiestrogenic	Cancer, heart disease
Cruciferous vegetables	Indoles, isothiocyanates—increase activities of enzymes of detoxication	Cancer
Evening primrose oil	γ linolenic acid—inhibits arachidonic acid metabolism	Heart disease, inflammation
Seafood	Eicosapentaenoic acid, docosahexaenoic acid, linolenic acid—inhibit arachidonic acid metabolism	Heart disease, diabetes, some other diseases, cancer
Allium vegetables	Allylic sulfides—increase activities of enzymes of detoxication; inhibit platelet aggregation	Cancer, heart disease, antibacterial
Grapes, nuts	Resveratrol, ellagic acid—increase activities of enzymes of detoxication	Cancer, heart disease
Turmeric	Curcumin—increases activities of enzymes of detoxication	Cancer, antibacterial
Licorice	Unknown—increases activities of enzymes of detoxication	Cancer
Peppermint	Menthol	Muscle-relaxing
Parsley	Myristicin	Diuretic, vasodilating, chemoprotective
Citrus fruits	Limonene, hesperetin, naringenin, nobiletin—increase activities of enzymes involved in detoxication	Cancer, heart disease
Cranberry juice	Unknown, condensed tannins	Urinary infection
Yogurt	Lactobacilli	Antidiarrheal, antibacterial, antimutagenic, heart disease, cancer
Tomatoes, autumn olive	Lycopene	Cancer, heart disease
Yellow, green vegetables	Lutein, zeaxanthin	Macular degeneration
Nuts	Flavonoids, phytosterols	Cancer, heart disease
Berries	Antioxidants	Various diseases
Cherries	Anthocyanins	Various diseases
Lemon grass	Unknown	Heart disease
Shiitake mushrooms	Lentinan, eritadenine	Immunomodulatory, antimicrobial
Olive oil	Oleic acid, antioxidants	Cancer, heart disease
Bitter melon	Unknown	Diabetes
Cinnamon	Methylhydroxychalcone polymer	Diabetes
Flaxseed	ALA, lignans	Cancer, heart disease

29.3.1   FOODS RICH IN FIBER

For many years, dietary fiber was not considered to have a significant nutritional value. But in the early 1970s, dietary fiber was the hottest new prospect in nutrition science; enthusiasts believed that a lack of fiber could explain every ill that plagues the populations in Western countries—from constipation to heart disease and cancer. Most research works were done (and are being done) to determine the possible benefits of fiber in the prevention of various diseases. The recommendation has been to include more fiber-rich foods in our diet. Although fiber is not the magic bullet it was believed to be, it does seem to offer benefits in some cases.

Fruits, vegetables, and legumes are major sources of dietary fiber, which has been hypothesized to be protective against a range of diseases such as cancer, atherosclerosis, diabetes, and obesity. All dietary fiber components have physical and chemical properties that contribute to their functionality in providing positive health benefits. Dietary fiber increases fecal bulk and decreases transit time. Thus, by diluting any toxicant present and by shortening the period of contact time, the interaction between carcinogens and the intestinal epithelium is reduced. Fiber appears to be protective against certain types of xenobiotics. It may bind carcinogens and bile acids. Certain types of fiber are fermented by the intestinal microflora and produce short-chain fatty acids, one of which, butyrate, is antineoplastic. The epidemiological data linking high-fiber diets to reduced risk of colon cancer are quite strong.

Fiber-rich whole grain products, flaxseed (linseed), fruits, berries, and soy products are the sources of lignans (which belong to a family of compounds with properties similar to phytoestrogens). They are formed in the intestine by the bacterial action on plant-derived precursors and possess both estrogenic and antiestrogenic biological properties. They are excreted in the urine at concentrations that are directly related to dietary fiber intake. Their chemical structures are similar to that of diethylstilbestrol, the synthetic nonsteroidal estrogen. Enterolactone and enterodiol are the major lignans in human urine and both bind (although with relatively low affinity) to estrogen receptors and exert some weak estrogenic bioactivity; however, in so doing, they cause antiestrogenic effects. In limited studies, they appear to have tumor-inhibitory properties, particularly as antiestrogens.[5] Generally, in countries where fiber intake is high, breast cancer rates are relatively low and vice versa; however, high-fiber diets are also low in fat and high in fruit and vegetable consumption. More studies are needed to determine the role of dietary fiber per se in the prevention of breast cancer.

In large epidemiological studies, a high-fiber intake has been associated with a decreased risk of CHD in both men and women. Soluble fibers in particular are thought to exert a preventive role against heart disease as they appear to have the ability to lower serum total and LDL cholesterol levels. Some of the better food sources of soluble fiber are fruits, vegetables, legumes, oatmeal, and psyllium. The latter is a plant whose stalks contain tiny seeds (also called psyllium) covered by husks. About 71% of the weight of psyllium (seeds) is soluble fiber; in contrast, only 5% of oat bran by weight is made of soluble fiber. A number of studies have demonstrated that rats fed controlled diets supplemented with psyllium fiber experience a significant decrease in serum cholesterol levels. Many studies in humans have also shown psyllium to be an effective agent in reducing serum cholesterol. Indeed, it is now recognized that soluble fiber is a valuable intervention to decrease serum cholesterol in clinically significant amounts, thereby reducing a known risk factor for CHD. In fact, in 1998, the Food and Drug Administration (FDA) approved labels on cereals supplemented with psyllium, which state "regular consumption of psyllium as part of a low-fat diet can reduce cholesterol levels." The average intake of fiber in the United States is only about 12–15 g daily. This consumption falls below current recommendations of the World Health Organization of 25–40 g of fiber daily. An increased intake of foods high in dietary fiber, especially cereal products, may be protective against CHD.

29.3.2 SOYBEANS

Soybeans are rich in good-quality proteins and some vitamins and have a low content of saturated fat. They contain lunasin,[11] a 43-amino acid peptide, which has anticancer and anti-inflammatory properties. They are a unique source of a group of phytochemicals called isoflavones. These compounds are thought to exert a myriad of biological effects and it has been hypothesized that they reduce the risk of a number of chronic diseases. In the United States and in most Western nations, the consumption of soy products is quite low in contrast to many Asian nations. For example, Japanese people consume 10-fold or greater amounts of soy as compared to

United States citizens. Differences in urinary excretions of isoflavones (reflection of consumption of foods containing isoflavones) between Asian and American populations are striking; Asians excrete 2000–3000 nmol of isoflavones per day, while Americans excrete 30–40 nmol of these compounds per day.

Isoflavones are particularly good candidates for the cardioprotective effect of soy because of their many chemical and biological similarities to estrogen. Epidemiological evidence has suggested that the populations consuming soy in fairly high amounts have a lower incidence of CHD mortality. Several clinical studies have found that the consumption of soy protein decreases blood concentrations of LDL and total cholesterol and triglycerides. Based on this evidence, the FDA in October 1999 approved a health claim for soy protein: "25 g per day may lower serum cholesterol as part of a heart healthy diet." Twenty-five grams of soy protein contains about 45 mg of isoflavones (although not part of seed protein, isoflavones bind strongly to them). In postmenopausal women, the phytoestrogens may have an estrogen effect leading to a reduction in menopausal symptoms and a reduced incidence of osteoporosis and CHD. Phytoestrogens include isoflavones (soybeans), coumestans (alfalfa, broccoli, spinach), and lignans (produced by colonic bacteria from dietary precursors in cereal grains, beans, peas, and berries). In a recent study, a careful inspection of the diets of nearly 1000 older women in Massachusetts found their average intake of these phytoestrogens to be less than 1 mg daily, which is less than 5% of the phytoestrogen intake reported for Asian populations. Soybeans and soy products like tofu are concentrated sources of phytoestrogens. By contrast, foods common in western diets are lower in these compounds.

Epidemiological evidence shows that Japanese women and vegetarians who eat a diet low in fat and high in phytoestrogens have a lower incidence of breast cancer, while Japanese men with a similar diet have a lower mortality rate from prostate cancer than do their American counterparts.

One phytoestrogen with a relatively high degree of biological activity is Equol, which is formed from the isoflavone compound present in soybeans. The consumption of a diet that contains cooked soy protein usually causes a 50- to 100-fold increase in urinary Equol excretion, compared with one containing textured soya. Although Equol has a low affinity for estrogen receptors relative to that of estradiol, the high (3.5–7 mg/day) concentration of the phytoestrogen produced when a dietary precursor such as soya is consumed may exert a dampening effect on total estrogen bioactivity at target cell sites; in so doing, it may have a beneficial effect on hormone-mediated cancer risks.

Other major isoflavones in soybeans are genistein and daidzein. They possess antiestrogenic, antioxidant, and antifungal properties. The first two properties are proposed to be anticarcinogenic. Genistein slows the growth of breast cancer cells that depend on estrogen for growth. This phytoestrogen shows promise as a natural anticancer agent.

It has been suggested that about 25–30 g of soybeans per day may provide health benefits. Traditional soy foods include cooked and roasted soybeans, soy milk, tempeh (fermented soybean cake with smoky meaty taste), tofu (a protein-rich curd made from hot extracts of soybeans), soy sauce, and some others. Except for soy sauce, these foods are good sources of isoflavones. To include these products (equivalent to 25–30 g of soybeans) into diets is a challenge to consumers. However, the food industry is responding with new soy products that should make such dietary changes possible.

Soy products such as tofu, tacos, burgers, and baby formula have swept the nation as a healthy source of high protein with a reputation for being all natural and good. But there are opposing viewpoints on the benefits of soy products. Some researchers are suggesting that there may be a downside to this "miracle food." Soybeans can cause allergy in some individuals, especially children. Soy may prevent breast cancer in some women but the effect of isoflavones in individuals at high risk for estrogen-dependent breast cancer appears to be different. Studies demonstrate a link between soy and fertility problems in certain animals. And one study has shown that men consuming more than two portions of soya-based foods a week had lower sperm count.[8] Genistein inhibits the activity of thyroid peroxidase, an enzyme needed for the formation of thyroid hormone. However, clinical studies in which subjects consumed 25–50 g of soy protein/day generally show little or no change in thyroid function. Soy may have a connection to accelerated aging of the brain in the elderly.[23] Soy infant formula is a life saver for the 3–4% of babies who are allergic to or cannot digest milk sugar. But the long-term effect of phytoestrogen exposure at this early age is not known. Research in this field is continuing and should answer the questions on the safety of soy products.

29.3.3 CRUCIFEROUS VEGETABLES

Cruciferous vegetables such as cabbage, cauliflower, broccoli, Brussels sprouts, and watercress contain little fat, are low in energy, and are good sources of vitamins and minerals. They have a fiber content of about 30% of their dry weight. These vegetables are unique in their high content of glucosinolates, which, on hydrolysis, yield a number of breakdown products, mostly isothiocyanates that are biologically active. Several of these isothiocyanate derivatives (e.g., phenylethyl isothiocyanate, sulforaphene, and indole-3-carbinol) have been shown to protect against carcinogens in various in vitro and animal testing systems. Epidemiological studies have revealed an inverse association between the ingestion of cruciferous vegetables and stomach cancer, cabbage and cauliflower ingestion and lung cancer, and broccoli ingestion and all cancers. Cabbage intake has been assessed with the greatest number of studies showing this effect.

In 1982, the National Research Council on Diet, Nutrition, and Cancer found that "there is sufficient epidemiological evidence to suggest that consumption of cruciferous vegetables is associated with a reduction in the incidence of cancer at several sites in humans." The committee recommended the consumption of these vegetables for cancer prevention. The glucosinolate content of these vegetables is influenced by genetic factors, growing conditions, and maturity at time of harvest. For example, among the 76 broccoli varieties evaluated, scientists found a 30-fold variation in both sulforaphene levels and enzyme induction potential. Breeders may be able to develop new varieties with greater levels of the protective compounds. Eating such improved broccoli might stimulate an enhanced chemoprotective response against cancer development.

The organosulfur compounds have been shown to increase the activity of enzymes involved in the detoxication of carcinogens and other foreign compounds. Isothiocyanates are ideal anticancer agents because some of them inhibit the phase I enzymes that metabolically activate carcinogens, damage DNA, and initiate malignancy. Many are also inducers of phase II enzymes, which eliminate carcinogens by detoxication. The balance between phase I and phase II enzymes is a major determinant of the outcome following exposure to carcinogens. One particular isothiocyanate, sulphoraphane, appears to be an exceptionally potent inducer of detoxication enzymes. Another component of cruciferous vegetables, indole-3-carbinol, has been shown to affect estrogen metabolism in human beings. Specifically, the estradiol hydroxylation pathway may be affected such that more of the less potent form of estradiol is formed. This may protect against estrogen-related cancers such as breast and endometrial cancers.

Recent work suggests that broccoli is especially good for the stomach. Sulphoraphane appears to easily kill the peptic ulcer-causing bacterium *Helicobacter pylori*, which is notoriously difficult to eradicate even with a combination of two or three antibiotics.[16,39] Moreover, tests in mice suggest that the compound offers formidable protection against stomach cancer, the second most common form of cancer worldwide. Investigators are preparing to start a clinical trial in Japan to test the broccoli sprouts' effectiveness in people infected with *H. pylori*. About 80% of Japanese adults have this microbe in their stomachs—one reason that gastric cancer is the no. 1 cancer killer in Japanese women and no. 2 after lung cancer in Japanese men. If upcoming human tests confirm the findings, a daily snack of tangy broccoli sprouts could become a medically indicated staple—especially in Asia where ulcer bacteria and stomach cancer occur in epidemic proportions.

29.3.4 Tomatoes, Autumn Olive Berries

Tomatoes have become a staple for humans in many parts of the world. Based on the production of vegetables and melons, the quantity of tomatoes and tomato products consumed in the United States is second only to potatoes. Tomatoes have modest to high concentrations of several nutrients. Tomato juice is ranked third as the highest contributor of vitamin C after orange juice and grapefruit juice, and ninth as the highest contributor of potassium in the American diet. Tomato is a source of lycopene, a red-colored carotenoid that is a potent antioxidant and quencher of singlet oxygen.

Other sources of dietary lycopene are pink grapefruit, watermelon, apricot, guava, and papaya. More than 80% of lycopene consumed in the United States is derived from tomato products. The ripeness of the fruit can cause variations in lycopene concentration in these foods. Varieties of tomatoes that are redder possess a lycopene concentration of about 5 mg/100 g, whereas yellow varieties have a lycopene content of about 0–5 mg/100 g. Cooking results in minimal losses and its bioavailability and absorption can be enhanced by an additional ingestion of some fats.[9]

Lycopene is a predominant carotenoid in human plasma with a concentration range between 0.22 and 1.06 nmol/ml. It is present in highest concentrations in the testes followed by the adrenals, liver, prostate, and other tissues. Lycopene has generated widespread interest as a possible deterrent to heart disease and cancer.[15] Available evidence suggests that lycopene, in addition to being an antioxidant, may inhibit cholesterol synthesis. Also, the risk of myocardial infarction is reduced in persons with higher adipose tissue concentrations of lycopene.

Epidemiological data support an association between the intake of tomato-based foods and a lower risk of cancer. The strongest relationships are found for cancers of the prostate, lungs, and stomach. Even two servings a week of a rich source of bioavailable lycopene such as tomato sauce is related to a substantially lower risk of prostate cancer. Supplementation of 15 mg of lycopene twice daily to prostate cancer patients appears to provide benefits, although much additional clinical studies are necessary. Recent studies have found that people who ate at least one serving of a tomato-based product per day had 50% less chance of developing cancer of the digestive tract, and older Americans may be less likely to die from all types of cancer.

Autumn olive (*Eleagnus umbellata*) is a nitrogen-fixing shrub covered with silvery green leaves and a profusion of red berries in late September and October. There are a few reports of people eating these sweet tart, pea-sized berries. Recently, it has been reported that this fruit contains lycopene levels ranging from 15 to 54 mg/100 g, compared with an average of 3 mg/100 g for fresh tomatoes, 10 mg/100 g for canned tomatoes, and 30 mg/100 g for tomato paste. These berries may be an excellent source to get lycopene economically because the plant thrives in poor soil.

29.3.5 Yellow and Dark Green Vegetables

Vegetables such as spinach, collard green, kale, mustard greens, broccoli, parsley, and dill are rich sources of yellow carotenoids, lutein and zeaxanthin. These two carotenoids are found in the eyes' lenses and are often referred to as macular pigment (MP). No other carotenoids, including β-carotene and lycopene (the two major carotenoids in the blood) are found in the lenses. Lutein and zeaxanthin are selectively accumulated in the retina from plasma and are particularly dense in the macula. These yellow pigments can filter visible blue light and protect the underlying tissues from phototoxic damage. This has been proposed as a factor, especially in the pathophysiology of age-related macular degeneration (ARMD).

Epidemiological studies have shown that a high dietary intake of lutein and zeaxanthin was associated with a 43% lower risk for ARMD. In other studies, people 55 years of age and older who ate five to six servings of spinach or collard greens a week were one-eighth as likely to suffer from macular degeneration (a leading cause of blindness) as those who ate one serving or less a month. An increased dietary intake of these carotenoids has been shown to increase their levels in plasma and MP density.

Cataracts are common in older adults, affecting 55–85% of people over 75 years of age. So identification of dietary strategies to delay their onset could have tremendous influence on the health of older people and on health care costs. Recent studies also suggest that lutein may be a potent protective factor against the progression of atherosclerosis.

Egg yolk contains large amounts of highly absorbable lutein and zeaxanthin compared with other common dietary sources of these carotenoids. The benefits of introducing these carotenoids into the diet with eggs are counterbalanced by a potential elevation of LDL cholesterol from the added dietary cholesterol. Yolk from a large egg contains, on average, about 0.3 mg of lutein and 0.22 mg of zeaxanthin. The corresponding values for spinach (1/2 cup, 60 g) are 10.5 and 0.3 mg and for corn (1 cup, 150 g) are 0.4 and 0.3 mg. A typical diet high in fruits and vegetables would be expected to contain about 2.3 mg/day lutein and 0.3 mg/day zeaxanthin.

29.3.6 GRAPES

The benefits of drinking a glass of wine have been touted over the past decade after the discovery of the "French paradox."[33] Epidemiological studies have shown that France has lower rates of heart diseases despite high-cholesterol diets. Much attention in explaining the French paradox has focused on the practice of the French consuming wine, particularly red wine,[32] with their meals. This cardioprotective effect is partly attributable to alcohol's ability to increase the concentration of high-density lipoprotein (HDL) cholesterol, a well-defined negative risk factor. Although the exact mechanisms by which wine consumption could offer protection against heart disease are not fully understood, a large body of literature suggests that some phytochemicals in grapes may account for the beneficial effects. Grapes are known to contain a variety of flavonoids (e.g., catechins, anthocyanins, etc.) and nonflavonoids. Of the nonflavonoids, resveratrol, a phytoalexin, has sparked much interest for its potential health-promoting effects. It is an antioxidant, it inhibits eicosanoid formation and platelet aggregation, and it modulates lipoprotein metabolism.

Recent work has shown that resveratrol has anticancer activity. It induces phase II enzymes of detoxication. Resveratrol inhibits the development of precancerous lesions in carcinogen-treated mouse mammary glands in culture; inhibits tumor formation in a mouse skin cancer model; and causes leukemic cells to differentiate into normal-looking blood cells.

Resveratrol is present mainly in grape skins, mulberries, and peanuts. An ounce of red wine provides about 160 mg of resveratrol and an ounce of peanuts provides 75 mg of resveratrol. Resveratrol merits further investigation as a potential cancer chemoprotective agent in humans.

29.3.7 BERRIES

29.3.7.1 Cranberries

Conventional wisdom has long held that drinking cranberry juice helps to fight urinary tract infections. A few yeas ago, scientists found an explanation. Certain components of cranberries interfere with the ability of *Esherichia coli* to adhere to uroepithelial cells, a prerequisite for the development of infections. Recently, researchers have identified and isolated condensed tannins from cranberries and found them to inhibit *E. coli* from adhering to cell surfaces in laboratory tests. This microbial antiadhesion effect may show promise in other parts of the body, including the oral cavity and gastrointestinal tract. A new study suggests that bacterial infection and the associated influx of white blood cells into the urine can be reduced by nearly 50% in elderly women, who drank 300 ml of cranberry juice cocktail each day over the course of the 6-month study.[3] It may also provide benefits related to antioxidant activity. Cranberry juice contains a chemical that is able to inhibit and even reverse the formation of plaque that causes tooth decay. Mouthwashes containing this compound are being developed to prevent periodontal disease. Cranberries are abundant sources of anthocyanins that may help prevent cancer, heart disease, and other diseases.[14,27]

29.3.7.2 Caneberries, Other Berries

Caneberries is an umbrella term that includes familiar berries such as red and black raspberries, marionberries, evergreen blackberries, and boysenberries. This group of berries grows on leafy canes in temperate regions of the world. These berries are a source of dietary fiber and a number of vitamins and minerals. They also contain antioxidants. The caneberries, along with blueberries and strawberries, contain ellagic acid, a plant phenol that is related to coumarins. Ellagic acid also occurs in high concentrations in grapes and nuts. It is a chemopreventive agent based on the fact that it induces glutathione S-tranferase (GST) and epoxide hydrolase, the enzymes of detoxication. It has shown inhibitory effects against chemically induced carcinogens in animal studies.

Strawberries contain fusetin, a flavonoid that has several properties of a neurotrophic factor. Researchers have recently found that fusetin protects and promotes survival of cultured neurons and enhances memory in healthy mice by increasing activation of the transcription factor cAMP response element-binding protein (CREB), which is involved in the physical changes in the brain underlying the development of long-term memory.[29] This is the first time that the function of a defined natural product has been characterized at the molecular level in the central nervous system. A synthetic form of fusetin may soon be available as a supplement. Eating strawberries sounds like an enjoyable alternative to popping a pill, but one would have to consume a large number of strawberries to get an adequate amount of fusetin used in laboratory experiments. Besides strawberries, fusetin is found in tomatoes, onions, oranges, apples, peaches, grapes, kiwi, and persimmons. Blueberries contain a compound called pterostilbene that has the potential to be developed into a natural medicine for lowering blood cholesterol, particularly for people who do not respond well to conventional lipid-lowering drugs.[24] Pterostilbene increases LDL receptors in rat-liver cells in vitro. The compound is similar to resveratrol, an antioxidant in grapes and red wine that is also a cholesterol buster.

Blueberries were found to have the highest antioxidant activity of 40 fruits, juices, and vegetables measured in a test tube assay; concord grape juice had two-thirds the potency of blueberries and strawberries were about half as potent.

29.3.8 Cherries

Tart cherry is touted for its various health benefits. It contains anthocyanins, which have antioxidant properties. In addition, it contains a number of compounds that inhibit cyclooxygenase activity and exhibit other pharmacological effects such as antiallergic, antiviral, anti-inflammatory and anticarcinogenic activities. The compounds also may prevent cardiovascular diseases and slow the aging process. Tart cherries added to ground beef at 4.5% by weight inhibits both the oxidation of lipids (spoilage) in raw and fried patties and the formation of heterocyclic aromatic amines in fried patties. Hence, the consumption of cherries might be beneficial in protecting humans against various chronic diseases.

29.3.9 Citrus Fruits

Citrus fruits are known for their high content of vitamin C. They also contain flavonoids, limonene, coumarins, and several other compounds. The most prevalent flavonoids are hesperetin in orange and naringenin in grapefruit found in fruit tissue and peels largely as their glycosides, hesperidin and naringin, respectively. Hesperidin gives orange juice its cloudy appearance and naringenin is responsible for the bitter taste of grapefruit. In tangerine, there are two main flavonoids, tangeretin and nobiletin. Hesperetin and naringenin are structurally similar to the isoflavone genistein found in soybeans. Like genistein, hesperetin and naringenin exhibit hypolipidemic effects in cholesterol-fed rats. This suggests that oranges and grapefruits and their juices could have cholesterol-lowering potential.

Naringenin and hesperetin also show antitumor activities in experimental animals. Most recently, it has been observed that naringenin, when administered to test tube cultures of estrogen-sensitive human breast cancer cells, is almost eight times more potent at halting the cell's growth than genistein. Naringenin is less effective than genistein, however, at slowing the growth of breast cancer cells that depend on estrogen for growth. Tangeretin and nobiletin are found to be about 250 times more potent than genistein in estrogen-insensitive cells and five times more potent in estrogen-dependent cancer cells. Delivered together, or with certain other fruit flavonoids, they are still more potent. They also appear to increase the efficacy of tamoxifen, the leading drug for halting breast cancer recurrence.

Several citrus flavonoids inhibit certain cytochrome P-450 enzymes. This is important because some of these enzymes can turn procarcinogens to carcinogens. One cytochrome P-450 enzyme, 1B1, is present in high levels in breast and prostate cancer cells but is rarely seen in normal cells. Hesperetin blocks cytochrome P-450 1B1, reducing the chances of formation of carcinogens from procarcinogens. Hesperetin's effect on this enzyme might lead to the development of alternatives to traditional cancer chemotherapy.

Epidemiological survey data have found the intake of citrus fruits to be beneficial for cancer prevention. Thus, orange juice and grapefruit juice are not just breakfast juices rich in vitamin C, but also have anticancer prospects.

Limonene, a monoterpene used for many years as a flavoring agent, induces GST and suppresses tumor growth in experimental animals exposed to direct-acting carcinogens as well as procarcinogens. It may also suppress the proliferation of tumor cells. Limonene is found in the essential oils of citrus fruits and the most abundant source is orange peel oil, which is 90–95% limonene by weight. Limonene is also found in the essential oils of cherry, spearmint, and dill.

29.3.10   Evening Primrose Oil and Olive Oil

29.3.10.1   Evening Primrose Oil

Evening primrose seed oil is a relatively unique plant oil in that it contains a high proportion of γ linolenic acid (GLA). The oil of borage seed, principally grown in western Canada, and black currant seed oil are also rich in GLA. The advantage of consuming oils rich in GLA is that this fatty acid bypasses the rate-limiting desaturase step of linoleic acid metabolism. GLA is easily converted to dihomo GLA (DHGL), which can generate beneficial eicosanoids such as prostaglandin (PG) El with anti-inflammatory potential, and may inhibit the production of eicosanoids derived from arachidonic acid (AA). Dietary supplementation with GLA has been shown in several experimental animal models to suppress acute and chronic inflammation as well as joint tissue injury.

29.3.10.2   Olive Oil

Olive oil is derived from the fresh ripe fruit and comprises about 20% of olive by weight. The oil has a unique fatty acid composition: its oleic acid content ranges from 56 to 84%, the saturated fatty acids palmitate and stearate are present in small amounts, and linoleate may compose 3–21% of the total fatty acid content. The taste of olive oil is influenced by many factors: soil, climate, variety of olive, vintage, harvest time, and method of processing, such as cold pressing, which uses stone wheels and generates no heat. The term extra virgin refers to a grade of olive oil, usually indicating the highest quality. Extra virgin olive oils are naturally low in levels of free oleic acid—less than 1%. This is the oil that is extracted under light pressure during processing and not further refined. Virgin olive oil has two to three times the free acid of an extra virgin oil. Most oils in the market are expressed under heavy pressure and undergo further refinement.

The interest in the health benefits of olive oil is due to the low incidence of cardiovascular disease and cancer, particularly breast cancer, in cultures where Mediterranean diet is consumed. This diet consists of ample fresh fruits, vegetables, grains, and legumes, which are low in meat and high in olive oil. The lower incidence of cardiovascular disease has been attributed to the relatively high oleate in olive oil. The virgin oil also contains significant amounts of antioxidant polyphenolic compounds, which may allow for the protection against LDL cholesterol oxidation.

Epidemiological studies have yielded consistent results on the inverse relation of monounsaturated fatty acids or olive oil consumption and the incidence of breast cancer. Recent studies also suggest that olive oil may protect against other types of cancer. The antioxidants present in the oil may also play an important role as they apparently do for heart disease. The extraction of these compounds and the use of experimental and clinical trials may provide a better insight into the role of these compounds in promoting health benefits.

29.3.11 Garlic and Related Vegetables

Garlic, onion, ginger, scallion, leeks, and chives belong to the allium vegetable family and are notable for their content of compounds such as diallyl sulfide and allyl methyl trisulfide. Garlic is a common plant used as food in all parts of the world. Actual garlic intakes are not known with certainty, especially because it is not typically considered in dietary assessment surveys. Intakes vary from region to region and from individual to individual. Average intakes in the United States may be around 0.6 g/week while intakes in some parts of China may be as much as 15 g/day. Since ancient times, it has been used as a folk medicine for a variety of human illnesses. Garlic has been used for the prevention and treatment of an impressive range of diseases from plague to heart disease and cancer, as well as for warding off evil spirits. At the present time, garlic is promoted as a "miracle" nutrient and the world's most ancient and versatile and enjoyable medicine.[31] Garlic is rich in vitamins and antioxidants, and garlic extracts are fashionable nutrient supplements. While some of the therapeutic claims are myths, others have a scientific basis for their actions. During the last few years, this folk medicine has been subjected to scientific investigations. Recent research has focused on garlic's cancer-protective and cardiovascular-protective effects.

The principal active ingredient in garlic is allicin, a sulfur-containing compound. This and other allyl sulfur compounds have been reported to possess a variety of health benefits. Notable among these are antimicrobial, anticarcinogenic, and protective benefits against cardiovascular disease. Considerable evidence indicates that garlic extracts can inhibit a range of gram-negative and gram-positive bacteria, and serve as an antifungal agent. The antibacterial activity of these compounds may serve to inhibit the bacterial conversion of nitrate to nitrite in the stomach. They may reduce the amount of nitrite available for reaction with secondary amines to form nitrosamines, which are known to be carcinogenic. These allium compounds have been shown to induce GST, an enzyme in the phase II reaction of detoxication. An inverse relationship between garlic intake and gastric cancer mortality in humans has been reported. Those consuming 20 g of garlic per day have a 10 times lower incidence of gastric cancer mortality than those who consume less garlic (2 g). While these are massive intakes, the influence of lower intakes remains to be determined.

In humans, garlic supplementation can lower cholesterol and triglyceride levels in the blood. Allicin, as well as extracts of garlic, onion, and ginger, has been shown to inhibit platelet aggregation by blocking thromboxane synthetase and thus reducing thromboxane A2 generation from AA. Also, epidemiological data in certain ethnic and geographical groups have shown that those who consume liberal quantities of garlic, onion, and ginger have a lower incidence of cardiovascular diseases. Studies in humans and animals have shown beneficial effects of garlic and its preparations in the control of hypertension. For centuries, it has been used for treating hypertension in China and Japan and is officially recognized for this purpose by the Japanese Food and Drug Administration.

The active component in garlic, onion, and ginger affects cyclooxygenase and lipoxygenase pathways and provides relief in rheumatoid arthritis by reducing pain and by improving the movement of joints in patients suffering from arthritis.

The nontoxic nature of garlic in its usual dosage has been established by its long use as an edible plant. However, in higher doses and in raw form, garlic may cause contact dermatitis and irritation of the digestive mucosa.

Garlic has recently received significant attention as a functional food both in the popular press and scientific journals. It is available in various forms in health food stores, drug stores, and even in some supermarkets. It seems reasonable to conclude that the ancient belief of the beneficial effects of garlic, at least as far as cancer and heart disease are concerned, may indeed have a scientific basis. Two or more cloves of garlic, as well as liberal use of onions and ginger daily, may help.

29.3.12 NUTS

Nuts are part of the meat alternate group and are a rich source of important nutrients: protein, fat, vitamin E, folic acid, and some other nutrients. Nuts are rich in unsaturated fatty acids and dietary fiber. An ounce of peanuts or mixed nuts provide 2.4–2.6 g of dietary fiber. In addition, nuts may be a source of healthful, biologically active phytochemicals (e.g., ellagic acid, flavonoids, phytosterols, and tocotrienols).

Epidemiological studies suggest that frequent consumption of nuts[25] may provide some protection against CHD. Nuts have a strong inverse relationship to the risk of myocardial infarction or dying in CHD. The proteins in nuts are relatively rich in arginine, a precursor of nitric oxide, which is a potent endogenous vasodilator that acts much like nitroglycerine. Nitric oxide may have other anti-atherogenic properties as well, such as inhibiting platelet aggregation. Folic acid in nuts may help lower blood homocysteine level. High levels of homocysteine have been linked to increased CHD risks. Human nutrition studies have shown that nuts cause a reduction in total and LDL cholesterol. Most studies used whole nuts with a wide range of intakes, between 35 and 110 g/day, during the dietary intervention.

Phytosterols are known to lower blood cholesterol by inhibiting dietary and biliary cholesterol absorption. The favorable fatty acid profile (oleic acid and linoleic acid) in nuts contributes to cholesterol lowering and, hence, CHD risk reduction. Dietary fiber and bioactive constituents (antioxidants) in nuts may confer additional protective effects.

Nuts contain many different flavonoids, including quercetin and kaempferol, which have been shown to decrease the in vitro proliferation of human cancer cell lines. Phytosterols may confer protection against cancer by inhibiting cell division and stimulating tumor cell death. Peanuts are one of the few plant foods shown to contain resveratrol, which has been shown to act as an antioxidant and antimutagen.

There is significant evidence that nuts may have beneficial effects on health through a variety of mechanisms regulated by many nut constituents. In 2003 the U.S. FDA approved that packages of nuts may state on their labels that "scientific evidence suggests but does not prove that eating 1.5 ounces per day of most nuts as part of a healthy overall diet low in saturated fat and cholesterol may reduce the risk of heart disease." It was the first qualified health claim approved by the FDA under the new program that will give consumers more labeling information about the potential health impact of their food. The FDA only approved the health claim for almonds, hazelnuts, peanuts, pecans, some pine nuts, pistachios, and walnuts, as these nuts contain <4 g of saturated fat per 50 g. However, this does not mean one should restrict only to these nuts. In addition to nuts, seeds such as flaxseeds, pumpkin seeds, and sunflower seeds may offer the same heart health benefits.

Each nut has its own virtues; walnut is an excellent source of ω-3 oils, which are scarce in the average American diet; almond is high in vitamin E. But given the calories (one ounce of nuts averages 170 calories, 15 g fat and 2 g saturated fat) moderation is required. The recommended portion is equal to a third of a cup or a large handful per day as part of a healthy diet.

29.3.13 TEA

Tea is the most popular beverage consumed worldwide. Of the total amount of tea produced and consumed in the world, 78% is black, 20% is green, and <2% is oolong tea. Black tea is the type typically used in the United States, Europe, India, and Africa; whereas green tea is consumed primarily in China, Japan, and a few countries in North Africa and the Middle East. The use of oolong tea is confined to southeastern China and Taiwan.

The tea leaves contain more than 35% of their dry weight in polyphenols. To produce green tea, freshly harvested leaves are rapidly steamed or pan-fried to inactivate enzymes, and then air-dried at high temperature. This prevents fermentation and produces a dry stable product. Green tea contains polyphenolic compounds, which include flavanols, flavonoids, and phenolic acids. Most of the polyphenols in green tea are flavanols, commonly known as catechins; the major catechins in green tea are epicatechin, epicatechin-3-gallate, and epigallocatechin-3 gallate (EGCG), accounting for its characteristic color and flavor. It has been estimated that one cup of green tea can contain 100–200 mg of catechins. Black tea is derived from aged leaves that have undergone enzymatically catalyzed aerobic oxidation and chemical condensation, particularly of the catechins. Consequently, the catechin levels are lower in black tea than in green tea. During the production process, some catechins are converted to theaflavin and thearubigin—the major polyphenols in black tea. They give black tea its characteristic color and flavor. Theaflavin concentrations are directly correlated with black tea quality. To produce oolong tea, fresh leaves are subjected to a partial oxidation stage before drying. Normal oolong tea is considered to be about half as fermented as black tea.

Tea is second only to water as the most consumed beverage in the world. In addition to the enjoyable aspects, tea provides a natural source of compounds that protect against a wide array of diseases.[40] It is the richest source of flavonoids and contributes, based on the amount of tea consumed, as high as 70% of dietary flavonoids. It also contains other beneficial compounds (e.g., vitamins, manganese, and fluoride). Tea is thought to have a greater antioxidant capacity than most vegetables, and is more potent than vitamins C and E and β-carotene. The possible beneficial health effects of tea consumption have been suggested and supported by some studies, but others have found no beneficial effects.

Tea may have antimicrobiological properties. There is evidence that ordinary tea may prime the immune system to fend off attacks from bacteria and other pathogens. Drinking 20 ounces of tea every day for at least 2 weeks is shown to double or triple the immune system's output of an infection-fighting substance called interferon γ. Apparently the body metabolizes the tea into molecules that mimic the surface protein of bacteria, jump-starting the immune system so that when real bugs show up, they can be more easily displaced. Microorganisms that cause diarrhea are affected by tea. It plays an important role in improving beneficial intestinal microflora. Tea polyphenols help inhibit the growth of bacteria that cause bad breath. Bad breath is due to sulfur compounds, such as hydrogen sulfide, produced by anaerobic bacteria. The bacteria thrive in oxygen-short places like the back of the tongue and deep gum pockets. The amino acid, theanine, found exclusively in the tea plant, boosts mental alertness.[35] It can also provide potential health benefits associated with its content of fluoride. Cardiovascular health appears to be better in tea drinkers than nontea drinkers. Several epidemiological studies have suggested that drinking either green or black tea provides a degree of protection against cardiovascular diseases. Drinking at least three cups of green or black tea a day can significantly reduce the risk of stroke.

A study has shown that adding milk to tea will block the normal healthful effects that tea has in protecting against cardiovascular disease.[28] This is because casein from milk binds to tea components that cause the arteries to relax, especially EGCG. Other studies have found little or no effect of milk on the observed increase in total plasma antioxidant activity after tea consumption.[34] Green tea with high EGCG content is not typically consumed with milk.

Tea and tea preparations inhibit tumorigenesis in a variety of animal models. A growing body of evidence suggests that a moderate consumption of tea may protect against several forms of cancer. Green tea contains EGCG. This polyphenol is not present in black tea. Recently, it has been suggested that EGCG binds urokinase, a proteolytic enzyme that is usually overexpressed in human cancers. Invading cancer cells use it to attack tissues and organs, enabling the cancer to metastasize. The enzyme is also involved in the formation of new blood vessels around developing tumors. Inhibiting urokinase decreases the size of tumors and, in some cases, it has led to a complete disappearance of cancer in mice. A cup of green tea contains about 150 mg of EGCG. Those who take two or more cups of tea each day can get a sizable amount of this cardiovascular disease and cancer-preventive agent.[26] But habitually drinking hot tea at a temperature of 65–70°C is associated with the risk of developing esophageal cancer, compared with individuals who prefer their tea at less than 65°C, according to a recent study. Those who drink tea very hot at more than 70°C increase their risk of developing esophageal cancer eightfold.

29.3.14 Chocolate

Chocolate is a product derived from cocoa (cacao) mixed with fat (i.e. cocoa butter and/or plant oils) and sugar. Pure unsweetened chocolate contains primarily cocoa solids and cocoa butter in varying proportions. Much of the chocolate consumed today is in the form of sweet chocolate, combining chocolate with sugar. Milk chocolate is sweet chocolate that additionally contains milk powder or condensed milk. White chocolate is formed from a mixture of cocoa butter, sugar, and milk but no cocoa solids and has, therefore, an off-white color. Dark chocolate[30] is sweetened chocolate with high content of cocoa solids. It is chocolate without milk, although in the United States it is added in most commonly found chocolates. Dark chocolate with its high cocoa content is a rich source of epicatechin and gallic acid, which are thought to possess cardioprotective properties. Dark chocolate contains a large number of antioxidants (nearly eight times the number found in strawberries). Epicatechin binds to milk protein and is not absorbed. Therefore, it is better to take chocolate without milk.

Eating dark chocolate has been shown to lower blood pressure in mildly hypertensive subjects. Chocolate is found to exhibit biochemical effects similar to aspirin in reducing platelet clumping. A recent study found that survivors of heart attack who ate chocolate at least two or three times a week reduced their risk of death by a factor of up to three times compared to survivors who did not eat chocolate. Theobromine, a cocoa-derived product, suppresses persistent coughing. Other suggested benefits of chocolate include anticancer, brain stimulator, and antidiarrheal effects.

It is still hard to think of chocolate as a health food. A 40 g chocolate provides about 210 calories and 17 g fat, 8 g of which is saturated. The amount of chocolate needed to have health benefits would provide a large quantity of calories which, if unused, would promote weight gain.

29.3.15 Miscellaneous Foods and Their Active Components

In the East, some varieties of edible mushrooms have been used to maintain health, dating back more than 2000 years. One variety, known as Shiitake (in Japan), is the second most commonly produced edible mushroom in the world. It contains proteins (26% of dry weight), linoleic acid, and some vitamins and minerals. Besides its nutritive content, several important compounds have been recently isolated from Shiitake, which have immunomodulatory, lipid-lowering, and antimicrobial properties. These include lentinan and eritadenine. Of these, eritadenine is the most studied. There are also a few other varieties of mushroom with these and other health benefits without any significant toxicity.

Turmeric is a spice isolated from the rhizome of the *Curcuma longa* plant. It is commonly used in Indian cuisine for its color and flavor. In ancient medicine, turmeric was used to treat contusions, sprains, and bruises, and as an astringent and antiseptic. The active principles of turmeric have been identified as yellow-colored phenolic compounds curcumin I and curcumin III. Curcumins exhibit COX2 inhibitor activity and are potent anti-inflammatory agents. They suppress the tumor's production of growth factors, induce GST in mice, and inhibit carcinogenesis in experimental animals. Turmeric's broad spectrum of action as an anti-inhibitor and antipromoter makes it an ideal functional food for the prevention of cancer. Turmeric is found to reduce death rates in mice with a genetic defect that causes cystic fibrosis in humans. Turmeric in daily amounts of 0.5–1 g has been consumed without any adverse effects.

Cinnamon, a spice, contains several bioactive substances. One of them, methylhydroxychalcone polymer (MHCP) has recently been found to increase glucose metabolism roughly 20-fold in the test tube assay of fat cells. Cinnamon makes fat cells much more responsive to insulin. Whether it is effective in patients with diabetes remains to be determined.

Bitter melon, also known as karela in India, is a common vegetable native to all tropical countries. Its scientific name is *Momordica charantia*. It has been used to reduce blood glucose in diabetic patients in some parts of Asia and South America for centuries. Bitter melon extracts have been shown to lower blood glucose and to improve glucose tolerance in clinical and experimental studies.

Lemon grass oil, a widely used flavoring in Asian cooking, contains a substance that inhibits cholesterol biosynthesis. In one recent study, feeding 140-mg capsules of the oil daily for 3 months to patients with hypercholesterolemia caused a decrease of about 10% in their serum cholesterol level.

Extracts of licorice have been used both as a medicine and as a flavoring for foods, particularly candies. Extracts cause the induction of GST, suggesting a detoxication potential and anticarcinogenic effect. The essential oil of peppermint contains menthol and several other compounds and flavonoids, which have been reported to have muscle-relaxing effects. Some compounds isolated from parsley have been reported to have diuretic, vasodilating, and spasmolytic functions. Another compound, myristicin, is a potent chemoprotective[45] agent.

Cilantro, also known as coriander leaves, has a distinct aroma due to its concentrated essential oils. The fresh leaves are often sprinkled over the tops of dishes. It contains dodecenal, which has the ability to kill certain bacteria such as Salmonella that cause food borne illness. Cilantro is thought to help regulate blood sugar. It has also been suggested that the chemicals in cilantro can bind heavy metals and other toxins to aid in removing them from the body.

Flaxseed is an oil seed that contains 41% fat, 28% dietary fiber, and 21% protein. Although not widely consumed by humans, it is a rich source of α linolenic acid (ALA) and contains the highest amount of lignans of any plant source examined. Flaxseed is known to lower blood cholesterol; to protect against heart diseases, stroke, and certain types of cancer; and to mediate immune response. Both ALA and lignans have been hypothesized as the chemoprotective agents in flaxseed because they are precursors of biologically active compounds. A regular intake of two tablespoons, 450 g of ground flaxseed, can deliver physiological quantities of ALA and lignans.

29.4   NEED FOR ADDITIONAL RESEARCH

In the past few years, much information has accumulated on the health effects of plant foods such as cereals, legumes, nuts, fruits, and vegetables. These foods are rich in several nutrients as well as many other classes of phytochemicals. These compounds have been shown to modulate detoxication enzymes, stimulate the immune system, inhibit platelet aggregation, modulate cholesterol synthesis, reduce blood pressure, and provide antioxidant, antiviral, and antibacterial effects. Epidemiological data support the association between a high intake of fruits and vegetables and a low risk of chronic diseases. The data also support the association between a regular consumption of certain foods and a low incidence of specific diseases.

Several health-promoting phytochemicals in foods have been identified. An extensive study of phytochemcials in cell culture systems and animal models has provided a wealth of information on the mechanisms by which a diet high in fruits and vegetables may lower the risk of chronic diseases in humans. However, it is not always clear whether the effects in animals often observed with high doses of single compounds can be readily extrapolated to humans. Controlled intervention studies in humans can help establish the benefits of phytochemical supplements. The concept that certain foods can provide health-enhancing and disease-preventing properties is being accepted by a growing number of individuals. This knowledge continues to be supported by research that demonstrates that dietary habits are intrinsically linked to health promotion and disease prevention.[41] What is also becoming increasingly apparent is that not all individuals respond identically to dietary intervention. It is important to understand how a person's hereditary material (DNA) and associated regulatory genes involved with absorption, transport, and metabolism may influence the overall response to dietary intervention strategies.

Until additional information on phytochemicals (e.g., dosage, effects of long-term use) is known, it is best to place emphasis on whole foods rather than individual dietary components. Many phytochemicals give fruits and vegetables their colors, which provide an easy way to communicate an increased diversity of fruits and vegetables to the public and to ensure that a wide variety is consumed daily.

29.5   SEAFOOD

The important role of seafood, which is rich in eicosapentaenoic acid (EPA) and docosahexaenoic acid (DHA), became evident as a result of epidemiological studies and observations on Greenland Eskimos. Cardiovascular disease, diabetes, and psoriasis in particular were rare in this population despite the fact that their diet is high in fat. Eskimos consume a high amount of EPA (6 g day) and DHA (9 g/day) compared to Danes, who consume only 0.5 g/day EPA and 0.4 g/day DHA. Danes have a relatively higher incidence of cardiovascular disease and diabetes. Both EPA and DHA (in the form of fish) lower blood triglyceride levels. They cause a decrease in platelet aggregation as a result of a decreased formation of TXA2 and an increased formation of TXA3. Both EPA and DHA lower blood pressure in patients with mild to moderate hypertension, probably because of the decrease in PGE2 and related metabolites. These fatty acids also decrease the production of proinflammatory leukotriene (LT) B4. The administration of fish oil diminishes the severity of arthritis. Clinical investigations and animal experiments have demonstrated that increasing the dietary intake of EPA and DHA in the form of fish or fish oil can alter the spectrum of biologically active eicosanoids and can induce an antithrombotic and anti-inflammatory state that is beneficial to health.

Fish oil intake in animal cancer model studies appears to reduce tumor development and growth. The benefits of ω3 fatty acids in fish oil are believed to be due to a number of factors that include the formation of eicosanoids that participate in immune surveillance, inflammation, and cellular proliferation; the modification of the normal environmental and hormonal receptors; and the changes in cell membrane structure, which affects cell signaling. The eicosanoid modification hypothesis has been used to explain the low cancer rates among Greenland Eskimos and other northern fish-eating cultures such as the Japanese. Diets high in DHA even in the presence of moderate amounts of linoleate (which appears to promote tumor growth) have been shown to reduce tumor promotion in animals.

The availability of the ethyl esters of individual ω3 fatty acids for human use should encourage further research to identify their specific metabolic actions and therapeutic potentials.

29.6   USE OF BIOTECHNOLOGY IN THE FOOD INDUSTRY

The classical methods of biotechnology for foods such as food fermentation and conventional agricultural breeding programs have been known for many years. Now it is possible by genetic engineering technique, which is the ability to transfer individual genes from one living organism to another, to manipulate genes in plants and animals to produce new food ingredients.[12] This technique is also used to produce a variety of plants with enhanced yield, decreased time to maturity, and increased tolerance to herbicides, pesticides, and viruses. In Japan, rice is produced with an enzyme that removes the allergen, globin, while retaining 80% of the nutritious rice seed protein. Its taste is that of ordinary rice and it prevents allergy in sensitive individuals. For unexplained reason, allergy to rice has become common in Japan. Rapeseed oil normally contains high erucic acid, which adversely affects the heart. It has been possible to manipulate the genes in this plant to produce seeds with very low erucic acid and high oleic acid. The oil is marketed in this country as canola.

Plants make vitamin A precursors and other carotenoids as well as vitamin E (tocopherols) in plastids, including chloroplasts, where they function as pigments and antioxidants in photosynthesis. These same antioxidant properties are important in human nutrition beyond RDAs. Extra carotenoids and tocopherols reportedly enhance cardiovascular health, prevent cancer, and slow the aging process. Because rice is an important food staple worldwide, it is an important target for nutritional improvement. A rice grain is mostly endosperm tissue whose specialized plastids store starch. Endosperm does not make chlorophyll or carotenes; therefore, rice grain is mostly white. In underdeveloped countries, vitamin A deficiency is a serious public health problem. Millions of children in these countries go blind each year because their diet is low in fruits and vegetables. To increase the availability of carotenoids, researchers have recently used recombinant DNA technology to create β-carotene-containing rice as a means to fight vitamin A deficiency.[44] Transgenic rice grains are golden yellow. Just 300 g of rice each day should prevent vitamin A deficiency.

Canola oil is very low in carotenes. A recombinant DNA technique has produced transgenic seeds that contain a small amount of lycopene and a great amount of α-carotene and β-carotene. Oils extracted from these seeds can provide the RDA for vitamin A. The total carotenoids in seeds increased 50-fold compared to controls—and more than in tomato or carrot.

In the United States, vegetable oils provide about 60% of the dietary vitamin E. α tocopherol is the most active form of vitamin E, but in general, vegetable oils are rich in the precursor γ tocopherol, which is 10% as active as the α isomer. With the use of recombinant DNA technology, it has been possible to alter the composition of these seeds to contain more than 95% of tocopherol in the form of the α isomer, leading to a fivefold increase in vitamin E activity. Similar techniques have produced new carotenoids called torulene and astaxanthin. The latter is responsible for the characteristic pink coloring of salmon, trout, and shrimp. This carotenoid is currently marketed commercially for use in salmon farming. Astaxanthin is also of interest for potential medical applications because it has been shown to boost immune function in humans, reduce oral cancer in rats, and inhibit breast cancer in mice.

Biotechnology is likely to have a major impact in the development of food products with health benefits such as vegetable oils rich in monounsaturated fatty acids and fruits and vegetables rich in disease-preventing phytochemicals.

29.6.1 Controversy Related to Genetically Modified Foods

Genetically modified foods were first put in the market in the early 1990s and the average growth of GM crop production has increased about 10% per year. As of 2006 land area being used to cultivate GM crops all over the world totaled about 252 million acres. There are at least 23 countries that plant GM crops and the United States has over 53% share of the global biotech crop production. The United States is followed by Argentina, Brazil, and Canada. Soybean is the principal GM crop grown all over the world followed by maize, cotton, and canola.

Proponents of GM technology claim several successes. These include pest and disease resistance, selective herbicide resistance, improved storage and nutritional quality, reduction in cost of bringing crop to market and increased food supply for a booming world population. Rice is produced with built-in vitamin A that can help prevent blindness in children suffering from vitamin A deficiency. A tomato is produced that softens more easily, allowing it to develop longer on the vine and keep longer on the shelf. Potatoes are produced that absorb less oil when frying and strawberry crops are created that survive frost.

But many people do not like the idea of transferring animal genes into plants and vice versa. Scientists argue that there is enough food in the world and that the hunger crisis is caused by problems in food distribution and politics, not production. There is growing concern that introducing foreign genes into food (plant and animal) may have an unexpected negative impact on health. A study has shown adverse effects on the gastrointestinal tract of rats fed GM potatoes. It is believed by some that GM foods cause the development of disease that may be immune to antibiotics. Many children in the United States and Europe have developed in recent years life-threatening allergies to peanuts and other foods. There is a possibility that introducing genes into a plant may create a new allergen or cause an allergic reaction in susceptible individuals. Not much is known about the long-term effects of GM crops.

The most common GM crops in the United States are soybeans, corn, cotton, and canola. In 1999 >40% of corn, >50% of cotton, and >45% of soybean planted in the United States were genetically modified. Many processed food products contain soybean or corn ingredients (e.g. soy protein, high fructose corn syrup). It is estimated that 60–75% of processed food in grocery stores include at least one ingredient from GM food. And yet only 40% of people in the United States know that some of the foods they are buying and eating are genetically modified. Additionally, 1 out of 4 people incorrectly believe that such foods are not being sold in the United States.

The majority of Americans are eating GM foods without their knowledge, because food labels do not list GM ingredients.[37] The general public has shown less resistance to the introduction of GM foods. The majority of Europeans oppose GM foods and this is true in some other parts of the world as well. Zambia has banned GM foods. Europe requires mandatory food labeling of GM foods and the European Union (EU) has established a 1% threshold for contamination of unmodified foods with GM products. At least 22 countries have announced plans to institute some form of mandatory labeling.

Manufacturers in many countries including in the United States do not voluntarily mention on labels that foods have genetically modified ingredients, because they think that this would affect their business. Environmental and consumer groups would like the U.S. FDA to follow the lead of the EU, Japan, and other countries by requiring labels on GM foods to allow consumers to know what they are buying. The FDA claims that such mandatory food labels are not necessary because GM food "poses no inherent safety risk." Until further studies can show that GM foods and crops do not pose serious threats to human health the debate over the use of GM foods is likely to continue.

29.6.2 GENETICALLY ALTERED ANIMALS GET CLOSER TO THE TABLE

Genetically engineered (GE) animals have been under development for decades. By inserting DNA segments from one species into another, biotech developers can introduce new traits into an animal. The benefits of GE animals are said to be huge and the possibilities endless. GE animals may be able to produce proteins or antibodies for drugs or vaccines. A drug called ATryn (a brand name for the anticoagulant antithrombin) is produced in the milk of GE goats. This is the first medicine produced by using GE animals. On February 6, 2009, the FDA approved the drug for the treatment of patients with hereditary antithrombin deficiency who are undergoing surgery or childbirth. The judgment in favor of using the drug produced by the goats paves the way for the approval of other GE animals, regardless of their intended use. For example, GE pigs could produce meat with high amounts of heart-healthy ω3 fatty acids or produce transplantable tissues.

The FDA is seriously considering whether to approve the first genetically engineered animal that people would eat—Atlantic salmon that contains growth hormone gene from a Chinook salmon as well as a genetic on-switch from the ocean pout fish, a distant relative of the salmon. It can grow at twice the normal rate. A public meeting to discuss the salmon was held in September of 2010. Some consumers and environmental groups are likely to raise objections to approval. Even within the FDA there is a debate as to whether the salmon should be labeled as GE (GE crops are not labeled in the United States). Salmon's approval would open a path for companies developing GE animals, like cattle resistant to mad cow disease or pigs that could supply healthier bacon. Cereal grains fed to pigs contain between 50% and 75% phosphorus in the form of phytate. Pigs do not digest phytate. It passes through the digestive tract and is concentrated in the manure. Because of poor digestibility, supplemental phosphorus is included in the feed to meet the dietary requirement of this nutrient for optimal growth. Farmers also use pig manure as a fertilizer. When the manure is spread on land, there is a buildup of phosphorus in the soil. When it rains it can leach into ponds, lakes, and rivers. With excess phosphorus, there is increased algal growth, leading to decreased oxygen concentration in the water. This can result in the death of fish and other aquatic animals. Researchers at the University of Guelph, Ontario, Canada, have developed environmentally friendly pigs to help pig farmers comply with nutrient management laws, which limit how much phosphorus can be applied to agricultural fields. The "enviropig" produces an enzyme, phytase, in the salivary gland. It is stable to gastric proteases. It helps the pigs digest phosphorus-rich phytate in animal feed, reducing the amount of phosphorus in their manure. This also eliminates the need for supplemental phosphorus in the diet.

How consumers will react is not clear. Some public opinion surveys have shown that Americans are more wary about GE animals than about the GE crops now used in a large number of foods. But other polls suggest that some Americans would accept the animals if they offered environmental or nutritional benefits. The safety of genetically altered foods should be looked at more carefully to determine whether they pose health risks. Any breeding technique that alters a plant or animal— whether by genetic engineering or other techniques—has the potential to create unintended changes in the quality or amounts of food components that could harm health. Documented adverse health effects from transgenic food have not been observed in humans, even though such foods have the potential to create toxins or allergens. In order for consumers to ultimately accept the technology, there are social, ethical, environmental, and religious issues that need to be considered. There is a need for laws that require labeling of GE products so consumers can decide for themselves whether to purchase the products.

29.7   DIETARY MODULATION OF COLONIC MICROORGANISMS

The bacteria that reside in the human intestinal tract may be divided into species that exert either harmful or beneficial effects on the host. Some bacteria (e.g., bifidobacteria, lactobacilli) produce short-chain fatty acids and vitamins, stimulate the immune system, improve digestion and absorption, and inhibit the growth of pathogenic bacteria. These are examples of health-promoting effects. Some bacteria contain enzymes that convert procarcinogens to carcinogens and produce fermentation products such as ammonia and phenols, which may be harmful to the host.

It is becoming increasingly accepted that colonic microorganisms may play an important role in the maintenance of health. There is, therefore, an interest in the manipulation of the composition of the gut flora toward a more salutary regimen; that is, an increase in the number and activities of bacterial groups such as bifidobacterium and lactobacillus, which are perceived as having health-promoting properties. Russian bacteriologist Elie Metchnikoff won a Nobel Prize in the early 1900s for linking yogurt consumption to the longevity that Balkan people enjoyed.

One approach has been the addition of live cultures to foodstuffs such as milk to produce yogurt by fermentation. The rationale is that a number of exogenous bacterial additions remain in a viable form during transit through the gastrointestinal tract and become active upon reaching the colon, where appropriate conditions exist for their growth to occur. Bacteria added to foodstuff for this purpose are termed probiotic bacteria. A probiotic is a viable microbial dietary supplement that beneficially affects the host through its effect in the intestinal tract.[6]

We are not born with probiotics; they come from our environment. Babies encounter their first friendly—health promoting—microbes in breast milk. Other familiar sources include yogurt, buttermilk, fermented cheese, and fermented soybeans. These microbes thrive on nondigested oligosaccharides (prebiotics) found in foods such as onions, asparagus, tomatoes, garlic, artichokes, honey, and bananas.

Studies suggest that probiotics can help ward off bladder infections and ease the inflammation caused by food allergies, Crohn's disease, ulcerative colitis, and irritable bowel syndrome.[13,36] Among hospitalized infants those given formula enriched with bifidobacteria (the bacteria found in breast milk) are less likely to develop infectious diarrhea. Lactobacillus can lower the risk of respiratory infections in children. Probiotic pills are available in the market. They have almost no side effects, but as dietary supplements they are not subject to rigorous quality-inspection or labeling rules. Many times the microbe advertised in the label may not be in the pill. One can add probiotic naturally to a diet by using yogurt or a similar item. The procedure for making yogurt is given at the end of this section.

Yogurt has been used as food in some parts of the world for centuries. The preparation of yogurt from milk involves introducing a nonpathogenic bacterial (lactobacillus) culture that produces an acid taste and changes the consistency of milk. The same nutrients are present in yogurt as in milk, except for the partial breakdown of lactose into its components, glucose and galactose. Because milk and yogurt buffer stomach acids, bacteria in yogurt survive passage to the more distal portion of the gastrointestinal tract. The bacteria become metabolically active upon reaching the colon. They produce lactic acid as the metabolic end product. This lowers the pH of the medium and thus exerts an antibacterial (inhibitory) effect on a range of gram-positive and gram-negative pathogenic bacteria. The consumption of yogurt results in the predominance of beneficial strains over potentially harmful species in the colon.

A large portion of the world adult population is deficient in intestinal lactase. The failure to digest lactose leads to its presence in the large intestine, providing a substrate for colonic bacteria. The ingestion of milk by lactase-deficient individuals causes bloating, flatulence, and diarrhea. The consumption of yogurt by these individuals improves their ability to digest milk. This is attributed to the ability of lactase-producing yogurt cultures to deliver lactase to the small intestine, facilitating the digestion of lactose in situ. The effectiveness of yogurt cultures in promoting lactose digestion is perhaps the best documented health effect of the bacteria associated with yogurt. Yogurt is an excellent alternative to milk as a calcium source for milk-intolerant individuals. Yogurt and extracts thereof have been shown to be antimutagenic against a range of mutagens and promutagens in microbial and mammalian cell systems. Certain epidemiological studies have suggested that consumption of yogurt and fermented milk may reduce the incidence of colon and breast cancers. Yogurt causes a reduction of plasma cholesterol, cancer suppression, and immune system stimulation. Yogurt also has beneficial effects on diarrhea, constipation, control of intestinal pathogens, and inactivation of toxic compounds. Thus, consumption of milk fermented with lactobacilli is likely to prolong one's life.

29.7.1 Preparation of Yogurt at Home

Yogurt is a dairy product produced by bacterial fermentation of milk. Fermentation of lactose produces lactic acid, which acts on milk protein to give yogurt its texture and its characteristic tang. It can be made from whole, low fat, or skim milk including milk reconstituted from dry milk powder.

Heat a quart of milk to near boiling (about 85°C) to kill undesired bacteria and to change milk proteins so that they set together rather than form curds. Transfer it to a glass container with cover and allow it to cool to slightly above room temperature (37°C). Add one tablespoon of the starter (previously prepared or purchased yogurt). Mix gently and keep the container in a warm place. Yogurt should be ready in 6–8 h. It can remain at room temperature for a day and then should be kept in a refrigerator for up to 2 weeks. The higher the content of fat the tastier is the yogurt. The taste varies slightly with the source of milk (cow, water buffalo, goat) and the starter used. For example, yogurt purchased at a Middle Eastern store differs slightly from yogurt obtained at a regular grocery store. Yogurt can be eaten plain, flavored, or with fruits that can be added before the start of fermentation.

For making buttermilk whip the desired amount of yogurt in a blender with salt, sugar, cumin, fresh ginger powder, and/or cilantro can be added as per the preference.

Lassie is a yogurt-based beverage originally from the Indian subcontinent. Take one cup of yogurt and four strawberries and whip the mixture to make strawberry lassie. Mango or other fruit can replace strawberry. Sweeten to taste.

Yogurt is easy to prepare at home, is inexpensive, and is a reliable source of healthy bacteria.

Tea Intoxication—A Case

A 44-year-old male presented with muscle cramps. During the taking of the patient history, the patient admitted that he had been drinking 4 L/day black tea during the past 25 years. His preferred tea brand was Gold Teafix (Tekanne, Austria). Because this type of tea occasionally gave him gastric pain, he decided to try Earl Grey tea (Twinnings, London, UK), which he thought would be less harmful to his stomach.

A week after he made the change to Earl Grey, he experienced repeated muscle cramps for a few seconds in his right foot. The cramps became more intense as he continued the consumption of the new tea. After three weeks, the cramps occurred in the left foot and after five weeks, muscle cramps had spread toward the right hands and the right calf. Additionally, he noted distal paresthesias in all limbs and a feeling of pressure in his eyes, associated with blurred vision, particularly in darkness. Neurological examination revealed that he had reduced visual acuity and fasciculations in the right tibialis anterior and adductor pollicis. Other neurological and ophthalmological tests, the usual blood and urine tests, and liver and kidney function tests were normal. Other tests excluded the possibility of motor neuron disease, polyneuropathy, myopathy, neuromyotonia, Stiffman syndrome, and Machado–Joseph disease.

Because the symptoms appeared to be due to tea, the patient completely stopped drinking Earl Grey tea, reverting to pure black tea again. Within one week, his symptoms completely disappeared. The patient liked Earl Grey tea and wanted to find out whether a small amount was safe. He tried various volumes of Earl Grey tea and found that the symptoms did not appear as long as he consumed no more than 1 L/day Earl Grey tea. However, he decided to go back to drinking only pure black tea but reduced the intake to 2 L/day. After six months, his neurological examination, nerve conduction studies, and electromyography were normal and he had no complaints.

Earl Grey tea is composed of black tea and the essence of bergamot oil, an extract from the rind of bergamot orange that has a pleasant, refreshing scent, which suits it well for use in candies, medicines, and perfumes. Bergamot oil is the aromatic base for eau de cologne. The oil contains bergapten, bergamottin, and citropten, which are also found in grapefruit juice, celery, parsnips, and Seville orange juice. Until a few years back, the oil was widely used as an ingredient in cosmetics but has been restricted or banned in most countries because of certain adverse effects. Bergamot oil has a strong phototoxic effect. It also has a hepatotoxic effect and may cause contact allergy.

The adverse reactions of bergamot oil observed in the patient are due to the effect of bergapten as a selective axolemnal potassium channel blocker, reducing potassium permeability at the nodes of Ranvier in a time-dependent manner.[46] It leads to a hyperexcitability of the axonal membrane and phasic alterations of potassium currents, causing fasciculations and muscle cramps. This is a very interesting case that makes the point that although tea may have health-promoting properties, excessive intake may cause stomach pain. As is true for all nutrients, just because a nutrient is good, more of it is not necessarily better. It can cause problems. There is an increasing interest in tea as a functional food. Various kinds of tea with different flavors are available to improve the taste. The case described here makes the point that tea, if flavored and consumed in extraordinarily high quantities for better health, can lead to health problems.

Topical bergamot oil has been used to treat psoriasis in conjunction with ultraviolet light. It is also used topically for vitiligo and mycosis fungoids. More recently, bergamot oil preparations have been gaining renewed popularity in aromatherapy, a form of alternative medicine involving the application of essential oils often in combination with massage to achieve therapeutical effects. Bergamot oil possesses photosensitive and melanogenic properties because of the presence of bergapten. However, bergapten is also potentially phototoxic and photomuta-genic. Therefore, there is a need for the public to be made aware of these potential dangers and there is a necessity for strict government surveillance and scrutiny of these increasingly popular preparations.

REFERENCES

1. Anderson, A. J., and T. J. Hanna. 1999. Impact of non-digestible carbohydrates in serum lipoproteins and risk for cardiovascular disease. *J Nutr* 129:1457S.
2. Aslami, F., A. Pourshams, D. Nasrollahdeh et al. 2009. Tea drinking habits and esophaseal cancer in a high risk area in northern Iran. *Brit Med J* 338:b929.
3. Avorn, J., M. Monane, J. H. Gurwitz et al. 1994. Reduction of bacteria and pyuria after ingestion of cranberry juice. *J Am Med Assoc* 271:751.
4. Balentine, D. A., M. Albano, and M. G. Nair. 1999. Role of medicinal plants, herbs, and spices in protect-ing human health. *Nutr Rev* 57:S41.
5. Bowen, P. E. 2001. Evaluating the health claim of flaxseed and cancer. *Nutr Today* 36(7):144.
6. Broussard, E. K., and C. M. Surawicz. 2004. Probiotics and prebiotics in clinical practice. *Nutr Clin Care* 7(3):104.
7. Caragay, A. B. 1992. Cancer preventative foods and ingredients. *Food Technol* 46:65.
8. Chavarro, J. E., T. L. Toth, S. M. Sadio, and R. Hauser. 2008. Soy food and isoflavone intake in relation to semen quality parameters among men from an infertility clinic. *Hum Reprod* 23:2384.
9. Clinton, S. K. 1998. Lycopene: Chemistry, biology, and implications for human health and disease. *Nutr Rev* 56:35.
10. Craig, W. J. 1999. Health promoting properties of common herbs. *Am J Clin Nutr Suppl* 70:491S.
11. De Lumen, B. O. 2008. Lunacin: A cancer-preventive soy peptide. *Nutr Rev* 63(1):16.
12. Dellapenna, D. 1999. Nutritional genomics: Manipulating plant micronutrients to improve human health. *Science* 285:375.
13. Doron, S., and S. L. Gorbach. 2006. Probiotics: Their role in the treatment and prevention of disease. *Expert Rev Anti Infect Ther* 4(2):261.
14. Duthie, S. J., A. M. Jenkinson, A. Crozier et al. 2006. The effects of cranberry juice consumption on antioxidant status and biomarkers relating to heart disease and cancer in healthy human volunteers. *Eur J Nutr* 45(2):113.
15. Dwyer, J. H., M. Navab, K. M. Dwyer, K. Hassan, P. Sun, A. Shircore, S. Hama-Levy et al. 2001. Oxygenated carotenoid lutein and progression of early atherosclerosis. *Ciculation* 103:2922.
16. Fahey, J. W. 2002. Sulforaphane inhibits extracellular, intracellular, and antibiotic-resistant strains of Heicobacter pylori and prevents benzo[a]pyrene-induced stomach tumors. *Proc Natl Acad Sci* 99:7610.
17. Goldberg, I., ed. 1994. *Functional Foods: Designer Foods, Pharmafoods, Nutraceuticals*. New York: Chapman and Hall.
18. Halliwell, B. 2007. Dietary polyphenols: Good, bad or indifferent for your health? *Cardiovasc Res* 73:341.
19. Hassler, C. M. 1998. Functional foods: Their role in disease prevention and health promotion. *Food Technol* 52(11):63.
20. Hassler, C. M., R. L. Huston, and E. M. Caudill. 1995. The impact of nutrition labeling and education. Act on functional foods. In *Nurition, Labeling Handbook*, ed. R. S. Shapiro, 471–93. New York: Marcel Dekker Inc.
21. Hathcock, J. N. 1993. Safety and regulatory issues for phytochemical sources: "Designer Foods." *Nutr Today* 27(6):23.
22. Hendrich, S., K. Lee, X. Xu, and H. Wang. 1994. Defining food components as new nutrients. *J Nutr* 124:1789S.
23. Hogervorst, E., T. Sadjimim, A. Yasufu et al. 2008. High tofu intake is associated with worse memory in elderly Indonesian men and women. *Dement Geriatr Cogn Disord* 26(1):51.
24. Kenyon, N. 1997. Cultivated blueberries. The good-for-you blue food. *Nutr Today* 32(3):122.
25. Kris-Etherton, P. M., G. Zhao, A. E. Binkoski, S. M. Coval, and T. D. Etherton. 2001. The effect of nuts on coronary heart disease risk. *Nutr Rev* 59:103.
26. Kuriyama, S., T. Shimazu, K. Ohmon et al. 2007. Green tea consumption and mortality due to cardiovas-cular disease, cancer and all causes in Japan. The Ohsaki Study. *J Am Med Assoc* 297:360.

27. Leahy, M., R. Roderick, and K. Briliant. 2001. The cranberry—promising health benefits, old and new. *Nutr Today* 36(5):254.

28. Lorenz, M., N. Jochmann, A. Von Krosigk et al. 2007. Addition of milk prevents vascular protective effects of tea. *Eur Heart J* 28:219.

29. Maher, P., T. Akaishi, and K. Abe. 2006. Flavonoid fisetin promotes ERK-dependent long-term potentiation and enhances memory. *Proc Natl Acad Sci* 103:16568.

30. McShea, S., E. Ramiro-Puig, S. B. Munro et al. 2008. Clinical benefit and preservation of flavonoids in dark chocolate manufacturing. *Nutr Rev* 66:630.

31. Mindell, E. 1994. *Garlic: The Miracle Nutrient*. New Canaan, CT: Keats Publishing.

32. Opie, L. H., and S. Lecour. 2007. The red wine hypothesis: From concepts to protective signaling molecules. *Eur Heart J* 28:1683.

33. Providencia, R. R. 2006. Cardiovascular protection from alcoholic drinks: Scientific basis of the French Paradox. *Rev Port Cardiol* 25:1043.

34. Reddy, V. C., G. V. Vidya Sagar, D. Sreeramulu et al. 2005. Addition of milk does not alter the antioxidant activity of black tea. *Ann Nutr Metab* 49:189.

35. Rezai-Zadeh, K., D. Shytle, T. Sun et al. 2005. Green tea epigallocatechin 3-gallate (EGCG) modulates amyloid precursor protein cleavage and reduces cerebral amyloidosis in Alzheimer transgenic mice. *J Neurosci* 25:8807.

36. Robertfroid, M. B. 2000. Prebiotics and probiotics: Are they functional foods? *Am J Clin Nutr Suppl* 71:1682S.

37. Smyth, S., and P. W. B. Philips. 2003. Labeling to manage marketing of GE foods. *Trends Biotechnol* 21:389.

38. Steinmetz, K. A., and J. D. Potter. 1996. Vegetables, fruits, and cancer prevention: A review. *J Am Diet Assoc* 96:1027.

39. Talalay, P., and J. W. Fahey. 2001. Phytochemicals from cruciferous plants protect against cancer by modulating carcinogen metabolism. *J Nutr* 131:3027S.

40. Trevisanato, S. I., and Y. Kim. 2000. Tea and health. *Nutr Rev* 58:1.

41. Walker, A. R. P. 1995. Dietary advice: From folklore to present beliefs. *Nutr Rev* 53:8.

42. Wattenberg, W. R. 1992. Inhibition of carcinogenesis by minor dietary constituents. *Cacer Res Suppl* 52:2085S.

43. Wildman, R. E. C., ed. 2001. *Hadbook of Nutraceuticals and Functional Foods*. Boca Raton, FL: CRC Press.

44. Ye, X., S. Al-Babili, A. Kloti, J. Zhang, P. Lucca, P. Beyer, and I. Potrykus. 2000. Engineering the provitamin A (β-carotene) biosynthetic pathway into (carotenoid-free) rice endosperm. *Science* 287:303.

45. Zheng, G. Q., P. M. Kenney, and L. K. T. Lam. 1992. Myristicin: A potent chemoprotective agent from parsley leaf oil. *J Agric Food Chem* 40:107.

CASE BIBLIOGRAPHY

46. Finsterer, J. 2002. Earl Grey tea intoxication. *Lancet* 359:1484.

30 Alternative Medicine
Dietary Supplements

The lay press is replete with articles touting the benefits of alternative therapies. In general, the value of these alternative treatments has been determined only by anecdotal reports. In fact, many can be harmful and even fatal.

Alternative medicine represents a subset of practices that are not an integral part of the prevailing health care system in the United States. However, they are still used by patients to supplement their health care, and they encompass a broad spectrum of beliefs and practices. Many are well known; others are exotic or mysterious, and some are dangerous. Several types of therapies fall into this category, including acupuncture, aromatherapy, Ayurvedic medicine, body work, chiropractic, detoxication therapy, chelation therapy, herbal therapy, and many others, a few of which are listed in Table 30.1. The most common forms of treatment are chiropractic, acupuncture, homeopathy, yoga, and dietary supplements (vitamins, other chemicals, and herbs). Several synonyms are used to describe these therapies, such as alternative, unconventional, unorthodox, and unscientific.

It is widely accepted that a patient's emotional state can affect the course of the disease. Laughter therapy has been found to be a benefit to human health for some time and recently it has become popular as part of a healthy lifestyle.[33] Some of the benefits attributed to laughter include improved immunological and endocrinological responses and improved pain tolerance. There is also a growing field of health care known as music therapy,[32] which uses music to heal. Studies have found that music therapy is effective at promoting relaxation, relieving anxiety and stress, treating depression, and management of pain. Scientific evidence also suggests that faith brings us health. People who attend religious services are known to fare better than people who do not attend.

In recent years, the use of alternative therapies has increased significantly (from 33.8% of the U.S. adult population in 1990 to 42.1% in 1997). According to one study in 1997, some 83 million Americans (more than 40% of the adult population) sought treatment by herbalists, chiropractors, and other unconventional practitioners.[31] People paid more visits to these practitioners (429 million) than to primary care physicians (388 million). The cost of the entire endeavor was more than $27 billion. The U.S. sale of herbal products alone reached $3.24 billion, and is growing by more than 20% a year. The most frequent users of alternative therapies are educated, upper-income Caucasian Americans in the 25–49-year-old age group. In a recent study, faculty members of a major health science center in Florida were asked what types of alternative therapies they personally used. In this survey, 52% of faculty physicians reported some personal use of one or more types of alternative therapies. Only about 38.5% of those who use these therapies discuss them with their physicians.[12]

A 2007 survey of more than 32,000 Americans, which for the first time included children, found that the use of complementary and alternative therapies held steady among adults for the last 5 years. Nearly 12% of children in the U.S. use alternatives to traditional medicine. Many of the alternative treatments have not been scientifically validated and those that have been rigorously tested have overwhelmingly been found to be ineffective.

In 1992, recognition of the rising use of herbal medicines, as well as other nontraditional remedies, led to the establishment of the Office of Alternative Medicine within the National Institutes of Health. This office has since been supporting studies of alternative therapies. Its other goal has been to modify the concept of "alternative" to "complementary" in describing therapies that might be included in conventional medical practice. In 1998, the office was re-established as the National

TABLE 30.1
Some Common Alternative Therapies

Acupuncture	Chiropractic	Magnetic field therapy
Alexander technique	Detoxification therapy	Meditation
Aroma therapy	Diet	Mind/Body medicine
Ayurvedic medicine	Flower remedies	Naturopathic medicine
Biofeedback training	Herbal medicine	Nutritional supplements
Body work	Homeopathy	Sound therapy
Cell therapy	Hypnotherapy	Traditional Chinese medicine
Chelation therapy	Juice therapy	Yoga

Center for Complimentary and Alternative Medicine. It funds research in this field including support for clinical trials. Many of the country's leading hospitals and research institutions are studying herbs, acupuncture, and other therapies as rigorously as they would study a new drug.

Little is known about the safety, efficacy, mechanism of action, and cost effectiveness of alternative treatment. Of greater concern is the use of various herbs and chemicals. It is beyond the scope of this chapter to review all the therapies mentioned. Instead, the focus is on dietary supplements, one of the most common forms of alternative health care practices. In this chapter, issues concerning the safety and efficacy of supplements, beneficial and adverse effects of a few popular herbs and supplements, reasons why people use alternative therapies, and the role of healthcare professionals are discussed.

30.1   HISTORY OF SUPPLEMENT REGULATION IN THE UNITED STATES

Regulatory laws were initiated in the United States with the Adulteration of Food and Drink Act of 1872. This law provided for the inspection and analysis of food primarily with regard to preservatives. Penalties for violations were also included. In 1906, the Pure Food and Drug Act was passed by Congress. This law contained what were regarded as rather weak enforcement statutes and relatively minimal fines for violations, and was really more a labeling law than anything else. Foods and drugs involved in interstate commerce were required to be labeled[4] with their exact contents; false labeling was prohibited, but false health claims were not. In addition, imported and special, distinctive product names exempted some products from evaluation under the law.

Little legislation pertaining to nutritional supplements was enacted until the Food, Drug and Cosmetic Act of 1938. This law required for the first time that manufacturers had to submit a new drug application (NDA) to the Food and Drug Administration (FDA) that detailed the composition, use, labeling, and safety for a new pharmaceutical, although there was no requirement for effectiveness.

Between 1936 and 1941, various Enrichment Laws were passed at the federal level as public health measures in order to prevent specific nutrient deficiencies. These laws specified that white bread be enriched with thiamin, riboflavin, niacin, and iron, that table salt must contain iodine to prevent goiters, and that milk must contain vitamin D in order to prevent rickets (osteomalacia). Minimum daily requirements for many nutrients were initially established in 1941, followed by Recommended Daily Allowances (RDAs) in 1943. The Food Additive Amendment was passed in 1958. This essentially shifted the burden of proof that a food additive was safe from the FDA to the manufacturer, and specified that an additive could not be added until the FDA was convinced it was safe. This amendment included the Delaney clause, which prohibited the use of any food additive that contained a carcinogenic substance with regard to either humans or animals.

From 1962 to January 1, 1973, the FDA made numerous attempts to protect consumers and prohibit false claims by nutritional supplement manufacturers. These were generally blocked in court or in Congress until specific product composition specifications and product labeling for vitamin and mineral supplements were permitted to go into effect.

The FDA regained some regulatory power in 1990 with the passing of the Nutritional Labeling and Education Act (NLEA). This law empowered the FDA to require that any health claim for a nutritional supplement had to undergo rigorous validation. Following the L-tryptophan-related deaths in 1989, the FDA established a task force to evaluate the regulation of nutritional supplements. This task force recommended that supplements be regulated like drugs when they are used for any purpose other than for food additives.

In 1993, the FDA began scrutinizing the herbal and dietary supplement industry. This triggered a massive letter-writing campaign organized by the multibillion-dollar dietary supplement industry. Consumers were urged to "write to your congressman to exempt herbs and other supplements from FDA regulation or kiss your supplement goodbye." Public response was overwhelming. Congress reportedly received more mail on this subject than any other issue since the Vietnam War. It led to the passage of Dietary Supplement Health and Education Act (DSHEA) in 1994 that severely limited the FDA's ability to regulate the dietary supplement industry. It classified herbal medicines (along with vitamins, minerals, amino acids, etc.) as dietary supplements. Since then, these products have flooded the market.

The DSHEA requires no proof of efficacy, no proof of safety, and sets no standards for quality control for products labeled as dietary supplements. If the question arises, the burden of proof lies with the FDA to prove a product is unsafe, rather than a manufacturer proving it is safe. In contrast, regulatory agencies in Germany, France, United Kingdom, and Canada enforce standards of herb quality and safety assessment on manufacturers.

30.2   SAFETY AND EFFICACY OF SUPPLEMENTS

The DSHEA defines supplements, places the responsibility for ensuring safety on manufacturers, and identifies how the product literature may be used. These products can be labeled with information regarding their effects on the structure and function of the body. However, disease claims are not allowed. This legislation forbids companies to imply that a product treats or prevents a disease. They cannot say, for instance, that a substance reduces the risk of prostate cancer, but they can state that a product helps support healthy prostate function or aids in maintaining normal urine flow. The companies are required to include on their label the following: "This statement has not been evaluated by the Food and Drug Administration. This product is not intended to diagnose, treat, cure or prevent disease."

Currently there are no government standards on the quality of herbal products (and other supplements) sold in the United States (Table 30.2). Herbs may be sold to manufacturers as whole plants or plant parts, cut pieces, or ground particles. Because of the lack of requirements for quality control, safety, or efficacy, consumers cannot determine if an herb's active ingredients are actually

---

TABLE 30.2
Quality Control Problems with Dietary Supplements

1. There are no government standards on the quality of herbal products and other dietary supplements. Products are not subject to FDA approval.
2. Manufacturers have no regulatory responsibility to ensure safety of their products. Unlike drugs, herbs do not need to be proven safe and effective to be marketed. This lack of regulation may pose a significant risk for the consumer.
3. The dosage of active ingredients necessary for effectiveness and toxicity has not been determined for most products.
4. Adulteration, substitution, and contamination may be possible. Additives may be used, yet not listed on labels.

contained in the product, if the ingredient is bioavailable, if the dosage is appropriate, if the next bottle they buy will have the same components, or what else is in the pill besides the claimed ingredients. Adulteration and substitution of the active ingredient(s) are more likely to occur with the more expensive plant materials. Dietary supplements vary tremendously in content, quality, and safety. They comprise multiple products, including herbs, plants, and minerals, which are formulated into tablets, powders, or liquids for ease of use. They are widely available in stores and have gained acceptance by the American public as a form of alternative medicine. Asian patent medicines may contain toxic ingredients, such as heavy metals, as well as prescription drugs or unapproved ingredients that may not be identified on the label. Some have caused serious illness[1] in unsuspecting consumers.

There have been a number of reports of poor quality among some dietary supplements (Table 30.3). Among them are tablets or capsules without labeled amounts of the supplement, lack of standardization, tablets not disintegrating, or the presence of harmful contaminants. Examples include melatonin (two out of nine products did not disintegrate), ginseng (25% of the products contained no ginseng, while in 60% of the products the active ingredient in each pill varied by as much as a factor of 10 among brands that were labeled as containing the smallest amount, with some brands containing none), and St. John's Wort showed a 17-fold difference between capsules containing the smallest amount of hypericin and those containing the largest amount. In still another report, only 7 of 16 dehydroepiandrosterone (DHEA) products were found to have a DHEA content within the typical product specifications of 90–110% of the label claim. No DHEA was detected in one product and only trace amounts were detected in two other products. Recently, a team from the University of California at Los Angeles examined eight major brands of commonly used herbal supplements in the United States. They found widely varying amounts of the active ingredients listed on the labels. This study focused on five different supplements, including ginseng and St. John's Wort. Some samples contained as much as 260% or as little as 44% of the amount of the compound listed on the label.

Herbal remedies may be sold without any explanation of their mechanism of action. For example, the herbal mixture called PC SPES (PC for prostate cancer, SPES for the Latin word hope) contains a substantial amount of estrogen activity. This substance is promoted as supporting the immune system in patients with PC that is refractory to treatment with estrogen. Estrogens can have substantial toxic effects. Without knowing it, many patients end up ingesting varying amounts of hormones in addition to the estrogen treatment prescribed for them by their physicians. Unregulated, commercially available dietary supplements may have biological activity that can affect various diseases, standard medical therapy, and general health.

Using herbs may be chancy. Just because herbs are labeled "natural," it does not necessarily mean they are without risks. They do not undergo rigorous testing demanded by the FDA for other drugs. So little is known about their effectiveness, optimum dosage, side effect, or interaction with

TABLE 30.3
Examples of Variability in the Quantity of the Known Ingredients

1. Melatonin—Two of nine products did not disintegrate, which means ingredients are not available for absorption and metabolism.
2. Ginseng—25% of the products contained no ginseng, while in 60% of the products the active compounds (panaxocides) in each pill ranged from 0.26 to 6.85 mg in a 250-mg sample, with some brands containing none.
3. St. John's Wort—A 17-fold difference between capsules containing the smallest amount of the active ingredient (hypericin) and those containing the largest amount.
4. DHEA—Only 7 out of 16 products were found to have DHEA content within the typical product specifications of 90–110% of the label claim. No DHEA was detected in one product and only trace amounts were detected in two other products.

other medications. In addition, they are subject to few controls on quality and purity. Unlike foods and drugs, herbal products do not require good manufacturing practices (GMPs).[35] These ensure that products meet specific quality standards, are not adulterated and misbranded, and contain the ingredients at doses stated on the label. The only actual determination may tell whether the concentration specified is accurate. Herbal manufacturers have little incentive to do so. It is costly and there is no pressure from the government for quality control. Without GMP herbal products are also at risk of adulteration and contamination.

Most herbal medicines are probably harmless. In addition, they seem to be used primarily by people who are healthy and believe the remedies will help them stay that way or by people who have common relatively minor problems such as backache or fatigue. Most such people would probably seek out conventional doctors if they have indications of serious diseases such as cancer, etc. However, some people may depend on herbs and other alternative therapies exclusively, thereby putting themselves in greater danger.

Because of consumers' concerns on the quality of dietary supplements manufacturers are trying to get a seal of approval on their products. Several new seals of approval are vying to cut through the clutter of competing products in the largely unregulated $17 billion dietary supplement industry. At least four outfits, U.S. Pharmacopeia (USP), NSF International, ConsumerLab.com, and Good Housekeeping, have begun or ramped up issuing official-looking stamps on herbs, vitamins, and other supplements that meet certain standards (Table 30.4).

Generally, the programs test and certify that the ingredients listed on the label accurately reflect the make-up of the pills inside the bottle. Most also purport to ensure that a substance is free of common contaminants, including heavy metals and pesticides. When a consumer sees that a supplement is verified, the natural assumption is that its efficacy and what is being claimed is verified, and that is just not true; seals do not conclusively answer the most important questions on shoppers' minds: Is the product safe and does it work? In addition, most of the programs require dietary supplement companies to pay for the privilege of being tested and certified or to put the stamp of approval on their packaging. Nevertheless, the new programs may help curb the Wild West nature of the dietary supplement industry and give consumers a little more information to decide which brand to buy.

TABLE 30.4
Seals of Approval and What They Mean

USP	Has been setting standards for prescription and over-the-counter drugs since 1820. Verifies the product was manufactured in a clean and professional environment; label reflects what is in the bottle, free of common contaminants; dissolves properly. Does not verify health claims.
NSF	Founded by a group of University of Michigan professors in 1944 to set standards in the food service industry. It launched its dietary supplement program about a year ago. Has certified over 60 products. Label reflects what is in the bottle; free of common contaminants. (Products that pass the test are posted on its Web site www.nsf.org.) Does not verify health claims.
ConsumerLab.com	Founded in 1999 by former FDA chemist and a doctor. Examines certain popular classes of supplements—ginseng, for example—without charging manufacturers. Companies can pay between $2,500 and $4,000 to make sure their product is included in testing, and they must pay to use the seal in advertising and on their bottles. (Products that pass the test are posted on its Web site consumerLab.com.) About 400 products have earned the seal. Label reflects contents; free of common contaminants; dissolves properly.
Good Housekeeping	Reviews manufacturing processes, but conducts only limited testing. Only those companies that agree to buy advertising in its magazine are considered for the seal. Label reflects the amount of active ingredient in bottle; requires manufacturers to back up health claims by submitting evidence, e.g., article accepted in a peer-reviewed scientific journal.

30.3 GERMAN COMMISSION E REPORT

The prevalence of dietary supplement use in Europe far exceeds that of the United States. The herbal medicines are standardized and prescribed by about 70% of the German physicians, and paid for by the German government's health insurance. Many different herbal drugs (approximately 1400), which correspond to 600–700 different species of plants, are available.

In 1978, the German Federal Health Agency established a special committee of medical experts known as Commission E to study the safety and efficacy of herbal medicines. By 1994, Commission E had published about 400 monographs. An English translation of the German Commission monographs on medicinal plants for human use is available through the American Botanical Council. The monographs include information on nomenclature, constituents, side effects, dosage, and action of herbs. Practitioners in the United States can now use these monographs as a source of information regarding herbal remedies.

In Germany, herbal medicines cannot be marketed until they are considered to be safe and "have reasonable proof of efficacy." An indication in a Commission E monograph is considered to represent such a proof. This standard is not as rigorous as that used by the U.S. FDA for drugs and food additives.

30.4 BENEFICIAL EFFECTS

About one-third of all FDA-approved drugs used in conventional medicines have their origin from plants.[9] Reserpine, used for the treatment of high blood pressure, was originally extracted from *Rauwolfia serpentina*. Digitalis, used as a heart stimulant, was derived from the foxglove plant. Salicylic acid (a component of aspirin) was obtained from willow tree bark to help relieve fever. Ma huang, which contains ephedrine, was used for the treatment of asthma. Taxol, a new chemotherapeutic agent, was obtained from the bark of the Pacific yew (*Taxus brevifolia*) and the needles of other yew species. The active ingredients from plants known to offer health benefits were identified and synthesized, and their mechanisms of actions studied. Safe, effective, and toxic doses of each of the active ingredients were established and only then were they approved as drugs. Studies on the identification of active principles of several other medicinal plants are currently in progress.[20,25] A few examples are given below.

Cranberry juice is known to help prevent urinary tract infections. At one time it was thought to work by acidifying the urine or by the excretion of hippuric acid. Recently, researchers have identified condensed tannins in cranberries (as well as blueberries) that fight infections in the urinary tract by inhibiting the adherence of *Escherichia coli* to uroepithelial cells, a prerequisite for the development of infection. Cranberry products can now be considered a safe prophylactic therapy that may help reduce the frequency of urinary tract infections in susceptible individuals. However, cranberry juice contains traces of quinine, which is known to cause immune-mediated thrombocytopenia. Recently, a 68-year-old man was reported to have thrombocytopenia linked to cranberry juice.

Moxibustion, a traditional Chinese practice that uses heat from burning herbs to stimulate acupuncture points, can help move a fetus into the proper position for head-first delivery. A study was done on 260 Chinese women, pregnant for the first time, whose fetuses were still in the breech or upright position after 33 weeks. Half of the women received daily moxibustion treatment on their little toes for 1–2 weeks. The others got the same care, minus moxibustion. The fetuses in the treatment group became more active and 75% of them (vs. 48% of the controls) righted themselves in time for a normal delivery. If further studies confirm the findings, moxibustion could become a part of Western obstetrics, helping to reduce our high rate of caesarian birth. That would be good for the mother, baby, and insurance companies. Chinese herbs may hold similar promise for treating irritable bowel syndrome that affects one in five Americans. Researchers in Australia reported that patients who took cocktails of powdered herbs for 16 weeks enjoyed nearly three times more relief than those who took placebo.

30.5 SUPPLEMENTS

A few of the popular herbal and nonherbal supplements are discussed below. Other commonly used herbal supplements, valerian, St. John's Wort, mu tong, saw palmetto, and don quai and nonherbal supplements copper, creatine, chromium, and tryptophan are presented in the next section.

30.5.1 SUPPLEMENTS FOR WEIGHT LOSS

A number of weight loss supplements are available in drug stores, supermarkets, health food stores, and online. Most have not proved effective and some may have serious adverse effects.[29]

Ephedra sinica is a plant native to Asia. It is high in physiologically active alkaloids (95% of which is ephedrine). It is often combined with caffeine or herbs containing caffeine such as guarana. Clinical trials have shown modest weight loss (2 pounds per month) but are associated with a number of adverse effects, including high blood pressure, heart attack, and stroke. In 2004, the United States Food and Drug Administration (FDA) banned supplements containing ephedra because they present unreasonable risk of illness or injury.

Hoodia is a plant from Southern Africa that is used as a natural appetite suppressant. There have been no clinical trials using this supplement and more than half of all hoodia products sold are found to contain no active ingredient.

Bitter orange weight loss products refer to extracts from the fruit or rind of *Citrus aurantium*, one of several orange species. They contain a group of adrenergic amines with structures similar to ephedrine and norepinephrine. These chemicals may speed up heart rate and raise blood pressure. There have been isolated case reports of stroke and myocardial infarction. Bitter orange gained popularity after ephedra was banned.

Conjugated linoleic acid (CLA) is a fatty acid found naturally in small amounts in milk and meat. Our daily diet contains approximately 200 mg CLA. The dose for weight loss is about 3 g/day. There is evidence that it inhibits triglyceride formation, increases loss of fat mass, and increases lean tissue mass. Experiments in humans have shown a modest weight loss compared to placebo. But others have raised concerns that it may worsen insulin sensitivity and the lipid profile in people who are overweight. There are many other supplements for weight reduction including chitosan, green tea, and caffeine. But it is best to follow a healthy diet and lifestyle that includes physical activity.

30.5.2 COENZYME Q10

This is one of the ubiquinones, so named because of their presence in almost all cells of the human body. Coenzyme Q10 functions in mitochondria as a link between flavin-containing dehydrogenases and cytochrome b of the electron transport chain. It is an essential cofactor and participates in ATP production within mitochondria, and as an antioxidant in membranes. It is used widely for a variety of ailments including cardiac disease, diabetes, hypertension, and muscle dystrophy. One of its most common uses, however, is in the treatment of cardiovascular disease. Whether it offers benefits beyond the present therapy is unknown.

The adverse effects of coenzyme Q10 include gastritis, loss of appetite, and diarrhea. When taken in amounts greater than 300 mg per day it can elevate serum aminotransferases. Oral hypoglycemic agents and the HMG-CoA reductase inhibitors such as lovastatin reduce serum coenzyme Q10 levels. Coenzyme Q10 can reduce the body's response to warfarin.

30.5.3 DEHYDROEPIANDROSTERONE

Dehydroepiandrosterone (DHEA) is a precursor hormone secreted by the adrenal cortex. It is rapidly converted to the sulfate, DHEA sulfate (DHEAS). The secretion of DHEA by adrenal glands increases during 6–8 years of age and maximum levels are typically observed between ages 20 and 30.

After that time the levels of DHEA and DHEAS decline with age. Peak DHEA levels occur at 25 to 30 years of age and decline progressively by 25% per decade of life until age 70. DHEA levels in men are higher than those in women at every decade of life until age 65. It has been estimated that greater than 50% of the total androgen of adult males is derived from DHEA. In women, the formation of peripheral estrogens from DHEA may be as high as 75% before menopause and 100% after menopause. DHEA is the current hot performance enhancing substance. It is being touted as an antidote for aging, an elixir for the "fountain of youth" and a superhormone to burn fat, build muscle, strengthen the immune system, retard memory loss, prevent type 2 diabetes, and even prevent or delay Parkinson's disease. There is no convincing evidence for the beneficial effect of DHEA on aging, obesity, or any disease process. The companies that sell it over the counter at health and nutrition centers and via the Internet tout its ability to boost strength and muscle-building ability by hiking the "body's level of testosterone." It can be converted to testosterone but there is no evidence that it helps athletic performance. Not much is known about the interaction of DHEA with other drugs or about potential adverse effects associated with its chronic use. There has been one report of transient hepatitis associated with DHEA use by a woman. There is concern that this supplement might increase the risk of breast and endometrial cancer in women and prostatic cancer in men. Young athletes may be at risk for serious side effects such as elevated blood lipids, liver problems, and testicular hypertrophy.

30.5.4 ECHINACEA

Echinacea, the top-selling herbal product in the United States, is at the forefront of the herbal revolution, with annual sales of more than $300 million. Extracts, teas, tinctures, tablets, and ointments containing various parts of the plant have been used since the 1600s by Native Americans for a variety of medical problems, from gums and coughs to bowel troubles and snakebites. Recent clinical studies have focused on the treatment and prevention of upper respiratory infections. It has at least six different active ingredients and there is controversy over which chemical is most effective. It does appear to exert its effect through immune system modulation, thus indirectly providing anti-infective effect.

30.5.5 GINSENG

Ginseng, the dried roots of several species of Panax and other closely related plants, are sold under the general name ginseng. It is one of the most popular and expensive herbs in the world. It is widely believed to be a panacea.[14] The root of *Eleutherococcus senticosus* Maxim is sold as Siberian ginseng or ginseng. For centuries, ginseng has been the panacea in China and Korea for most ills. It is regarded as a strong aphrodisiac. The root is currently advertised as a performance and endurance enhancer. As such, ginseng is believed to increase resistance to stress, build general vitality, and strengthen overall body functions.

No adverse reactions have been reported with the oral use of Panax ginseng. There are reports of ginseng abuse syndrome consisting of hypertension, nervousness, insomnia, and diarrhea. However, because of the poor study design these reports have been discredited.

30.5.6 GINKGO

Ginkgo biloba is used in China to treat cognitive deficits, including Alzheimer's-type dementia and peripheral vascular disease. The active ingredients, flavonoids and terpenes, are believed to act as free radical scavengers, protecting vascular walls and nerve cells, as well as inhibiting platelet-activating factors, thus reducing clotting. It is promoted as improving cognitive function and blood flow. Early studies suggested the gingko supplements could boost mental function in people with and without mild dementia. However, the most recent study on 230 individuals over age 60 found that gingko worked no better to improve memory than dummy pills over a 6-week period. It does not prevent or delay the progression of dementia or Alzheimer's disease, according to a clinical trial involving thousands of volunteers between the ages of 75 and 96 who took the tablets twice a day for 6 years.[13] The most popular use in Western countries includes disorders associated with cerebral insufficiency and peripheral vascular disease. Ginkgo is well tolerated in small amounts, but should be used with caution in patients who are on anticoagulants. There are at least four reports of spontaneous bleeding associated with the use of this supplement.

It may interact with aspirin and cause ocular hemorrhage. Therefore, patients with cardiovascular disease who are prescribed aspirin should avoid this supplement. Patients who take drugs with anticoagulant or antiplatelet effects should be cautioned about potential interaction with this herb.

30.5.7   GLUCOSAMINE AND CHONDROITIN SULFATE

Glucosamine is an amino monosaccharide utilized for the biosynthesis of glycoproteins and glycosaminoglycans. Chondroitin sulfate (CS) is most abundant in the articular cartilage and consists of repeating units of glucosamine and amino sugars. Both glucosamine and CS are formed endogenously from glucose via the hexosamine pathway.

Glucosamine has been promoted for use alone and in combination with CS to treat and prevent osteoarthritis (OA). Glucosamine is claimed to increase cartilage formation and CS is commonly advocated to decrease cartilage breakdown. Both glucosamine and CS are widely available through health food stores and pharmacies. In supplements, glucosamine comes from crab shells and CS from cow cartilage.

Many poorly designed studies evaluating the safety and efficacy of glucosamine and CS for OA have observed improved joint mobility. A recent meta-analysis found similar results, but also noted that studies overestimated the biological effects. Two fairly well-designed, randomized, double-blind placebo-controlled trials have shown improvements in symptoms scores and pain after 6 to 8 weeks of glucosamine administration. In a 6-month study combination of glucosamine and CS appeared to relieve knee pain associated with moderate-to-severe arthritis, but not with mild pain.[8] They appear to have few side effects. There is a need for larger, long-term studies, and few are underway in this country.

Should arthritis sufferers rush out to buy this stuff? Well, the substances are not a cure. The risks of long-term use are unclear, ideal doses have not been determined, and the quality of supplements varies widely. Moreover, no one thinks these substances will prove able to restore cartilage that is eroded. They may, however, protect cartilage and even slow its loss. Glucosamine and CS are among the top 10 nutritional supplements in terms of annual sales. Americans shelled out $734 million for the products in 2004.

30.5.8   KAVA

Kava has gained widespread popularity as an anxiolytic and sedative. Results from chemical trials suggest that kava has a therapeutic potential in the symptomatic treatment of anxiety. The active constituents, kava lactones, have experimentally been found to have skeletal muscle relaxant, anticonvulsant, and local anesthetic properties. Kava may be a beneficial herbal medicine for mild stress or anxiety with minimal abuse potential. However, the potential for adverse effects from doses higher than recommended (140–250 mg/day) and drug interactions are of concern. Kava is contraindicated in Parkinson's disease. On rare occasions, kava may cause at least one side effect, liver inflammation or damage. Recently, Britain has pulled kava from shelves, while Germany and Switzerland are considering doing the same thing after reports of 30 cases of serious liver damage.[6] In Germany, three people needed liver transplant and one person died of liver failure. There have been no reports of any problems in North America, but the FDA is investigating the supplement.

30.5.9   Ma Huang

This herb is also known as ephedra. The active principles include the alkaloids ephedrine and pseudoephedrine. The herb can directly and indirectly affect the central nervous system, increase systolic and diastolic pressure, increase heart rate, cause peripheral vasoconstriction and bronchodilation. Ma huang is commonly found in herbal weight-loss products referred to as herbal fen-phen. Ma huang does elevate metabolism and reduce appetite, but sometimes at the cost of raising blood pressure and causing a heart attack or stroke. In Chinese medicine, it is used for colds, flu, fever, chills, headaches, edema, and as a diuretic. It is promoted in this country as an enhancer of athletic performance and body-building efforts, decongestant, bronchodilator, and stimulant.

Ma huang can cause dizziness, motor restlessness, anorexia, and nausea. Concomitant use of ephedra with caffeine increases the stimulatory effects and risks, especially in people with cardiac, thyroid, or circulatory ailments. The FDA has advised consumers not to use ephedrine-containing products marketed as alternatives.

Herbal ecstasy is advertised as a safe organic alternative to illicit street drugs and sold in record stores, nightclubs, etc. The product contains ma huang and kola nut, guarana, and green tea (all of which contain caffeine).

30.5.10   Melatonin

Melatonin is a naturally occurring hormone derived from serotonin and secreted by the pineal gland. It is produced abundantly throughout life. The level drops slightly before puberty and declines steadily into old age. Melatonin secretions are primarily controlled by daylight and darkness and correspond to typical sleep–wake cycle hours. Darkness stimulates melatonin release. Secretion increases progressively after the onset of darkness, usually between 9 p.m. and 4 a.m.; peak melatonin levels occur between 2 a.m. and 4 a.m. It is being heralded as the "all-natural nightcap" and the "hormone of darkness." It is being touted as a natural hypnotic, an agent to combat jet lag, a drug to treat bipolar disorder and anorexia nervosa, an oral contraceptive, and an antiaging drug. A few studies suggest that low doses of melatonin supplement can hasten sleep, alleviate jet lag, and be an effective oral contraceptive.

An estimated 20%–40% of adults[5] experience insomnia in any given year, according to the American Academy of Sleep Medicine. People over 50, and many women of any age, are most likely to suffer from problems including having trouble falling asleep, waking up too early, or waking at night and not getting back to sleep. Even people who usually sleep soundly can become sleep deprived while traveling or when their careers require them to work overnight. How well melatonin aids sleep is still an open question. Most of the studies testing its efficacy involved fewer than 30 subjects and are not considered conclusive. Two meta-analyses—studies that combined results of smaller studies to draw a larger conclusion—reached opposing conclusions. In the latest finding researchers found that melatonin was significantly better than a placebo in aiding sleep efficiency. However, the hormone helped only during the hours when the subjects would not normally be sleeping—suggesting that only people with jet lag or with unusual work hours will benefit from melatonin.

The side effects of melatonin include depression and nausea. There is concern that high doses, while causing no immediate harm, could have unknown long-term effects. Even 1 mg, the smallest commercially available dose, is at least three times higher than the normal amount in the body.

30.5.11   SAMe

S-adenosylmethionine (SAMe) is formed in all cells of the body. It plays an essential role in many biochemical reactions involving enzymatic methylation. It contributes to the synthesis, activation, and/or metabolism of hormones, neurotransmitters, nucleic acids, proteins, phospholipids, and some drugs. Once SAMe donates its methyl group, it breaks down to form homocysteine, which at higher levels is a risk factor for heart disease and stroke. In pregnancy, high plasma homocysteine raises the risk of spina bifida and other birth defects. SAMe synthesis and reduction of homocysteine are closely linked to vitamin B_{12} and folate metabolism. Deficiency of these vitamins results in decreased SAMe concentration in the central nervous system. SAMe entered the U.S. market in early 1999 although it is approved as a drug in some countries. It is used orally for treating depression, liver disease, heart disease, arthritis, Parkinson's disease, and Alzheimer's disease and for slowing the aging process and several other conditions. In people with OA, SAMe is reported to be as effective as nonsteroidal anti-inflammatory drugs (NSAIDs). It exerts analgesic and anti-inflammatory effect and promotes stimulation of cartilage growth and repair. It compares favorably with tricyclic antidepressants and may have faster onset of effect. It may normalize liver function in patients with cirrhosis, hepatitis, and cholestasis. It may also prevent or reverse liver damage caused by certain drugs. SAMe is the fourth most popular dietary supplement in retail chains.

Oral SAMe appears to be safe with few side effects such as nausea at higher doses. In one reported case, SAMe did induce mania in a patient with no history of mania. No information is available on the interaction of SAMe with other supplements and drugs.

30.6 ADVERSE EFFECTS OF DIETARY SUPPLEMENTS

Dietary supplements, once limited primarily to vitamins and minerals, have grown into a multibillion-dollar business.[21,30,34] Today, millions of Americans use some form of dietary supplement on a regular basis. Congress's Government Accountability Office estimates that consumers spent $31 billion in 1999 on dietary supplements and "functional foods." A recent survey shows that 63% of consumers took a vitamin, mineral, or herbal supplement in the past 3 months. Many take all of them at once. What is more, only about one-third of patients tell their doctors they are taking supplements. Even if they do, doctors admit that they do not know anything about those products in terms of their pharmacology. That is because, unlike prescription drugs, the FDA requires no scientific studies on safety and effectiveness before supplements are put on the market. Dietary supplement information is readily available from unqualified nonmedical sources. Often, patients ask the local health food store sales clerks, who get their information from the manufacturer. The manufacturer is interested primarily in selling the product, however, and inaccurate and unapproved claims are common. Accurate information about some supplements is available in the basic science and biomedical literature, but not much is available in medical journals. More studies are now being reported in medical journals so physicians will have access to up-to-date information.

A large number of doctors are concerned about consumers mixing and concentrating vitamins, herbs, and traditional remedies for daily use. These can have serious effects.[11]

The current U.S. regulatory mechanism provides little assurance that commercial herbal preparations have predictable pharmacological effects and that product labels provide accurate information. The potency of herbal medications can vary from manufacturer to manufacturer and from lot to lot within a manufacturer. Plants may be misidentified or deliberately replaced with cheaper or more readily available alternatives. Herbal medications, especially those of Eastern origin, can be adulterated with heavy metals, pesticides, and even conventional drugs. Because there is no mechanism for postmarketing surveillance, the incidence and the exact nature of adverse events is unknown.

More than 5000 suspected herb-related adverse reactions were reported to the World Health Organization before 1996. Between January 1993 and October 1998, 2621 adverse events, including 101 deaths associated with dietary supplements were reported to the FDA. For every adverse event in its files, the FDA estimates 100 more go unreported because there are no central mechanisms for mandatory reporting as there are for conventional medications. Other factors that contribute to underreporting are that physicians do not always recognize adverse events associated with herbal medical use and that patients are reluctant to report and seek treatment for adverse reactions. Ephedra (ma huang) products have been among the most controversial and lucrative of all supplements. More than 1200 complaints about the hundreds of ephedra products on the market fill FDA files, including reports of 70 deaths. Dietary supplements containing ma huang are widely consumed in the United States for purposes of weight reduction and energy enhancement.

In response to growing concern about the safety of ephedra-containing supplements, the FDA requested an independent review of 140 of its adverse-event reports to assess causation and determine the level of risk these products pose to consumers. Among these 140 cases, the independent investigators found 104 descriptions of strokes, heart attacks, seizures, hypertension, and more that were likely or probably related to ephedra. There were 10 reports of cardiac arrest and sudden deaths. The review concluded that given these side effects ma huang (ephedra) supplements should not be used without medical supervision.[17]

Ephedra supplements are raising the greatest worry in the medical community at this time, but other herbal remedies are also of some concern. Recently, it has been reported that colchicine was present in placental blood from patients taking ginkgo supplements. Colchicine was found in these tablets. These supplements should be avoided by women who are pregnant and those who are trying to conceive because colchicine is an alkaloid with teratogenic activity. A few examples of adverse effects related to other herbs and nonherbal supplements are described below.

30.6.1 Herbal Ecstasy and Parkinson's Syndrome

Ecstasy is a mixture of herbal stimulants including ma huang (which contains ephedrine), kola nuts, guarana, and green tea (all of which contain caffeine). It is advocated as a safe, all-natural energy source with no side effects, as well as being a safe alternative to illicit street drugs. Recently, a case of Parkinson's syndrome involving Ecstasy was described in the literature.[22] A 29-year-old male had taken Ecstasy 10 times during the preceding year. He also admitted taking creatine regularly and had started DHEA for a week when he felt lightheaded. He then went to a medical center for treatment of slight clumsiness of his upper and lower extremities. During the next four weeks he began to have difficulty walking and lost his ability to write and drive. Parkinsonism was diagnosed as a result of a delayed neurotoxic effect of the ingredient(s) in Ecstasy on the substantia nigra and striatum. Neurotoxicity to the serotonergic system in the brain can cause permanent physical and psychiatric problems. A detailed review of the literature has revealed over 87 Ecstasy-related fatalities.[19]

30.6.2 Asian Herbal Medicines and Adverse Effects

Many patent medicines marketed in Asian countries contain toxic ingredients such as heavy metals, as well as prescription drugs or unapproved ingredients that may or may not be identified on the label. Some have caused serious illness in unsuspecting consumers.

30.6.2.1 Chinese Medications with Undeclared Prescription Drugs

Chinese herbal medications ("Chinese black balls") are sold under various names, including Miracle Herb, Tung Shuch, and Chuifong Toukuwan. These are small black balls marketed for liver and kidney ailments, spasms, muscle aches, and rheumatism, as well as for other indications, at dosages of 6–12 pills daily. The only ingredients listed are 20 or more herbs. However, laboratory analysis revealed the presence of at least two prescription drugs. Some patients taking the medication had to be rushed to the emergency room because of complications, some life threatening, associated with these pills. Two of these cases[16] are described below.

> *Patient 1:* A 71-year-old white woman presented with a history of intermittent black stools of two months' duration, and a one-day history of "coffee-ground" emesis, with marked epigastric pain. Laboratory data and esophagogastroduodenoscopy demonstrated an ulcer, as well as esophagitis. She also had severe erosion of the antrum. She was started on

amoxicillin and omeprazole, and her condition responded well to this therapy. Analysis of the pills revealed the presence of diazepam (a hypnotic-sedative) and mefenamic acid (an NSAID). It was determined that ingestion of 12 pills a day would itself exceed the recommended maximum daily dose of mefenamic acid.

Patient 2: A 58-year-old Cambodian woman with a history of chronic sleeplessness and symptoms of depression took at least five pills at 7 PM on the day of presentation. She became somnolent and nonresponsive over the next 2 hours. She was taken to the emergency room and treated with charcoal. Urine toxicology screen was positive for benzodiazepines. Determination of diazepam in the pill revealed that ingestion of 5 pills was the equivalent to 7 mg of diazepam.

Two other patients taking these pills were also on prescription medications. These cases illustrate the adverse effects associated with adulterated preparations, particularly if taken concomitantly with other prescribed drugs.

30.6.2.2   Indian Herbal Medicine and Lead Intoxication

A 43-year-old man had type 2 diabetes for 6 years. He was hospitalized because of a 3-day history of epigastric pain, right upper quadrant pain, and constipation. The pain was intermittent and not associated with nausea, vomiting, fever, or eating. Among the laboratory findings were a low hemoglobin level (8.9 g/dl), a very high urinary coproporphyrin level (16,470 Ag/day, normal <180 Ag), and lead (6751 Ag/day, normal <80 Ag). About 3 months before admission, the patient had begun taking two tablets daily of an Indian herbal preparation for diabetes, and gradually increased the dosage to eight tablets daily. Toxicological examination of the tablets showed that each tablet contained 10 mg of lead. Thus, the patient's cumulative lead intake before hospitalization was approximately 4 g.

A diagnosis could not be made early because the patient did not tell the physician that he was taking these pills. Also, the possibility that the pills contained lead was not considered. Had the physician known that the patient was taking an herbal preparation, the possibility of some kind of intoxication might have been considered earlier.

30.6.3   VALERIAN AND WITHDRAWAL SYMPTOMS

For centuries, the root of valerian, a pink-flowered perennial growing wild in temperate areas of America and Europe, has been a popular calming and sleep-promoting agent. In the United States, valerian was approved for use in flavoring foods and beverages, such as root beer. Taken orally, valerian is used for restlessness and sleeping disorders. No serious effects have been reported. The sedative properties of valerian are attributed to the volatile oil (valerenic acid) and valeprotriate fractions. Valerenic acid inhibits the catabolism of γ aminobutyric acid, a neurotransmitter.

A 58-year-old North Carolina man with a history of coronary artery disease and hypertension was admitted to the hospital for biopsy of a lung nodule. He unexpectedly suffered delirium and a racing heart, landing him in the intensive care unit. A doctor's inquiry revealed the patient's customary use of megadoses of the herbal sedative valerian, which abruptly ended in the hospital, triggered symptoms similar to valium withdrawal.[15] Valerian is a widely used herbal product with putative sedative, hypnotic, and anxiolytic benefits similar to the benzodiazepines.

30.6.4   ST. JOHN'S WORT AND ADVERSE REACTIONS

St. John's Wort is a perennial herb found in Europe and North America. Since the Middle Ages it has been used as a remedy for the treatment of depression and anxiety. One of the active ingredients, hypericin, appears to be a monoamine oxidase inhibitor. A number of clinical trials have reported efficacy in the short-term treatment of mild-to-moderate depression. It has been popular in Europe for the last 15 years as a natural remedy for depression. It is currently the leading treatment in Germany, where it is prescribed 20 times more than Prozac. Now, thanks to a number of books and articles touting the herb's properties, its popularity is spreading in the United States. Several clinical studies have shown that St. John's Wort is effective in battling mostly mild to moderate depression. However, a recent multicenter clinical trial concluded that this herb is not effective in the treatment of major depression. St. John's Wort can interact with sunlight, producing oxygen free radicals that damage myelin around the nerves. This can produce electrical activity that feels like tingling, needles, or pain. Also, its safety has recently been questioned, especially when taken in the presence of certain prescribed drugs.

30.6.4.1 Neurological Effects

A 20-year-old New Yorker, under treatment with a selective serotonin reuptake inhibitor, became agitated and confused, shouting in the hospital corridors. Psychiatrists later found that the patient had added St. John's Wort (nicknamed natural Prozac) to his prescription regimen. This combination unleashed a serotonin syndrome because of an overload of the neurotransmitter. If the patient had disclosed his self-treatment, or if the doctor had been more probing, these complications could have been prevented. Unfortunately, withholding information is more the rule than the exception.

There are reports of at least five cases of clinically diagnosed central serotonergic syndrome among elderly patients who combined prescription antidepressants with St. John's Wort. These patients developed dizziness, nausea, vomiting, confusion, and anxiety—all symptoms characteristic of central serotonin excess syndrome. The symptoms resolved two to four days after stopping all medications. The patients then resumed the prescription drugs without problems. There were also two cases of mania in young adults who were temporarily associated with this herb.

30.6.4.2 Enzyme Induction

St. John's Wort is a potent inducer of some hepatic enzymes involved in drug metabolism. It may reduce the efficacy of some drugs and make a patient a nonresponder. It may also cause increased toxicity of the drug after withdrawal of the herb. In this regard, there are two findings that have been reported most recently.

In one study, researchers at the National Institutes of Health evaluated the effect of St. John's Wort on plasma concentration of the administered HIV-1 protease inhibitor indinavir. They observed a large reduction in the concentration of indinavir by simultaneous ingestion of St. John's Wort. The results have important clinical implications for HIV-infected patients receiving these two agents because low plasma concentrations of protease inhibitors are a cause of antiretroviral resistance leading to failure of treatment.

In another report,[27] a 61-year-old patient who had a heart transplant 11 months earlier was admitted to the hospital for an elective endomyocardial biopsy. He had been maintained on a standard immunosuppressive regimen of cyclosporine, azathioprine, and corticosteroids. His plasma cyclosporine levels had remained stable throughout the preceding year. Three weeks before hospital admission, the patient started self-medication with St. John's Wort because of mild depression. On admission, he had nonspecific fatigue but was feeling well otherwise. Laboratory examination showed decreased concentrations of plasma cyclosporine, but no other abnormalities were noted. Endomyocardial biopsy revealed an acute cellular transplant rejection. Interaction of St. John's Wort with cyclosporine was suspected and the patient's self-medication was stopped. Cyclosporine dosages (along with other drugs) were increased for the next few days. This treatment resolved the episode of rejection. After stopping treatment with St. John's Wort, regular plasma cyclosporine levels remained within therapeutic range, with no further episode of rejection.

Another patient who had a heart transplant 20 months earlier and who had taken St. John's Wort for 3 weeks also had low plasma cyclosporine levels. Endocardial biopsy showed acute heart transplant rejection. This patient was also similarly treated with cyclosporine. No further episodes of rejection occurred.

The findings in these two patients strongly suggest that St. John's Wort ingestion caused the drop in plasma cyclosporine levels with the resultant episodes of rejection. These serious adverse reactions described above make it clear that even a folk medicine, regarded as safe and well-tolerated, can have a potential fatal risk.

30.6.5   MU TONG AND NEPHROPATHY

Mu tong is the name of a Chinese plant derived either from *Aristolochia monchuriensis* (AM) or various species of Akebia or Clematis. The plant derived from AM is called Guam Mu Tong and contains aristolochic acid, a nephrotoxin. The other varieties do not contain this toxin. Mu tong has been added in weight-reducing products because it is supposed to cause muscle relaxation and eliminate stress-related water retention. During 1991–1992, 30 women who were using a weight-reduction diet died of kidney failure.[36] Recently, two women in UK who were taking herbal tea containing mu tong had kidney failure requiring renal transplant. It has also been reported that some patients using mu tong-containing products have high incidence of uroepithelial cancer. The probable reason for the presence of toxin is lack of verification of the type of mu tong used. Incidences of this kind highlight the importance of developing and enforcing appropriate quality assurance procedures for herbal medicines.

30.6.6   SAW PALMETTO AND LIVER DISEASE

Saw palmetto is a dwarf palm tree native to the southeastern United States and West Indies. Extract of saw palmetto is widely used in Europe for the treatment of benign prostatic hyperplasia (BPH). Several studies suggest that this herb offers relief from the unpleasant symptoms of an enlarged prostate gland. It improves urine flow and urinary symptoms. In a recent double-blind study, the researchers matched the appearance and taste of the placebo capsules to the ones with saw palmetto (bitter taste and foul smell). Patients took the capsules for a year. The study found no significant difference between the placebo and the saw palmetto group. Because the previous evidence favoring saw palmetto included men with "mild to moderate" BPH and the new recent study included men classified as having a "moderate to severe" form of the disease, it remains possible that men with mild symptoms could see a benefit. Saw palmetto also has been used for colds, coughs, sore throat, and various other non-respiratory conditions. Saw palmetto is the third highest selling herbal supplement in the U.S. (after garlic and Echinacea). The active ingredient appears to have predominantly antiandrogenic activity, which is thought to be influential in the management of BPH. However, there is not sufficient long-term safety information available on saw palmetto.

A 65-year-old man with nocturia and hesitancy began taking prostata, which was ordered from a catalog. Two weeks later he developed jaundice and severe pruritus, and stopped taking this medication.[18] Prostata is a combination of zinc picolinate, pyridoxine, Panax ginseng, saw palmetto, and some other ingredients. Saw palmetto is presumably the most active ingredient providing estrogenic and antiandrogenic effects. Both estrogens and antiandrogens can be hepatoxic.

30.6.7   DONG QUAI AND HYPERTENSION

Dong quai is a popular Chinese herbal medicine derived from the dried root of *Angelica sinensis*. Women use this herb orally to treat various gynecological ailments such as palliation for dysmenorrhea, irregular menstruation, postpartum weakness, and uterine hypotonicity. The reputation of dong quai in traditional Chinese medicine is second only to ginseng, and it is considered the ultimate, all-purpose women's tonic herb. Dong quai has also been used to treat anemia, arthritis, abdominal pain, migraine headache, and many other conditions in both men and women. In the United States, it is among the 20 top-selling herbal medicines. Despite its long and well-documented use in Chinese medicine, the effectiveness of dong quai is supported more by anecdotes than science.

A 32-year-old woman, 3 weeks postpartum, had ingested soup prepared from dong quai. She was taken to the hospital emergency department because of an acute onset of headache, weakness, lightheadedness, and vomiting.[23] Her blood pressure was 195/85 mm Hg. (She had been normotensive during her uneventful term delivery.) She improved rapidly and was normotensive within 12 hours. The next day her 3-week-old breast-fed son was taken to his pediatrician for evaluation of possible hypertension. The infant's blood pressure was 115/69 mm Hg (normal for age 105/65). Breast-feeding was temporarily discontinued and his blood pressure normalized within 48 hours. A possible explanation for hypertension in this woman and her child is an adverse effect of dong quai soup, passed to the child via breast milk.

30.6.8 KOMBUCHA MUSHROOM AND COAGULATION DISORDER

The Kombucha mushroom is derived from the fermentation of several species of yeast and bacteria with black tea, sugar, and other ingredients. The resulting liquid is called Kombucha tea. In the popular press, advocates of Kombucha tea have attributed many therapeutic effects to the drink. These include prevention of cancer, relief of symptoms of arthritis, treatment of insomnia, and stimulation of regrowth of hair.

In 1996, two female patients died as a result of disseminated intravascular coagulability. Kombucha mushroom tea was suspected to be the cause.[10] In the same year there was an outbreak of skin lesions affecting 20 patients in Iran. They reported that they had applied the mushroom tea locally on the skin of various parts of the body as a painkiller. Six to seven days later, skin lesions developed. Cultures from the skin lesions confirmed the presence of *Bacillus anthracis*. Fortunately, the tea had been applied locally. If it had been taken orally, these patients might have developed intestinal anthrax, which has a high mortality rate.[28]

30.6.9 HERB–HERB AND HERB–DRUG INTERACTION

A 39-year-old white woman with a history of depression and migraine headaches was hospitalized in a disoriented, agitated, and confused state. On the recommendation of friends, she had been taking two tablets of St. John's Wort (for depression) plus a tablet of valerian daily for 6 months (to improve sleep). She had a pulse rate of 140 beats per minute and a blood pressure of 140/100 mm Hg. Her pupils were dilated at 6 mm and unreactive. Her blood glucose was 139 mg/dl, but other blood chemistry was normal. A toxicological screen was positive for opioids. Further history revealed recent ingestion of loperamide, an opioid-based antidiarrheal, over-the-counter drug. The use of this drug explains the positive finding of opioids on the toxicology screen, and diarrhea can be a side effect of St. John's Wort. Her delirium could be due to either a monoamine oxidase inhibitor-induced reaction to a drug or food product, an interaction between St. John's Wort and valerian, or possibly to interactions between these herbs and loperamide. Within 2 days the patient recovered from the delirium. This case illustrates possible risks of the concomitant use of herbal and over-the-counter drugs.

30.6.10 COPPER AND LIVER TOXICITY

Copper is an essential trace element that is involved in several important biochemical functions of the body. The safe and adequate dietary intake for this nutrient is considered to be about 1.5 to 3 mg per day. Dietary copper deficiency in humans is extremely rare because the amount of copper present in food is more than adequate to provide average needs.

An individual decided on his own that he was metal deficient. He began taking zinc, and after 8 months of failing to see any improvement, he started taking copper, which he obtained by mail order. The recommended dose was 3 mg, but he took 10 times this amount and continued taking this amount for 2 years. By that time, the patient "was not feeling so good," so he doubled the dose. He came to the hospital with malaise, jaundice, and abdominal swelling.[24] The usual causes of hepatitis were excluded and it was thought that he might have Wilson's disease. His urinary copper level was 204 Amol/l (normal 1.2–1.6 Am/l). The patient then went into acute hepatic failure and received a liver transplant, which was successful. When the copper in the patient's liver was measured, it was 3280 Ag/g (normal 20–50 Ag/g).

30.6.11 CREATINE AND RENAL FUNCTION

Creatine is formed in the liver and is also present in food. It is converted to creatine phosphate (CP) in muscle, where it serves as a reserve source of high-energy phosphate. Resting muscle contains six times as much CP as adenosine triphosphate (ATP), which provides energy for muscle activity. Whenever the expenditure of ATP exceeds its production, CP stores are used up in an attempt to replenish ATP supplies. Recent studies have shown that oral creatine supplementation increases its levels in muscle and affects short-term performance positively. Creatine, unlike some other ergogenic aids that fall into the class of controlled substances, is synthesized endogenously and is also provided in a meat-containing diet. No evidence of long-term chronic benefit or optimal duration for supplementation has been determined.

For more than a decade, creatine has been used in Europe as an ergogenic aid. This supplement hit the U.S. market about five years ago and has proliferated. It is promoted as a "natural muscle builder" and is boosted by endorsements from athletes. Many sports nutrition experts believe that the majority of world-class athletes use creatine. It is also in heavy use among athletes at the college level. However, the safety of oral creatine has been questioned, with the deaths of three college wrestlers linked to its use. A study of healthy, young men who consumed 20 g of creatine for 5 days, followed by 3 g per day for 58 days, showed no adverse effect on renal function. But recently, a publication appeared that described the occurrence of glomerulosclerosis in a patient with nephrotic syndrome, which reversed when creatine[26] was discontinued.

30.6.12 CHROMIUM PICOLINATE AND RENAL FAILURE

The trace mineral chromium, as part of glucose tolerance factor, is involved in the metabolism of glucose and fat by potentiating the effect of insulin. Proponents claim that chromium burns fat, builds lean muscle, and reduces food craving. It is one of the top-selling dietary supplements. People use it for weight loss, glycemic control in diabetes, and enhancing athletic performance. Chromium picolinate given orally can lead to cognitive perceptual and motor dysfunction at 200–400 Ag/day. It has been reported that at high doses it can damage chromosomes in hamster cells and could be carcinogenic. Theoretically, chromium can increase the risk of hypoglycemia. Vitamin C may increase chromium absorption.

Two cases of renal failure associated with chromium picolinate have been reported.[7] In one case, a 33-year-old woman ingested 1200–2400 mg per day of the supplement for 4 to 5 months to enhance weight loss. The other case involved a 49-year-old woman who took 600 mg per day of chromium picolinate for 6 weeks to lose weight. Following discontinuation of the supplement the condition of both patients improved.

30.6.13 TRYPTOPHAN, 5-HYDROXYTRYPTOPHAN, AND EOSINOPHILIA–MYALGIA SYNDROME

Tryptophan is an essential amino acid, and 5-hydroxytryptophan (5-HTP) is the intermediate metabolite of tryptophan in the formation of the neurotransmitter serotonin. Both tryptophan and 5-HTP are promoted as treatment for headaches, obesity, binge eating, insomnia, and depression.

Impurities in tryptophan (heterocyclic compounds) were implicated in an outbreak of the rare illness eosinophilia–myalgia syndrome (EMS), with about 30 deaths occurring in 1989.[2] Those deaths caused the FDA to ban the nonprescription sale of tryptophan, and this led to a dramatic drop in new cases of this unusual disorder. In 1991, there was one report of a family sickened with 5-HTP. Similar impurities have been found in some 5-HTP products. Research has not resolved whether EMS was actually caused by these impurities, but people should not consume 5-HTP until this issue is settled.

30.7 ALTERNATIVE MEDICINE AND CANCER

The use of alternative medicine by patients with cancer is common and widespread, but at this time, no alternative treatment has been proved to be an effective means of curing an existing cancer. For some people, alternative therapies may be helpful in relieving the stress and side effects of treatment. However, patients who decide against pursuing their doctors' recommended traditional treatments in favor of alternative therapies offered outside the mainstream medicines are likely putting themselves at risk and making the cancer harder to treat later on.

A 13-year-old boy was found to have localized osteogenic sarcoma. It was recommended that he receive radiation and chemotherapy, and he was told that, with this treatment, the expected 5-year event-free survival was about 65%. However, after initial treatment, the boy, on the advice of his parents, refused further chemotherapy, opting for herbal and other alternative remedies. He died less than a year after his diagnosis.

Another patient, a 15-year-old boy, received a diagnosis of Stage II-A Hodgkin's disease. He was told that he would have an 80% chance of survival if treated with radiation and chemotherapy. The patient, with the approval of his mother, elected instead to take Matol. This tablet contained the herb astragalus, in combination with a special extract of dairy colostrum from a "select herd of cows raised on strict organic conditions." The tablet, according to the manufacturer's promotional literature, is alleged to create a synergistic effect of the immune system, resulting in the elevation of natural killer cell activity.

The boy was encouraged to visit his physician regularly to monitor his condition. Four months later, both clinical and radiological evidence of marked disease progression was seen. The patient then requested previously recommended conventional remedies. This time, because of the progression of the disease, more intense therapy was needed.

30.8 SUPPLEMENTS AND THE ELDERLY—IS THERE A NEED?

The levels of many hormones decline with aging. At present it is uncertain whether replacement of these hormones will extend life and improve its quality or decrease lifespan. Estrogen replacement in women at menopause is perhaps the best example of this. Clearly estrogen can prevent the unpleasant effects of menopause and delay the rapid decline in bone mineral density (BMD) that occurs following menopause. However, despite the salutary effects of estrogen on lipids and endothelial function, the Heart Estrogen Replacement Study and the Women's Health Initiative Memory Study have suggested that estrogen replacement may increase early cardiovascular deaths in some women taking estrogen. Testosterone levels decline with aging in men. A number of studies have shown that testosterone replacement in older men increases muscle mass, strength, BMD, cognition, and function while having minimal deleterious effects. There are, however, no safety studies demonstrating the long-term effects of this hormone. Growth hormone, insulin-like growth factor, DHEA, and pregnenolone levels decline dramatically with aging. Although hormone replacement strategies have been shown in clinical trials to modify some of the physiological attributes associated with aging, negative side effects occur frequently with those interventions shown to have some benefits, such as growth hormone. At present, there is no evidence to support the use of these hormones as anti-aging supplements.

Numerous herbals are touted to improve quality of life or as longevity agents. Of these, there is some scientific evidence for the utility of ginkgo biloba for memory disorders, glucosamine and chondroitin for arthritis, and saw palmetto for benign prostate hyperplasia. But the long-term effects of these supplements and others like St. John's Wort, garlic, shark cartilage, and more is not known. In spite of considerable hype to the contrary, there is no evidence that currently existing so-called anti-aging remedies promoted by a variety of companies and other organizations can slow aging or increase longevity in humans. Exercise is perhaps the best anti-aging medicine. It is particularly useful to improve strength, enhance cognition, and decrease depression.

30.9   WHY PEOPLE USE ALTERNATIVE THERAPIES

There are multiple reasons why people use alternative therapies. Often cited is a sense of control, a mental comfort derived from taking action. Natural plant products are perceived to be healthier than manufactured medicines and there is dissatisfaction with conventional medicine. Patients feel that their doctors (a) do not listen or respect cultural beliefs/traditions, (b) are not knowledgeable or willing to discuss alternative therapies, including nutrition and dietary supplements, and (c) focus on the disease or condition rather than the individual patient. Traditional medicine is a Johnny-come-lately approach focusing on treating/curing disease after it has occurred. Many of the alternative therapies are portrayed as being preventative as well as for treatment and cure. Many patients who have chronic or incurable diseases, such as diabetes, arthritis, or depression, often believe that conventional medicine has failed them.

Evolution of the Internet with its information revolution has allowed patients to become more informed (or misinformed) about their health. Daily we are bombarded with newspaper reports, magazine articles, television and radio commercials, and product advertisements via direct mailings and by word of mouth from friends, relatives, and coworkers. Most of the alternative therapies that are noninvasive and do not require ingestion of supplements may be safe. Dietary supplements are of concern because they may be toxic in the amounts taken and/or may interact with prescribed medications.

Supplement users give a variety of reasons for taking them. Health maintenance and disease prevention are often cited as the reasons for dietary use. Some believe (correctly or not) that supplements decrease susceptibility to, or severity of, health problems, including serious illness, stress, colds, skin problems, heart disease, and cancer. Others believe that supplements increase their energy, and still others perceive that the frequent use of supplements will give them greater control over their health.

Despite enthusiasm for dietary supplements, they can be harmful in some cases. Some supplements pose greater concern than others. For example, there may be a relatively narrow range between recommended doses and toxic doses even for essential nutrients. While there is some evidence to indicate that β-carotene supplementation can reduce precancerous oral lesions, two studies indicate that relatively high doses are associated with increased risk of lung cancer among heavy smokers. Adverse effects can be due to direct toxicity (large doses of vitamins A, D, or B6), interaction with other medications (e.g., vitamin E potentiates the effect of warfarin), or a contaminant in the supplement, such as impurities in tryptophan, mentioned above.

30.10   THE ROLE OF PHYSICIANS

The adverse effects described above illustrate the point that although many herbs may be safe and effective complements to conventional medical treatment, they also can be dangerous. Clinicians are being confronted on a daily basis with patients taking herbal and nonherbal supplements. Morbidity and mortality associated with herbal medications may be more likely in the perioperative period because of physiologic alterations that occur. Such complications include myocardial infarction, stroke, bleeding, prolonged or inadequate anesthesia, organ transplant rejection, and interference

TABLE 30.5
Some Facts to Share with Patients

1. Not all that is natural is harmless.
2. If something is good for the health, it does not mean that more is necessarily better; it can be harmful.
3. Medical herbs and supplements may not only have potential benefits, but also the potential to interact with other drugs and cause toxic reactions.
4. Advice given in health food stores can be dangerously misleading.
5. Manufacturers have no regulatory responsibility to ensure safety of their products. There are no requirements for FDA approval.
6. Possibility of contamination, adulteration, and misidentification of plant species may exist.
7. Use of supplements should be avoided during pregnancy and lactation because of possible adverse effects on the fetus and the newborn.
8. Children and the elderly may be more prone to adverse effects from herbal treatments because of their decreased metabolizing ability.

with medications indispensable for patient care. Herbal supplements can pose greater health risk to seniors who are more likely to be on prescription drugs and have medical problems. These two factors can be adversely affected by supplements. Patients who use supplements are often misguided by misconceptions or inaccurate information. Frustrated patients who have chronic disease often seek herbal treatment. Manifestations of illness and organ dysfunction may result not only from disease or therapy that meets scientific protocols but also from herbs as well.

Recent evidence suggests that patients often do not report the use of dietary supplements on written medication questionnaires. It is imperative to ask patients about supplement use during the taking of the patient's medical history. Physicians are ideally situated to help their patients in integrating alternative modalities with conventional care and to assist them in making informed treatment decisions.

Patients need to understand (Table 30.5) that (a) if something is natural it is not automatically safe; (b) if something is good for health it does not mean that more is necessarily better; it can be harmful; (c) medical herbs and supplements may not only have potential benefits but also the potential to interact with other drugs and to cause toxic reactions; (d) important similarities and differences exist between FDA-approved drugs and supplements, particularly because supplements are not required to be proved either safe or effective prior to marketing; (e) lack of regulation in the supplement industry has resulted in contamination during manufacturing and misidentification of plant species; (f) use of supplements should be avoided during pregnancy and lactation because of possible adverse effects on the fetus and the newborn; and (g) children and the elderly may be more prone to adverse effects from herbal treatments because of their decreased metabolizing ability.

30.11   CONCLUSION

In reviewing the case for alternative therapies, a major fact emerges. Several of these therapies, if correctly administered and if due consideration is given to the effect of other elements applied at the same time, can be safe and effective complements to conventional medical treatments. However, many others are not. Some of these are outwardly dangerous to health and their use should be avoided or closely supervised. Some are ineffective and a waste of time and money, while still others may dangerously delay recourse to conventional medical treatment. One of the most serious herb–drug interactions is increased risk of bleeding when warfarin is combined with anticoagulant herbs; cases of bleeding have been reported with ginkgo, garlic, and dong quai. The soluble fiber guar gum and psyllium can slow or reduce the absorption of many drugs.

The fundamental principles of good nutrition are to eat a balanced variety of foods and maintain ideal body weight. Dietary supplements have become a large and lucrative business that promotes the idea that our food is somehow lacking in specific nutrients and that additional intake of any number of food components and herbs will treat or prevent specific diseases, improve athletic and sexual performance, and make us live longer. These claims are largely untested or unproven. Unfortunately, the DSHEA of 1994 prevents the FDA from monitoring the quantity and safety of dietary supplements before marketing. Even vitamins and mineral supplements may have unexpected results. Supplements do not even have to be dietary components to be sold as dietary supplements.

In short, they should not be administered indiscriminately. In the case of herbals and other dietary supplements, the FDA should be encouraged and permitted to look closely into their content, quality, dosage, and recommended application.

A Puzzling Cause of Hypokalemia—A Case

A 67-year-old man presented with progressive muscular weakness. A month earlier he had been diagnosed with hypertension but received no treatment. His blood pressure was 165/95 mm Hg (normal <130/85 mm Hg). He weighed 65 kg and was 1.64 m tall. Blood tests showed his plasma potassium to be 2.2 mmol/l (normal 3.5–4.5 mmol/l) and he had metabolic alkalosis. His urinary excretion of potassium was high (18 mmol/l; 24-h potassium excretion, 42 mmol). He said he did not experience nausea, vomiting, and diarrhea and was not using diuretics. Abdominal sonography did not reveal renal or adrenal abnormalities. He was prescribed oral potassium (potassium chloride) 48 mmol/day. One week later his plasma potassium was 2.3 mmol/l despite potassium supplementation. Additional laboratory tests showed he had normal plasma cortisol but plasma renin was 0.03 ng/l (normal 0.11–0.69 ng/l) and aldosterone 36 pmol/l (normal 111–860 pmol/l). The patient was again asked if he used any other drug and he admitted to taking daily powdered Chinese herbal formula (50 g dissolved in 600 ml water for the last 4 months to control BPH). A sample of the formula solution was tested by high-performance liquid chromatography and found to contain 0.56 mg/ml glycyrrhizic acid (GA). This amounted to 336 mg GA in 600 ml of herbal solution the patient was taking daily. He was asked to stop taking herbal formula and was prescribed 100 mg spirinolacton, an aldosterone antagonist, once daily. After 2 weeks his blood pressure and plasma potassium returned to normal and he lost 2 kg in weight as the concomitant sodium retention resolved. When seen again after 4 months, the patient had no complaints and had normal blood pressure and plasma potassium levels.

GA is a component of licorice and makes up from 4% to more than 20% of the licorice root. GA is more than 150 times sweeter than table sugar. Traditional Chinese medicine extensively calls for licorice as a herbal healing agent. Europeans use it as a soothing agent in cough suppressants and to help heal ulcers. In early Western medicines, licorice was used to relieve the symptoms of Addison's disease, which is caused by a deficiency of cortisol. Early herbalists knew that licorice treated these diseases, but it was not until the 1960s that hypertension researchers began to figure out why licorice was a boon.

It is now known that GA inhibits 11-β hydroxysteroid dehydrogenase (BHSD), which catalyzes the conversion of cortisol to cortisone. Cortisol interacts with the mineralocorticoid receptor as an agonist; cortisone does not. Because the circulating concentrations of cortisol are several times more than those of aldosterone, cortisol can have considerable mineralocorticoid activity in humans. Excess activity is prevented by the action of BHSD, which converts cortisol to its metabolite, cortisone. If the activity of this enzyme is impaired, cortisol assumes the role of aldosterone. Because cortisol secretion is not regulated by the renin–angiotensin system, a state of mineralocorticoid[37] excess at normal concentration of plasma cortisol results. This syndrome with all features of mineralocorticoid excess (hypokalemia, hypertension, and suppression of renin–angiotensin system), but without an increase of any known mineralocorticoid hormone is known as apparent mineralocorticoid excess. The patient described above had this syndrome as a result of excess licorice in herbal formula.

Licorice is used for flavoring cigarettes, cigars, and chewing tobacco. Beverage makers use licorice as a foaming agent. Pharmaceutical companies use the sweetness of licorice to mask the taste of bitter drugs. It is found in candy, alcoholic drinks, and several herbal medicines. The possibility of licorice intake should be considered by physicians in the taking of patients' histories especially in patients who present with hypokalemia in combination with hypertension.

REFERENCES

1. Beigel, Y., I. Ostfeld, and N. Schoenfeld. 1998. A leading question. *N Engl J Med* 339:827.
2. Belongia, E. A., C. W. Hedberg, G. J. Gleich, K. E. White, A. N. Mayeno, D. A. Loeering, S. L. Dunnette, P. L. Pirie, K. L. MacDonald, and M. T. Osterholm. 1990. An investigation of the cause of the eosinophilia–myalgia-syndrome associated with tryptophan use. *N Engl J Med* 323:357.
3. Brevoort, P. 1999. *Overview of the U.S. Botanical Market.* Washington, DC: Presented at Third Conference on Botanicals.
4. Buchman, A. L. 2002. Personal and government regulations of nutritional supplements: What we want and what we should expect. *J Lab Clin Med* 139:339.
5. Buscemi, N., B. Vandermeer, N. Hooton et al. 2006. Efficacy and safety of exogenous melatonin for secondary sleep disorders and sleep disorders accompanying sleep restriction: Meta-analysis. *BMJ* 332:385.
6. CBC News Online Staff. 2001. Britain pulls herbal drug kava kava. CBC News. http://cbc.ca/cgi-bin/templates/views.cgi?/category-Consumers&story-/news/2001/12/21/Consumers/kavakava 011221
7. Cerfulli, J., D. W. Grabe, I. Gauthier, M. Malone, and M. D. McGoldrick. 1998. Chromium picolinate toxicity. *Ann Pharmacol* 32:428.
8. Clegg, D. O., D. J. Reda, C. L. Harris et al. 2006. Glucosamine, chondroitin sulfate, and the two in combination for painful knee osteoarthritis. *N Engl J Med* 354:795.
9. Craig, W. J. 1999. Health promoting properties of common herbs. *Am J Clin Nutr* 70(Suppl):491s.
10. Currier, R. W., J. Goddard, and K. Buechler. 1996. Unexplained severe illness possibly associated with consumption of Kombucha tea—Iowa, 1995. *J Am Med Assoc* 275:96.
11. Dalton, L. 2002. Licorice. *Chem Eng News* 80(23):37.
12. Davis, H. A., R. B. Phillips, and R. S. Eisenberg. 2005. Trends in use of complementary and alternative medicine by U.S. adults: 1997–2002. *Altern Ther Health Med* 11(1):42.
13. Dekowsky, S. T., J. D. Williamson, A. L. Fitzpatrick et al. 2008. Ginkgo biloba for prevention of dementia. A randomized controlled trial. *J Am Med Assoc* 300:2253.
14. Ernst, E. 2002. The risk–benefit profile of commonly used herbal therapies: Ginkgo, St. John's Wort, ginseng, echinaecea, saw palmetto, and kava. *Ann Int Med* 136:42.
15. Garges, H. P., I. Varis, and P. M. Doraiswamy. 1998. Cardiac complications and delirium associated with valerian root withdrawal. *J Am Med Assoc* 280:1566.
16. Gertner, E., P. S. Marshall, D. Filandrinos, A. S. Potek, and T. M. Smith. 1995. Complications resulting from the use of Chinese herbal medications containing undeclared prescription drug. *Arthritis Rheum* 38:614.
17. Gordon, J. S. 2004. Banning ephedra: Good call, poor vision. *Altern Ther Health Med* 10:18.
18. Hamed, S., S. Rojter, and J. Vierling. 1997. Protracted cholestatic hepatitis after the use of Prostata. *Ann Intern Med* 127:169.
19. Kalant, H. 2001. The pharmacology and toxicology of "ecstasy" (MDMA) related drugs. *Can Med Assoc J* 165:917.
20. Mar, C., and S. Bent. 1999. An evidence based review of the ten most commonly used herbs. *West J Med* 171:168.
21. Massey, P. B. 2002. Dietary supplements. *Med Clin North Am* 86(1):127.
22. Mintzer, S., S. Hickenbottom, and S. Gilman. 1999. Parkinsonism after taking ecstasy. *N Engl J Med* 340:1443.
23. Nambiar, S., R. H. Schwartz, and A. Constantine. 1999. Hypertension in mother and baby linked to ingestion of Chinese herbal medicine. *West J Med* 171:152.
24. O'Donahue, J., M. Reid, A. Varghese, B. Portmann, and R. Williams. 1999. A case of adult chronic copper self-intoxication resulting in cirrhosis. *Eur J Med Res* 4:252.
25. O'Hara, M. 1998. A review of twelve commonly used medicinal herbs. *Arch Fam Med* 7:523.

26. Pritchard, N. R., and P. A. Kalra. 1998. Renal dysfunction accompanying oral creatine supplements. *Lancet* 351:1252.
27. Ruschitzka, F., P. J. Meier, M. Turina, T. F. Luscher, and G. Noll. 2000. Acute heart transplant rejection due to St. John's Wort. *Lancet* 355:548.
28. Sadjadi, J. 1998. Cutaneous anthrax associated with the Kombucha mushroom. *J Am Med Assoc* 280:1567.
29. Saper, R. B., D. N. Eisenberg, and R. S. Phillips. 2004. Common dietary supplements for weight loss. *Am Fam Physician* 70:1731.
30. Sardesai, V. M. 2002. Herbal medicines. Poisons or potions? *J Lab Clin Med* 139:343.
31. Sardesai, V. M., and T. Myers. 2001. Nutrient supplements in clinical care. *Nutr Clin Pract* 16:35.
32. Sendelbach, S. E., M. A. Halm, K. A. Doran et al. 2006. Effects of music therapy on physiological and psychological outcomes for patients undergoing cardiac surgery. *J Cardiovasc Nurs* 21(3):194.
33. Takeda, M., R. Hashimoto, T. Kudo et al. 2010. Laughter and humor as complementary and alternative medicines for dementia patients. *BMC Complement Altern Med* 10:28.
34. Tolston, L. G. 2001. Herbal remedies: Buyers beware! *Nutr Today* 36(4):223.
35. U.S. Food and Drug Administration. 1997. Current good manufacturing practice in manufacturing, packing or holding dietary supplements; proposed rule. *Fed Reg* 62:5700–9.
36. Vanherweghem, J. L., M. Depierreaux, C. Tielemans, D. Abramowicz, M. Dratwa, M. Jadoul, C. Richard et al. 1993. Rapidly progressive interstitial fibrosis in young women: Association with slimming regimen including Chinese herbs. *Lancet* 341:387.

CASE BIBLIOGRAPHY

37. Lin, S. H., and T. Chau. 2002. A puzzling case of hypokalemia. *Lancet* 360:224.

31 Gene–Nutrient Interaction— Molecular Genetics, Epigenetics, and Telomeres

31.1 GENE–NUTRIENT INTERACTION

The relation of genes to nutrition is obviously a two-way relationship. Thus, not only genes profoundly affect nutrient metabolism, but also, in turn, nutrients regulate gene expression. Before discussing their interrelationship a brief review of molecular genetics follows.

31.1.1 MOLECULAR GENETICS

The basic tenet of molecular genetics—often referred to as "the central dogma"—is that deoxyribonucleic acid (DNA) encodes ribonucleic acid (RNA), which in turn encodes the amino acid sequence of proteins. The flow of genetic information between DNA, RNA, and protein is illustrated in Figure 31.1. This is a simplified view of the function of the genome, a term that means all of the DNA in an organism.

Genetic information is encoded in the sequence of a linear polymer of purine and pyrimidine bases termed DNA. This genetic message codes for the building and operation of the human body. The message is written in an alphabet that uses only four letters: A, C, G, T. Each of the letters represents one of the four bases that are chemical building blocks of DNA. A stands for adenine, C for cytosine, G for guanine, and T for thymine.

31.1.2 DNA STRUCTURE

The structure of DNA is a double helix, composed of two polynucleotide strands that are coiled about each other in a spiral. The nucleotides, which spell out the genetic message, are arranged in a linear sequence of the double-stranded helical DNA molecule.[23] The two strands of DNA are complementary copies of each other to form two antiparallel polynucleotide strands. The nucleotides on one strand pair with the complementary nucleotides on the other strand; adenine is paired with thymine and guanine is paired with cytosine. Each strand has a sugar phosphate backbone linked by phosphodiester bond from the 5′ position of one deoxyribose (sugar) to the 3′ position of the next. At the end of the strand is either a 5′ phosphate group (5′ end) or a 3′ phosphate group (3′ end). One strand of DNA (sense strand) contains the genetic information in a 5′ to 3′ direction in the form of the four nucleotide bases A, G, C, and T. Its partner strand (antisense strand) has the complementary sequence; A is paired with T and G is paired with C. Hydrogen bonds exist between the bases to stabilize the pairing. The double-stranded DNA structure is essential for replication (the duplication of DNA) to ensure that each dividing cell receives an identical DNA copy.

Human DNA is estimated to consist of about 3 billion base pairs (bp) per haploid genome. Because humans are diploid organisms two copies of DNA exist. Therefore, the actual number of base pairs is 6 billion. The DNA, about 6 ft long in each eukaryotic cell, must be compressed to fit within the nucleus, which is only a few micrometers in diameter. DNA is condensed by the formation of nucleosomes, groups of small proteins (histones) around which 160–180 bp of DNA

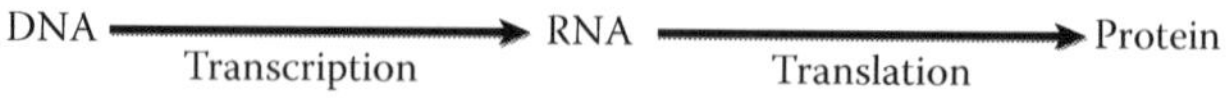

DNA ⟶ RNA ⟶ Protein
Transcription   Translation

FIGURE 31.1   The central dogma of biological information.

are wrapped. Nucleosomes are wound into a left hand helix for further condensation of DNA. Nucleosomes then fold in upon one another forming chromatin fiber. This fiber then buckles and coils resulting in the formation of chromosomes.

31.1.3   CHROMOSOMES

DNA is packaged into chromosomes, which are physical structures in the cell nucleus consisting of DNA complexed with a set of lysine and arginine rich proteins called histones. The combination of DNA and histones is called chromatin. The packaging is very efficient. It allows a large amount of DNA to be located within a small space. The DNA is in the form of supercoils—like a rubberband that is tightly wound until it compacts upon itself. It is then folded into the chromatin assembly by the binding of basic histone proteins. Histones may act to regulate the availability of a particular segment of DNA for gene activity.

There are 23 pairs of chromosomes per somatic nucleus: 2 pairs of autosomes numbered by descending size and one pair of sex chromosomes (XX, female; XY, male). The majority of genetic material is stored on chromosomes within the nucleus of the cell (the remainder being in the mitochrondria). During mitosis the chromosomes are unwound; the DNA helix is split apart and copied. Each replicated strand creates a complimentary copy of the original double helix, allowing the transmission of a complete set of genetic information into each daughter cell. In meiosis, a reduction division of genetic information occurs. Homologous chromosomes are allowed to segregate into a gamete. Thus, a diploid germ cell gives rise to a haploid sperm, or egg that contains an assortment of one of each of the 23 pairs of homologous chromosomes in the parental cell. During fertilization, sperm and egg unite to create a zygote with a complete set of 46 chromosomes.

31.1.4   GENETIC CODE

The genetic message is read not as a single letter, but rather it is grouped into a three-letter word. The 20 amino acids found in the proteins of humans are spelled out using the four nucleotide bases. A sequence of three bases is called a codon; each codon codes for a specific amino acid. Because 64 combinations of bases are possible ($4 \times 4 \times 4$), the code is redundant, meaning that some amino acids are coded for by several different combinations of bases. The positions indicating where a polypeptide starts and where it ends are also defined by triplet codons. For example, ATG is found at the start, and the end or stop codons are TAA or TAG or TGA.

31.1.5   GENE STRUCTURE AND FUNCTION

The word "gene" is derived from the Greek word *genesis* ("birth") or *genos* ("origin"). It originally arose as a derivative of *pangene*, a term used to describe entities involved in pangenesis, Darwin's hypothetical mechanism of heredity. The term "gene" was first used by Wilhelm Johannsen in 1909 based on a concept Mendel had developed in 1866. In pea plants, Mendel showed that certain traits (such as height or flower color) do not appear blended in offspring. Instead these traits are passed on as distinct,[34] discrete entities. Furthermore, he demonstrated that variations in such traits are caused by variations in heritable factors.

In its simplest form, a gene is a segment of a DNA molecule containing the specific code for the amino acid sequence of a polypeptide chain and the regulatory sequence necessary for expression. A gene product is usually a protein, but can occasionally consist of a RNA that is not translated. The human genome contains enough base pairs to make a million average-size proteins, but there are only about 20,000–25,000 genes. Genes are composed of coding spaces (exons)[32] intercepted by noncoding sequences (introns), as shown in Figure 31.2. Only about 10% of the entire human genome is composed of exons.[32]

Gene expression refers to the process whereby a gene gives rise to its product, namely, its unique polypeptide. It consists of three phases: transcription, translation, and post-translational modification. This is a highly controlled process. Transcription is the process whereby messenger (m) RNA is synthesized in the nucleus using a strand of the double helix DNA as a template. The mRNA and other RNAs are then transported from the nucleus to the cytoplasm where the RNA sequence is decoded or translated to determine the sequence of amino acids in the protein being synthesized. The process of translation occurs in ribosomes. Translation involves transfer (t) RNAs, which provide the molecular link between the coded base sequence of the mRNA and the amino acid sequence of the protein. Many proteins undergo extensive post-translational modifications. The polypeptide chain that is the primary translation product is folded and bonded into a specific three-dimensional structure that is determined by the amino acid sequence itself. Two or more polypeptide chains, products of the same gene or of different genes, may combine to form a single, mature protein complex that can perform a specific cell function. Other modifications may involve cleavage of the protein to remove specific amino-terminal sequences, addition of phosphate, or various amino acid modifications.

Some genes, the so-called housekeeping genes, are turned on all of the time and provide the common proteins for cell structure, cellular organelles, and metabolic enzymes that perform basic cell function.[30] For other genes, expression is tightly controlled with particular genes being turned on or off in particular cells at specific times in development or in response to physiological signals. The control gives those cells their tissue-specific characteristics to perform the unique function of that organ. Therefore, in most cells, a small proportion of genes are actively transcribed. This specificity explains why there is a large variety of different cell types making different protein products, even though almost all cells have exactly the same DNA sequence. For example, the globin genes are transcribed only in the progenitors of red blood cells (to form hemoglobin), and the low density lipoprotein receptor genes are transcribed only in liver cells.

To initiate mRNA transcription, RNA polymerase II binds to a specific segment of the gene called the promoter site (Figure 31.2) on the DNA. The promoter is a nucleotide sequence that lies just upstream or at the 5′ end of the gene sequence. The transcription initiation site is located within the promoter. Many different proteins participate in the process of transcription. Some of these proteins are required for the transcription of all structural genes. These are called general transcription factors. Others, labeled specific transcription factors, have more specialized roles, activating only certain genes at certain stages of development. The transcription activity of specific genes can be greatly increased by interaction with sequences called enhancers, which may be located thousands of bases upstream or downstream of the gene. Enhancers are bound by a specific

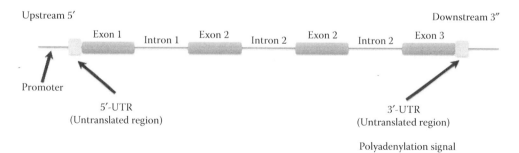

FIGURE 31.2 Schematic representation of gene structure. A gene is a segment of DNA that contains genetic information. Structural genes are composed of both coding regions called exons and noncoding regions called introns. Each gene sequence contains various regulatory sequences. The most common of these is the promoter element that typically resides upstream at the 5′ end of the gene sequence.

class of transcription factors, termed activators. Activators bind to a second class of transcription factors, called co-activators, which in turn bind to the general transcription factors. This chain of interactions, from enhancer to activator to co-activator to the general transcription factor complex and finally to the gene itself, increases the transcription of specific genes at specific points in time. There are also other DNA sequences, known as silencers, which help to repress the transcription of genes through a similar series of interactions.

31.1.6 Genetic Variations

Humans display a remarkable degree of genetic variation. This is seen in traits such as height, blood pressure, and skin color. Included in the spectrum of genetic variation are disease states such as cystic fibrosis.[30]

All genetic variations originate from the process known as mutation, which is defined as a change in DNA sequence. One important type is the base-pair substitution in which one base pair is replaced by another. Mutations may be harmless (in the sense that they do not cause disease), either because they occur in introns or because of the redundancy of the genetic code; these mutations do not change the amino acid sequence and thus have no consequence. Such mutations are called silent substitution. Nonsilent substitution consists of two base types: 1) missense mutation and 2) nonsense mutation. A missense mutation causes a change in a single base in the DNA sequence, resulting in a codon that codes for a different amino acid. This can make the resulting protein nonfunctional. Such mutations are responsible for diseases such as sicke-cell disease. Nonsense mutations involve nucleotide base substitution in one of the three stop codons. Because sop codons terminate translation of mRNA, these mutations result in a premature termination of the polypeptide chain. Conversely, if the stop codon is altered so that it encodes for an amino acid, an abnormally elongated polypeptide is produced. Disorders such as thalasemias result from nonsense mutations. Alterations in amino acid sequences can have profound consequences, and many of the serious genetic diseases are the result of such alterations.

Mutations in enhancers, silencers, or promoter sequences, as well as genes that encode transcription factors, can lead to faulty expression of genes and consequently to genetic diseases.

As a result of mutation a gene may differ among individuals in terms of its DNA sequence. The differing sequences are referred to as alleles. Individuals have two copies (alleles) of each gene and receive one copy of each gene from the germ cells of each parent. A gene's location on a chromosome is termed a locus. If an individual has the same allele in both members of a chromosome pair, he or she is said to be homozygous. If the alleles differ in DNA sequence the individual is heterozygote. The alleles that are present at a given locus are referred to as the individual's genotype (genetic constitution of an individual). The phenotype is what is actually observed physically or clinically by the interaction of genes and environment.

Most changes in the DNA sequence do not lead to disease. These changes are called polymorphisms. By convention, a polymorphism is a difference in DNA sequence between individuals that occurs in >1% of the population. Since only about 1%–2% of the human genome contains sequence for genes, the great majority of polymorphisms will not directly affect gene function although a polymorphism falling within a regulatory region in the genome might have functional significance.

Autosomal involves traits that are encoded by the 22 pairs of autosomes. X-linked inheritance refers to genes located on the X chromosome. Autosomal recessive diseases require the inheritance of an abnormal copy of the gene from both the mother and the father. For example, a child with sickle cell disease (SCD) will have inherited two copies of the mutation that causes SCD. Both parents will be carriers but are normally not affected. Cystic fibrosis is another well-known example in which phenotypically normal parents are only recognized to be carriers of a mutant allele when they have a child who has inherited the dysfunctional forms of the gene from both parents.

Dominant inheritance occurs when one member of a gene pair contains a mutation in that gene, and the mutation is associated with symptoms of a condition or a disease. The genes that are associated with most dominantly inherited traits are located on the autosomes; they are, therefore, referred to as autosomal dominant traits. Examples of autosomal dominant diseases include Huntington's disease and many of the recognized cancer predisposition syndromes.

Sex-linked disease means that the disease gene is located on a sex chromosome. Most sex-linked disorders result from a mutated gene on the X chromosome. The majority of these conditions are recessive, but there are also X-linked disorders that follow a dominant pattern of inheritance. With X-linked inheritance women typically do not manifest disease even when they inherit a mutant gene because the normal copy of the gene on their other X chromosome compensates. Men with only a single X chromosome are not protected by a normal gene copy and therefore manifest disease. Hemophilia A is an example of sex-linked disease.

Other disorders, including common diseases such as diabetes mellitus and hypertension may involve the interactive effects of multiple genes. This is referred to as polygenic or multifactorial inheritance.

31.1.7 Mitochondrial DNA and Inheritance

In addition to the DNA found in the nucleus of the cell, a relatively small amount of DNA exists in the mitochondria. Mitochondrial DNA (mDNA) is a small, double-stranded closed-circular molecule containing 16,569 nucleotides.

The mDNA codes for proteins that are required for proper mitochondrial function, primarily proteins involved in oxidative phosphorylation. Unlike nuclear DNA, mDNA contains no noncoding regions and the mitochondrial genes contain no introns. Furthermore, the mDNA is not packaged through interaction with histone proteins. The mutation rate for mDNA is about 10 times higher than that of nuclear DNA. This is caused by a lack of DNA repair mechanisms in the mDNA and possibly also by damage from free oxygen radicals released during the oxidative phosphorylation process.

The mDNA exhibits two critical differences from the nuclear genome that accounts for unusual patterns of inheritance of mitochondrial genetic traits. These are maternal transmission and heteroplasmy—occurrence of two or more populations of genetically distinct mDNAs in a cell.

The mDNA is transmitted only from the egg of the mother. The mitochondria in spermatozoa are located in the tail which is discarded at fertilization. Although all of the children of women with a mitochondrial mutation might be expected to inherit the mutation, there is usually a wide range of variation in expression. This is due to a phenomenon of heteroplasmy. Unlike the nuclear genome, which is represented by one complete copy per cell, there are hundreds of mDNA molecules in each cell. Mitochondria separate passively when a cell divides, in contrast to the orderly separation of chromosomes in the nuclear genome during cell division. If some of the mitochondria contain a mutation and others do not, the result can be unequal distribution of mutant and nonmutant mitochondria to daughter cells. This can translate into offspring who inherit the mutation to different degrees. In somatic cells, it results in some tissues having a preponderance of mutant or nonmutant mDNA molecules and consequent tissue-specific effects of the mitochondrial mutations. This heterogeneity is an important cause of variable expression in mitochondrial diseases. The larger the population of mutant mDNA molecules, the more severe the expression of the disease.

The number of mitochondria in human cells varies according to the type of cell. For example, neural cells have more mitochondria than skin cells and, therefore, disorders caused by mitochondrial mutations often affect the neuromuscular systems.

A number of clinical disorders have been identified that are due to mutations within mitochondrial genes. As might be expected these traits are associated with failure of mitochondrial energy production. Mitochondrial mutations are also involved in some common human diseases. A mitochondrial deletion causes a form of deafness. Mitochondrial defects may also be associated with some cases of Alzheimer's disease. It has also been suggested that mDNA mutations that accumulate free radicals through the life of an individual could contribute to the aging process.

31.2   EFFECTS OF NUTRIENTS ON GENE EXPRESSION

The formation of purine and pyrimidine bases in the DNA and RNA require the participation of folic acid, vitamin B_{12}, and other nutrients. Mechanisms that regulate gene expression play a critical role in the function of genes.[5] The transcription of genes is controlled by a group of DNA-binding proteins (transcription factors) that determine which regions of the DNA are to be transcribed. Nutrients bind to these proteins to form nutrient–protein complexes that target small (8–15 nucleotides) DNA regions. Transcription control is exerted by that portion of the DNA called the promoter region to which transcription factors bind. Several nutrients have a role in the transcription process. In many instances, the specific DNA-binding protein contains zinc. Zinc binds to histidine and cysteine residues in the linear portions of these proteins. This binding results in the formation of a loop "finger" in the protein that permits the folded region to bind DNA sequences in the promoter region. Thus without zinc the transcriptor factors cannot bind and stimulate transcription of gene. Nutrients such as vitamins A and D and some hormones have their effects on expression of specific genes because they bind to these zinc fingers that in turn bind to specific DNA sequences.

The gene remains turned-on directing the synthesis of more protein until something causes it to be switched off. A common mechanism of gene regulation is negative feedback. The presence of a large amount of the protein product from the gene can interfere with the binding of transcription factors (inducers) that originally turned the gene on. When this happens the gene is turned off. There are several nutrients that also control the transcription or translation processes. For example, dietary cholesterol exerts an inhibitory effect on transcription of the gene for hydroxymethylglutaryl CoA reductase, a key enzyme in cholesterol synthesis. Alterations in the diet have stricking effects on the expression of a number of genes. Polyunsaturated fatty acids regulate the expression of many genes that are involved in lipid metabolism. Vitamin A, in the form of retinoic acid, modulates the expression of a variety of genes that encode for many types of proteins, including growth factors, transcription factors, and enzymes. Copper appears to stimulate transcription of super oxide dismutase gene.

Nutrients and hormones may affect the synthesis of specific proteins by regulating several steps in the translation and post-translational processing.[12,35] For example, cellular iron concentration directly affects the translation and stability of mRNA for ferritin and transferrin receptor proteins. The synthesis of proteins in the translation process depends on the availability of constituent amino acids and energy. The changes required in the post-translational process are dependent on the availability of vitamins K, C, and several other nutrients. Thus nutrients serve as regulators of the gene expression.

31.3   GENETIC VARIATION AND NUTRITION

Genetic predisposition is known to contribute to variations in the incidence and prevalence of chronic nutritional diseases among individuals, families, and nations. The lifetime risk of non-insulin-dependent diabetes mellitus is about 40% in children with one diabetic parent. Studies in the U.S. have shown that 50% of the variance in plasma cholesterol concentration is genetically determined. Also 30%–60% of the variations in blood pressure are genetically determined. Studies in coronary artery disease (CAD) suggest 15% variance in the United Kingdom, whereas it is 51% in the Hawaiian population, indicating significant differences between populations. The variance in bone density is genetically determined. Osteoporosis is a metabolic bone disease with strong genetic predisposition.

Mutations in the genes are known to cause several disorders. Some of the disorders can be treated nutritionally. Well-known are the single gene disorders that are expressed as phenylketonuria (PKU), lactose intolerance, and celiac disease. A diet restricted in phenylalanine largely circumvents the neurological damage in classic PKU. Lactose intolerance can be managed by dietary lactose exclusion and celiac disease by dietary exclusion of gluten-containing foods.

In several metabolic disorders, there is altered binding of a cofactor (often a vitamin) to the mutant enzyme. It may be possible to provide a large excess of the cofactor and overcome the altered binding ability to the enzyme impaired by mutation. Examples are biotin in some types of multiple carboxylase deficiencies and vitamin B_1 with some forms of lactic acidosis. In fact, the vitamin responsive inborn errors are among the most successfully treated of all genetic diseases. The vitamins used are remarkably nontoxic, generally allowing the safe administration of amounts several times greater than those required for normal nutrition.

31.4   EPIGENETICS

The word epigenetics encompasses all of the layers of genetic control in cells that do not entail changes in DNA sequences. It was first coined by the British embryologist Conrod H. Waddington in the early 1940s, when he defined it as "the interactions of genes with their environment that bring the phenotype into being." It literally means "outside conventional genetics" and is now recognized as one of the most important mechanisms in regulating gene function and is responsible for the preservation patterns of gene expression for different cell types. Epigenome is a parallel to the word "genome" and refers to the overall epigenetic state of a cell. The way that each cell or organization determines its path through development, aging, or even disease is encoded not only in the genome but also in the epigenome code that defines whether or when a gene will be programmed to be active or silent despite the same DNA sequence. The changes may remain through cell division for the remainder of the cell's life and may also last for multiple generations. However, there is no change in the underlying DNA sequence of the organism. Instead non-genetic factors cause the organism's genes to behave (or express themselves) differently.

A lot of epigenetic activity involves the most subtle of chromatin modifications.[16,40] Researchers have identified a number of epigenetic pathways such as DNA methylation and histone modifications. One of the most prevalent modifications is the addition of a single methyl group at those cytosine nucleotides along chromatin's DNA that are right next to a guanine, so-called CpG pairs. Lots of such DNA methylations along a stretch of chromatin usually mean that any genetic sequences in the same stretch are marked as "do not transcribe."

Another subtle but consequential chemical change is the addition of acetyl groups to chromatin's protein complexes, nucleosomes. Histones influence how tightly or loosely packed the chromatin is during the phase when gene transcription occurs. DNA is negatively charged due to the phosphate group in its phosphate–sugar backbones and positively charged histones bind with DNA tightly. Acetylation of lysine residues at the N-terminus of the histone proteins removes positive charges thereby reducing the affinity between histones and DNA. With enough histone acetylation the DNA loosens from the nucleosomes, thereby becoming accessible to RNA polymerase and transcription factors in the promoter regions that start the gene-to-protein process. Therefore, in most cases, histone acetylation enhances transcription while histone deacylation represses transcription. Histones also can be phosphorylated, methylated, and otherwise modified with small molecule and larger sized chemical marks whose gene controlling consequences researchers now are studying.

All of these modifications contribute to the transcriptional activation or inactivation of gene sequences in the DNA. These modifications to both DNA and to the histones are heritable through both mitosis and in some cases meiosis (sperm and egg formation). The epigenome is crucial to the regulation of gene expression by regulating which genes are able to be transcribed in certain cell types. In cells, where certain genes are not transcribed, they can be highly condensed as heterochromatin leaving room for the genes that are necessary in that cell type.

Epigenetics provides an extra layer of transcriptional control that regulates how genes are expressed.[39] These mechanisms are critical components in the normal development and growth of cells. Epigenetic abnormalities have been found to be causative factors in cancer, genetic disorders,[16,39] pediatric syndromes, neurodevelopmental disorders, cardiovascular disease, autoimmunity, and other disorders.[13,3] In cancer cells, hypermethylation is frequently detected in the promoter regions of genes that process proliferation, apoptosis, and DNA repair. Silencing of genes that regulate these processes can, therefore, promote tumor formation and growth.

Unlike genetic mutations that are almost impossible to reverse, epigenetic aberrations are potentially reversible and thus have many and varied medical applications. Drugs are being developed that can treat illness simply by silencing bad genes and jump-starting good genes.[44] The first epigenetic drug, Azacitidine, was approved by the FDA in 2004. It works by removing methyl groups from the DNA in chromatin. It is used for treating a family of blood disorders, myelodysplastic syndromes, which leave patients anemic, fatigued, weak, and at risk for developing leukemia. Another drug, valproic acid, inhibits an enzyme that adds acetyl group to histone. It is used to treat HIV and for increasing the effectiveness of radiation therapy for certain brain tumors. The effects of diet and environment are discussed in the next section.

31.4.1 EFFECTS OF ENVIRONMENTAL FACTORS ON GENE EXPRESSION

Most human diseases are related in some way to the loss or gain in gene functions. Regulation of gene expression is a complex process. In addition to genetic mechanisms, epigenetic causes are gaining new perspectives in human diseases related to gene deregulation. The epigenome is particularly susceptible to deregulation during gestation, neonatal development, puberty, and old age. Nevertheless, it is most vulnerable to environmental factors during embryogenesis because the DNA synthetic rate is high and DNA methylation patterning and chromatin structure required for normal tissue development is established during early development.

Nutrition is the major environmental factor that alters expression of the fetal genome and may have lifelong consequences.[24,44] This phenomenon termed "fetal programming" has led to the recent theory of "fetal origins of adult disease." Alterations in fetal nutrition and endocrine status may result in developmental adaptations that permanently change the structure, physiology, and metabolism of the offspring, thereby predisposing individuals to metabolic, endocrine, and cardiovascular disease in adult life.

Epidemiologic studies have shown that if pregnant women eat poorly, their children would be at significantly higher than average risk for cardiovascular diseases as adults. A Dutch famine near the end of World War II led to an increased incidence of schizophrenia in adults who had been food deprived during the first trimester of their mothers' pregnancy. Malnutrition among the pregnant women in the south during the Civil War and the Depression has been proposed as an explanation for the high incidence of stroke among subsequent generations. Scientists looked at the historical records of annual harvests from a small Swedish community that depended entirely on local food production. They found that food availability between the ages of 9 and 12 years for the paternal grandfather affected the lifespan of his grandchildren. Shortage of food for the grandfather was associated with extended lifespan of his grandchildren and abundance of food was associated with shortened lifespan mostly due to diabetes and heart disease. Dietary interventions in animal models have provided considerable evidence to suggest that nutritional imbalances and metabolic disturbances during critical time windows of developmental programming may have a persistent effect on the offspring. A few examples are given below.

31.4.2 EFFECT OF SUPPLEMENTS DURING PREGNANCY

There is a saying, "If you don't like your hair, blame your mother." In a study of nutrition's effect on development, researchers were able to change the coat color of baby mice by feeding their mothers dietary supplements. Both mice and humans have a gene called agouti. When a mouse's agouti gene is not completely methylated the mouse has a yellow coat color, is obese, and is prone to diabetes and cancer. When the agouti gene is methylated (as in normal mice) the coat color is brown, the mouse is skinny, and it has a low disease risk. Researchers gave four methyl group-generating dietary supplements (folic acid, vitamin B_{12}, betaine, and choline) to some pregnant yellow mice. Mice receiving supplements gave birth to pups predominantly with brown coats. They had reduced incidence of obesity, diabetes, and cancer and remained healthy that way for life. In contrast, pregnant yellow mice that did not receive supplements gave birth to pups predominantly with a yellow coat. The nonsupplemented mice were not deficient in these nutrients. Extra supplementation caused methylation of the agouti gene and silenced it or reduced its expression. These results indicate that an individual's adult health is influenced by early prenatal factors.

31.4.3 EFFECT OF MALNUTRITION DURING PREGNANCY

Researchers recently found that rat fetuses receiving poor nutrition in the womb became genetically primed to be born lacking proper nutrition.[22] As a result of this genetic adaptation nutritionally deprived rats did not grow to the same size as their larger counterparts. These smaller rats were also at higher risk for a host of health problems such as diabetes, growth retardation, obesity, and cardiovascular disease throughout their lives. The lack of nutrients then causes the gene responsible for the promotion of IGF-1 to significantly reduce the amount of IGF-1 produced in the body both before and after birth.[18] IGF-1 promotes normal development and growth in rats and humans. Therefore, it is imperative to insure that the gene is *not* compromised in any way what would result in reducing the amount of IGF-1, particularly in the embryonic and infant stages of life. Because, we are indeed "what our mother ate … or did not eat."

31.4.4 EFFECT OF TRAFFIC POLLUTANTS DURING PREGNANCY

A study of umbilical cord blood from mothers living in New York City has shown that exposure to traffic pollutants in the womb may increase the child's risk of developing asthma later in life. The suspected pollutants are polycyclic aromatic hydrocarbons (PAHs), the by-products of incomplete combustion of carbon-containing fuels such as gasoline. When mothers are exposed to PAHs during pregnancy, the methylation of specific genes are affected in the developing fetus. This is associated with four times greater incidence of asthma symptoms in children prior to age five. The levels of PAHs are high in the air in heavy traffic areas, posing health risks for inner city neighborhoods, and residential communities in proximity to major highways. It should be noted that asthma in particular has been on the rise, especially in urban areas due to increasing air pollution, which affects the fetus.

31.4.5 EFFECT OF ENVIRONMENTAL CHEMICALS DURING PREGNANCY

Many xenobiotics, ubiquitously present in the environment have estrogenic, and/or other properties, and function as endocrine disrupters. Recently, the yellow mouse model was used to evaluate the effects of maternal exposure to bisphenol A (BPA) on the fetal epigenome. BPA is a chemical used to make polycarbonated plastic. It is found in many consumer products including water bottles, baby bottles, tin cans, and dental sealants, and now even on cash register receipts.

When pregnant agouti mice were fed BPA more yellow unhealthy babies were born than normal. Exposure to BPA during early development had caused decreased methylation of the agouti gene. But when the BPA exposed pregnant yellow mice were fed nutritional supplements (folic acid, vitamin B_{12}, betaine, and choline) or the phytoestrogen genistein, the mother gave birth to puppies that were predominantly brown.[13,20] The maternal nutrient supplementation had counteracted the negative effect of BPA exposures so the mother's diet can affect the child's epigenetic outcome.

Vinclazolin, a widely used pesticide and endocrine disrupter, can alter DNA methylation in exposed laboratory animals. Embryonic exposure to this pesticide at the time of gonadal sex determination in rats has been shown to promote an epigenetic transgenerational disease state of subfertility and spermatogenic defects. Altered DNA methylation is involved.

31.4.6 Exposure to Environmental Chemicals and Obesity

In the early 1970s, diethylstilbestrol (DES) was used in the U.S. and other countries as a drug to reduce the risk of miscarriage in women. Additionally, the drug was fed to farm animals to enhance meat production, which led to low level exposure of DES in the general population. In later years, it was discovered that the daughters whose pregnant mothers were treated with DES had increased risk of abnormal development of the uterus and cervix and increased risk of developing adenocarcinoma. The use of DES is currently forbidden.

We are exposed to numerous chemicals in the environment. The level of exposure is considered to be below the safe permissible level set by appropriate government agencies. But we are now learning what long-term low-dose exposure can do. The recent epidemic of chronic diseases now being observed in children such as obesity, type 2 diabetes, and childhood asthma may be due to exposure to environmental chemicals.

Obesity is the fastest rising health concern in the U.S., and some scientists do not think that our diet and exercise habits have changed enough in the last few decades to be the cause of our high levels of obesity. The prevalence of obesity in infants under 6 months has risen 73% from 1980 to 2006. Babies are eating only formula or breast milk and exercise is not much of a factor at this early age. Research has shown that the current obesity epidemic coincides with an increase in environmental chemicals being released into the environment over the past 40 years. Environmental chemicals, especially hormone disrupters, are a possible third component in the obesity epidemic along with diet and exercise at least for people under the age of 50.[28] Older people were not as exposed to as many chemicals in their early life.

Indeed, studies have shown that rats and mice fed low doses of BPA during early development become more obese as adults[24] than those that were not fed chemicals.[27] Research has also shown that prenatal exposure to BPA at human-relevant doses accelerated weight gain of the female offspring compared to offspring of mothers not exposed to BPA. Precursor cells grown in cultures in the presence of BPA and other pollutants are converted to fat cells. Government agencies have put a limit on exposure levels of various toxic chemicals. Recent animal studies have shown that even lower doses of some chemicals such as BPA may affect epigenetically to some degree. The cumulative exposure effect of several chemicals in low doses on epigenome is not known. There is a need for more studies in this area.

One other point regarding methyl group-generating nutritional supplements: As stated above, these supplements methylate some genes. Folic acid and other water-soluble vitamins are considered safe, and many take larger amounts of folic acid because it is generally considered nontoxic. To prevent or reduce the incidence of neural tube defects, many common foods are enriched with folic acid to ensure adequate intake of this nutrient by women of childbearing age. However, there is no data available on the impact of excess folic acid during pregnancy. It is possible that folic acid could methylate an important gene(s) and silence its expression at a critical time of early development, and this would therefore be detrimental to the developing fetus and/or infant. There is no data to show the effects of excess folic acid in pregnant women. Just because something is good, more is not necessarily better.

31.4.7 Effect of Father's Exposure to High-Fat Diet on Female Offspring

Having either parent obese is an independent risk factor for childhood obesity in offspring. The effect of diet-induced maternal obesity on adiposity and metabolism in offspring is well established, but the contribution of obese fathers is unclear. Recent studies have shown that male rats fed a high-fat diet had daughters with diabetes-like β-cell dysfunction, showing for the first time that the environment of the parent can influence the phenotype of the offspring.[29] The underlying mechanisms appear to include epigenetic modifications, possibly hypomethylation. A father's bad habits may have an insidious long-term effect on their unborn daughters.

31.5   TELOMERE

31.5.1   STRUCTURE AND FUNCTION

Telomere is a segment of DNA located at the end of chromosome tip. Its name is derived from the Greek words telos—"end" and meros—"part." The DNA that forms the telomere consists of the sequence 5′-TTAGGG-3′, which is referred to as "telomeric repeat" since it is tandomly repeated. It reads as TTAGGG.TTAGGG.TTAGGG. … and so on. Although the bulk of telomeric DNA is double-stranded, the extreme terminus is a single-stranded G-rich 3′-overhang that serves as a template for elongation and forms a telomeric "T-loop." This loop is stabilized by certain telomeric-binding proteins.

The telomeres protect the ends of chromosomes from recombination and degradation and are involved in replication and stability.[1,33] One of the most important functions is to facilitate replication of the linear DNA without loss of essential genetic material. The enzymes that replicate DNA are not 100% efficient and a small amount of DNA gets lost from the end of each strand during replication. A portion of telomeric material at the end of a DNA strand is lost during cell division rather than important coding DNA. Telomeres also play a significant role in determining the number of times that a normal cell can divide.

The enzyme telomerase, a specialized reverse transcriptase, is important for long-term cell proliferation and genome stability, because it elongates telomeric DNA. Thus depending on the cell type telomerase partly or completely counteracts the progressive shortening of telomeres that otherwise occurs. Telomerase is less active in cells that divide less often. Telomere length and telomerase activity are implicated in human health and disease. Studies during the last decade have found links between shorter telomeres and risks for several diseases.[7] Elizabeth Blackburn, Jack Szostack, and Carol Greider were awarded the 2009 Nobel Prize in Physiology and Medicine for their elucidation of the structure and maintenance of telomeres.

31.5.2   LENGTH

Telomere length varies greatly between species from approximately 300 to 600 bases in yeast to many kilobases in humans. In human leukocytes, the length of telomeres ranges from about 8000 base pairs at birth, 3000 base pairs as people age, and as low as 1500 base pairs in elderly people. Telomere length is dictated in part by heredity and partly by environmental and epigenetic factors. There is some evidence that suggests that telomere length is paternally inherited. Sperm cells show increasing telomere length with age. The father's age can affect telomere length in blood of the offspring. Male and female children have an average of 22 more base pairs in the DNA nucleotide sequence for each year older their father was at conception, which can add on as much as 20% of the length of the average telomere. There is no significant correlation between maternal age and male and female offspring. In general, females have longer telomeres than males.

Each time a somatic cell divides and the DNA within the cell is copied, the telomeres shorten. This process continues until the telomeres reach a critical length called the Hayflick limit (after the scientist who discovered it) at which point the cell stops dividing. When a cell stops replicating, it enters into a period of decline known as cellular senescence, which is the cellular equivalent of aging. As an example, under normal aging this critical length limit of telomere may be reached (arbitrary) at the age of 80 years (Figure 31.3). Immortal cancer cells escape telomere loss by switching on a gene that expresses telomerase.

31.5.3   TELOMERE LENGTH AND HEALTH

A study has linked the length of telomeres with rate of survival among people over 60 years of age. Researchers measured telomere lengths in a group of subjects who donated blood in the mid-1080s. They then compared the telomere length to survival data they had gathered on those subjects.

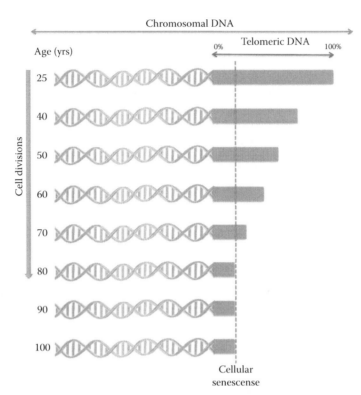

FIGURE 31.3 Telomere length reduction—normal aging. The critical telomere length limit for cellular senescence is seen at age 80 years.

They found that subjects with shorter telomeres were more than three times as likely to have died of heart disease and more than eight times as likely to have died of infectious diseases as their counterparts with longer telomeres.[8] Other preliminary epidemiologic studies also have related shorter telomeres with higher mortality and higher risk of some age-related chronic diseases. From these studies, the general idea is that telomeres may be a "biological clock" that reflects an individual's physiological age/health more accurately than chronological age. In other words, the longer the telomeres, the healthier the cells and slower the aging process. A recent study that focused on Ashkenazi Jews[3,4] found that those who live the longest inherit a hyperactive version of telomerase that rebuilds telomeres and keeps their length long (see Chapter 14).

Another study in 38 sex- and age-matched controls were reported recently. A total of 19 "healthy" centenarians with physical function in the independent range and the absence of hypertension, congestive heart failure, myocardial infarction, peripheral vascular disease, cancer, stroke, chronic obstructive pulmonary disease, and diabetes were compared to 19 centenarians with physical function limitations and two or more of the above conditions. Healthy centenarians had significantly longer telomeres than did unhealthy centenarians.[37] These findings are in support of the concept that one's functional health may be associated with telomere length rather than chronological age.[8]

Systemic telomere length has been proposed as a marker of biological aging. Blood leukocyte telomere length (LTL) is the generally preferred measure of systemic telomere length.

Advocates of human life extension promote the idea of lengthening the telomeres in certain cells through temporary activation of telomerase by drugs or possibly permanently by gene therapy. They reason that this would extend human life. So far, these ideas have not been proven in humans. But one study has successfully reversed the signs of aging in laboratory mice by activating telomerase. Telomerase-based therapies for extending lifespan are likely to come in the next few years. But experts have raised questions whether telomerase can be used as an anti-aging therapy. They raise the possibility that shortening telomerase length in old age may be a protection against some aspects of age-related diseases such as cancer. Mice with elevated levels of telomerase have higher cancer incidents and hence do not live longer.[42] Inhibition of telomerase activity remains a very interesting approach for cancer treatment. Most tumors express telomerase and inhibition of telomerase remains a very interesting approach for cancer treatment.

31.5.4 Factors That Accelerate Telomere Attrition

As stated above, shortening of telomeres is found to correlate with general aging, i.e., as people get older the LTL gets shorter. Males appear to lose telomere length faster than women. LTL is emerging as a prognostic marker of disease risk. In addition, a number of diseases[1] such as cardiovascular disease, hypertension, type 2 diabetes,[1] and osteoporosis are known to accelerate telomere shortening. Oxidative stress, inflammation, increased plasma cholesterol, triglycerides and homocysteine, and exposure to pollutants[21] also contribute to telomere attrition. Chronic stress is associated with telomere attrition and risk for several diseases including cardiovascular disease and poorer immune function.[14] Smoking significantly decreases telomere length. Each pack-year smoked corresponds to on average an additional 5 bp decrease in telomere length compared with the rate of overall cohort.

It is commonly thought that heavy drinking leads to premature aging and early onset of age-related diseases. Studies have shown that heavy alcohol consumption (four drinks or more per day) accelerates telomere shortening. LTL in alcohol abusers is found to be about half as much as in non-abusers.

Obesity is an important risk factor for many age-related diseases. A study on 1122 white women (age 18–76 years) has found that telomere length decreases steadily with age at a mean rate of 27 bp per year. Telomere length of obese women was found on average to be 240 bp shorter than women with normal bodyweight. In another study, telomere length was measured in subcutaneous adipose tissue cells in 21 nonobese and 51 obese subjects.[25] Telomere lengths were negatively associated with body mass index (BMI), systolic blood pressure, and blood triglycerides. After controlling for age, fasting glucose, triglycerides, and smoking habits, BMI was found to contribute 16% of telomere length variance.[38] A study on 647 women aged 34–74 years showed that higher BMI and hip circumference were inversely associated with telomere length. Studies in children (age 5–12) also showed LTL was significantly shorter in obese boys compared with their lean counterparts but not in girls. In boys, there was also association of LTL to blood pressure and waist circumference. The effects in obese boys suggest clinical implications as to the contribution of these parameters in premature aging. These findings support the hypothesis that obesity may accelerate aging and highlights the importance of maintaining desirable weights in children and in adults.

In general, those who have certain chronic diseases or follow unhealthy lifestyle described above will experience accelerated telomere attrition (Table 31.1). The telomere critical length limit for cellular senescence will be reached earlier in life. As an example, this point is shown (arbitrary) at the age of 70 years in Figure 31.4.

31.5.5 Factors That Slow Telomere Attrition

After its discovery in 1984 by Blackburn and Greider, telomerase gained a reputation as a fountain of youth. There is an association between short telomeres and early death. People with rare diseases characterized by shortened telomeres or telomerase mutations seem to age prematurely. In a recent study, when mice were engineered to lack telomerase completely, their telomeres shortened progressively and they aged much faster than normal mice. They were also barely fertile. They suffered from age-related conditions such as osteoporosis, diabetes, and neurodegeneration and died young. But when the inactivated telomerase was switched back by feeding a chemical, the animals bounced back to normal health. They regained their fertility and age-related conditions reversed. Thus, telomerase may be considered a serious antiaging intervention. But other researchers question

TABLE 31.1
Factors Affecting Telomere Attrition

Factors That Accelerate Attrition	Factors That Slow Attrition
Cardiovascular disease	Increase in dietary fiber
Poor lipid profile	Limit dietary linoleic acid
Type 2 diabetes	Vitamin D supplementation
Osteoporosis	Multivitamin supplementation
Inflammation	ω_3 fatty acid supplementation
Oxidative stress	Liberal intake of fruits, vegetables
Psychosocial stress	Decrease intake of processed meat
Increased plasma homocysteine	Low fat intake
Exposure to pollutants	Liberal use of tea
Smoking	Increased physical activity
Alcohol abuse	Healthy lifestyle
Obesity, high waist circumference	
Unhealthy lifestyle	

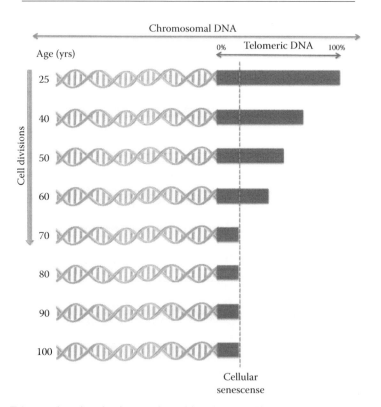

FIGURE 31.4 Telomere length reduction—aging with unhealthy lifestyle. The critical telomere length for cellular senescence is seen at age 70 years.

whether mice lacking telomerase are a good model for human aging. And increasing telomerase activity in humans by taking a pill could potentially encourage the growth of tumors. This remains a concern because cancer cells turn on telomerase to make themselves virtually immortal.

So those hoping for the fountain of youth will have to wait a little longer while scientists determine the benefits and risks of telomerase activation by drugs in humans. The aging process is complex, and the telomere is just one element that contributes to its course. Instead of a pill, one can follow a healthy lifestyle to protect one's telomere length and health.

Evidence assembled over the last few years shows that telomere shortens with age and the average telomere length acts as a biomarker for biological aging. Research on the anti-aging potential of telomere manipulation has focused on telomerase that adds DNA bases to telomeres, thus continually renewing telomere length. There is scientific evidence pointing to an important role for telomerase activity and telomere length in the causes of human disease. Regularly new studies are published demonstrating the correlation between telomere and health. Studies in humans suggest that by making simple lifestyle changes, it may be possible to increase telomere length or at least reduce the rate of telomere shortening and thus improve health and possibly increase longevity.[26] Based on reported studies, a few of the lifestyle changes that may have a positive impact on health are described below and also are presented in Table 31.1.

31.5.5.1 Dietary Fiber, Linoleic Acid

A study examined the relationship between diet and lifestyle factors and telomere length in over 2000 women participating in the Nurses' Health Study. High dietary fiber intake was associated with longer telomere length and cereal fiber was found to be particularly effective. Linoleic acid is a dietary essential nutrient but consuming high amounts of this fatty acid has been found to shorten telomere length in women. So, it is best to limit the amount to the recommended daily allowance.

31.5.5.2 Vitamin D

Decreased levels of vitamin D are associated with increased risk of autoimmune diseases such as multiple sclerosis, rheumatoid arthritis, and type 1 diabetes, and administration of vitamin D has been shown to reduce the risks of these diseases. Recently in a study of more than 2100 female twin pairs ages 19–79 (mean age 49.1 years) scientists measured blood 25-hydroxyvitamin D (vitamin status), C-reactive protein (an inflammatory biomarker), and LTL. They found that after adjusting the results for age of the volunteers, women with the highest vitamin D levels had the longest telomeres and lowest levels of inflammation and body stress.[6] The difference (on telomeres) between the highest and the lowest tertiles of vitamin was 92.6 bp. That was equivalent to 4.2 years of telomeric age. These results demonstrate that people with the highest levels of vitamin D may age more slowly than people with lower levels of vitamin D.

31.5.5.3 ω_3 Fatty Acids

Increased dietary intakes of ω_3 fatty acids are associated with prolonged survival in patients with CAD.[17] However, the mechanisms underlying the protective effect are poorly understood. Researchers recruited 608 outpatients with stable CAD in a study between 2000 and 2002 and measured LTL at baseline and again after 5 years of follow-up. They also assessed baseline blood levels of eicosapentaenoic acid (EPA) and docosahexaenoic acid (DHA) as percentage of total fatty acids. Patients were divided into quartiles on the basis of ω_3 fatty acids with means of 2.3%, 3.3%, 4.3%, and 7.3% in the four groups, respectively. The optimum level of ω_3 fatty acids is thought to be around 7%–8%. Most people on a Western diet have considerably below this level. There was an inverse relationship between baseline blood levels of ω_3 fatty acids and the role of telomere shortening. Those with the lowest quartile of EPA and DHA experienced the fastest rate of telomere shortening and those with the highest quartile experienced the lowest rate of telomere shortening over 5 years, with linear trend across the quartile.

31.5.5.4 Green Tea, Fat

An association between green tea and longer telomere length has been reported recently. In an epidemiologic study, 976 Chinese men and 1030 Chinese women aged 65 years and older were evaluated. In addition to daily food intake questionnaires, their LTL was measured. The research was to identify any dietary or other lifestyle factors that might be associated with lengthening of telomeres.

After adjusting for other health, lifestyle, and nutritional factors known to be associated with telomere length the researchers found that consumption of tea was associated with longer telomeres in elderly Chinese men.[10] The difference in telomere length between those who drank an average of 4 cups per day and those who drank an average of quarter cup per day was equivalent to a potential lifespan difference of 5 years between the two groups of men. The effect of green tea on telomere length in the elderly Chinese women was less significant in this study. According to these researchers, it may be related to hormones or other factors in women. Therefore, frequent consumption of green tea appears to be linked to longer telomeres at least in elderly Chinese men. Among other dietary constituents studied, dietary fat was found to be inversely associated with telomere length in both men and women.

31.5.5.5   Multivitamins

A cross-sectional analysis of data from 586 participants in the Sister Study, an ongoing risk-enriched prospective cohort of healthy sisters (ages 35–74 years) found that the use of multivitamins was associated with longer telomeres.[43] Compared with nonusers, the women who took daily multivitamin pills had on average 5.1% longer telomeres (273 bp), which can be translated to a difference of a potential 9.8 years of age-related telomere loss.

31.5.5.6   Processed Red Meat

Researchers studied cross-sectional association between telomere length and dietary patterns that were associated with markers of inflammation. They collected data from 840 white, black, and Hispanic adults from the Multi-Ethnic Study of Atherosclerosis. After adjustment for age, other demographics, lifestyle factors, and intake of other foods or beverages, only processed meat intake was found to be inversely associated with telomere length.

31.5.5.7   Lifestyle Changes

A study was done to determine the effect of lifestyle changes on telomere length.[31] Investigators used 30 men with low risk prostate cancer. They were asked to make several lifestyle changes: eating a diet low in sugar and rich in whole food, fruits, and vegetables with only 10% calories derived from fat and engaging in moderate exercise, relaxation, and breathing exercises. Blood telomerase activity was measured at baseline and again after 3 months. Telomerase activity increased 29% in these volunteers and presumably telomere length. This suggests that these lifestyle changes may reduce the rate of telomere attrition in the general population.[27] But to be on a diet restricted to 10% of calories from fat may be difficult. This is an interesting study and needs to be repeated with varying amounts of fat.

31.5.5.8   Physical Activity

A sedentary lifestyle increases telomere attrition and may accelerate the aging process. Researchers studied 2401 white twin volunteers (2152 women and 249 men) using questionnaires on physical activity level, smoking status and socioeconomic status, and LTL that was adjusted for age and potential confounders. LTL was significantly positively associated with increasing physical activity in leisure time, an association that remained significant after adjustment for age, sex, BMI, smoking, socioeconomic status, and physical activity at work. LTLs of the most active subjects were 250 nucleotides longer than those of the less active subjects (7.1 and 6.9 kb, respectively).[11,41] The most active people had telomere of a length comparable to those found in inactive people who were up to 10 years younger on average.[11] Physically activity may help people to reduce stress levels.

The studies described support the concept that diet and lifestyle are modestly related to telomere length. There are a number of steps people can take to slow telemere attrition, protect the way the genetic material functions, and stay healthy longer. Some forms of meditation may have salutary effects in telomere length.[15] With a healthy lifestyle the critical telomere length limit for cellular senescence may reach much later in life. This is shown at age 90 (arbitrary) years in Figure 31.5. The research supports the

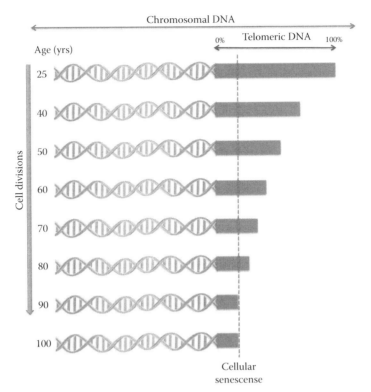

FIGURE 31.5 Telomere length reduction—aging with healthy lifestyle. The critical telomere length limit for cellular senescence is seen at age 90 years.

effectiveness of whole foods, low refined sugar, and a low-fat diet, enhanced by supplementation with antioxidants to minimize oxidative stress and inflammation, and thus telomere attrition. Combining the health effects of regular exercise with a plant-based diet in a comprehensive lifestyle plan appears to increase telomerase activity and improve telomere length. Some experts in this field believe that by taking necessary steps the lifespan can be increased by several years.

Most of the studies are based on LTL measurements with the expectation that telomere attrition in other tissue cells follows that pattern. Some studies described above are only done on men (e.g., lifestyle changes), while other studies are only done on women (e.g., vitamin D) and it is likely that similar effects will be seen in both sexes, but there may be exceptions. For instance, the effect of green tea is seen in older men but not in older women. This is an exciting new field, and more research is needed in the area of telomere and disease not only to determine association with some factors to LTL but also to confirm a causal relationship.

31.6 LONGEVITY BASED ON WALKING SPEED

Unrelated to telomeres, but of recent interest relative to predicting longevity, recently an analysis of nine studies involving more than 34,000 people 65 years old and older has shown that faster walking speeds were associated with living longer.[9,36] Those who walked slower than 2 feet per second had an increased risk of dying. Those who walked 3.3 feet per second or faster survived longer. In addition, the scientists found that predicting survival based on gait speed was as accurate as predictions based on age, sex, chronic conditions, smoking history, blood pressure, BMI, and hospitalization.

According to these researchers, walking is a reliable tool to measure well-being because it requires body support, timing and power, and places demands on the brain, spinal cord, muscles, joints, heart, and lungs. Slowing down is associated with getting older. By age 80 gait speed is about 10%–20% slower than in young adults. The measurement of walking speed is inexpensive.

Both telomere length and walking speed are considered to be useful for predicting longevity. Therefore, they must have a common relationship. Older people with varying walking speeds should have proportional differences in their LTL. It would be interesting to experiment further to determine this relationship between longevity and walking speed.

DEFINITIONS

Allele: An alternative form of a gene that may occupy a given locus.

Autosomes: All chromosomes other than the X and Y chromosomes.

Chromosome: A highly ordered structure composed of DNA and proteins that carries the genetic information. In humans, there are 46 chromosomes ordered in pairs.

Dominant allele: An allele that is expressed when present at only a single copy (i.e., it dominates over the other allele present).

Gene: A sequence of nucleotides that represent a functional unit of inheritance.

Heterozygous: The two alleles are different.

Homozygous: Both alleles at a locus are the same.

Locus: Position of a gene on a chromosome.

Mutation: A permanent heritable change in the sequence of DNA.

Recessive allele: An allele that is only expressed when homozygous.

X-Linkage: The distinctive inheritance pattern of alleles at loci on the X chromosome.

Epigenetics: Study of changes in phenotype (appearance) or gene expression caused by mechanisms other than changes in the underlying DNA sequence.

REFERENCES

1. Al-Attas, O., N. Al-Daghni, A. Bamakhramah et al. 2010. Telomere length in relation to insulin resistance, inflammation and obesity among Arab youth. *Acta Paediatr* 99:896.
2. Amato, I. 2006. Pulling gene's strings. *Chem Eng News* 84(29):13.
3. Atzmon, G., M. Cho, R. M. Cawthon et al. 2010. Evolution in health and medicine Sackler colloquium: Genetic variation in human telomerase is associated with telomere length in Ashkenazi centenarians. *Proc Natl Acad Sci U S A* 107(Suppl 1):1710.
4. Aubert, G., and P. M. Lansdorp. 2008. Telomere and aging. *Physiol Rev* 88:557.
5. Berdanier, C. D. 2000. Nutrient–gene interaction. *Nutr Today* 35(1):8.
6. Brent Richards, J., A. M. Valdes, J. F. Gardner et al. 2007. Higher serum vitamin D concentrations are associated with longer leukocyte telomere length. *Am J Clin Nutr* 86:1420.
7. Caldado, R. T., and N. S. Young. 2009. Telomere diseases. *New Engl J Med* 361:2353.
8. Cawthon, R. M., K. R. Smith, E. O'Brien et al. 2003. Association between telomere length in blood and mortality in people aged 60 years or older. *Lancet* 361:360.
9. Cesari, M. 2011. Role of gait speed in the assessment of older patients. *J Am Med Assoc* 305:91.
10. Chan, R., J. Woo, E. Suen et al. 2010. Chinese tea consumption is associated with longer telomere length in elderly Chinese men. *Br J Nutr* 103(1):107.
11. Cherkas, L. F., J. L. Hunkin, B. S. Kato et al. 2008. The association between physical activity in leisure time and leukocyte telomere length. *Arch Int Med* 168:154.
12. Clark, S. D., and S. Abraham. 1992. Gene expression: Nutrient control of pre- and post-translational events. *FASEB J* 6:3146.
13. Dolinoy, D. C., D. Huang, and R. L. Jirtle. 2007. Maternal nutrient supplementation counteracts Bisphenol A-induced DNA hypomethylation in early development. *Proc Natl Acad Sci U S A* 104:13056.
14. Epel, E., J. Daubenmier, J. T. Moskovitz et al. 2009. Can meditation slow rate of cellular aging? Cognitive stress, mindfulness, and telomeres. *Ann NY Acad Sci* 1172:34.
15. Epel, E. S., J. Lin, F. S. Dhabher et al. 2010. Dynamics of telomerase activity in response to acute psychological stress. *Brain Behav Immun* 24:531.
16. Esteller, M. 2008. Epigenetics in cancer. *N Engl J Med* 358:1148.

17. Farzaneh, R., J. Lin, E. S. Epel et al. 2010. Association of marine omega-3 fatty acid levels with telomeric aging in patients with coronary heart disease. *J Am Med Assoc* 303:1250.

18. Fu, Q., X. Yu, C. W. Callaway et al. 2009. Epigenetics: Intrauterine growth retardation (IUGR) modifies the histone code along the rat hepatic IGF-1 gene. *FASEB J* 23:2438.

19. Goldberg, A. D., C. D. Allis, and E. Bernstein. 2007. Epigenetics: A landscape takes shape. *Cell* 128:635.

20. Heindel, J. J. 2008. Animal models for probing the developmental basis of disease and dysfunction paradigm. *Basic Clin Pharmacol Toxicol* 102(2):76.

21. Hoxha, M., L. Dioni, M. Bonzini et al. 2009. Association between leukocyte telomere shortening and exposure to traffic pollution: A cross-sectional study on traffic officers and indoor office workers. *Environ Health* 8:41.

22. Kaati, G., L. O. Bygren, M. Pembrey, and M. Sjostrom. 2007. Transgenerational response to nutrition, early life circumstances and longevity. *Europ J Human Genet* 15:784.

23. Korf, B. R. 2007. *Human Genetics and Genomics*. 3rd ed. Madden, MA: Blackwell Publishing.

24. Liotto, N., M. Miozzo, M. L. Giani et al. 2009. Early nutrition: The role of genetics and epigenetics. *Pediatr Med Chir* 31(2):66.

25. Navarrete, J. M., F. Ortaga, M. Sabater et al. 2010. Telomere length of subcutaneous adipose tissue cells is shorter in obese and formerly obese subjects. *Int J Obesity* 34:1345.

26. Nettleton, J. A., A. Diez-Roux, N. S. Jenny et al. 2008. Dietary patterns, food groups, and telomere length in the multi-ethnic study of atherosclerosis. *Am J Clin Nutr* 88:1405.

27. Newbold, R. A., E. P. Banks, W. N. Jefferson, and J. J. Heindel. 2008. Effects of endocrine disrupters on obesity. *Int J Andrology* 31:201.

28. Newbold, R. A., E. P. Banks, R. J. Snyder et al. 2007. Developmental exposure to endocrine disrupters and the obesity epidemic. *Reprod Toxicol* 23:296.

29. NG, S. F., C. Y. Ruby, D. Lin et al. 2010. Chronic high-fat diet in fathers programs beta-cell dysfunction in female rat offspring. *Nature* 467:963.

30. Nussbaum, R. L., R. R. McInnes, H. F. Willai, and A. Hamosh, eds. 2007. *Genetics in Medicine*. 7th ed. Philadelphia, PA: Saunders Elsevier.

31. Ornish, D., J. Lin, J. Daubenmier et al. 2008. Increased telomerase activity and comprehensive lifestyle changes: A pilot study. *Lancet Oncol* 9(11):1048.

32. Pearson, N. 2006. Genetics: What is a gene? *Nature* 441:398.

33. Riethman, H. 2008. Human telomere structure and function. *Annu Rev Genomics Hum Genet* 9:1.

34. Seringhaus, M., and M., Gerstein. 2008. Genomics confounds gene classification. *American Scientist* 96(6):466.

35. Simopoulos, A. P. 1995. Genetic variation and nutrition. *Nutr Today* 30(4):157.

36. Studenski, S., S. Perera, K. Patel et al. 2011. Gait speed and survival in older adults. *J Am Med Assoc* 305:50.

37. Terry, D. F., V. E. Nolan, S. L. Anderson et al. 2008. Association of longer telomeres with better health in centenarians. *J Geront A Biol Sci Med Sci* 63(8):809.

38. Valdes, A. M., T. Andrews, J. P. Gardner et al. 2005. Obesity, cigarette smoking and telomere length in women. *Lancet* 366:662.

39. Van Vliet, J., N. A. Oates, and E. Whitelaw. 2007. Epigenetic mechanisms in the context of complex diseases. *Cell Mol Life Sci* 64:1531.

40. Weihold, R. 2006. Epigenetics: The science of change. *Environ Health Perspect* 114:A160.

41. Werner, C., T. Fürster, T. Widmann et al. 2009. Physical exercise prevents cellular senescence in circulating leukocytes and in the vessel wall. *Circulation* 120:2438.

42. Willeit, P., J. Willeit, A. Mayr et al. 2010. Telomere length and risk of incident cancer and cancer mortality. *J Am Med Assoc* 304(1):69.

43. Xu, Q., C. G. Parks, L. A. DeRoo et al. 2009. Multivitamin use and telomere length in women. *Am J Clin Nutr* 89:1857.

44. Zeisel, S. H. 2009. Epigenetic mechanisms for nutrition determinants of later health outcomes. *Am J Clin Nutr* 89:1488S.

32 Personalized Nutrition and Personalized Medicine

32.1 PERSONALIZED NUTRITION

Traditional nutrition research uses epidemiological, clinical, and physiological studies to identify how deficiencies in certain nutrients translate into compromised health. It builds on these findings to explore how dietary choices in general help explain differences in health from one population to another. The United States Department of Agriculture, the Department of Health and Human Services, and various special interest organizations provide dietary guidelines to promote health and to reduce risk for major chronic diseases through diet and physical activity. Major causes of morbidity and mortality are related to poor diet and a sedentary lifestyle. Some specific diseases linked to poor diet and physical inactivity include cardiovascular disease (CVD), type 2 diabetes, hypertension, osteoporosis, and certain cancers.

But general health and disease-specific dietary guidelines do not take into account physiologic differences in how individuals respond to nutrient intakes. These differences in response may greatly affect the efficacy of these recommendations at the individual level. For example, in some people inappropriate choices of food can enhance the risk of diseases such as atherosclerosis and diabetes, but other individuals can tolerate such foods without much problem. One individual may consume a few more calories but still can maintain weight while another individual gains weight with same amount of food consumption. Some eat cholesterol-rich foods and still show low blood cholesterol while others are sensitive to such foods. Some who eat meat regularly may be susceptible to cancer while others are not affected. One chain smoker may stay relatively healthy and another may get lung cancer. A similar phenomenon is observed in dosage and tolerance to prescribed drugs. These differences are attributed to specific enzymes and/or other causes.

The incidence and prevalence of chronic diseases varies among individuals, families, and nations. Genetic predisposition, and environmental factors including diet and quality of care all contribute to these variations. Advances in genetics and molecular biology indicate that susceptibility to chronic diseases such as CVD hypertension, diabetes, and so on to a great extent is genetically determined. Because of genetic variations, not everybody is susceptible to chronic diseases to the same extent.

In 2003, after more than a decade of research the Human Genome Project was completed by the U.S. Department of Energy and the National Institutes of Health. The goals of the project were to learn the order of the three billion units of DNA that go into making a human genome, as well as to identify all the genes located in the genome. One of the hopes of the project was to pinpoint specific genes that cause common diseases. The answer is more complex, with many diseases the result of multiple genes interacting. Nevertheless, the information garnered from the Human Genome Project has the potential to forever transform health care. It has sparked a great deal of research on individual variations in gene sequences, particularly single nucleotide polymorphisms (SNPs)—pronounced "snips"—and their role in chronic diseases and predicting individual responses to drugs (pharmacogenetics). Nutritional genomics is the off-shoot of this genetic revolution that includes nutrigenomics and nutrigenetics.

32.1.1 Single Nucleotide Polymorphism

Single nucleotide polymorphisms are the most common variations that exist in the human genome. Each person's genetic material contains a unique SNP pattern that is made up of many different genetic variations. SNPs are considered distinct from rare mutations in that a SNP by definition must occur in at least 1% of the population. Most of these sequence alterations may occur in noncoding regions and may have no significance; others may lead to alterations in the amino acid sequence of the gene product, leading to a functional change in the protein; and still others may alter the promoter region, thus having an impact on efficiency of transcription of the gene.

Most SNPs are not responsible for a disease state. Instead, they serve as biological markers for pinpointing a disease on the human genome map, because they are usually located near a gene found to be associated with a certain disease. Occasionally, a SNP may actually cause a disease, and therefore, can be used to search for and isolate a disease-causing gene.

Technology is available to decode hundreds of "marker" SNPs in a person's DNA all at once using a so-called gene chip." By applying gene chips to thousands of people, some affected with a disease and some without the disease, researchers have been able to figure out that some "marker" SNPs are highly associated with disease (though the association is typically not perfect and associations do not imply causality). Some common variants may have minimal impact on a gene's function by "turning the dial" on the gene's activity and very slightly changing that activity. These variants are not strong enough to cause disease by themselves. Instead each needs to be combined with several other variants in other genes, or with environmental factors (diet, smoking, etc.) in order for the disease to occur. For example, for some people, blood cholesterol goes up only with dietary intake of saturated fatty acids and/or cholesterol.

Nutrients and some other food components interact and alter gene expression.[26] Genetic polymorphisms affect the metabolism of dietary factors which in turn affect the expression of genes involved in a number of important metabolic processes. Genetic polymorphisms in the targets of nutrient action such as receptors, transporters, or enzymes could alter molecular pathways that influence the physiological response to dietary intervention. Some enzymes are involved in phase I and phase II detoxication reactions as discussed in Chapter 28. Variations in genes that produce these enzymes can affect the elimination of toxic substances from the body. So, different outcomes result according to the genetic makeup of people. Understanding these mechanisms can help people make up for inherited weakness or genetic flaws by eating differently and when necessary, taking supplements. Personalized nutrition is the concept of adapting food to individual needs.

32.1.2 Nutrigenetics and Nutrigenomics

Nutrigenetics or the science of personalized nutrition is the study of how genes and nutrients interact to promote health or disease.[38] It also includes understanding how gene and protein expression are affected by the presence or absence of specific nutrients, whether and how diet-regulated genes play a role in disease, the degree to which an individual diet affects the risk of disease given his or her genetics, and whether one's diet may be altered to maintain the balance between health and disease.

The terms nutrigenetics and nutrigenomics are often used interchangeably. However, traditionally these terms have different meanings. While nutrigenetics focuses on SNPs and nutritional implications associated with these variations, nutrigenomics contemplates the effects of nutritional compounds on the expression of the multitude of human genes, proteins, and metabolites. Nutrigenomics elucidates how diet influences our genome, and as a result, our body. The goal of both disciplines is the same: optimizing of health through personalization of diet.

Some examples of the effects of food components based on SNPs are given below.

32.1.2.1 Lipoproteins and Cardiovascular Disease

32.1.2.1.1 *Apolipoprotein E*

The most common gene affecting low density lipoprotein (LDL) cholesterol levels is apolipoprotein E (APO E). In humans, APO E is a 299 amino acid polypeptide synthesized primarily in the liver. APO E in serum is associated with chylomicrons, very low density lipoprotein (VLDL), and high density lipoprotein (HDL), and serves as a ligand for the LDL receptor and the LDL receptor-related protein. The APO E gene is polymorphic with three alleles: e2, e3, and e4 on chromosome 19 producing respectively three isoforms of the protein E2, E3, and E4. The e2 and e4 variants differ from the more common e3 allele by a single amino acid substitution, which affects ligand binding of the triglyceride-rich lipoprotein and HDL to the hepatic LDL and APO E receptor. APO E3 contains cysteine at 112 and arginine at 158. APO E2 has cysteine at both positions and E4 has arginine at both sites. The most common form, e3 occurs in approximately 78% of the Caucasian population, while e4 has a frequency of 15% and e2 a frequency of 7%. The APO E gene polymorphism also has a strong effect on the level of its gene product: e2 is associated with high concentrations of APO E and e4 with lower concentrations.

APO E plays a major role in regulating blood cholesterol.[11] Several studies have established that the e4 allele is associated with higher levels of LDL cholesterol and e2 with lower levels of LDL cholesterol than the e3 allele.[24] The response to diet appears to be determined by the genetic variant of APO E. On a low fat/high cholesterol diet individuals with APO e4 phenotype respond with an increase in blood cholesterol, whereas those with APO e2/e2, e3/e2, and e3/e4 do not show an increase. On a low fat/low cholesterol diet, all variants show a decrease in serum cholesterol. The magnitude of LDL cholesterol lowering is twice as great in males as in female subjects. The lowering of LDL cholesterol in APO e3/e4 male subjects is about 23%, which is significantly greater than that observed in APO e3/e3 (14%) or APO e3/e2 (13%) suggesting that male subjects with APO e3/e4 are more responsive to diets restricted in saturated fat and cholesterol than APO e3/e3 subjects.

APO e4 is associated with hypercholesterolemia, whereas APO e2 protects against high plasma cholesterol. However, in the presence of obesity, hyperthyroidism, and diabetes, APO e2 is associated with the development of Type III hyperlipidemia and the accumulation of chylomicrons and VLDL remnants in plasma. Increase in either energy intake, *trans* fatty acids intake, or carbohydrate intake (particularly in women) leads to hypertriglyceridemia. Women of the APO e3/e2 phenotype stand to benefit the least from a high polyunsaturated (P): saturated (S) fatty acids (P:S) diet because of the reduction in the more protective HDL, whereas men of the APO e4/e3 phenotype show the greatest improvement in the LDL:HDL ratio. Therefore, a general recommendation to increase PUFA content of the diet to decrease plasma cholesterol and risk of coronary artery disease does not seem to be appropriate for women with the APO e3/e2 phenotype.

The presence of small, dense LDL particles is associated with increased risk of coronary artery disease and the particle size of LDL is dependent on genetic factors and dietary fat composition. A monounsaturated fat diet increases LDL size in APO e3/e3 subjects but decreases LDL size in APO e4/e3 subjects. Therefore, each individual has to be examined and guided individually when dietary recommendations are made.

Oat bran is known to decrease serum cholesterol. Recent studies have shown that individuals with APO e3/e3 phenotype show hypocholesterolemic effect after taking oat bran for 4 weeks. But no change is noted for individuals with APO e4/e4 or e4/e3 phenotype.[41] Thus, specific genetic information is needed to define the optimal diet for an individual. There is a negative association with alcohol intake and LDL cholesterol in men with the e2 allele but a positive association with e4 allele. No significant associations are seen in men and women with e3 allele. The effect of moderate alcohol intake in raising plasma HDL is stronger in subjects without e4 allele than with e4 allele.[6,9]

People with e4 allele are at increased risk of developing diabetes. Presence of at least one copy of e4 allele reverses the usual protective effect of moderate drinking and it vastly increases the risks of smoking. But e4 allele is extremely susceptible to environment. The increased diabetes risk is found only in people who are overweight. Therefore, all of the genetic predisposition for heart disease that comes with e4 can be removed by eliminating smoking, giving up alcohol, eating a diet low in saturated fat, and doing regular exercise. The APO e4 allele also increases the risk for Alzheimer's disease, but there is not much that can be done to prevent it.

32.1.2.1.2 Apolipoprotein A-IV

Apolipoprotein A-IV (APO A-IV) is secreted by the small intestine and is involved in the metabolism of chylomicrons and HDL. The gene for the protein is located on chromosome 11. The protein displays two codominant alleles 1 and 2. The 2 allele is caused by a single base substitution of guanine for thymine in codon 360. This substitution leads glutamate to histidine change and significantly alters its biophysical properties. Approximately one person in seven in the United States carries the APO A-IV 2 allele as heterozygous. Increasing dietary cholesterol intake from 200 mg to 1100 mg/day by an individual with APO A-IV 1/1 (homozygous for the common allele) increased total cholesterol by about 22 mg/dl and only by 6 mg in APO A-IV 1/2 group. The mean plasma LDL cholesterol increased by 19 mg/dl in the APO A-IV 1/1 group and only by 1 mg in APO A-IV 1/2 group. No changes in triglycerides or HDL levels were observed. These results show the effects of genetic variation on the response to dietary cholesterol.[21]

32.1.2.2 Folic Acid Requirements

The enzyme 5, 10 methylenetetrahydrofolate reductase (MTHFR) is involved in folate metabolism. It catalyzes the conversion of 5, 10 methylenetetrahydrofolate to 5 methyltetrahydrofolate (MTHF), and the predominant circulating form of folate. The MTHF participates in the conversion of homocysteine to methionine. Abnormalities of MTHFR are associated with increased plasma levels of homocysteine. Hyperhomocysteinemia is an established risk factor for coronary artery disease,[19] stroke, and thromboembolism. Hyperhomocysteinemia during pregnancy is a risk factor for delivery of infants with neural tube defects (NTDs) and recurrent embryo loss. It may also play a role in preeclampsia (high blood pressure (BP) in pregnancy). It is estimated that folic acid, if taken daily in sufficient amounts can reduce NTD occurrence as much as 50–70%.

The MTHFR gene is located on chromosome 1 and two common alleles have been described. The C677T allele is a single base pair mutation in which cytosine is replaced by thymine at the base pair 677, resulting in an amino acid substitution (alanine to valine) in the enzyme. Functionally, the encoded protein has a reduced enzyme activity at and above 37 °C and the C677T mutation is often termed "thermolabile." The homozygotes and heterozygotes have about 70% and 35% reduced MTHFR activity in vitro, respectively. Homozygosity for the C677T allele is associated with elevated plasma homocysteine levels predominantly in individuals who have a low plasma folate levels. The variant enzyme has a reduced affinity for its riboflavin cofactor than the wild type. It is associated with low folate status and altered distribution of folate within the cell.[3]

A second allele is A1298C in which adenine is replaced by cytosine at the base pair 1298, resulting in glutamate to alanine substitution. The A1298C allele leads to decreased MTHFR activity, although not to the same extent as the C677T allele. Individuals who are homozygous for this allele have about 40% reduced enzyme activity in vitro but do not appear to have higher plasma homocysteine levels than controls. However, individuals who are compound heterozygous for the C677T and A1298C, which produce a C677T/A1298C genotype, have a 40–50% reduction in MTHFR activity and a biochemical profile similar to those seen among C677T homozygous with increased plasma homocysteine and decreased folate levels.

Homozygosity for C677T polymorphism is associated with high CVD risk, particularly among those with low folate intake. Paradoxically, the C677T allele is associated with a lower risk of colorectal cancer.[20,37] The lower risk was only noted when dietary intake of folate, and vitamins B_{12} and B_6 was adequate. The inverse association (a higher risk of cancer) seems to be stronger in individuals over 60 years old with low intake of these vitamins compared with the controls. The Physicians Health Study has confirmed that individuals with homozygosity for C677T allele and with lower intake of folate are especially sensitive to the carcinogenic effect of alcohol in colorectal cancer. Alcohol causes malabsorption of folate and increased excretion and abnormal metabolism of this nutrient. Therefore, consumption of excess amounts of alcohol may be counter indicated in homozygotes of this allele in terms of risk of developing colorectal cancer, especially if folate intake is low. Researchers in the Nurses' Health Study also have shown increased risk for breast cancer in individuals taking less folic acid compared to those whose folate intake is adequate.

The frequency of the C677T allele shows geographic and ethnic variation. It appears to be high in Italy (44%) and in white Hispanics from California (42%) and relatively low in African Americans (14%).

Individuals who are homozygous for these variants may have a higher requirement for folate (and possibly for vitamins B_2, B_6, and B_{12}) than other individuals. Interventions with folic acid can modulate the deleterious effect of this polymorphism as measured by an ability to raise tissue folate and lower plasma homocysteine. The recommended dietary allowances for folate and other nutrients are derived from population-based studies on supposedly normal people. Being designed for the majority of people, they do not cover small groups with special needs such as those with metabolic or genetic abnormalities or disorders.

If genetic variants that cause altered nutrient status are common as the description above suggests there may not be such a thing as "normal population" with respect to nutrient requirements. In order to provide the best recommendations for everyone, it is necessary to include the impact of genetic variation and to consider requirements for each individual, given their specific profile.

32.1.2.3 Hereditary Hemochromatosis

Hereditary hemochromatosis (HH) is one of the most common genetic disorders in the United States. It causes the body to absorb and store too much iron. The extra iron builds up in organs and damages them. Without treatment, the disease can cause these organs to fail.

Healthy people usually absorb about 10% of the iron contained in the food they eat to meet the body needs. The body has no natural way to eliminate the excess iron, so it is stored in the body tissues, especially the liver, heart, and pancreas.

Hereditary hemochromatosis is mainly associated with a defect in the gene called HFE located on chromosome 6.[1,2] The gene product is thought to be a major regulator of intestinal iron absorption. It is a cell-surface protein that binds to the transferrin receptor, overlapping the binding site for transferrin and inhibiting transferrin-mediated iron uptake. This interaction is thought to be involved in a cell's ability to sense iron levels. This function is disrupted in individuals with mutation in HFE, resulting in inappropriate increase in iron absorption from the small intestine.

The most common mutation responsible for HH is the substitution of cysteine for tyrosine at the 282nd amino acid in the protein sequence and is known as C282Y. When C282Y is inherited from both parents, iron is overabsorbed from the diet and hemochromatosis results. A person who inherits a defective gene from one parent is a carrier but usually does not develop the disease. Carriers, however, may have a slight increase in iron absorption. A number of less pathogenic (in terms of iron status) mutations also exist in addition to C282Y. They usually cause little increase in iron absorption.

Hereditary hemochromatosis most often affects Caucasians of Northern descent, although other ethnic groups also are affected. About 5 people in 1000 (0.5%) of the U.S. Caucasian population carry two copies of the hemochromatosis gene and are susceptible to developing the disease. One person in eight is a carrier of the abnormal gene. The disease is less common in African Americans, Hispanic Americans, Asian Americans, and American Indians. Although both men and women can inherit the gene defect, men are about five times more likely to be diagnosed with the effects of HH than women. Symptoms usually develop between ages 40 and 60 years in males, and somewhat later in females, after menopause.

Excessive iron stores in the organs first produce only non-specific symptoms, but left untreated, patients develop hepatic fibrosis or cirrhosis, diabetes mellitus, congestive heart failure, and other problems.

Diagnosis in patients with symptoms is usually based on a serum transferrin iron saturation of greater than 60% for men and greater than 50% for women on at least two different determinations, in the absence of other causes of primary and secondary iron overload disorders. Identification of type(s) of mutations present in affected individuals is important. It allows predictive testing in their at-risk siblings and children. Treatment of hemochromatosis is by phlebotomy at regular intervals.[28,29]

People diagnosed with HH must follow a special diet to help maintain a lower serum ferritin. They should refrain from using iron supplements including multivitamins that contain iron. A low-iron diet is not necessary, but red meat should be consumed in moderation. They should minimize alcohol use because alcohol and iron are synergistic.

Hemochromatosis is often undiagnosed and untreated. It is considered rare and physicians may not consider testing for it. The initial symptoms can be diverse and vague and can mimic the symptoms of many other diseases. If the iron overload is diagnosed and treated before organ damage has occurred, a person can live a normal healthy life. Since the genetic defect is common and early detection and treatment are effective, widespread screening for hemochromatosis would be cost-effective.

32.1.2.4 Hypertension

Hypertension or high BP is a major risk factor for CVD, stroke, and chronic renal disease. About 29% of adult Americans have hypertension (systolic BP $\geq$ 140 mm Hg, diastolic BP $\geq$ 90 mm Hg) and another 30% have prehypertension (systolic BP 121–139 mm Hg and diastolic BP 81–89 mm Hg). Prehypertensive individuals have a high probability of developing hypertension and carry on excess risk of CVD as compared to those with a normal BP (systolic <120 mm Hg and diastolic <80 mm Hg).

Hypertension develops as the consequence of a complex interplay over time between susceptibility genes and environmental factors.[14] Of the environmental factors, diet has a predominant role in BP homeostasis. Hypertension in persons younger than 55 years is four times more common in individuals with a family history of hypertension than those with no family history for it. Estimates of genetic contribution to BP variations range from 30% to 60%. However, the genetic contribution to hypertension is complex. Rather than a single gene BP is influenced by the interaction of multiple genes and environment.

Most of the available evidence has focused on genetic factors that influence the BP response to salt intake.[34] Several genotypes that influence BP have been identified. Most of these genotypes influence the renin-angiotension-aldosterone systems (RRAS) or renal salt handling. Several of the genes encoding members of the RAAS pathway exhibit polymorphisms that influence functions.

Plasma angiotensinogen levels correlate with BP and track through families suggesting that angiotensinogen may have a role in essential hypertension. Studies have indicated that A for G nucleotide substitution in the promoter region of the angiotensinogen gene-6 nucleotide upstream from the start site of the transcription results in increased plasma angiotensin levels and also influences salt sensitivity to raising BP. Salt sensitivity is defined as a greater than 10% increase in BP following a high salt diet.

Researchers studied three forms of variations of the gene referred to as AA, AG, and GG to determine the effect of salt restriction on BP. Those who had AA or AG gene were found to be salt sensitive—meaning that they fared better in lowering their BP through salt restriction. Individuals with GG genotype were salt insensitive.[40] Similar BP results were obtained with weight loss. Individuals who carried the AA or AG did lower their BP on the weight-loss diet, but individuals with GG did not. The AA genotype conferred excess risk of hypertension and was associated with increased responsiveness to diet. Knowledge of a patient's genotype may assist physicians in assessing prior risk of a pathophysiologic outcome and in tailoring therapy.

32.1.2.5 Osteoporosis

Osteoporosis is a skeletal disorder characterized by an increased risk of fracture. It represents a major public health concern that is expected to increase in importance as life expectancy increases and the population ages. The lifetime risk of suffering an osteoporosis-related fracture exceeds 40% in women and 15% in men.

There is compelling evidence to suggest that both the development of bone to peak bone mass at maturity and subsequent loss depends on the interaction between genetic, hormonal, nutritional, and other environmental factors.[30] The major part (or 80%) of the age specific variation in bone turnover and bone density is genetically determined. But the genetic element has been difficult to characterize because bone growth is controlled by many genes, including those for various hormones, growth factors, signaling molecules, and structural components of bone and cartilage.[32]

The notion of genetic determinant is of little value unless the specific genes that are involved can be identified. Most work in this area of osteoporosis research has focused on candidate gene approach, which has identified several candidate genes for osteoporosis.[4,7] Advances in knowledge about the genetic basis of osteoporosis are important because they offer the prospect of fracture risk and the opportunity to identify diet and molecules that will be used as targets for the design of new drugs for the prevention and treatment of bone disease. Some of the more important candidate genes that have been studied (especially genes where a gene-nutrient interaction is likely or possible) are discussed below.

32.1.2.5.1 VDR

One of the first genes to be associated with the common form of osteoporosis is that for vitamin D receptor (VDR). A strong relationship was reported between VDR alleles and bone density in twin and non-twin Caucasian populations in Australia. Several Japanese studies have reported differences in bone density response to 1, α hydroxylated vitamin D metabolites. The "bb" genotype, which is most common in Japanese cohorts (approximately 75% of the subjects) were more responsive to vitamin D metabolites compared with the "Bb" genotype, which either did not respond as well or actually worsened with the treatment. The "Bb" genotype is the most common (about 50%) in Caucasian populations. So VDR genotype differences could contribute to the variable and generally less impressive responses to vitamin D metabolites in Caucasian as opposed to Japanese studies. A Dutch study of simple vitamin D supplementation in the prevention of hip fracture found that the bone density response to the supplement varied according to VDR genotype. Bone density increased significantly in the "BB" and "Bb" genotype subjects (>4%) but not in "bb" genotype subjects (0.3%). These two groups of studies (Japanese and Dutch) in different racial groups suggest that "BB" and "Bb" subjects may respond positively to simple vitamin D but not to 1, α hydroxylated vitamin D. By contrast "bb" subjects may respond positively to 1, α hydroxylated vitamin D but not to simple vitamin D.

32.1.2.5.2 CYP1A1

The gene called CYP1A1 makes an enzyme that detoxifies foreign substances as well as estrogen as a normal part of maintaining estrogen balance. Several variants of the gene exist and one variant is known to be present in 19% of the general population. Women having this variant of the gene have significantly lower blood estrogen levels, higher urinary estrogen metabolite, and exhibit lower than normal bone density of the upper femur near the hip joint.[25] The presence of this variant produces an enzyme that breaks down estrogen faster than usual leading to low estrogen levels. This puts a woman at risk for osteoporosis. Resveratrol, a substance present in grapes and some other foods has been found to inhibit the expression of CYP1A1. This substance may have therapeutic potential for bone health.

32.1.2.5.3 Duffy Antigen Receptor for Chemokines (DARC)

A gene called Duffy antigen receptor for chemokines (DARC) negatively regulates bone mineral density (BMD) in mice. The protein encoded by DARC (Duffy protein) binds to chemokines—or small signaling proteins—that are included in osteoclast formation. Osteoclasts break down bone in a process called bone resorption releasing important minerals such as calcium and phosphorus in the blood. They cause reduction in BMD.[10] There are differences between African Americans and Caucasians that could be associated with this gene. African Americans exhibit higher BMD compared to Caucasians. Also African Americans generally do not have the Duffy protein on red blood cells while Caucasians do. The potential genetic association between DARC gene variation and these traits in humans certainly make it worthy of further investigation.

32.1.2.5.4 COL1A1

COL1A1 is one of the two genes that code for the two polypeptides in collagen. The polymorphic sequence in the COL1A1 gene binds a transcription factor, and therefore, variations in the sequence may alter the synthesis of collagen. A study on post-menopausal women in the Netherlands has shown a relationship between the presence of a specific allele of this gene and reduction in bone density and a predisposition to fractures.

32.1.2.6 Perilipin and Obesity

Perilipin is a protein which in humans is encoded by the perilipin gene. The protein plays a significant role in determining whether fat is stored in the body or released for energy. The more perilipin is produced the more fat is stored. Women with two specific variants (AG and AT) tend to have a higher percentage of body fat and greater waist circumference than women with the other two possible variants. These inherited alleles are significant markers of obesity in women.[39] Variants TC and GA help protect their carriers from developing diabetes regardless of their body weight. Learning more about these genetic variations could eventually help create new—perhaps personalized—treatment for obesity and diabetes.

32.1.2.7 Tea Consumption and Protection from Cancer

Green tea contains catechol-containing potent antioxidants known to help prevent heart disease and certain cancers, but only some women seem to show reduction in breast cancer from drinking it. The antioxidants are rapidly metabolized by catechol-o-methyl transperase (COMT). There are two forms of the gene for COMT—low activity form and high activity form. A case-control study found that higher intake of green tea was associated with lower breast cancer risk only in women who had inherited at least one copy of the low activity form of COMT, suggesting that those who are less efficient at eliminating antioxidants may be more likely to benefit from green tea consumption. Individuals with high activity COMT allele would have rapid elimination of tea antioxidants and would have less protective effect of tea consumption.[16]

32.1.3 PERSONALIZED DIETARY RECOMMENDATIONS

Much of the variability in risk of chronic disease results from interactions between individual genomic variations and environmental exposures, including diet. Identification of specific gene-nutrient interactions opens up possibilities for a more individualized approach to dietary recommendations based on genotype and more effective strategy for disease prevention through dietary modification. In a limited number of cases, diet-gene interactions are well defined. For example, variations in the MTHFR gene affects MTHFR activity, which results in increased requirement for folate to normalize blood homocysteine levels. Also, the HFE gene variation affects susceptibility to iron overload and the individuals with variations in this gene have to be on a low iron diet. Individuals with APO e4 variant can reduce the risk for CVD by consuming a diet low in saturated fat and exercising. However, for most diet-gene interactions, their impact on whole body metabolism and functional nutrient status and the subsequent effects on chronic disease risk are poorly characterized. There is a need to identify SNPs in key target genes that result in proteins with altered functions as well as to determine how variations in candidate genes and/or proteins modify phenotype. The current dietary advice is rather generalized and takes a one size fits all approach. It is a good strategy to use nutritional genomics for general dietary advice depending on variations in specific alleles. If a person's genetic information indicates a higher than average risk of developing a particular disease the person may modify a diet and lifestyle or sometimes be prescribed a medication to better regulate the aspects of health and wellness over which he or she has control. The person may benefit in the long run after making preventive lifestyle choices that will help counter the biological risk. The field is still in its infancy and a lot more research is needed to determine whether personalized nutrition advice based on genetic data in the prevention of nutrition associated diseases will work in practice.

Personalized nutrition is the concept of adapting food to individual needs. While it has become apparent that people respond differently to diet depending on their genetic makeup, lifestyle, and environment the related knowledge and understanding remain fragmented; we all know that even when people are eating the same diets, some will become overweight, some will develop heart disease, and some will develop allergies, while others will not. There is increasing consumer awareness of understanding and assessing individual health status and nutritional needs. Ongoing research in this field will help identify just how diet affects our genes and why individuals vary in their response to different nutrients and diets. The time will come when it will be possible to use genomic testing to screen individuals for genes related to particular diseases and conditions and to determine an individual's health-promoting diet. It may even become commonplace for health care professionals to give tailor-made dietary advice to an individual's needs as determined by the information from the individual's genes.

32.2 PHARMACOGENETICS

Foods we ingest contain thousands of complex compounds that must be processed. Some are not absorbed from the gastrointestinal tract, but most are absorbed, distributed, and metabolized (biotransformed) to a variety of products that are utilized immediately, stored, or excreted. Drugs that are administered to achieve a specific effect on the human body also undergo biotransformation and humans vary in the efficiency and speed at which they do this. Moreover, the response of a drug's target (e.g. enzymes and receptors) can also vary among individuals.

The study of how genes influence the individual's response to drugs is called pharmacogenetics.[17] It largely focuses on specific genes, such as those involved in the expression of drug-metabolizing enzymes. Pharmacogenomics deals with the entire human genome, including genes for numerous proteins in the body, such as transporters, receptors, and the entire signaling networks that respond to drugs and move them through the system. Even though individual differences in drug response can result from the effects of age, sex, disease, or drug interactions genetic factors also influence both the efficiency of a drug and the likelihood of an adverse reaction.[15,22]

Though the field of pharmacogenetics seems to be brand new, it is more than a half century old. In 1950s, scientists first identified deficiencies in enzymes that explained adverse reactions to drugs and that they could be inherited. For example, early research showed that 10% of African Americans serving in the Korean War became anemic after ingesting an anti-malarial drug, primaquine, which rarely, if ever, caused problems for Caucasian soldiers. The anemic reaction was determined to be caused by a deficiency of glucose 6-phosphate dehydrogenase (G6PDH), and it was found to be common in people of African descent but not so among Caucasians. It was discovered later that G6PDH helps protect red blood cells against certain chemicals. Lacking that protective effect, those with enzyme deficiency (variant form) are vulnerable to deleterious effects when exposed to certain chemicals.

Since that time, numerous other enzyme variants have been identified and found to cause adverse reactions to certain drugs. Such adverse reactions were identified until recently by trial and error methods. Specifically, a drug was administered and the individual's metabolite of that drug was tracked by recording the amount of by-product in their urine. In some cases, the plasma drug level at a certain time after administration was measured to determine speed of inactivation. It was discovered that a common genetic variation in a phase II pathway of drug metabolism, *N*-acetylation, could result in striking differences in the half-lives and plasma concentrations of drugs metabolized by N-acetyl transferase. Such drugs included the anti-tuberculosis agent isoniazid, the hypertensive agent hydralazine, and the anti-arrhythmic drug procainamide and this variation had clinical consequences in all cases. The bimodal distribution of plasma isoniazid concentrations in subjects with genetically determined fast or slow rates of acetylation in one of those early studies strikingly illustrates the consequences of inherited variations in this pathway for drug metabolism. These early examples of the potential influence of inheritance on the effect of a drug set the stage for subsequent studies of genetic variations in other pathways of drug metabolism.

Over the past decade, ambitious efforts have been undertaken to advance the knowledge of pharmacogenetics. This has been driven, in part, by the expectation that through the use of pharmacogenetics, we will be able to profile DNA differences among individuals and thereby predict responses to different medicines. For example, a genetic profile may predict who is more or less likely to respond to a drug or to suffer an adverse event. Such a profile would greatly personalize an individual's health care and could substantially change the way the medicine is practiced.

Once the drug is administered, it is distributed to its site of action, where it interacts with the target, undergoes metabolism, and is excreted. If the drug is less efficiently metabolized, it will remain in circulation and continue to act for longer time. On the other hand if it is metabolized faster, its level at the target site will be lower.

The cytochrome P450, or CYP for short, is the name of a large family of genes that code for enzymes involved in the metabolism of drugs, chemicals, and biochemicals. These drug-metabolizing enzymes are involved in degrading the majority of prescribed drugs. So our personal CYP complement is crucial to determining what effect drugs have on us, what dosages are appropriate, and what dangers the drugs pose. Eighty percent of the most serious adverse reactions to medicines appear to involve drugs that are metabolized by the CYP enzyme systems.[27] Understanding individual variations in CYP genes has become possibly the main focus of attention for researchers developing personalized therapeutics. So far 57 genes for CYP enzymes have been identified and variants of some of these enzymes have already been linked with the inability of some commonly prescribed drugs to be effective in some patients. One member of this family, CYP2D6, represents one of the most intensively studied and best understood examples of pharmacogenetic variations in drug metabolism.[45] More than 70 alleles have been described, some of which lead to no activity, reduced activity, or enhanced activity. Based on the ability of drug metabolism, four phenotypic subpopulations of metabolizers exist: poor metabolizers (PMs), intermediate metabolizers (IMs), extensive metabolizers (EMs), and ultrarapid metabolizers (UMs). Importantly, their frequency varies according to racial background. Subjects with UMs have two copies of the CYP2D6 gene. Such subjects can have inadequate therapeutic response to standard doses of the drugs metabolized by CYP2D6. In general, the rule is that the faster one metabolizes the drug, the larger the dose one should receive.

Although the occurrence of multiple copies of this gene is relatively infrequent among Northern Europeans, in East Africans the allele frequency can be as high as 28%. Approximately 5–10% of white subjects were found to have a relative deficiency in their ability to oxidize the anti-hypertensive drug debrisoquine and anti-arrhythmic drug sparteine metabolized by CYP2D6 and 1% of Japanese are deficient in this enzyme. Individuals with poor metabolism of these two drugs had lower urinary concentrations of metabolites and higher plasma concentrations of the parent drug than did those with extensive metabolism. Furthermore, the drugs had an exaggerated effect in these subjects. Family studies demonstrated that poor oxidation of these drugs was inherited and the subjects had two copies of the gene or genes that encoded an enzyme with decreased CYP2D6 activity or with no activity.

Similar approaches were subsequently applied to other isoforms CYP2C9,[18] which metabolizes warfarin and CYP2C19, which metabolizes mephenytoin, an anticonvulsant. About 20% of Japanese are PMs of S-mephenytoin whereas less than 5% of Caucasians are so affected. Table 32.1 shows the most common CYP variant alleles, enzyme activities, and allele frequencies in various racial groups.

TABLE 32.1
Common CYP Variant Alleles, Enzyme Activities, and Frequencies in Various Racial Groups

Gene	Allele	Enzyme Activity	Frequency Caucasians (%)	Frequency African American (%)	Frequency Asian (%)
CYP2C9	*2	Reduced	8–19	2.9	<1
	*3	Reduced	3–16	2	2–5
CYP2C19	*2	Reduced	14	16	32
	*3	Reduced	<1	<1	8
CYP2D6	*3	None	2	1	<1
	*4	None	18	2	<1
	*6	Reduced	2	1	1

Three examples on the effects of variations on the drug action are described below to illustrate the concepts and to demonstrate the potential contribution of pharmacogenetics to medical practice. They are warfarin, which involves two major genes for estimating optimal dosage; codeine, a pro-drug, which has to be converted to morphine for its action; and herceptin, which acts on the basis of gene variations in tumor.

32.2.1 WARFARIN

Warfarin, an anticoagulant, consists of equal amounts of S- and R-enantiomers; S-warfarin accounts for about 80% of warfarin's anticoagulant activity and undergoes hydroxylation by CYP2C9 (Figure 32.1). R-warfarin is metabolized by CYP1A2 and CYP3A4. Warfarin is one of the most commonly prescribed oral anticoagulants for short- and long-term management of thromboembolic and hemostatic disorders such as deep-vein thrombosis, pulmonary embolism, prevention of myocardial infarction, and stroke. It is very effective but also causes a high rate of adverse reactions. It is a difficult drug to manage due to its narrow therapeutic index and wide interindividual variability in anticoagulant response and maintenance dose. One of the side effects of the drug is an increased risk for bleeding. Too much of the drug can lead to serious bleeding events, while too little may allow a dangerous blood clot to form. Therefore, correct dosing is central to successful patient management.[31] The major genes implicated in targeting and metabolism are those that produce vitamin K epoxide reductase (VKOR) complex (VKORC1), which determines the effectiveness of the circulating dose, and CYPS2C9, which metabolizes warfarin and is involved in how much of the activated drug circulates in the blood. Common genetic variations in these two genes have

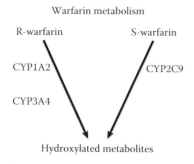

FIGURE 32.1   R-warfarin is metabolized by CYP1A2 and CYP3A4 and the more potent S-warfarin is metabolized by CYP2C9 to the hydroxylated products.

been discovered to significantly decrease warfarin maintenance dose requirements. Warfarin acts by inhibiting VKOR, which interferes with recycling of vitamin K and decreases its availability for the synthesis of vitamin K-dependent clotting factors II, VII, IX, and X as well as protein C and S (Figure 32.2).

VKOR is encoded by the VKORC1 gene, which has multiple polymorphisms that affect its expression.[44] In particular, a polymorphism within the promoter (−1639G>A) decreases expression of the gene: a heterozygous or homozygous adenine (A) at position 1639 in the VKORC1 promoter significantly reduces VKORC1 expression compared with individuals who are homozygous for a guanine (G) at that position. The variant reduces the amount of VKOR and leads to decreased levels of vitamin K-dependent clotting factors. This results in increased sensitivity to warfarin. Patients with −1639A genotype will require a lower dose of warfarin compared to the −1639G genotype. The frequency of the lower dose, warfarin-sensitive homozygous VKORC1 −1639A genotype is approximately 14–17% in Caucasians, 72–78% in Asians, and 4–5% in African Americans. The high frequency of this promoter polymorphism in Asians is thought to explain the majority, but not all the warfarin sensitive phenotypes in this population. They need dose adjustment to optimize their response to warfarin.

CYP2C9 is the main enzyme involved in the metabolism and clearance of warfarin. Two common variant alleles in the CYP2C9 gene, CYP2CP*2 and CYP2C9*3, produce enzymes with decreased activity to 12% and 5%, respectively. This reduces the rate of warfarin clearance, leading to a lower maintenance dose requirement. Patients with one or more of these variants usually take longer to metabolize the drug. In addition, they have increased risk for certain drug interactions. Numerous drugs are metabolized by CYP2C9 and if co-prescribed with warfarin, may reduce warfarin metabolism through competition. Other drugs inhibit or induce CYP2C9 activity. These effects may be further complicated by the presence of CYP2C9 variants. The two variants are found in approximately 20–30% of Caucasians and in 5% or less of Asians and African Americans. They need lower doses of warfarin.

In recent years, underlying genetic factors have been shown to account for approximately 35–40% of the variation observed in how patients respond to warfarin. Each year about two million people begin warfarin therapy to prevent or treat blood clots and as many as 43,000 patients experience the drug's life-threatening bleeding complications that require emergency treatment. In light of the potential dire consequences of incorrect warfarin dosing, the Food and Drug Administration

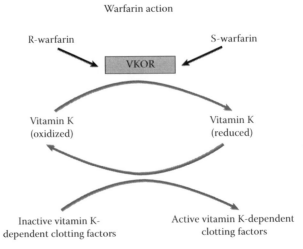

FIGURE 32.2 Warfarin inhibits vitamin K epoxide reductase (VKOR), which is expressed by vitamin K epoxide reductase (VKOR) complex (VKORC1) gene. By impairing the regeneration of the reduced form of vitamin K, warfarin inhibits vitamin K-dependent carboxylation of blood clotting factors.

(FDA) recently approved updated labeling for Coumadin (Bristol-Myers), the brand name version of warfarin, to highlight the importance of warfarin pharmacogenetic testing and to suggest that physicians incorporate the information obtained from such testing into warfarin dosing decisions. Shortly after the FDA approved the updated labeling, it cleared the first genetic test for warfarin sensitivity and other manufacturers have announced plans to submit similar tests to the FDA. The warfarin genetic test detects the common variants in CYP2C9 and VKORC1 genes and identifies patients who require a lower maintenance dose of warfarin and are at increased risk for bleeding events. Using the pharmacogenetics-based dosing has the potential to increase the safety and efficacy of warfarin therapy. In the latest significant development in this area, Roche Diagnostics recently received clearance in both the United States and the European Union for its AmpliChip, a microarray-based diagnostic test for detecting genetic variations that can influence drug efficacy and adverse drug reactions. It reveals which variants people have for two of the most significant genes CYP2C9 and CYP2D6.

32.2.2 Codeine

Codeine is a drug that must be converted from an inactive form to the active form (morphine) by CYP2D6 enzyme for therapeutic effect to occur. Patients with polymorphism of the CYP2D6 gene, which results in increased production of the enzyme are ultra rapid metabolizers and are more likely to develop adverse effects and toxicity (of morphine) when taking a standard dose of codeine, including impaired breathing and sedation. In contrast patients with decreased CYP2D6 production are PMs and will show little or no conversion of codeine to morphine.[43] They will not experience any pain relief, but will become nauseated due to the higher amounts of codeine in their body. As many as 7% of Caucasians may have a defective gene resulting in reduced pain relief due to poor metabolism of the drug. Genotyping of this enzyme has helped predict adverse effects in sensitive patients, leading to publication of dosage recommendations for codeine in this subset of the population.

32.2.3 Herceptin

One drug already on the market requires administration of a test before it can be prescribed. The drug is herceptin, an engineered monoclonal antibody that is used as a treatment for metastatic breast cancer. It is only prescribed for patients whose tumors overexpress the human epidermal growth factor receptor (HER2) protein, about 25–30% of women with breast cancer. This overproduction of HER2 protein is believed to lead to continuous growth-promoting signals being transmitted to affected cells as a key part of the development of cancer. Herceptin binds to the HER2 protein and mediates anticancer effects through a combination of mechanisms. The preliminary test ensures that the drug is targeted at these patients who can benefit.[33] The test is not a true pharmacogenetic test, because it measures protein expression in a tumor rather than the underlying genetic makeup of the patient. For women who would not benefit and could face only side effects, the drug is avoided.

Note regarding the above three examples: It is now established that many of the genes that encode proteins involved in pharmacology of xenobiotics display genetic polymorphisms. The polymorphisms, in turn, alter the functionality of the proteins and lead to dramatic phenotype differences in response to medicine or susceptibility to carcinogens. Pharmacogenetic testing provides information about individual genetic variation affecting drug response and helps clinicians tailor pharmacotherapy for each patient.

32.3 PERSONALIZED MEDICINE

Traditionally, personalized medicine has been practiced using patient's clinical signs and symptoms, data from laboratory and imaging evaluations, and family history to diagnose and treat disease. This is a reactive approach to treatment (treatment or medication starts after the signs and symptoms appear). Family history is a crude but time honored form of genetic screening. Since a person's genes are shared with his or her relative, family history provides the clinician with information on the impact that a substantial subset of an individual's genetic makeup might have on one's health. Also family members often share environmental factors such as diet. Thus, relatives provide information about the shared genes and shared environmental factors. Family medical history can identify people with a higher than usual chance of having common disorders such as heart disease, high BP, stroke, certain cancers, and diabetes. These complex disorders are influenced by a combination of genetic factors, environmental conditions, and lifestyle choices. A family history also can provide information about the risk of rarer conditions caused by mutations in a single gene such as cystic fibrosis. Researchers have identified several genetic or biochemical markers for dozens of rare conditions that can be treated nutritionally with some success.

It is long recognized that individuals differ in their therapeutic responses to medicines, in terms of efficiency and susceptibility to adverse events. While there are many factors that can influence therapeutic response, including patient compliance, correct diagnosis, and environmental factors such as drug interactions and drug-food interactions, it is becoming increasingly clear that genetic variations also influence drug response. These genetic influences encompass differences in drug-metabolizing enzymes to variations in drug targets and associated pathways.

Throughout the world hundreds of thousands of patients die each year due to adverse drug reactions, and many more are hospitalized but eventually recover. It is believed that many of these adverse reactions are due to genetic variations. As described earlier about 10% of African Americans experience adverse effects when administered an antimalarial drug. Antidepressants are notorious in that they achieve successful therapy in only 30% of patients, so the majority of users are exposed to the risk of side effects that, in their case, may be the only effects they experience. Patients with variations in CYP2C9 and/or VKORC1 gene require a much smaller maintenance dose of warfarin.

Personalized medicine is about making the treatment as individualized as the disease. It involves identifying genetic, genomic, and clinical information that allows accurate predictions to be made about a person's susceptibility of developing disease, the course of disease, and its response to treatment. Personalized medicine is a young but rapidly advancing field of health care.[12] It is not yet an established part of clinical practice, but a number of medical schools have personalized medicine programs such as testing patients genetically to determine their likelihood of having a serious reaction to some cancer drugs.

Physicians can now individualize therapy in the case of a few drugs. As our knowledge of genetic variations affecting proteins involved in uptake, distribution, metabolism, and the action of various drugs improve our ability to test for that variation and as a result to select the best drug for each patient should also increase. Now, in the era of human genomics, we have the means to assess an individual's genotype at all relevant loci and to characterize the genetic underpinning of each person's unique "chemical individuality." When the genetic variants relevant to maintaining health and preventing or treating illness in each individual are known, and when that knowledge is used in making important clinical decisions as a routine part of medical care, we will have entered the era of personalized medicine.

Personalized medicine will make it possible to give the appropriate drug and dosage to the appropriate patient, at the appropriate time. The benefits of this approach are in its accuracy, efficacy, safety, and speed.

32.4 GENETIC TESTING BENEFITS AND CONCERNS

Research into the identification of genes and their variations correlating with disease or inherited disorders has resulted in the availability of genetic tests. Evaluation of the benefits and risks of genetic testing is an important factor in the process of considering the ethics of its use.[13]

Genetic information can help in the diagnosis of a current health condition or provide insight into future health. Increased genetic testing makes it more likely that scientists will come up with early life saving therapy for a wide range of diseases with hereditary links. Genetic testing will also help doctors catch problems early, perhaps leading to preventive treatment. Genetic testing has potential benefits whether the results are positive or negative for a gene mutation. Test results can provide a sense of relief from uncertainty and help people make informed decisions about managing their health care. For example, a negative result can eliminate the need for a check up and screening tests in some cases. A positive result can direct a person towards available prevention and treatment options. Newborn screening can identify genetic disorders early in life, so treatment can be started as early as possible. The tests can also be used to give personalized advice about what to eat and drink to stave off diseases such as CVD, hypertension, diabetes, cancer, and other chronic diseases.

One of the most serious limitations of these tests is the difficulty of interpreting positive results because some people who carry a disease-associated mutation never develop a disease. It is believed that some mutations work together with other unknown mutations or with environmental factors to trigger the disease. Some tests give only a probability percentage that one will develop the disorder.

Consideration of the benefits of genetic testing is sometimes difficult. For example, when a therapy is available for a genetic disease, conducting a test is helpful. But if the treatment is not available, the value of having genetic information becomes more questionable. Susceptibility testing is another area that raises possible ethical issues for patients and clinicians. Susceptibility implies that the test does not provide the final answer regarding a disease, but rather that additional factors are involved. Polymorphic variants of the APO E gene have been found to be associated with variations in blood lipids, which may in turn influence risk for heart disease. Clinicians and patients may wish to learn which APO E variants they have to help determine their susceptibility to CVD, and the likelihood that altering their lifestyle risk factors or using pharmaceutical therapy might help prevent CVD. When deciding to test for APO E gene variants, however, there are additional consequences which must be considered, particularly the fact that the same gene variant may play multiple roles in health and disease. Studies have shown that the APO e4 allele is associated with increased risk for Alzheimer's disease. So the patient may get unwanted additional information. There are no medicines at this time that are known to prevent this disease.

The availability of genetic testing at a relatively lower cost has led to intense debate about the psychological, social, legal, and ethical consequences of genetic testing. The first is the concern over the patient's privacy as more and more genetic data are generated and stored over the Internet. Personal information is relevant not only to the individual who gets the test done but for some family members. For example, if one receives information on one's breast cancer risk and shares it with others it can also mean sharing information about the daughter's risk of breast cancer—even though she never consented to have that information shared. Society may single out people with specific biomarkers and distinct clinical features into a small subset of the population. DNA analyses in combination with the Internet create an unregulated market and new opportunities for invasion of privacy.

Physicians and society at large are concerned about the effect genetic knowledge will have on the well-being of individual persons and groups. There is a fear that genetic information will be used in ways that can discriminate people to deny them access to health insurance and employment. In the United States, the Genetic Information Nondiscrimination Act (GINA) was passed in Congress in 2008 to prohibit the improper use of genetic information in health insurance and employment. The Act prohibits insurance companies from denying coverage or charging that person a high premium based solely on a genetic predisposition to developing a disease in the future. The legislation also bans employers from using the individual's genetic information when making hiring, firing, job placement, or promotion decisions. Usually to obtain a genetic test health care professionals such as doctors acquire permission from patients and order the desired test. The American Medical Association recommends that the physician be involved in ordering the test and interpreting the results. Direct-to-consumer (DTC) genetic testing is available directly to the consumer without having to go through a health professional. There are a lot of DTC tests available in the market. Some tests are from well-established companies that provide an honest risk assessment of developing a serious disease and others are from questionable companies. The cost of genetic sequencing has come down and several companies are popping up on the Internet hoping to cash in on the increasing demand for personal genetic information. For a few hundred dollars, consumers can send their saliva samples to obtain a personalized genetic profile that will tell them about their ancestry, their risk of developing particular diseases, and various traits such as their food preferences.

Although the FDA regulates test kits as medical devices to ensure that they are safe and that they mean what they say they do, most genetic tests are considered laboratory-developed tests, which are not subject to FDA regulations. One company had planned to sell the kits over-the-counter in a chain of drug stores. But the FDA said the kit has not proven effective. The drug store chain decided not to sell the kits.

Because of the fragmented and complex regulatory environment for DTC genetic testing, the quality of tests varies from one lab to another. Consumers do not have a reliable way of knowing which labs are good and which ones are not. Also, scientists have found that even when the genotyping is accurate, the interpretation of the results varies from one service to another. An increasing number of people are raising concerns about these DTC genetic tests and are calling for more government oversight. They question the technical performance of the tests, their clinical utility, and the likelihood that they will make a difference in an individual's health. Some also worry about privacy and who should have access to a person's genetic information.

Scientists believe that genetic testing will eventually become an integral part of health care. In a few cases, testing has played a role in reducing adverse effects, or in determining proper dose of drugs, for various cancers and CVD. And many more gene-based therapies are on their way. There is growing consumer demand for genetic tests. It is likely that the FDA will move to regulate some aspects of the test.

REFERENCES

1. Adams, P. C., and J. C. Burton. 2007. Hemochromatosis. *Lancet* 370:1855–60.
2. Bomford, A. 2002. Genetics of hemochromatosis. *Lancet* 360:1673–81.
3. Boto, L. D., and Q. Yang. 2000. 5, 10-Methylenetetrahydrofolate reductase variants and congenital anomalies. A HuGE Review. *Am J Epidemiol* 151:862–77.
4. Cashman, K. D., and K. Seamans. 2007. Bone health, genetics and personalized nutrition. *Genes Nutr* 2:47–51.
5. Ciolino, H. P., P. J. Daschner, and G. C. Yeh. 1998. Resveratrol inhibits transcription of CYP1A1 in vitro by preventing activation of the aryl hydrocarbon receptor. *Cancer Res* 58:5707–12.
6. Corella, D., K. Tucker, C. Lahoz et al. 2001. Alcohol drinking determines the effect of the APO E locus on LDL-cholesterol concentrations in men: The Framingham Offspring study. *Am J Clin Nutr* 73:736–45.
7. Cummings, S. R., and I. J. Melton. 2002. Epidemiology and outcomes of osteoporotic fractures. *Lancet* 359:1761–7.
8. De Wardener, H. E., and G. A. MacGregor. 2002. Harmful effects of dietary salt in addition to hypertension. *J Hum Hypertens* 16:213–23.
9. Djousse, L., S. Pankow, D. K. Arnett et al. 2004. Apolipoprotein E polymorphism modifies the alcohol-HDL association observed in the National Heart, Lung, and Blood Institute Family Heart Study. *Am J Clin Nutr* 80:1639–44.
10. Edderkaoui, B., D. J. Baylink, W. G. Beamer et al. 2007. Identification of mouse Duffy antigen receptor for chemokines (Darc) as a BMD QTL gene. *Genome Res* 17:577–85.
11. Eichner, J. E., S. T. Dunn, G. Perveen et al. 2002. Apolipoprotein E polymorphism and cardiovascular disease: A HuGE review. *Am J Epidemiol* 155:487–95.
12. Erickson, B. E. 2008. Barriers to genetic-based medicine. *Chem Eng News* 86(27):20.
13. Erickson, B. E. 2009. Genetic testing goes mainstream. *Chem Eng News* 87(39):54.
14. Hajja, I., and T. A. Kotchen. 2003. Trends in prevalence, awareness, treatment and control of hypertension in the United States, 1988–2000. *J Am Med Assoc* 290:199–206.
15. Innocenti, F. 2005. *Pharmacogenomics*. Totowa, NJ: Humana Press.
16. Inoue-Choi, M., J. Yuan, C. S. Yang et al. 2010. Genetic association between the COMT geneotype and urinary levels of tea polyphenols and their metabolites among daily green tea drinkers. *Int J Epidemiol Genet* 1(2):114.

17. Issa, A. M. 2008. Clinical applications of pharmacogenomics to adverse drug reactions. *Expert Rev Clin Pharmacol* 1:251–60.

18. Kirchheiner, J., and J. Brockmoller. 2005. Clinical consequences of cytochrome P450 2C9 polymorphisms. *Clin Pharmacol Ther* 77:1–16.

19. Ma, J., M. J. Stampfer, C. Hennekens et al. 1996. Methylenetetrahydrofolate reductase polymorphism, plasma folate, homocysteine, and risk of myocardial infarction in U.S. physicians. *Circulation* 94:2410–6.

20. Mah, J., M. J. Stampfer, E. Giovannucci et al. 1997. Methylenetetrahydrofolate reductase polymorphism, dietary interactions, and risk of colorectal cancer. *Cancer Res* 57:1098–102.

21. McCombs, R. J., D. E. Marcadis, J. Ellis, and R. B. Weinberg. 1994. Attenuated hypercholesterolemic response to a high-cholesterol diet in subjects heterozygous for the apolipoprotein A IV 2 allele. *N Engl J Med* 331:706–10.

22. McLoyd, H. L., and W. E. Evans. 2001. Pharmecogenomics: Unlocking the human genome for drug therapy. *Annu Rev Pharmacol Toxicol* 41:101–21.

23. Moolchan, E. T., F. H. Franken, and M. Jaszyna-Gasior. 2006. Adolescent nicotine metabolism: Ethnoracial differences among dependent smokers. *Ethn Dis* 16:239.

24. Moreno, J. A., F. Perez-Jimènez, C. Marin et al. 2004. The effect of dietary fat on LDL size is influenced by apolipoprotein E genotype in healthy subjects. *J Nutr* 134:2517–22.

25. Napoli, N., D. T. Villarreal, S. Mumm et al. 2005. The effect of CyP1A1 gone polymorphisms on estrogen metabolism and bone density. *J Bone Miner Res* 20:232–9.

26. Ordovas, J. M., and V. Mooser. 2004. Nutrigenomics and nutrigenetics. *Curr Opin Lipidol* 15:101–18.

27. Pirmohamed, M., and B. K. Park. 2003. Cytochrome P450 enzyme polymorphisms and adverse drug reactions. *Toxicology* 192:23–32.

28. Powell, L. W. 2002a. Diagnosis of hemochromatosis. *Semin Gastrointest Dis* 13:80–8.

29. Powell, L. W. 2002b. Hereditary hemochromatosis and iron overload disease. *J Gastroenterol Hepatol* 17(Suppl):S191–5.

30. Ralston, S. H. 2007. Genetics of osteoporosis. *Proc Nutr Soc* 66:158–65.

31. Reynolds, K. R., R. Valdes Jr., B. R. Hartung, and M. W. Linder. 2007. Individualizing warfarin therapy. *Personal Med* 4:11–31.

32. Riancho, J. A., M. T. Zarrabeitia, and J. G. Macias. 2008. Genetics of osteoporosis. *Aging Health* 4:365–76.

33. Roses, A. D. 2004. ERBB2 and herceptin for breast cancer: An example of pharmacogenomics. *Nat Rev Genet* 5:645–56.

34. Sanada, S., J. Yatabe, S. Midorikawa et al. 2006. Single-nucleotide polymorphisms for diagnosis of salt-sensitive hypertension. *Clin Chem* 52:352–60.

35. Schwahn, B., and R. Rozen. 2001. Polymorphisms in the methylenetetrahydrofolate reductase gene: Clinical consequences. *Am J Pharm* 1:189–201.

36. Seeman, E. 2002. Pathogenesis of bone fragility in women and men. *Lancet* 359:1841–50.

37. Sharp, L., and J. Little. 2004. Polymorphisms in gene involved in folate metabolism and colorectal neoplasia: A HuGE review. *Am J Epidemiol* 159:423–43.

38. Simopoulos, A. P. 2004. Genetic variation: Nutritional implications. *World Rev Nutr Diet* 93:1–28.

39. Soenen, S., E. C. Mariman, N. Vogels et al. 2009. Relationship between perilipin gene polymorphism and body weight and body composition during weight loss and weight maintenance. *Physiol Rev* 96:723.

40. Svetkey, L. P., T. J. Moore, D. G. Simons-Morton et al. 2001. For the DASH collaborative research group: Angiotensinogen genotype and blood pressure response in the Dietary Approaches to Stop Hypertension (DASH) Study. *J Hypertens* 19:1949–56.

41. Uusitupa, M. I. J., E. Ruuskanen, E. Makinen et al. 1992. A controlled study on the effect of beta-glucan-rich oat bran on serum lipids in hypercholesterolemic subjects: Relation to apolipoprotein E phenotype. *J Am Coll Nutr* 11:651–9.

42. Weinshilboum, R. 2003. Inheritance and drug response. *N Engl J Med* 348:529–37.

43. Williams, D. G., A. Patel, and R. E. Howard. 2002. Pharmacogenetics of codeine metabolism in an urban population of children and its implications for analgesic reliability. *Br J Anesthesiol* 89:839–45.

44. Yuan, H. Y., J. J. Chen, M. T. Lee et al. 2006. A novel functional VKORC1 promoter polymorphism is associated with inter-individual and inter-ethnic differences in warfarin sensitivity. *Hum Mol Genet* 14:1745–51.

45. Zanger, U. M., S. Raimundo, and M. Eichelbaum. 2004. Cytochrome P450 2D6: Overview and update on pharmacology, genetics, biochemistry. *Arch Pharmacol* 369:23–37.

Index

An environmentally friendly book printed and bound in England by www.printondemand-worldwide.com

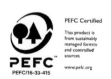

PEFC Certified

This product is
from sustainably
managed forests
and controlled
sources

www.pefc.org

PEFC/16-33-415

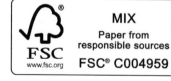

MIX

Paper from
responsible sources

FSC® C004959

This book is made entirely of sustainable materials; FSC paper for the cover and PEFC paper for the text pages.

#0324 - 231214 - C0 - 254/178/38 [40] - CB